drug information

A GUIDE FOR PHARMACISTS

Notice

drug information

A GUIDE FOR PHARMACISTS

seventh edition

Editors

Patrick M. Malone, PharmD, FASHP
Drug Information Consultant
Kirkland, Washington
Associate Dean Emeritus
College of Pharmacy
University of Findlay
Findlay, Ohio

Meghan J. Malone, PharmD, BCACP
Pharmacist
Swedish Medical Group
Seattle, Washington

Benjamin A. Witt, PharmD, MBA, BCPS
Drug Information Pharmacist
Cleveland Clinic
Cleveland, Ohio

David M. Peterson, PharmD, BCPS
Drug Information Specialist
University of Utah Health
Salt Lake City, Utah

New York • Chicago • San Francisco • Athens • London • Madrid • Mexico City • Milan
New Delhi • Singapore • Sydney • Toronto

Drug Information: A Guide for Pharmacists, Seventh Edition

1 2 3 4 5 6 7 8 9   LCR   27 26 25 24 23 22

ISBN   978-1-260-46030-8
MHID   1-260-46030-4

This book was set in Century Old Style by MPS Limited.
The editor was Michael Weitz.
The production supervisor was Catherine H. Saggese.
Project management was provided by Poonam Bisht and Adwiti Pradhan, MPS Limited.

This book is printed on acid-free paper.

Library of Congress Control Number: 2021947443

Contents

Chapter Three. Drug Information Resources **61**
Meghan K. Lehmann and Anthony Trovato

Chapter Four. Drug Literature Evaluation I:
Controlled Clinical Trial Evaluation **121**
Jennifer Phillips, Amy Heck Sheehan, Jacob Gettig, and Michael G. Kendrach

Chapter Five. Drug Literature Evaluation II:
                    Beyond the Randomized Controlled Trial **219**
Stacy L. Haber, Jason C. Cooper, Christopher S. Wisniewski, and
Cydney E. McQueen

Chapter Six. The Application of Statistical Analysis
                  in the Biomedical Sciences **297**
Ryan W. Walters

Chapter Seven. Pharmacoeconomics 407
James P. Wilson and Karen L. Rascati

Chapter Eight. Evidence-Based Clinical Practice Guidelines. 445
Jeanine P. Abrons and Pavnit Kukreja

Chapter Eleven. Legal Aspects of Drug Information 529
Martha M. Rumore

Chapter Twelve. Ethical Aspects of Drug Information Practice 601
Elyse A. MacDonald

Chapter Fifteen. Pharmacy and Therapeutics Committee 699
Patrick M. Malone, Mark A. Malesker, Indrani Kar, Danial E. Baker, and
Sunil Kumar Jagadesh

Chapter Sixteen. Drug Evaluation Monographs 775
Patrick M. Malone, Mark A. Malesker, Indrani Kar, Danial E. Baker, and
Sunil Kumar Jagadesh

Chapter Seventeen. Drug Shortages and Counterfeit Drugs 821
Erin R. Fox

Chapter Eighteen. Quality Improvement and the
Medication Use System 835
Jennifer K. Thomas and Rachel Digmann

Chapter Nineteen. Medication Safety I: Adverse Drug Reactions. . .895
Kelly Besco and Megan E. Keller

Chapter Twenty. Medication Safety II: Medication Errors. 933
Katie Johnson and Liz Hess

Chapter Twenty-One. Policy, Procedure, and Guideline Development 979
Whitney Mortensen, Gregory Heindel, and Conor Hanrahan

Chapter Twenty-Two. Project Management 995
Conor Hanrahan and Candice Burns Wood

Chapter Twenty-Three. Investigational Drugs 1013
Bambi J. Grilley

Chapter Twenty-Four. Regulatory Affairs and Pharmaceutical Industry 1059
Jennifer L. Dill and Daniel A. Kapp

Chapter Twenty-Five. Assessing Drug Promotions. 1107
Genevieve Lynn Ness and Robert D. Beckett

Contributors

Jeanine P. Abrons, PharmD
Clinical Assistant Professor
The University of Iowa
College of Pharmacy
Department of Pharmacy Practice &
  Science
Iowa City, Iowa
Chapter 8

Danial E. Baker, PharmD, FASHP,
FASCP
Regents Professor of Pharmacotherapy
J. Roberts and Marcia Fosberg Distinguished
  Professor in Pharmacy
Director, Drug Information Center
Washington State University
College of Pharmacy and Pharmaceutical
  Sciences
Spokane, Washington
Chapters 15, 16

Robert D. Beckett, PharmD, BCPS
Associate Professor of Pharmacy Practice
Manchester University
College of Pharmacy
Fort Wayne, Indiana
Chapter 25

Kelly Besco, PharmD, FISMP, CPPS
Medication Safety Officer
OhioHealth Pharmacy Services
2751 Tremont Road
Columbus, Ohio
Chapter 19

Jason C. Cooper, PharmD
Clinical Specialist, Drug Information
  Services
Medical University of South Carolina
MUSC Drug Information Center
Charleston, South Carolina
Chapter 5

Rachel Digmann, PharmD, BCPS
Senior Director, Measure Operations &
  Analytics
Pharmacy Quality Alliance
Alexandria, Virginia
Chapter 18

Jennifer L. Dill, PharmD
Clinical Coordinator, Drug Information &
  Drug Policy
The University of Kansas Health System
Kansas City, Kansas
Chapter 24

Erin R. Fox, PharmD, BCPS, FASHP
Senior Director, Drug Information and
    Support Svcs.
University of Utah Health
Salt Lake City, Utah
Chapters 14, 17

Brent I. Fox, PharmD, PhD, FASHP
Associate Professor, Health Outcomes
    Research and Policy Director of Student
    Affairs
Auburn University
Harrison School of Pharmacy
Auburn, Alabama
Chapter 28

Jacob Gettig, PharmD, MPH, MEd, BCPS, CHCP
Associate Dean of Assessment and
    Postgraduate Affairs and Professor of
    Pharmacy Practice
Midwestern University College of Pharmacy
Downers Grove, Illinois
Chapter 4

Bambi J. Grilley, RPh, RAC, CCRA, CCRC, CIP
Director, Clinical Research and Early Product
    Development and Assistant Professor,
    Pediatrics
Center for Cell and Gene Therapy
Baylor College of Medicine
Houston, Texas
Chapter 23

Stacy L. Haber, PharmD
Director, Midwestern University, Drug
    Information Center/Professor, Department
    of Pharmacy Practice
Midwestern University College of Pharmacy,
    Glendale Campus
Glendale, Arizona
Chapter 5

Conor Hanrahan, PharmD, MS, BCPS,
Medication Policy, Outcomes and
    Stewardship Director
Intermountain Healthcare Pharmacy
    Services
Salt Lake City, Utah
Chapters 21, 22

Gregory Heindel, PharmD, BCPS
Clinical Specialist, Drug Information/Policy
University of North Carolina Hospitals
Department of Pharmacy
Chapel Hill, North Carolina
Chapter 21

Liz Hess, PharmD, MS, FISMP, CPPS
Pharmacy Program Coordinator, Medication
    Use Safety & Quality
University of Kentucky HealthCare
Lexington, Kentucky
Chapter 20

Brian S. Hoffmaster, PharmD, MBA, BCPS
Drug Information Pharmacist/Associate
    Professor of Pharmacy Practice
Cleveland Clinic/Northeast Ohio Medical
    University
Cleveland, Ohio/Rootstown, Ohio
Chapter 9

Joshua C. Hollingsworth, PharmD, PhD
Discipline Chair for Pharmacology
Biomedical Sciences/Affiliate Assistant
    Professor
Health Outcomes Research and Policy
Auburn University
Edward Via College of Osteopathic Medicine
Auburn, Alabama
Chapter 28

Sunil Kumar Jagadesh, MD
Nephrologist/Assistant Professor, School of
  Medicine
Creighton University Medical Center
Omaha, Nebraska
Chapters 15, 16

Katie Johnson, PharmD, BCPS, CPHIMS
Pharmacy Program Coordinator, Medication-
  Use Safety & Technology
University of Kentucky HealthCare
Lexington, Kentucky
Chapter 20

Joseph K. Jordan, PharmD, BCPS
Professor of Pharmacy Practice/Drug
  Information Specialist
Butler University College of Pharmacy and
  Health Sciences/ Indiana University Health
  Department of Pharmacy Practice
Indianapolis, Indiana
Chapter 2

Daniel A. Kapp, PharmD, BCPS
Clinical Pharmacist, Drug Policy Program
University of Wisconsin Health
Middleton, West Virginia
Chapter 24

Indrani Kar, PharmD
Clinical Pharmacy Specialist—Drug Policy/
  Formulary
University Hospitals
Cleveland, Ohio
Chapters 15, 16

Megan E. Keller, PharmD, BCACP, CDE
Medication Safety/Antimicrobial Stewardship
  Pharmacist
OhioHealth Pharmacy Services
Columbus, Ohio
Chapter 19

Michael G. Kendrach, PharmD, FASHP
Executive Associate Dean, Associate Dean
  for Academic Affairs and Professor
Samford University
McWhorter School of Pharmacy
Birmingham, Alabama
Chapter 4

Pavnit Kukreja, PharmD
Scientific Director, US Medical Affairs,
  Neuroscience
AbbVie
Chicago, Illinois
Chapter 8

Meghan K. Lehmann, PharmD, BCPS
Coordinator, Drug Information Services
Cleveland Clinic
Cleveland, Ohio
Chapter 3

**Elyse A. MacDonald, PharmD,
MS, BCPS**
Pharmacy Manager, Investigational Drug
  Service
University of Utah Health
Huntsman Cancer Hospital
Salt Lake City, Utah
Chapter 12

**Mark A. Malesker, PharmD, FCCP,
FCCP, FCCM, FASHP, BCPS**
Professor of Pharmacy Practice and
  Medicine
Creighton University
School of Pharmacy and Health
  Professions
Omaha, Nebraska
Chapters 15, 16

Patrick M. Malone, PharmD, FASHP
Drug Information Consultant
Kirkland, Washington
Associate Dean Emeritus
College of Pharmacy
University of Findlay
Findlay, Ohio
Chapters 13, 15, 16

Meghan J. Malone, PharmD, BCACP
Pharmacist
Swedish Medical Group
Seattle, Washington
Chapter 13

J. Russell May, PharmD, FASHP
Assistant Dean for Extended Campuses and
  Clinical Professor
University of Georgia
College of Pharmacy
Augusta, Georgia
Chapter 1

Dianne May, PharmD, BCPS, FCCP
Clinical Professor
University of Georgia
College of Pharmacy
Augusta, Georgia
Chapter 1

Michelle W. McCarthy, PharmD, FASHP
Coordinator, Pharmacy Education, Training,
  and Development Programs
University of Virginia Health System
Department of Pharmacy Services
Charlottesville, Virginia
Chapter 30

Cydney E. McQueen, PharmD
Clinical Associate Professor, Division of
  Pharmacy Practice and Administration
UMKC School of Pharmacy
Kansas City, Missouri
Chapter 5

**Whitney Mortensen, PharmD, MBA,
BCPS**
Drug Information Services Manager
Intermountain Healthcare
Pharmacy Services
Salt Lake City, Utah
Chapter 21

Genevieve Lynn Ness, PharmD
Director, Christy Houston Drug Information
  Center
Associate Professor in Pharmaceutical, Social
  and Administrative Science
Belmont University
College of Pharmacy
Nashville, Tennessee
Chapter 25

Heather A. Pace, PharmD
Clinical Pharmacist
Utilization Management
Drug Information
Kansas City, Missouri
Chapter 27

David M. Peterson, PharmD, BCPS
Drug Information Specialist
University of Utah Health
Salt Lake City, Utah
Chapter 10

Jennifer Phillips, PharmD, BCPS, FCCP, FASHP
Professor of Pharmacy Practice
Midwestern University College of Pharmacy,
  Downers Grove Campus
Downers Grove, Illinois
Chapter 4

Karen L. Rascati, PhD
Professor, Health Outcomes
The University of Texas at Austin
Austin, Texas
Chapter 7

Martha M. Rumore, PharmD, JD, MS, LLM, FAPhA
Of Counsel
Sorell, Lenna & Schmidt, LLP
Rego Park, New York
Chapter 11

Amy Heck Sheehan, PharmD
Professor of Pharmacy Practice/Drug
  Information Specialist
Purdue University College of Pharmacy/
  Indiana University Health
Indianapolis, Indiana
Chapters 2, 4

Morgan L. Sperry, PharmD
Clinical Associate Professor/Director, Drug
  Information Center
UMKC School of Pharmacy
Kansas City, Missouri
Chapter 27

Suzanne M. Surowiec, PharmD, BCACP
Associate Professor of Teaching in Pharmacy
  Practice
University of Findlay
Findlay, Ohio
Chapter 26

Jennifer K. Thomas, PharmD
Medication Quality & Safety Sr. Pharmacist
Qlarant
Columbia, Maryland
Chapter 18

Anthony Trovato, PharmD, BCPS
Drug Information Specialist
University of Utah Health
Salt Lake City, Utah
Chapter 3

Linda S. Tyler, PharmD, FASHP
Professor (Clinical), Department of
  Pharmacotherapy
College of Pharmacy, University of Utah
  Health
Salt Lake City, Utah
Chapter 14

Eric D. Vogan, MSPH
Manager, Reporting and Analytics
Cleveland Clinic
Lyndhurst, Ohio
Chapter 29

Ryan W. Walters, MS, PhD
Assistant Professor, Department of
  Medicine
Creighton University Medical Center—
  Bergan Mercy
Omaha, Nebraska
Chapter 6

Marc A. Willner, PharmD, CPHIMS
Lead Pharmacy Informatics Specialist
Cleveland Clinic
Cleveland, Ohio
Chapter 29

James P. Wilson, PharmD, PhD, FASHP
Associate Professor
The University of Texas at Austin
Health Outcomes Division
Austin, Texas
Chapter 7

Christopher S. Wisniewski, PharmD, MSCR, BCPS
Professor, Department of Clinical Pharmacy
  & Outcome Sciences
Medical University of South Carolina
Charleston, South Carolina
Chapter 5

Benjamin A. Witt, PharmD, MBA, BCPS
Drug Information Pharmacist
Cleveland Clinic
Cleveland, Ohio
Chapter 9

Candice Burns Wood, MSMIS, PAL, PSM, PSPO
Enterprise Solutions Architect
MetaBank
Sioux Falls, South Dakota
Management Consultant
Verity
Glenwood, Iowa
Chapter 22

Reviewers

Ellena Anagnostis, PharmD, MS, BCPS
Clinical Specialist, Drug Information
Program Director, PGY2 Medication-Use
  Safety and Policy Pharmacy Residency
Thomas Jefferson University Hospital
Philadelphia, Pennsylvania

Stephen Andrews, PharmD, BCPS
Drug Information Specialist
University of Utah Health
Salt Lake City, Utah

Elizabeth Bald, PharmD
Assistant Professor (Clinical), Department
  of Pharmacotherapy/Clinical Pharmacist
University of Utah College of Pharmacy/
  Madsen Family Health Clinic
Salt Lake City, Utah

Bruce A. Bouts, RPh, MD, FACP
Chair, P&T Committee
Blanchard Valley Regional Health Center
Findlay, Ohio

Jamie N. Brown, PharmD, FCCP, BCPS, BCACP
Drug Information/Investigational Drug
  Service Program Manager
Durham VA Health Care System
Durham, North Carolina

Lorrie Burns, PharmD, CPPS
Medication Safety Pharmacist
OhioHealth Riverside Methodist
  Hospital
Columbus, Ohio

Delia Carias, PharmD, BCPS, DPLA
Medication Use Policy Coordinator
St. Jude Children's Research Hospital
Memphis, Tennessee

Joseph T. DiPiro, PharmD
Dean/Archie O. McCalley Chair
Virginia Commonwealth University
School of Pharmacy
Richmond, Virginia

Akesha Esther Edwards, PhD, PharmD
Assistant Professor of Pharmaceutical
  Sciences
The University of Findlay
College of Pharmacy
Findlay, Ohio

Amanda Hansen, PharmD, MHA, FACHE, FASHP
Senior Director of Pharmacy
Cleveland Clinic
Cleveland, Ohio

Seth W. Hartman, PharmD, MBA
Director, Pharmacy Informatics
University of Chicago Medicine
Chicago, Illinois

Randy C. Hatton, PharmD, FCCP
Clinical Professor/Track Director Online
 Master's Program, Patient Safety in
 Medication Use
University of Florida College of Pharmacy/
 Department of Pharmaceutical Outcomes
 and Policy
Newberry, Florida

Darren Hein, PharmD
Assistant Professor, Pharmacy Practice
Creighton University
Center for Drug Information & Evidence-
 Based Practice
School of Pharmacy and Health Professions
Omaha, Nebraska

Megan Holsopple, PharmD, BCPS
Clinical Director, Innovation and Research
RxRevu Inc.
Denver, Colorado

Michelle Jeon, PharmD, BCACP
Assistant Professor of Pharmacy Practice
University of Health Sciences & Pharmacy in
 St. Louis
St. Louis, Missouri

Ellen A. Keating, PharmD, MS, BCPS
Medication Use Policy Coordinator
OSU Wexner Medical Center
Columbus, Ohio

Ken Kester, PharmD, JD
System Director of Telepharmacy
CommonSpirit Health
Lincoln, Nebraska

Wesley T. Lindsey, PharmD
Associate Clinical Professor/Drug
 Information and Learning Resource Center
Auburn University
Harrison School of Pharmacy
Auburn, Alabama

Scott Nelson, PharmD, MS
Assistant Professor, Biomedical Informatics/
 Assistant Clinical Director, HealthIT
Vanderbilt University Medical Center
Nashville, Tennessee

Linda K. Ohri, PharmD, MPH
Associate Professor, Emeritus
Creighton University
School of Pharmacy and Health Professions
Omaha, Nebraska

Terry L. Seaton, PharmD, BCCP, BCPS
Professor, Department of Pharmacy Practice/
 Clinical Pharmacist
St. Louis College of Pharmacy/Mercy
 Clinics—East Communities
St. Louis, Missouri

Emily Shor, PharmD
PGY-2 Internal Medicine Pharmacy
St. Louis College of Pharmacy/Veterans
 Affairs St. Louis Healthcare System
St. Louis, Missouri

John E. Stanovich, RPh
Special Assistant to the Dean
The University of Findlay
Findlay, Ohio

Joseph S. Van Tuyl, PharmD, BCCP
Associate Professor
St. Louis College of Pharmacy at UHSP
St. Louis, Missouri

Kristina E. Ward, PharmD, BCPS
Clinical Professor and Vice Chair of
  Pharmacy Practice and Director, Drug
  Information Services
University of Rhode Island College of
  Pharmacy
Kingston, Rhode Island

**Terri Warholak, PhD, RPh, CPHQ,
FAPhA**
Assistant Dean, Academic Affairs and
  Assessment
The University of Arizona College of
  Pharmacy
Tucson, Arizona

Geralyn Waters, PharmD, BCPS
Clinical Pharmacy Specialist, Drug Policy
  Development Specialist
UC Health
Cincinnati, Ohio

**Cindy J. Wordell, PharmD, BCPS,
FASHP**
Assistant Director of Pharmacy/
  Medication Policy and Clinical
  Services
Thomas Jefferson University Hospital
Philadelphia, Pennsylvania

Preface

Twenty-five years ago, drug information was in a very different place. Most drug information references were paper, communication was orally or via memos/letters (email was rarely available), the first web browser (Mosaic) was new, the number of medically related websites could be counted on one hand and most health care professionals had not seen any of them, and the only book on the practice of drug information was about 15 years old and had not been comprehensive when it was new. Even so, it was obvious that drug information was important and likely to become more so. It was with the hope of having a tool to use by both practitioners and students to learn the skills necessary to find and use drug information that this book was being developed. Over the years since, the tools available to practitioners, skills necessary, and functions performed in the field of drug information have rapidly evolved, resulting in a much longer and comprehensive book than was first even imagined.

Change continues to happen in the book. Perhaps the most obvious upon picking up the book is a continuing change in editors. Sharon Park, who edited the sixth edition, is no longer involved with the book. However, we have two new editors—Ben Witt and Dave Peterson, who we would like to welcome.

One constant in the book has been the focus on providing training in drug information management. It has been tested and refined continuously, based on experience in both practice and the classroom. In this seventh edition, the goal of this book continues to be to educate both students and practitioners on how to efficiently research, interpret, evaluate, collate, and disseminate information in the most usable form. While there is no one right method to perform these professional responsibilities, proven methods are presented and demonstrated. Also, seldom-addressed issues are covered, such as the legal and ethical considerations of providing drug information.

However, other significant changes have been made to the seventh edition that allow it to continue to expand, updating information from previous editions, and move into new areas. This includes new chapters on peer review and media relations. In addition, the chapter on pharmacy informatics from previous editions has been expanded to be two separate chapters, dedicating a new chapter to the use of large volumes of data for decision-making and how data will shape the future of pharmacy practice.

As in the past, the book begins by introducing the concept of drug information, including its history, and providing information on various places drug information specialists may be employed. This is followed by information on how to answer a question, from the process of gathering necessary background information, through determining the actual information need, to answering the question. The chapter on drug information resources includes descriptions of the most commonly used references and contains information on apps available for practitioners. The drug literature evaluation chapters have been updated and expanded to cover newer concepts, such as adaptive clinical trials. Chapters from the previous edition have been updated and rearranged in a way to make the subjects flow better. As always, numerous practical examples are provided through the chapters and in the appendices.

With the veritable Niagara Falls of drug, medical and pharmacy information available, much of which is complex, health care professionals have an increasing need for information management skills. This book will assist health care professionals and students with improvement in drug information skills and allow individuals to evolve into new roles for the advancement of the profession and patient care. The authors and editors of this book hope you, the reader, enjoy your journey toward expertise in drug information management.

Editors of Previous Editions

- Patrick M. Malone, PharmD, FASHP (Editor-in-Chief, editions 1–6)
- Karen L. Kier, PhD, MSc, RPh, BCPS, BCACP (editions 1–5)
- Kristen Wilkinson Mosdell, PharmD, BCPS (editions 1–2)
- John E. Stanovich, RPh (editions 1–5)
- Meghan J. Malone, PharmD, BCACP (editions 5-6)
- Sharon K. Park, PharmD, MEd, BCPS (edition 6)

Chapter One

Introduction to the Concept of Drug Information

J. Russell May • Dianne May

Learning Objectives

After completing this chapter, the reader will be able to:

- Define the term "drug information" and how it has changed into what is now contemporary practice.
- Identify the drug information services provided by pharmacists and drug information specialists.
- Describe the skills needed to perform drug information responsibilities.
- Identify major factors that have influenced the ability to provide drug information.
- Describe how the expanding integration of information technology has changed the methods of searching, analyzing, and providing drug information to patients and health care professionals.
- Describe practice opportunities in drug information for pharmacists.

Key Concepts

❶ Drug information may be patient-specific or developed for a given patient population.

❷ Drug information provision has evolved over the past 60 years as focus has shifted to development of safe and effective medication-use policies and processes, advancements in pharmacy informatics, focus on formulary management, evidence-based practice, drug shortages, and incorporation of new environments of care.

❸ With electronic medical records and order entry systems, drug information specialists can take a leadership role in incorporating automated interventions and decision support that improve safety and provide education at the point of prescribing.

❹ Pharmacists providing drug information must keep abreast of advancements in information technology.

❺ Biomedical literature evaluation skills are essential for all health care professionals.

❻ Leadership and career opportunities exist in a variety of settings for a drug information pharmacist.

Introduction

The United States health care system continues to undergo important changes, which are offering challenges and opportunities for health care professionals, insurers, caregivers, and consumers. Several factors are driving these changes, including regulations in health care (e.g., value-based care, rising prescription drug prices, and expanding health coverage options), continued pressure to reduce health care costs, and need to improve efficiency, quality, and safety of care.[1,2] The appropriate use of medications continues to be an essential element in this process because it represents a significant portion of the health care dollars spent in the United States.

Total health care spending in the United States in 2018 was $3.6 trillion. Pharmaceutical expenditures grew to $507.9 billion in 2019, representing a 5.4% increase from 2018.[2] Within nonfederal hospitals, prescription expenditures approached $36.9 billion in 2019.[2] In clinics, the prescription expenditures were even higher at $90.3 billion, which represents an increase of 11.8% from 2018.[2] The use of "**specialty drugs**," which are high-cost medications used to treat complex chronic conditions such as hepatitis C, cancer, cystic fibrosis, rheumatoid arthritis, and pulmonary arterial hypertension, have contributed greatly to the increased prescription expenditures especially in the clinic setting.

The availability of patient-, disease-, and medication-specific information, and a knowledgeable decision-maker are integral components of providing a system that supports the safe and appropriate use of medications in contemporary practice. Pharmacists can serve as leaders in the development of safe and effective medication-use policies and processes, selection of drug information resources, analysis and dissemination of medication-related information.

The provision of **drug information** is a fundamental responsibility of all pharmacists. ❶ *Drug information may be patient-specific or developed for a given patient population,* such as development of therapeutic guidelines, communication of a national quality initiative, or coordination of an adverse drug event reporting and monitoring program. Drug information can be disseminated through multiple avenues including presentations, publications, newsletters, websites, or even lay public or social media coverage. Delivery may be face-to-face, by phone or email, or online with programs such as Microsoft Teams or Zoom®. Changes within health care are driving increased opportunities for providing drug information, including national efforts to expand access to care while reducing health care costs, the rise in the self-care movement, and the integration of new health information technologies (e.g., electronic health record [EHR] and computerized provider order entry [CPOE], telemedicine, social media, and changes in environment of care). Opportunities for provision of drug information continue to grow in areas within the health care environment including managed care organizations, pharmaceutical industry, medical and specialty care clinics, scientific writing and medical communication companies, and the insurance industry (see Chapters 24, 26, and 27).

The term "drug information" may have different meanings to different people depending on the context in which it is used. It is sometimes used interchangeably with the term "medication information" which could be defined as information found in a reference, or verbalized by an individual, that pertains to medications. Individuals put the term "drug information" in different contexts by associating it with other words such as (1) specialist/practitioner/pharmacist/provider; (2) center/service/practice; and (3) functions/skills. The first group of words implies a specific individual, the second group implies a place, and the third implies activities and abilities of individuals. These terms may refer to either the provision of information for a specific patient or in the context of addressing medication-use issues for a population (e.g., individuals defined by a set of common characteristics, such as a policy on medication use developed by pharmacists working in the emergency department of a health care system).

Pharmacy informatics emphasizes the use of technology and automation as an integral tool in effectively organizing, analyzing, managing, and communicating information on medication use in patients.[3] It refers to the management and integration of medication-related data, information, and knowledge that spans across systems and supports the medication-use process.[3] With the mandated integration of EHR and CPOE, there is greater opportunity to provide medication information at the point of care, and be able to assess outcomes more readily.[4] The impact of new technologies and opportunities in pharmacy informatics in current and future practice will be discussed in later chapters (see Chapters 28 and 29).

The goals of this chapter are to define drug information, to describe how the role of the pharmacist has evolved in providing drug information, to discuss factors contributing to that evolution, and to describe opportunities to use drug information skills, either as a generalist or in a specialty practice.

The Beginning

The term "drug information" was developed in the early 1960s and used in conjunction with the words "center" and "specialist." In 1962, the first drug information center was opened at the University of Kentucky Medical Center.[5] The purpose of this center was to provide comprehensive drug information for staff physicians, dentists, and nurses. Another goal was to take an active role in the education of health professional students including medicine, dentistry, and nursing, and specifically influence pharmacy students in developing their roles as medication consultants. Several other drug information centers were established shortly thereafter. The first formal survey, conducted in 1983, identified 54 pharmacist-operated centers in the United Status.[6] The number of formal drug information centers continued to grow, with the highest number reported in 1986 with 127 drug information centers in existence.[7] In 2018, there were 82 reported pharmacist-operated drug information centers in the United States.[8]

The individual responsible for operating the center was called the drug information specialist. The expectation was that drug information would be stored in the center and retrieved, selected, evaluated, and disseminated by the specialist. As practice progressed, some drug information centers evolved to drug information services where drug information activities were provided outside a formalized center. In addition, other specific functions evolved over time as listed in Table 1-1.[9] A drug information center or specialist may be involved in one or all these functions. Detailed information regarding these activities is provided in subsequent chapters.

In the 1960s, the availability of new medications (e.g., neuromuscular blockers, first-generation cephalosporins) provided challenges for health care professionals to keep abreast of current information and make appropriate decisions for their patients. Part of the problem was finding a way to effectively communicate the wealth of information to those needing it. The information environment relied heavily on the print medium for storage, retrieval, and dissemination of information. MEDLARS® (Medical Literature Retrieval and Analysis System) was developed by the National Library of Medicine in the early 1960s.[10] While it provided a computerized form of searching, requests for searches were submitted by mail and results returned by mail. The ability to transmit such information over telephone lines (online technology) was not available until 1971 when MEDLINE® was introduced and was limited to libraries. During this time, the drug information specialist was viewed as a person who could bridge the gap and effectively communicate drug information. Direct access by other health care professionals was allowed in 1981, if they completed a week-long training class offered only in three cities. Of course, methods for accessing information have evolved tremendously with the creation of the Internet, mobile technologies, and applications (apps), and the integration of the EHR.

CHAPTER 1. INTRODUCTION TO THE CONCEPT OF DRUG INFORMATION

TABLE 1–1. DRUG INFORMATION SERVICES[9]

- Support clinical services with drug information when more research is required
- Answer questions regarding medications from patients' caregivers, and health care professionals (Chapter 2)
- Coordinate pharmacy and therapeutics committee activity (Chapter 15)
- Develop and educate health care professionals on medication-use policies
- Critically evaluate the literature to make formulary and patient-specific decisions (e.g., drug monograph, class review) (Chapters 4–6)
- Provide poison information
- Publish or edit information on appropriate medication use through newsletters, journal columns, websites, email, social media, etc. (Chapters 10 and 13)
- Provide education (e.g., in-services, classes, experiential education, journal club) for health care professionals, students, and patients (Chapters 9 and 30)
- Participate in health outcome initiatives
- Coordinate formulary management initiatives
- Maintain current print and online drug information resources
- Develop criteria/guidelines for medication use
- Analyze the clinical and economic impact of drug policy decisions
- Manage medication-use evaluation and other quality assurance/improvement activities
- Manage drug shortages (Chapter 17)
- Manage investigational medication use (e.g., institutional review board activities, information for practitioners) (Chapter 23)
- Coordinate ADE reporting and monitoring programs (Chapters 19 and 20)
- Consult on pharmacy informatics projects in the health care system setting (Chapter 28)
- Ensure and implement changes to medication-use policies and formulary decisions via informatics system
- Develop clinical decision support tools for CPOE including order sets and alerts

Early reports that examined the training requirements for drug information specialists recommended the following courses be added or strengthened in the pharmacy school curricula: biochemistry, anatomy, physiology, pathology, biostatistics, and experimental design (with some histology, embryology, and endocrinology incorporated into other courses).[11] In today's pharmacy curricula, most of these topics receive considerable emphasis or are incorporated in prepharmacy requirements. In addition to these subjects, incorporation of evidence-based practice and patient- and family-centered care into pharmacy school curricula became a priority. The governing bodies of pharmacy all stress the need for evidence-based practice expertise and educating patients and health care providers regarding the appropriate use of medications.[12-14] Today, pharmacists use knowledge and skills to make clinical decisions about medication use in specific patients or a group of patients in conjunction with other health care professionals. Training and expertise in evidence-based practice have led pharmacists to take a leadership role in publishing in the area of therapeutic guidelines, drug policies, and outcome analyses. These activities illustrate how pharmacists play a major role meeting the needs of individual patients and large patient groups.

The Evolution

Looking at the evolution of drug information practice from the perspective of drug information centers and from the perspective of practicing pharmacists is useful. Calculating accurate numbers of drug information centers nationally or internationally (e.g., Puerto Rico, Japan, Saudi Arabia, Africa) is difficult, because no agency or organization is responsible for maintaining a list. Well-defined criteria are not established for using the titles of drug information center/service. Some centers specialize in a particular area of drug information, and the name of the center may reflect that specific function (e.g., Center for Drug Evaluation and Research, Center for Clinical Outcomes Research and Education, Center for Drug Policy, Drug Information Center, and Poison Control Center). Some centers limit their practice to a subset of clients (e.g., pharmacists, physicians, nurses, attorneys, faculty, or consumers) based on their source of funding (e.g., pharmaceutical manufacturer, government, college of pharmacy, managed care organization, law firm, law enforcement agency, or fee-for-service). Some drug information centers are available for all consumers, 7 days a week, 24 hours a day, as is the case for a poison control center. The center may provide services via telephone, website, face-to-face, email, or other methods.

IMPACT OF DRUG INFORMATION SERVICE

A study published in 2009 examined 89 drug information centers for changes in number or type of questions, and time spent on activities compared to 5 years earlier.[15] Eighty-four percent of the drug information centers operating 5 years earlier were still in existence when the paper was published. There was an increase in time spent educating students (53%) and supporting adverse drug reaction reporting initiatives (44%). Seventy percent reported an increase in the number of complex questions, with 53% documenting an increase in the time required to answer questions.

When studying the availability of drug information centers in the hospital setting, a 2013 survey examining over 1400 U.S. general and children's medical-surgical hospitals found that 54.5% of surveyed hospitals with more than 600 beds had a formal drug information center.[16] Formal drug information centers were found in 1.6–17.6% of hospitals with less than 600 beds.[16] Regardless of hospital size, 97.2% of hospitals reported having a pharmacist available to answer drug information questions as the most frequent method for providing objective drug information to prescribers.[16]

A few studies have described the economic benefit of maintaining a drug information center or related activity in an academic institution or hospital. One such study examined the economic impact of drug information services responding to patient-specific requests.[17] The resultant cost-benefit ratio was found to be 2.9:1 to 13.2:1. Most of the cost savings resulted from decreased need for monitoring (e.g., laboratory tests) or decreased need for additional treatment related to an adverse effect. Other studies examined the drug cost avoidance and revenue associated with the provision of investigational drug services, which may or may not be the responsibility of the drug information center.[18,19] In one study, the annualized drug cost avoidance plus revenue was 2.6 million dollars.[18] Although some of these studies were completed several years ago, the basic premise of the design and results are applicable today and can be used to assess the value of a particular center or service based on location, clientele, and funding. Other literature also exists that evaluates the economic benefits of clinical pharmacy services in hospitals and community pharmacies.[20] This work may help provide a framework for how to assess the value of a drug information service.

DRUG INFORMATION SERVICE—FROM CENTERS TO PRACTITIONERS

The responsibilities of individual pharmacists providing drug information have changed substantially over the years. The impetus for this change was provided not only by the development of drug information centers and the clinical pharmacy concept, but also by the Study Commission on Pharmacy.[21] This external group was established to review the state of the practice and education of pharmacists and report its findings. One of the findings and recommendations stated that:

> ... among deficiencies in the health care system, one is the unavailability of adequate information for those who consume, prescribe, dispense, and administer drugs. This deficiency has resulted in inappropriate drug use and an unacceptable frequency of drug-induced disease. Pharmacists are seen as health care professionals who could make an important contribution to the health care system of the future by providing information about drugs to consumers and health care professionals. Education and training of pharmacists now and in the future must be developed to meet these important responsibilities.

The report of the Commission was issued in 1975 and, since that time, drug information practice has changed both for drug information centers and individual pharmacists. The development of clinical pharmacy has helped move pharmacy forward in recognizing its capabilities to contribute to the care of patients. Clinical pharmacy was thought of primarily as an institutional patient care process and did not gain widespread acceptance outside of hospitals until much later as pharmacists' direct care responsibilities spread to the ambulatory and community pharmacy environments.

EVOLVING ROLE OF PHARMACISTS AS MEDICATION EXPERTS IN HEALTH CARE

Pharmacists are now involved in many patient care areas (e.g., hospitals, primary care and specialty clinics, long-term care, and home health care) where they frequently answer drug information questions, participate in evaluating a patient's medication therapy, conduct medication-use evaluation activities, and coordinate medication policy and formulary management activities. Over time, the activity of the pharmacist as a medication expert for patients has gained acceptance and spans the continuum of care. There is much emphasis on pharmacists in community and ambulatory settings to counsel patients, answer drug information questions, review patient medication regimens for potential problems (medication therapy management), and assist patients in managing their chronic diseases. The **patient-centered medical home** (PCMH) philosophy has become a widely accepted model for how primary care should be organized and delivered throughout the health care system. While not a particular building or place, the patient-centered medical home model is considered to be comprehensive, team-based, coordinated, and accessible. As a component, the health care team helps improve the quality of care through access to information technology and other tools, to help make sure that both patients and families are making informed choices about their health. Drug information should be provided when needed, and in a culturally and linguistically appropriate manner. Proficiency in finding and evaluating the literature helps the pharmacist become an integral part of the patient-centered care model. Other organizations, including the Joint Commission of Pharmacy Practitioners, have formalized the concept of patient-centered care with the adoption of the **Pharmacists' Patient Care Process** (PPCP) which is now widely accepted by pharmacy organizations and accrediting bodies including those charged with training future pharmacists (e.g., Accreditation Council for Pharmacy Education [ACPE] and American Society of Health-System Pharmacists [ASHP]).[13]

PHARMACISTS AS EDUCATORS OF DRUG INFORMATION

Providing drug information may be on a one-on-one basis or may occur using a more structured approach, such as a presentation to a class of patients with diabetes or a group of nurses in the practice facility. In either case, the pharmacist educates those who are the beneficiaries of the drug information. There is a well-described systematic approach to answering drug information questions (see Chapter 2). One must obtain the necessary background information including pertinent patient factors, disease factors, and medication-related factors to determine the true question. Good problem-solving skills are required to fully assess the situation, develop a search strategy (see Chapter 3), evaluate the information (see Chapters 4 and 5), then formulate and communicate a response. Good communication skills are essential to respond in a clear and concise manner, using terminology that is consistent with the patients', caregivers', or health care professionals' level of understanding. Table 1-2 lists the drug information skills that a pharmacist should possess when confronted with a drug information question.

TABLE 1–2. DRUG INFORMATION SKILLS FOR ANSWERING QUESTIONS USING A SYSTEMATIC APPROACH

1. Access available information (e.g., drug information database, patient's medical records) and gather situational data needed to characterize question or issue
2. Assess the level of urgency, detail, and extent of the needs for information
3. Formulate appropriate question(s)
4. Use a systematic approach to find needed information
5. Evaluate information critically for validity and applicability
6. Develop, organize, and summarize response for question or issue
7. Communicate clearly and effectively when speaking or writing, at an appropriate level of understanding
8. Anticipate other information needs and follow-up

Pharmacists may also participate in precepting students in patient care or pharmacy environments. In any of these roles, the pharmacist must use appropriate drug information retrieval and evaluation skills to make sure that the most current and accurate information is provided to make decisions about medication use for those they are serving. This role of the pharmacist as a drug information provider continues to be an important component of the Center for the Advancement of Pharmaceutical Education (CAPE) educational outcomes. These outcomes are initiated and maintained by the American Association of Colleges of Pharmacy (AACP) to help transform the pharmacy curriculum to support education of the future.[22]

FACTORS INFLUENCING THE EVOLUTION OF THE PHARMACIST'S ROLE AS A DRUG INFORMATION PROVIDER

❷ *Drug information provision has evolved over the past 60 years as focus has shifted to development of safe and effective medication-use policies and processes, advancements in pharmacy informatics, focus on formulary management, evidence-based practice, drug shortages, and incorporation of new environments of care.*

Medication Safety: Adverse Drug Events (ADEs)

An estimated 1.3 million emergency room visits and 350,000 hospitalizations annually are attributed to adverse drug events (ADEs) with an annual extra cost of 3.5 billion dollars to the health care system.[23,24] Many of these events are considered preventable. These numbers are probably even higher in the elderly population because of age-related physiological changes, coexisting conditions, and polypharmacy.[25] Pediatrics is another population of concern. A medication-related cause was found in approximately 8% of emergency department visits by pediatric patients with 67% of them deemed preventable.[26] The prevention of ADEs will continue to be a significant health care issue in the future.

One of the primary drug information roles for pharmacists in the beginning was collecting and evaluating ADEs.[5] This role will continue to expand due to an anticipated increase in the number of ADEs in the future. Reasons for this increase include: (1) the availability of new medications and new indications, (2) the growing elderly population, (3) increased use of medications for disease prevention, and (4) improved insurance coverage for medications. Pharmacists perform this function in institutional health systems, managed care, or the pharmaceutical industry (see Chapters 19, 20, and 24). To illustrate how a central area for reporting ADEs, such as a drug information center in an institutional health system, can be beneficial, consider the following unpublished example from an academic medical center.

> The drug information center received three reports of patients developing methemoglobinemia within a 2-week period. The offending agent was suspected to be benzocaine spray. Upon investigation, the drug information pharmacist recognized that all reports had one thing in common, the administering nurse. The pharmacist witnessed the administration of the medication by the nurse the next time it was ordered for a patient. Instead of a single brief spray as directed by the prescribing information, several sprays were used resulting in a potentially toxic dose of medication. A series of in-services for nurses was developed by the drug information pharmacist. No reports of benzocaine-induced methemoglobinemia were reported at the institution since.

The role of the drug information specialist in the pharmaceutical industry, as it relates to reporting ADEs, is especially important in postmarketing surveillance activities. Because of the specific definition of a study population using inclusion and exclusion criteria in a new medication trial, many ADEs go undetected until the agent is commercially available and used in a broader population. By quickly identifying potential problems and communicating them to health care professionals, patient safety may be improved. The training and expertise of the drug information pharmacist qualifies them to play a major role in this process.

The importance of maintaining a comprehensive, multidisciplinary, ongoing program for monitoring, reporting, and resolving drug-related problems, and developing mechanisms to prevent future ADEs will continue to be an important element of managing medication use. The drug information pharmacist can provide leadership and innovative techniques to improve the overall ADE monitoring and reporting program (e.g., establishment of a multidisciplinary adverse drug reaction conference was an innovative way to increase awareness and reporting of adverse drug reactions at one health system).

Integration of New Health Information Technologies

The effort to nationally modernize health care using information technology dates back to the Institute of Medicine's (IOM; name recently changed to the National Academy of Medicine, NAM) 2001 report.[27] Implementation of health information technologies in health care over the past 10 years has been expedited with policies such as the Health Information Technology for Economic and Clinical Health (HITECH) Act and EHR incentive programs through Centers for Medicare & Medicaid Services (CMS).[28] Pharmacists can play an integral role in implementing information technology that improves quality of care, patient safety, efficiencies and leads to economic benefit. Future trends in information technology are likely to involve or affect such things as **digital health**, population health management, interoperability (e.g., sharing digital patient data across critical systems and functional teams), EHR optimization, data security, value-based care, virtual care, and **clinical decision support**.[29]

Pharmacy Informatics

Pharmacy informatics emphasizes the use of technology and automation as an integral tool in effectively organizing, analyzing, managing, and communicating information on medication use in patients. It refers to the management and integration of medication-related data, information, and knowledge that spans across systems and supports the medication-use process.

Several key advancements in health information technologies include the use of CPOE, electronic order sets with clinical decision support, **smart pumps**, and barcoding. With the mandated integration of EHR and CPOE, there is greater opportunity to provide information on medications for individual patients at the point of care and to be able to assess outcomes more readily. In fact, the Joint Commission of Pharmacy Practitioners' "Pharmacists' Patient Care Process" takes full advantage of advancements in health information technologies to make communication between health care professionals more efficient and effective.

❸ *With electronic medical records and order entry systems, drug information specialists can take a leadership role in incorporating automated interventions and decision support that improve safety and provide education at the point of prescribing.*

Can we move this up to make one paragraph with the preceding information use of **computer-based clinical decision support systems** (CDSS) (see Chapter 28) that provide patient information with recommendations based on the best evidence has shown to be valuable in the patient care setting, including a reported decrease in length of hospital stay.[30,31] In one study examining the value of using a decision support program to assist physicians in using anti-infective agents, the length of hospital stay of patients with caregivers using the recommendations was compared with a group of patients with caregivers who did not always use the recommendations, and compared against a group of patients who were admitted to the unit 2 years before the intervention program.[30] The length of hospital stay was statistically different with an average of 10 days, 16.7 days, and 12.9 days, respectively. Drug information pharmacists can also play an instrumental role in developing and maintaining electronic order sets to be used within CPOE and medication libraries used with smart pump technology.

Although technology affords remote-site access to drug information resources, pharmacists must have the skills to perceive, assess, and evaluate the information, and apply the information to the situation. One of the most rapidly changing technologies in health care is information technology. ❹ *Pharmacists providing drug information must keep abreast of advances in information technology* in an effort to integrate new and valuable systems in a timely and efficient manner. The need for this type of training is emphasized in a NAM report.[32]

Pharmacists' participation in the use of "big data" (e.g., large and complex datasets) will become very important as it may lead to more confident decision-making, improved operational efficiency, and optimized outcomes (see Chapter 29).[33,34]

Drug Information Resources and Apps

Even though the amount of literature is much larger today than in the past, it is more manageable (see Chapter 3). The Internet allows the user to easily access the scientific literature, government publications, news reports, clinical guidelines, and other useful items, frequently without cost to the health care professional or the consumer. Handheld devices (e.g., smartphones, tablets) allow health care professionals to have a full range of applications (e.g., decision support tools, medical references) available at the point of care. These offer the convenience of collecting and accessing information from a device that can be carried in a user's pocket. These systems can be used more conveniently than a desktop computer for online searching, calculations, patient tracking, laboratory order entry, and results. They are also convenient for providing medication profiles, setting up appointments, and searching drug information databases. Patients and health care professionals can find information on nearly every disease and treatment, and virtual health communities and forums provide a mutually supportive environment for patients and their families, and friends. The use of social media (e.g., Twitter®, Facebook®, and LinkedIn®), web forums, and blogs has simplified the way in which peers can exchange news and share opinions. Several professional organizations (e.g., ASHP) have used technology to maintain awareness of important news affecting pharmacy and the health care environment (e.g., regulatory and health policy issues, pandemic-related issues), drug shortages, and meeting notifications. Live continuing education is offered at a health care professional's computer desktop through webinars. With the ever-growing access to information through media outlets, pharmacists should develop relationships with these media outlets (e.g., newspaper, television, etc.) to ensure that the drug information reported by these groups is accurate and useful for patients (see Chapter 14).

Drug Information Availability

There is an increasing need by health care professionals, as well as consumers, to get more information about medications sooner. Information is needed quickly when a new medication becomes commercially available because of the potential for health and cost implications, when a product is withdrawn from the market for safety reasons, or when data from a new study is released that could have an impact on how a common disease is treated. The lag time that occurs with the print format may not be acceptable for many direct patient care issues. The Internet allows medical information to be available sooner to both health care professionals and the public. The availability of electronic journals and texts has minimized the need to travel to a library. Online repositories for articles, such as BioMed Central (https://www.biomedcentral.com/) and PubMed Central® (https://www.ncbi.nlm.nih.gov/pmc/), allow individuals to access millions of articles quickly, easily, and free of charge. The majority of printed medical textbooks with an online version require a subscription; however, there are exceptions (e.g., https://www.merckmanuals.com where two editions of Merck Manuals can be viewed and searched for free; one for health care professionals and one for patients, parents, or caregivers). Registries of ongoing clinical trials, such as ClinicalTrials.gov (https://www.clinicaltrials.gov), provide information on the purpose and criteria for participation in an ongoing clinical trial. This has allowed pharmacists to anticipate new therapies, and perhaps help their patients receive medications not yet FDA-approved through enrollment in a clinical trial.

Accuracy of Drug Information on the Internet

In addition to health care professionals, patients are also accessing information from the web, using sites that are sponsored by a variety of companies and individuals with diverse interests. In one survey, 85% of physician respondents had experienced a patient bringing Internet information to a visit.[35] Information that is either incomplete or inaccurate may be more harmful than useful. In one study, medication information on Wikipedia was found to be narrower in scope and had more errors of omission than the comparator database on the web (e.g., Medscape Drug Reference, which is a free, online, evidence-based, peer-reviewed database).[36]

There is some effort toward helping consumers accurately assess the quality of information on the Internet. Health on the Net (http://www.hon.ch) is a nonprofit, nongovernment organization that uses criteria to assess the quality of a website. The organization will give a seal of approval to those sites that apply and meet the quality criteria. If misinformation or inaccurate information is found on the web, organizations exist to monitor fraud (e.g., Quackwatch®, https://quackwatch.org).

Some drug information centers have created their own websites to (1) post information about their center and services; (2) provide links to related sites considered to be of acceptable quality; (3) accept adverse drug reaction reports; (4) serve as a convenient means of receiving and answering drug information questions; and (5) provide information regarding formulary changes, institution-specific therapeutic guidelines, and medication policy initiatives.[37,38] Some drug information pharmacists have developed guiding principles to help evaluate health care resources from various sources including print, online databases, mobile applications, and social media.[39]

Focus on Evidence-Based Medicine and Drug Policy Development

The pharmacist's ability to apply their drug information skills to medication policy decisions will be of growing importance in this changing health care environment. This includes identifying trends of inappropriate medication use and providing supporting scientific evidence to help change behavior. Continued growth in national health expenditures has raised the interest of government, insurance agencies, health care professionals, and the public in identifying strategies to control spending while maintaining access to quality health care. For 2015–2025, health spending is projected to grow at an average rate of 5.8% per year.[40] Because drug expenditures are the largest component of the pharmacy operating budget and a significant portion of the entire health system budget, the pharmacy budget frequently attracts significant attention from leadership. In recent years, there has been a shift from a fee-for-service, inpatient focus, to a capitated, managed care, ambulatory focus.

Managed care, a process seeking to manage the delivery of high-quality health care in order to improve cost-effectiveness, is an ever-increasing portion of health care delivery. Today, providers are relying less on impressions of what may be happening in a practice setting and more on data that is actually being collected in that same group of patients (e.g., number of patients receiving appropriate dose of medications). Goals are set for a particular group of patients (e.g., all patients receive beta-blocker therapy after a myocardial infarction) based on evidence found in the scientific literature.

Evidence-Based Outcomes

The connection of applying the scientific information to the patient care setting is made through evidence-based medicine. Evidence-based medicine (see Chapter 8) is an approach to practice that integrates current clinical research evidence with pathophysiological rationale, professional expertise, and patient preferences to make decisions for a population.[41] **❺** *Biomedical literature evaluation skills are essential for all health care professionals.* Pharmacists, for example, need to have a solid understanding of drug information concepts and skills, be able to evaluate the medication-use issues for a group of patients, be able to search, retrieve, and critically evaluate the scientific literature, and apply the information to the targeted group of patients. Evidence-based medicine techniques are used in health care organizations to develop and implement various quality assurance tools (e.g., therapeutic guidelines, clinical pathways, and medication-use evaluations) in an effort to improve patient outcomes and decrease costs across the health care system. The goal is to support the appropriate use of medications including correcting the overuse, underuse, or misuse of medicines. In the United States, the NAM designated evidence-based patient-centered health care delivery as a key feature of high-quality medical care.[27] The process of evidence-based medicine requires that systems be developed to measure and report processes and outcomes that can be used to drive quality improvement efforts. As an example, data can be collected and analyzed by a drug information specialist using scientific methods to support the decision-making process in a managed care organization.[42]

Outcomes research is a type of investigation that uses scientific rigor to determine which interventions are most effective for certain types of patients and under certain circumstances. This contrasts with traditional randomized controlled studies to determine *efficacy*, which examines the success of treatments in controlled environments. Outcomes research, taking place in real-life settings, is called *effectiveness* research. The branch of outcomes research, pharmacoeconomics, provides tools to assess cost, consequences (e.g., quality of life, patient functionality, patient preferences), and efficiency (see Chapter 7).[43,44] These types of publications can help guide the health care professional in developing guidelines on appropriate medication use in their practice setting.

Sophistication of Medication Therapy

The sophisticated level of medication therapy that occurs today provides pharmacists much more opportunity to:

- Lend their expertise in assessing drug information needs of health care professionals, patients, or family members.
- Provide literature to help choose the best medication to use within a class.
- Convey the appropriate information to help patients correctly and safely use the more potent medications.
- Address administration and delivery issues.

Keeping up with new developments in medication therapy is increasingly difficult for health care professionals. Over 7000 compounds are in various stages of clinical drug development.[45] Nearly 75% of the projects in the clinical-study pipeline involve medications that attack a disease in a way that is unique to any other existing medicine. Several of the medications in the different stages of development could have a substantial impact on clinical practice and drug expenditures once they are commercially available. For instance, over 1600 of these medications are anticancer agents, which could have an impact on life expectancy, quality of life, and the related expenses associated with the potential need for increased ancillary care, additional physician office visits, or hospitalization.[45] Pharmacists need to proactively monitor these pipeline medications to provide adequate time to identify the patient population that will most benefit from the new medication and to help anticipate the cost of treating these patients compared to traditional therapy. See Chapter 21 for more information on medication policy, procedure, and guideline development.

The use of **pharmacogenomic** profiling is expanding with approximately 72 genes affecting over 270 medications now recognized as actionable in the clinic setting.[46] As the types and sophistication of medication therapy continues to evolve, this will present challenges for patients, family members, and health care providers seeking information on these emerging therapies. In addition, specific gene therapy is being developed (e.g., therapy to treat spinal muscular atrophy in children). The ability to assess drug information needs, search, analyze and retrieve appropriate literature, and apply the information to patients will be important.

Rise in the Self-Care Movement

Consumers have a continually growing desire for information about their medications (see Chapter 27). The growth of the self-care movement, the increased focus on health care costs, and the improved accessibility of health information are some of the factors that have influenced patients to participate more fully in health care decisions, including the selection and use of medications. **Direct-to-consumer advertising (DTCA)** campaigns appear in virtually all mediums including magazines, television ads, web-based ads (e.g., through email, search engine marketing, or banner-style ads on specific websites), and radio reports (see Chapter 25). Patients will need assistance interpreting this DTCA to determine what information is applicable to their medical condition. While DTCA may be beneficial to patients by helping them feel empowered to have a more active role in their health care, it may lead to patients requesting medications that are more expensive or that are not the best choice for them.

Health information is one of the most frequently searched topics on the Internet. A report from the Pew Research Center stated approximately 60% of Americans sought health information online in the past year.[47] About 81% of Americans own a smartphone and the majority of these owners use their phone to look up health information.[48] When a patient finds information about medications that they are either taking or considering, from the Internet, through the lay press, or by DTCA, a pharmacist can help patients critically assess the drug information that they find and add to the information based on specific patient-related needs (see Chapter 27).

Growing Use of Complementary and Alternative Medicine

The use of **complementary and alternative medicine** (CAM), which includes herbal supplements, dietary supplements, meditation, chiropractic care, and acupuncture, is widespread. The need to critically assess information regarding CAM has become increasingly important, with approximately 38% of U.S. adults aged 18 years and over, and approximately 12% of children, using some form of CAM.[49] The 2007 National Health Interview Survey (NHIS), a nationwide government survey, found that the highest rates of use were among people aged 50–59 years (44%).[50] The NHIS data also revealed that approximately 42% of adults who used CAM in the past 12 months disclosed their use of CAM to their health care provider.[50] In a more recent survey, 42% of responding hospitals indicated that they offer one or more complementary or alternative medicine therapies.[51]

Because many adults also use nonprescription medications, prescription drugs, or other conventional medical approaches to manage their health, communication between patients and health care professionals about CAM and conventional therapies is vital to ensuring safe, integrated use of all health care approaches. The changing environment affords the pharmacist many opportunities to use the full spectrum of drug information skills. Factors such as the integration of new technologies, the focus on evidence-based medicine and drug policy development, the sophistication of medication therapy, and the rise in self-care movement require that all health care professionals have a strong foundation in drug information concepts.

EDUCATING STUDENTS ON DRUG INFORMATION CONCEPTS

The education of pharmacists continues to evolve in scope and depth. Many of the areas identified earlier as needed by the drug information specialist are now incorporated into pharmacy curricula and taught to all student pharmacists. In 1991, a consensus conference in New Mexico was held to define a set of objectives for didactic and experiential training in drug information for the year 2000.[52] Twenty-three educators and practitioners participated in the conference. Several key concepts were developed including: (1) drug information should be a required component of the pharmacy curriculum and include both didactic and competency-based experiential components, (2) drug information concepts and skills should be spread throughout the curriculum, beginning the day the students enter pharmacy school, and (3) problem solving should be a major technique in drug information education, with the goal of developing self-directed learners. Developing these skills should provide the foundation for the pharmacist to be a lifelong learner and problem solver. Based upon the work of this conference, as well as changes in the health care system and the movement toward outcome-based education, many colleges of pharmacy have redesigned their curricula to provide a more comprehensive and integrated approach to teaching drug information concepts and skills.[53,54] The CAPE outcomes, which are guidelines used for pharmacy education, continue to include drug information skills for all student pharmacists.[22] In one survey published in 2006, all pharmacy schools offered didactic drug information education to first professional year students either as a stand-alone course (70%) or integrated throughout the professional curriculum.[54] Fifty-one of the 60 colleges offered an advanced pharmacy practice experience in drug information, and 62% of these had it as an elective. However, 58% of respondents felt that they had an inadequate number of drug information training sites. Communication skills are taught formally to facilitate the pharmacist's ability to transmit information to both health care professionals and patients.

In 2009, the American College of Clinical Pharmacy (ACCP) Drug Information Practice and Research Network (DI PRN) published an opinion paper that provided recommendations regarding the curriculum and instructional methods for teaching drug information in both colleges of pharmacy and advanced training, to help meet the needs of the changing health care environment and the changing culture of drug information practice.[55] In a follow-up survey examining which recommendations were included in U.S. pharmacy college curricula in the areas of drug information, literature evaluation, and biostatistics, only 47% (9/19) of the core concepts outlined in the opinion paper were included in curricula of all responding institutions.[56]

This supports the need to continually re-evaluate and update the curriculum that focuses on drug information concepts because of changes in the health care environment. Of note, many respondents identified the areas of evidence-based medicine, medication safety, and pharmacy informatics as areas of expanded focus. The evolution in technology and social media has changed the way faculty teach, how students learn, and the way faculty and students communicate in colleges of pharmacy. An academic technologist can support the college faculty and staff in the use of learning management systems, distance education programs, and classroom technology. The COVID-19 pandemic has expedited this process and made this support a necessity.

Upon graduation, a pharmacist can choose to enter the workforce or continue their education in a practice-based residency or fellowship. Postgraduate training through residencies and fellowship experiences can help prepare a pharmacist to be a skilled clinical practitioner, researcher, educator, and leader in the profession of pharmacy. Drug information and medication policy development are integrated throughout the postgraduate year 1 (PGY1) residency standards. Currently, there are 70 ASHP-accredited specialty practice (PGY2) residencies in areas affiliated with drug information including 34 Medication-Use Safety and Policy, 33 Pharmacy Informatics, and 3 Population Health Management and Data Analytics[57] (https://accreditation.ashp.org/directory/#/program/residency). In addition, there are several specific drug information specialty residencies that are still available; however, they are not ASHP-accredited. All programs were designed for those who practice in health systems. Individuals who specialize in drug information can practice in a variety of different areas (e.g., scientific writing and medical communications). See Chapter 30 for more information.

Opportunities in Drug Information Specialty Practice

As the role of the practicing pharmacist has changed regarding drug information activities, so has the role of the specialist. The role of the drug information specialist has evolved and may include individuals who specifically answer questions in a call center to those who focus on development of medication policies and provide information on complex drug information questions. ❻ *Leadership and career opportunities exist in a variety of settings for drug information specialists,* including health system pharmacies, contract drug information centers, pharmacy informatics, managed care organizations (e.g., health maintenance organizations [HMOs]/pharmacy benefit management organizations [PBMs]), scientific writing and medical communications, poison control, pharmaceutical industry, government (e.g., U.S. Food and Drug Administration), and academia. A drug information specialist can be involved in multiple activities in practice settings described in the next sections.

HEALTH SYSTEM DRUG INFORMATION SERVICES

Opportunities exist for drug information specialists in most health system pharmacies. For example, roles covered by a drug information specialist in health systems often include managing the formulary system, medication safety programs, medication usage evaluation, and medication policy development and management (see Chapters 15–18).

Drug information specialists are in an enviable position to provide a service that will improve patient outcomes and decrease health care costs through the provision of unbiased information that supports rational, cost-effective, patient- and disease-specific medication therapy. With formulary management, more emphasis will be needed on evaluating nontraditional medications such as herbal and natural products, compounded products, and biosimilars to determine if they have a place on the formulary. Formulary management software will need to be evaluated and implemented, and automated formulary restrictions and decision support will need to be developed. In addition, drug shortages and counterfeit medications will need to be addressed (Chapter 17). Drug information specialists will also be tasked with deciding what drug information resources are to be used by health care professionals in the health system, publishing drug information newsletters, and managing websites.

CONTRACTED DRUG INFORMATION CENTER (FEE-FOR-SERVICE)

Another way to deliver evidence-based drug information services is by contracting with a drug information service with formally trained drug information specialists.[58]

Potential clients include the following: managed care groups, contract pharmacy services, federal or state government, pharmacy benefits managers, buying groups, attorneys, pharmaceutical industry, individual hospitals, large health systems, chain pharmacies, independent pharmacies, nursing home chains, and medical education companies. Several different fee structures have been used, including a fee per request price structure, hourly rate fees, fees per contracted item (e.g., drug monograph), or an annual flat fee.[58] A client may be charged a simple fee per question or may be offered a detailed menu of services with the final cost dependent on the number and types of services chosen by the contracting party.

Services provided within these contracts may include:

- Providing answers to medication information requests
- Preparing new drug evaluation monographs or class reviews
- Developing medication-use evaluation criteria
- Preparing pharmacoeconomic evaluations
- Developing guidelines for a particular disease
- Writing a pharmacotherapy publication (e.g., website, blog, newsletter)
- Providing continuing education programming

Additional services that the center may make available are access to in-house question files for sharing of information on commonly asked questions, and direct access to the center's Internet home page for review of medication-use evaluations, formulary reviews, and newsletters. One center reports information on drug shortages to ASHP through a grant.[59] This type of involvement by drug information centers may lead to other opportunities to provide expertise such as contributing to national guidelines.[60] Frequently, the contracting drug information center also has responsibilities for pharmacy services (e.g., drug information, medication policy) as part of an entire health system or based out of a college of pharmacy.

PHARMACY INFORMATICS IN A HEALTH SYSTEM

The majority (92%) of published articles on health information technology's effect on outcomes (quality, efficiency, and provider satisfaction) reached positive conclusions.[61] There are tremendous opportunities for a **pharmacy informatics specialist**—an individual that has advanced drug information skills with a keen understanding of computer and information technology. Postgraduate year 2 (PGY-2) residencies are available in pharmacy informatics. This individual can help support patient care activities by improving the efficiency of workflow, by increasing access to patient-specific information and the medical literature through technology by remote-site availability. This individual may also be involved in the area of institutional medication policy management. The role of a pharmacist as an informatics specialist has been clearly described in the successful implementation of CPOE system in an academic medical center setting.[62] The role goes beyond the implementation phase and includes system maintenance (e.g., formulary updates, revised clinical decision support as new guidelines and medical evidence are published, developing specialized smart pump libraries) (see Chapter 28).[63]

MANAGED CARE PHARMACY

With total U.S. drug expenditures for pharmaceuticals increasing annually, there are tremendous opportunities for the drug information specialist to provide leadership in the development and implementation of mechanisms to support the cost-effective selection and use of medications in managed pharmacy organizations.[2] With the appropriate training (e.g., specialized residency in drug information practice or managed care pharmacy) and expertise, opportunities are growing for the drug information specialists in the insurance industry, HMOs, PBM companies, state and national government agencies (e.g., Medicaid, Medicare), as well as other groups interested in the cost-efficient use of medications. A list of residencies in managed care pharmacy is available through the Academy of Managed Care Pharmacy (AMCP; https://www.amcp.org). A drug information specialist may be involved in several activities, which include providing medication-use evaluation assessments, encouraging the use of cost-effective alternatives, providing medication and practice-related information, managing formularies, providing information to support formulary guidelines, and developing disease management program.

POISON CONTROL

Poison information is a specialized area of drug information with the pharmacist typically practicing in an accredited poison information center or an emergency room. Specialized training in toxicology, such as a toxicology fellowship, would be advisable. In drug information centers, health care professionals generate most consultations, whereas, in a poison control center, most are generated from the lay public. Poison control centers must be prepared to provide information on management of any poison situation, including household products, poisonous plants and animals, medications, and other chemicals. Because of the type of information that the specialist provides, nearly all requests for information to a poison control center are urgent. A specialist in poison information requires expertise in clinical toxicology to be able to obtain a complete history that correctly assesses the potential severity of exposure. They need to know where and how to search for this type of information and be able to develop an appropriate plan for intervention. They also need to be able to communicate the plan in a comprehensive, concise, and accurate manner to a consumer at an appropriate level of understanding.

PHARMACEUTICAL INDUSTRY

The pharmaceutical industry provides many career opportunities for pharmacists in a variety of areas, including information technology, training and development, scientific communications, post-marketing research, regulatory affairs, professional affairs, medical information services, medical liaison, drug discovery, product development, and clinical research.[64] Each position listed above requires a different skill set, which may differ between companies, depending on the infrastructure and mission of the individual companies.

A pharmacist with specialized drug information expertise or training can answer drug information questions, report and monitor ADEs, and provide information support to other departments within the company. A pharmacist, who is often referred to as a medical science liaison, can help educate health care professionals about a particular group of products or provide academic support or partnership for educational initiatives. They may interact with sales and marketing, participate with regulatory affairs issues, and handle product complaints. Regulatory affairs specialists help ensure that medications under development meet the state and federal regulations that have been developed to protect the public. Pharmacists may be called on to review adverse effects identified in clinical studies and communicate this and other information to the appropriate research and development team.

In addition to providing written information on the medication product produced by the manufacturer, there are opportunities to provide additional information at pharmacy and therapeutics committees or state's drug use review (DUR) boards. Pharmaceutical companies have extensive scientific data on their products; some of which are not available through other published sources or may require a formal FOIA (Freedom of Information Act) request.

Pharmacists with specialized drug information training can take a leadership role in evaluating current research, serving as an associate in managing ongoing research, or designing studies to help answer questions about new indications for future use of the product. The area of postmarketing research is a growing area that offers tremendous opportunity for pharmacists to share their knowledge of the health care environment, research design, technology, and economics from the perspective of the pharmaceutical industry. As the sophistication of medication products and information management (e.g., electronic **new drug application** [NDA]) has increased, so have the opportunities for pharmacists to practice in the pharmaceutical industry and focus on using the skills of a drug information specialist and clinical specialist. Postgraduate residencies and fellowships, which are typically shared with a college of pharmacy, are available to help strengthen some of the drug information skills needed to work in the pharmaceutical industry. Other positions (e.g., drug discovery, product development, clinical research) require an advanced degree of study (e.g., M.B.A., Ph.D.). See Chapter 24 for more information.

ACADEMIA

The drug information specialist can provide leadership in the pharmacy curriculum, including both didactic and experiential training. In addition to teaching drug information skills that are required across practice sites, the specialist also serves as collaborator with other faculty on cases and activity designed to reinforce drug information skills for students. Approximately one-third of drug information centers are funded by a college of pharmacy.[8] This environment allows the student to be prepared to efficiently and accurately provide information to the appropriate audience, while emphasizing both didactic and competency-based experiential training.

As the prevalence of evidence-based practice increases, the importance of teaching drug literature evaluation skills increases. Courses incorporating biomedical literature evaluation, formulary management, and the development and management of medication-use policies will be best taught by drug information specialists in academia (see Chapter 30).

SCIENTIFIC WRITING AND MEDICAL COMMUNICATION

Medical education and communications companies, separate from the pharmaceutical industry, may provide educational programming for health care professionals and consumers to meet continuing education needs (e.g., symposia, workshops, monographs), or nonaccredited or promotional activities (e.g., sales training, publication planning, journal articles).[65,66] These individuals may write, edit, or develop medication-related materials by gathering, organizing, interpreting, and presenting information for either health care professionals or the public. Examples of these materials include patient education materials, journal articles, regulatory documents, poster presentations, grant proposals, sales and marketing of pharmaceuticals, drug evaluation monographs for health care systems.

In addition to having good writing skills, the pharmacist also needs to have scientific expertise and literature evaluation skills. More than 77% of medical education and communication companies employ at least one licensed health care professional. These professionals may have several positions including director and scientific writer. Pharmacists in this capacity would work closely with editors, graphic designers, website strategists, meeting planners, and scientists. This type of information may be communicated in a variety of ways including orally, in print format, and electronically on the web. Medical communication fellowships are available to help provide a solid foundation through experiences to various aspects of the medical communication industry.

Summary and Direction for the Future

All pharmacists must be effective drug information providers regardless of their practice site. It is one of the most fundamental responsibilities of a pharmacist. Developing the skills of an effective drug information provider is the foundation for the pharmacist to be a lifelong learner and problem solver. The literature is a valuable component of both processes and will allow the individual pharmacist to adapt to the needs of a continually changing health care system.

Opportunities abound for pharmacists to use drug information skills in all practice settings either as a generalist or a specialist practitioner. Drug information specialists will still be needed to operate the drug information centers, to provide leadership in the area of pharmacy informatics, managed care organizations, poison control, pharmaceutical industry, scientific writing and medical communications, and in academia.

Self-Assessment Questions

1. The first drug information center was opened in 1962 at:
   a. The University of Iowa
   b. The Ohio State University
   c. The University of Kentucky
   d. Misr International University in Cairo, Egypt
   e. None of the above

2. Formal drug information centers are found more often in hospitals of the following size:
   a. <100 beds
   b. 100–150 beds
   c. 200–300 beds
   d. 301–400 beds
   e. >600 beds

3. In current practice, the term "drug information" is used:
   a. To convey the management and use of information on medication therapy
   b. To prevent confusion with information on drugs of abuse
   c. To signify the broader role that all pharmacists take in information provision
   d. a and b
   e. a and c

4. There is evidence that the cost-benefit ratio of drug information services ranges from:
   a. 1:1 to 1.5:1
   b. 1.6:1 to 2:1
   c. 2.9:1 to 13.2:1
   d. 14:1 to 20:1
   e. >25:1

5. The cost-benefit ratio of a drug information services related to patient-specific requests largely resulted from savings by:
   a. Decreasing the books in the library by increasing the use of electronic sources
   b. Decreasing the need for drug monitoring
   c. Decreasing the need for additional treatment related to an adverse event
   d. Preventing adverse drug reactions
   e. Both b and c are correct

6. What was the approximate cost for pharmaceutical expenditures in the United States in 2019?
   a. $100.5 billion
   b. $200.3 million
   c. $300.7 billion
   d. $507.9 billion
   e. $10.2 trillion

7. Which of the following are essential drug information skills in contemporary practice?
   a. Evaluate the medical literature critically for validity and applicability.
   b. Use a systematic approach to find needed information.
   c. Communicate clearly when writing and/or speaking at an appropriate level for understanding.
   d. Anticipate drug information needs.
   e. All the above.

8. What percentage of medication-related emergency department visits by pediatric patients is thought to be preventable?
   a. 1%
   b. 2%
   c. 67%
   d. 95%
   e. 99%

9. The drug information pharmacist's role in pharmacy informatics should include:
   a. Incorporating automated interventions at the point of physician order entry
   b. Writing code for CPOE systems
   c. Developing and maintaining electronic order sets
   d. a and b
   e. a and c

10. With pharmacogenomics profiling, approximately how many medications are now recognized as actionable in the clinic setting?
   a. 81
   b. 20
   c. 1000
   d. 270
   e. 940

11. What percentage of pharmacy schools offer didactic drug information education as either a stand-alone course or integrated throughout the curriculum?
   a. 100%
   b. 80%
   c. 75%
   d. 60%
   e. 50%

12. According to the Pew Research Center, what percentage of Americans own a smartphone?
   a. 10%
   b. 25%
   c. 51%
   d. 62%
   e. 81%

13. Which of the following changes have influenced the role of the drug information specialist?
   a. Rise in self-care movement
   b. Development of evidence-based medicine
   c. Expansion of social media
   d. Focus on medication safety
   e. All the above

14. For pharmacies in organized health care settings, the largest component in the pharmacy operating budget is:
    a. Personnel
    b. Drugs
    c. Clerical supplies
    d. The drug information center
    e. Intravenous (IV) room equipment

15. Which of the following is true regarding complementary and alternative medicine (CAM)?
    a. CAM is not used in children.
    b. The use of CAM has been growing nationally.
    c. Only 5% of hospitals have some sort of CAM option for patients.
    d. It is easy to find complete and accurate information on CAM.
    e. Drug information centers never answer questions regarding CAM.

REFERENCES

1. 2019 Health care regulatory outlook changes in health care laws and regulations [Internet]. London (UK): Delloitte [cited 2019 Oct 21]. Available from: https://www2. deloitte.com/us/en/pages/regulatory/articles/health-care-regulatory-outlook.html.
2. Tichy EM, Shumock GT, Hoffman JM, Suda K J, Rim M H, Tadrous M, Stubbings Jo A, Cuellar S, Clark J S, Wiest M D, Matusiak L M, Hunkler R J, Vermeulen L C. National trends in prescription drug expenditures and projections for 2020. Am J Health-Syst Pharm. 2020;77:1213-30.
3. Section of Pharmacy Informatics and Technology's glossary of informatics terms [Internet]. Bethesda (MD): American Society of Health-System Pharmacists [cited 2019 Oct 23]. Available from: https://www.ashp.org/Pharmacy-Practice/Resource-Centers/ Informatics/General-Pharmacy-Informatics.
4. Centers for Medicare & Medicaid Services. Electronic health records [Internet]. [cited 2019 Oct 23]. Available from: https://www.cms.gov/Medicare/E-Health/EHealthRecords/index.
5. Parker PF. The University of Kentucky drug information center. Am J Hosp Pharm. 1965;22:42-7.
6. Amerson AB, Wallingford DM. Twenty years' experience with drug information centers. Am J Hosp Pharm. 1983;40:1172-8.
7. Rosenberg JM, Martino FP, Kirschenbaum HL, Robbins J. Pharmacist-operated drug information centers in the United States—1986. Am J Hosp Pharm. 1987;44(2):337-44.
8. Grossman S, Nathan JP, Ipema HJ, Ness GL, Tierno HE, Gabay MP, Calip GS Survey of drug information centers in the United States—2018. Am J Health-Syst Pharm. 2020;77(1):33-8.
9. Ghaibi S, Ipema H, Gabay M. ASHP guidelines on the pharmacist's role in providing drug information. Am J Health-Syst Pharm. 2015;72:573-7.

10. Mehnert RB. A world of knowledge for the nation's health: The U.S. National Library of Medicine. Am J Hosp Pharm. 1986; 43:2991-7.

11. Francke DE. The role of the pharmacist as a drug information specialist and clinical specialist. Am J Hosp Pharm. 1966;23:49.

12. Accreditation Council for Pharmacy Education. Accreditation standards and key elements for the professional program in pharmacy leading to the doctor of pharmacy degree [Internet]. Chicago (IL): Accreditation Council for Pharmacy Education [cited 2019 Oct 23]. Available from: www.acpe-accredit.org/pdf/Standards2016FINAL.pdf.

13. Joint Commission of Pharmacy Practitioners. Pharmacists' patient care process [Internet]. [cited 2019 Oct 23]. Available from: https://jcpp.net/wp-content/uploads/2016/03/PatientCareProcess-with-supporting-organizations.pdf.

14. Haines ST, Pittenger AL, Stolte SK, Plaza CM, Gleason BL, Kantorovich A, McCollum M, Trujillo JM, Copeland DA, Lacroix MM, Masuda QN, Mbi P, Medina MS, Miller SM Core entrustable professional activities for new pharmacy graduates. Am J Pharm Educ. 2017;81(1):Article S2.

15. Rosenberg JM, Schilit S, Nathan JP, Zerilli T. Update on the status of 89 drug information centers in the United States. Am J Health-Syst Pharm. 2009; 66:1718-22.

16. Pedersen CA, Schneider PJ, Scheckelhoff DJ. ASHP national survey of pharmacy practice in hospital settings: prescribing and transcribing—2013. Am J Health-Syst Pharm. 2014;71:924-42.

17. Kinky DE, Erush SC, Laskin MS, Gibson GA. Economic impact of a drug information service. Ann Pharmacother. 1999;33:11-6.

18. LaFleur J, Tyler LS, Sharma RR. Economic benefits of investigational drug services at an academic institution. Am J Health-Syst Pharm. 2004;61:27-32.

19. Brown JN, Tillman F, Jacob S, Britnell SR. Economic outcomes associated with an investigational drug service within a Veteran's Affairs health care system. Contemp Clin Trials Commun. 2019;14:100354.

20. Gammie T, Vogler S, Zaheer-Ud-Din B. Economic evaluation of hospital and community pharmacy services. Ann Pharmacother. 2017;51(1):54-65.

21. Study Commission on Pharmacy. Pharmacists for the future. Ann Arbor (MI): Health Administration Press; 1975. p. 139.

22. Medina MS, Plaza CM, Stowe CD, Robinson ET, DeLander G, Beck DE, Melchert RB, Supernaw RB, Roche VF, Gleason BL, Strong MN, Bain A, Meyer GE, Dong BJ,Rochon J, Johnston P. Center for the advancement of pharmacy education 2013 educational outcomes. Am J Pharm Educ. 2013;77(8):Article 162.

23. Shehab N, Lovegrove MC, Geller AI, Rose KO, Weidle NJ, Budnitz DS. US emergency department visits for outpatient adverse drug events, 2013-2014. JAMA. 2016;316:2115-25.

24. Institute of Medicine. Committee on Identifying and Preventing Medication Errors. Preventing medication errors. Washington (DC): The National Academies Press; 2006.

25. Budnitz DS, Lovegrove MC, Shehab N, Richards CL. Emergency hospitalizations for adverse drug events in older Americans. N Engl J Med. 2011;365:2002-12.

26. Zed PJ, Black KJL, Fitzpatrick EA, Ackroyd-Stolarz, S., Murphy, N. G., Curran, J. A., MacKinnon, N. J., Sinclair, D. Medication-related emergency department visits in pediatrics: a prospective observational study. Pediatrics. 2015;135(3): 435-43.

27. Committee on Quality of Health Care in America, Institute of Medicine. Crossing the quality chasm: a new health system for the 21st century. Washington (DC): National Academic Press; 2001.

28. Centers for Medicare and Medicaid Services. An introduction to the Medicare EHR Incentive Program for eligible professionals [Internet]. 2013 March 20 [cited 2019 Oct 31]. Available from: https://www.cms.gov/regulations-and-guidance/legislation/ehrincentiveprograms/downloads/ehr_medicare_stg1_begguide.pdf.

29. HealthData Management. 12 trends that will dominate healthcare IT in 2019 [Internet]. [cited 2019 Oct 31]. Available from: https://www.healthdatamanagement.com/list/12-trends-that-will-dominate-healthcare-it-in-2019.

30. Evans RS, Pestotnik SL, Classen DC, Clemmer T P, Weaver L K, Orme J F Jr, Lloyd J F, Burke J P. A computer-assisted management program for antibiotics and other anti-infective agents. N Engl J Med. 1998;338:232-8.

31. Hunt DL, Haynes RB, Hanna SE, Smith K. A computer-assisted management program for antibiotics and other anti-infective agents. JAMA. 1998;280;1339-46.

32. Institutes of Medicine. Health professions education: a bridge to quality. Washington (DC): National Academy Press; 2003.

33. Stokes LB, Rogers JW, Hertig JB, Weber RJ. Big data: implications for health system pharmacy. Hosp Pharm. 2016;51(7):599-603.

34. Hernandez I, Zhang Y. Using predictive analytics and big data to optimize pharmaceutical outcomes. Am J Health-Syst Pharm. 2017;74:1494-500.

35. Murray E, Pollack L, Donelan K, Catania J, Lee K, Zapert K, Turner R. The impact of health information on the Internet on health care and the physician-patient relationship: national U.S. survey among 1,050 U.S. physicians. J Med Internet Res. 2003;5:e17.

36. Clauson KA, Polen HH, Boulos MN, Dzenowagis JH. Drug information: scope, completeness, and accuracy of drug information in Wikipedia. Ann Pharmacother. 2008;42:1814-21.

37. Belgado BS. Drug information centers on the Internet. J Am Pharm Assoc. 2001;41:631-2.

38. Costerison EC, Graham AS. Developing and promoting an intranet site for a drug information service. Am J Health-Syst Pharm. 2008;65:639-43.

39. Phillips JA, Hanrahan CT, Brown JN, May D, Britnell SR, Ficzere CH. Guiding principles for evaluating tertiary health care resources: The A2C2QUIRE framework. J Am Coll Clin Pharm. 2020;3:485-93.

40. Centers for Medicare and Medicaid Services. National Health Expenditure Projections 2015-2025 [Internet]. [cited 2019 Oct 31]. Available from: https://www.cms.gov/Research-Statistics-Data-and-Systems/Statistics-Trends-and-Reports/NationalHealthExpendData/Downloads/Proj2015.pdf.

41. Ellrodt G, Cook DJ, Lee J, Cho M, Hunt D, Weingarten S. Evidence-based disease management. JAMA. 1997;278:1687-92.

42. Avorn J. In defense of pharmacoepidemiology embracing the yin and yang of drug research. N Engl J Med. 2007;357(22):2219-21.

43. Vermeulen LC, Beis SJ, Cano SB. Applying outcomes research in improving the medication-use process. Am J Health-Syst Pharm. 2000;57;2277-82.

44. Top 10 areas of research: report on the most popular fields of drug development. Med Ad News. 2003;137;S22.

45. PhRMA. In the pipeline—what's next in drug discovery [Internet]. [cited 2019 Oct 31]. Available from: https://www.phrma.org/en/science/in-the-pipeline.

46. U.S. Food and Drug Administration. Table of pharmacogenomics biomarkers in drug labeling [Internet]. [cited 2019 Oct 31]. Available from: https://www.fda.gov/drugs/science-and-research-drugs/table-pharmacogenomic-biomarkers-drug-labeling.

47. Pew Research Center. Majority of Adults Look Online for Health Information [Internet]. 2013 Feb 1 [cited 2019 Nov 1]. Available from: https://www.pewresearch.org/daily-number/majority-of-adults-look-online-for-health-information.

48. Pew Research Center Mobile Fact Sheet [Internet]. [cited 2019 Oct 31]. Available from: https://www.pewresearch.org/internet/fact-sheet/mobile/.

49. Barnes PM, Bloom B, Nahin R. Complementary and alternative medicine use among adults and children: United States, 2007. Natl Health Stat Report. 2008;(12):1-23.

50. Complementary and alternative medicine: What people aged 50 and older discuss with their healthcare providers. AARP and NCCAM Survey Report 2010 [Internet]. 2013 Mar 9 [cited 2019 Oct 31]. Available from: https://nccam.nih.gov/news/camstats/2010.

51. American Hospital Association. More hospitals offering complementary and alternative medicine services. Washington (DC) [Internet]. 2011 Sep 15 [cited 2019 Oct 31]. Available from: https://www.aha.org/presscenter/pressrel/2011/110907-pr-camsurvey.pdf.

52. Troutman WG. Consensus-derived objectives for drug information education. Drug Inf J. 1994;28:791-6.

53. Gora-Harper ML, Brandt B. An educational design to teach drug information across the curriculum. Am J Pharm Educ. 1997;61:296-302.

54. Wang F, Troutman WG, Seo T, Peak A, Rosenberg JM. Drug information in doctor of pharmacy programs. Am J Pharm Educ. 2006;70:51.

55. Bernknopf AC, Karpinski JP, McKeever AL, Peak AS, Smith KM, Smith WD, Timpe EM, Ward KE. Drug information: from education to practice. Pharmacotherapy. 2009;29:331-46.

56. Phillips JA, Gabay MP, Ficzere C, Ward KE. Curriculum and instructional methods for drug information, literature evaluation, and biostatistics: survey of US pharmacy schools. Ann Pharmacother. 2012;46:793-801.

57. American Society of Health-System Pharmacy Residency Directory [Internet]. [cited 2021 May 6]. Available from: https://accreditation.ashp.org/directory/#/program/residency.

58. Gabay M. Generate revenue with drug information services. Pharm Purchas Prod. 2013;10(5):50,52.

59. Fox ER, Tyler LS. Managing drug shortages: seven years' experience at one health-system. Am J Health-Syst Pharm. 2003;60:245-53.

60. Fox ER, McLaughlin MM. ASHP guidelines on managing drug product shortages. Am J Health-Syst Pharm. 2018;75:1742-50.
61. Buntin BM, Burke MF, Hoaglin MC, Blumenthal D. The benefits of health information technology: a review of the recent literature shows predominately positive results. Health Aff. 2011:30(3):464-71.
62. Cooley TW, May D, Alwan M, Sue C. Implementation of computerized prescriber order entry in four academic medical centers. Am J Health-Syst Pharm. 2012;69:2166-73.
63. Traynor K. Pharmacy informatics aids cancer center care. Am J Health-Syst Pharm. 2012;69:2125.
64. Riggins JL. Pharmaceutical industry as a career choice. Am J Health-Syst Pharm. 2002;59:2097-8.
65. Overstreet KM. Medical education and communication companies: career options for pharmacists. Am J Health-Syst Pharm. 2003;60:1896-7.
66. Moghadam RG. Scientific writing: a career for pharmacists. Am J Health-Syst Pharm. 2003;60:1899-900.

SUGGESTED READINGS

1. Tichy EM, Shumock GT, Hoffman JM, Suda KJ, Rim MH, Tadrous M, Stubbings JA, Cuellar S, Clark JS, Wiest MD, Matusiak LM, Hunkler RJ, Vermeulen LC. National trends in prescription drug expenditures and projections for 2020. Am J Health-Syst Pharm. 2020;77:1213-30.
2. Ghaibi S, Ipema H, Gabay M. ASHP guidelines on the pharmacist's role in providing drug information. Am J Health-Syst Pharm. 2015;72:573-7.
3. Fox BI, Flynn AJ, Fortier CR, Clauson KA. Knowledge, skills and resources for pharmacy informatics education. Am J Pharmaceut Educ. 2011;75(5):Article 93.
4. Bernknopf AC, Karpinski JP, McKeever AL, Peak AS, Smith KM, Smith WD, Timpe EM, Ward KE. Drug Information: from education to practice. Pharmacotherapy. 2009; 29:331-46.
5. Costerison EC, Graham AS. Developing and promoting an intranet site for a drug information service. Am J Health-Syst Pharm. 2008;65:639-43.
6. Wang F, Troutman WG, Seo T, Peak A, Rosenberg JM. Drug information in doctor of pharmacy programs. Am J Pharm Ed. 2006;70:51.
7. Zeind CS, Blagg JD, Amato MG, Jacobson S. Incorporation of Institute of Medicine competency recommendations with doctor of pharmacy curricula. Am J Pharm Ed. 2012;76(5):Article 83.

Chapter Two

Formulating an Effective Response: A Structured Approach

Amy Heck Sheehan • Joseph K. Jordan

Learning Objectives

After completing this chapter, the reader will be able to:

- Develop strategies to overcome the impediments that prevent health care professionals from providing effective responses and recommendations.
- Outline the steps that are necessary to identify the actual drug information needs of the requestor.
- List and describe the four critical factors that should be considered and systematically addressed when formulating a response.
- Define analysis and synthesis, and describe their application in the process of formulating responses and recommendations.
- List the elements and characteristics of effective responses to medication-related queries.

Key Concepts

❶ Rational pharmacotherapy can be promoted by ensuring that drug information is correctly interpreted and appropriately applied.

❷ The absence of sufficient background information and pertinent patient data can greatly impair the process of information synthesis and the ability to formulate effective responses.

❸ Critical information that defines the problem and elucidates the context of the question is not readily volunteered, but must be expertly elicited.

❹ Providing responses and offering recommendations without knowledge of pertinent patient information, the context of the request, or how the information will be applied can be potentially harmful.

❺ Formulating the response requires the use of a structured, organized approach whereby critical factors are systematically considered and thoughtfully evaluated.

❻ Approaching a question haphazardly, or prematurely fixating on isolated details, can misdirect even the most skilled clinician.

❼ Responses to drug information queries often must be synthesized by integrating data from diverse sources through the use of logic and deductive reasoning.

Introduction

Health care professionals are asked to provide responses to a variety of drug information questions every day. Although the type of requestor, query, and setting can vary, the process of formulating responses remains consistent. This chapter introduces an organized, structured approach for formulating effective responses and recommendations to drug information questions.

As the medical literature expands, access to drug information resources by health care professionals and the public continues to grow. Yet many professionals and consumers lack the necessary skills to use this information effectively. **❶** *Rational pharmacotherapy can be promoted by ensuring that drug information is correctly interpreted and appropriately applied.* This presents an opportunity and a challenge for pharmacists who are true drug therapy experts and play a broader role in patient care.

Regardless of specialty or practice site, health care professionals with the responsibility for overseeing the safe and rational use of medications must strive to develop expertise in applied pharmacotherapy. Whether working in a community setting, nursing home, outpatient clinic, hospital, or in any other practice site, pharmacists and other health care professionals can apply their skills and knowledge for the optimal care of patients. The pharmacist should not be relegated to the role of information dispenser or gatekeeper, but they should instead extend their knowledge of drugs and therapeutics to the clinical management of individual patients or the care of large populations.

Steps for Answering a Question

ACCEPTING RESPONSIBILITY AND ELIMINATING BARRIERS

Health care professionals should recognize that their responsibility extends beyond simply providing an answer to a question. Rather, it is to assist in resolving therapeutic dilemmas or managing patients' medication regimens for their entire therapeutic outcome. Knowledge of pharmacotherapy alone does not ensure success. Moreover, isolated information is not sufficient for formulating responses to questions or ensuring proper patient management. In fact, it is uncommon to find comprehensive answers in the literature that completely and effectively address specific situations or circumstances that clinicians encounter in their daily practices. Responses and recommendations must often be thoughtfully synthesized using information and knowledge gathered from a number of diverse sources. To effectively manage the care of patients and resolve complex situations, added skills and competence in problem solving and direct patient care are also necessary.

In order to provide meaningful responses and effective recommendations to drug information questions, real or perceived impediments must first be overcome. One such impediment is the false perception that many drug information questions do not pertain to specific patients. Another is the perception that the seemingly casual interactions with requestors and the lack of formal, written consultation somehow preclude the need for in-depth analysis and extensive involvement in patient management. Oversimplification of these interactions with requestors and failure to identify the context of the question or recognize its significance can jeopardize the clinical management of patients. ❷ *The absence of sufficient background information and pertinent patient data can greatly impair the process of information synthesis and the ability to formulate effective responses.*

IDENTIFYING THE GENUINE AND PRECISE NEED

Evolution of the Systematic Approach

Historically, the approach to answering drug information queries has centered on the use of a systematic method first described by Watanabe and subsequently modified by others.[1,2] This simple approach relied on the collection of basic information to document and categorize the request and to subsequently develop an organized strategy for formulating cogent responses. The American Society of Health-System Pharmacists (ASHP) guidelines on the pharmacist's role in providing drug information have outlined a nine-step, systematic approach for responding to drug information requests which includes identifying the requestor, defining the true question, obtaining background information, categorizing the question, performing a systematic search, analyzing the information, disseminating the information, documenting the response, and performing a follow-up assessment.[3] Although this structure remains theoretically useful from a training standpoint, if strictly applied without proper context and guidance, it has the potential to artificially fragment the process and disrupt the natural exchange of information. Additionally, the specific approach used to respond to a drug information request should be flexible, depending on the given practice setting and specific scenario. The full process outlined above may not be practical in certain direct patient care settings or when an urgent response is necessary. The Pharmacists' Patient Care Process (PPCP) has also been used as a more general model by colleges and schools of pharmacy to provide students with a systematic, patient-centered approach to improving medication outcomes across various practice settings.[4] This approach is similar to the ASHP guidelines and Watanabe's method. The PPCP includes collection of all necessary information in order to understand the clinical status of the patient, followed by analysis of data, development and implementation of an evidence-based plan, and appropriate follow-up. A documentation form (see Appendix 2-1) may be useful to guide the process of data collection and ensure that all relevant information is considered.

Eliminating Potential Barriers

Ultimately, the success of providing an effective response will depend largely on maintaining the flow of information with minimal distractions and unnecessary or ill-timed questions. The goal should be to remove obstacles, such as those provided by lack of background or situational information, when communicating with clinicians to determine the actual informational needs, also referred to as the ultimate question. This is particularly relevant in clinical settings where most queries are not purely academic or general in nature. In fact, it is rational to assume that queries from health care providers will invariably involve specific patients and unique clinical circumstances. For example, a physician who asks about the association of liver toxicity with atorvastatin is probably not asking this question whimsically or out of curiosity. The physician most likely is caring for a patient who has developed signs or symptoms of hepatic impairment possibly associated with the use of this medication. Although other reasonable scenarios, albeit less likely, could have prompted this question, it would be most prudent nonetheless to consider the possibility of a patient-specific drug-induced liver injury.

Eliciting Critical Information

Even questions that are not related to patient care (refer to Case Study 2-1 as an example) must be viewed in their proper context. Requestors of information are typically vague in verbalizing their needs and generally provide adequate information only when specifically asked and/or thoughtfully prompted. Although these requestors may seem confident about their perceived needs, they may be less certain after further probing. Requestors, regardless of background, are often uncertain about the nature and extent of information that should be disclosed in order to derive the most optimal assistance. ❸ *Critical information that defines the problem and elucidates the context of the question is not readily volunteered, but must be expertly elicited.* This can be accomplished using effective questioning strategies (asking logical questions in a logical sequence) and other means of information gathering that are essential for formulating informed responses. Failure of the requestor to disclose critical information or clarify the question does not obviate the need for such information or relieve the pharmacist of the duty to collect it. Although it is easy to assign blame to the requestor for failing to disclose all the necessary information, it is ultimately the responsibility of the provider of the response to obtain this information completely and efficiently.

Case Study 2–1

■ INITIAL QUESTION

What is the molecular weight of fosamprenavir calcium?

■ POTENTIAL RESPONSE IN THE ABSENCE OF RELEVANT BACKGROUND INFORMATION

Fosamprenavir is an oral antiretroviral agent that is indicated for the treatment of human immunodeficiency virus (HIV-1) infection in combination with other antiretroviral agents.[5,6] The molecular weight of fosamprenavir is 623.7 g/mol.[6]

■ PERTINENT BACKGROUND INFORMATION

The requestor is a basic scientist who is conducting an in vitro experiment to evaluate the pharmacologic effects of fosamprenavir. She would like to know the molecular weight of fosamprenavir so that she can perform appropriate calculations specified for this experiment.

■ PERTINENT PATIENT FACTORS

N/A

■ PERTINENT DISEASE FACTORS

N/A

■ PERTINENT MEDICATION FACTORS

Fosamprenavir is a prodrug that is converted in vivo to the pharmacologically active form, amprenavir.[5,6] Fosamprenavir is available for prescription use in the United States as 700-mg oral tablets and 50 mg/mL oral suspension. Amprenavir has been discontinued and is no longer commercially available in the United States.

■ ANALYSIS AND SYNTHESIS

Considering that fosamprenavir is a prodrug that must be converted to a pharmacologically active compound in *vivo*, and given that this researcher wishes to conduct an in vitro study, the researcher should use the active form of the drug in the experiment. Therefore, the true information need is the molecular weight of amprenavir rather than fosamprenavir.

■ RESPONSE AND RECOMMENDATIONS

Fosamprenavir is an oral antiretroviral agent indicated for the treatment of human immunodeficiency virus (HIV-1) infection in combination with other antiretroviral agents.[5,6] Because fosamprenavir is a prodrug that requires conversion to the active form, the requestor was advised to consider using amprenavir in the experiment. The molecular weight of amprenavir is 505.6 g/mol, and is available for purchase from several chemical vendors.[7]

■ CASE MESSAGE

This example illustrates the importance of collecting pertinent background information, even for seemingly uncomplicated questions. The question as originally posed related simply to the physicochemical properties of the drug; after obtaining additional information, the question ultimately pertained to both the drug's physicochemical properties and pharmacokinetics/pharmacology.

Failure to understand exactly how the information that is provided will be used could result in an inaccurate or misleading response. In this case, providing the molecular weight without alerting the requestor that in vitro fosamprenavir is pharmacologically inactive would have resulted in wasted time and money, and the results of the experiment would likely have been invalid.

Good communication skills (both listening and questioning) are essential for gathering relevant information, discerning the real question, and identifying the genuine needs of the requestor. ❹ *Providing responses and offering recommendations without knowledge of pertinent patient information, the context of the request, or how the information will be applied can be potentially harmful.* For assistance in identifying some of the questions that should be posed, please refer to Appendix 2-2. Even well-equipped drug information centers with trained staff are not immune to this problem. A study of the quality of pharmacotherapy consultations provided by drug information centers in the United States found that the centers generally failed to obtain pertinent patient data, thereby risking incorrect responses and inappropriate recommendations.[8]

Verifying the Context of Question

Some health care professionals may be quick to attempt to answer questions without adequately understanding the context or unique circumstances from which they evolved. They focus exclusively on the answer and ignore or fail to obtain key information needed to establish the framework of the question. In essence, this can result in a correct response being provided to address an incorrect question. For example, in a question about the dose of an antibiotic, an incorrect response can be formulated and inappropriate recommendations made if one fails to consider such factors as the patient's age, sex, condition being treated, end-organ function, weight and body composition, concomitant diseases (e.g., cystic fibrosis), possible drug interactions, site of infection, spectrum of activity of the antimicrobial, resistance patterns, or other factors such as pregnancy or dialysis.

Before attempting to formulate responses, one must consider several important questions to ensure that they understand the context of the query and the scope of the issue or problem (see Table 2-1). Without this information, there is a risk of providing general responses that do not address the needs of the requestor. More concerning, however, is that the information provided can be misinterpreted or misapplied. This not only compromises one's credibility, but also can jeopardize patient care. Pharmacists must recognize the value and potential benefits of their contributions as members of the health care team. Lack of confidence in communicating with requestors can be a limiting factor. Because a telephone call from another health care provider or even a face-to-face interaction may not be perceived as a formal request for a consult, the significance of such apparently informal daily interactions can easily be overlooked. Interactions with physicians and other health

TABLE 2-1. QUESTIONS TO CONSIDER BEFORE FORMULATING A RESPONSE

Are the requestor's name, profession, and affiliation known?

How can the requestor be contacted (e.g., pager, email, cellphone)?

Does the question pertain to a specific patient? If so, has pertinent patient history been obtained?

Is there a clear understanding of the question or problem?

Has the true information need (i.e., ultimate question) been determined?

Why is the question being asked? Why now?

What are the unique circumstances that generated the query?

Are the requestor's expectations understood?

Has pertinent background information been obtained?

What information is actually needed?

When is the information needed and in what format (e.g., verbal, written)?

How will the information provided be used or applied?

How has the problem or situation been managed to date?

Are there alternative explanations or management options that should be explored?

care providers present valuable opportunities for direct involvement in patient care. The lesson often missed is that there is a fine line between a simple, seemingly general drug information question and a meaningful pharmacotherapy consult. Knowing the context of the question, obtaining the pertinent patient data and background information, and understanding the true needs of the requestor often can be the difference.

Case Study 2–2

■ INITIAL QUESTION

Can you tell me the recommended dose of azithromycin for gastroparesis?

■ POTENTIAL RESPONSE IN THE ABSENCE OF RELEVANT BACKGROUND INFORMATION

Azithromycin is structurally similar to erythromycin, a macrolide that has been used historically for short-term management of gastroparesis. While erythromycin is noted to reduce symptoms from delayed gastric emptying in either the intravenous (IV) or oral formulation, current guidelines from the American Gastroenterology Association (AGA) do not address the role of azithromycin.[9] A search of tertiary and secondary sources did note a few reports of using IV or oral formulations of azithromycin at doses of 250–500 mg daily.[10-14]

◼ PERTINENT BACKGROUND INFORMATION

The requestor is an internal medicine physician who is managing a patient with diabetic gastroparesis. A nurse recently informed the internal medicine team of a nationwide erythromycin shortage. The physician would like to know if azithromycin is an alternative to erythromycin, and, if so, what the appropriate dose would be for this specific patient.

◼ PERTINENT PATIENT FACTORS

CD is a 53-year-old female. She is presenting today to the office with reported history of abdominal pain, persistent nausea, occasional vomiting, decreased appetite, and flatulence for past 2 months. Currently the patient is receiving as-needed metoclopramide 10 mg by mouth (PO) 10 minutes after meals.

Past Medical History

- Type 2 diabetes mellitus × 13 years
- Peripheral neuropathy × 5 years
- Diabetic gastroparesis × 2 years
- Hypertension × 8 years

Social History

- Negative for ethanol
- Negative for tobacco or illicit drugs

Current Medications and Supplements

- Insulin glargine 15 units subcutaneously at bedtime
- Insulin lispro 5 units subcutaneously 15 minutes before each meal
- Lisinopril 10 mg PO daily
- Hydrochlorothiazide 50 mg daily
- Metoclopramide 10 mg PO 10 minutes after meals as needed
- Atorvastatin 40 mg PO every evening
- Acetaminophen 1000 mg PO every 6 hours as needed for pain
- Centrum® Women daily multivitamin
- Fish oil supplement

Allergies and intolerances

- Morphine

Laboratory Results

- Temperature 98°F, blood pressure (BP) 151/84 mmHg, heart rate (HR) 91 BPM, respiratory rate (RR) 18/min, O$_2$ saturation 93%
- Serum creatinine (SCr) 1.3 mg/dL, blood urea nitrogen (BUN) 22 mmol/dL

- White blood cells (WBC) 5.4×10^9 per liter
- Blood glucose (BG) 88 mg/dL, A1$_C$ 9.4% (3 months ago)
- Low-density lipoprotein (LDL) 126 mg/dL, high-density lipoprotein (HDL) 44 mg/dL, triglycerides (TG) 155 mg/dL

■ PERTINENT DISEASE FACTORS

Gastroparesis is characterized by delayed gastric emptying and is most commonly associated with diabetes mellitus. The incidence increases with the duration of diabetes and the presence of complications such as retinopathy, neuropathy, or nephropathy. Common symptoms of this condition include nausea, vomiting, abdominal pain, and fullness. Treatment of gastroparesis generally involves modifications to diet and pharmacotherapy with prokinetics, antiemetics, and nonopiate analgesics.[9]

■ PERTINENT MEDICATION AND SUPPLEMENT FACTORS

Erythromycin is a macrolide antibiotic with known prokinetic effects resulting from stimulation of motilin receptors in the gut. Azithromycin is also a macrolide antibiotic but is more commonly used for infection-related conditions as opposed to gastrointestinal motility. As compared with erythromycin, azithromycin has less drug interactions and a longer half-life. While large trials comparing erythromycin and azithromycin for the treatment of gastroparesis were not located, there are some smaller trials comparing manometry results with both agents.[11-13] The administration of IV azithromycin 250 mg infused over 30 minutes was found to have a greater effect in the postprandial period than a dose of IV erythromycin 250 mg infused over 20 minutes.[11,12] Due to the long half-life of the agent, the authors argue that the product can be given once daily compared with the four times daily regimen of erythromycin. In addition, at higher doses of 500 mg of IV azithromycin infused over 30 minutes, a greater effect on manometry readings was noted.[13] A case report describing the effectiveness of azithromycin in an elderly woman with diabetic gastroparesis notes successful resolution of symptoms after a 3-day regimen of 500 mg IV azithromycin followed by a 14-day regimen of 500 mg PO azithromycin.[14]

■ ANALYSIS AND SYNTHESIS

As CD is already on the first-line agent for gastroparesis (i.e., metoclopramide) and is still symptomatic, erythromycin would be an option to improve gastric emptying and symptoms from delayed gastric emptying. However, CD is not optimally taking the metoclopramide since she is taking it after meals instead of the recommended before meals. This should be pointed out since this may be contributing to symptoms. Since erythromycin is unavailable at the present time, azithromycin is an additional option based on similar effects seen in manometry studies.

RESPONSE AND RECOMMENDATIONS

Metoclopramide is a first-line agent for treatment of diabetic gastroparesis at a dose of 10 mg up to four times daily before meals and at bedtime.[9] Taking the medication after meals, instead of the recommended 30 minutes before meals, will decrease the efficacy of the prokinetic agent. Before making additional changes to CD's regimen, it is worth adjusting the metoclopramide dosing.

CASE MESSAGE

This question highlights the importance of skillful problem solving. As always, collecting appropriate background information and patient data is critical. Analyzing this information before synthesizing a logical response is paramount for effective patient management. The question as originally presented related to medication dosing; after obtaining additional information, the question broadened to the appropriate management of the patient's condition, with a need to optimized use of the first-line agent. In this case, failure to recognize that the patient was inappropriately taking metoclopramide could lead to potentially unnecessary addition of therapy for her diabetic gastroparesis.

In the absence of information that provides the proper context, a question about the half-life of a medication appears rather simple. However, if the question were posed for the purpose of assisting the requestor in determining a sufficient washout period for a crossover study, one would be remiss if factors, other than the half-life of the parent compound, were not considered. Proper determination of a washout period also would mandate consideration of other factors such as the activity and half-lives of known metabolites; the presence of potentially interacting medications; the effects of age, illness, or end-organ function; the persistence of pharmacodynamic effects of the medication beyond its detection in the plasma (e.g., omeprazole); and the effect of administration route on the apparent half-life (e.g., transdermally administered fentanyl).

The case studies in this chapter emphasize the importance of looking beyond the initial question and recognizing that the requestor's needs often go well beyond a

TABLE 2–2. IMPORTANT QUESTIONS NOT POSED BY THE REQUESTOR

Initial query posed by requestor: Do any of the following antibiotics cause tooth discoloration—amoxicillin, nitrofurantoin, and sulfamethoxazole-trimethoprim?

What is the incidence of antibiotic-induced tooth discoloration?

Are specific antibiotic agents (i.e., amoxicillin, nitrofurantoin, or sulfamethoxazole-trimethoprim) more likely to cause tooth discoloration than others?

Are there any known predisposing factors?

Is the pathogenesis of this adverse effect understood?

How does the tooth discoloration typically present?

Are there any characteristic subjective or objective findings?

Does tooth discoloration caused by antibiotics differ from that caused by other medications, or other etiologies?

Is the tooth discoloration dose related?

How severe can it become?

Is antibiotic tooth discoloration reversible?

How is antibiotic-induced tooth discoloration usually managed?

Are there other antibiotics available that can be used in place of the patient's current agents?

Are there alternative explanations for the tooth discoloration in this patient (including other medications, medication combinations, or underlying medical conditions)?

What complications, if any, can be expected?

superficial answer to the primary question. Pharmacists should always anticipate additional questions or concerns, including those that are not directly asked or addressed by the requestor. These questions nonetheless must be considered if a clinical situation is to be managed optimally. In Case Study 2-3, as an example, a question is posed about antibiotics as a possible cause of tooth discoloration. Although the requestor may neglect to provide clarifying information or pose insightful questions that further inform the case, additional related issues and complementary questions should nonetheless be considered, as these will likely be critical in determining the ultimate success of the response (see Table 2-2). Failure to address such questions will undoubtedly result in either an incorrect or inadequate response.

Case Study 2–3

■ INITIAL QUESTION

Do any of the following antibiotics cause teeth discoloration— amoxicillin, nitrofurantoin, and sulfamethoxazole-trimethoprim?

◼ POTENTIAL RESPONSE IN THE ABSENCE OF RELEVANT BACKGROUND INFORMATION

An extensive search of tertiary and secondary literature sources noted that tooth discoloration has been seen rarely with amoxicillin.[15] However, with dental hygiene practices such as brushing or professional cleaning, this discoloration may be reversible. No documentation was found of tooth discoloration with nitrofurantoin or sulfamethoxazole-trimethoprim.

◼ PERTINENT BACKGROUND INFORMATION

The requestor is a urology nurse practitioner who is caring for a patient with vesico-ureteral reflux (VUR). The patient had been receiving ½ teaspoon of sulfamethoxazole-trimethoprim for about 8 months when his parent noticed darkening of his two teeth. The clinician would like to use an antibiotic prophylaxis for VUR but wants to make sure that tooth discoloration is unlikely with choice.

◼ PERTINENT PATIENT FACTORS

AB is a 10-month old male with VUR.

Past Medical History

- Febrile urinary tract infection (UTI)

Social History

- N/A

Current Medications and Supplements

- Trimethoprim/sulfamethoxazole (40–200 mg/5 mL) 2.5 mL daily × 8 months [stopped]
- Patient is currently breastfed
- Liquid multivitamin supplement (Poly-Vi-Sol® with iron) 0.5 mL by mouth once daily

Allergies and Intolerances

- N/A

◼ PERTINENT DISEASE FACTORS

VUR involves the retrograde passage of urine from the bladder into the upper urinary tract. Patients with VUR who develop bladder infection are at increased risk for febrile UTIs compared with patients without VUR. The management of VUR involves preventing recurring febrile UTIs, preventing renal injury from potential kidney infections (e.g., acute pyelonephritis), and minimizing morbidity of treatment.[16-18] Antibiotic prophylaxis has been given for several decades under the idea that sterilizing the urine will lead to less kidney infections and in turn, less kidney scarring. Children younger than 1 year of age are recommended to receive antibiotic prophylaxis since they are more likely to suffer morbidity with acute kidney infections than older children.[18]

Tooth discoloration is described as either extrinsic (i.e., outer surface) or intrinsic (i.e., within enamel). Extrinsic discoloration can be seen with tea, coffee, tobacco, and some medications such as mouth rinses and iron salts. In contrast to intrinsic stains, extrinsic stains can usually be removed with tooth brushing or dental scaling and polishing.[15]

■ PERTINENT MEDICATION AND SUPPLEMENT FACTORS

Reports of tooth discoloration with amoxicillin, but not trimethoprim-sulfamethoxazole or nitrofurantoin were found in the primary and tertiary literature. A review of the patient's current medication and supplements reveals an iron-containing multivitamin. Iron-containing products have more reports of tooth discoloration than amoxicillin.[15]

Trimethoprim-sulfamethoxazole and nitrofurantoin have traditionally been used for VUR prophylaxis at one-half to one-fourth of the usual therapeutic doses for treating acute infections. Amoxicillin is not traditionally used secondary to concerns of increased likelihood of resistant organisms.[16-18]

■ ANALYSIS AND SYNTHESIS

As AB is less than 1 year of age and has a history of febrile UTI, it is recommended to receive antibiotic prophylaxis. Trimethoprim-sulfamethoxazole and nitrofurantoin are the most common antibiotics recommended. While AB has been on trimethoprim-sulfamethoxazole for 8 months, there is no record of having received dental cleaning during this time. Amoxicillin and nitrofurantoin are other options for VUR prophylaxis, although amoxicillin has reports of tooth discoloration. A more likely causative factor is the liquid multivitamin containing iron. Iron supplements are usually not needed in children who are breastfed or who get iron-fortified infant formula. Since AB is still being breastfed, there is likely not a need for the iron supplement.

■ RESPONSE AND RECOMMENDATIONS

A review of AB's current medications reveals one agent, a liquid multivitamin containing iron, which has been reported to cause extrinsic tooth discoloration. This discoloration is usually reversible with tooth brushing and polishing.[15] Trimethoprim-sulfamethoxazole has not previously been reported to cause tooth discoloration but it cannot be ruled out as a possible cause. The practitioner was advised to consult a dentist for cleaning of the extrinsic discoloration and to discuss discontinuing the iron-containing multivitamin supplement with the parents. If the staining returns after discontinuation of the iron supplement, then transition to nitrofurantoin could be considered.

■ CASE MESSAGE

This question highlights the importance of skillful problem solving. As always, collecting appropriate background information and patient data is critical. Analyzing this information before synthesizing a logical response is paramount for effective patient management. While the classification of the original drug information request (adverse effect) did not change in the process of addressing the question, obtaining an accurate medication list broadened the list of potential list of medications that could be associated with the adverse effect in this particular patient. In this case, failure to recognize that the patient was receiving a liquid multivitamin with iron could have led to possible suboptimal antibiotic prophylactic therapy for VUR.

To expertly address requests for drug information, clinicians also must depend on their patient care skills, problem-solving skills, insight, and professional judgment. Computer databases and other specialized information sources can assist in identifying critical data, but overreliance on such resources without careful attention to pertinent background information and patient data can mislead even the most experienced clinician.

Formulating the Response

BUILDING A DATABASE AND ASSESSING CRITICAL FACTORS

Formulating a response comprises a series of steps that must be performed completely, objectively, and in a logical sequence. The steps in the process include obtaining pertinent background information, identifying other relevant factors and unique or special circumstances, assembling and organizing a database of the patient information, gathering information about relevant disease states, and collecting medication information. ❺ *Formulating the response requires the use of a structured, organized approach whereby critical factors are systematically considered and thoughtfully evaluated.* Table 2-3 outlines in detail the specific types of information that may need to be considered for each of the

TABLE 2–3. FACTORS TO BE CONSIDERED WHEN FORMULATING A RESPONSE

Pertinent Background Information, Special Circumstances, and Other Factors

Setting

Context

Sequence and time frame of events

Rationale for the question

Event(s) prompting the question

Unusual or special circumstances (including medical errors)

Acuity and time constraints

Scope of question

Desired detail or depth of response

Limitations of available information or resources

Completeness, sufficiency, and quality of the information

Applicability and generalizability of the information available to address the question

Patient Factors

Demographics (e.g., name, age, height, weight, gender, race/ethnic group, and setting)

Primary diagnosis and medical problem list

Allergies/intolerances

End-organ function, immune function, nutritional status

Chief complaint

History of present illness

Past medical history (including surgeries, radiation exposure, immunizations, psychiatric illnesses, and so forth)

Family history and genetic makeup

Social history (e.g., alcohol intake, smoking, substance abuse, exposure to environmental or occupational toxins, employment, income, education, religion, travel, diet, physical activity, stress, risky behavior, and compliance with treatment regimen)

Review of body systems

Medications (prescribed, nonprescription, and complementary/alternative)

Physical examination

Laboratory tests

Diagnostic studies or procedures

Disease Factors

Definition

Epidemiology (including incidence and prevalence)

Etiology

Pathophysiology (for infectious diseases consider site of infection, organism susceptibility, resistance patterns, and so forth)

Clinical findings (signs and symptoms, laboratory tests, diagnostic studies)[a]

Diagnosis

Treatment (medical, surgical, radiation, biologic and gene therapies, other)

Prevention and control

Risk factors

continued

TABLE 2–3. FACTORS TO BE CONSIDERED WHEN FORMULATING A RESPONSE (*CONTINUED*)

Disease Factors (*continued*)
Complications
Prognosis

Medication Factors
Name of medication or substance (proprietary, nonproprietary, other)
Status and availability (investigational, nonprescription, prescription, orphan, foreign, complementary/alternative)
Physicochemical properties
Pharmacology and pharmacodynamics
Pharmacokinetics (liberation, absorption, distribution, metabolism, and elimination)
Pharmacogenomics
Indications (Food and Drug Administration [FDA] approved and unlabeled)
Uses (diagnosis, prevention, replacement, or treatment)
Adverse effects
Allergy
Cross-allergenicity or cross-reactivity
Contraindications and precautions
Effects of age, organ system function, disease, pregnancy, extracorporeal circulation, or other conditions or environments
Mutagenicity and carcinogenicity
Effect on fertility, pregnancy, and lactation
Acute or chronic toxicity
Drug interactions (drug–disease, drug–drug, or drug–food)
Laboratory test interference (analytical or physiologic effects)
Administration (routes, methods)
Dosage and schedule
Dosage forms, formulations, preservatives, excipients, product appearance, delivery systems
Monitoring parameters (therapeutic or toxic)
Product preparation (procedures, methods)
Compatibility and stability

[a]Factors such as disease or symptom onset, duration, frequency, and severity must always be carefully assessed.

four critical factors depending on the nature of the query. A more thorough list of possible background questions is found in Appendix 2-2. It should be noted that only some of this information may be pertinent for a given query or case scenario.

For patient-related questions, development of a patient-specific database is one of the first steps in preparing a response. This requires the collection of pertinent information from the patient, caregivers, health care providers, medical chart, and other patient records. A comprehensive medication history also is essential. This database would invariably include information that overlaps with the medical and nursing databases.

Case Study 2–4

■ INITIAL QUESTION

What is the maximum dose of rizatriptan?

■ POTENTIAL RESPONSE IN THE ABSENCE OF RELEVANT BACKGROUND INFORMATION

Rizatriptan is an oral selective serotonin 5-HT$_{1B/1D}$ receptor agonist indicated for the acute treatment of migraine headache.[19] The recommended dose for acute migraine is 5–10 mg. If the migraine resumes or symptoms have not subsided within 2 hours, a second dose may be administered. The maximum daily dose is 30 mg in a 24-hour time period.[19]

■ PERTINENT BACKGROUND INFORMATION

The requestor is a medical resident who is caring for a patient with migraine headaches. The patient has experienced an increased intensity and frequency of migraines over the past several months. She reports that she has experienced two to three migraines per week over the past month. The patient uses 5 mg of rizatriptan for treatment of acute migraine attacks. This has worked in the past. However, recently she has required a second dose for complete resolution of symptoms. The medical resident would like to know if higher doses of rizatriptan have been studied. He is planning to increase the patient's dose of rizatriptan to provide more rapid relief to the patient.

■ PERTINENT PATIENT FACTORS

EF is a 27-year-old woman who has suffered from migraine headaches for the last 7 years. She presents today complaining of increased frequency and intensity of migraine headaches over the past month. The migraines are now affecting her job performance as a teacher, and she has recently missed several days of work.

Past Medical History

- Recurrent migraine headaches
- Depression

Social History

- EF is a kindergarten teacher and lives with her husband
- EF denies alcohol and tobacco use

Current Medications

- Rizatriptan 5 mg orally for acute migraine
- Bupropion 150 mg twice daily
- Loratadine 10 mg daily

Allergies/Intolerances

- Nonsteroidal anti-inflammatory drugs (NSAIDs) (anaphylaxis)

■ PERTINENT DISEASE FACTORS

Migraine is characterized by episodic attacks of severe headaches that are associated with throbbing pain, nausea, vomiting, and photophobia, with or without aura.[20] If not treated, the duration of a migraine headache can range from 4 hours to several days. Recommended treatments for the management of acute migraine include acetaminophen, NSAIDs, selective serotonin 5-$HT_{1B/1D}$ receptor agonists, antiemetics, and dihydroergotamine.[21] For patients who experience greater than six migraines per month or have very severe symptoms that are not relieved by acute treatment, use of preventive treatments are recommended.[22] First-line preventive treatments with established efficacy include antiepileptic drugs (e.g., valproate, topiramate) and beta-adrenergic blocking agents (e.g., metoprolol, propranolol).[23]

■ PERTINENT MEDICATION FACTORS

The recommended dose of rizatriptan for treatment of migraine in adults is 5–10 mg. If the migraine resumes or symptoms have subsided with 2 hours, a second dose may be administered. The maximum daily dose is 30 mg in a 24-hour time period.[19] A dose of 10 mg may provide greater efficacy over a dose of 5 mg. However, adverse events of selective serotonin 5-$HT_{1B/1D}$ receptor agonists have been shown to be dose-related. In clinical trials, patients who received 40 mg of rizatriptan reported dizziness and somnolence.[19]

■ ANALYSIS AND SYNTHESIS

Although increasing EF's dose of rizatriptan to 10 mg may provide greater efficacy for acute migraine relief, doses above this level are associated with a higher incidence of adverse effects. Review of EF's migraine history reveals that she is a candidate for preventive treatment. Addition of a preventive treatment will likely have a greater clinical impact than increasing the rizatriptan dose by reducing the frequency of migraine headaches that she has been experiencing.

■ RESPONSE AND RECOMMENDATIONS

The practitioner was advised that the maximum dose of rizatriptan during a 24-hour period is 30 mg. Although it may be reasonable to increase EF's dose for acute migraine relief to 10 mg, EF should also be started on a preventive treatment, such as valproate, to minimize the frequency of migraine headaches that she has been experiencing. Because the patient is of childbearing potential, the specific choice of a preventive treatment should be discussed with the patient with consideration of any plans to become pregnant.

■ CASE MESSAGE

This example demonstrates the importance of understanding proper context of the query. In this case, the pharmacist must collect critical background information to determine the actual drug information needed. The question originally appeared to be related directly to drug dosing. However, once information related to the critical factors was gathered, the true information need became clear: how to optimally manage the patient's disease state. Had the pharmacist failed to collect pertinent patient information, the physician may have increased the dose of rizatriptan after being told that the maximum dose is 30 mg in a 24-hour time period. Given this patient's migraine history, it would be more important to offer a clinical recommendation: also consider the addition of a preventive treatment in order to minimize the total number of migraine attacks. Moreover, larger doses of this medication are associated with a higher incidence of adverse effects.

Once these data are collected and carefully assembled, they must be critically analyzed and evaluated in the proper context before final responses and recommendations are synthesized. Background reading on topics related to the query (e.g., diseases, medications, and laboratory tests) is often essential. This process also often involves careful evaluation of the literature (see Chapters 4 and 5). To effectively perform the steps outlined previously, one must begin with a broad perspective (i.e., observing the big picture) to avoid losing sight of important information. ❻ *Approaching a question haphazardly, or prematurely fixating on isolated details, can misdirect even the most skilled clinician.*

ANALYSIS AND SYNTHESIS

Analysis and **synthesis** of information are among the most critical steps in formulating responses and recommendations. Together, they assist in forming opinions, arriving at judgments, and ultimately drawing conclusions. Analysis is the critical assessment of the nature, merit, and significance of individual elements, ideas, or factors. Functionally, it involves separating the information into its isolated parts so that each can be critically assessed. Analysis requires thoughtful review and evaluation of the quality and overall weight of available evidence. Although this process requires consideration of all relevant positive findings, pertinent negative findings should not be overlooked.

Once the information has been carefully analyzed, synthesis can begin. Synthesis is the careful, systematic, and orderly process of combining or blending varied and diverse elements, ideas, or factors into a coherent response. ❼ *Responses to drug information queries often must be synthesized by integrating data from diverse sources through the use of logic and deductive reasoning.* This process relies not only on the type and quality of the data gathered, but also on how the data are organized, viewed, and evaluated. Synthesis, as it relates to pharmacotherapy, involves the careful integration of critical information about the patient, disease, and medication along with pertinent background information to arrive at a judgment or conclusion. Synthesis can give existing information new meaning and, in effect, create new knowledge. The use of analysis and synthesis to formulate a response is similar to assembling a jigsaw puzzle. If the pieces are identified and then grouped, organized, and assembled correctly, the image will be comprehensible. However, if too many of the pieces are missing—as may be the case if patient information or if supporting evidence is incomplete or absent—or are not arranged logically (e.g., when information is not evaluated, interpreted, or applied correctly), formulating a cogent response may prove difficult or altogether impossible.

RESPONSES AND RECOMMENDATIONS

An effective response obviously must adequately address and answer the question. It should also be tailored to the specific requestor. For example, a nurse with a straightforward question may need a very different type of response compared to a prescriber with a more complicated question. Other characteristics of effective responses and recommendations are outlined in Table 2-4. The response to a question must include a restatement of the request and clear identification of the problems, issues, and circumstances. The response should begin with an introduction to the topic and systematically present the specific findings. Pertinent background information and patient data should be succinctly addressed. Conclusions and recommendations are also included in the response along with pertinent reference citations from the literature. In formulating responses, one

TABLE 2-4. DESIRED CHARACTERISTICS OF A RESPONSE

Timely

Current

Accurate

Complete

Concise

Supported by the best available evidence

Well-referenced

Clear and logical

Objective and balanced

Free of bias or flaws

Applicable and appropriate for specific circumstances

Answers important related questions

Addresses specific management of patients or situations

Considers local regulations, policies, and formulary (if applicable)

should disclose the available information that is most relevant to the question and present all reasonable options and alternatives along with an explanation and evaluation of each. Specific recommendations must be scientifically sound, evidence-based, clearly justified, and well documented. A carefully written record of the response must be maintained for follow-up and legal reasons. The records may be confidentially maintained in a patient's medical record or in the provider's secure electronic database.

FOLLOW-UP

When recommendations are made, follow-up always should be provided in a timely manner. Follow-up is required for assessment of outcomes and, when necessary, to re-evaluate the recommendations and make appropriate modifications; it is also a hallmark of a true professional and demonstrates a commitment to patient care. Furthermore, follow-up allows the provider of the information to know if their recommendations were accepted and implemented. Finally, follow-up also allows the provider to receive valuable feedback from other clinicians and to learn from the overall experience.

Conclusion

Formulating effective responses and recommendations requires the use of a structured, organized approach whereby critical factors are systematically considered and thoughtfully evaluated. The steps in this process include organizing relevant patient information, gathering information about the disease states and affected body systems, collecting medication information, obtaining pertinent background information, and identifying other relevant factors that can potentially influence outcomes. Once these data are collected and carefully assembled, they must be critically analyzed and evaluated in the proper context. Responses and recommendations are synthesized by integrating information from diverse sources through the use of logic and deductive reasoning.

Self-Assessment Questions

1. Which of the following best describes the pharmacist's responsibility during the process of responding to drug information questions?
   a. Coordinating purchase of appropriate drug information resources
   b. Educating clinicians about appropriate drug information resources
   c. Ensuring that drug information is correctly interpreted and applied
   d. Providing clinicians with ready access to electronic resources

2. Which of the following steps of the systematic approach is conducted after providing a response to a drug information request?
   a. Categorizing the question
   b. Identifying the requestor
   c. Follow-up on patient outcomes
   d. Analyzing the information

3. Which of the following strategies can help clinicians overcome barriers when collecting pertinent patient information for responses to drug information responses?
   a. Advanced training in literature searching
   b. Accepting responsibility for patient outcomes
   c. Acknowledging most requests are not patient specific
   d. All the above

4. Which of the following factors can greatly impair a clinicians' ability to formulate an effective response for a drug information request?
   a. Absence of sufficient background information
   b. Lack of specialty training in drug information
   c. Absence of specialty board certification
   d. Lack of dedication to patient care

5. Which of the following statements are correct regarding the steps of the systematic approach for responding to drug information requests?
   a. The full approach may not be practical for certain practice settings.
   b. The steps must always be completed in a specific order.
   c. It is acceptable to skip collecting pertinent background information.
   d. All the above.

6. Which of the following can improve the process of data collection when a clinician is receiving a drug information request?
   a. Minimizing distractions to information flow
   b. Using a standard data collection form for all requests
   c. Using effective questioning strategies
   d. All the above

7. Which of the following factors are important to consider when responding to a question regarding an adverse drug event?
   a. Incidence of adverse drug event
   b. Sequence and time frame of events
   c. Predisposing factors for adverse event
   d. All the above

8. Which of the following is the first step in preparing an effective response to a patient-specific drug information request?
   a. Development of a patient-specific database
   b. Critical analysis of relevant literature
   c. Synthesis of information from diverse resources
   d. Use of deductive reasoning and logic

9. Which of the following steps of the systematic approach to responding to drug information requests involves careful evaluation and interpretation of available information?
   a. Evaluate
   b. Categorize
   c. Analyze
   d. Disseminate

10. Which of the following are the four critical factors to be considered when formulating a response to a drug information request?
    a. Disease incidence, severity, duration, and prognosis
    b. Primary, secondary, and tertiary literature resources
    c. Patient, disease, medication, and pertinent background
    d. Identity, question category, documentation, and follow-up

11. Which of the following statements is true regarding the process of eliciting critical background information from a requestor?
    a. The requestor should be blamed for failure to disclose critical information.
    b. Communication skills are essential for gathering relevant information.
    c. It is the requestor's responsibility to provide relevant background information.
    d. Gathering background information is not essential to formulation of a response.

12. Which of the following are potential consequences of providing responses and offering recommendations without knowledge of pertinent patient information?
    a. General response that does not meet the needs of the requestor
    b. Damage to the clinician's reputation
    c. Patient harm or death
    d. All the above

13. Which of the following involves integration of information about the patient, disease, and medication to arrive at a judgment or conclusion?
    a. Synthesis
    b. Analysis
    c. Research
    d. Integration

14. Which of the following are desired characteristics of a well-formulated drug information response?
    a. Timely, accurate, and complete
    b. Applicable and appropriate for specific circumstance
    c. Supported by best available evidence
    d. All the above

15. Which of the following assumptions is appropriate when receiving a drug information question from health care professional?
    a. Question is usually academic or general in nature.
    b. Commonly prompted by drug company representatives.
    c. Likely involves specific patients and unique clinical circumstances.
    d. All the above.

REFERENCES

1. Watanabe AS, Conner CS. Principles of drug information services. Hamilton (IL): Drug Intelligence Publications Inc.; 1978.
2. Galt KA, Calis KA, Turcasso NM. Clinical skills program: module 3 drug information. Bethesda (MD): American Society of Health-System Pharmacists Inc.; 1995.

3. Ghaibi S, Ipema H, Gabay M, American Society of Health-System Pharmacists. ASHP guidelines on the pharmacist's role in providing drug information. Am J Health-Syst Pharm. 2015;72(7):573-7.

4. The Joint Commission of Pharmacy Practitioners. The pharmacists' patient care process [Internet]. c2014 [cited 2019 Aug 27]. Available from: https://jcpp.net/patient-care-process/.

5. McEvoy GK, editor. AHFS drug information 2019. Bethesda (MD): American Society of Health-System Pharmacists; 2019.

6. Lexiva [package insert]. Cambridge (MA): Vertex Pharmaceuticals Inc.; 2019.

7. National Center for Biotechnology Information. PubChem Open Chemistry Database CID=65016 [Internet]. Bethesda (MD): U.S. National Library of Medicine; c2005–2017 [cited 2019 Aug 27]. Available from: https://pubchem.ncbi.nlm.nih.gov/compound/65016.

8. Calis KA, Anderson DW, Auth DA, Mays DA, Turcasso NM, Meyer CC, Young LR. Quality of pharmacotherapy consultations provided by drug information centers in the United States. Pharmacotherapy. 2000;20(7):830-6.

9. Camilleri M, Parkman HP, Shafi MA, Abell TL, Gerson L. Clinical guideline: management of gastroparesis. Am J Gastroenterol. 2013;108:18-37.

10. Potter TG, Snider KR. Azithromycin for the treatment of gastroparesis. Ann Pharmacother. 2013;47:411-5.

11. Larson JM, Tavakkoli A, Drane WE, Toskes PP, Moshiree B. Advantages of azithromycin over erythromycin in improving the gastric emptying half-time in adult patients with gastroparesis. J Neurogastroenterol Motil. 2010;16:407-13.

12. Chini P, Toskes PP, Waseem S, Hou W, McDonald R, Moshiree B. Effect of azithromycin on small bowel motility in patients with gastrointestinal dysmotility. Scand J Gastroenterol. 2012;47:422-7.

13. Moshiree B, McDonald R, Hou W, Toskes PP. Comparison of the effect of azithromycin versus erythromycin on antroduodenal pressure profiles of patients with chronic functional gastrointestinal pain and gastroparesis. Dig Dis Sci. 2010;55:675-83.

14. Sutera L, Domingues LJ, Belvedere M, Putignano E, Vernuccio L, Ferlisi A, Fazio G, Costanza G, Barbagallo M. Azithromycin in an older woman with diabetic gastroparesis. Am J Ther. 2008;15:85-8.

15. Kumar A, Kumar V, Singh J, Hooda A, Dutta S. Drug-induced discoloration of teeth: an updated review. Clin Pediatr. 2012;51:181-5.

16. Roberts KB, for the Subcommittee on Urinary Tract Infection, Steering Committee on Quality Improvement and Management. Urinary tract infection: clinical practice guideline for the diagnosis and management of the initial UTI in febrile infants and children 2 to 24 months. Pediatrics. 2011;128:595-610.

17. Peters CA, Skoog SJ, Arant BS, Copp HL, Elder JS, Hudson RG, Khoury AE, Lorenzo AJ, Pohl HG, Shapiro E, WT Snodgrass, Diaz M. Summary of the AUA guideline on management of primary vesicoureteral reflux in children. J Urol. 2010;184:1134-44.

18. Tullwus K. Vesicoureteral reflux in children. Lancet. 2015;385:371-9.

19. Maxalt [package insert]. Whitehouse Station (NJ): Merck & Co Inc.; 2019.

20. Charles A. The evolution of a migraine attack: a review of recent evidence. Headache. 2013;53(2):413.

21. Marmura MJ, Silberstein SD, Schwedt TJ. The acute treatment of migraine in adults: the American Headache Society Evidence Assessment of Migraine Pharmacotherapies. Headache. 2015;55(1):3-20.
22. Lipton RB, Bigal ME, Diamond M, Freitag F, Reed ML, Steward WF, The American Migraine Prevalence and Prevention Advisory Group. Migraine prevalence, disease burden, and the need for preventive therapy. Neurology. 2007;68:343-9.
23. Silberstein SD, Holland S, Freitag F, Dodick DW, Argoff C, Ashman E. Evidence-based guideline update: pharmacologic treatment for episodic migraine prevention in adults: report of the Quality Standards Subcommittee of the American Academy of Neurology and the American Headache Society. Neurology. 2012;78(17):1337-45.

3

Chapter Three

Drug Information Resources

Meghan K. Lehmann • Anthony Trovato

Learning Objectives

After completing this chapter, the reader will be able to:

- Differentiate between primary, secondary, and tertiary sources of biomedical information.
- Select appropriate resources for a specific information request.
- Describe the role of Internet- and mobile-based resources in the provision of drug information.
- Explain the advantages and disadvantages of print- versus Internet- or mobile-based resources for drug information.
- Evaluate tertiary resources to determine appropriateness of information.
- Describe appropriate search strategy for identification of drug information.
- Recognize alternative resources for provision of drug information.
- Describe reliable health information resources for patients and consumers.
- Explain the role and progress of drug information resources retrieved from mobile applications and their potential impact on patient care.

Key Concepts

❶ There are three types of information sources in biomedical literature: primary, secondary, and tertiary resources.

❷ Tertiary resources contain information that has been filtered and summarized by the author or editor to provide a quick and concise overview of a topic.

❸ Secondary resources are mainly in the form of searchable databases that enable location and retrieval of primary or tertiary resources.

④ Several types of publications are considered primary, including controlled trials, cohort studies, case series, and case reports.

⑤ Knowing the most appropriate resource for information retrieval is the first step in the provision of quality drug information.

⑥ Secondary resources provide access to primary (e.g., clinical trials) and some tertiary (e.g., narrative reviews) literature found in journals.

⑦ Various secondary electronic resources index and abstract information from journals, meetings, publications, or other sources, differently; therefore, a practitioner should search various secondary resources in order to perform a comprehensive search.

⑧ Drug or health information retrieved from Internet-based or online media needs to be evaluated for accuracy, comprehensiveness, and mode of maintenance (e.g., recent updates, qualifications of those performing updates).

Introduction

The quantity of medical information and medical literature available continues to grow at an astounding rate. Over 3 million articles are published annually from 33,100 active scholarly peer-reviewed English-language journals.[1] The number of articles published grows by about 4% each year, whereas the number of journals increases by about 5%. The U.S. National Library of Medicine (NLM) processes about 3.3 billion online searches per year from users seeking medical and health-related information via PubMed®.[2]

The introduction of tablets, smartphones, and Internet resources has radically changed the methods by which information is accessed. Mobile devices increase point-of-care accessibility to information, providing fast and convenient access to useful resources needed for answering drug information (DI) questions.[3,4] They can also help health care providers access information via a large number of downloadable mobile applications (apps) that can be accessed even when not connected to the Internet.

Mobile devices and digital technologies have also vastly increased the accessibility of health information to patients, caregivers, and consumers. Approximately 90% of American adults use the Internet to access information.[5] In a 2018 Consumer Survey on Digital Health, 56% of consumers referred to medical-related websites for information about managing their health, while 46% utilized mobile applications.[6] Social media sites were used as sources of medical and health information by 35% of consumers. It was estimated that for 2018, 50% of the more than 3.4 billion smartphone and tablet users would have downloaded mobile health applications, including health care professionals, consumers, and patients.[7]

Due to this access and trend of using online information by patients, health care professionals are faced with not only answering health- and medication-related questions, but also with staying current and vigilant on the latest information regarding medical practice and treatments. Not all published information is accurate or reliable, and some resources are more reputable, more current, and easier to use than others.

As new therapies become available to treat many conditions, health care professionals, especially pharmacists, are being asked daily to provide responses to numerous DI requests for a variety of requesters. It is tempting to select the easiest, most familiar resources to find information without ensuring or checking the original source of the information. However, doing so may increase the possibility of missing new resources, limit the comprehensiveness of the information found, or potentially include incorrect or outdated information. In clinical practice, providing inaccurate or outdated information may lead to suboptimal patient outcomes and harm; thus, caution should be used when accessing information from various online or mobile-enabled media. See Chapter 11 for more information on legal aspects of DI practice. With the large number of medical- and health-related websites, mobile applications, and social media outlets available, health care providers must be diligent about selecting and utilizing high-quality, accurate, and reliable resources when researching DI requests.

For these reasons, using the systematic approach (see Chapter 2) can help practitioners develop effective and streamlined search strategies when answering DI questions. While the amount of DI and the means of accessing such information have changed dramatically over the years, the process of evaluating and providing accurate DI has not. This chapter discusses various DI resources that are reliable, current, and professionally prepared for everyday use by clinicians.

Types of Biomedical Resources

Health care professionals must be knowledgeable and proficient with the different types of biomedical resources when developing search strategies and finding reliable and current information in an efficient manner. Without this skill, they may be unable to use the abundant and helpful resources available to their advantage and may waste time and energy, and not obtain appropriate information. ❶ *There are three types of information sources in biomedical literature: primary, secondary, and tertiary resources.* They are synonymously referred to as primary, secondary, or tertiary literature or references. Definitions of the three types may vary depending on discipline, and a reference may serve as more than one type of resource depending on the scenario (e.g., a narrative or systematic review serves as a secondary resource in one scenario and as a tertiary resource in another).

Typically, the most appropriate and efficient first step to finding information is to consult **tertiary resources** before searching in other types of resources. ❷ *Tertiary resources contain information that has been filtered and summarized by the author or editor to provide a quick and concise overview of a topic.* Some examples of tertiary resources include textbooks, **compendia**, systematic and narrative review articles in journals, **clinical guidelines**, and other general information (see below for more detail). Some tertiary resources are available as electronically searchable online applications (e.g., Clinical Pharmacology, IBM® Micromedex®, Lexicomp®), whereas online access for others is via electronic books (e-books). These resources will provide the practitioner with a general overview needed to familiarize the reader with a topic. This is also an opportunity for the practitioner to learn general information about the disease or drug in question and use the information to form a more structured and productive search. The types and usability of tertiary resources will be discussed later.

After evaluation of the information found in tertiary resources, a practitioner can use a **secondary resource** to find additional resources and gain more insight on the topic. ❸ *Secondary resources are mainly in the form of searchable databases that enable location and retrieval of primary or tertiary resources.* This category of resources is similar to an old cataloging system. There are various secondary resources available either as paid (e.g., CINAHL, EBSCOhost, Excerpta Medica, International Pharmaceutical Abstracts, Ovid MEDLINE®) or free (e.g., PubMed®) subscriptions to many health care professionals. Using a secondary resource allows for more efficient and expedient searching for either primary literature (e.g., a clinical trial) or tertiary literature (e.g., a narrative review) for a given topic. Of note, some disciplines classify narrative and systematic reviews as secondary resources because they summarize and help identify primary resources related to a specific topic. For simplicity purposes, we classify them as tertiary resources throughout the book. More information is provided in the "Tertiary Resources" and "Secondary Resources" sections of this chapter.

Primary resources include clinical research studies and reports, both published and unpublished. ❹ *There are several types of publications that are considered primary, including controlled trials, cohort studies, case series, and case reports.* Primary resources often provide the most in-depth information about a topic, and allow the reader to analyze and critique the study methodology to determine if the results and conclusions are valid (see Chapters 4 and 5 for more information on critiquing the primary literature). Typically, primary resources require strong literature evaluation skills and a longer time commitment to review to accurately assess the value and application to health care. They may be available freely (e.g., open-access articles) or by paid subscription (e.g., New England Journal of Medicine).

Often, a search for information does not require the use of all three types of resources. ❺ *Knowing the most appropriate resource for information retrieval is the first step in the provision of quality drug information.* For example, a question regarding commercial availability of a product formulation or mechanism of action could quickly be found in a tertiary resource, such as the product's prescribing information (i.e., package insert). The information found there may be sufficient to conclude the search and provide a response. However, a question regarding the clinical trials supporting off-label use in a specific population will likely require a search of primary literature.

The type of requestor may also substantially influence the resources used to respond to a question. Generally, a request from a consumer or patient could more appropriately be answered from available tertiary resources than from a clinical trial. However, if the requestor is a prescriber requesting detailed information about the management of a specific disease state and role of investigational therapies, provision of primary literature may be appropriate.

Tertiary Resources

BENEFITS OF TERTIARY RESOURCES

Tertiary sources provide information that has been filtered and summarized by the author or editor to provide a general overview of a topic. Thus, these resources are convenient, easy to use, and are familiar to most practitioners. As mentioned earlier, some examples of tertiary resources include textbooks, compendia, review articles in journals, clinical guidelines, and other general information. Although some tertiary references are limited to print versions, many are available via online access, downloadable applications, or as e-books. These references may often serve as an initial place to identify information, since they provide a fairly complete and concise overview of information available on a specific topic. Most of the basic information needed by a practitioner can be found in these sources, making these excellent first-line resources when dealing with a DI question.

LIMITATIONS OF TERTIARY RESOURCES

Many tertiary resources are available in both hard copy (print) and electronic formats (e.g., e-books, electronically searchable DI databases). An advantage of electronic formats includes the ability to easily search for specific terms of interest. Searching for specific terms in print references can be more challenging. Ease of searching print references depends on the table of contents and indexes and the ability of the practitioner to decipher under which sections the authors have included specific pieces of information.

Another major drawback to hard copy tertiary resources is the lag time associated with updating information. Medical information changes very rapidly; thus, information may become outdated shortly after publication or even before publication. Electronically available tertiary resources, such as e-books and DI databases (e.g., IBM® Micromedex®, Lexicomp®), have helped this situation in some cases; however, the time required for updated information to be compiled, reviewed, and summarized results in an inherent delay in communicating new information. It is also possible that complete or detailed information in a tertiary resource may be lacking, due either to space limitations of the resource, incomplete literature searches by the author or other reasons. Even though electronic resources may be updated more frequently, they may be more expensive to purchase or subscribe to than to buy a print version of the same resource. Practitioners must weigh these advantages and disadvantages when deciding which references to purchase (i.e., print or electronic). Table 3-1 lists some questions to consider when evaluating tertiary literature.

Other potential limitations of tertiary information include errors in transcription, human bias, incorrect interpretation of information, or a lack of expertise by authors. It is also important to note that, DI databases, both print and electronic, may contain different information among them for similar sections or topics. An example might be a drug's indications for use; some references and databases only include the same language as the drug's prescribing information (e.g., package insert), whereas some contain more in-depth literature evaluation pertaining to off-label uses. One resource may be favored over the other depending on the question asked. Therefore, it is important to become familiar with the expertise, scope, and other characteristics of each database before using them, as discussed below. Over time, practitioners get familiar with and comfortable at using one or two preferred resources only; however, because of inherent differences in the extent and quality of information among tertiary resources, it is critical to always consult and review more than one resource when possible before providing clinical recommendations.

TABLE 3–1. EVALUATION OF TERTIARY LITERATURE

Does the author have appropriate experience/expertise to publish in this area?

Does the resource contain relevant information to answer the question asked?

Is it the most updated version of the resource?

Is the information contained within the reference appropriate to answer the category of drug information question asked?

Is the information likely to be timely, based on publication date?

Is information supported by appropriate citations?

Does the resource appear free from bias and blatant errors?

Is the reference peer-reviewed?

SELECTING TERTIARY RESOURCES

It is impossible to acquire all available resources that are useful in all areas of clinical practice. It is also impractical to choose only one resource for a practice setting, because each resource may possess different levels of accuracy, comprehensiveness, focus, currency, and ease of use. Differences in practice setting, available funding, patient populations seen, and types of information most needed all impact which tertiary resources should be available at a specific practice site. The legal requirements for information sources available at a practice setting vary from state to state, but rarely will the minimally required resources be sufficient to meet all information needs in a practice.

Another important factor in the selection of appropriate tertiary resources includes selecting a resource focused on the type of information needed for a specific request or situation. For example, a well-written, comprehensive therapeutics text may have very limited use in providing information regarding pharmacokinetics of a specific drug. For this reason, it is important to consider the type of information most needed in a particular practice setting to ensure that appropriate tertiary resources are available.

FORMAT OF TERTIARY RESOURCES

Electronic resources are often preferred due to their ease of use (a keyword search and an instant return of search results) and quicker access to information. They may include information on several different topics within a single resource, allow multiple searches to be performed simultaneously, and often contain more recent information on a topic than is found in the hard copy version of a reference. Additionally, many electronic networked resources allow use of the same resource at more than one location and by more than one user at a time. This allows many practitioners to access information from a variety of physical locations rather than being restricted to only medical libraries or DI centers. Mobile apps have no geographic restriction to accessing and retrieving information once downloaded.

Many textbooks are now being combined into electronic packages, for example, the McGraw-Hill Professional product AccessPharmacy® (https://accesspharmacy.mhmedical. com/). The combination of multiple resources in one package may make selection of resources for a practice site much easier, but also costlier. As these combination packages increase in popularity with students and universities, the expectations that practitioners have for access to resources in work settings will also likely continue to increase.

TERTIARY RESOURCES FOR MOBILE DEVICES

The incorporation of mobile devices into clinical practice settings has prompted an expanding choice of DI databases for that medium. Many of the major compendia available

electronically also offer a product for a mobile device (e.g., Facts & Comparisons®
eAnswers, IBM® Micromedex®, Lexicomp®). It is important to recognize that the information available in a mobile app version of a database may differ from that available in the
online or hardcopy forms. Specifically, online versions may provide more scope and completeness of information compared with their mobile versions. In addition, the specific
functionality of an app and the way that one accesses information for an app may differ
from online versions.

GENERAL MEDICATION INFORMATION

Examples of available general pharmacy practice tertiary references commonly used by
DI specialists and health care professionals are listed below. Each includes a summary of
the resource's features as well as links to the resource (if available), or to the publisher's
website. A more comprehensive and inclusive list of resources and their categories is
available in Table 3-2.

This list reflects only a limited number of resources available because it is impossible to compile a complete list of all resources that are useful in all areas of practice.
The list is in alphabetical order for ease of organization, not by rank of importance. The
Basic Resources for Pharmacy Education listing distributed by the American Association
of Colleges of Pharmacy (AACP),[125] and Doody's Core Titles (https://www.doody.com/
dct/) are helpful compilations of available resources for clinicians and students that may
be consulted to determine possible references that should be obtained for a particular
practice site.

AHFS® Drug Information

American Society of Health-System Pharmacists (https://www.ashp.org), https://www.
ahfsdruginformation.com. The American Hospital Formulary Service® (AHFS®) Drug
Information resource contains information for both prescription and nonprescription
medications. Medications are categorized using AHFS® Pharmacologic-Therapeutic
Classification©. Within each major class (e.g., 4.00 Antihistamine Drugs) are subclasses
(e.g., 4:04 First Generation Antihistamines). Within each subclass are individual monographs containing information on both the Food and Drug Administration (FDA)-approved
and off-label uses of medications. Information about dosing in specific populations is
also included, as is a wide variety of general information about medications (e.g., dosing, administration, pharmacology, drug interactions, adverse reactions, and stability).
Information about orphan drugs is also included. AHFS® Drug Information is available in
a print version that is updated annually. It is available online and as a mobile application as
well, including an excerpted format (AHFS DI® Essentials™), and as a part of a subscription
in databases, such as Lexicomp®. AHFS® Drug Information and AHFS DI® Essentials™

TABLE 3–2. USEFUL RESOURCES FOR COMMON CATEGORIES OF DRUG INFORMATION

Category	Resource
General medication information	Major compendia (AHFS® Drug Information,[8] Clinical Pharmacology Online,[9] DRUGDEX®[10] [IBM® Micromedex®], Facts & Comparisons® eAnswers,[11] Lexi-Drugs™[12] [Lexicomp®, Drug Information Handbook], and Martindale: The Complete Drug Reference[13]),[a] prescribing information, PDR[14,b]
Adverse effects	Clin-Alert®,[15] Drug-Induced Diseases,[16] Meyler's Side Effects of Drugs,[17] Side Effects of Drugs Annual,[18] Reactions Weekly,[19] major compendia,[a] prescribing information, PDR,[14,b] FDAble (MedWatch),[20] ISMP Medication Safety Alert!® Acute Care[21]
Compatibility, stability, and compounding	Gahart's Intravenous Medications: A Handbook for Nurses and Health Professionals,[22] ASHP Injectable Drug Information,[23] King Guide to Parenteral Admixtures,[24] Trissel's™ 2 Clinical Pharmaceutics Database,[25] Extended Stability for Parenteral Drugs,[26] Trissel's Stability of Compounded Formulations,[27] Remington: The Science and Practice of Pharmacy,[28] USP-National Formulary (USP-NF),[29] prescribing information, Pediatric Injectable Drugs: The Teddy Bear Book[30]
Compounding, formulations	Handbook of Drug Administration via Enteral Feeding Tubes,[31] Remington: The Science and Practice of Pharmacy,[28] Merck Index,[32] A Practical Guide to Contemporary Pharmacy Practice,[33] USP-NF,[29] Trissel's Stability of Compounded Formulations,[27] Extemporaneous Formulations,[34] Pediatric Drug Formulations[35]
Dietary and herbal supplements	Natural Medicines,[36] NIH's Dietary Supplement Label Database,[37] MedlinePlus,[38] Natural Products Database,[39] FDA,[40] PDR[14,b]
Diseases, diagnoses	Pharmacotherapy: A Pathophysiologic Approach,[41] Pharmacotherapy Principles and Practice,[42] Applied Therapeutics: The Clinical Use of Drugs,[43] The Merck Manual of Diagnosis and Therapy,[44] Harrison's Principles of Internal Medicine,[45] Goldman-Cecil Medicine,[46] Textbook of Therapeutics,[47] Conn's Current Therapy,[48] Medscape,[49] DynaMed®,[50] UpToDate®[51]
Drug availability, shortages, and pricing	Red Book,[52] Clinical Pharmacology,[9] Lexi-Drugs™,[12] Medi-Span Price Rx,[53] FDA Drug Shortages website,[54] ASHP Drug Shortage website[55] (see Chapter 15)
Drug identification	IDENTIDEX®,[56] Clinical Pharmacology,[9] Drugs.com,[57] Lexi-DrugID,[58] Facts & Comparisons® eAnswers,[11] Merck Manual Professional Version,[59] PDR[14,b]
Drug interactions	Clin-Alert®,[15] The Top 100 Drug Interactions: A Guide to Patient Management,[60] Lexicomp®,[61] Stockley's Drug Interactions,[62] major compendia,[a] prescribing information
Drug use in renal dysfunction	Major compendia,[a] Drug Prescribing in Renal Failure: Dosing Guidelines for Adults (Aronoff),[63] Demystifying Drug Dosing in Renal Dysfunction,[64] Dialysis of Drugs,[65] prescribing information
Geriatric pharmacotherapy	Geriatric Dosage Handbook,[66] major compendia,[a] prescribing information
Infectious diseases	Infectious Diseases Society of America website (https://www.idsociety.org/),[67] Kucers The Use of Antibiotics,[68] Red Book® Report of the Committee on Infectious Diseases,[69] Sanford Guide,[70] Centers for Disease Control and Prevention website (https://www.cdc.gov),[71] Mandell, Douglas, and Bennett's Principles and Practice of Infectious Diseases,[72] CDC Yellow Book,[73] Hospital-specific Antibiogram

continued

TABLE 3–2.   USEFUL RESOURCES FOR COMMON CATEGORIES OF DRUG INFORMATION   (*CONTINUED*)

Category	Resource
International drugs	Drug Information Handbook with International Trade Names Index,[74] Clinical Pharmacology,[9] DRUGDEX®,[10] Martindale: The Complete Drug Reference,[13] Index Nominum International Drug Directory[75]
Investigational drugs	FDA website (https://www.fda.gov),[40] ClinicalTrials.gov,[76] MedlinePlus,[38] manufacturer websites
Laboratory tests	Basic Skills in Interpreting Laboratory Data (ASHP),[77] Mosby's Manual of Diagnostics and Laboratory Test (Pagana),[78] Guide to Diagnostic Tests (Nicoll),[79] Laboratory Tests and Diagnostic Procedures[80]
Latex content	LatexDrugs.com,[81] prescribing information, manufacturer
Method/Rate of administration	Prescribing information, ASHP Injectable Drug Information,[23] major compendia,[a] Gahart's Intravenous Medications: A Handbook for Nurses and Health Professionals[22]
Nonprescription drugs	Handbook of Nonprescription Drugs,[82] product labeling, major compendia[a]
Pediatric pharmacotherapy	The Harriet Lane Handbook,[83] Pediatric and Neonatal Dosage Handbook,[84] Nelson Textbook of Pediatrics,[85] Neofax,[86] Red Book®: Report of the Committee on Infectious Diseases,[69] major compendia,[a] prescribing information
Pharmaceutical calculations	Learning and Mastering Pharmaceutical Calculations[87] Pharmaceutical Calculations (Zatz),[88] Pharmaceutical Calculations (Ansel),[89] Lexicomp®[61]
Pharmaceutical industry	FirstWord Pharma,[90] IPD Analytics,[91] Pink Sheet[92]
Pharmaceutical manufacturers	Clinical Pharmacology,[9] Red Book,[52] major compendia,[a] PDR[14,b]
Pharmacokinetics	Winter's Basic Clinical Pharmacokinetics,[93] Applied Biopharmaceutics and Pharmacokinetics,[94] Martindale: The Complete Drug Reference,[13] major compendia,[a] Applied Clinical Pharmacokinetics[95]
Pharmacology	Goodman & Gilman's: The Pharmacological Basis of Therapeutics,[96] Basic & Clinical Pharmacology (Katzung),[97] Brody's Human Pharmacology: Mechanism-Based Therapeutics,[98] Principles of Pharmacology (Golan)[99]
Pharmacotherapeutics	Pharmacotherapy: A Pathophysiologic Approach,[41] Pharmacotherapy Principles and Practice,[42] Applied Therapeutics: The Clinical Use of Drugs[43]
Pharmacy law	Pharmacy Practice and the Law,[100] Guide to Federal Pharmacy Law,[101] State Board of Pharmacy websites
Pregnancy and lactation	Drugs in Pregnancy and Lactation (Briggs),[102] LactMed,[103] Medications and Mother's Milk,[104] Drugs During Pregnancy and Lactation,[105] REPROTOX,[106] major compendia[a]
Toxicology	PubChem,[107] LiverTox,[108] POISINDEX®,[109] Lexi-Tox™,[110] Goldfrank's Toxicologic Emergencies,[111] Casarett & Doull's Toxicology: The Basic Science of Poisons,[112] Safety Data Sheets
Veterinary medicine	Textbook of Veterinary Internal Medicine,[113] Veterinary Pharmacology and Therapeutics (Riviere),[114] The Merck Veterinary Manual,[115] Plumb's Veterinary Drug Handbook,[116] Plumb's Veterinary Drugs website (https://www.plumbsveterinarydrugs.com),[117] Exotic Animal Formulary,[118] FDA Center for Veterinary Medicine,[119] Animal Drugs@FDA,[120] Pet Coach,[121] Pet Place,[122] Pets with Diabetes,[123] USP Standards for Veterinary Drugs[124]

[a]Major compendia include AHFS® Drug Information, Clinical Pharmacology Online, DRUGDEX® (IBM® Micromedex®), Facts & Comparisons® eAnswers, Lexi-Drugs™ (Lexicomp®; Drug Information Handbook), and Martindale: The Complete Drug Reference.
[b]Physicians' Desk Reference/Prescribers' Digital Reference (online).

are also available online through AHFS® Clinical Drug Information™ (AHFS® CDI™). This database incorporates real-time drug and safety updates, and includes information about drug shortages. It is also available in a mobile version.

Clinical Pharmacology

Elsevier's Gold Standard, http://www.clinicalpharmacology.com. This electronic database contains monographs of prescription and nonprescription products as well as some herbals and nutritional supplements. It also includes information about investigational drugs. Tools within the database allow users to screen for drug interactions, create comparison tables for drug products, determine intravenous (IV) compatibility (based on Trissel's 2™ Clinical Pharmaceutics Database) and search for tablets by description or imprint codes. Patient education handouts and FDA-required Medication Guides are included. It also has a Resource Center that provides drug class summaries, lab values and ranges for both adult and pediatric patients, and contact information for pharmaceutical manufacturers. It is available online or as a mobile application; however, it is not available in print.

ClinicalTrials.gov

This free access website (https://www.clinicaltrials.gov) is maintained by the NLM through the National Institutes of Health (NIH) and serves as a main registry for publicly and privately supported clinical studies of human participants conducted throughout the world. Health care professionals can locate clinical research currently ongoing or to be conducted in the future, and register their research as investigators. The trial results are not always fully added to the database and require an additional search via secondary resources such as PubMed®. Since not all clinical trials, particularly those with negative results, are published, this can be a valuable source for professionals to try to locate unpublished data.

DailyMed

NLM, https://dailymed.nlm.nih.gov/. This free electronic resource contains over 110,000 drugs in their monograph format as approved for marketing by the FDA (i.e., prescribing information). Basic searches can be done using medication names, National Drug Codes (NDCs), drug classes, or keywords. An advanced search option allows health care professionals to conduct more refined searches using Boolean Logic (i.e., "and," "or," "in," "not in") and by searching for keywords within specific categories (e.g., benzyl alcohol "in" inactive ingredients). The resource contains photos of current medication package labels and archives of old prescribing information and labels. In addition to prescribing information, it provides links to MedlinePlus, ClinicalTrials.gov, and PubMed® entries for the searched medication. It also provides a link to biochemical data for the medication. Links to the FDA Safety Recalls site, to report adverse events through FDA's MedWatch, and to lactation information through the NLM's LactMed are provided. It is current and cross-references with FDA's website to provide FDA guidances. This resource includes DI for both humans and animals.

Drugs.com

Drugs.com, https://www.drugs.com. This free online resource includes drug monographs (searchable as a keyword or by choosing from an alphabetical list), tablet/capsule identifier, interactions checker, information about recalls and shortages, and news related to medication approvals, including newly FDA-approved medications, new indications and dosage forms for existing medications, and first-time generic approvals. A pipeline section provides information about agents for which New Drug Applications or Biologics License Applications have been submitted to the FDA. It also has a disease and condition index, symptom checker, and a treatment options section searchable by disease state. The professional version provides more detailed information sourcing from reliable sources such as AHFS® DI, IBM® Micromedex®, and FDA. It is also available as a mobile application.

Epocrates®

Epocrates, https://online.epocrates.com. This family of electronic resources includes both free mobile and online products. These resources include information about drugs (e.g., monographs, interaction checker, safety data, tablet/capsule identification) and diseases (e.g., epidemiology, prognosis, treatment). It also includes some clinical calculators (e.g., anion gap, creatinine clearance, ideal body weight).

Facts & Comparisons® eAnswers

Wolters Kluwer Clinical Drug Information, Inc., http://online.factsandcomparisons.com. This reference contains monographs for prescription and nonprescription drugs organized by therapeutic or pharmacologic classes. Drugs within the same class are grouped together, allowing for easy comparison. The reference also includes an Off-Label Drug Facts database, pregnancy and lactation information, Risk Evaluation and Mitigation Strategy (REMS) program requirements and links to associated Medication Guides, a Natural Products database, links to hundreds of Black Box Warnings, a list of do not crush or chew medications, immunization schedules, a manufacturer index, patient education handouts, and information for various patient assistance programs. There are also interactive modules for determining product availability and potential alternatives, drug interactions, drug identification, clinical calculators, Trissel's™ 2 Clinical Pharmaceutics Database for checking IV compatibilities, and Martindale: The Complete Drug Reference™. The Drug Comparison tool creates side-by-side tables of full monographs or specific data points (e.g., indications, adverse reactions, or drug interactions) to help discern differences between or among agents within the same class or different classes of agents. A Drug Reports feature allows searching for drugs based on known conditions or symptoms (e.g., contraindicated for a specific condition).

Handbook of Nonprescription Drugs: An Interactive Approach to Self-Care

American Pharmacists Association®, https://www.pharmacist.com. This book is organized by body system, focusing on those disease states for which self-care may be appropriate. Information is provided about FDA-approved dosing, comparative efficacy of various over-the-counter (OTC) agents, as well as contraindications for self-treatment, drug interactions, patient education, and product administration illustrations. It also includes information on nutritional supplements, medical foods, nondrug and preventive measures, and complementary therapies. Treatment algorithms and patient care cases are included. The book is also available online through https://www.PharmacyLibrary.com. The online version includes monthly content updates and additional case studies.

Index Nominum: International Drug Directory

MedPharm Scientific Publishers GmbH, http://www.drugbase.de/en/databases/indexnominum.html. Edited by the Swiss Pharmaceutical Society. This DI reference is an international database containing information on over 5100 drugs available in 166 countries, including international nonproprietary names (INN), synonyms, and global proprietary names as well as chemical structures and therapeutic classes. It is available online as part of the IBM® Micromedex® suite of references (subscription dependent).

Lexicomp®

Wolters Kluwer Clinical Drug Information, Inc., http://online.lexi.com. This resource allows for integrated searches of various products (depending on subscription purchased) and includes a variety of references such as Lexi-Drugs™, Geriatric Lexi-Drugs™, Pediatric & Neonatal Lexi-Drugs™, Pregnancy & Lactation database, Lexi-Tox™, Drug Allergy and Idiosyncratic Reactions, Summary Pharmacogenomics and Pharmacogenomics database, Natural Products database, Martindale: The Complete Drug Reference™, and Trissel's™ 2 Clinical Pharmaceutics Database. Lexicomp® has also partnered with AHFS® (described above) to offer an electronic subscription combining their two databases in a seamless search. Components of Facts & Comparisons® eAnswers, such as the Drug Comparison tool, and UpToDate® have also been incorporated. Additional features include a drug-drug interaction and drug-allergy checker, solid oral dosage form identifier, clinical calculators, patient education handouts on medications, procedures, and conditions, and The 5-Minute Clinical Consult, a database of 900 medical conditions and information about their diagnosis and medical management. Each Lexi-Drugs™ reference provides monograph-based general DI, including dosing, administration, adverse reactions, pharmacokinetics, drug interactions, clinical practice guideline references, available dosage forms, and pricing.

There are accompanying print versions for some of the Lexi-Drug™ references, including Adult Drug Information Handbook and Pediatric & Neonatal Dosage Handbook. Lexi-Drugs™ and its companion resources are available via mobile applications but require an additional subscription.

Martindale: The Complete Drug Reference/MedicinesComplete

Pharmaceutical Press, https://www.pharmpress.com. This reference is considered one of the most comprehensive and trusted information sources on a variety of domestic and international drugs, including over 6300 drug monographs in print and over 7500 online, covering over 40 countries. It also includes treatment reviews, with references from published articles. Proprietary names and manufacturer contact information are available for a variety of countries. Information about herbals, diagnostic agents, radiopharmaceuticals, pharmaceutical excipients, toxins, and poisons is also included. This information is available in hardcopy and via online (MedicinesComplete) subscription. It is also included with some database subscriptions, such as Lexicomp®, Facts & Comparisons® eAnswers, and IBM® Micromedex®.

Medscape

WebMD®, http://www.medscape.com. This electronic resource is published by WebMD® and references over 200 medical journals and textbooks. It is a free subscription service that allows the health care professional to register their information preferences, sending the latest information within a particular specialty area. It also provides a free weekly emailed newsletter with the latest highlights within the field. It includes clinical information as well as financial, managed care, and medical practice information, and provides simplified monographs for DI as well as a drug interaction checker, solid oral dosage form identifier, and clinical calculators. Continuing education activities are available, including activities for continuing medical education (CME) and continuing pharmacist education (CPE) credit. Information is available in several languages. This resource is also available as a mobile application.

IBM® Micromedex®

IBM Watson Health, http://www.micromedex.com. This electronic resource contains multiple references within the database including DI presented both in condensed summary monographs (i.e., Quick Answers) and detailed monographs (i.e., In-Depth Answers/DRUGDEX®) providing FDA-approved indications, off-label uses, pharmacokinetic data, safety information, and pharmacology. Interactive tools are available to assess for drug-drug/allergy/food/ethanol/lab/lactation/pregnancy interactions, and intravenous incompatibilities (via Trissel's™ 2 Clinical Pharmaceutics Database). It includes a toxicology-related tool that allows identification of drugs based on imprint codes and discussion of overdose management. Patient-education materials are available via its CareNotes® reference. IBM® Micromedex® is available online and as a suite of multiple mobile applications (e.g., IBM® Micromedex® Drug Information, IBM® Micromedex® IV Compatibility, IBM® Micromedex® Drug Interactions).

IBM® purchased Truven Health Analytics in 2016. IBM® Micromedex® with Watson™ gives users access to the DI normally available through Micromedex®, but combined with IBM® Watson™ artificial intelligence (Watson™ Assistant). Watson™ Assistant is integrated within IBM® Micromedex® and functions like a conversational search engine. Users can ask Watson™ Assistant questions, the more specific the question, the more specific the response. Watson™ Assistant uses the cognitive computing IBM® cloud to gather information in response to a user's question, and it may ask follow-up questions to refine its search. The program currently only retrieves information from certain portions of drug monographs, including drug class, dosing and administration, medication safety, mechanism of action, pharmacokinetics, drug interactions, and IV compatibility. It cannot currently retrieve information from some of the specialty resources within Micromedex® (e.g., Index Nominum, Martindale, NeoFax®, POISINDEX®, REPRORISK®). However, it does provide links to the DrugPoint and DRUGDEX® monographs, so users can click and look within the specialty references. IBM® Micromedex® states that the system learns from user interaction, and the feature will become more advanced over time.

MPR®

Haymarket Media, Inc., https://www.empr.com. This resource (also known as the Monthly Prescribing Reference®) is available in print, online, and as a mobile app. The online and mobile versions are free; however, the print version requires a subscription. In the online version and mobile app, DI is searchable by brand name, generic name, therapeutic category, and manufacturer. Updates on investigational drugs, new drugs and medical devices, comparative treatment charts and algorithms, and patient fact sheets are also included.

Physicians' Desk Reference® / Prescribers' Digital Reference (PDR®)

PDR®, https://www.pdr.net. This resource is one of the oldest DI references and a compilation of prescription products' official prescribing information (i.e., package inserts). It also contains some information about nonprescription medications, herbals, and dietary supplements. It is available online or as mobile application (mobilePDR®) and is available without a subscription after a free registration via the website. In addition to prescribing information, the site contains links to issued FDA Drug Safety Communications and "Dear Healthcare Professional" letters released searchable by drug. PDR® Updates include recent FDA-approvals and labeling updates. The mobile version includes a drug interaction checker, solid oral dosage form identifier, and the ability to compare drug products.

R2 Digital Library

Rittenhouse Book Distributors, https://www.r2library.com/. The R2 Digital Library is an online database with searchable access to thousands of allied health, medical, nursing, pharmacy, and veterinary books from over 70 health sciences publishers. A free, 30-day trial is available for users who want to explore the database prior to subscribing.

U.S. Food and Drug Administration (FDA)

This free access website (https://www.fda.gov) provides very comprehensive information regarding drugs, vaccines, biologics and biosimilars, blood products, medical devices, food and dietary supplements, veterinary products, cosmetics, and tobacco products. It provides updates on drug recalls, drug shortages, medication safety information and adverse drug events (e.g., Drug Safety Communications), drug approvals, changes to drug labeling, REMS program requirements and Medication Guides, and documents exchanged between the manufacturer and FDA during the drug approval process or when manufacturing issues have been identified (i.e., Warning Letters). FDA-approved DI is searchable at Drugs@FDA by using brand, generic, or application number. The Orange Book is a helpful resource within the website that lists approved drug products with therapeutic equivalent evaluations. It also includes information about individual medication patents and exclusivity. Another useful reference available through the site is The Purple Book which can be used to determine if a biological product is biosimilar to or interchangeable with a reference biological product. The site also contains guidance for pharmaceutical industry documents and consumer information. Several different features and components of the website are available as mobile apps (e.g., Drugs@FDA, drug shortages).

USP Dictionary of United States Adopted Names (USAN) and International Drug Names

U.S. Pharmacopeial Convention, https://www.usp.org. This is the official resource for determining accepted adopted generic and chemical names of over 6000 U.S. drugs as well as international nonproprietary names. Additionally, useful information such as chemical structures, molecular weights, Chemical Abstracts Services (CAS) registry numbers, pronunciations, pharmacologic or therapeutic categories, and manufacturers are provided. This resource is available online (subscription required) and is updated annually in January.

ADVERSE EFFECTS

Clin-Alert®

SAGE Publishing, https://journals.sagepub.com/home/CLA. This bimonthly publication primarily focuses not only on providing summaries of adverse drug reactions, but also includes information regarding drug interactions, medication errors, and market withdrawals. Other covered topics include food-drug interactions and dietary supplement information. In addition to a summary of the reaction or interaction, information regarding management of the event, pertinent lab data, and potential legal implications are often discussed. It also includes a "First Report" notice feature, which notes when the adverse reaction described is the first documented report of the adverse event with a particular medication. It is available in print and online.

Drug-Induced Diseases

American Society of Health-System Pharmacists, https://www.ashp.org. This reference provides information on the contributing factors, prevention, detection, and management of diseases induced by medications. It is organized into sections by body system, each with chapters about specific diseases or conditions. It also includes chapters on the regulatory and legal aspects surrounding drug safety and drug-induced diseases, and the epidemiology and public health impact of these diseases. This resource is available in both print and e-book versions.

FDAble

FDAble, LLC, https://www.fdable.com. This online resource allows a search for adverse drug events reported to the FDA's MedWatch, FDA Adverse Event Reporting System (FAERS), Manufacturer and User Facility Device Experience (MAUDE), and Vaccine Adverse Event Reporting System (VAERS). The resource contains over 12 million adverse drug event cases, about 95,000 vaccine adverse event cases, and over 6.5 million medical device adverse event cases. It provides up to 30 events specific to a drug, device, or vaccine for free; obtaining more than 30 events requires a user to send a report request with a fee. An event report includes suspected drug, adverse reaction, patient outcomes, patient's age and gender, and event date. Returned reports permit manipulation of data, including filtering and sorting.

ISMP Medication Safety Alert!® Acute Care

Institute for Safe Medication Practices (ISMP), https://www.ismp.org/newsletters/acute-care. This online resource is published as a digital newsletter every 2 weeks (25 issues per year). This resource is intended for acute care practitioners and contains medication safety and adverse event data voluntarily reported by hospitals and pharmacies. Because it is published so frequently, the newsletter helps practitioners stay abreast of medication safety issues occurring at other institutions. The ISMP also forwards adverse event data to the FDA in a standardized format. The newsletter requires a yearly subscription and is distributed via email.

Meyler's Side Effects of Drugs: The International Encyclopedia of Adverse Drug Reactions and Interactions

Elsevier, https://www.elsevier.com. As one of the most comprehensive resources on adverse drug effects, this reference provides a critical review of international literature for adverse reactions and interactions with thorough referencing. General monographs for classes of agents are complemented by monographs for individual drugs that are listed in alphabetical order by generic name. Within each monograph may be general information about the drug followed by adverse reactions broken down by organ system. Additional information about susceptibility factors, long-term effects, effects on pregnancy and lactation, and management and monitoring are provided. Drug interactions with other drugs, alcohol, food, and procedures are also described. It is available in print and as an e-book. Updates are published every year as the Side Effects of Drugs Annual. Note that the books are not completely comprehensive. In any edition, it may refer back to previous editions for further information on a topic.

Side Effects of Drugs Annual

Elsevier, https://www.elsevier.com. This reference is updated annually and serves as a companion to the book Meyler's Side Effects of Drugs. A team evaluates international literature published each year to identify new information about adverse drug reactions and interactions and summarizes that information in this resource. It is available in print and as e-book. All previous volumes can be accessed electronically using ScienceDirect® (https://www.sciencedirect.com).

DIETARY AND HERBAL SUPPLEMENTS

Dietary Supplement Label Database

The NIH Office of Dietary Supplements and U.S. NLM, (https://www.dsld.nlm.nih.gov) publish and maintain this free online database. Information is derived directly from dietary supplement product labels, and includes names and amounts of active ingredients, inactive ingredients, formulation, percent daily value of nutrients, dietary claims made, directions for use, warnings, and intended target consumer. Photographs of the product label are included, as is manufacturer information. Searches can be performed by ingredient, product, or manufacturer. There are also searches based on three special patient populations: pregnancy and lactation, children, and seniors.

Natural Medicines™

Therapeutic Research Center, https://naturalmedicines.therapeuticresearch.com. This resource is available online and in a mobile device format, and is one of the most comprehensive resources on dietary and herbal supplements. It includes detailed summary monographs for over 1200 natural medicines and over 200 complementary and alternative therapies with evidence-based ratings for safety and efficacy and references. Additional features include patient handouts, disease state searching, an interaction checker, adverse effects checker, safety during pregnancy and lactation, and a nutrient depletion checker that identifies nutrients that are decreased by prescription and nonprescription medications. Commercially available products are also assigned a Natural Medicines Brand Evidence-based Rating™ (NMBER™) based on scientific evidence for safety, effectiveness, and product quality.

Natural Products Database

Wolters Kluwer Clinical Drug Information, Inc., http://online.factsandcomparisons.com. This resource provides detailed information about the chemistry, pharmacology, and toxicology of a number of natural products, based on references to primary literature. Summaries of relevant clinical trials by disease state or condition are also available. Patient education handouts are included. This is available online through Facts & Comparisons® eAnswers and as a mobile app.

DRUG IDENTIFICATION (U.S. AND FOREIGN)

Identidex

IBM Watson Health, http://www.micromedex.com. This electronic resource can be accessed via IBM® Micromedex® and allows search by either description (e.g., color, shape, pattern) or imprint code. It provides information on dosage form, color, shape, active and inactive ingredients, manufacturer, NDC numbers, and available container sizes. It includes product images.

Lexi-Drug ID

Wolters Kluwer Clinical Drug Information, Inc., http://online.lexi.com. This resource is accessed through Lexicomp® and allows for identification of oral dosage forms (both solid and liquid), topical dosage forms (e.g., creams, ointments, gels), aerosols, suppositories, and injections. When searching solid oral dosage forms one or more descriptions such as imprint, dosage form, shape, or color can be entered. Drug names, manufacturers or labelers, and NDCs can also be searched. It includes a picture of the product.

DRUG INTERACTIONS

Clin-Alert®

SAGE Publishing, https://journals.sagepub.com/home/CLA. Please see the description under the "Adverse Effects" section.

Stockley's Drug Interactions

Pharmaceutical Press, https://www.pharmpress.com/. This international print resource includes in-depth information on interactions among drugs, herbal medicines, foods, drinks, and drugs of abuse. It includes an assessment of clinical evidence, clinical importance of interactions, and guidance on managing the interaction in practice. The online version is available via the MedicinesComplete database (http://www.medicinescomplete.com).

The Top 100 Drug Interactions: A Guide to Patient Management

H&H Publications, http://www.hanstenandhorn.com. This pocket-sized print reference describes approximately 10,000 common drug interactions and their management, including potential alternatives. It also includes an extensive table of drugs and the cytochrome P450 enzyme(s) by which they are metabolized, and enzymes the drugs may inhibit or induce.

Case Study 3–1

A 25-year-old patient has recently been started on duloxetine for treatment of generalized anxiety disorder. She is taking no other medications. She has been experiencing headaches recently and wants to know if this might be drug related.

- *What are appropriate tertiary resources to consult for a response to this request?*

DRUG PRICE

Red Book®

IBM Watson Health, https://www.ibm.com/us-en/marketplace/micromedex-red-book. This reference includes pricing and availability information for prescription and nonprescription medications, nutraceuticals, bulk chemicals, medical devices, and supplies. Searching can be done by product name, active ingredient, NDC, or manufacturer name. Additionally, information such as dosage form, route of administration, strength, package size, NDC, and manufacturer are provided. This resource is available electronically within IBM® Micromedex®. The online version is updated daily. It can also be purchased as a raw data file with updates delivered weekly, monthly, quarterly, or annually.

PHARMACOKINETICS

Applied Biopharmaceutics and Pharmacokinetics

McGraw-Hill Education, https://www.mheducation.com/. This book describes the role of pharmacokinetics as it relates to drug development and to patient care. This covers the clinical application of pharmacokinetics and addresses the impact of pharmacogenetics on drug metabolism. Chapters include examples and practice problems. This book is also included in the AccessPharmacy® electronic subscription.

Applied Clinical Pharmacokinetics

McGraw-Hill Education, https://www.mheducation.com/. This resource emphasizes the practical issues of drug dosing for patients with changes in pharmacokinetics and pharmacodynamic parameters, especially antibiotic drugs, anticonvulsants, cardiovascular agents, and immunosuppressants. Chapters include practice questions. It is available as part of the AccessPharmacy® suite of electronic textbooks.

Concepts in Clinical Pharmacokinetics

American Society of Health-System Pharmacists, https://store.ashp.org/Default.aspx?TabID=251&productId=624898817. This print resource describes basic principles of pharmacokinetics and pharmacodynamics using a simplified approach, and includes clinical cases and practice problems. It is also available as an e-book.

PHARMACOLOGY

Goodman & Gilman's: The Pharmacological Basis of Therapeutics

McGraw-Hill Education, https://www.mheducation.com/. The focus of this classic pharmacology book is to provide a correlation between principles of pharmacology and contemporary clinical practice. It also provides information about pharmacokinetics and pharmacodynamics for a number of drugs. Pharmacogenetics and drug poisoning and toxicity information is also included. The book makes extensive use of charts and tables to convey information. This book is also included in the AccessPharmacy® electronic subscription.

Basic & Clinical Pharmacology

McGraw-Hill Education, https://www.mheducation.com/. This book, organized by therapeutic class of agents, provides general discussion of pharmacology principles as well as more detailed discussion of specific agents. Figures and tables are frequently used to illustrate difficult material. Patient cases are included with most chapters. To remain current, this resource is updated every 2–3 years. This book is also included in the AccessPharmacy® electronic subscription.

Brody's Human Pharmacology: Mechanism-Based Therapeutics

Elsevier, https://www.us.elsevierhealth.com. This book is designed with a student focus and emphasizes therapeutic impact of pharmacology through systems-based learning. Students can use Student Consult, an interactive learning platform, which provides exam questions, videos, animations, and colorful illustrations. The book is organized by organ system impacted. Each chapter includes a "Clinical Relevance for Healthcare Professionals" section. The book is also available as an e-book.

Principles of Pharmacology: The Pathophysiologic Basis of Drug Therapy

Wolters Kluwer, https://shop.lww.com. This textbook is designed for students and uses clinical vignettes to illustrate therapeutic problems. Chapters are listed by organ systems with illustrations that highlight key points and drug summary tables that contain essential elements. This resource is also available as an e-book.

PHARMACY LAW

Information about individual state pharmacy law is best obtained through the individual state boards of pharmacy. A listing of state board website URLs is available from https://nabp.pharmacy/boards-of-pharmacy/. The Code of Federal Regulations containing aspects of federal law is available from https://www.ecfr.gov/. One general text about federal law is listed below.

Pharmacy Practice and the Law

Jones & Bartlett Learning, http://www.jblearning.com/. This print resource contains information about federal laws and regulations impacting pharmacy practice, specifically about drug development, production, marketing, and dispensing. Some state regulations are also included, as is information about pharmacist liability and risk management strategies. Various summaries of case law are provided. It is also available as an e-book.

PREGNANT AND LACTATING WOMEN

Drugs in Pregnancy and Lactation

Wolters Kluwer, http://www.lww.com. This reference (often referred to as Briggs) focuses on the use of both medications and drugs of abuse in pregnant or lactating women. Fetal risk summaries are provided via evaluation of the literature regarding the safety of fetal exposure. Animal literature is provided in cases where human literature is lacking. Breastfeeding summaries include literature describing the excretion of medications into breast milk and effects of exposure in nursing infants. Each drug monograph includes a use in pregnancy recommendation and a use in breastfeeding recommendation. It is available in print and as an e-book. Quarterly updates are provided online. The online version is incorporated into tertiary databases such as Lexicomp® and Fact & Comparisons® eAnswers.

Drugs and Lactation Database (LactMed)

NLM, https://www.nlm.nih.gov. A peer-reviewed and fully referenced free database of drugs and chemicals to which breastfeeding mothers may be exposed; accessible through Bookshelf, an online searchable collection of scholarly literature in biology, medicine, and life sciences, including books, reports, and databases (https://www.ncbi.nlm.nih.gov/books/NBK501922/). Among the included data are maternal and infant levels of drugs, possible effects on breastfed infants and on lactation, and alternate drugs to consider. LactMed is updated monthly. This database is also available as a mobile app.

Hale's Medications & Mothers' Milk

Springer Publishing Company, https://www.halesmeds.com. This comprehensive reference contains evidence-based information describing the transmission of maternal drugs into breast milk. Each drug monograph includes a summary of available literature, adult concerns (common adverse effects), typical adult dosage, pediatric concerns, suggested infant monitoring parameters, and alternative medication, if available. Lactation risk categories range from L1 Compatible to L5 Hazardous. It is available as a mobile app, in print, and as an e-book.

Reprotox®, ReproCollection™ System

IBM Watson Health, http://www.micromedex.com. Retrieved through IBM® Micromedex® system, it provides comprehensive information on general toxicity, fertility, male exposures, genetic influences, teratogenic agents, and lactation, and helps clinicians to evaluate human reproductive risks of drugs, chemicals, and physical/environmental agents. It is only available online.

Case Study 3-2

A mother has been breastfeeding her child for 6 months. The mother has recently been prescribed fluconazole for treatment of Candidiasis infection.

- *What sources should be consulted to determine the appropriateness of this choice?*
- *What additional patient information might be helpful to know prior to researching the patient's question?*

SPECIAL POPULATIONS (GERIATRIC, PEDIATRIC)

Geriatric Dosage Handbook

Wolters Kluwer, http://online.lexi.com. The monographs in this resource contain traditional sections of DI, but focus on dosing recommendations for geriatric patients. There is a special section of each monograph addressing concerns specific to the geriatric population. Limited references to primary literature are provided. This reference is also available online and as a mobile app.

The Harriet Lane Handbook

Elsevier, https://www.us.elsevierhealth.com. This resource, assembled by medical residents and reviewed by faculty at The Johns Hopkins Hospital, contains a succinct discussion of common diseases and conditions of newborn to adolescent patients. A significant portion of the book is dedicated to pediatric medication dosing. This resource also contains information about common side effects, therapeutic monitoring, and dosage forms available and includes a variety of topic areas, such as palliative care, genetics, and toxicology. It is available in print and as an e-book. This e-book is available for mobile devices and as part of a supplemental reference in online databases such as Clinical Pharmacology. There is a separate print publication that focuses on antimicrobial therapy.

Pediatric & Neonatal Dosage Handbook

Wolters Kluwer, http://online.lexi.com. The monographs in this resource contain traditional sections of DI, but focus on detailed dosing recommendations for pediatrics. It also includes information about common extemporaneous preparations for pediatric use. Limited references to primary literature are provided. This reference is also available online and for mobile devices.

Pediatric Injectable Drugs: The Teddy Bear Book

American Society of Health-System Pharmacists, https://store.ashp.org/Default.aspx?TabID=251&productId=613654675. This resource includes evidence-based information on pediatric intravenous infusions. It focuses on issues surrounding intravenous access sites, limited fluid amounts, and pediatric dosing. It has been around for more than 20 years and is available in print and as an e-book.

Red Book: Report of the Committee on Infectious Diseases

American Academy of Pediatrics, http://www.aap.org. The Committee on Infectious Diseases of the American Academy of Pediatrics provides recommendations for the care of pediatric patients with infectious diseases. This resource includes disease summaries, epidemiologic data, treatment recommendations, and immunization information.

The resource is available in print, online, and via a mobile app. The print version is updated every 3 years; the online version and the mobile app are updated more frequently with topics including current disease outbreak information and changes to immunization schedules.

STABILITY / COMPATIBILITY / COMPOUNDING

ASHP Injectable Drug Information

American Society of Health-System Pharmacists, https://store.ashp.org/Store/Product Listing/ProductDetails.aspx?productId=765323999. This resource includes compatibility and stability for various parenteral medications. Information is primarily provided in charts and tables, making finding information relatively quick. The resource also provides information about routes of administration and commercially available strengths. This resource is available in print and via an interactive mobile app.

King Guide to Parenteral Admixtures

King Guide Publications, Inc., http://www.kingguide.com. This resource is one of the oldest and most comprehensive compatibility references. It focuses on compatibility and stability information for parenteral medications, and includes data from more than 3000 references. It is available in a loose-leaf edition and as an online, stand-alone database.

Trissel's™ 2 Clinical Pharmaceutics Database

This resource is an online database containing data from over 4700 parenteral drug compatibility studies. The database is searchable by either parenteral drug or by IV solution, and contains admixture, syringe, and Y-site compatibility data. The database is integrated into some of the major online compendia (e.g., Lexicomp®, IBM® Micromedex®).

Trissel's Stability of Compounded Formulations

American Pharmacists Association Publications, https://www.pharmacist.com. This reference is only available in print and provides stability information on nonsterile medications compounded as enteral, topical, ophthalmic, oral, and other special formulations. It summarizes published stability data for efficient evaluation, and provides proper storage and packaging information.

Extemporaneous Formulations for Pediatric, Geriatric, and Special Needs Patients

American Society of Health-System Pharmacists, https://store.ashp.org/Store/ProductListing/ProductDetails.aspx?productId=597629134. This resource contains a compilation of published formulations with recipes and stability data for nonsterile compounds. Most recipes are for oral formulations not commercially available that may be useful in pediatric, geriatric, or special needs patient populations. Information on legal and technical compounding issues is also provided. It is available in print and as an electronic copy.

Merck Index

Merck & Co., Inc., https://www.rsc.org/merck-index. This resource is one of the oldest resources focusing on chemicals and drug ingredient information. It provides descriptions of the chemical and pharmacological information about a variety of chemicals, drugs, and biologicals. Data include CAS number, chemical structure, molecular weight, and physical data, including solubility, which may be useful in compounding. This reference is available in print and online (The Merck Index Online via the Royal Society of Chemistry).

Remington: The Science and Practice of Pharmacy

Pharmaceutical Press, http://www.pharmpress.com. This classic book contains information about all aspects of pharmacy practice. There is discussion of social issues impacting pharmacy as well as information about the basics of pharmaceutics, manufacturing, pharmacodynamics, nuclear pharmacy, and medicinal chemistry. Information includes common compounding techniques and ingredients. The book is divided into two volumes, and is also available online.

USP-NF (United States Pharmacopeia and National Formulary)

United States Pharmacopeial Convention, https://www.usp.org. This resource, available in print and online formats, contains the official substance and product standards. It also contains official preparation instructions for a limited number of commonly compounded products.

THERAPY EVALUATION / DRUG OF CHOICE

Applied Therapeutics

Lippincott Williams & Wilkins, https://www.lww.com. This resource includes information about disease states and treatment options. Information is presented in the form of cases with follow-up discussion to help readers apply therapeutic knowledge in clinical contexts. Cases contain information on diseases, treatment options, drug interactions, pharmacogenomics, and other drug-related topics. It is available in print and as an e-book. A handbook version is also available that lists information in bulleted and tabular formats for quick access.

Centers for Disease Control and Prevention (CDC)

A division of the Department of Health and Human Services, the CDC (https://www.cdc.gov) is the frontline information medium in the U.S. for any diseases affecting a large patient population such as infectious diseases or other epidemics. It includes data and statistics regarding various diseases and conditions, and practice recommendations for emergency preparedness and natural disasters. CDC also publishes a weekly epidemiological report, Morbidity and Mortality Weekly Report (MMWR), based on data received from state health departments. It is CDC's main vehicle for disseminating public health information and recommendations. MMWR is available for free via email subscription. CDC-INFO on Demand includes valuable information that can be shared with patients. The resource is also available as a mobile app. CDC also publishes the Epidemiology and Prevention of Vaccine-Preventable Diseases, or "Pink Book," which contains detailed information on vaccine-preventable diseases and vaccine recommendations. CDC publishes the Yellow Book (Health Information for International Travel) every 2 years, which contains current travel vaccine recommendations and destination-specific disease prevention strategies. These resources are available in print and online. There is also an interactive mobile app (PneumoRecs VaxAdvisor) containing a clinician's guide to CDC's pneumococcal vaccine recommendations, and a mobile app containing general vaccine schedule recommendations.

Goldman-Cecil Medicine

Elsevier, https://www.us.elsevierhealth.com. This resource is one of the oldest and most respected textbooks in internal medicine. It provides detailed information on disease etiology, clinical presentation, diagnosis, treatment, and prognosis. Information is organized by disease state and color-coded to increase ease of use. It is available in print, online as an e-book, and as a mobile application. It is also incorporated in databases such as ClinicalKey®. The electronic versions are updated continuously to include the most recent guideline and treatment information.

Harrison's Principles of Internal Medicine

McGraw-Hill Education, https://www.mheducation.com/. This resource serves as a fairly comprehensive introduction to clinical medicine. It includes comprehensive information on diseases including pathophysiology, differential diagnosis, and disease management. It is divided into sections by clinical specialty, and is available in text and electronic formats. It is also included in the AccessMedicine® and AccessPharmacy® electronic suite of resources.

The Merck Manual of Diagnosis and Therapy

Merck & Co. Inc., https://www.merck.com. This source provides a quick summary of disease state information, including pathology, symptoms, diagnosis, and treatment. It is also available online as a free resource at https://www.merckmanuals.com and as a mobile app.

Medscape

WebMD®, https://www.medscape.com. Refer to the "General Medication Information" section.

Pharmacotherapy: A Pathophysiological Approach

McGraw-Hill Education, https://www.mheducation.com/. This textbook (commonly referred to as DiPiro) focuses on the management of a variety of disease states. It includes information on epidemiology, etiology, presentation, treatment, and outcomes. It is available in text and electronic formats. There are also the accompanying books Pharmacotherapy Casebook: A Patient-Focused Approach and Pharmacotherapy Handbook. These resources are also included in the AccessPharmacy® electronic subscription.

Pharmacotherapy Principles and Practice

McGraw-Hill Education, https://www.mheducation.com/. This book focuses on the management of a variety of disease states, centering on the diseases most likely to be seen by pharmacists, nurse practitioners, and physician assistants. It is more concise than Pharmacotherapy: A Pathophysiological Approach; it also contains various features to help student learning. Information provided about disorders includes epidemiology, etiology, presentation, treatment, and treatment outcomes. This is available in text and electronic formats. This resource also has accompanying textbook, Pharmacotherapy Principles and Practice Study Guide. It is also available as an add-on reference for AccessPharmacy®.

TOXICOLOGY

Casarett and Doull's Toxicology: The Basic Science of Poisons

McGraw-Hill Education, https://www.mheducation.com. This resource includes information on toxicology concepts and mechanisms and substance-specific toxicity. It presents information from general principles to organ-specific toxicology. This resource is available in print and online as part of the AccessPharmacy® suite of resources.

Goldfrank's Toxicologic Emergencies

McGraw-Hill Education, https://www.mheducation.com. The book is one of the most comprehensive resources focusing on poisoning and overdose. It discusses the clinical application of toxicology and poisoning, and provides a case study approach to medical toxicology and poison management. It is available in print and online through the AccessPharmacy® suite of resources.

Lexi-Tox™

Wolters Kluwer, https://www.wolterskluwercdi.com/lexicomp-online/. This resource is accessed through Lexicomp® and contains information on toxic agents including chemical, pharmaceutical, nuclear, biologic, and terrorism agents, along with toxic bite information (i.e., envenomation). It also includes information on nontoxic agents, antidotes and decontaminants, household products, toxicology-specific calculations, and a drug identification tool.

POISINDEX®

IBM® Micromedex®, https://www.micromedexsolutions.com. The POISINDEX® System includes information on the toxicology, range of symptoms, and treatment options for thousands of biological, commercial, and pharmaceutical substances. It is available online through the IBM® Micromedex® online database.

Safety Data Sheets

Safety data sheets (SDS), formerly referred to as material safety data sheets (MSDS), are documents containing data on the hazardous classification, composition, physical and chemical properties, handling and storage, disposal and transport, and exposure/first aid measures for medications and chemicals. These sheets are created using a standard format as mandated by the Occupational Safety & Health Administration (OSHA) of the U.S. Department of Labor. Sheets are available through product manufacturers and various tertiary databases (e.g., Lexicomp®, IBM® Micromedex®).

Case Study 3–3

A pharmacy student is on a clinical rotation and there is a patient who has overdosed on gabapentin. She is curious about the toxic effects of gabapentin.

- *Which resources would be useful for her project?*
- *What search terms might she utilize?*

Secondary Resources

❻ *Secondary resources provide access to primary (e.g., clinical trials) and some tertiary (e.g., narrative reviews) literature found in journals.* Practitioners can use secondary resources to stay abreast of recently published literature or to find published literature related to a specific topic. Indexing and abstracting are two common terms used when discussing secondary resources; the two terms differ slightly. **Indexing** consists of providing bibliographic citation information (e.g., title, author, citation of the article), while **abstracting** also includes a brief description (or abstract) of the information provided by the article or resource. There is a delay between article publication and indexing and abstracting within secondary databases; the delay may vary depending on the database. Published articles in the process of being indexed are often referred to as "in-process" citations. **❼** *Various secondary electronic resources index and abstract information from journals, meetings, publications, or other sources, differently; therefore, a practitioner should search various secondary resources in order to perform a comprehensive search.* Secondary resources also index and abstract different journals and publications based on their scope. For example, PsychINFO predominantly indexes and abstracts primary and tertiary resources focused on psychology-related topics and psychiatric illnesses and treatments. Practitioners should be sure to search multiple secondary resources to ensure all relevant information is captured.

A user will follow a similar strategy when searching most databases, with small changes to reflect differences in database systems. However, there are several challenges in searching secondary databases. Systems use different standardized terms when indexing articles, so users must determine what terms each database uses in order to conduct a successful search. For example, the disease commonly known as cystic fibrosis was indexed by one secondary database under the official term, fibrocystic disease of the pancreas. A practitioner searching for articles on cystic fibrosis might miss a number of pertinent references without reviewing the official **indexing terms** of that disease prior to searching. Therefore, it is important to recognize that different databases may require the use of different search terms.

Most computerized databases also include a free-text search option, which is useful when searches with index terms do not identify relevant articles. This option is also useful when a term is newly emerging or before an official index term is defined. Keep in mind that searches using only official index terms might exclude in-process citations relevant to the topic of interest.

The need to utilize a variety of terms when developing a search strategy is illustrated in the following sample question: "Is axicabtagene ciloleucel (Yescarta®) effective in the treatment of large B-cell lymphoma in adolescents?" It is first important to identify the key terms. These terms might include axicabtagene ciloleucel, large B-cell lymphoma, and adolescents. However, some databases may not recognize the term "adolescent," and instead use the term "pediatric" or "child." Additionally, the use of the term "pediatric" may refer to the medical specialty caring for pediatric patients, rather than treatment in the pediatric patient population. Therefore, users should verify the meaning of different search terms within each database when performing searches.

The NLM uses **Medical Subject Heading (MeSH)** indexing terms to ensure that searches retrieve the most appropriate content. MeSH terms are a set of specific medical words used when indexing articles in MEDLINE®. MeSH terms define or categorize a topic and automatically map certain words to a standardized indexing term. For example, when one enters the keywords "low blood sugar" using MeSH, the system will automatically map "low blood sugar" to hypoglycemia, instead of the words as three separate terms. This automatic mapping capability is helpful when a keyword can be interpreted in multiple ways, and searches may include irrelevant articles. For example, when one enters the keyword "cold" in the general search box, it will generate a large list of articles that interpreted the word as either temperature OR the illness (e.g., common cold). Searching for "cold" using the MeSH terminology allows users to include either temperature OR the illness in search results, instead of both. One additional point to bear in mind when performing electronic searches is that the same search phrase could be indexed under a variety of search terms or spellings. For example, if looking for information regarding the herbal product ginkgo, it may be helpful to search under the botanical name, common name(s), as well as common alternative spellings. Thus, a possible search strategy may be to use the terms "ginkgo," "ginkgo biloba," the Latin name "Ginkgoaceae," as well as the misspelled word "gingko." This same principle holds true when considering disease states whose names have changed over time. As databases and resources continue to modify search features, there are more Google-like search engines that allow for natural language searching.

In 2014, it was identified that the MeSH database only contained 26 pharmacy-specific terms, whereas other health professions, such as nursing and dentistry, had 94 and 145 specific terms, respectively.[126] Additionally, pharmacy terms were broader compared to those for the other disciplines. As the MeSH thesaurus is used to index and catalogue articles, the lack of appropriate pharmacy-specific MeSH terms and granularity could result in inaccurate or incorrect indexing. This could impact the completeness of literature retrieval for pharmacy-related searches. As a result, 16 additional pharmacy-specific MeSH terms were submitted to the U.S. NLM for consideration. In its 2017 annual MeSH Headings update, the NLM added two of these proposed terms ("Faculty, Pharmacy" and "Pharmacy Research"), and a new third term ("Nuclear Pharmacy").[127] The NLM recommended that other proposed pharmacy-specific MeSH terms could be created by combining already existing terms (e.g., "Pharmacy" and "Informatics"). Seven additional pharmacy-related terms were added with the 2019 New MeSH Heading release.[128] When conducting primary literature searches involving pharmacy topics, one must keep in mind that the MeSH database lacks standardized pharmacy-specific terminology, which could result in inconsistencies with indexing. If desired MeSH terms cannot be located, one should attempt to combine already existing MeSH terms and/or search by keywords so all related literature is captured.

Electronic searches generally use the Boolean operators AND, OR, and NOT (see Figure 3-1) to combine search terms, although natural language searching is becoming more available, as is seen in a typical Google search. The operator AND will combine two terms, returning only citations containing both of those concepts or terms. Most databases will automatically combine terms using AND if a term is not specified in the search. Combining two terms with the operator OR will result in an equal or greater number of returns since it will include any citation where either term is used. Use NOT with caution; it will always decrease the number of returns since it eliminates any references with that term. It may eliminate relevant articles simply because the term appears somewhere in the article.

For example, in the axicabtagene ciloleucel example earlier, the appropriate search terms (axicabtagene ciloleucel AND diffuse large B-cell lymphoma) may be used with the AND operator. However, if the requestor wanted information regarding use of either axicabtagene ciloleucel or tisagenlecleucel (Kymriah®) in this disease state, then OR might be used. See Figure 3-2 for a graphic presentation of this search. A search using OR will return a number of results equal to or greater than a search using AND. OR might also be useful when searching for a term with synonyms, for example, plasmablastic lymphoma OR diffuse large B-cell lymphoma. The operator NOT would be helpful if a user wants to exclude certain topics, for example, a specific disease state. In this case, a search might be performed for large B-cell lymphoma NOT acute lymphoblastic leukemia. Since the use of the term "NOT" will exclude any article mentioning acute lymphoblastic leukemia, an article focused on treatment of large-B-cell lymphoma with a small section about acute lymphoblastic leukemia would also be excluded. Parentheses can also be used to further streamline a search. In this example, a search may be performed for axicabtagene ciloleucel AND (plasmablastic lymphoma OR diffuse large B-cell lymphoma). This

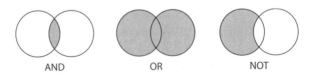

AND   OR   NOT

Figure 3–1. Boolean operators.

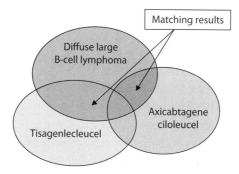

Figure 3–2. Diffuse large B-cell lymphoma AND (tisagenlecleucel OR axicabtagene ciloleucel).

would retrieve articles that contain the drug of interest as well as either of the two disease-related MeSH terms of interest. Of note, grouping terms together with parenthesis anytime OR or NOT is used in searches with three or more terms can be particularly important. The search will produce different results based on the grouping of terms and the placement of the operators. An additional example of search strategy using Boolean operators is provided in Appendix 3–1.

Some databases will also use the terms "WITH" or "NEAR." These operators are similar to AND; however, they require the terms to be within a set number of words of each other. These terms may be useful when other searches are identifying a large number of articles where both terms are mentioned, but not in conjunction with each other.

Most databases allow results to be restricted via use of limits or filters. For example, this may include language of publication, year of publication, type of article (e.g., human study, review, case report, randomized, clinical trial), or type of journal where a publication is found. Additional limits are available in certain databases. Limits are most helpful when the initial search terms return a large number of possible matches. However, using too many limits with the initial search may eliminate pertinent articles or citations. Keep in mind that the way articles were originally indexed also affects how easily limits or filters can be applied. Filters or limits may be misapplied by either the practitioner or the person who originally indexed the article within the database.

Listed below are some examples of secondary databases and types of literature that they index. Detailed information about PubMed® (https://pubmed.ncbi.nlm.nih.gov/) is found in Appendix 3-1.

BIOSIS Previews

Clarivate Analytics, https://clarivate.com/webofsciencegroup/solutions/webofscience-biosis-previews/. This is a comprehensive database of biological and biomedical information. BIOSIS also covers abstracts from conferences relating to basic sciences. This is most helpful when seeking more basic science information about activity of compounds on a cellular level.

ClinicalKey®

Elsevier, https://www.elsevier.com/solutions/clinicalkey. ClinicalKey® is a clinical search engine available from Elsevier that features its full-text books and journals, abstracts indexed in MEDLINE®, images, videos, practice guidelines, and clinical trials. Searches can be refined by using filters, including by specialty, study type, and date. Its Clinical Overviews summarize the latest evidence-based information on various disease states, incorporating guidelines, diagnosis, treatment options, prognosis, prevention, and references. Drug information monographs about U.S. prescription drugs, herbal supplements, vitamins, nutrition, and OTC products contained within Clinical Pharmacology are powered by ClinicalKey®. ClinicalKey® also contains patient education handouts that can be customized in various languages and font sizes, and also allow addition of individual-tailored information or instructions. New information is indexed daily. It is also available as an app, ClinicalKey® Mobile. Both the database and application require paid subscriptions.

Cochrane Library

John Wiley & Sons, Inc., https://www.cochranelibrary.com/. This database is comprised of three individual databases: the Cochrane Database of Systematic Reviews (CDSR), the Cochrane Central Register of Controlled Trials (CENTRAL), and Cochrane Clinical Answers (CCAs). All are searchable within the same library. The CDSR contains systematic reviews (i.e., Cochrane Reviews, Systematic Reviews from Epistemonikos), editorials, and supplements prepared by the Cochrane Review Group. The evidence-based reviews are based on extensive analysis of current literature (see Chapter 8 on evidence-based medicine). The CENTRAL database contains abstracts of controlled trials mainly from PubMed®, Embase®, ClinicalTrials.gov, and the World Health Organization's International Clinical Trials Registry Platform. It is published monthly. The CCAs are short summaries of Cochrane Reviews. Their purpose is to help practitioners make point-of-care clinical decisions. They are written in a user-friendly, question-and-answer format.

Cumulative Index to Nursing and Allied Health Literature (CINAHL)

EBSCO, https://www.ebsco.com/products/research-databases/cinahl-complete. This is an indexing service that covers thousands of journals primarily in the fields of nursing and allied health. It is useful when seeking information about patient care from the perspective of allied health professionals. It is updated monthly and contains full text of many articles. This database does not use a specific vocabulary for indexing terms, and searches are conducted with user-defined keywords.

Current Contents Connect

Clarivate Analytics, https://clarivate.com/webofsciencegroup/solutions/webofscience-current-contents-connect/. This electronic service is updated daily and offers an overview of very recently published literature as it relates to scientific information. There are multiple content editions to which users can subscribe, including Clinical Medicine and Life Sciences subgroups which are likely the most useful for health care practitioners, and focus on useful information about recent drug research or developments.

Embase®

Elsevier, https://www.embase.com. Embase® is a comprehensive abstracting service covering biomedical literature worldwide. Embase® is comprised of three databases: Embase® Classic (1947–1973), Embase® (1974–present), and MEDLINE®. It contains greater coverage of international publications, and there is less lag time between publication and inclusion (indexing) than in other secondary databases. It is useful when seeking information about conference abstracts, medical devices, dietary supplements, or medications available in other countries. Users can also search for literature based on the PICO (patients, intervention, comparator, and outcome) elements (see Chapter 8 for more information regarding PICO). Articles in Embase® are indexed using a standardized database of terms referred to as **Emtree terms**. Elsevier created the Emtree database based on the MeSH database, but modified terms to be more intuitive for those performing searches. This database is available through subscription only.

Google Scholar

Google, https://scholar.google.com. Google Scholar is a free Internet search engine designed to retrieve scholarly materials available online, in a variety of professional areas including health care. It contains all the articles indexed in MEDLINE®, plus additional scholarly journal articles and publications. Google Scholar is different from Google because it provides only scholarly publications. Because of its powerful keyword search capability, it is useful when searches in other secondary resources have been unsuccessful. Some articles that are unavailable in full text in other secondary databases are available via Google Scholar. Search results via Google Scholar are listed by how many times a particular article was cited by other publications, whether scholarly or not. This can be troublesome when looking for recently published articles on a particular topic. It also allows connections to article retrieval systems, such as OhioLINK (https://www.ohiolink.edu/).

International Pharmaceutical Abstracts (IPA)

Clarivate Analytics, https://clarivate.com. Access to the database is available through a number of third-party vendors (e.g., EBSCOhost, OVID, ProQuest). Coverage dates back to 1970 and includes drug-related information, including drug use and development. This database also abstracts a variety of meeting presentations. The name of this database is a misnomer as it contains many full-text articles. The main focus of this database is pharmacy information, including pharmacy administration, clinical services, and compounding or stability information, making it the most comprehensive global database for pharmacy-specific information. This database does not use a specific vocabulary for indexing terms, and searches are conducted with user-defined keywords.

Journal Watch®

Massachusetts Medical Society, https://www.jwatch.org. Journal Watch® is an abstracting service associated with the New England Journal of Medicine. It includes recent information, summarized by physicians, from a variety of medical literature. A general newsletter covering major medical stories and additional newsletters in specific specialty areas are published. This is most helpful when monitoring for new clinical trials involving specific medications.

MEDLINE®

NLM, https://www.nlm.nih.gov. MEDLINE® is part of the NLM PubMed® program. MEDLINE® includes more than 5200 medical journals in 40 different languages. Coverage includes basic and clinical sciences as well as nursing, dentistry, veterinary medicine, and many other health care disciplines. A number of online secondary databases index journal articles from the MEDLINE® database (e.g., Embase®, Google Scholar, PubMed®). MEDLINE® is the main component of PubMed® (https://pubmed.ncbi.nlm.nih.gov/), although PubMed® also contains citations from other life science and biomedical journals not contained in MEDLINE®. PubMed is maintained by the NLM and access is free. Google Scholar access is also free, whereas other databases providing access to MEDLINE® are maintained by private companies and are associated with a subscription fee. As mentioned in the Secondary Resources introduction, articles in MEDLINE® are indexed using the standardize MeSH database of terms. A sample search is provided in Appendix 3–1.

Nexis Uni™

LexisNexis Academic & Library Solutions, https://www.lexisnexis.com. This indexing and abstracting service provides coverage of a variety of types of information, including medical, legal, and business news. Some publications are available book through this service. This resource is helpful when attempting to locate information about recent medical news or research.

Trip Database

Trip Database Ltd., http://www.tripdatabase.com. The Trip (Turning Research Into Practice) database provides advertisement-free, unbiased search results using the online searching capabilities through millions of articles. Users can search for literature based on the PICO format or an advanced search. Its search results are listed by evidence type (e.g., clinical trials, guidelines, systematic reviews) and include many guidelines sorted by the country of publication. It is one of the most comprehensive and evidence-based resources for retrieving medical literature. It is available free online.

Case Study 3–4

A physician requests information about the use of fludarabine and busulfan prior to hematopoietic stem cell transplant. She wants to know if there are data supporting this regimen in this setting.

- *What resources might be good places to look for this information?*
- *What search terms should be used?*
- *Should limits be utilized?*

Primary Resources

Primary literature includes clinical research studies and reports, both published and unpublished. Not all literature published in a journal is classified as primary literature; for example, review articles or editorials are not primary literature. There are several types of publications considered primary, including controlled trials, cohort studies, case series, case reports, and meta-analyses. Although meta-analyses are classified here as primary resources, some classify them as secondary or tertiary resources. We classify them here as primary resources since they provide new quantitative data analyses regarding clinical questions. Additional information about study designs commonly found in medical literature (including differences between narrative reviews, systematic reviews, and meta-analyses) and how to evaluate them is found in Chapters 4 and 5.

There are several advantages to using primary literature as a resource. Primary literature gives practitioners access to detailed information on specific interventions in various patient populations. Practitioners evaluate the original literature on a topic and assess the validity and applicability of study results. Therefore, practitioners must develop strong medical literature evaluation skills to effectively use primary literature as resources in practice (discussed in Chapters 4 and 5). In general, primary literature acts as a supplement to research when tertiary resources provide insufficient information. There are, also, some disadvantages to the primary literature. Using primary literature alone can be difficult due to the difficulty in performing a search to identify appropriate articles and the time needed to evaluate the potentially large volume of available articles. Also, practitioners may draw misleading conclusions if only certain trials are evaluated without the context of other research (i.e., without a comprehensive search and literature evaluation).

It is also difficult to determine which journals are most essential to pharmacy practice due to the rapidly increasing number of specialty journals being published. Appendix 3–2 provides a listing of selected core holdings for a college of pharmacy, and several commonly mentioned journals in medicine. While this list may be more extensive than what is required in most practice settings, it does provide a core listing of journals. Each practice setting requires slightly different primary literature based on the specific areas that are of greatest importance to that facility, and the patients cared for in that location.

OBTAINING THE PRIMARY RESOURCES

Once literature has been identified in a secondary searching database, practitioners can obtain the full-text articles in various ways. Many electronic secondary resources link users directly to the article of interest. For example, PubMed® links users to open-access journal publications and articles of NIH-funded research through PubMed® Central (https://www.ncbi.nlm.nih.gov/pmc/). Some resources, such as Google Scholar, may link into other article retrieval systems, such as OhioLINK (https://www.ohiolink.edu/).

Many articles are not available via open-access routes; in those cases, alternative techniques may be needed. Once a citation is identified, utilizing a local library catalog is a good next step. Often a local library may carry the journal needed or may be affiliated with other facilities that can provide that article. Articles are often available for a fee via the publisher website.

Case Study 3–5

A physician is seeking information about the use of cannabidiol (CBD) in the management of pain. He sees a large number of patients in his practice and is seeking information about efficacy, safety, and appropriate dosing of this product.

- *What are the advantages and disadvantages of tertiary resources in responding to this request?*
- *What are the advantages and disadvantages of primary literature in this scenario?*

Alternative Resources

INTERNET SEARCHES

At times, even well-designed searches of standard medical literature do not yield sufficient information to make clinical decisions or recommendations. In these cases, practitioners may need to use alternative resources. One method of identifying relevant resources might be a general Internet search for information. This can be useful as a starting point for questions about uncommon diseases, unfamiliar terms, drugs in development, or marketed OTC products and combination dietary supplements. For example, natural products may contain multiple herbal or vitamin supplements in combination. If a requestor asks about the use of a herbal supplement called Usana Hepasil DTX™ in cirrhosis, it would be difficult to search for information unless the requestor was able to provide a full list of product ingredients. Requestors may not have that information; therefore, it may be necessary to search for a manufacturer website to identify the specific product ingredients, and to look for information on the individual components. An Internet search is also helpful in identifying information or specific product claims provided by the manufacturer. Internet searches may be useful to find information on topics recently in the news, where information is changing more rapidly than standard paper resources can be updated.

It is important to remember that different search engines use different techniques to identify webpages, and that no search engine identifies all websites. Some search engines are geared toward scholarly content (e.g., Google Scholar, https://scholar.google.com) or scientific research, rather than general information. In order to efficiently perform a search, practitioners should consider which search engine would most likely index the desired material.

There are several caveats to finding information on the Internet. The first is to carefully evaluate the quality of all information provided. There are millions of websites, and there are no true quality assurance measures in place to ensure the reliability of information. ❽ *Drug or health information retrieved from Internet-based or online media needs to be evaluated for accuracy, comprehensiveness, and mode of maintenance (e.g., recent updates, qualifications of those performing updates).* There are some general tenets to keep in mind when evaluating this type of literature. Generally, sites maintained by educational institutions, not-for-profit medical organizations, or a division of the U.S. government are more likely to contain high-quality information, whereas information maintained by a company selling or promoting a specific product may be more questionable. Some websites are maintained by individuals or organizations with questionable viewpoints.

In order to assess the quality of online information, several standards and programs now exist. These include organizations such as the Health on the Net

(HON code, https://www.hon.ch), which clearly defines standards to evaluate the quality of information available via a website. These organizations do not evaluate every website available; a website must request an evaluation. Many websites do not request an evaluation; therefore, the lack of a quality seal does not necessarily indicate that the information is of low quality.

Practitioners should use the following criteria when determining the quality of online material:

- Is the source credible, without a vested interest in promoting one particular treatment or product?
- Is the information accurate and current?
- Does the site link to other nonaffiliated sites that provide consistently good information?
- Is the information appropriately detailed and referenced?
- Is it possible to identify the author of the site to contact with additional questions or comments?

Information on evaluating health-related content on websites is discussed further in Chapter 5. In addition, the NLM posted a video and frequently asked questions to help determine high-quality sites (https://medlineplus.gov/evaluatinghealthinformation.html).

OTHER INFORMATION SOURCES

Occasionally, sufficient information to address a DI request cannot be obtained from standard resources and may require the use of alternative sources. If a question involves, for example, a recent news story reporting the removal of a medication from the market, a logical first place to find initial information would be to identify the original news story. This can be done by searching various newswire services such as PR Newswire, major news network websites such as CNN, or even general Internet search engines (Table 3-3). LexisNexis™, https://www.lexisnexis.com, indexes a variety of newswire stories as well as transcripts of news reports. While this news story may not provide all the information needed, it can serve as a starting point for researching additional information. LexisNexis™ requires a paid subscription.

In some cases, there may be such limited information available that it would be wise to seek out an expert in the field, for example, for a question about the use of heparin in a troche dosage form. In these cases, it may be prudent to contact persons performing research in this area or practitioners who are currently using that therapy. These experts may help identify unpublished information or resources missed during an initial search. Practitioners can identify experts via specialized medical organizations, leadership of medical societies, or by identifying persons who have authored numerous papers on a specific medication or medical condition.

TABLE 3–3. MAJOR ONLINE NEWS SOURCES

News source	Website address
ABC News	www.abcnews.go.com
The Associated Press	www.ap.org
BBC	www.bbc.com
Bloomberg	www.bloomberg.com
CBS News	www.cbsnews.com
The Chicago Tribune	www.chicagotribune.com
CNN	www.cnn.com
The Economist	www.economist.com
Fox News	www.foxnews.com
The Guardian	www.theguardian.com/us
Google News	https://news.google.com/
MSNBC	www.msnbc.com
NBC News	www.nbcnews.com
The New York Times	www.nytimes.com
NPR	www.npr.org
PBS	www.pbs.org
Pink Sheet	https://pink.pharmaintelligence.informa.com
PR Newswire	https://pr.prnewswire.com/prnewswire
Reuters	www.reuters.com
The Wall Street Journal	www.wsj.com
The Washington Post	www.washingtonpost.com
USA Today	www.usatoday.com
Yahoo News	www.yahoo.com/news/

Note: These resources are subject to bias in selection of content presented and in how information is presented. Some are available for free, while some require a paid subscription.

When looking for recent recommendations regarding treatment of a specific disease state, it may be helpful to identify an organization affiliated with that disease. For example, when looking for treatment recommendations for management of irritable bowel syndrome it might be appropriate to contact the International Foundation for Functional Gastrointestinal Disorders (https://www.iffgd.org/), the American Gastroenterological Association (https://gastro.org/guidelines), or the American College of Gastroenterology (https://gi.org/guidelines/) to obtain information about current practice standards, as well as possible emerging therapies.

When seeking information about a specific drug therapy, it may be helpful to contact the product manufacturer via their medical information department. A manufacturer may have unpublished data on file that it is willing to share. This resource could be especially helpful for obtaining difficult-to-access literature, temperature excursion data, product access and availability information, or for identifying a possible rare adverse drug reaction.

Finally, experts in the field can also be useful alternative resources. They may have insight into clinical information or data that have not yet been published, or that were recently presented at a national meeting.

Case Study 3–6

A patient tells you she saw a news story that said all patients should stop taking their Xarelto® and switch to the "new Xarelto®." She tells you she is not planning to take it anymore and wants the physician to find a different medication. She is indignant that you as a health care professional did not know this was going on.

- *Where might you find a copy of the news story that this patient saw to help her better understand what the news reporter was trying to convey?*

Consumer Health Information

Consumers may also benefit from some free online resources they can search and access from home or through a personal mobile device, or text and online resources available through a local library. Some resources are published by organizations that produce references for health care professionals, while lay press companies publish others. There is great variation in the quality of information provided from resource to resource. In addition, some of the most popular resources may not be written at an appropriate level for a consumer to understand or may not provide helpful information for the patient. For this reason, it is important to discuss with patients what other resources they are using to find additional drug and medical information. Opening a dialogue with patients about this topic is fairly simple and can consist of open-ended questions such as "Where else have you found information on your disease state?" or "What other material have you read about your medication/disease state?"

If being asked to recommend a source of online information for a patient, one can confidently recommend health care organizations (e.g., Mayo Clinic or Cleveland Clinic Health Library) or disease or professional societies (e.g., American Diabetes Association or American Academy of Pediatrics), all of which usually provide helpful, high-quality disease-specific and health information geared for the average consumer. The NLM also publishes information for patients and consumers about using online health resources appropriately. For example, MedlinePlus (https://medlineplus.gov/evaluatinghealthinformation.html) provides guidance on how to locate reliable online health information and how to evaluate and understand online resources and provided information. The National Institutes of Health also published via several of its offices information regarding how to find and evaluate online resources. One example of this is from the National Center for Complementary and Integrative Health (https://nccih.nih.gov/health/webresources).

In addition to these resources aimed at consumers, there are consumer-specific sections of many tertiary resources discussed earlier. Electronic resources such as IBM® Micromedex®, Lexicomp®, Facts & Comparisons® eAnswers, ASHP's SafeMedication.com, or Clinical Pharmacology online have subsections dedicated to consumer-level information available for a practitioner to print and provide to the patient. Of note, online resources such as Wikipedia and blogs are not appropriate and reliable sources for health-, medical-, or medication-related topics for consumers; they often lack scientific rigor and review for accuracy and comprehensiveness, and they may not be updated as new evidence-based information becomes available. In addition, information contained in such sources can be easily changed or manipulated by anyone who reads them.

Below is a brief explanation of some widely used and reliable free online resources specifically designed for patients and consumers.

Centers for Disease Control and Prevention (CDC)

The CDC (https://www.cdc.gov) is the frontline information site for any diseases of interest affecting a large patient population, such as infectious illnesses and other epidemics. The CDC website includes information about diseases, conditions, healthy living (e.g., obesity, tobacco use, food safety, immunizations), information for international travelers (e.g., diseases endemic to other countries, immunization recommendations when traveling outside of the U. S., and travel warnings based on outbreaks, natural disasters, or threats), and emergency preparedness. It has an "A-Z Index" for easy searching, and the website is also available in Spanish. Telephone numbers are provided that can offer language assistance services for 16 different languages, and patient information sheets for certain topics are available in 64 different languages.

ClinicalTrials.gov

This website (https://www.clinicaltrials.gov) is maintained by the NLM through the National Institutes of Health and serves as a main registry for publicly and privately supported clinical studies of human participants conducted in the world. Patients or family members can find clinical studies that are currently ongoing or studies that will be conducted in the future, and register patients as participants. Searches can be done by disease state, drug intervention, location, or study sponsor. The trial results are not always fully added and may require health care professionals to effectively search for them using secondary resources discussed above.

Food and Drug Administration

This website contains information for both consumers (https://www.fda.gov/consumers) and patients (https://www.fda.gov/patients). The consumer site provides very comprehensive health and safety information regarding drugs, medical devices, women's and minority health-related topics, and major recalls of drugs and food. It also provides information on veterinary medicine, vaccines, cosmetics, and tobacco products. The patient site provides drug and device approval information, information about expanded access, investigational new drugs, and off-label use of medications.

Myhealthfinder.gov

This website (https://health.gov/myhealthfinder) is hosted and maintained by the Office of Disease Prevention and Health Promotion within the U.S. Department of Health and Human Services. It contains health topics that may be relevant to any consumers, including nutrition and physical activity, pregnancy, parenting, healthy living tips, and directories for health care providers and services near consumers. It is also available in Spanish.

KidsHealth.org

This website (https://kidshealth.org) provides doctor-approved health information about children from before birth through adolescence. Created by The Nemours Foundation's Center for Children's Health Media, KidsHealth covers diverse topics including information specifically for kids, teens, parents, and educators.

MedlinePlus

Supported by reliable information generated from the NLM, this website (https://medlineplus.gov/) is a highly regarded information medium for consumers seeking health information. It includes information about wellness and health, diseases and disorders, medications, and dietary supplements. Additional features include videos about body systems and how diseases and conditions affect them, a medical encyclopedia, explanations of medical tests and why they are ordered, directories to locate health care providers near consumers, and information on clinical trials through ClinicalTrials.gov. Information is available in several different languages.

More resources to assist patients and consumers with questions related to medical information can be found in Table 3-4 and in Chapter 27.

Staying Current

The rate at which medical knowledge expands has been accelerating over the past several decades.[129] With such rapid expansion of medical and scientific knowledge, it is essential for practitioners to find efficient and effective ways to keep abreast of newly published literature. Practitioners can use various tools such as list servers, professional email subscriptions, and professional social media accounts to stay current.

List servers are an excellent medium for practitioners to post, read about, and comment on current issues within the profession. Practitioners can solicit advice from other institutions and gain valuable insight regarding current practice challenges. List servers are available through various professional organizations or even through group purchasing organizations. For example, a drug information list server is available through ASHP Connect (https://connect.ashp.org/). Practitioners can subscribe to list servers focused on specialized practice areas (e.g., ambulatory care, inpatient care, small and rural hospital care) and receive regular email updates with recent list server activity.

Many professional organizations curate relevant, newly published literature and medical news stories. Practitioners can subscribe and have literature and news compilations delivered directly to them via email. Receiving email summaries is less tedious and time-consuming than collecting publications and news stories individually. Useful pharmacy-specific subscriptions include APhA Pharmacy Today©, ASHP Daily Briefing©, and Pharmacy Learning Network©, but there are more general medical subscriptions as well (e.g., Monthly Prescribing Reference® [MPR], NEJM Catalyst©). There are also administrative-focused subscriptions for leadership and management (e.g., Becker's Hospital Review©, Advisory Board©). Practitioners can also subscribe to government websites for notifications on clinical or regulatory guidance updates (e.g., CDC's MMWR, FDA Guidance Documents, FDA MedWatch Alerts). Some organizations also pay for subscriptions to more comprehensive pharmacy and medical news resources (e.g., IPD Analytics©, Pink Sheet©).

Users can connect and interact with other experts via social media. They can network via nonpharmacy platforms (e.g., LinkedIn©, Twitter©), or via social media platforms created by professional organizations (e.g., AACP Connect©, APhA Engage©, ASHP Connect©). Practitioners can build a professional network and easily share health- or pharmacy-related literature and news. Once practitioners build a professional network,

TABLE 3–4. ONLINE CONSUMER INFORMATION SOURCES

Title	Author/Owner	Website	Features
Centers for Disease Control and Prevention	Centers for Disease Control and Prevention	https://www.cdc.gov	Contains information about the treatment and prevention of infectious diseases and epidemics, healthy living information, and information about travelers' health.
Complementary and Integrative Health	National Center for Complementary and Integrative Health	https://nccih.nih.gov	A government-maintained resource describing complementary alternatives (e.g., dietary supplements) to conventional medicine.
DailyMed	U.S. National Library of Medicine	https://dailymed.nlm.nih.gov/	Contains about 110,000 drug listings as submitted to the Food and Drug Administration. Includes drug information based on drug classes.
Dietary Supplements Fact Sheets	National Institute of Health Office of Dietary Supplements	https://ods.od.nih.gov/	Compiles accurate and current information about the efficacy and safety of dietary supplements including scientific facts.
FamilyDoctor.org	American Academy of Family Physicians	https://familydoctor.org/	Provides information on various topics related to disease prevention and wellness for all consumer age ranges.
Healthfinder.gov	National Health Information Center	https://www.healthfinder.gov/	Provides information on a variety of health topics, maintained by the Office of Disease Prevention and Health Promotion. Also provides information in Spanish.
HealthyChildren.org	American Academy of Pediatrics	https://www.healthychildren.org/	Provides unbiased, accurate information focused on pregnancy and children from newborn to young adults. Information is available also in Spanish.
Informedhealth.org	Institute for Quality and Efficiency in Health Care	https://www.informedhealth.org/	Established in Germany in 2004, provides independent and evidence-based health information that includes advantages and disadvantages of treatment options.
KidsHealth	The Nemours Foundation	https://kidshealth.org	Provides health information about children from before birth through adolescence for parents and educators.
Merck Manual Consumer Version	Merck	https://www.merckhomeedition.com	A consumer-based version of the Merck Manual. It includes a variety of medical topics and interactive features such as videos and self-assessment tools. It is also available in Spanish.

continued

TABLE 3–4. ONLINE CONSUMER INFORMATION SOURCES *(CONTINUED)*

Title	Author/Owner	Website	Features
MedlinePlus	U.S. National Library of Medicine	https://medlineplus.gov/	Contains information about wellness and health, diseases and disorders, medications, and dietary supplements.
Mental Health Information	National Institute of Mental Health	https://www.nimh.nih.gov/health/topics/index.shtml	Provides information regarding a variety of mental health topics, clinical trial information, educational resources, and contact information for assistance.
National Cancer Institute	National Cancer Institute/National Institutes of Health	https://www.cancer.gov/	Provides helpful and accurate information regarding cancer research, diagnoses, prevention, and treatment.
National Institute on Aging	National Institute on Aging/National Institute of Health	https://www.nia.nih.gov/	Contains reliable and current information on aging research and health and wellness for older adults.
NetWellness	University of Cincinnati, The Ohio State University, Case Western Reserve University	https://www.netwellness.org/	A global, community service providing quality, unbiased health information assembled by university faculty.
SafeMedication	American Society of Health-System Pharmacists	http://www.safemedication.com/	Provides a patient version of AHFS® Drug Information Resource, as well as tips about medication administration.
St. Jude Children's Research Hospital	St. Jude Children's Research Hospital	https://www.stjude.org/	Contains information about childhood cancers and other life-threatening disorders, including treatment options and ongoing clinical research.
U.S. Food and Drug Administration	U.S. Food and Drug Administration	https://www.fda.gov/consumers	Contains information about drugs, medical devices, vaccines, food, pet food, and cosmetics. Also includes information about recalls.
WebMD	WebMD	https://www.webmd.com/default.htm	Provides information on a variety of health topics and medications. Contains interactive videos and self-assessment tools.
Womenshealth.gov	Office on Women's Health, U.S. Department of Health and Human Services	https://www.womenshealth.gov/	Contains information about conditions and diseases of special interest to women, including drug use during pregnancy and lactation. Information is also available in Spanish.

they have access to newly published literature and news stories at their fingertips just by scrolling through a platform's news feed.

Reference Budget Considerations

As described throughout this chapter, there are numerous resources, both print and online, available to assist health care professionals with answering drug- and medical-related questions. Some of these resources are free of charge; however, many of them come with a cost, so there are factors to consider when deciding which references to have available in your personal library, or accessible to your department or to all health care providers within the institution. The patient population(s) served and medical specialties practiced at your institution should be considered when determining the types of resources to have available. Online versions of tertiary references are often preferred because they are updated more frequently than their printed counterparts, and they can be accessed by numerous users at once from various locations (though multiuser subscriptions are often significantly more expensive than single-user subscriptions). However, they can be costly. Many of these resources contain several databases and tools within, and also have add-on module options. In order to help contain costs, thoughtful consideration should be placed on which components of the resource are actually needed, will get used by practitioners, and don't overlap with other resource offerings that are already available at your site. Requesting a limited number of users, if possible, or negotiating health system-wide contracts may also help lower subscription costs. Regarding secondary resources, some databases provide access to citations and abstracts for free (e.g., PubMed® and Google Scholar), whereas others are associated with subscription fees (e.g., Embase® and IPA). PubMed® Central and Google Scholar also provide free access to select full-text articles. Again, the needs of the institution and patient population(s) seen will help determine which are most appropriate. Some primary literature articles are available for free via open-access journals; however, additional paid subscriptions will need to be obtained in order to successfully respond to all DI requests. Pricing will vary from journal to journal. For tertiary, secondary, and primary references it may be helpful to collaborate with your institution's medical library to avoid risk of having duplicate subscriptions and to share resource costs, if possible. In some cases, institutions may participate in a group to provide additional resources at a more reasonable price, such as OhioLINK (https://www.ohiolink.edu/) or the Utah Academic Library Consortium (https://ualc.net/). A listing of over two hundred such consortia can be found at the International Coalition of Library Consortia (https://icolc.net/). Available resources should be assessed annually to ensure that most up-to-date versions are obtained, and to ensure that they continue to meet the needs of the institution. This review will also provide an opportunity to identify resources that are infrequently used that could perhaps be removed from your armamentarium or replaced with something more useful.

Conclusion

Medical information is changing rapidly, and the amount of information is growing at a faster rate than health care professionals can keep pace in this digital technology era. More DI resources are becoming available online or via mobile access in addition to or replacing print versions. The information in this chapter helps provide guidance as to where specific types of DI might be found and how to begin a search for DI, targeting the tertiary and secondary resources.

Practitioners must not, however, be satisfied with merely identifying sources for DI. Understanding where to access information is only the first step in the provision of quality DI. Information must be interpreted and evaluated to become knowledge. It is this unique knowledge that will enable practitioners to optimize patient care. Therefore, health care professionals need to stay current and vigilant about the effective methods of retrieving and evaluating medical information for efficient patient care. The next several chapters will provide additional guidance on how to interpret and apply the information that is gathered.

As technological advances continue and more information becomes available regarding medications and their appropriate place in therapy, the need for pharmacists' expertise in DI will continue to grow. With the increased emphasis on interprofessional practice in all clinical settings, all health care professionals should develop skills in retrieving and interpreting medical literature to provide optimal patient care.

Self-Assessment Questions

1. A physician asks for a tertiary reference that discusses the results of a new drug's efficacy and safety in treating migraine headache. Which of the following is a tertiary resource in biomedical literature?
   a. A research article describing a clinical trial
   b. A review paper describing several clinical trials
   c. A case report of one patient's experience
   d. MEDLINE®

2. A pharmacy technician calls you with a patient-specific drug information request: "An elderly patient is asking if it is okay to take oxycodone, acetaminophen, omeprazole, and clonazepam together." Which of the following categories of drug information resources is most appropriate for an efficient search of references?

   a. Drug interaction
   b. Drug stability
   c. Adverse drug reaction
   d. Indication

3. A physician calls and asks "my patient takes cannabidiol (CBD) oil every day. Does that interact with his abiraterone and prednisone?" What would be the most appropriate DI reference to use for this question, given the product of interest?

   a. Handbook of Nonprescription Drugs
   b. Geriatric Dosage Handbook
   c. Natural Medicines
   d. The Harriet Lane Book

4. A nurse calls and asks, "can I administer ceftriaxone IV and Lactated Ringers solution together via y-site"?" What would be the most appropriate DI reference to answer this question?

   a. Merck Index
   b. AHFS® Drug Information
   c. Neofax
   d. ASHP Injectable Drug Information

5. A medical assistant in the travel clinic calls and asks about the recommended vaccines for a patient traveling to Indonesia. Which reference would contain information on recommended travel vaccines?

   a. DrugPoint
   b. The FDA website
   c. Lexi-Drugs™
   d. CDC's Yellow Book

6. Which of the following is a secondary resource that can assist in finding original research papers?

   a. Lexi-Drugs™
   b. IBM® Micromedex®
   c. PubMed®
   d. DailyMed

7. A patient walks up to your pharmacy counter and asks "My doctor told me to take over-the-counter Prilosec®. How much should I take?" Which of the following is the most appropriate tertiary resource for this question?
   a. Handbook of Nonprescription Drugs
   b. USP-NF
   c. Natural Medicines
   d. The Merck Manual

8. A nurse practitioner calls your drug information center to ask if ranitidine can affect platelet counts. Which of the following is the most appropriate tertiary resource for this question?
   a. Stockley's Drug Interactions
   b. PubMed®
   c. Red Book
   d. Meyler's Side Effects of Drugs

9. Which of the following electronic databases would provide the largest international biomedical journal coverage?
   a. EMBASE®
   b. MEDLINE®
   c. International Pharmaceutical Abstracts
   d. PsychINFO

10. A pregnant woman is concerned about potential adverse effects of her current medication to her baby. She is currently taking fexofenadine and sertraline. Which of the following is the most appropriate resource to determine if the medications are potentially harmful to the fetus?
    a. Briggs Drugs in Pregnancy and Lactation
    b. Meyler's Side Effects of Drugs
    c. Remington: The Science and Practice of Pharmacy
    d. POISINDEX®

11. When evaluating the quality of tertiary biomedical resources, which of the following is **NOT** an appropriate question to consider?
    a. Is the information likely to be timely based on publication date?
    b. Are there enough photos and animations to assist in understanding?
    c. Is information supported by appropriate citations?
    d. Does the resource appear free from bias and blatant errors?

12. A patient was admitted to your emergency department (ED) with chest pain while visiting his daughter in the United States. He brought with him a few medications from his home country and your ED team is to trying to find similar therapy here. Which of the following resources would be most appropriate to help the ED team?
    a. Clin-Alert®
    b. The Harriet Lane Handbook
    c. Martindale: The Complete Drug Reference
    d. Lexi-Drugs™

13. Miss Jones calls the pharmacy to say that she accidently threw away the step-by-step administration instructions that came with her albuterol inhaler and wonders if they are available online. Which consumer-focused resource contains administration instructions for several different formulations of medications?
    a. REPROTOX
    b. Wikipedia
    c. Healthfinder.gov
    d. SafeMedication.com

14. Which of the following is true when considering drug information (DI) resources for mobile devices?
    a. Current standards and regulations on mobile applications for DI are not adequate.
    b. Mobile application versions of DI database are identical to their online databases.
    c. Health care providers rarely use mobile devices for retrieving DI.
    d. There are too few mobile applications available to use.

15. Which of the following is a benefit of using tertiary resources?
    a. They are quickly outdated.
    b. They provide a comprehensive and quick overview of a topic.
    c. Their contents are filtered by other experts and therefore are not biased.
    d. They are typically shorter than primary resources.

REFERENCES

1. Johnson R, Watkinson A, Mabe M. The STM report: an overview of scientific and scholarly journal publishing [Internet]. The Netherlands: International Association of Scientific, Technical and Medical Publishers; 2018 Oct [cited 2019 Aug 18]; [about 214 p.]. Available from: https://www.stm-assoc.org/2018_10_04_STM_Report_2018.pdf.
2. MEDLINE PubMed Production Statistics [Internet]. Bethesda (MD): U.S. National Library of Medicine; 2018 [cited 2019 Aug 18]. Available from: https://www.nlm.nih.gov/bsd/medline_pubmed_production_stats.html.

3. Aungst TD. Medical applications for pharmacists using mobile devices. Ann Pharmacother. 2013;47(7-8):1088-95. Referenced in PubMed PMID: 23821609.

4. Aungst TD, Clauson KA, Misra S, Lewis TL, Husain I. How to identify, assess and utilise mobile medical applications in clinical practice. Int J Clin Pract. 2014;68(2):155-62. Referenced in PubMed PMID: 24460614.

5. Pew Research Center. Internet/Broadband fact sheet [Internet].Washington (DC): Pew Research Center; [updated 2019 Jun 12; cited 2019 Aug 18]. Available from: https://www.pewinternet.org/fact-sheet/internet-broadband/.

6. Safavi K, Kalis B. Accenture 2018 consumer survey on digital health [Internet]. Arlington (VA): Accenture; 2018 Mar 6 [cited 2019 Aug 18]. Available from: https://www.accenture.com/t20180306t103559z__w__/us-en/_acnmedia/pdf-71/accenture-health-2018-consumer-survey-digital-health.pdf.

7. U.S. Food and Drug Administration. Mobile medical applications [Internet]. Silver Spring (MD): The U.S. Food and Drug Administration; [updated 2018 Sep 4; cited 2019 Aug 18]. Available from: https://www.fda.gov/medical-devices/digital-health/mobile-medical-applications.

8. AHFS Drug Information® 2019. Bethesda (MD): American Society of Health-System Pharmacists (ASHP); 2019.

9. Clinical pharmacology [Internet]. Tampa (FL): Gold Standard, Inc.; 2019 [cited 2019 Aug 30]. Available from: http://www.clinicalpharmacology.com.

10. DRUGDEX® [Internet]. IBM Watson Health, Greenwood Village, Colorado, USA; 2019 [cited 2019 Jul 5]. Available from: https://www.micromedexsolutions.com/.

11. Facts & Comparisons® eAnswers [Internet]. St. Louis (MO): Wolters Kluwer Health; 2019 [cited 2019 Jul 5]. Available from: http://online.factsandcomparisons.com.

12. Lexicomp® Lexi-Drugs [Internet]. St. Louis (MO): Wolters Kluwer Health; 2019 [cited 2019 Jul 5]. Available from: http://online.lexi.com.

13. Brayfield A. Martindale: the complete drug reference. 39th ed. East Smithfield (London, UK): Pharmaceutical Press; 2017.

14. Prescribers' Digital Reference [Internet]. Whippany (NJ): PDR, LLC; 2019 [cited 2019 Jul 5]. Available from: https://www.pdr.net/.

15. Clin-Alert®. Thousand Oaks (CA): SAGE Publishing; 2019 [cited 2019 Aug 30]. Available from: https://journals.sagepub.com/home/CLA.

16. Tisdale JE, Miller DA. Drug-induced diseases: prevention, detection, and management. 3rd ed. Bethesda (MD): American Society of Health-System Pharmacists; 2018.

17. Aronson JK. Meyler's side effects of drugs: the international encyclopedia of adverse drug reactions and interactions. 16th ed. Amsterdam: Elsevier; 2015.

18. Ray SD. Side effects of drugs Annual 41: a worldwide yearly survey of new data and trends in adverse drug reactions. 41st ed. Amsterdam: Elsevier; 2019.

19. Reactions Weekly. London (UK): Springer Nature; 2019 [cited 2019 Aug 30]. Available from: https://www.springer.com/journal/40278.

20. FDAble [Internet]. Silver Spring (MD): The U.S. Food and Drug Administration; 2019 [cited 2019 Aug 18]. Available from: http://www.fdable.com.

21. ISMP Medication Safety Alert!® Acute Care Newsletter. Horsham (PA): Institute for Safe Medication Practices (ISMP); 2020 [cited 2020 Mar 29]. Available from: https://www.ismp.org/newsletters/acute-care.

22. Gahart BL, Nazareno AR, Ortega MQ. Gahart's 2020 intravenous medications: a handbook for nurses and health professionals. 36th ed. St. Louis (MO): Elsevier (Mosby); 2019.

23. ASHP injectable drug information. 2021 ed. Bethesda (MD): American Society of Health-System Pharmacists; 2021.

24. King JC, Catania PN. King guide to parenteral admixtures. King Guide Publications; 1971-2019 [cited 2019 Aug 30]. Available from: https://www.kingguide.com.

25. Trissel's™ 2 Clinical Pharmaceutics Database [Internet]. St. Louis (MO): Wolters Kluwer Health; 2019 [cited 2019 Aug 31]. Available from: https://www.wolterskluwercdi.com/drug-reference/apps/iv-compatibility/.

26. Bing CD, Nowobilski-Vasilios A. Extended stability for parenteral drugs. 6th ed. Bethesda (MD): American Society of Health-System Pharmacists; 2017.

27. Trissel LA, Ashworth LD. Trissel's stability of compounded formulations. 6th ed. Washington (DC): American Pharmacists Association; 2018.

28. Allen LV, Adejare A, Desselle SP, Felton LA. Remington: the science and practice of pharmacy. 22nd ed. Philadelphia: Lippincott Williams & Wilkins; 2012.

29. USP 42–NF 37: the official compendia of standards. Rockville (MD): The United States Pharmacopeial Convention; 2019.

30. Phelps JP, Hagemann TM, Lee KR, Thompson AJ. Pediatric injectable drugs: the teddy bear book. 11th ed. Bethesda (MD): American Society of Health-System Pharmacists; 2018.

31. White R, Bradnam V. Handbook of drug administration via enteral feeding tubes. 3rd ed. East Smithfield (London, UK): Pharmaceutical Press; 2015.

32. O'Neil MJ. Merck Index: an encyclopedia of chemicals, drugs and biologicals. 15th ed. Whitehouse Station (NJ): Royal Society of Chemistry; 2013.

33. Thompson JE, Davidow LW. A practical guide to contemporary pharmacy practice. 3rd ed. Philadelphia (PA): Lippincott Williams & Wilkins; 2009.

34. Jew RK, Soo-Hoo W, Erush SC, Amiri E. Extemporaneous formulations for pediatric, geriatric, and special needs patients. 3rd ed. Bethesda (MD): American Society of Health-System Pharmacists; 2016.

35. Nahata MC, Vinita BP. Pediatric drug formulations. 7th ed. Cincinnati (OH): Harvey Whitney Books; 2019.

36. Natural Medicines [Internet]. Stockton (CA): Therapeutic Research Faculty; 2019 [cited 2019 Aug 18]. Available from: https://naturalmedicines.therapeuticresearch.com.

37. Dietary Supplement Label Database [Internet]. Bethesda (MD): National Institutes of Health Office of Dietary Supplements and the U.S. National Library of Medicine; 2019 [updated 2019; cited 2019 Aug 18]. Available from: https://www.dsld.nlm.nih.gov.

38. MedlinePlus [Internet]. Bethesda (MD): U.S. National Library of Medicine; 2019 [updated 2019; cited 2019 Aug 30]. Available from: https://medlineplus.gov/.

39. Natural Products Database [Internet]. St. Louis (MO): Wolters Kluwer Health; 2019 [cited 2019 Jul 5]. Available from: http://online.factsandcomparisons.com.

40. U.S. Food and Drug Administration [Internet]. Silver Spring (MD): U.S. Food and Drug Administration; 2019 [cited 2019 Aug 18]. Available from: https://www.fda.gov/.

41. DiPiro JT, Talbert RL, Yee GC, Matzke GR, Wells BG, Posey LM. Pharmacotherapy: a pathophysiologic approach. 10th ed. New York: McGraw-Hill; 2016.

42. Chisholm-Burns MA, Schwinghammer TL, Malone PM, Kolesar JM, Lee KC, Bookstaver PB. Pharmacotherapy principles and practice. 5th ed. New York: McGraw-Hill; 2019.

43. Zeind CS, Carvalho MG. Applied therapeutics: the clinical use of drugs. 11th ed. Philadelphia (PA): Lippincott Williams & Wilkins; 2017.

44. Porter RS. The Merck manual of diagnosis and therapy. 20th ed. Whitehouse Station (NJ): Merck Research Laboratories; 2018.

45. Jameson JL, Fauci AS, Kasper DL, Hauser SL, Longo DL, Loscalzo J. Harrison's principles of internal medicine. 20th ed. New York: McGraw-Hill; 2018.

46. Goldman L, Schafer AI. Goldman-Cecil medicine. 25th ed. Philadelphia (PA): Saunders Elsevier; 2015.

47. Helms RA, Quan DJ. Textbook of therapeutics: drug and disease management. 8th ed. Philadelphia (PA): Lippincott Williams & Wilkins; 2006.

48. Kellerman RD, Rakel D. Conn's current therapy 2019. Philadelphia (PA): Saunders Elsevier; 2019.

49. Medscape [Internet]. New York: WebMD®, LLC.; 2019 [cited 2019 Aug 18]. Available from: http://www.medscape.com.

50. DynaMed® [Internet]. Ipswich (MA): EBSCO Health; 2020 [cited 2020 Mar 29]. Available from: https://www.dynamed.com/.

51. UpToDate® [Internet]. St. Louis (MO): Wolters Kluwer Health; 2020 [cited 2020 Mar 29]. Available from: https://www.uptodate.com/home.

52. Red Book Online [Internet]. Armonk (NY): IBM Watson Health; 2019 [cited 2019 Aug 18]. Available from: https://www.ibm.com/us-en/marketplace/micromedex-red-book.

53. Medi-Span [Internet]. St. Louis (MO): Wolters Kluwer Health; 2019 [cited 2019 Aug 30]. Available from: http://www.wolterskluwercdi.com/medispan-clinical/.

54. U.S. Food and Drug Administration. FDA Drug Shortages [Internet]. Silver Spring (MD): U.S. Food and Drug Administration; 2019 [cited 2019 Aug 29]. Available from: https://www.accessdata.fda.gov/scripts/drugshortages/default.cfm.

55. University of Utah Drug Information Service. Current Drug Shortages [Internet]. Silver Spring (MD): American Society of Health-System Pharmacists; 2019 [cited 2019 Aug 29]. Available from: https://www.ashp.org/drug-shortages/current-shortages.

56. IBM Micromedex® Identidex® [Internet]. IBM Watson Health, Greenwood Village, Colorado, USA; 2019 [cited 2019 Jul 5]. Available from: https://www.micromedexsolutions.com/.

57. Drugs.com [Internet]. Dallas (TX): Drugsite Trust; 2019 [cited 2019 Aug 30]. Available from: https://www.drugs.com/.

58. Lexicomp® Lexi-DrugsID [Internet]. St. Louis (MO): Wolters Kluwer Health; 2019 [cited 2019 Jul 5]. Available from: http://online.lexi.com.

59. Merck Manuals Professional Version [Internet]. Kenilworth (NJ): Merck & Co., Inc.; 2019 [cited 2019 Aug 30]. Available from: https://www.merckmanuals.com/professional/druginformation/pill-identifier.

60. Hansten PD, Horn JR. The top 100 drug interactions: a guide to patient management. Freeland (WA): H&H Publications; 2019.

61. Lexicomp® [Internet]. St. Louis (MO): Wolters Kluwer Health; 2019 [cited 2019 Jul 5]. Available from: http://online.lexi.com.

62. Preston CL. Stockley's drug interactions. 12th ed. East Smithfield (London, UK): Pharmaceutical Press; 2019.

63. Aronoff GR, Bennett WM, Berns JS, Brier ME, Kasbekar N, Mueller BA, Pasko DA, Smoyer WE. Drug prescribing in renal failure. 5th ed. Philadelphia (PA): American College of Physicians; 2007.

64. Nemecek BD, Hammond DA. Demystifying drug dosing in renal dysfunction. 1st ed. Bethesda (MD): American Society of Health-System Pharmacists; 2019.

65. Bailie GR, Mason NA. Dialysis of drugs. Saline (MI): Renal Pharmacy Consultants, LLC; 2018.

66. Semla TP, Beizer JL, Higbee MD. Geriatric dosage handbook. 21st ed. Hudson (OH): Lexicomp®; 2016.

67. Practice Guidelines: IDSA Infectious Diseases Society of America; 2019 [updated 2019; cited 2019 Aug 29]. Available from: https://www.idsociety.org/practice-guideline/practice-guidelines/.

68. Grayson ML, Cosgrove SE, Crowe SM, Hope W, McCarthy JS, Mills J, Mouton JW, Paterson DL, editors. Kucers' the use of antibiotics. 7th ed. Boca Raton (FL): Taylor & Francis Group; 2018.

69. Red Book 2018: Report of the Committee on Infectious Diseases. 31st ed. Elk Grove Village (IL): American Academy of Pediatrics; 2018.

70. Gilbert DN, Chambers HF, Eliopoulos GM, Saag MS, Pavia AT, editors. The Sanford guide to antimicrobial therapy 2019. 50th ed. Sperryville (VA): Antimicrobial Therapy, Inc.; 2019.

71. Centers for Disease Control and Prevention [Internet]. Atlanta (GA): Centers for Disease Control and Prevention; 2019 [cited 2019 Aug 29]. Available from: https://www.cdc.gov/.

72. Bennett JE, Dolin R, Blaser MJ. Mandell, Douglas, and Bennett's principles and practice of infectious diseases. 9th ed. Philadelphia (PA): Saunders Elsevier; 2019.

73. Centers for Disease Control and Prevention. CDC yellow book: health information for international travel. New York: Oxford University Press; 2019.

74. American Pharmacists Association. Drug Information Handbook with International Trade Names Index. 27th ed. Hudson (OH): Lexicomp®; 2018.

75. Swiss Pharmaceutical Society. Index nominum: international drug directory. 19th ed. Stuttgart (Germany): Medpharm Scientific Publishers; 2008.

76. ClinicalTrials.gov [Internet]. Bethesda (MD): U.S. National Library of Medicine; 2019 [cited 2019 Aug 18]. Available from: https://www.clinicaltrials.gov.

77. Lee M. Basic skills in interpreting laboratory data. 6th ed. Bethesda (MD): American Society of Health-System Pharmacists; 2017.

78. Pagana KD, Pagana TJ. Mosby's manual of diagnostic and laboratory tests. 6th ed. Amsterdam: Elsevier; 2017.

79. Nicoll D, Lu CM, McPhee SJ. Guide to diagnostic tests. 7th ed. New York: McGraw-Hill; 2017.

80. Chernecky CC, Berger BJ. Laboratory tests and diagnostic procedures. 6th ed. Philadelphia (PA): Saunders Elsevier; 2012.

81. LatexDrugs.com [Internet]. Hurricane (WV): 2RPh; 2019 [cited 2019 Aug 30]. Available from: www.latexdrugs.com.

82. Krinsky DL, Ferreri SP, Hemstreet B, Hume AL, Newton GD, Rollings CJ, Tietze KJ. Handbook of nonprescription drugs: an interactive approach to self-care. 19th ed. Washington (DC): American Pharmacists Association; 2017.

83. Hughes HK, Kahl LK. The Harriet Lane handbook. 21th ed. Philadelphia (PA): Elsevier; 2017.

84. Taketomo CK, Hodding JH, Kraus DM. Pediatric and neonatal dosage handbook. 25th ed. Hudson (OH): Lexicomp; 2018.

85. Kliegman R, St. Geme J, Blum NJ, Shah SS, Tasker RL, Wilson KM, Behrman RE. Nelson textbook of pediatrics. 21th ed. Philadelphia (PA): Elsevier; 2020.

86. Neofax® [Internet]. Armonk (NY): IBM Watson Health; [cited 2019 Aug 30]. Available from: https://www.ibm.com/products/micromedex-neofax-pediatrics.

87. Ferencz N. Learning and mastering pharmaceutical calculations. 1st ed. Bethesda (MD): American Society of Health-System Pharmacists; 2017.

88. Teixeira MG, Zatz JL. Pharmaceutical calculations. 5th ed. Hoboken (NJ): Wiley & Sons, Inc.; 2017.

89. Ansel HC, Stockton SJ. Pharmaceutical calculations. 15th ed. St. Louis (MO): Wolters Kluwer Health; 2016.

90. FirstWord Pharma [Internet]. New York (NY): Doctor's Guide Publishing Limited; 2019 [cited 2019 Aug 30]. Available from: http://firstwordplus.com.

91. IPD Analytics [Internet]. Adventura (FL): IPD Analytics; 2019 [cited 2019 Aug 31]. Available from: https://www.ipdanalytics.com/.

92. Pink Sheet: Pharma Intelligence. London (UK): Informa plc; 2019 [cited 2019 Aug 29]. Available from: https://pink.pharmaintelligence.informa.com/.

93. Beringer PM. Winter's basic clinical pharmacokinetics. 6th ed. Philadelphia (PA): Lippincott Williams & Wilkins; 2017.

94. Shargel L, Yu AB. Applied biopharmaceutics and pharmacokinetics. 7th ed. New York: McGraw-Hill; 2016.

95. Bauer LA. Applied clinical pharmacokinetics. 3rd ed. New York: McGraw-Hill; 2014.

96. Brunton LL, Hilal-Dandan R, Knollman BC. Goodman & Gilman's: the pharmacological basis of therapeutics. 13th ed. New York: McGraw-Hill; 2018.

97. Katzung BG. Basic and clinical pharmacology. 14th ed. New York: McGraw-Hill; 2018.

98. Wecker L, Taylor DA, Theobald RJ. Brody's human pharmacology: mechanism-based therapeutics. 6th ed. Philadelphia (PA): Elsevier; 2019.

99. Golan DE, Armstrong EJ, Armstrong AW. Principles of pharmacology: the pathophysiologic basis of drug therapy. 4th ed. Philadelphia (PA): Lippincott Williams & Wilkins; 2016.

100. Abood RR, Burns KA. Pharmacy practice and the law. 9th ed. Burlington (MA): Jones and Bartlett Publishers; 2020.

101. Reiss BS, Hall GD. Guide to federal pharmacy law. 9th ed. Delmar: Apothecary Press; 2016.

102. Briggs GG, Freeman RK. Drugs in pregnancy and lactation: a reference guide to fetal and neonatal risk. 10th ed. Philadelphia (PA): Lippincott Williams & Wilkins; 2014.

103. LactMed [Internet]. Bethesda (MD): U.S. National Library of Medicine; 2020 [updated 2020; cited 2020 Mar 29]. Available from: https://www.ncbi.nlm.nih.gov/books/NBK501922/?report=classic.

104. Hale TW. Medications and mother's milk 2019. 18th ed. New York: Springer Publishing Co.; 2019.

105. Schaefer C, Peters P, Miller RK. Drugs during pregnancy and lactation. 3rd ed. Waltham (MA): Elsevier; 2015.

106. REPROTOX [Internet]. Washington, DC: The Reproductive Toxicology Center; 2019 [cited 2019 Aug 30]. Available from: https://www.reprotox.org/.

107. PubChem [Internet]. Bethesda (MD): U.S. National Library of Medicine; 2020 [updated 2020; cited 2020 Mar 29]. Available from: https://pubchem.ncbi.nlm.nih.gov/.

108. LiverTox [Internet]. Bethesda (MD): U.S. National Library of Medicine; 2020 [updated 2020; cited 2020 Mar 29]. Available from: https://www.ncbi.nlm.nih.gov/books/NBK547852/.

109. POISINDEX® System [Internet]. IBM Watson Health, Greenwood Village, Colorado; 2019 [cited 2019 Aug 30]. Available from: https://www.micromedexsolutions.com/.

110. Lexicomp® Lexi-Tox™ [Internet]. St. Louis (MO): Wolters Kluwer Health; 2019 [cited 2019 Aug 31]. Available from: http://online.lexi.com.

111. Nelson LS, Howland MA, Lewin NA, Smith S, Goldfrank LR, Hoffman RS. Goldfrank's toxicologic emergencies. 11th ed. New York: McGraw-Hill; 2019.

112. Klaassen C. Casarett & Doull's toxicology: the basic science of poisons. 9th ed. New York: McGraw-Hill; 2019.

113. Ettinger SJ, Feldman EL, Cote E. Textbook of veterinary internal medicine. 8th ed. Philadelphia (PA): Elsevier; 2017.

114. Riviere JE, Papich MG. Veterinary pharmacology and therapeutics. 10th ed. Hoboken (NJ): Wiley-Blackwell; 2018.

115. Merck veterinary manual [Internet]. Whitehouse Station (NJ): Merck & Co, Inc.; 2019 [cited 2019 Aug 31]. Available from: https://www.merckvetmanual.com/.

116. Plumb DC. Plumb's veterinary drug handbook. 9th ed. Hoboken (NJ): Wiley-Blackwell; 2018.

117. Plumb's veterinary drugs [Internet]. Tulsa (OK): Brief Media; 2019 [cited 2019 Aug 21]. Available from: https://www.plumbsveterinarydrugs.com/.
118. Carpenter JW, Marion C. Exotic animal formulary. 5th ed. Philadelphia (PA): W.B. Saunders; 2017.
119. U.S. Food and Drug Administration Center for Veterinary Medicine [Internet]. Silver Spring (MD): The U.S. Food and Drug Administration; 2019 [cited 2019 Aug 31]. Available from: https://www.fda.gov/animal-veterinary.
120. Animal Drugs@FDA [Internet]. Silver Spring (MD): The U.S. Food and Drug Administration; 2019 [cited 2019 Aug 31]. Available from: https://animaldrugsatfda.fda.gov/.
121. PetCoach.com [Internet]. Rhinelander (WI): Drs. Foster & Smith Inc.; 2019 [cited 2019 Aug 31]. Available from: https://www.petcoach.co/.
122. PetPlace.com [Internet]. Stamford (CT): The IHC Group; 2019 [cited 2019 Aug 31]. Available from: https://www.petplace.com.
123. Pets with Diabetes [Internet]. Petdiabetes.com; [date unknown] [cited 2019 Aug 31]. Available from: http://www.petdiabetes.com.
124. USP Standards for Veterinary Drugs [Internet]. Bethesda (MD): United States Pharmacopeia; 2019 [cited 2019 Aug 31]. Available from: https://www.usp.org/chemical-medicines/veterinary-drugs.
125. American Association of Colleges of Pharmacy. Basic resources for pharmacy education 2019 [Internet]. Arlington (VA): American Association of Colleges of Pharmacy; 2019 Jul [cited 2019 Aug 29]; [about 50 p.]. Available from: https://connect.aacp.org/HigherLogic/System/DownloadDocumentFile.ashx?DocumentFileKey=3d70ed16-cb20-c959-26fe-ddcd6f768c8d.
126. Minguet F, Van Den Boogerd L, Salgado TM, Correr CJ, Fernandez-Llimos F. Characterization of the Medical Subject Headings thesaurus for pharmacy. Am J Health-Syst Pharm. 2014;71(22):1965-72. Referenced in PubMed PMID: 25349242.
127. Fernandez-Llimos F, Minguet F, Selgado TM. New pharmacy-specific Medical Subject Headings included in the 2017 database [Letter]. Am J Health-Syst Pharm. 2017;74(15):1128-9. Referenced in PubMed PMID: 28743776.
128. New MeSH Headings for 2019. Bethesda (MD): U.S. National Library of Medicine; 2018 Dec [cited 2019 Aug 18]. Available from: https://www.nlm.nih.gov/mesh/2019/download/2019NewMeShHeadings.pdf.
129. Densen P. Challenges and opportunities facing medical education. Trans Am Clin Climatol Assoc. 2011;122:48-58. Referenced in PubMed PMID: 21686208.

SUGGESTED READINGS

1. MEDLINE®: Description of the Database [Internet]. Available from: https://www.nlm.nih.gov/bsd/medline.html.
2. PubMed® Overview [Internet]. Available from: https://pubmed.ncbi.nlm.nih.gov/about/.
3. PubMed Central (PMC) Overview [Internet]. Available from: https://www.ncbi.nlm.nih.gov/pmc/about/intro/.

Chapter Four

Drug Literature Evaluation I: Controlled Clinical Trial Evaluation

Jennifer Phillips • Amy Heck Sheehan • Jacob Gettig • Michael G. Kendrach

Learning Objectives

After completing this chapter, the reader will be able to:

- Identify skills health care practitioners need to evaluate medical literature and apply it to patient care.
- Describe special characteristics of a controlled clinical trial that distinguish this research design as the prototype for clinical research.
- Prepare a null hypothesis (H_0) based upon the clinical trial objective(s) and endpoint(s).
- Differentiate between the types of data, measures of central tendency, and measures of variability.
- Differentiate between Type I and Type II errors; discuss methods to reduce the possibility of either of these errors occurring.
- Interpret *p* values and 95% confidence interval (CI); discuss whether to reject or fail-to-reject the H_0 by using these clinical trial results.
- Calculate and interpret relative risk (RR), relative risk reduction (RRR), absolute risk reduction (ARR), and number needed to treat (NNT).
- State whether statistical significance and clinical difference are present using the clinical trial results.
- Explain the purpose and usage of editorials, letters to the editor, and secondary journals in critiquing clinical trials and the application of results into practice.
- Identify key features of adaptive clinical trials and noninferiority trials.

Key Concepts

1. Practitioners need to be able to efficiently locate, critically analyze, and effectively communicate data from the primary literature to patients, other health care professionals, and the public.

2. A controlled clinical trial is the gold-standard study design to measure and quantify effect differences between an intervention and a control.

3. The entire published study should be read and thoroughly evaluated; decision-making should not rely solely on reading abstracts.

4. The results of a controlled clinical trial should be extrapolated to the type of patient enrolled in the study, and readers should be aware of the limitations of surrogate endpoints and subgroup analyses.

5. Randomization is an essential component of all controlled clinical trials that significantly differentiates them from other study designs.

6. The controlled clinical trial primary endpoint should be appropriate for the study purpose and measured using valid techniques and methods.

7. An appropriate sample size in a controlled clinical trial is vital for the study results to have any significant meaning; conducting a power analysis is important to determine a suitable sample size.

8. Correctly interpreting p values is crucial to evaluating a controlled clinical trial; not all statistically significant p values are clinically important. The magnitude of difference in effect between the intervention and control cannot be determined with the p value.

9. The use of 95% CI can assist the reader in assessing the magnitude of difference in effect between the intervention and control.

10. Calculating measures of association (RR, ARR, RRR, NNT) for nominal data provides further information to interpret controlled clinical trial results

11. Nonstatistically significant results do not equate to the intervention and control being the same or equal.

12. All controlled clinical trial results need to be assessed to determine the clinical relevance of the intervention versus control.

13. Controlled clinical trial investigators and authors should disclose any funding sources and potential conflicts of interest.

14. Editorials, letters to the editor, and commentary publications can assist in interpreting controlled clinical trial results.

Introduction

The health care professions are dynamic, with new information constantly emerging. Therefore, staying up to date on treatments, data, and guidelines requires that health care practitioners regularly use the biomedical/pharmacy literature in their daily practice. In 2018, there were 59 new molecular entities and 21 biological agents approved by the Food and Drug Administration (FDA).[1] In that same year, 33,100 peer-reviewed English-language journals were responsible for publishing over 3 million articles, which represents an estimated annual growth rate of 4% per year.[2]

Practitioners must keep current with new advances in order to remain competent, trustworthy health care professionals. ❶ *Practitioners need to be able to efficiently locate, critically analyze, and effectively communicate data from the primary literature to patients, other health care professionals, and the public.* Therefore, drug literature retrieval and evaluation skills are necessary to prepare the health care practitioner for practice.

Practitioners need to be able to carefully review and critique the literature instead of just accepting the authors' conclusions. Many studies have very positive conclusions but include study design errors that limit the clinical usefulness of the results. Also, health care–related presentations may contain biases and/or inaccuracies, while textbooks/review articles may contain misinterpreted, outdated, and/or noncomprehensive information. Due to the important contribution all practitioners have in patient care, they need to have skill in identifying the strengths and limitations of the biomedical literature. This chapter is devoted to explaining and discussing core concepts for critiquing one essential type of biomedical literature—the controlled **clinical trial.**

Biomedical/Pharmacy Literature

Three types of literature serve as information resources for practitioners: tertiary, secondary, and primary (see Table 4-1).[3] Readers are referred to Chapter 3 in this text for more in-depth discussions of these literature types.

Primary literature, specifically controlled clinical trials, serve as the foundation for clinical practice by providing data that enables evidence-based decision-making. Although vast amounts of primary literature are published each year, individuals can efficiently locate information specific and useful to their needs by incorporating appropriate search techniques.[4,5] ❷ *A controlled clinical trial is the gold-standard study design to measure and quantify effect differences between an intervention and a control.* The FDA requires clinical trials to be conducted and the results submitted before a new molecular entity

TABLE 4–1. THREE TYPES OF LITERATURE

Literature Type	Description	Examples
Tertiary	Established knowledge	Textbooks, review articles, UpToDate, WebMD°, Lexicomp°
Secondary	Indexing/abstracting services (i.e., databases)	PubMed° or MEDLINE°, Embase°, International Pharmaceutical Abstracts (IPA), CINAHL (Cumulative Index to Nursing and Allied Health) InfoTrac OneFile, Academic LexisNexis°
Primary	Original research	Controlled clinical trials, case-control studies, crossover trials, case reports

(i.e., medication) can be marketed and/or receive new indications for use.[6] Newly published information may support, contradict, or serve as the root for altering existing practice regimens. As a result, practitioners need to effectively critique clinical trials. Proper interpretation of clinical trials is vital to providing appropriate health care. This chapter focuses on how to analyze controlled clinical trials, and Chapter 5 outlines strategies to evaluate other types of primary literature.

In general, the goal of a controlled clinical trial is to compare the effects of an investigational (intervention) group to a control group, which can be either a placebo (i.e., "placebo-control") or another intervention (i.e., "active-control").[7,8] While in many studies this "intervention" is a new medication, it does not have to be. Other types of interventions that can be used in a controlled clinical trial include different medication dosing regimens, dietary changes, surgery, behavioral processes, exercise programs, diagnostic procedures, radiation therapy, or educational interventions.

Once published, health care professionals review and use information from clinical trials to make decisions regarding proper care for patients (i.e., to use or not use the investigational intervention).[7] Although the origins of the controlled trial date back to the eighteenth century, a formalized process of conducting controlled clinical trials was not implemented until the late 1940s, and the process of using results from clinical trials to make recommendations ("evidence-based medicine") was not popularized until the 1990s.[9,10] While the use of clinical trials to guide patient treatment has become the "norm," it is important to remember that not all clinical trials are of the same quality and relying on results from poorly designed clinical trials may not be in the best interest of patients. The literature is replete with both poorly designed and well-designed clinical trials and it is the obligation of the end user (in this case, the health care practitioner) to be able to distinguish between the two. Thus, having strong literature evaluation skills is important for all health care practitioners involved in the patient care process.

The journals in which clinical trials are published usually choose to present the trial in an orderly format to facilitate reading and improve the readers' comprehension of the study, results, and conclusions. Table 4-2 displays the style in which a clinical trial usually

TABLE 4–2. FORMAT AND CONTENT OF CONTROLLED CLINICAL TRIALS

Controlled Clinical Trial Section	Type of Information Presented
Abstract	Brief overview of the research project
Introduction	Research background
	What is already known
	Rationale for study
	Objective/hypotheses
Methods	Study design
	Study setting
	Population to be sampled
	Inclusion and exclusion criteria
	Intervention and control groups
	Randomization
	Blinding
	Endpoints/outcomes
	Follow-up procedure
	Sample size calculations/power analysis
	Statistical analysis
Results	Subject characteristics
	Subject dropouts/adherence
	Endpoints quantified
	Statistical significance
	Safety assessments
Discussion	Interpretation of results
	Clinical significance
	Other study results compared
	Limitations
	Conclusion/application to practice
Acknowledgments	Other contributors
	Funding source
	Peer-review dates/manuscript acceptance date (not all trials)
References/Bibliography	Citations for information included from other resources (e.g., trials and reports)

appears in resources.[9,11] This chapter discusses the information presented in these sections according to the CONSORT (Consolidated Standards of Reporting Trials) format. The CONSORT format was designed to improve the quality of reporting clinical trials in the published literature, since inadequate reporting methods hinder the interpretation of results produced by clinical trials. While many journals adhere to the CONSORT recommendations, it is not mandatory for journals to use this format, and other journals may choose to use a different organizational format. Further information about CONSORT may be found in Chapter 13. Other research types (e.g., case-control study) may use a publishing format similar to a controlled clinical trial.[10] Therefore, one should not assume all publications that use this format are controlled clinical trials. Rather, the end user should evaluate the methods section of each publication to deduce which type of research design was used by the author.

Health care practitioners use evidence from clinical trials to make patient care decisions.[12,13] As stated previously, the controlled clinical trial is the most robust method to measure and quantify differences in effects between a therapy under study and the control group.[7,11,14] Clinical studies are perpetually being initiated, but not every study is published in the primary literature.[15,16] There are several reasons for this. First, the trial may have been submitted for publication, but the journal editor or peer reviewers may have recommended not publishing it due to poor research design or perceived lack of audience interest in the topic. In some cases, the researcher may not submit the research for publication consideration due to lack of time or publishing experience. Finally, the clinical trial may have been submitted and accepted but awaiting publication; a lag time is common for many articles submitted for publication.

Readers of the biomedical literature also need to consider the issues of publication bias when searching for evidence. Usually, one clinical trial does not provide sufficient evidence to justify a clinical recommendation. It is prudent to consider all data when making decisions, since conclusions may differ between trials. Thus, while "positive studies" (i.e., those that show a difference between an intervention and a comparator) tend to be published more frequently, journal editors have an obligation to publish negative studies (i.e., those that do not show a difference between an intervention and a comparator), as well. This concept is gaining appreciation among journals and clinicians. Results of these studies are important in formulating practice patterns. Failure by investigators, authors, and journal editors to publish negative studies contributes to publication bias.[17,18]

The intent of this chapter is to equip the reader with the skills necessary to correctly critique clinical trials in order to properly apply the results and conclusions to clinical scenarios. In addition to the discussions of critiquing clinical trials from this chapter, readers should refer to chapters addressing the evaluation of other study types (Chapter 5) and the principles of evidence-based medicine (Chapter 8) when providing patient care.

Approach to Evaluating Research Studies (True Experiments)

Many different research designs are published, but the most common of these are studies in which an intervention (e.g., drug therapy) is directly compared to a control (e.g., placebo, other active treatment), and differences between these are measured. Examples of studies include clinical trials (e.g., evaluation of drug A vs. drug B in humans), stability of compounded drug formulations (e.g., suspension made from drug tablets), compatibility of intravenous drug admixtures, and drug pharmacokinetic interactions. Regardless of the study design and objective, fundamental elements should be reported in all studies, including: appropriate qualifications of the investigators conducting the research; valid investigational methods; proper research techniques; and appropriate analysis and interpretation of the results. A checklist for pertinent information to be included in a clinical trial is located in Appendix 4-1. Answering the questions contained in Appendix 4-1 can allow readers to determine the strengths and limitations of a clinical trial. The remainder of this chapter discusses the questions presented in the Appendix plus techniques for critiquing a clinical trial.

JOURNALS AND PEER REVIEW

Health care practitioners need to regularly access information in published professional journals to assist them in keeping current in their practice responsibilities.[19] Misleading information may be available from many sources; thus, it is important for health care practitioners to independently evaluate and critique information from clinical trials when making patient care decisions.[20]

Incorporating peer review into the publication process is an important way to reduce erroneous or misleading research from reaching the health care community. Reliable journals typically employ a peer-review process. Simply defined, the peer-review process involves sending a draft version of the study or article to a group of individuals with expertise on the topic or in the field under study.[21] These individuals read the manuscript, comment upon the strengths and limitations, and offer a recommendation to the journal editor regarding accepting or rejecting the manuscript for publication. The peer reviewers' comments are sent to the authors who use them to make revisions that improve the quality of the manuscript. In some cases, manuscripts may be rejected as being too flawed or inappropriate for the journal.

Although the peer-review process increases the time required before publication, the goal is to reduce the publication of manuscripts that have inappropriate methods/design, are poorly written, and/or do not meet the needs of the journal's readership.[22] However, the peer-review process does not always prevent publication of articles with deficiencies, and readers should assess the quality of each published article.[23,24] Regardless of whether a clinical trial is published in a peer-reviewed or non-peer-reviewed journal, the article needs to be appropriately evaluated for biases, and the methods and results must be interpreted accurately. Although the value of the peer-review process has been debated, studies have demonstrated improved journal article quality after the peer-review process.[21,25,26]

Two journal sections can be checked for information addressing whether the peer-review process is used: the instructions for authors and the journal's scope/purpose. Additional details on the peer-review process are available in Chapter 10.

As readers become more familiar with the professional literature, they will find certain journals are often cited and have a reputation for high-quality publications, such as New England Journal of Medicine and Annals of Pharmacotherapy. One method that is often used to evaluate the importance of a publication is the impact factor.[27] The impact factor takes into account the number of times that articles published in a specific journal are cited by other articles relative to the number of articles published within that journal. Thus, journals with higher impact factor values are generally considered to be of relatively higher importance. Another way to evaluate the quality of a journal is to assess how many article retractions or errata are published; journals with a high number of retractions or errors may indicate a less robust peer-review process compared to those with less retractions. This information can be found in Medline.[28] While the quality of a journal can be considered in the evaluation of literature, it is important to consider that poor articles can still be found in well-respected journals and excellent articles are published in other journals.[29,30]

PUBLICATION TYPES

Research results can be published in other venues besides journals. A very common publication type is meeting abstracts. Research presented during a professional organization's meeting, whether as a platform or poster presentation, is usually available to meeting attendees in the form of a published abstract. While these abstracts usually undergo a peer-review process prior to presentation and publication, readers should still be cautious of using information contained within the abstract because the entire study details are not available to the reader.

Journal supplements are another common publication type for research. The purpose of such supplements is to publish a collection of articles related to a specific topic in a separate journal issue.[21] Many, but not all supplements, are sponsored by an outside entity (e.g., pharmaceutical company) which serves as another source of revenue for the journal. The articles should undergo peer review using the same rigorous process, but readers should refer to the journal's website to obtain the policies regarding the peer-review process for journal supplements. Journal supplements can serve as a venue for organizations to publish disease state practice guidelines.

AUTHORSHIP

Other factors to evaluate in a published study are the investigators' credentials and practice site(s). Investigators with proper training and experience in their area of study are viewed as more credible. The location where the clinical trial was conducted should not be used to immediately endorse or condemn the quality of the research, other than it should be a site that has the capability to perform the study (i.e., have the resources to properly and completely perform the necessary study methods). The quality of the research must be evaluated because even prestigious institutions can conduct poor clinical trials. Also, persons involved with the study need to be ethical and responsible to protect patients enrolled in the study.[29] Persons with specialized credentials in biostatistics may contribute with statistical analysis of the data. Furthermore, all authors listed should have made substantial contributions to the research and/or publication. The Recommendations for the Conduct, Reporting, Editing, and Publication of Scholarly Work in Medical Journals,[30] prepared by journal editors, explicitly outlines the criteria for persons to be listed as authors for a published article. Further information about the requirements for authorship are found in Chapter 13.

Articles with authors who are employees of a pharmaceutical company should be more selectively analyzed, since there may be concern about potential bias or conflicts of interest. The pharmaceutical industry must conduct research for new therapies to be introduced to the marketplace and many companies collaborate with academic researchers.[25,31] The concern regarding influence from the pharmaceutical industry on health care providers has not gone unnoticed, particularly involving practitioners conducting research for the pharmaceutical industry. In response, many journals now require authors to declare any conflicts of interest with the research and outside interests.[21,32] A **conflict of interest** is possible even when investigators may not consider that their relationship affects their scientific judgment.[21] Authors need to declare if they have received honoraria or research grants from pharmaceutical companies, or are members of an industry speaker's bureau. Readers should be informed of potential investigator bias. However, immediately discarding or discounting clinical trials in which investigators declare relationships with the pharmaceutical industry is premature. Many investigators are required to obtain external funding for research projects and academic promotion. Clinical trials that have researchers with relationships with multiple pharmaceutical companies may not be considered overtly biased. Investigators have an ethical obligation to submit credible research results for publication.[21] Biases may be present, but readers with the skills to identify study strengths and limitations can still use the clinical trial results appropriately.

TITLE

A title should be reflective of the work, unbiased, specific, and concise (i.e., usually less than or equal to 10 words or 40 characters) but not too general or detailed. Interrogative sentences should be avoided. Declarative statements that overemphasize a conclusion are not preferred for scientific articles.[33] The title should include key words that are both sensitive (easing the task of locating the appropriate articles) and specific (excluding those not being searched for), allowing easier electronic retrieval of the article.[21] Furthermore, randomized controlled trials should be identified as such in the title. It is important to note that each journal may have more specific requirements for word count, phrasing, and other logistics for the title as well as other sections within an article.

The following is an example of what could be considered a biased study title: "Improved bronchodilation with levalbuterol compared with racemic albuterol in patients with asthma."[34] The title implies that levalbuterol is better than racemic albuterol. Upon further assessment of study results, although the average change in lung function parameters was slightly greater with levalbuterol, no significant differences were reported in the trial.[34] Thus, the reader could have been misled had they only read the title. A suggested unbiased title for this trial is: "Comparison of levalbuterol and racemic albuterol bronchodilation in patients with asthma: a randomized clinical trial."

ABSTRACT

An abstract is a concise overview of the study or a synopsis of the major principles of the article. ❸ *The entire published study should be read and thoroughly evaluated; decision-making should not rely solely on reading abstracts.* Although format may vary among publishers, abstracts typically include information addressing the article objective, methods, results, and conclusions.

If the abstract is prepared for a published article, it should be used by readers to obtain an immediate overview of the article to determine if the entire article should be read.[32,36] Results of published studies illustrate the dangers of reading only the abstract.[37,38] These studies provided evidence of omissions and discrepancies between the abstract and the manuscript in medical, psychology, and pharmacy journals. In some instances, these differences can be significant. For instance, in one analysis of abstract accuracy, the authors found a 48% 15-year survival mentioned in the abstract, whereas in the text, the 15-year survival was cited as 58%.[35] If the abstract is prepared for a poster or podium presentation at a professional conference, it may not have a resulting published article. In this instance, the reader may use the information within the abstract only but may need to contact the author to clarify missing or incomplete data. Informative abstracts may entice some individuals to read the study; thus, abstracts should be thorough, complete, and use unbiased statements. Abstracts should be consistent with the manuscript and should not present biased and/or inaccurate information.[40–42] For further information regarding abstracts and preparation, refer to Appendix 13-2.

Many journals now require abstracts to be prepared in an organized format (i.e., structured abstract) and usually contain less than or equal to 500 words. Structured abstracts may be organized differently and have different titles for sections, but should include the following information: background for the study, the study's purpose, the basic procedures (i.e., participant selection, setting, measurements, and analysis), results or main findings of the study that include enough information to ascertain statistical and/or clinical significance, and main conclusions. In addition, any funding sources should be listed after the abstract so that the reader may evaluate potential for conflicts of interest.[43] Structured abstracts are more informative, easier to read, and generally preferred by readers compared to unstructured abstracts.[40,41] However, structured abstracts usually require more journal space.

INTRODUCTION

The introduction section identifies a "research gap" and outlines the purpose of the study.[10,44] The research gap may be a lack of data available to answer a question, or it may involve conflicting data on a specific issue. Every clinical trial is designed to answer one or more research questions.

The introduction section should capture the readers' interest. Usually, readers are first briefly educated on prior research in the field and the issues that were the basis for conducting the study. The investigators should explain how the clinical trial will overcome the shortcomings of the prior research, if applicable.

The study objective is often stated within the last paragraph, and often within the last sentence, of the introduction. Well-written studies provide a clearly stated research purpose, and this statement should be understood by the reader before continuing with the remaining article content. Studies with a clear purpose statement enable the reader to better assess research methods and determine how to use the results of the study.

Once the clinical trial objective is determined, the investigators need to formulate a **research hypothesis** and a **null hypothesis**. A research hypothesis (also known as the **alternative hypothesis**, H_A) states that there is a difference between the therapy under investigation and the control, while the null hypothesis (H_0) states that there is no difference between these two groups (see next paragraph for an example). After the study is completed, the researchers analyze the data and the research hypothesis is either accepted (which is also stated as rejecting the null hypothesis, H_0) or rejected (which is also stated as accepting H_0). A research and null hypothesis may not be explicitly stated in the introduction section of clinical trials, but the methods should be written clearly enough to allow the reader to determine the alternative and null hypotheses.

Example:

The Improved Reduction of Outcomes: Vytorin Efficacy International Trial (IMPROVE-IT) will be used to illustrate some of the material included thus far in this chapter. In this trial, the researchers assessed whether ezetimibe (Vytorin) added to statin therapy was associated with a reduction in cardiovascular mortality in patients who had an acute coronary syndrome and whose LDL cholesterol values were within guideline recommendations. Specifically, simvastatin 40 mg plus ezetimibe 10 mg was compared to simvastatin 40 mg plus placebo.[45]

The investigators noted in the introduction section that the rationale for conducting this clinical trial was that no evidence had been published to determine whether ezetimibe added to simvastatin would improve cardiovascular events. The research hypothesis of the IMPROVE-IT trial would be: "There is a difference in the incidence of cardiovascular events in patients receiving combination therapy with ezetimibe and simvastatin compared to simvastatin monotherapy." The H_0 for this clinical trial was: "There is no difference in the incidence of cardiovascular outcomes between combination therapy with ezetimibe and simvastatin compared to simvastatin monotherapy." After reading the IMPROVE-IT trial introduction, the reader has a clear understanding of the study rationale and purpose: the results of this trial should provide health care providers with evidence to prescribe combination therapy with ezetimibe and simvastatin or simvastatin monotherapy after acute coronary syndrome in patients with LDL cholesterol levels within the guideline recommendations.

As with all sections of a clinical trial, the introduction needs to be carefully read. Authors may set the stage by presenting only selective (i.e., not comprehensive) information and/or weak references (to be discussed later in the chapter) to support the rationale for conducting the study. Information presented may use biased wording and predispose the reader to believing the prior research was insignificant in providing evidence applicable to practice.

METHODS

Following a well-designed plan is essential for the clinical trial results to be acceptable and useful to practitioners. The design of a study (i.e., methods) is important for the results to be valid, just as abiding by construction blueprints is vital to building a house. The methods section of a clinical trial contains a large amount of information that describes the type of subjects enrolled, the comparative therapy description, outcome measures, and planned statistical analyses. Flaws within the design of a clinical trial limit the application and significance of the results. Poor study design leads to reduced study **internal validity**, thus resulting in limited external study validity (see Table 4-3).[46] The methods section must thoroughly describe the process by which the study was conducted, and it should be written with sufficient detail to allow the study to be easily replicated by another investigator. A reader should devote most of the time used to assess the trial in this section.

Clinical trials present the study methodology with a standardized format[10] that allows study details to be quickly located. The methods section should include the trial design, participants, interventions, outcomes, sample size, randomization sequence generation, allocation concealment mechanisms (e.g., mechanisms used to generate random

TABLE 4–3. INTERNAL VERSUS EXTERNAL VALIDITY OF CLINICAL TRIALS

Term	Meaning	Application
Internal validity	Quality of the study design	Strong design should translate into reliable results
External validity	Ability to apply results in practice	Study results meaningful to practitioners and can be used for patient care

allocation sequence), blinding, and statistical methods. Readers of the biomedical literature should understand the overall design to appropriately critique clinical trials and use
the study results for patient care activities.

Study Design

Several study designs are available for investigators to select from when conducting
research. The study questions that researchers wish to answer dictate which study design
is selected to conduct the research.[42,47] Both investigators and readers of the literature
need to identify the strengths and limitations of the research designs. Although many
study designs are available, this chapter only discusses controlled clinical trials. For additional information on other study designs, the reader is referred to Chapter 5.

A simple description of a controlled clinical trial is that it prospectively measures a
difference in effect between two or more interventions (e.g., drug therapy). The groups
are similar and treated identically except for the interventions that are being investigated. The subjects in the study are assigned to one of the groups and monitored.[7,11,13,48]
This study type, called parallel design, is the primary study design encountered in the
literature.

Controlled clinical trials offer investigators the most rigorous method of establishing
a cause-and-effect relationship between treatment and outcome.[11] Simply explained, the
treatment under study is the cause, and the result of giving the treatment is measured as
the effect. The effect of the treatment being studied is compared to the effect of the other
group(s). Consequently, investigators can use a clinical trial to claim that a treatment has
an effect that may be important in modifying disease outcomes. In addition, the magnitude (i.e., size) of the difference in the effect between the groups can be estimated.[11]

An example of a controlled clinical trial measuring a cause-and-effect is a study that
compared simvastatin 80 mg plus placebo or with ezetimibe 10 mg in patients with familial
hypercholesterolemia. The study objective was to compare simvastatin plus ezetimibe
(cause) to simvastatin plus placebo and measure the change in intima-media thickness of
the walls of the carotid and femoral arteries (effect).[39] The study results documented that
simvastatin plus ezetimibe did not result in a significant change in intima-media thickness
compared to simvastatin plus placebo.

A clinical trial also quantifies the differences in the effect, such as atorvastatin compared to simvastatin in lowering LDL-C.[49] Atorvastatin 10 mg daily was compared to

simvastatin 20 mg daily to measure the difference in average LDL-C reduction by these two agents. After 6 weeks of therapy, the average LDL-C level was lowered slightly more with atorvastatin than simvastatin (−37% vs. −35%). Thus, the results of this study can be used to determine the magnitude of difference in LDL-C lowering by atorvastatin 10 mg daily compared to simvastatin 20 mg daily and determine which medication to use in clinical practice.

Patient Inclusion/Exclusion Criteria

❹ *The results of a controlled clinical trial should be extrapolated to the type of patient enrolled in the study, and readers should be aware of the limitations of* **surrogate endpoints** *and subgroup analyses.* The **inclusion criteria** lists subject demographics that must be present for a subject to be enrolled into the trial. **Exclusion criteria** are characteristics that prevent subject enrollment into the trial or necessitate withdrawal from the study, if exclusion criteria are later determined to be present.[10] Diagnostic criteria for conditions under study and definitions of the inclusion/exclusion criteria must be included in an article reporting study results. For instance, if subjects with hypertension are the target group to be enrolled in a trial, hypertension needs to be defined in terms of the minimal and maximum systolic blood pressure (SBP) and diastolic blood pressure (DBP). Clinical characteristics of study participants should reflect the disease under investigation, but the existence of complex and/or extensive comorbid conditions (e.g., terminal cancer, pregnancy, numerous other disease states) in study patients may prevent an accurate measurement of differences in effect between the groups. The decision to include or exclude subjects with complex and/or extensive comorbid conditions is challenging and must balance the need for including subjects representative of real patients with the need to accurately assess a new treatment. Whenever possible and appropriate, typical individuals with the condition being assessed, who in all probability will receive the therapy in real practice, should be represented in the trial. This includes ensuring a realistic representation of gender, race, and other demographics. Subjects with one or more (but not numerous) other disease states and taking other medications are usually enrolled in the clinical trial to ensure the study sample is representative of typical patients intended to receive the therapy under investigation.

The inclusion/exclusion criteria are pertinent to the extrapolation of the study results (i.e., applying the study results into practice [**external validity**]).[50] Trial results are only applicable to the type of subject included in the study. The investigators of the IMPROVE-IT trial enrolled men and women with acute coronary syndrome.[45] Additionally, patients were at least 50 years of age and were required to have an LDL-cholesterol level of 50 mg/dL. Thus, the results of IMPROVE-IT cannot be extrapolated to patients who are younger than 50 years of age since only those who were at least 50 years of age with acute coronary syndrome were included in this clinical trial.

Researchers are careful in deciding which subjects to include and exclude in the clinical trial. Standard types of subjects disqualified are pregnant and lactating females, and children. Also, most clinical trials will not enroll subjects with severe health conditions that may alter the medication's pharmacokinetics and/or pharmacodynamics (e.g., renal and/or hepatic dysfunction) because differences in the outcome effect are likely in these subjects compared to those without these conditions. Generally, the inclusion criteria attempt to include subjects who are homogeneous and are similar to patients commonly seen in practice.[52] However, one criticism of clinical trials is that the patient sample in the clinical trial does not match all of the patient types encountered in clinical practice. There are inherent advantages and disadvantages to stringent inclusion criteria. Tight criteria may reduce the number of people who will be able to participate in the trial or exclude patients who may be at risk for treatment complications. In other scenarios, subjects most likely to receive benefit may be selected for inclusion; the patient population may be restricted to those with advanced disease; or patients noncompliant to therapy may be excluded, etc. If the inclusion criteria are loose, more patients reflective of those encountered in clinical practice may be recruited; however, if a heterogeneous patient population is included, with various disease states, it may be difficult to determine which intervention works the best.[52]

Although investigators should attempt to establish inclusion and exclusion criteria that select a representative study sample, readers of clinical trials need to be conscious of the potential for **selection bias** in those criteria. Selection bias can occur due to various reasons and seriously affect the study results. Selection bias can be intentionally or unintentionally introduced into a study. In general, a selection bias occurs when subjects meet the inclusion and exclusion criteria, but are not enrolled into the study.[51] The investigators may prevent a subject from being enrolled since this person may either positively or negatively alter the results.[7,13,50,53]

Although it is difficult for the reader to detect the above form of selection bias, the following paragraphs describe selection biases that can be more readily identified but are not present in all clinical trials. One common form of selection bias is requiring the subjects to complete a **run-in phase** (also called lead-in phase) before being officially enrolled in the study. This phase is usually short in duration (e.g., 2–4 weeks) and observes subjects' responses to a placebo or the therapy under investigation. The investigators should inform the reader of the intent of the run-in phase. Typical reasons include identifying subjects who may or may not adhere with the therapy regimen, experience side effects from the therapy, or do not meet prespecified criteria (e.g., blood pressure less than a set value). Afterward, these identified subjects are excluded from study participation even though they met the original inclusion criteria. The run-in phase produces a bias by selecting a group of subjects who do not completely represent the population, since a selected group of the subjects meeting the study inclusion criteria are not included in the study, and their run-in phase results are not included in the final analysis.[54] In addition, a run-in phase can delay the time from identifying candidates to actually enrolling into the clinical trial, which can increase the chance of patients withdrawing from the study.[48]

The following examples explain a selection bias by a run-in phase. Subjects meeting the hypothetical trial inclusion criteria complete a 4-week run-in phase in which a new therapy under investigation is given to all persons. Individuals experiencing side effects to the new therapy during the run-in phase are not allowed to be enrolled into the study. By excluding those persons eliminated after the run-in phase, the incidence and severity of the side effects of the therapy are not accurately measured during the actual study since subjects experiencing the side effects during the run-in phase were not enrolled in the study. A second example is where researchers may include a run-in phase in which only those persons achieving a preset goal are allowed to be included in the study. For instance, only subjects achieving at least a 25% reduction in LDL-C after a 4-week phase with a new therapy are enrolled in the 12-week study comparing the new therapy to placebo. By only including those with a favorable response, the final average reduction in LDL-C with the new therapy is falsely elevated since subjects without the initial 25% LDL-C reduction were not allowed into the study. If these individuals were included in the 12-week trial, the final average reduction in LDL-C most likely would have been substantially lower than actually measured.

Inclusion of a run-in phase in a study is not always considered to be a study limitation.[55] The investigators may stop a therapy previously prescribed to the subjects and give a placebo during the run-in phase. This allows the effects of the prior therapy to diminish and is intended to prevent interference with the effects of the therapy under investigation. If a study does include a run-in phase to allow prior therapy washout, the run-phase duration should be based upon the therapy elimination rate. Furthermore, investigators may design a clinical trial to enroll a very specific type of subject, which can be considered a selection bias in the inclusion criteria. For instance, a trial was designed so that only subjects who experienced a gastrointestinal (GI) bleed with aspirin alone were enrolled.[56] The investigators specifically selected a unique group of subjects (having a GI bleed due to aspirin). The combination of aspirin plus esomeprazole was compared to clopidogrel to determine which therapy had a lower recurrence of GI bleeding. Even though the trial results indicated that the aspirin plus esomeprazole combination has a lower GI bleeding recurrence rate, this does not mean this drug combination should be used instead of aspirin alone in all patients who require aspirin therapy. The results of this trial can only be used for selected patients who had a GI bleed while taking aspirin and need to continue antiplatelet therapy.

Investigators should also explain the process of recruiting subjects and define the time period during which the recruitment occurred.[10] Sponsors of clinical trials and investigators typically recruit subjects for clinical trials by four main strategies: (1) sponsors may offer financial and other incentives to investigators to increase enrollment;

(2) investigators may target their own patients as potential subjects; (3) investigators may seek additional subjects from other sources (e.g., physician referrals and disease registries); or (4) sponsors and investigators may advertise and promote their studies. The most common means for advertising recruitment to clinical trials is through newspapers, radio, Internet, television, or posters on public transportation and in hospitals.[57] The methods in which investigators recruit subjects may have implications on the generalizability of the research results to the population (i.e., external validity). Newspaper and Internet advertisements are common; however, there are inherent problems with this form of advertisement. Survey results indicate that most people who read the newspapers are older in age, Caucasian, wealthier, and more educated than the average American. **Gender bias** can also affect recruitment rates as it has been documented that female readers consider newspaper advertising to be more important than male readers.[58] Lack of representation by ethnic minorities, elders, and females represents a significant health burden as health care disparities are predominant in these patient populations. These disparities may persist if adequate clinical trial recruitment strategies are not developed. Community partnered research efforts may help increase clinical trial recruitment in these critical patient populations.[53]

Internet recruitment has similar problems. Typically, minority and elderly individuals are less familiar and have less access to the Internet. A study described the process of registering persons with cancer for clinical trials via the Internet or a telephone call center. Most of the subjects registered via the Internet compared to the telephone call center (88% vs. 12%). The majority of subjects who registered were female (73% vs. 27% male), Caucasian (88.9%), and received colorectal cancer screening (59%); the median age was 49 years. No differences with respect to ethnicity or gender were observed for patients registering via the Internet compared to the call center; however, subjects registering via the Internet were significantly younger than those registering through the call center.[55,59] Recruitment via the Internet may offer some benefits, although the lack of uniformity with respect to access may increase the difficulty of applying these results to all populations. Other areas of significant concern with Internet recruitment includes the potential for security lapses for personal data. However, when conducted appropriately, Internet recruitment can be an efficient and economical method for clinical trial recruitment.[59] Another important issue that affects the recruitment of patients is the increasing number of clinical studies that are outsourced to other countries due to costs associated with conducting clinical trials in the United States. Although outsourcing clinical trials to other countries may decrease the problems associated with insufficient recruitment of patients who enroll in clinical trials, the results may not be able to be applied due to the differences in the population studied versus the patients in the practitioners' population.[60] Potential ethnic differences may affect the way drugs are handled in the body (e.g., overall response, drug distribution, metabolism, excretion). Therefore, readers of clinical studies that included foreign patients need to ensure that the results of the study are generalizable to the patient population in which they serve. However, clinical trials including a majority of foreign patients should not be viewed with a bias. Various factors have led to more clinical research conducted in foreign countries including governments competing for clinical research to be conducted in their country, increased number of health care specialists plus improving medical infrastructure, and changes in regulations.[61]

Intervention and Control Groups

Once the subjects are enrolled in the clinical trial, they will be assigned to either the intervention or control group. The intervention group receives the therapy under investigation (e.g., medication, procedure). The intervention is compared to a control so that the fundamental principle of a controlled clinical trial can be accomplished, measuring cause and effect. The control group can consist of no therapy (e.g., placebo), another therapy (a.k.a. **active control** [e.g., exercise]), or compared to existing data (i.e., historical data). Both the intervention and control groups are to be as similar as possible in all respects (e.g., average age, number of males/females, medication use, existing disease states) other than the treatment received. Afterward, the investigators quantify and measure the difference(s) in effect(s) between the group assigned to the intervention and the group assigned to the control group. Any identified differences in the measured effect can be attributed to the intervention rather than other factors (i.e., confounders).[62,63]

A key term in the phrase "controlled clinical trial" is the word "control." A control is another therapy that serves as the measuring point for the effect of the intervention. Without a control, the effects measured by the intervention may be secondary to chance or falsely quantified, consistent with reports documenting placebo effects (i.e., measured change even though no therapy was given).[64] For example, investigators of a study reported that oxandrolone caused an average increase in body weight in patients with chronic obstructive pulmonary disease (COPD).[65] However, all the subjects were treated with oxandrolone and no control group was included in the study. Although patients gained weight, oxandrolone may not be the sole reason for this effect. Weight gain may have occurred naturally, even without the medication or by some unidentified reason. The results of this noncontrolled clinical trial may underpin the rationale for a clinical trial to evaluate the mechanism or magnitude of weight gain with oxandrolone. However thus, a noncontrolled clinical trial cannot be used as evidence that weight gain was solely attributed to this drug. The results of studies designed without a control can be useful, but since no control group was present, readers cannot be certain that oxandrolone caused the weight gain, even if caloric intake and exercise were held constant, because other variables that may cause weight gain were unaccounted.

Researchers can select from a few different types of controls, including historical, placebo, or active. Historical controls are described as data that have been collected prior to the beginning of a clinical trial. Investigators conduct the study with the intervention group, and compare the results to the existing data.[66] One advantage of using historical controls is that only one group needs to be enrolled, which may result in less time, expense, etc. Another advantage is the usefulness of studying a disease with a low incidence or prevalence or a disease with high incidence of death or other serious sequelae in which some form of therapy should not be denied to a patient. Disadvantages include a tendency to overestimate the effect of the intervention,[67] lack of homogeneity between patients in the trial and historical controls, and differences in therapeutic procedures or techniques from one study period to the next.[68] (Please refer to Chapter 5 for discussions of observational trials, which may use historical controls.) Historical controls are not used very often in published clinical trials, but are acceptable in selected situations. For example, the use of a placebo group is not considered ethical in clinical trials evaluating new therapies in patients with epilepsy. Due to the morbidity and/or mortality associated with an uncontrolled seizure disorder, this patient type should not be denied therapy in order to investigate a new therapy. Thus, investigators may assess a new therapy in these patients and compare the research results to a historical control group.[69]

An intervention under investigation is compared to a placebo in many clinical trials to document and measure the pharmacological effect of the intervention. These studies are generally conducted as a requirement by the FDA to document that drug therapy is better than no therapy (placebo) for a given disease state.[70] Those trials reporting a significant difference in effect of the intervention compared to placebo could be used to support the use of the intervention in treating patients. Simvastatin was compared to placebo to determine if the incidence of death would be lower in subjects with a history of angina pectoris or myocardial infarction (MI).[71] Before this study was conducted, health care providers did not have any information indicating that simvastatin would benefit or harm patients with this medical problem. At the time this trial was designed and initiated, persons with angina pectoris or history of MI were not routinely treated with a HMG-CoA reductase inhibitor (i.e., statins); thus, a placebo was selected as the control. However, the place in therapy for the intervention may be difficult to determine when a placebo is the control. For example, in this case, although simvastatin lowers LDL-C greater than placebo,[70] investigators are unable to determine the relative effectiveness and/or safety of simvastatin compared to other drugs that also lower LDL-C.

Not all clinical trials will have a placebo as the control group for various valid reasons. For example, including a placebo as one of the groups in a trial may decrease the willingness of subjects to participate; some may not wish to be treated with placebo.[72] But more importantly, denying therapy that has been documented to reduce morbidity and/or mortality to patients with selected diseases may be unethical. These studies would not include a placebo as the control but, instead, may use active control (i.e., standard therapy).[68]

For example, cancer trials may not include a placebo as the control if another potentially effective therapy is available.

After a new therapy is compared to a placebo, a trial using an active therapy as the control can be used to assess the difference in effect between the groups. Readers should be aware that clinical trials with a placebo as the control may yield a larger treatment effect than if an active therapy was selected as the control group.[73,74] For instance, the difference in LDL-C reduction is expected to be significantly greater with a new statin versus placebo than it would be if compared to another statin or other lipid-lowering agent. The treatment effect may appear substantial versus placebo but could be minimal compared to another active drug used as the control. Also, it is possible that the new treatment may be inferior in efficacy and/or safety compared to an active drug, even though the new treatment appears better in comparison to a placebo. An appropriate control needs to be included in the study for the results to be applicable for practice. The use of a historical control or placebo is acceptable in some clinical studies (as described above). Further, studies may be designed with a control that is no longer the preferred treatment after the trial results are published. The study may have been designed and initiated based upon either recommendations of the FDA or before new therapy recommendations were available.

Investigators need to choose an appropriate medication and dosing regimen (i.e., dose, frequency) as the control.[75] Standard references should be consulted to ensure appropriate dosing regimens were included in the trial to reduce the chance of obtaining biased results. A trial concluding that a new analgesic relieved pain better than morphine 0.05 mg intravenously (IV) every 24 hours postsurgery in otherwise healthy adult subjects is biased in favor of the new analgesic because an insufficient morphine dose was used as the control. However, at times, investigators may not know the equivalent dosing regimen of the intervention relative to the control. Investigators directly comparing rosuvastatin 10 mg daily to atorvastatin 10 mg daily for 12 weeks reported a greater reduction of mean LDL-C with rosuvastatin (43% vs. 35%, $p < 0.001$).[76] Other studies comparing these two medications have reported average LDL-C levels are similar with atorvastatin doses two times that of the rosuvastatin dose.[77] Thus, concluding rosuvastatin is a superior LDL-C lowering agent to atorvastatin, based solely upon the results of a single trial evaluating both agents dosed 10 mg once daily, is incorrect. A more appropriate conclusion is that these two agents do not have an equivalent pharmacological effect or potency at this dose.

Institutional Review Board (IRB)/Subject Consent

Research projects that use humans as study subjects must be approved before investigators enroll subjects into the trial. The Institutional Review Board (IRB) is the group charged with ensuring that the study subjects are protected and not exposed to unnecessary harm or unethical medical procedures,[78,79] including vulnerable populations (e.g., pediatrics, pregnant women, impaired persons).[80] The name of the actual group may differ from place to place (e.g., local ethics committee), although the purpose of the committee remains to protect study subjects. This committee consists of both health care and non-health-care professionals; people specialized in ethics also need to be included.[80] The rules and regulations of human research require the study to be assessed prior to the initiation of the project.

Another primary responsibility of the IRB is to approve the informed consent form.[73,83,73,83] Before agreeing to participate in a trial, each subject is presented with an informed consent form that notifies the subjects of the study procedures, their rights and responsibilities of participating in the study, plus at least eight major points that include risks, benefits, compensation, voluntary participation, and right to withdraw from the study without any penalty. In addition to the content of the informed consent form, the IRB provides investigators with suggestions on how to write the form in language that laypersons can comprehend.[75,81,73,84-89,84-89] Additional information regarding the role of the IRB and investigator in clinical trial research can be obtained at http://phrp.nihtraining.com/. Also, the reader may refer to Chapter 23 "Investigational Drugs" for further information. According to the Recommendations for the Conduct, Reporting, Editing, and Publication of Scholarly Work in Medical Journals,[36] articles describing clinical trials using humans as research subjects are required to include a statement that the research was approved by the IRB (or other committee that protects subjects) and consent was obtained from the subject to participate in the research project.[21] Readers of the medical/pharmacy literature should expect to read IRB/ethics approval information within the published studies. Trials not including the IRB/informed consent information should be questioned.

Blinding

Since clinical trials measure differences in effect between groups, outside influences (i.e., biases) should be minimized. This is especially important in studies measuring subjective outcomes (e.g., pain, depression scores). **Blinding** is a technique in which subjects and/or the investigators are unaware of who is in the intervention or control group. Blinding techniques are incorporated to reduce possible bias (defined as "differences between the true value and that actually obtained [are] due to all causes other than sampling variability").[13] Patients knowing they are taking a placebo to reduce depression symptoms are likely to report no change or worsening of the disease. The results in such a situation are biased, since the subjects knowingly are taking a substance that does not reduce symptoms. Therefore, blinding techniques are important to reduce the influence of bias on measuring a difference in effect between the intervention and control. Four types of blinding can be used in a clinical trial (see Table 4-4). The specific blinding type usually is

TABLE 4–4. TYPES OF BLINDING

Type of Blinding	Definition
No blinding (open-label)	Investigators and subjects are aware of the assignment of subjects to the intervention or control group.
Single	Either investigators or subjects, but not both, are aware of the assignment of subjects to the intervention or control group.
Double	Both investigators and subjects are not aware of the assignment of subjects to the intervention or control group.
Triple	Investigators, subjects, and trial personnel involved with data analysis and interpretation are not aware of the assignment of subjects to the intervention or control group.

dictated by the effect being measured during the trial (e.g., subjective or objective) or the procedure(s) under study (e.g., surgery vs. medication).

Single-blinding and nonblinding techniques are primarily incorporated in clinical trials that have study objectives not conducive to blinding (e.g., surgery vs. medication). Some trials may include a procedure that is difficult to blind (e.g., surgery) and it may not be ideal to include a placebo procedure because sham surgery may increase risks of death or infection-related complications.[75] The use of placebo/sham procedures for clinical trials is controversial and possibly unethical if the investigators do not thoroughly discuss the rationale for including and/or not using other methods to blind the trial.[85] A clinical trial designed to compare surgery to a medication is an example of using nonblinding methods since both the investigators and subjects know to which group the subjects have been assigned.

Single-blinding can be described as either the investigator or subjects knowing who is receiving the intervention or control, but not both parties. An example of single-blinding of investigators is when one group of subjects is administered a medication subcutaneously once daily versus the other group who took an oral anticoagulation medication. The subjects would not be subjected to blinding since the risk of injecting a saline solution subcutaneously (e.g., pain, bleeding, infection) poses ethical concerns, and does not provide added benefit to the patient. The investigators would measure the occurrence of a blood clot, an objective outcome that cannot be biased or influenced by the subjects. The subjects' knowledge of which therapy they were receiving is unlikely to influence the incidence of the blood clots. Since the investigators do not know which therapy each subject received, the potential for the results to be biased is minimized. There are also cases in which the subjects were blinded, but not the investigator.

Double-blinding, where neither the investigator nor patient knows which treatment the patient is receiving, is considered the gold-standard blinding technique, and is most commonly used in clinical trials.[14] As a general rule, regardless whether the outcome is a subjective or objective measure, the study should be double-blinded. A clinical trial measuring an objective outcome usually assesses other outcome measures, such as the incidence and severity of side effects, which may be biased if double-blinding was not incorporated into the trial. For instance, double-blinding was used in the IMPROVE-IT trial[51] to not only minimize biases in liver enzyme levels and creatine kinase levels (objective measurements) but also side effects (subjective assessments) in patients assigned to intervention or control.

To ensure blinding remains intact, the therapy each group receives should have the same frequency of administration, appearance, size, taste, smell, and other variables perceptible to investigators and subjects. Double-dummy methods are included in clinical trials when two therapies being compared are not the same (e.g., different routes of administration, different formulations). Patients receive two formulations, one active and one control, to ensure that blinding is maintained.[7] For example, investigators of a clinical trial evaluating the blood pressure lowering effects of amlodipine (a tablet) and the combination product of amlodipine plus benazepril (a capsule) should administer amlodipine tablets plus placebo capsules to those subjects randomized to amlodipine therapy and amlodipine/benazepril capsules plus placebo tablets to the other subjects. A similar situation may present in clinical trials in which the formulations being compared are administered via different routes. Investigators comparing the efficacy of a once-daily oral contraceptive tablet to an intramuscular contraceptive agent administered every 3 months may allocate an intramuscular placebo to those patients randomized to once-daily oral contraceptives and a once-daily placebo tablet to those patients randomized to the intramuscular contraceptive. Each patient receives a formulation that represents each therapy, and both subjects and investigators would be less likely to determine which formulation is active.

Sometimes it is necessary to triple-blind a study. In addition to the trial investigators and subjects, other personnel involved with the trial (e.g., data collection, analysis, or monitoring; drug administration or dispensing) can have opinions regarding the outcome of the therapy being studied based on their interaction with the subjects involved in the trial or their experience with the intervention and/or control being assessed. These opinions may cause inappropriate data collection, measurement, analysis, and/or interpretation of the results by the study personnel. Also, data collection personnel having a bias for or against the intervention may not maintain consistent data collection procedures if they know group assignment of study subjects. This may result in an inappropriate interpretation (e.g., overestimation of the treatment effects) of the study results.[7,29,69] Therefore, it is often necessary to blind these other individuals. Although triple-blinding is commonly used in controlled clinical trials, many publications that follow a triple-blind design erroneously report their design as "double-blind" when describing their methods.

Randomization

❺ *Randomization is an essential component of all randomized controlled clinical trials that significantly differentiates them from other study designs* (e.g., case-control, cohort).

With simple randomization, all subjects in a clinical trial have an equal chance to be in the intervention or control group.[81,91] Results obtained from randomized trials are more dependable than nonrandomized trials. Bias causes nonrandomized trials to overestimate the treatment effects of the intervention compared to the control.[67] Randomization minimizes the risk of bias and allows investigators to achieve more reliable results, but it is necessary to remember not all randomized trials are without faults.

Subjects are eligible for randomization after meeting the trial inclusion criteria. Subjects are randomized to prevent investigators from purposely or unintentionally assigning selected persons to one group over another (i.e., individuals with more comorbidities in the control vs. healthier individuals in the intervention group). Randomization minimizes bias by lowering the potential for an imbalance of risk factors or prognostic variations between the intervention and control groups. A difference in effect measured by a clinical trial may result from many causes, and the intervention is only one of these variables. Disparities between the groups at baseline may cause a false result instead of measuring differences in effect between the intervention and the control.[67] Therefore, to assure that the difference is truly due to the intervention, the groups need to be as similar as possible to control for any confounding variables. Measuring differences in the effect between the intervention and control group requires the groups to be as similar in as many characteristics as possible (e.g., age, gender, severity of illness) so that outside factors (i.e., confounders) do not influence the results. Baseline discrepancies between the groups do not allow true differences in effect between the intervention and controls to be measured and quantified. If unbalanced factors are present between the two groups, the outcome measure is biased, and the treatment effect may be either under- or overestimated.[62]

Besides reducing bias,[86] an additional reason to include randomization in a clinical trial is to ensure validity of statistical tests. Most statistical tests require subjects to be randomized so that similar groups are being compared and selected statistical tests can determine whether certain subject characteristics are equivalent between groups.[12]

Randomization Techniques

Many randomization techniques are available and range from very simple to complex processes. Specific randomization methods include simple randomization (e.g., coin toss) or more advanced techniques (e.g., **stratification**). The nature of the study and outcomes measured influence the randomization procedure. The randomization procedures should be unbiased and prevent subjects or investigators from knowing the group assignment of study subjects.[7]

Simple randomization is an easy technique to implement and can be performed by various methods. Study subjects may be randomized according to prespecified criteria (e.g., day of the week, subject birthday, or subject medical record number), but this method is unreliable since the number of subjects in the groups can become imbalanced. For example, if investigators assign all subjects with an office visit on a specific day of the week to one group (i.e., control), then these subjects did not have equal opportunity to be assigned to either group. This may decrease the ability of investigators to detect differences in effects between the two groups. Few trials use simple randomization techniques due to the limitations of this method.[12] Although the mentioned simple randomization techniques do have limitations, a random number table can be considered useful since the table allows for each study subject to have equal opportunity to be assigned to either group.

Stratification is a more sophisticated randomization procedure designed to achieve similarities in baseline patient characteristics between groups. Known factors (e.g., age, smoking, presence of other disease states) that may influence a study outcome are identified and used to determine to which group subjects will be assigned to prevent a significant imbalance of these factors among the groups, while all subjects with any specific factor have an equal chance of being in each group[87] Since these patient factors can affect the outcome being measured, stratified randomization is a technique that enables these factors to be comparable between the study groups.[12]

The person randomizing study participants should receive only the participant information used for the randomization process. Extra and unnecessary patient information could bias the randomization process. Unduly influencing the randomization sequence by randomizing subjects to either therapy based on some preference can occur with the extra personal information.[12] Thus, to minimize these issues, investigators should only provide the pertinent subject information that will allow randomization of the subject to either the intervention or control group.

Patients may also be allocated to groups via a block randomization process. Block randomization allows for a balance of groups between the intervention and control. For instance, if there are four patients in each group, the group will be balanced every time the fourth patient is enrolled in the study. There are six ways in which four patients can be allocated to a group with two As and two Bs per group. The allocation sequence could be: 1. AABB; 2. ABAB; 3. ABBA; 4. BBAA; 5. BABA; or 6. BAAB. Block randomization is helpful when interim analyses are planned throughout the study duration because it ensures an equal balance between groups, thus not leading to disproportional group sizes and possible bias.[91] The disadvantage to this strategy is that the person who is responsible for treatment allocation can predict every fourth sample. To counter this effect, the allocator may hide the block size from the executer and use randomly mixed block sizes (e.g., 2, 4, 6).[88]

Although most trials have an equal allocation of subjects, there are times when an unequal allocation (e.g., 2:1 ratio of treatment to control) is used.[89] If cost is a factor, an unequal allocation allows randomization to favor the least expensive trial arm and more patients to be included in the study. There are also times in which unequal randomization is favored when a new technology or treatment is available. Allocating more patients to the new treatment/technology will allow clinicians to find out more about the newer technology in relation to the existing technology. If prior research indicates that a high incidence of adverse effects are observed with one of the therapies in the study, investigators may use an unequal randomization allocation to spare this group from additional adverse effects in the study. In addition, if a higher dropout rate is expected in one group versus another, an investigator may opt to have more subjects in one group compared to another.[81] Allocating more subjects to the intervention group also allows additional subjects to receive the presumed "beneficial" treatment option. Readers should keep in mind that unequal allocation of subjects in studies may predispose the evaluation to bias and may reduce statistical power.[89] Investigators should provide a well-justified rationale for unequal allocation of study subjects.

Endpoints

Clinical trials measure some effect caused by the intervention and control in order to compare these groups.[8,29,82] All trials specify one effect caused by the intervention and control as the **primary endpoint**, which can be referred to as what the investigators measured to achieve the study objective. Since significant time, money, and effort are devoted to conducting a clinical trial, researchers usually measure **secondary endpoints** in addition to the primary endpoint. These secondary endpoints are important but not considered to be the primary purpose of the study. The selected primary endpoint should be a routine and useful measure for the study.[29,82] For example, a trial evaluating the cholesterol-lowering effect of an HMG coenzyme A reductase inhibitor compared to placebo selected a change in average LDL-C value, which is an appropriate measure for the primary endpoint to satisfy the study objective. Measuring the change in average triglyceride value may be a secondary endpoint. Measuring a change in serum creatinine between losartan and captopril to improve heart failure (HF) symptoms[83] is not ideal, since serum creatinine is not the predominant parameter used in practice to monitor the progression or improvement in HF status.

❻ *The primary endpoint of the controlled clinical trial should be appropriate for the study purpose and measured using valid techniques and methods.* Investigators may combine a group of endpoint measures into one primary endpoint, referred to as a **composite endpoint**. The group usually consists of clinical outcomes directly related to morbidity and mortality as opposed to a pharmacological action (e.g., reduction in any incidence of stroke/MI/cardiovascular-related death vs. lowering cholesterol levels). The investigators select a group of endpoints that can occur during therapy and are considered clinically important. For example, after experiencing an MI, a therapy is prescribed to reduce the occurrence of multiple adverse outcomes that may accompany an MI (e.g., reinfarction, death, hospitalization), not just one clinical outcome. The rationale for measuring composite endpoints is to increase power by examining several important endpoints at the same time rather than a single endpoint, which may be difficult to assess statistically because it occurs infrequently (e.g., death).[73,90]

The use of composite endpoints is not without debate.[73,90,92] In addition to reporting the composite endpoint, the results of the individual components of the composite should also be reported separately and analyzed.[90,97] Investigators may claim the investigational therapy is better than the control based upon the overall result of the composite endpoint, even though the investigational therapy was shown to significantly affect only one or a few (but not all) of the composite endpoint components. Also, the most important component of the composite (e.g., death) may not be affected by the intervention under study. Due to the issues of using composite endpoints, researchers are in the process of designing new methods to assess the individual components of the composite endpoint (e.g., assigning weights to each endpoint) to better gauge the clinical trial results.[96,97]

The following example explains some of the issues encountered with composite endpoints. The investigators of the Efficacy and Safety of Subcutaneous Enoxaparin in Non-Q-Wave Coronary Events (ESSENCE) trial used a composite primary endpoint, which consisted of death, MI (or reinfarction), or recurrent angina after 14 days of follow-up.[98] The incidence of the primary endpoint was lower with enoxaparin (intervention) than unfractionated heparin (control) (16.6% vs. 19.8%, respectively; $p = 0.02$) in patients with angina at rest or non-Q-wave MI. However, only one of the three components of the composite endpoint was significantly different with enoxaparin, recurrent angina (12.9% vs. 15.5%, respectively; $p = 0.03$).[98] As seen by the percentages, the majority of primary endpoint composite (~78%) consisted of this single event, which is the least robust of the three outcomes.[99] Although lowering the incidence of recurrent angina is clinically important, this outcome is not as severe as death or reinfarction. The composite endpoint effect of enoxaparin appears to be superior to heparin even though the incidence of two of the three components of the composite endpoint indicates no difference between these two drugs. Enoxaparin was considered to be a useful therapy in this patient type, but further research was recommended to determine if the therapy reduces the occurrence of death and MI in these patients.[100]

Endpoint definitions and valid measuring techniques need to be determined prior to the start of the clinical trial and incorporated in the study design.[7,29] By doing so, the investigators ensure consistent measurement of endpoints and reduce study variances or biases. To illustrate, the IMPROVE-IT trial primary endpoint was "a composite of cardiovascular death, nonfatal MI, unstable angina requiring rehospitalization, coronary revascularization (≥ 30 days after randomization), or nonfatal stroke."[45] If the reader is informed of the measurement types and methods under investigation, he/she may judge whether practical methods were used to measure the endpoints and determine if the study can be replicated by future investigators or by individuals wanting to implement the trial results into practice to actual patients. Endpoints involving human judgment (e.g., cause of stroke) may also contribute to the complexity of analyzing and interpreting study results if strict criteria or a blinded clinical events committee designed to produce valid recommendations are not incorporated and utilized during the trial.[107] Sponsors of clinical studies may elect to establish a blinded clinical events committee. This committee is responsible for reviewing endpoints in a clinical trial to determine whether the endpoints meet the criteria that were specified before the study.[93]

A final type of endpoint that may be seen is a surrogate endpoint. This will be discussed later in the chapter.

Follow-Up Schedule/Data Collection/Adherence

A study should be conducted for an appropriate duration, and data need to be consistently collected throughout the entire trial. A magical number of weeks or months has not been established as a rule for all clinical trials, but the length of the study (i.e., follow-up time) should be an ideal representation to answer the question being researched.[29] Statins usually exert the maximum cholesterol-lowering effect after approximately 6 weeks of stable dosing.[101] Thus, the results of a study directly comparing LDL-C reduction between atorvastatin 10 mg once daily and simvastatin 20 mg once daily for 6 weeks would be considered acceptable.[49] However, in this same example, if the primary endpoint of the trial was to determine whether atorvastatin or simvastatin was superior for reducing the incidence of MI, a much longer follow-up period would be needed because MI is an infrequent event.

A number of trials do not have an extensive follow-up time and the reader may have difficulty interpreting the results for clinical practice. For example, a study evaluated the efficacy and safety of liraglutide versus placebo over 12 weeks in patients with poorly controlled type 1 diabetes.[102] Although liraglutide caused a reduction in body weight and insulin requirements, the clinical effects and tolerability of the medication beyond 12 weeks could not be assessed due to the short duration of the trial. Since diabetes is a chronic disease and the duration of drug therapy will exceed 12 weeks,[103] a longer study duration would help address the long-term clinical effects of this drug in practice.

Monitoring trial results at predetermined intervals is important throughout the duration of the study. The Code of Federal Regulations and good clinical practice guidelines for clinical research state subject monitoring is required during the clinical investigation.[29] Larger trials may have a clinical trial investigator subgroup who serve as the data and safety monitoring board members. These individuals are blinded to subject groupings and are responsible for reviewing the results obtained while the trial is ongoing. Interim analyses of study results may indicate that the intervention produces either a favorable outcome or increased risk over the control before the established duration of the study has been completed. Typically, the protocol for discontinuing the clinical trial early is established prior to enrolling study subjects.[99]

If the study were discontinued because patients in the intervention group were experiencing significant harm compared to the control group, subjects randomized to the intervention would be at greater risk for experiencing the harmful events if the trial was allowed to continue. Conversely, if the intervention was shown to be more beneficial than the control, the investigators would be denying useful therapy to those subjects randomized to the control if the trial continued.

Prior to the start of the study, data collection methods are established to ensure incomplete follow-up by trial personnel and subjects at each follow-up time is minimized. In addition, investigators should ensure that trial personnel are properly trained and have sufficient resources to complete data collection.[104]

Another data collection and follow-up issue is measuring the adherence of therapy in study participants.[29] This includes medication dosage unit counts, serum drug levels, or regular follow-up communications (e.g., telephone conversations). Subjects not complying with the therapy regimen may cause inaccuracies and less reliable data. Insufficient and/or inappropriate data collection methods and nonadherence usually lead to biased results that may limit generalizability of results to clinical practice. On the other hand, a trial in which patients are extremely compliant with therapy may overestimate the benefits of treatment in a population that is unable to attain this level of compliance.

Sample Size

❼ *An appropriate* **sample size** *for a controlled clinical trial is vital for the study results to have any significant meaning; conducting a* **power** *analysis is important to determine a suitable sample size.* Sample size (denoted by the letter N) refers to the number of subjects randomized into a study and is of considerable importance to the validity of the study results. Financial and logistical limitations may prevent all subjects with the specific inclusion criteria from being enrolled into the study.[29] For example, investigators may want to evaluate a new drug to treat hypertension. It would be impossible to enroll all people around the world with hypertension into this clinical trial. In response, investigators will enroll a representative group (i.e., sample) of individuals from all those with hypertension (i.e., population). Researchers do not wish to include too few or too many subjects in the trial. Obviously, having only one subject in each group is insufficient to determine differences in effect between groups since chance alone may be the reason for a difference found (if any). On the other hand, having too many subjects can be excessive, costly, and may expose some subjects to unnecessary experimental treatment. The sample size should not be determined on the basis of convenience, arbitrarily, or by the number of easily recruited subjects.[94]

The number of subjects to enroll in a clinical trial is dependent upon the expected magnitude of difference (i.e., effect size) in the endpoint effect between the intervention and control. The effect size is estimated based on the results of previously conducted trials or other research assessing the intervention. In general, an inverse relationship exists between the sample size and the effect size. A large sample size is needed to detect a small difference in effect between the intervention and control outcome, while a smaller sample size can detect larger differences between groups.[111] For example, large sample size is needed to detect differences in blood pressure between two antihypertensive therapies (small difference in blood pressure reductions), while a smaller sample size is needed to measure the difference in relieving postoperative pain between morphine and placebo (large difference in pain relief).

Researchers use various procedures from table/charts to manual calculations to estimate the necessary sample size for a particular trial.[63,94] Regardless of the method selected, the sample size must be calculated prior to initiating the clinical trial. A study lacking a sample size calculation may be biased since the reader is not informed of the basis on which the investigators determined the number of subjects to enroll. The sample size must be calculated based upon the estimated differences in the primary endpoint between the intervention and control groups. For example, the IMPROVE-IT investigators[45] used a statistical model approach based on pooled blinded endpoint rates in previous trials; they assumed a mean absolute reduction of 15 mg/dL in LDL-C in the combination group (ezetimibe/simvastatin) would result in a 9.375% reduction in the primary endpoint incidence of CV death, major coronary events, or nonfatal stroke at 2 years.[105]

If investigators intend to measure differences for secondary endpoints, the sample size calculation for these endpoints needs to be included in the article. Larger sample sizes more reliably measure and detect a true difference in effect (if one exists) between the intervention and control.[95] Consequences of an insufficient sample size (i.e., too small or too large) are discussed later in the **Type I error** and **Type II error** section of this chapter and in Chapters 5 and 6.

The importance of an appropriate sample size is demonstrated in the following example. Investigators conducted a small study (51 patients) to compare renal plasma flow between fenoldopam mesylate to 0.45% sodium chloride infusion in patients receiving radiocontrast for angiography. The investigators concluded fenoldopam was a promising agent since fewer subjects receiving fenoldopam developed radiocontrast-induced nephropathy (RCN) at 48 hours than those treated with 0.45% sodium chloride infusion (21% vs. 41%, respectively).[112] One primary contributor to the large difference in results was the small number of subjects enrolled; the incidence of RCN is increased by 4% for each subject developing this outcome. Even though the percent difference was 20% (41% minus 21%), this represents a difference of only five subjects developing RCN. After the results of this large reduction in RCN were released, clinicians began to frequently administer fenoldopam to these patients.[106] However, the CONTRAST study (Evaluation of Corlopam in Patients at Risk for Renal Failure—A Safety and Efficacy Trial) was designed to determine if fenoldopam reduces RCN in patients after receiving iodine-based dye during cardiac angioplasty,[106] but this study had a much larger sample size (157 patients in the fenoldopam group and 158 in the placebo) compared to the previous study evaluating fenoldopam therapy. At 48 hours, RCN incidence was 19.9% versus 15.9% with fenoldopam and placebo, respectively. At 96 hours, the incidence was 33.6% versus 30.1%, respectively. Based upon the results of this clinical trial, the incidence of RCN was numerically higher with fenoldopam than placebo (but not statistically different). By conducting a study with a larger sample size, the treatment effect of fenoldopam was more accurately measured compared to the study of only 51 subjects.

Statistical Analysis

Within controlled clinical trials, the use of statistics is a means to analyze sample data and apply it to the population. Readers should be familiar with and have a basic understanding of the most common tests used in clinical trials. Some statistical analyses can be easily conducted using simple computer programs, while others require specialized training and extensive skill. Typically, a biostatistician is consulted as one of the trial investigators to assist in selecting an appropriate test and perform the statistical analysis.[96,107] However, even with biostatisticians evaluating the data, study results may be biased by using incorrect statistical analyses.[115]

The purpose of statistical analysis of the study data is to collect sufficient evidence to reject the null hypothesis (H_0) in favor of accepting the research hypothesis (H_A).[115,117] Appropriate tests are selected prior to the start of the study based upon the type of data that will be collected and analyzed. Readers must be able to identify different types of data before assessing the validity of a statistical test for a given controlled trial.

There are four types of data (see Table 4-5)[109]: **nominal**, **ordinal**, **interval**, and **ratio** (the latter two are usually referred collectively as continuous). Nominal data are

TABLE 4–5. TYPES OF DATA

Type of Data	Definition	Examples
Nominal	Categorical data Data placed in one category, but not more than one category	Yes/No; alive/dead; colors of cars in a parking lot into five categories of either red, white, blue, black, or other
Ordinal	Ranking, ordered	Likert scale; visual analog scale; pain scale
Interval	Data with measurable equal distances between points, but no absolute zero	Temperature in degrees Fahrenheit
Ratio	Data with measurable equal distances between points and an absolute zero	Temperature in degrees Kelvin, blood pressure, cholesterol levels, white blood count

categorical without any sense of order; these data only can be categorized into one of the possible groups (e.g., either dead or alive, but not both), hence mutually exclusive. Ordinal data (i.e., ranking) are categorical data with an intrinsic order but no equal intervals between units. Pain severity (or other type of subjective data) measured by a scale is a typical example of ordinal data. For example, a five-point pain scale with a score of 0 indicates no pain, while a score of 5 indicates severe pain. A one-point change in pain intensity on this five-point pain scale is not necessarily the same from one-to-two as from four-to-five on the scale. Interval and ratio data both have measurable and equal intervals between data points, but interval data have no absolute zero (e.g., Fahrenheit temperature) while an absolute zero point (e.g., white blood cell count) is a characteristic for ratio data. Identification of the type of data allows a reader to determine correct statistical tests were selected and that correct data collection methods were employed.

The type of data collected dictates the use of inferential or descriptive statistical methods. **Inferential statistics** (e.g., Student's t test, chi-square test) are used to draw conclusions based upon the sample, for the application of the trial results to the population.[116,117] In other words, data are analyzed to make a conclusion of the study results from the sample that is then extrapolated to the population. **Descriptive statistics** describe the characteristics of the sample (e.g., average subject age, baseline endpoint values, number of subjects with another disease present) and the results in some studies (e.g., X% had an adverse effect). Descriptive data are typically presented as measures of central tendency (e.g., **mean** [average], **median**, **mode**) and/or measures of variability (e.g., range, standard deviation, variance) (see Table 4-6).[118] Refer to Chapter 6 for further information on descriptive and inferential statistics.

A trial that measured change in LDL-C provides a good example to explain the terms in Table 4-6. Two-hundred subjects were enrolled in a clinical study to compare LDL-C reduction between simvastatin and placebo. The LDL-C is measured in all subjects at the

TABLE 4–6. DATA PRESENTATION METHODS

Type of Data	Mode	Median	Mean	Range	Interquartile Range	Standard Deviation
Nominal	X					
Ordinal	X	X		X	X	
Interval and Ratio	X	X	X	X	X	X

Note: Mode = most frequently occurring data point; Median = midpoint of the data (point at which 50% of the data lie above and the other 50% below); Mean = average of the data points; Range = officially the difference between the smallest and largest data point in the data set, although usually described by listing the smallest and largest data points (e.g., "The range is from 5 to 9"); interquartile range = difference between the scores at the 75th and 25th percentile; SD = degree in which individual data points deviate from the mean value of the data set.

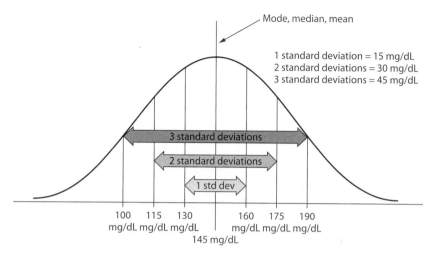

Figure 4–1. Histogram of LDL-C with standard deviation (SD) ± 15 mg/dL.

beginning of the trial. The values are then plotted using a histogram (see Figure 4-1). A mark is placed on the graph for each subject with a specific LDL-C value. Taller columns denote LDL-C values measured in a greater number of subjects whereas shorter columns denote LDL-C values measured less frequently in the sample. All plotted LDL-C values would form a bell-shaped curve (also known as a normally distributed data set) if the sample of subjects was randomly taken from the population. The values for the terms in Table 4-6 can be calculated after the investigators obtain all LDL-C values. As seen from the graph, the mode (most commonly occurring LDL-C value), median (point at which 50% of the LDL-C values lie above and below), and the mean (average) LDL-C are the same. The mean, median, and mode equal an LDL-C of 145 mg/dL. The range for the LDL-C values can be determined by identifying the lowest and highest LDL-C value. The data also can be organized into quartiles, four groups containing 25% of the data points. The data are arranged from the lowest to highest value; afterward, the data points are divided into four groups: 25th, 50th, 75th, and 100th percentile. Therefore, a LDL-C value that corresponds to the 75th percentile would be in the upper limit of this third quartile of the distribution. The upper limit of the 50th quartile would equal the median value for the data set. The interquartile range is the difference between the scores at the 75th and 25th percentile.[118]

Since many trials present the results as a mean, a more detailed discussion of this measure of central tendency is warranted. Using the LDL-C example, the mean LDL-C value is calculated using all the measured values. However, the mean does not inform the reader of the diversity in the set of values. Thus, a standard deviation (SD) is calculated using all of the LDL-C values. The SD is presented with the mean value of the sample (e.g., 145 ± 15 mg/dL, where the first number is the mean and the latter number is the SD).

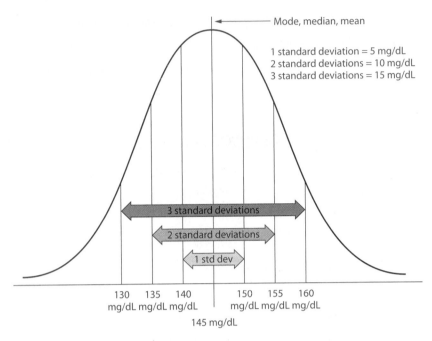

Figure 4–2. Histogram of LDL-C with standard deviation (SD) ± 5 mg/dL.

The SD describes the dispersion of LDL-C values around the mean and allows a difference to be observed between data samples with the same mean. Figure 4-2 displays a set of LDL-C values taken from a different sample of subjects. The mean LDL-C is the same as Figure 4-1, but the SD or spread of values is relatively narrow.

The presentation of the mean ± SD allows the readers to calculate the percentage of LDL-C values within portions of the graph. Figure 4-3 illustrates the distribution of LDL-C within one, two, and three SDs from the mean in a normally distributed data set. In normally distributed data, ~68% of the LDL-C values will be in ±1 SD, ~95% in ±2 SDs, and ~99% in ±3 SDs. Using Figure 4-1, the average LDL-C is 145 ± 15 mg/dL. Based upon these numbers, 68% of the LDL-C values are in the range of 130–160 mg/dL, 95% between 115 and 175 mg/dL, and 99% between 100 and 190 mg/dL. In Figure 4-2, the mean ± SD is 145 ± 5 mg/dL with corresponding values of: 140–150 mg/dL, 135–155 mg/dL, and 130–160 mg/dL, respectively. Notice that even though the mean body weight in both data sets is the same, 95% of the LDL-C values are in the range of 115–175 mg/dL in Figure 4-1 but between 135 and 155 mg/dL in Figure 4-2. The SD allows for the readers to assess more than just the mean for a set of data.

Although SD is commonly used, some investigators may present the standard error of the mean (SEM) which is calculated as the SD divided by the square root of the sample

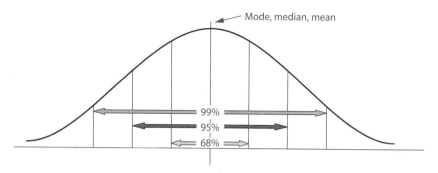

Figure 4–3. Histogram of normal distribution with standard deviations.

size (SD / $\sqrt{n}$).[117, 118, 120, 121] While standard deviation measures the deviation of the individual values from the mean of the sample, SEM measures the deviation of the individual sample means from the mean of the population.[117] The SEM identifies the variability in the population; 95% of the time, the true mean of the population lies within two SEM of the sample mean.[121] As seen by the SEM formula, the SEM is smaller than the SD which implies a smaller dispersion of the data points away from the mean. Investigators may present the SEM instead of SD so that readers observe a small dispersion of the data from the mean instead of a large variance seen with if the SD was presented. At times, SEM is used appropriately (more than one clinical trial), but it is most often used incorrectly.[121] Readers should be aware of these distinctions and interpret the data accordingly.

Inferential statistics are used to determine if a statistical difference is present between the intervention and control groups. A **p value** is calculated based upon trial results and statistical tests; afterward, the p value is compared to the **alpha (α) value** established prior to the beginning of the trial (see statistical significance vs. clinical difference later in this chapter for further discussion).[116-117] The selection of the statistical test depends upon a few factors, which include data being parametric (i.e., normal distribution) versus nonparametric, type of data (e.g., continuous, ordinal), and number of groups compared (see Chapter 6 for more details). Typically, continuous data are assessed via parametric statistics; common tests are Student's t test, analysis of variance (ANOVA), and analysis of covariance (ANCOVA). Nonparametric tests are used for nominal and ordinal data; examples are chi-square (χ^2) test and Mann-Whitney U test.[116,117] A multitude of other statistical procedures are available. An analysis of all research articles in six common pharmacy journals published during 2001 identified chi-square (χ^2) test, Student's t test, and analysis of variance (ANOVA) as the three most common statistical tests used.[127] Chapter 6 in this textbook is devoted to a more in-depth discussion of statistical analyses.

Other statistical terms encountered while reading clinical trials are independent versus paired and one-tailed versus two-tailed statistical analysis. A paired analysis compares the same subject to themselves or to a similar matched subject.[110, 117] For example, measuring the mean change in LDL-C from baseline to 12 weeks within the same subject receiving simvastatin would be a paired analysis. Analyzing the difference in mean LDL-C reduction after 12 weeks between a group receiving simvastatin and another receiving atorvastatin requires an independent test because the groups are independent of one another.

Two-tailed (also known as two-sided) statistical tests are used for trials in which investigators are not sure in which direction the primary endpoint will be affected by the intervention. These tests analyze results in both directions for positive or negative effects in comparison to the control.[95] Two-tailed tests are more common because the direction of change is not known prior to the analysis.[23,95] For example, a two-tailed test is used for an investigational drug compared to placebo to treat elevated LDL-C. The investigators do not know the effect of the intervention on the LDL-C levels (i.e., the levels can increase or decrease relative to the placebo). A one-tailed test is primarily used in a study in which the direction of the effect of the intervention and active control (e.g., another medication, but not placebo, such as a noninferiority study) are known or can only go in one direction. The intent of this study type is to more precisely measure the difference in effect between the two groups. Some investigators have used a one-tailed test to determine differences in LDL-C changes in patients receiving statins. Prior research has documented the effects of atorvastatin or simvastatin on LDL-C reduction compared to other medications or placebo. Since these research results are available, a one-tailed test could be used to increase the statistical accuracy of detecting a difference between the two statins in lowering LDL-C.

Type I and II Errors/Power Analysis

A clinical trial is conducted to test a research hypothesis that a difference in effect exists between the intervention and control treatments. Investigators develop a null hypothesis (H_0; no difference between the groups) and research hypothesis (H_A; a difference is present between the groups) before the trial begins. The trial is conducted and the investigators measure the difference in effect between the groups (if any). Differences observed between groups could be due to the intervention or happen by random chance (error).[108,115] Hypothesis testing is conducted to examine how likely any observed difference between the intervention and control is due to chance if the H_0 were true. As the trial results diverge farther and farther from the finding of no difference, the H_0 is rejected (i.e., failure to accept the H_0) between the intervention and control group.[108,115]

Two types of error are possible in hypothesis testing (see Table 4-7). A Type I error can occur when the H_0 is falsely rejected and the H_A is falsely accepted. In other words, the investigators are stating a difference in effect was measured even though there really is no difference between the intervention and control groups (also known as a false-positive

TABLE 4–7. TYPE I AND TYPE II ERRORS POSSIBILITIES

Error Type	Action/Decision	Interpretation
Type I	Statistical difference found even though it is not really present; Reject H_0	H_0 is really true, but was rejected, which leads to a false-positive result. The probability equals the α error rate. There is one reason for a Type I error: chance.
Type II	No statistical difference calculated, even though there is one. Fail-to-reject ("accept") H_0	H_0 is really false, should be rejected but was accepted, which leads to a false-negative result. The probability equals the β-error rate. There are two reasons for a Type II error: chance or small sample size.

finding).[95,118] On the other hand, a Type II error can occur when H_0 is falsely accepted and the H_A is falsely rejected. In this case, the investigators are stating no difference in effect is present between the intervention and control even though there really is a difference between the groups (also known as a false-negative finding).[95,118]

Investigators attempt to control for Type I and II error occurrence by setting limits on the probability of these occurring. The only reason that a Type I error can occur is by chance. Since no research is error-proof, methods usually are developed to allow up to an X% (typically 5%) probability that chance was the reason a difference in effect was measured between the intervention and control. The process of setting the probability of a Type I error (false-positive result) is termed as establishing the alpha [α] value.[95,104,118] The α is a measure of how willing the researchers are to accept the chance of making a Type I error.[115] This is also referred to setting the statistical significance to 0.05 but can also be phrased as setting the α at 0.05. Alternatively, trials may state that p values < 0.05 are considered statistically significant. Most clinical trials use an α of 0.05; however, a few trials may use a more conservative α of 0.01. This latter rate indicates the investigators are more stringent by reducing the possibility of a Type I error to 1%. However, setting $\alpha = 0.1$ is too relaxed and permits the Type I error possibility to be very high (at 10%). An α at 0.05 indicates that a difference in effect being measured between the groups can be due to chance in one of 20 trials.[104] An α of 0.002 indicates that a difference in the measured effect between groups can be due to chance in two out of 1000 trials. When researchers are interpreting the results of the study, they will compare the probability of making an error (p value) to the acceptable rate of error (alpha). Thus, the smaller the p values, the less likely that chance (error) was the reason for finding the differences. The p value can also be expressed as the probability of rejecting a true H_0.[116] This last statement will be explained in the statistical significance section later.

The probability of making a Type II error is referred to as beta [β].[95,111] Although investigators want to avoid a Type II error, appropriately designed clinical trials allow this error (false-negative) to occur no greater than 20% of the time.[111] Investigators attempt to balance the possibility of a Type I and Type II error knowing that decreasing the probability of one error may increase the probability of the other error occurring. Even though investigators want to avoid making both a Type I and Type II error, a Type II error is more acceptable than a Type I error for a few reasons. A Type II error may be easier to determine than a Type I error and may be identified by studies with no power analysis and/or too small of a sample size.[115] Type I errors have the potential of being more dangerous to patients (see next paragraph). Therefore, the α value is set lower than the β value.

Making a Type I error means a difference in effect was measured by chance but really no difference in effect exists between the two groups. The danger of using a therapy no different than the control is more serious when the control is a placebo versus an active therapy. A Type II error indicates no difference was measured between the two groups. If the control group is another therapy, then the intervention is shown to be no different. If the control is a placebo, then the intervention may not be considered an effective option to treat patients. Although the false-negative result is a concern (i.e., a useful therapy may be not used), this is less severe than a false-positive results (i.e., using a therapy that really is no different in effect than the placebo-control but was found to be different by chance).

A Type II error may occur by random chance or small sample size, the latter of which is usually the reason for the error.[95] The ultimate goal of each clinical trial is to ensure the difference in effect size is properly measured between the intervention and control groups, and this requires a sufficient sample size.[63] One method for the investigators to ensure a sufficient number of subjects are enrolled in the trial is by conducting a power analysis. The power of a study is defined as the ability to detect a difference in the outcome between the intervention and control if a difference truly exists. Power is calculated from the β-error rate (power = $1 - \beta$).[94,111] As seen from this formula, the lower the β-error rate, the higher the power. Increasing the sample size then reduces the β-error rate, increases study power, and reduces the chance of a false-negative result.[94] In addition, the magnitude of difference in the effect that can be detected between the intervention and control group is related to the sample size; smaller differences in the effect between the intervention and control can be detected with larger sample sizes.[94]

Estimating the absolute difference (δ) in effect between intervention and control is essential to ensure that the clinical trial has the power to detect differences.[12] This value is not as easily determined as the two other rates; the δ is usually based upon prior or preliminary research results or even consensus discussion among the researchers (i.e., educated guess).[94] As an example, the IMPROVE-IT investigators used prior research results to assume that the difference in the incidence of the primary endpoint between groups was 9.375%.[45]

The sample size needed is influenced by the α, β, and δ values. The purpose of the sample size calculation is to provide sufficient power to be able to reject the H_0 established for the clinical trial's primary endpoint.[63] Hopefully, a clinical trial with an appropriate sample size will not lead to an erroneously detected difference in effect when there is no real difference (Type I error) and also maintain a degree of certainty that the true difference in effect was not missed (Type II error).[104] In theory, a trial with an appropriate sample size increases the precision of estimating the difference in effect (effect size) between the intervention and control.[7] The total number of subjects completing the trial should be similar to the actual sample size calculation for the study to have appropriate power.[94] Normally, the investigators will increase the sample size by some factor above the number calculated to be necessary to account for subject attrition and therapy non-adherence (previous research can be helpful in determining that number). In addition, investigators can use the study results to conduct an after-the-study calculation to confirm that an appropriate sample size was included in the trial.

RESULTS

Clinical trial results are presented after the methods section. This section contains **primary** and **secondary endpoint** results and other useful information, which includes subject baseline characteristics, participant flow, data analysis procedure, and safety information. Critical appraisal of the section allows the reader to verify if the study objective was met and evaluate the other types of outcomes that may have occurred. Data are frequently tabulated or arranged in histogram or line graph format to provide readers a visual representation of results that may be minimally discussed within the text of the manuscript. Readers should carefully examine all charts and graphs paying close attention to the scale of the horizontal and vertical axis. The results of a controlled clinical trial should only be extrapolated to the patient type enrolled in the study, and readers should be aware of the limitations of surrogate endpoints and subgroup analysis results.

Subject Baseline Characteristics

The first type of information provided in the results section describes the subjects actually enrolled and randomized in the clinical trial.[9] A general overview of the average subject is described and usually presented in a table of demographic information.[131] Typical information in the table includes mean age, gender ratio, measures of disease severity, comorbid disease states, and/or drug therapy use among the study participants at the time of enrollment that could affect the interpretation of the primary endpoint. Any additional lifestyle factors that can affect the endpoint(s) or trial outcome(s) may also be described, such as the number of subjects who smoke, amount of caffeine intake, etc.

Subject baseline characteristics need to be compared between treatment groups to ensure the groups are as similar as possible. The groups should not have any significant differences if proper randomization techniques are incorporated by the study investigators, but a few differences can still occur due to chance.[7] Statistically significant dissimilarities between the groups that could contribute to differences in the study outcome should be closely scrutinized. If subject baseline differences are substantial, a confounding variable is present, and the study investigators must analyze the results to determine if the differences have affected the outcome of the study. Otherwise, interpretation of the study results may be flawed.

An example of baseline subject demographics is illustrated by select patient information from the IMPROVE-IT trial.[45] The simvastatin monotherapy and simvastatin-ezetimibe groups both had a similar number of males (75.9% and 75.5%, respectively) and subjects with a diagnosis of hypertension (61.3% and 61.6%, respectively). Mean age, ethnicity, and region of origin also were evenly matched. The disproportion of females and Whites enrolled in the study may be concerning to the beginning reader. However, it is more important in this study that no differences exist between the two groups. Sometimes the disproportion of gender enrollment in a trial reflects the true prevalence in the population at large (e.g., more males with cardiovascular disease). Nevertheless, for trials that involve disease states in which gender is not a prespecified risk factor, each group should consist of similar proportion of male and female subjects and not be skewed in one direction for any risk factor, as this sample-based anomaly could affect interpretation and application of study results.

Subject Dropouts/Adherence

Data describing subject follow-up (i.e., subject dropout or attrition) and adherence should be presented. Subjects randomized in a clinical trial may not complete the entire duration of the study, at which time they are then termed a study dropout or lost to follow-up. Reasons vary for discontinuing study participation and include lack of desire to continue, subject relocation (e.g., moving to another city), difficulty finding transportation to clinic visits, subject protocol violation, side effects, and death. Subjects may also be noncompliant with study therapies. Failure to account for the number of dropouts and subject nonadherence can affect interpretation of trial results.[128] As a result, the investigators need to report the number of subjects and major reasons for discontinuing the study, adherence rates, and the techniques of assessing the data for the readers to draw appropriate conclusions about the intervention under study and subsequent trial results. This information is typically presented in a flow diagram that outlines the original number of subjects who were assessed for study eligibility, the number randomized to receive treatment in each group, the number who actually received the intervention, the number who were lost to follow-up or discontinued treatment, and the final number of subjects who were analyzed in each treatment group.[13] All too often clinicians and industry personnel focus on the efficacy of a medication, but practitioners in particular should clearly analyze the costs of better efficacy in terms of patient safety. Dropout data can be very revealing about the overall tolerability of a medication and illuminate important safety risks associated with emerging therapies compared to conventional therapies. However, studies may not be adequately powered to observe differences in safety outcomes, and readers should cautiously draw conclusions about overall adverse effects because of this limitation.

The impact of attrition on overall study results is dependent on the magnitude of subject discontinuations. A few subjects dropping out of the study may not cause a substantial difference in the results, whereas a sizable attrition rate may significantly alter the study results. No threshold of dropout/attrition rates have been established that deem trial results to be of no clinical value. Similar to demographic information, attrition rates should be analyzed to ensure study groups are similar. Attrition rates of 60% among both groups of a clinical trial, although not ideal, are much less concerning than a study with disparate attrition rates of 10% in one group and 50% in the other. Disproportionate attrition rates can be an indicator of significant medication adverse effects that warrant further investigation, particularly if safety endpoints were not a primary endpoint of the study.

Frequently, the study results will be analyzed using data collected from all randomized subjects, regardless of whether they completed the entire study duration (i.e., results from dropouts are not discarded, but are considered to be treatment failures). This technique is referred to as the **intention-to-treat** (ITT) principle (see Chapters 5 and 6 for more on ITT and **per-protocol** [PP]).[113,132] Even in cases where a subject may not have taken one dose of the medication under investigation, that subject's data are still included in the ITT analysis (i.e., once randomized, always analyzed). The ITT analysis more accurately mimics real-life application of an intervention into practice because, similar to real-life, all subjects in a clinical trial may not complete therapy as prescribed.[128] However, a concern with the ITT analysis is that data from subjects discontinuing a trial early may bias the analysis. This is of considerable importance for endpoint measurements that worsen over time or require prolonged therapy to observe a difference. For measures that may worsen over time (e.g., cognitive function in subjects with dementia), the last score obtained in a subject discontinuing the trial early may suggest a better response than the last score obtained if this subject discontinued later in the trial.[125] For endpoints which require several months to years to observe a treatment effect (e.g., mortality in subjects with cardiovascular risks), early treatment discontinuation could bias study bias results toward a conclusion of no difference.

At times, the study results are analyzed via both ITT and the PP procedure. The latter term refers to analyzing data only from subjects completing the trial according to protocol (e.g., subjects who withdrew prior to study completion are excluded from analyses). The advantage of this technique is for determining the effects of the intervention in subjects that followed the study protocol and completed the entire course of therapy. The ITT and PP analytical methods are simply models under which the study results are analyzed. The ITT analysis can be thought of a worst-case scenario model, whereas the PP analysis can be thought of as a best-case scenario model. The ITT analysis is typically favored by clinicians and readers when analyzing results due to the desire to determine whether statistically and clinically significant differences are present between the two groups under worst-case scenario conditions. Such results are much stronger than demonstrating statistical or clinical significance under best-case scenario conditions as patients in the greater population are not completely adherent to prescriber instructions. Study investigators will ideally present both ITT and PP results; the desire is to see no significant differences between the ITT and PP results. If a significant difference exists, this can be an indicator of differences in attrition rates between treatment arms that are represented in the ITT analysis. Furthermore, clinical trials including only the PP results should be scrutinized more because, without an assessment of results from all subjects, treatment effects may be overestimated in favor of a treatment arm with high attrition rates.

An example of analyzing study data according to ITT and PP methods follows with a study that assessed the effect of caffeine therapy on the Epworth Sleepiness Scale (ESS) score in patients with Parkinson's disease.[126] This scoring scheme is based upon questionnaire responses to eight items and the perceived propensity of patients to fall asleep based upon theoretical situations (0 = no chance of sleeping, 3 = high chance of sleeping; total score range: 0–24). The primary ITT analysis indicated that caffeine 200 mg twice daily ($n = 30$) had no significant effect on ESS scores compared to placebo ($n = 31$) at 6 weeks (difference of −1.71 points; 95% CI −3.57 to 0.13). However, statistical significance was determined by PP analysis for the same endpoint and treatment (difference of −1.97 points; 95% CI −3.87 to −0.05) leading the investigators to conclude that caffeine therapy produces marginal but insignificant improvement in daytime sleepiness in patients with Parkinson's disease. The difference in results between the ITT and PP populations are tied to the exclusion of four subjects who violated study protocol (two in each group). This exemplifies that even very small and equal subject attrition or exclusion can significantly affect study results, particularly in studies with small sample sizes, and underscores the importance of analyzing both ITT and PP study results to make the most measured conclusions regarding treatment effect.

Endpoints/Safety

A critical component of the results section is the primary endpoint results. These results can be displayed as tables, graphs, or other illustrations. The information should be presented clearly and completely, using transparent and unbiased methods. Results should include the effect size for each group including its precision using 95% CIs.[13] Endpoints that are binary should be reported using absolute and relative effects. Results of secondary endpoints should follow and are presented in a fashion similar to the primary endpoints; however, endpoints other than the primary endpoint may not be adequately powered to detect differences between the intervention and control. Additionally, if statistically significant results do occur with secondary endpoints, the results may be due to chance as multiple comparisons (commonly referred to as multiplicity) may increase the risk of Type I error. Endpoints other than the primary endpoints should be adequately powered to draw meaningful conclusions regarding use in practice and are generally considered hypothesis-generating.

If a clinical trial allows medication dose titration, the medication doses received by subjects in the intervention and control group must be evaluated. Readers of a clinical trial should analyze the final doses in each group at the end of the trial. For instance, the final medication dose of one group may be maximized while the other group did not receive maximum doses, and this could lead the investigators to make a conclusion based upon misleading information. Ideally, both groups should have similar dose titrations at the end of the study instead of one group receiving near the maximum daily dose versus the other group not requiring much of a dose increase.

Safety assessments or tolerability of all therapies should be included in the results section.[9] Investigators need to implement valid methods of defining, collecting, and analyzing these results. As with the secondary endpoints, the study may not be sufficiently powered to definitively quantify the safety/tolerability of the intervention. In addition, the frequency and severity of these results may be dissimilar to those observed in clinical practice. Investigators need to monitor the subjects closely and collect these data.[114] Other factors to be considered include the equipotency of doses of medications being studied, clinical trial duration, sample size, and exclusion of selected subjects, particularly exclusion of persons who are otherwise qualified to be part of the study according to the inclusion and exclusion criteria.

Surrogate Endpoints

Investigators of some clinical trials select a primary endpoint that can be classified as a surrogate endpoint which is described as "a measure of the efficacy of a treatment defined as laboratory values (e.g., HDL-C/LDL-C), symptoms (e.g., pain), or clinical parameters (e.g., blood pressure) that are employed as a substitute for a clinical endpoint (e.g., morbidity, mortality)."[123] Surrogate endpoints should be extensively studied and predictive of or correlated with the expected clinical endpoint.[134] The primary reason that surrogate endpoints are selected for clinical trials is to quickly measure an effect at a lower overall cost.[135] The established efficacy and other data collected from trials measuring surrogate endpoints provide the rationale for larger trials with clinical endpoints (e.g., MI, stroke, death) which typically are more costly and time-consuming. In certain circumstances, conducting a study using surrogate endpoints instead of clinical endpoints may be more ethical, particularly if a placebo is being used as the control therapy. The following conditions should be fulfilled before a surrogate endpoint is considered a valid substitute for a clinical endpoint: convenience (easily and readily assessable); well-established relationship between the surrogate and clinical outcomes (e.g., hemoglobin A_{1C} and risk/severity of diabetes); and determination of clinical benefit because of changes in the surrogate endpoint.[135]

The primary limitation of surrogate endpoints is illustrated by the following example. Investigators of the ILLUMINATE trial reported a significant increase in mean HDL-C with adding the investigational agent torcetrapib to atorvastatin versus atorvastatin alone (+72% vs. +2%, respectively, $p < 0.001$), and this was accompanied by a change in mean LDL-C (−25% vs. +3%, respectively, $p < 0.001$) after 12 months of therapy.[129] One would expect these two changes in cholesterol levels to reduce the risk of cardiovascular events (e.g., nonfatal MI, stroke). However, the incidence of a major cardiovascular event was significantly higher in patients treated with torcetrapib than atorvastatin alone (6.2% vs. 5%, respectively, $p = 0.001$). Thus, beneficial surrogate endpoint results do not always translate into positive clinical outcomes.

Subgroup Analysis

Investigators often analyze the results of subsets of study subjects, as divided into various groups that often include gender, age, and presence of concomitant diseases or other complicating factors (e.g., diabetes vs. no diabetes). Reasons to analyze the results in these subgroups vary but usually relate to an assessment of treatment effect in these specific patient types as opposed to the overall trial results from all randomized subjects.

Although the investigators may be able to obtain more information from a trial by using subgroup analysis, limitations and other issues need to be recognized by the reader.[119,122,136] Subgroup analysis should be defined prior to the initiation of the trial (i.e., *a priori*) and have documented justification (e.g., past studies suggest a benefit in that patient group). Additionally, data analysis should only be conducted from those studies in which the primary endpoint was statistically significant; otherwise, investigators may be perceived to be on a fishing expedition, searching for statistically significant results.[137,138] Furthermore, the investigator may have conducted a multitude of subgroup analyses and only reported the statistically significant results. As the number of statistical evaluations on a data set increases, the likelihood of finding a statistical difference by chance alone (i.e., Type I error) increases. Therefore, multiple subgroup analyses on the same data set should be avoided, unless authors can demonstrate that they have powered the endpoint for the multiple analyses a priori and/or have adjusted error rates statistically to control for multiple comparisons. Study power is reduced with subgroup analyses, since results from a smaller number of subjects are analyzed as compared to the entire trial sample. Additionally, to avoid making invalid conclusions based on subgroup analyses, the ITT data set of the trial should be utilized to ensure that all dropouts are included for all treatment arms. Subgroup analyses can be helpful in determining future research targets, but, unless powered appropriately, should not be used as a basis for therapeutic decision-making.

Subgroup analyses may lead trial authors to report potentially misleading claims. According to an evaluation of clinical trials published during 2007, 41% of these trials reported claimed subgroup effects.[136] However, the credibility of the claims was low. An illustration of this effect was documented by the African-American Antiplatelet Stroke Prevention Study (AAASPS)[124] which was conducted in response to the subgroup analysis of Ticlopidine Aspirin Stroke Study (TASS).[140] The TASS investigators documented a lower incidence of nonfatal stroke or death from any cause in subjects with recent transient or mild persistent focal cerebral or retinal ischemia taking ticlopidine compared to aspirin (17% vs. 19%; $p = 0.048$). The investigators also reported fewer cases of stroke and death with ticlopidine compared to aspirin in a subgroup analysis of African Americans enrolled in this trial. However, the AAASPS results documented a slightly higher incidence of the composite endpoint (recurrent stroke, MI, or vascular death) in patients taking ticlopidine compared to aspirin (14.8% vs. 12.4%; $p = 0.12$). Although the study designs were not identical, the AAASPS results demonstrate the limitations of selecting therapy based upon subgroup analyses. Thus, although subgroup analysis may document greater benefits in selected individuals, the differences in effect may be due to chance or other factors.

Case Study 4–1[141]

The REDUCE-IT study evaluated whether icosapent ethyl, which had been previously shown to reduce triglyceride (TG) levels, would reduce the risk of ischemic events in patients with established hypertriglyceridemia. Eligible subjects were those who were $\geq$ 45 years old with established cardiovascular disease or $\geq$ 50 years old and had diabetes mellitus and one additional risk factor. Eligible subjects also had to have a fasting TG level between 150 and 499 mg/dL and fasting LDL-C level of 41–100 mg/dL and be on a stable dose of a statin for a minimum of 4 weeks. A protocol amendment later modified the lower limit of eligibility for baseline TG levels to 200 mg/dL.

REDUCE-IT was a randomized, double-blind, placebo-controlled trial. Subjects randomized to the intervention arm received icosapent ethyl 2 g twice daily with food. Subjects were enrolled into the study from 2011 to 2015 across 473 study centers in 11 countries. The primary efficacy endpoint was a composite of cardiovascular death, non-fatal MI, nonfatal stroke, coronary revascularization, or unstable angina. An independent committee blinded to treatment assignment reviewed and adjudicated all events. The authors planned subgroup analyses of the primary efficacy endpoint across a number of variables, including but not limited to: risk stratum, geographic region, sex, race, and age.

Of 19,212 subjects screened, 8179 were randomized with 4089 subjects receiving icosapent ethyl and 4090 subjects receiving placebo. Baseline characteristics between the two groups were similar; median age was 64, and 28.8% of subjects were female. The median follow-up was 4.9 years.

At the close of the study, significantly fewer cardiovascular events occurred in subjects randomized to icosapent ethyl compared to placebo using the intention-to-treat principle. The primary efficacy endpoint occurred in 17.2% of subjects taking icosapent ethyl and 22.0% of subjects taking placebo (HR 0.75; 95% CI 0.68–0.83; $p < 0.001$). For the subgroup analysis, 19.3% of subjects in the secondary-prevention cohort taking icosapent ethyl experienced the primary endpoint versus 25.5% of subjects taking placebo in this cohort (HR 0.73; 95% CI 0.65–0.81) whereas 12.2% of subjects in the primary-prevention cohort taking icosapent ethyl experienced the primary endpoint versus 13.6% of subjects taking placebo in this cohort (HR 0.88; 95% CI 0.70–1.10). The p value for the difference in primary endpoint between the secondary prevention and primary prevention cohorts was 0.14.

1. This study used the intention-to-treat principle in its statistical analysis. What is the benefit of using this method of analysis in this study?
2. Identify the individual outcomes within the composite primary efficacy endpoint, and define the term "composite endpoint." What is a potential benefit and drawback of a composite endpoint?
3. The authors of the study estimated 7990 patients were necessary to achieve 90% power to detect a 15% lower risk of the primary composite endpoint in the treatment group versus the placebo group. If the authors had sought 85% power instead of 90% power, how would that have affected estimated sample size? What would happen to estimated sample size if the investigators decided to detect of 10% lower risk of the primary composite endpoint with icosapent ethyl? Justify your responses.
4. Interpret the primary endpoint's p value in terms of probability.
5. In this study, the authors perform many subgroup analyses. What are the advantages and disadvantages of subgroup analyses? What does the comparison of the secondary-prevention cohort versus the primary-prevention cohort tell us about the role of icosapent ethyl in the treatment of hypertriglyceridemia?

Ancillary versus Adjunctive Therapies

Clinical trials are designed to have almost identical groups with the only difference being the assignment to the intervention or control. At times, the study design may allow **ancillary therapy** to be included, in which subjects can take another therapy that can distort or confound study results.[62] The effect of the ancillary therapy on the study results needs to be assessed and included in the study evaluation. Readers should not confuse ancillary therapy with **adjunctive therapy**. All participants of a study receive an adjunctive therapy while an ancillary therapy may not be equally distributed between the intervention and control groups. Any significant difference in treatment effect between the groups should be due to the therapies under investigation and not an ancillary therapy. For example, a clinical trial investigated the effect of cinnamon extract on glycemic markers in patients with diabetes.[130] Study subjects received either cinnamon extract or placebo; all subjects were taking an adjunctive sulfonylurea agent each day. Although sulfonylureas can lower blood glucose levels, all subjects in the trial received this therapy. Since therapy to control blood glucose should not be withheld in patients with diabetes, the use of a sulfonylurea in this trial was appropriate and use was similar between the two groups. However, ancillary therapy would occur if patients were allowed to take any other agent that could alter blood glucose levels at their own discretion resulting in a difference between the two groups. This would introduce another difference between groups, besides one group taking the intervention and the other taking the control. If ancillary therapy is permitted within a clinical trial, study results should report the specific medications used, as well as the number of subjects in each group who used the medications.

Clinical Trial Result Interpretation

Statistical Significance versus Clinical Difference

❽ *Correctly interpreting p values is crucial to evaluating a controlled clinical trial; not all statistically significant p values are clinically important. The magnitude of difference in effect between the intervention and control cannot be determined with the p value.* Once the clinical trial is completed, the investigators calculate a *p* value for the endpoints using the collected study results and statistical tests. The *p* value is an abbreviation for probability value and is comparable to the alpha (α) value established prior to the beginning of a clinical trial. Alpha is the benchmark to which *p* values are compared to determine if statistical significance is present. A *p* value for the primary endpoint that is less than the α value indicates that the H_0 is rejected and a statistically significant difference is declared between the intervention and control groups. This also indicates chance alone was not likely the reason that a difference in effect was measured. The H_0 is accepted (failed to be rejected) when a *p* value equal to or greater than α is reported, and no statistically significant difference is declared.[108]

Statistical significance does not necessarily imply that there is a clinical difference in effect between the intervention and control groups.[135] (See next section regarding the assessment of clinical difference.) The reader needs to decide when determining if the intervention is worth using instead of the control therapy, and this is often dependent upon the judgment and experience of the reader (i.e., assessing both internal and external validity). Not all statistically significant studies have clinically different results (see Figure 4-4). A *p* value less than α only represents the probability that a true H_0 has been rejected. In other words, the *p* value answers the question, "What is the probability that the difference in effect between the intervention and control is due to chance?"[115] Alternatively stated, "What is the chance of observing this difference if there really was no difference between the two groups?"[95] Lower *p* values indicate a lower probability that chance alone could be the reason a difference in effect was measured between the intervention and control. Recall that a Type I error is possible after rejecting the H_0; the results may be statistically significant due to chance alone. Thus, the *p* value represents the probability of a Type 1 error for any given statistical comparison.

Another paramount issue in understanding clinical trials is that the *p* value does not express the *magnitude* of difference in the effect between the intervention and control.[108] Statistically significant results simply signify that the H_A is accepted. The H_A states a difference in the effect is present between the intervention and control. From this information, the reader cannot determine complex quantitative differences in effect (i.e., clinical difference between intervention and control groups).[95,116]

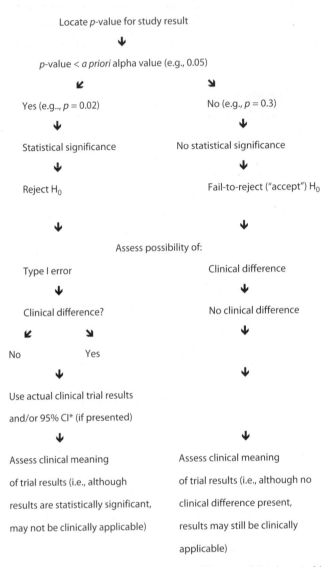

Figure 4–4. Determining statistical significance, clinical difference, and clinical meaningfulness.
* 95% Confidence Interval.

Specific p values should be stated in the text of the article (i.e., $p = 0.0012$ instead of $p < 0.05$) to be more informative and helpful to the reader.[95, 108] All p values should be presented in conjunction with associated endpoint results (i.e., investigators concluded that drug A lowered mean DBP more than placebo, -12 mmHg vs. -3 mmHg, respectively [$p = 0.001$] as opposed to investigators who concluded that drug A lowered mean DBP more than placebo [$p = 0.001$]). Readers should scrutinize study data that presents p values without endpoint results (naked p values). Such a situation should prompt the reader to ask if endpoint results were excluded because the magnitude of the difference in effect was minimal. Without the endpoint results being presented, statistical significance alone can be concluded with the p value; however, clinical differences cannot be assessed without accompanying endpoint results. See next sections for further discussion of this issue.

Assessing Clinical Difference

Two critical items needed to assess clinical difference between the intervention and control groups of a clinical trial are the p value and actual study results used to calculate the p value. A fundamental first step to determining clinical difference in a given trial begins with determining if statistical significance exists (i.e., $p <$ a priori alpha value) (see Figure 4-4). Clinical difference is predicated on statistical significance. In other words, clinical difference between the intervention and control cannot exist with study outcome data if the results are not statistically significant. The second step in assessing clinical difference is evaluating the results used to calculate the p value. The reader must analyze the magnitude of endpoint difference between the intervention and control results.[95,135] Once a reader determines that statistical significance is present with study data, no magical formula is available to conclude whether clinical difference exists between the intervention and control.[108] The remainder of the process is based upon clinical knowledge and experience. Determination of the presence of a clinical difference is based on the reader's opinion and clinical judgment. For example, an antihypertensive therapy lowers mean DBP by 14 mmHg versus 3 mmHg with placebo in subjects with a mean baseline DBP of 98 mmHg. In this case, the results are clinically different due to mean difference of 11 mmHg, and subjects are achieving goal DBP values from baseline (<85 mmHg). However, atorvastatin lowering mean LDL-C by 1.7% greater than simvastatin (37.1% vs. 35.4%; $p = 0.0097$[49]) cannot be considered clinically different in subjects with a mean baseline LDL-C of 181 mg/dL. The mean LDL-C was reduced by <2% with atorvastatin compared to simvastatin, a difference that most likely is not associated with effecting change in a clinical endpoint.

Some readers may consider the trial results to be clinically different while others may not. In fact, two people may have different conclusions after reading the same clinical trial. This situation is very common when interpreting clinical trials in health care practice. In response, readers must justify their own conclusion for or against a clinical difference. A few suggestions and examples are provided to assist in determining clinical difference.

Understanding the instrument that was used to measure the endpoint is important when assessing if there is a clinical difference between the intervention and control group in a clinical trial. Ordinal data typically use scales or ranking (e.g., pain, depression scales),[109] so understanding the minimum and maximum numbers on these scales is necessary to interpret data and determine if a clinical difference is present. For example, investigators of a hypothetical clinical trial may conclude that glucosamine sulfate 500 mg three times a day reduced pain greater than placebo in men with osteoarthritis (OA) of the knee. Assume that the pain intensity difference at rest was assessed using a 11-point visual analog scale (0 = no pain; 10 = worst pain imaginable) and that the authors chose an *a priori* alpha of 0.05. At the end of the trial, the median scores were 3.3 with glucosamine versus 3.6 with placebo ($p = 0.03$).[126] Although results were statistically significant between glucosamine and placebo, the magnitude of the difference in scores between groups is minimal at only 0.3 points on an 11-point scale. Stating that there is a clinical difference between glucosamine and placebo would be considered incorrect.

The effect of sample size on power must be considered when assessing for a clinical difference. Clinical trials with too large of a sample size (i.e., overpowered) may lead to smaller p values compared to those with smaller sample sizes.[94,108] The magnitude of the p value is dependent upon sample size; small differences in effect can be statistically significant with a large sample size.[95] Thus, statistically significant results can occur even though a small absolute difference in effect is present. An example of this issue is a clinical trial that compared esomeprazole ($n = 2624$) to lansoprazole ($n = 2617$). The primary endpoint—incidence of erosive esophagitis healing—was statistically significant in favor of esomeprazole (92.6% vs. 88.8%; $p = 0.0001$).[142] The investigators (and marketing advertisements) concluded esomeprazole is superior to lansoprazole, even though the absolute difference in healing was only 4% between these two drugs. In addition, a significant number of subjects in each group (>88%) experienced erosive esophagitis healing.

A data assessment technique that can be misleading is converting a continuous endpoint measure into a dichotomous value. One example involves a study that compared blood pressure (continuous variable) between rofecoxib (which was later withdrawn from the market) and celecoxib. Subjects with a blood pressure above a predefined cut-off point were classified as hypertensive. The variable was nominal data because subjects had a blood pressure either below or above this cut-off point. Significantly more subjects taking rofecoxib were diagnosed with systolic hypertension compared to celecoxib (17% vs. 11%, respectively; $p = 0.032$). However, when SBP was compared as a continuous variable, the change in mean SBP values was +2.6 mmHg versus −0.5 mmHg, respectively ($p = 0.007$).[143] Assessment of the two data sets together indicate that the magnitude of change in SBP caused by rofecoxib may not be clinically different from celecoxib. The actual SBP in the subjects taking rofecoxib may have just exceeded the cut-off hypertensive value (increase > 20 mmHg with absolute value > 140 mmHg) while it was just below this value for celecoxib (i.e., 141 mmHg vs. 139 mmHg, respectively). The absolute difference between these two blood pressure values was minimal (2 mmHg), but the number of subjects counted as hypertensive was more substantial (6%). The change in SBP between these two medications did not appear to be clinically different. Even though the measured endpoints between subjects randomized to the intervention were numerically close to the control, the subjects were categorized differently based upon cut-off blood pressure values. Thus, this form of data analysis and presentation introduces a potential source of bias into study results.

The foundation for determining clinical difference between an intervention and control is the p value and the magnitude of the study results. Other items that can assist the reader in this endeavor include 95% **confidence intervals** and calculating measures of association; both of these are described below. However, readers must remember that not all clinical trials may have these latter two items. Thus, the importance of analyzing and interpreting p values and the magnitude of difference between the intervention and control cannot be overemphasized.

Confidence Intervals

Many clinical trials include 95% CIs with the study results. ❾ *The use of 95% confidence intervals can assist the reader in assessing the magnitude of difference in effect between the intervention and control.* CIs provide information on the size of effect (e.g., mean reduction in DBP) of the intervention under investigation by presenting a range that likely covers the true but unknown value.[133,144] Although the basis of accepting or rejecting the H_0 rests upon the p value, a limitation of the p value is that the magnitude of difference in effect between the intervention and control groups of a clinical trial is not known, since it is not able to be determined based upon a statistical calculation.[123] The use of a CI can assist in judging the clinical usefulness of the study result.[128]

Clinical trials report the effect of an intervention as a point estimate, a single value that represents the effect determined in a particular trial (e.g., mean reduction in DBP). However, since this number is an estimate, the "true effect" may be a little higher or a little lower. For instance, if an angiotensin converting-enzyme (ACE) inhibitor lowered mean DBP by 8 mmHg, this value would be termed the point estimate. If the study was repeated, a similar, but not exact, reduction in mean DBP may occur (e.g., -10 mmHg, -12 mmHg). The presentation of the results only as a point estimate provides the reader with limited information. Clinical trials presenting 95% CI in conjunction with the point estimate enables the readers to determine the range of possible values for the treatment effect and further critique study results.

A CI provides an indication of the outcome within the population and is interpreted as a range of values in which the "true value" likely exists. The 95% CI for a mean is calculated using the standard error of the mean (SEM) from the trial sample. Recalling the formula for SEM, the standard deviation is divided by the square root of the sample size ($SD / \sqrt{n}$). A 95% CI is equivalent to approximately two SEMs from the sample mean, with an exact formula of: $CI = mean \pm 1.96 \times SEM$. The SEM is used instead of the SD because SEM is more reflective of population variance while SD is indicative of the dispersion within the sample.[108,144] A 95% CI is not the only CI reported in the literature, and readers of clinical trials need to recognize how this changes data interpretation. A 99% CI indicates more confidence that the true, but unknown, endpoint value is within this range compared to a 95% CI. Thus, the 99% CI range is wider than a 95% CI whereas a 90% CI range is narrower (i.e., less confident).[145]

A 95% CI for a point estimate is the most common method of data presentation. To illustrate using another example—investigators of a clinical trial reported that the mean reduction in DBP with an ACE inhibitor was −11.3 mmHg (95% CI, −14.4 to −8.2 mmHg) in subjects with a mean baseline DBP of 99 mmHg. This indicates that the investigators are 95% confident that the mean DBP reduction in the population is between −14.4 and −8.2 mmHg. The further away a value is from the point estimate within the 95% CI range, the lower the probability that this value is representative of the given population. Therefore, there is a lower probability for the mean reduction in DBP at the upper and lower end of the 95% CI range compared to numbers near the point estimate value.[117] A low probability exists that the ACE inhibitor lowers mean DBP in the population by only 8.2 mmHg compared to a higher probability that mean DBP reduction is closer to the point estimate of 11.3 mmHg. The same is true with the upper end of the 95% CI.

Within this same trial, the effect of the ACE inhibitor on DBP was compared to hydrochlorothiazide (HCTZ), and the mean DBP reduction with HCTZ was −9.9 mmHg (95% CI, −13.3 to −7.5 mmHg). The same principles are used to interpret this 95% CI as with the ACE inhibitor 95% CI; the investigators are 95% confident that the mean reduction of DBP in the population with HCTZ is between 7.5 and 13.3 mmHg. In addition, these two 95% CI ranges can be compared to determine any difference in effect between the two agents—ACE inhibitor and HCTZ. Since both 95% CI ranges (−11.3 to −8.2 mmHg and −13.3 to −7.5 mmHg) overlap considerably, no difference in effect between them can be concluded.[95,108] However, if no overlap of the 95% CI for the two groups were present (i.e., −11.3 to −8.2 mmHg for ACEI and −4.4 to −3.4 mmHg for HCTZ), then a clinical difference between the agents could have been concluded.

A 95% CI for the difference of point estimates between two groups may also be calculated and presented in a trial. In the above example, the point estimate of mean DBP reduction with the ACE inhibitor was −11.3 mmHg while it was −9.9 mmHg for HCTZ. The difference in mean DBP between these two equals −1.4 mmHg (−11.3 minus −9.9 = −1.4 mmHg). The 95% CI for the difference in the point estimates is calculated to be −3.9 to +1.1 mmHg. This is interpreted as being 95% confident that the difference in mean DBP reduction can be 1.1 mmHg greater with HCTZ (i.e., −13.1 mmHg for HCTZ vs. −12 mmHg for ACE inhibitor) or 3.9 mmHg greater with the ACE inhibitor (i.e., −16.9 mmHg for ACE inhibitor vs. −13 mmHg for HCTZ). Notice the upper end of the 95% CI of the difference in point estimates is a positive number (+1.1 mmHg). This does not indicate the mean DBP was increased, only that the *difference* in mean DBP lowering was 1.1 mmHg greater with HCTZ compared to ACE inhibitor (i.e., −12 minus −13.1 mmHg for ACE inhibitor and HCTZ, respectively). Also, if the number zero (value of equality for a difference in continuous variables) were included within the 95% CI, this would indicate with 95% confidence that there is no difference in mean DBP between these two groups (i.e., −13.2 minus −13.2 mmHg for both agents equals zero). If zero had not been within the 95% CI of the difference between the two point estimates, then a statistical difference in effect between the intervention and control could be concluded.

It is important to note that the "value of equality" depends on whether the data is a fraction or a subtraction. For example, if the RR—or any other type of data summary involving a fraction—(see next section) was calculated for a clinical trial and an accompanying 95% CI was presented, the number might look like this: RR 1.5 [95% CI 1.2–1.7]. In this instance, we would not want to see the value "1" within the CI because that is the value of equality for a fraction. That is, "1" is the number that indicates no difference between the groups.

The interpretation of clinical difference using 95% CI is dependent upon clinical experience and appropriate assessment. A 95% CI without a zero in the range does not always indicate a clinical difference between the intervention and control. For example, a 95% CI for mean DBP lowering in a trial comparing an ACE inhibitor and HCTZ was −1.9 to −0.5 mmHg. Even though this 95% CI range does not contain a zero, a mean difference of only 0.5–1.9 mmHg would not be considered clinically different.

Interpreting Risks and Number Needed to Treat

Another technique to critique and interpret clinical trial results is to calculate the measures of association: relative risk (RR), relative risk reduction (RRR), absolute risk reduction (ARR), and number needed to treat (NNT). ❿ *Calculating measures of association (RR, ARR, RRR, NNT) for nominal data provide further information to interpret controlled clinical trial results.* However, these calculations can only be performed with clinical trials designed to determine if there is a reduction in an outcome that occurs with modification of a risk factor when comparing the intervention to the control. Examples of outcomes could include the incidence of MI, stroke, hospitalization, or death. Since the endpoint is nominal and dichotomous (i.e., occurred or did not occur), the results can be set up in a table, as illustrated in Table 4-8. As seen from Table 4-8, the subjects randomized to the intervention experiencing the outcome are represented by "A," and those not

TABLE 4–8. PRESENTING NOMINAL DATA STUDY RESULTS

Group	Did an Adverse Event Occur?	
	Yes	No
Intervention	A	B
Control	C	D

experiencing the outcome are designated as "B." Subjects assigned to the control group who experience the outcome are designated by "C" while those who did not are designated as "D."[147]

Table 4-9 displays the formulas to calculate measures of association values and provides a description of each calculation. A description of interpreting these values follows. The RR is calculated as the proportion of the intervention group experiencing the outcome divided by the proportion of the control group experiencing the event. An RR equal to 1 indicates no difference between the intervention and control (i.e., the incidence of the outcome was not increased or decreased with the intervention compared to control). Anytime a numerator divided by a denominator calculates to 1, these two variables are equal. The RR < 1 signifies the intervention lowered the risk of the outcome compared to the control (i.e., protective effect); a lower proportion of the intervention group experienced the outcome compared to the control. An RR > 1 indicates the intervention increased the risk of the outcome; a greater proportion of the intervention group had the outcome compared to control. As an example, an RR of death equal to 0.70 was reported in a clinical trial in which subjects were randomized to either simvastatin ($n = 2221$) or placebo ($n = 2223$).[71] The RR was calculated by dividing the proportion of the subjects who died taking simvastatin ($n = 182$) by the proportion of those who died taking placebo ($n = 256$). The calculation of RR for this trial is: $(182/2221)/(256/2223)$. The RR of 0.70 indicates simvastatin lowered the risk of death by almost one-third of the baseline risk compared to placebo.

RRR indicates the relative change in the outcome rate between the intervention and control groups. For the aforementioned results, the RRR can be calculated using the following formula: ([control event rate (CER) – experimental event rate (EER)]/ CER) * 100%. This is sometimes reduced to 1 – RR. In both instances, the number would be 30%. The risk of experiencing death was 30% lower by treating these subjects with simvastatin instead of placebo.

ARR refers to a reduced outcome rate between the intervention and control groups. In contrast, absolute risk increase (ARI) refers to an increased risk of the outcome in question between the intervention and control groups. A higher proportion of subjects taking placebo died ($n = 256$ of 2223 or 11.5%) compared to those taking simvastatin (182 of 2221 or 8.2%). The ARR for death associated with simvastatin in this trial equals 3.3% (ARR = 11.5% – 8.2%); thus, 3.3% of the subjects receiving simvastatin were spared death compared to placebo.

The NNT of this study is calculated by taking the reciprocal of the ARR. In this case, it equals 30 (NNT = 1/0.033), meaning 30 subjects need to be treated for a median of 5.4 years with simvastatin instead of placebo to prevent one case of death. It is important to note the time period when reporting NNT. In this case, the trial had a median follow-up time period of 5.4 years.

Many clinical trials present an endpoint as a relative change, which can be a misleading value. For instance, the RRR of stroke associated with atorvastatin was 48% compared to placebo in this study. Although this value appears very beneficial to subjects at risk for stroke, the ARR may lead the reader to a different conclusion than the RRR value. The actual incidence of stroke was 1.5% (21 of 1428 subjects treated with atorvastatin) versus 2.8% (39 of 1409 subjects treated with placebo), which calculates to an absolute difference of 1.3% (ARR). Even though almost 50% less subjects (a relative difference) experienced a stroke with atorvastatin, this represents only a difference of 18 subjects in a group of just over 2800 subjects.[149] Thus, RRR may be a hyperbolic presentation of treatment effect compared to control.

All four measures of association can be calculated for clinical trials measuring nominal data, and they can be assessed together for the reader to determine the clinical difference in effect between the intervention and control. As seen by the simvastatin example above (Table 4-9), the same study result (e.g., death) can be presented using four different methods, each of which imparts different meanings. However, readers should not be misled by clinical trials that only present and discuss one of these values, which usually is the most appealing value (i.e., the one that seems to show the greatest difference). In fact, studies have documented that practitioners are more inclined to select a therapy when results are presented as RRR than if the same study result was presented as all four values (i.e., ARR, RR, RRR, NNT).[150] Thus, investigators may be biased and selectively present the most appealing of these four values to mislead the reader into concluding a greater difference in effect among the intervention and control, even though the difference may be minimal.

The same method for interpreting RR and associated CI can be used to interpret HR, which refers to whether the hazard of the adverse event (e.g., MI, hospitalization) is lowered or increased with the intervention compared to the control.[151] When interpreting RR (and HR), a calculated value of 1 signifies that the incidence of the adverse event is equal between the intervention and control (i.e., numerator and denominator are equal).[128] As previously mentioned, an RR < 1 signifies the intervention lowered the risk and an RR > 1 indicates the intervention increased the risk of the adverse event compared to the control. Therefore, investigators of a clinical trial presenting an RR (or HR) with a 95% CI that lies entirely on one side of 1 (i.e., up to 0.99 or 1.01 and upward) indicates a difference in effect between the intervention and control. The 95% CI range for death in the simvastatin study was 0.58–0.85[71] which means investigators are 95% confident that the RR associated with simvastatin is between 0.58 and 0.85 for the population. Since 1 (the number of equality) is not in this range, the investigators are 95% confident that the RR of experiencing the adverse event is reduced with simvastatin (i.e., statistical difference in effect).

Using another example, the calculated HR for the primary endpoint of coronary heart disease (CHD) was 1.82 with a 95% CI of 1.49–2.01. This information indicates that

TABLE 4–9. MEASURES OF ASSOCIATION DESCRIPTION AND FORMULAS[148]

Measure of Association	Description	Formula
RR (Relative Risk)	The ratio of risk of an event occurring in one group compared to another group.	[A / (A + B)] / [C / (C + D)] In other words, (% of intervention group with primary endpoint) / (% of control group with primary endpoint)
RRR (Relative Risk Reduction)	Percent of baseline risk removed The difference in event rates between two groups, expressed as a proportion of the event rate in the untreated group	1 — RR
ARR (Absolute Risk Reduction)	Percentage of subjects treated with the intervention spared the adverse outcome compared with the control	[C / (C + D)] — [A / (A + B)] In other words, (% of control group with primary endpoint) – (% of intervention group with primary endpoint)
ARI (Absolute Risk Increase)	Percentage of subjects treated with the intervention who experienced the adverse outcome compared with the control	[C / (C + D)] — [A / (A + B)] In other words, (% of control group with primary endpoint) – (% of intervention group with primary endpoint). The resulting calculation is typically a negative number.
NNT (Number Needed to Treat)	Number of subjects needed to be treated to prevent one adverse event. A time course is included that represents the mean (or median) duration of follow-up during the trial	1 / (ARR)
NNH (Number Needed to Harm)	Number of subjects needed to be treated to prevent for one adverse event to occur. A time course is included that represents the mean (or median) duration of follow-up during the trial. The value is referred to as NNH when the ARR is calculated as a negative number (i.e., ARI)	1/ (ARR)

the investigators are 95% confident that the risk of CHD is increased with the intervention versus placebo in the population since the HR is >1. However, a 95% CI containing the value of 1 indicates that the intervention may have neither lowered nor increased the risk (or hazard) of the adverse event. For instance, a HR for death due to other causes was calculated as 0.92 (95% CI, 0.74–1.14). The 95% CI range lies on both sides of 1 and indicates the risk of death could be lowered to 0.74 or increased to 1.14 with the intervention. Thus, the investigator (or reader) would conclude that the intervention is not statistically different than placebo in decreasing or increasing the risk of death.

No Difference Does Not Indicate Equivalency

● Remember, study results are not automatically clinically different when the p value is less than α. Clinical studies reporting p values greater than α translate into no statistical significance; thus, no clinically significant effect is declared between the intervention and control group. The H_0 is accepted (fail to be rejected) and the H_A is rejected.[114] The H_0 is written to state that no difference exists between the intervention and control. ⓫ *Nonstatistically significant results do not equate to the intervention and control being the same or equal.* The lack of a statistical difference could be due to a Type II error from random chance or a small sample size. In this latter instance, the clinical trial may not have been powered sufficiently to detect the difference. Usually, clinical trials in which the H_0 is accepted have too small of a sample size.[115]

Some studies may even be designed with an insufficient sample size so the investigators may claim equivalence between the intervention and active control after rejecting the H_0 even though a trial with an appropriate sample size could detect a difference. For instance, a study comparing the blood pressure–lowering effects of a new ACE inhibitor to a highly prescribed ACE inhibitor may use a small sample size to obtain study results that are not statistically different. Unfortunately, some readers may incorrectly conclude both ACE inhibitors are equivalent. This situation can occur in biased articles and/or presentations. However, the correct interpretation is that no difference was detected between groups. In other words, "absence of evidence is not evidence of absence."[94]

Assessing the Clinical Relevance of the Results

⓬ *All controlled clinical trial results need to be assessed to determine the clinical relevance of the intervention versus control.* In other words, what do these results mean to practice? Small treatment effects and/or differences may be statistically different but not lead to changes in clinical outcomes.[50,73,95] For example, in one study, an antihypertensive medication lowered mean DBP by 5 mmHg versus 2 mmHg for placebo ($p = 0.04$). The H_0 was rejected due to a statistical difference. However, mean baseline DBP was 98 mmHg, and this antihypertensive medication only lowered mean DBP to 93 mmHg, which is still classified as hypertensive.[139] Thus, practitioners would consider these results to be not clinically meaningful. Even though the results are statistically significant, the effect of the treatment was not useful to treat patients with hypertension.

Case Study 4–2[146]

VERO was a randomized double-blinded, double-dummy study that compared subjects taking 20 μg daily of subcutaneous teriparatide and once weekly oral placebo to subjects taking 35 mg once weekly of oral risedronate and daily subcutaneous placebo injections. The target population for the study included postmenopausal women older than 45 years of age who had a T score ≤ 1.50 standard deviations at the femoral neck, total hip, or lumbar spine. The screening period for subjects was 4 weeks, followed by a 24-month study period. The primary endpoint was new vertebral fracture. A number of secondary endpoints were studied as well, and they included, but were not limited to: new and worsened vertebral fracture, pooled clinical fracture, and nonvertebral fragility fracture.

In total, there were 683 subjects randomized to each treatment arm, and 680 subjects in each arm who started treatment. A total of 1013 (74.2%) of subjects completed the study. At 24 months, the incidence of the primary endpoint of new vertebral fractures was 5.4% in the teriparatide group and 12.0% in the risedronate group ($p < 0.0001$). In addition, the incidence of new vertebral fractures appeared to be significantly lower in the teriparatide group than the risedronate group as early as 12 months into the study period (3.1% vs. 6.0%, respectively; RR 0.52; 95% CI 0.30–0.91; $p = 0.019$). A number of secondary endpoints appeared to significantly favor teriparatide as well. There were no statistically significant differences in serious adverse drug events between the treatments; however, subjects in the teriparatide group experienced significantly more adverse events than those in the risedronate group included, but not limited to: pain, dizziness, and hypercalcemia.

1. This study employed double-dummy blinding. What is double-dummy blinding and was its use necessary?
2. The study was performed in 123 study centers across 14 countries in Europe, South America, and North America. Comment on the impact of this on external validity and internal validity of the results.
3. Calculate the RR for new vertebral fracture (primary endpoint) for the teriparatide group versus the risedronate group and interpret the value.
4. Calculate RRR for new vertebral fracture (primary endpoint) for the teriparatide group versus the risedronate group and interpret the value.
5. Calculate the ARR for new vertebral fracture (primary endpoint) for the teriparatide group versus the risedronate group and interpret the value.
6. Calculate the NNT for new vertebral fracture (primary endpoint) for the teriparatide group versus the risedronate group and interpret the value.
7. Interpret the hazard ratio and 95% CI for the secondary endpoint of first nonvertebral fragility fracture. (Assume teriparatide is the intervention and risedronate is the control.) HR 0.66; 95% CI 0.39–1.10.

DISCUSSION/CONCLUSION

The primary purpose of the discussion/conclusion is to evaluate and/or interpret the results of the clinical trial. This section typically begins with a summary of the key findings of the study, followed by potential explanations of the results, focusing on the internal and external validity of the outcomes.[9] The investigators should present an unbiased summary and interpretation of the results. A well-written discussion section should also include an analysis of how the trial results compare to other similarly designed studies as well as a critical analysis of the trial's limitations. Finally, an assessment of the clinical relevance of the clinical trial results and how they should be used in practice is beneficial to the reader. All this information allows the reader to understand the application of the clinical trial results in practice. The discussion/conclusion section of an article needs to be critically evaluated just as carefully as the other sections. No new information from the clinical study should be presented in this section that has not been presented elsewhere in the article and the author should not use biased wording.

Readers should determine the extent to which the study results compare with patients encountered in clinical practice. One of the most commonly cited criticisms of clinical trials is the lack of external validity of the results; this may be one explanation for the underuse of reportedly favorable treatment options in clinical trials by clinicians.[138] Although some investigators may report beneficial results of an intervention under investigation, the patient population in the clinical trial may be so dissimilar to patients encountered in practice that clinicians are not convinced that the favorable results will be beneficial in patients they treat. Several issues may potentially affect the external validity of a clinical trial and should be evaluated to assess the effects of the results in practice. These include the setting of the trial, selection of patients, characteristics of randomized patients, differences between the trial protocol and routine practice, outcome measures, follow-up, and adverse effects of treatment.[138] If the characteristics of the patients and setting are very different from those encountered in practice, the clinical usefulness of the reported information may be questionable.

All clinical trials have limitations which may vary from minor to those that seriously hinder the usefulness of results or completely invalidate the study. Potential limitations may include small sample size, short duration of follow-up, or use of an instrument that has not yet been validated or used extensively in clinical practice. The investigators should address methods to circumvent trial limitations in subsequent clinical studies. There is no minimum or maximum number of limitations that investigators should address; a thorough discussion of the limitations should be provided so that readers can determine the applicability of the trial results to their patient population.

The investigators should compare the current study to previously published studies relevant to the topic. According to the results of one study, discussion sections of trial reports were lacking complete analysis of previous clinical trial results.[119] A total of 33 randomized trials were identified in 19 issues of leading medical journals (e.g., Annals of Internal Medicine, JAMA). The authors of four reports claimed that their study was a first-of-a-kind study; however, reports of similar trials were located for one of these studies. In three of the reports, systematic reviews of earlier trials were mentioned; however, no attempts to incorporate the results of the new trial with the existing results were identified in the remaining 27 reports. The results of other trials should be included to allow the reader to assess the results of the current trial in context with previous trial results. The readers can determine if the study is a first-of-a-kind study that adds substantial information to a topic or is a "me-too" study that adds no new information to existing knowledge. The discussion section should also address future concerns and unanswered questions.

BIBLIOGRAPHY

References are a very important part of the manuscript. The reference or bibliography section is typically at the end of the manuscript and provides documentation to support the information provided in the manuscript or acknowledgment for the work of other authors.[33] Any material an author uses in the manuscript should have an appropriate citation. References should be recent and complete. Outdated articles should not be used unless the results of the article are pertinent to the manuscript. Readers should scan the references listed in the bibliography to determine if the authors used material from reputable sources. In addition, authors should refrain from extensively citing their own work.[154] References should be listed only once and typically are listed in numerical order as each appears in the manuscript. However, several referencing styles exist and are journal-dependent (refer to Appendix 13-3 for further information about referencing). At minimum, the information in the reference section should be sufficient to lead the reader to locating the same article. With electronic publication, reference numbers throughout the text will appear as hyperlinks to the references. For this reason, many publishers will request that weblinks and/or the direct-object identifier (DOI) be included at the end of the citation. Publishers of biomedical information may also request a PubMed identification number (PMID). Weblinks to the reference should be provided following the page number. The information should be listed in the following order: the phrase "Available from" followed by a colon, a space, and then the URL. A period should follow the URL only if it ends with a slash; otherwise, no punctuation is used. If the full content is not freely available (e.g., subscription only), the author should use the most accurate URL to lead the reader to the content. If the URL length is disrupting to the formatting, the URL may be separated by placing a space after a hyphen or slash in the address.[155] Readers use the references to verify the cited information and to locate additional references on a topic.[33]

ACKNOWLEDGMENTS

Individuals contributing to the clinical trial, but who do not meet the requirements for authorship, can be recognized in this section (see Chapter 13 for more information). Many journals have a prespecified amount of space for the acknowledgment section to which authors must adhere. Persons identified in this section may be those providing manuscript preparation, technical assistance, or donors of equipment or supplies. Medical writers or editors also may be listed if their contributions significantly strengthened the clarity of the content. A collaboration or group may receive recognition in the acknowledgment section. Authors must obtain written permission from persons acknowledged before listing in this section so readers do not infer endorsements of the data and conclusions from these contributors.[17,33]

Other types of information, such as financial support (see below for further information) and conflicts of interest, can also be included in this section. This can help the reader identify or reconcile sources of bias. Indicators that the manuscript underwent peer review, signified by a series of dates and titled received/revised/accepted, may also be included in the acknowledgments section. Typically, at least 4–8 weeks are between these stages since it is necessary to allow time for the reviewers to comment and the authors to revise and receive another review of the manuscript. Some journals only present the manuscript acceptance date which allows readers to determine the lag time between publication and article manuscript acceptance by the journal. A minimal time between the acceptance and publication date is beneficial since this increases content currency.

FUNDING

⑬ *Controlled clinical trial investigators and authors should disclose any funding sources and potential conflicts of interest.* Due to the enormous expense often required to conduct a clinical trial, investigators may seek financial assistance to conduct the research. Various funding sources are available that include pharmaceutical companies, government agencies (e.g., National Institutes of Health [NIH]), national organizations (e.g., American Heart Association), university grants (e.g., faculty development grants), and private donations. Although financial disclosure by industry and investigators is recommended, this may not occur. In 2010, the Patient Protection and Affordable Care Act (also known as The Sunshine Act) "required that pharmaceutical and medical industry manufacturers disclose their financial relationship with physicians."[156] Reporting of payments by pharmaceutical companies to physicians has been assessed in numerous studies. In general, reporting is difficult to evaluate because pharmaceutical companies and journals may have different financial-disclosure thresholds for what is considered a significant monetary payment; there can be variability in required reporting timeframes (distinct vs. unspecified); disclosures may differ depending on whether the requirement is a listing of *all* financial relationships versus those that are related to the research topic being evaluated; and there are inconsistencies in the categories of relationships (e.g., speaking, consulting, research, travel, expert witness) and how to report other nonmonetary support (e.g., meals, continuing education, gifts).[156] One study that evaluated the agreement between pharmaceutical disclosure and author self-disclosures for payments over $10,000 found that authors and industry only disclosed 19% and 12% of payments, respectively.[156]

During 2015, an estimated $58.8 billion was spent by the pharmaceutical companies for research and development including clinical drug trials. Current estimates indicate that the cost to develop a new medication is $2.6 billion, and only 12% of medications that make it into phase I clinical trials are deemed safe and effective enough to be approved by the FDA.[158] The pharmaceutical industry is responsible for a significant amount of the clinical research conducted worldwide, and new medications have reduced morbidity and mortality and improved quality of life for various disease states. Thus, readers of industry-sponsored research should not automatically disregard a clinical trial solely based upon a pharmaceutical company sponsoring the research. Readers should be cognizant of possible **conflicts of interest** defined as, "a set of conditions in which professional judgment concerning a primary interest (such as a patient's welfare) tends to be unduly influenced by a secondary interest (such as financial gain),"[159] that may result in potential bias. Conflicts of interest may arise because the industry may be prompted to publish articles as a means of making their product appear better for a disease state in relation to the standard of care. This research may result in methodological bias, premature termination of trials for nonscientific/unethical reasons, or reporting/publication bias.[160]

To counter this, investigators are encouraged to promote objectivity by designing studies that have clear methodology with outcome measures that are transparently reported to minimize different interpretations.[161] Many journals now include a funding and conflicts of interest section in the methodology of the manuscript. The role of the funding source in the design of the study, collection and analysis of data, and the interpretation study results should be included in this section. Further, this section should state whether the investigators made the decision about publication of the data and the role the investigators had in writing, editing, and approving the manuscript. The International Committee of Medical Journal Editors (ICMJE) has adopted a disclosure form for all their member journals to obtain financial associations of the authors submitting manuscripts. The form is posted on the ICMJE website (http://www.icmje.org/disclosure-of-interest/).[162]

The study design, results, data presentation, and conclusions should be assessed appropriately by the reader to determine if the funding source had any influences on the overall clinical trial. Pharmaceutical companies need to determine the clinical usefulness of newly developed medications, but they are also expected to profit from the new medication being approved by the FDA and marketed to prescribers. Pharmaceutical companies typically design a clinical trial according to FDA-approval standards (e.g., FDA Guidance for

Industry documents). However, the methods of presenting (i.e., results section), interpreting (i.e., introduction and/or discussion sections), and summarizing the data and results (i.e., conclusion) can be biased and are not governed by the regulations of the FDA. The reader is responsible for evaluating the quality of the research. Not all investigator-pharmaceutical industry relationships have the potential to cause a conflict of interest, but readers should decide if a publication is intentionally or unintentionally biased.

Unfortunately, there have been reports in the literature of selected pharmaceutical companies terminating studies for various reasons unrelated to efficacy or safety,[163] employing inappropriate comparators,[164] using inappropriate study samples,[165] and suppressing the results of negative studies.[166] Failure to publish study results based on the direction or strength of the study findings is known as **publication bias**.[167] This type of sponsored research usually yields larger treatment effects than not-for-profit funded studies.[73]

Trial registration with an official government entity is another method for the reader to discern if publication bias exists in favor of a particular interventional therapy. Specifically, the national clinical trials registry (http://www.clinicaltrials.gov)[168] hosted by the NIH is a very useful resource for the reader to determine if potentially negative study results are being excluded from discussion in clinical trials or promotional materials. The Food and Drug Administration Amendments Act of 2007 (also known as FDAAA 801) mandates registration and reporting of results from clinical trials utilizing certain drugs, biologics, and devices, regardless of study outcome.[169] ClinicalTrials.gov indexes more than 224,186 federally and privately funded clinical trials conducted in the United States and more than 192 countries. Furthermore, this resource provides the user details about a trial's purpose, guidelines for participation, study locations, and contact information for more details. This website can be searched by a variety of functions, including investigational agent or disease state. With this in mind, the national clinical trials registry is also a very useful tool for the practitioners who may need to identify treatment options for a patient unable to afford conventional intervention or who has a rare or terminal disease state and is seeking additional treatment options.[170]

COMMENTARIES/CLINICAL TRIAL CRITIQUES

Every journal should provide its readership the opportunity for correspondence to exchange ideas about a topic or relay new information about articles published in the journal.[17,33] **14** *Editorials, letters to the editor, and commentary publications can assist in interpreting controlled clinical trial results.* Commentaries can be essential in assisting readers with interpreting and/or critiquing articles published within journals by providing an analysis of strengths and limitations of the original research, an update to published information, or questions to the authors of the original research manuscript.

Editorials, defined as, "a written expression of opinion that may reflect the official position of the publication,"[33] are short essays from the editor or other experts in a particular field written to convey additional opinions about an article, typically, in the same issue of a journal. Editorials may not reflect the ideas/thoughts of the journal because these are opinions of the editorial author. Although editorials may contain bias, they may also provide insight into trial results and aid in the comprehension and clinical application of trial results. For instance, an editorial in response to IMPROVE-IT discussed many issues ranging from the large discontinuation rate (42%) in the groups, despite the fact that therapy for hyperlipidemia is long term, to the addition of other agents to lower LDL-C levels in combination with statins, potentially producing the same effect.

Several issues should be considered during the preparation or evaluation of editorials. Quality editorials are original; those editorials with nonoriginal ideas need to include a clear justification of why these ideas need repeating. The editorial objective should be clearly presented and reflect a complete message. The content should be significant to merit publication, applicable to practice, accurate, and thorough. The editorial points should be timely with respect to the publication in which the author is responding. Finally, the editorial author should state the facts clearly, and the material should be applicable to the readership of the publication.[152]

Original research reports are not necessarily accompanied by an editorial. Persons seeking an editorial associated with a clinical trial can locate one with a few methods. First, the journal issue that contains the clinical trial will list the editorial title in the journal issue's table of contents. Although not always present in clinical trials, a notation may be printed on the first page of the article referring the reader to another page (i.e., "For comment, see page..."; "Commentary, page ..."). Readers without access to the actual clinical trial or journal issue's table of contents can locate the trial citation in PubMed® (http://www.pubmed.gov) using the Single Citation Matcher. Those clinical trials with an accompanying editorial will contain a notation of Comment and an abbreviated journal citation (i.e., journal name, date, plus volume, issue, and page numbers). A reader may also search the clinical trial topic (i.e., via Medical Subject Heading [MeSH] term in PubMed®) and limit the search to the publication type of editorial.

Some journals/websites are published for the primary purpose of providing editorials/commentaries addressing published clinical trials. These resources are known as secondary journals and are independent of the journals that directly publish clinical trials.[19,49,171] Secondary journals assist busy practitioners by keeping them current regarding important and relevant studies and present key study information in a concise format. Clinical trials are usually presented in the format of a structured abstract instead of just copying and pasting the exact abstract prepared by the trial investigators. The prepared abstracts may present additional and/or more precise information. In addition, a commentary addressing the study strengths, limitations, and application into practice is authored by a leading practitioner in the field of study. Readers may find these resources helpful while critiquing the biomedical/pharmacy literature.

Examples of secondary journal websites include http://www.theheart.org and http://www.medscape.com. Typically, these publications provide an overview of the study followed by a commentary. Medscape is particularly useful for medication-related content since pharmacy-specific topics are addressed in a section of this website. ACP Journal Club is an online resource included in issues of Annals of Internal Medicine in which biomedical literature (i.e., original research, systematic reviews) is selected based on predefined criteria and summarized by an expert in the field in the form of structured abstracts followed by a commentary. More than 130 journals are reviewed and are selected due to their potential impact on clinical practice.[172] Another example is the New England Journal of Medicine (NEJM) Journal Watch, an online resource that is published at least monthly in print[173] and daily on the Internet. Updated information for over 10 specialty areas of medical practice obtained from over 250 medical journals and other vital medical news sources is provided by physicians with a commentary to help clinicians determine the impact of the research results on their practice.[173] Several specialty editions of Journal Watch are available including Journal Watch Cardiology, Journal Watch Emergency Medicine, Journal Watch Gastroenterology, and Journal Watch Infectious Diseases.[174]

Letters to the Editor

Letters to the editor can provide valuable insight on original research. These may be in the form of comments, addenda, or updates from previously published articles; alerts regarding potential problems in practice; observations/comments on trends in medication use; opinions on trends; or controversies in therapy or original research. Authors of letters to the editor must adhere to strict guidelines from journals regarding the length; number of authors, tables, and references; and format of the publication.[157] The primary content of letters to the editor is feedback from journal readers regarding previously published materials in the journal. Typically, these letters are published within 3–6 months of the original publication. The letters may disagree with the design, result interpretation, and/or conclusions of the publication. Letters may also request additional information that can be used to interpret, clarify, comprehend, and/or critique the information within the publication. Afterward, authors of the original publication may provide a response to published letters. The letters to the editor can serve as another source of valuable information or perspective for those using and critiquing the biomedical literature.

Specialized Types of Controlled Clinical Trials

NONINFERIORITY TRIALS

Description

Randomized controlled clinical trials are utilized to determine one of three different outcomes between comparative drugs: superiority, equivalency, or **noninferiority (NI)**.[175] All three trial designs involve a new test drug compared to an accepted active control or standard of care. In the case of superiority trials, as with many examples previously discussed in this chapter, the comparator is often placebo. The aim of a superiority trial is to determine that a drug is superior to a comparator.[176] In contrast, equivalency trials are designed to determine whether the new drug is therapeutically similar to the control and is used primarily to determine bioequivalence between two drugs. NI trials seek to show that any difference between two treatments is small enough to conclude the test drug has "an effect that is not too much less than the active control"[177] also referred to as the reference drug or standard treatment.[177-179] This section will focus on description, interpretation, and evaluation of NI trials.

There has been a dramatic increase in publication rate of NI studies since 1999.[178] Along with this increase, an understanding of several potential study design issues has become apparent including choice of reference drug, determining inferiority of the intervention, and optimal analytical approaches. Each issue requires rigor in design and conduct of these trials.[182,183]

An NI study design is often considered when superiority of a test drug over a reference drug is not anticipated.[184] In this case, the objective is showing the test drug to be statistically and clinically not inferior to the reference drug based on efficacy. The test drug could offer other potential advantages related to safety, tolerability, convenience, or cost. These ancillary benefits can justify use of the test drug to replace standard treatment if the intervention is deemed noninferior. NI trials are also considered when the use of a superiority trial would be unethical.[177] For example, it is unethical to use a placebo when there is available effective treatment that possesses an important benefit, such as preventing death or irreversible injury to the patient. For this reason, NI trials may provide an alternative method to superiority trials for meeting USFDA marketing approval requirements.[177] Between 2002 and 2009, 14% of approved New Drug Applications (NDAs) contained evidence from pivotal NI trials.[187] The percentage of NDAs using NI trials is likely higher now. Rather than going through the process of showing a new drug is therapeutically superior to the reference drug treatment or a placebo, pharmaceutical companies are choosing to use an NI design. This is a developmental strategy to confirm that the new drug has a valid therapeutic effect and that the drug's effect is not worse than the reference drug.[188,189] Often the anticipated key differentiating factor for the test drug in this situation is improved safety. For example, a new drug for cardiac arrhythmias is anticipated to have similar efficacy but fewer serious side effects than the standard treatment. It should be noted that NI design is not recommended when the reference drug treatment effect is not consistently superior to placebo (both statistically and clinically).[170]

Establishing the NI Margin

The NI margin is an important component of an NI trial and is a prespecified value used to determine if the test drug's treatment effect is not worse than the reference drug by more than this specific degree.[188,190] In other words, the NI margin is the extent to which the test drug's therapeutic effect can be less than the reference drug, but still be considered not worse.[192] For instance, if the reference drug's minimal treatment effect is a 5-mmHg decline in DBP compared to placebo, then the test drug could not be worse than this 5-mmHg reduction to be considered noninferior to the reference drug. If the results from the NI trial showed the test drug's treatment effect to be 4 mmHg, then the test drug would be considered potentially inferior to the reference drug.

A combination of statistical reasoning and clinical judgment is required to determine the NI margin.[183,204] The FDA guidance document defines the NI margin as the largest clinically acceptable difference (i.e., degree of inferiority) of the test drug compared to the reference drug.[177] Methods to determine the NI margin have been proposed; however, concern exists with the subjectivity and potential bias associated with any method that relies on an indirect comparison of historical data rather than a true placebo arm built into the NI study.[174,181,195,196]

A simple method to determine the NI margin is to look at the CI for the reference drug treatment effect (reference drug – placebo = treatment effect). This treatment effect is best determined from examining the historical reference drug versus placebo-controlled trials. A meta-analysis of several historical placebo-controlled trials is preferred over separate evaluation of individual studies to obtain the most accurate and representative overall treatment effect.[186] The CI around the mean reference drug treatment effect is used to establish the NI margin (see Chapter 6 for further understanding of CIs). The lower bound of that CI represents the smallest expected reference drug treatment effect. For example, if the CI around the mean reference drug treatment effect is 3–14 mmHg DBP, then the lower bound of that CI would be 3 mmHg. This lower bound can be used to set the NI margin; however, since a 3-mmHg DBP reduction may be considered marginal, a 5-mmHg change in DBP could be considered the smallest clinically significant change. Given this information, the NI margin can be set at 5 mmHg, but a more conservative NI margin would be 3 mmHg. Treatment effects are often small in placebo-controlled cardiovascular trials, and researchers want to preserve adequate treatment effect in NI studies.[180] To account for this, cardiovascular outcome trials often use 50% of the lower bound of the CI of the difference between the reference drug and placebo as the NI margin.

Contrast this with antibiotic trials in which treatment effects are often large between reference drugs and placebo. NI margins in antibiotic NI studies often range between 10% and 15% of an absolute risk difference.[180]

Interpretation of Results

The NI design focuses on the mean treatment difference between the test drug (intervention or new treatment) and the reference drug (comparator or standard treatment) (see Figure 4-5).[188] To determine NI, the CI around the mean treatment difference between the test drug and the reference drug is compared against the NI margin. If the CI around the mean treatment difference does not include or cross the NI margin, then the test drug is noninferior to the reference drug (see Scenario A in Figure 4-5). If noninferiority is determined, three assumptions may be made: (1) test drug exhibits noninferiority to the reference drug; (2) test drug performs better than placebo, if placebo were included as a comparator group; or (3) test drug may offer ancillary benefits and these could include safety, tolerability, convenience, or cost.[185] However, the test drug would be determined inferior if the entire CI around the mean treatment difference was located on the inferior side of the NI margin (see Scenario B in Figure 4-5). Conversely, and although there is some controversy to this discussed later in this section, the test drug could be determined

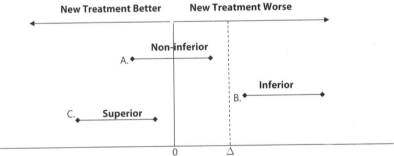

Figure 4–5. Noninferiority trial results scenarios.
Error bars indicate two-sided 95% confidence intervals (CIs) of the treatment difference between the new treatment (intervention) and standard treatment (comparator).

- Scenario A: The upper limit of the 95% CI of the treatment difference does not exceed the noninferiority margin (Δ); however, the 95% CI includes 0. Therefore, the new treatment appears to be noninferior to the standard treatment in this scenario.
- Scenario B: The entire 95% CI of the treatment difference exceeds the noninferiority margin (Δ) and lies in the "new treatment worse" zone. Therefore, the new treatment appears to be inferior to the standard treatment in this scenario.
- Scenario C: The entire 95% CI of the treatment difference lies in the "new treatment better" zone, and the 95% CI does not include 0. Therefore, the new treatment appears to be superior to the standard treatment in this scenario.

Adapted from Piaggio et al.[197]

superior if the entire CI around the mean treatment difference did not include 0 and therefore fell in the "new treatment better" zone (see Scenario C in Figure 4-5).

For example, an NI study of a new antihypertensive agent (test drug) compared to reference drug is published in the literature. The overall treatment effect of the reference drug compared to previous placebo-controlled studies is a 12 mmHg (CI 6–15 mmHg) reduction for a sitting DBP. The lower bound of that CI, or some percentage of that lower bound based on consideration of the clinical significance, can be used to establish the NI margin. In this case, the lower bound of the CI is 6 mmHg, a treatment effect that may be considered a clinically significant difference in sitting DBP. Given this, the NI margin is established as 6 mmHg sitting DBP. In other words, when the NI trial is completed, the test drug's lower bound of the CI associated with the mean treatment difference cannot include or cross the set NI margin of 6 mmHg on the graph (see Figure 4-6). If the test drug's lower bound of the CI includes (or crosses) the NI margin, this would suggest that the test drug failed to exhibit noninferiority to the reference drug (see Scenario A in Figure 4-6). This situation would be considered an inconclusive result unless the entire CI for the mean treatment difference is located on the inferiority side of the NI margin of 6 mmHg, confirming inferiority. Upon completion of the example antihypertensive NI study, the actual results confirm noninferiority of the new antihypertensive agent. The lower bound of the CI interval for the test drug treatment effect does not include (or cross) the NI margin (see Scenario B in Figure 4-6).

If an NI margin and/or CI are not provided, then noninferiority can still be determined if an α and p value have been given. To use p values for this purpose, there must be an understanding that the statistical rationale for NI trials differs from superiority trials.[180,198] Specifically, defining parameters for the null and alternative hypotheses (see previous section in this chapter and Chapter 6) are different from those used with superiority

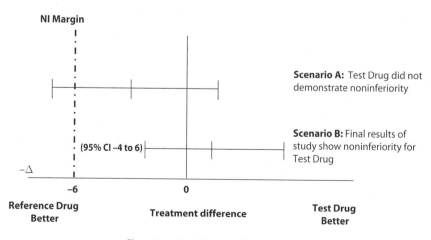

Figure 4–6. Noninferiority trial design example.

TABLE 4–10. DIFFERENCES IN DEFINING PARAMETERS FOR NULL AND ALTERNATIVE HYPOTHESES

Type of Trial	$p \geq 0.05$ ($\alpha = 0.05$) (not statistically sig) Fail to reject the H_0	$p < 0.05$ ($\alpha = 0.05$) (statistically sig) Reject the H_0 in favor of the H_A
Superiority trial	H_0 = No difference	H_A = Difference
Noninferiority trial	H_0 = Inconclusive	H_A = Noninferior

Note: H_0: null hypothesis.

trials.[188] In fact, the definitions for the two hypotheses are essentially reversed and rela-beled compared to superiority trial hypotheses (see Table 4-10).[185,186] The null hypothesis for a superiority trial postulates that there is no statistically significant difference between treatment groups, and the alternative hypothesis states there is a statistically significant difference between the treatment groups. With NI trials, the null hypothesis states the test drug fails to exhibit noninferiority to the reference drug within a certain margin (i.e., the NI margin).[184,188] The alternative hypothesis states that the test drug is noninferior to the reference drug (not significantly worse) within a certain margin (i.e., the NI margin). With NI trials, the null hypothesis must be rejected in favor of the alternative hypothesis to conclude noninferiority for the test drug. This requires a p value less than the set α. For example, if given an a priori α of 0.05, a p value < 0.05 would indicate noninferiority for the test drug. If the p value were ≥ 0.05, the null hypothesis would not be rejected, and the test drug would fail to exhibit noninferiority.

Some controversy exists whether an NI trial alone can show superiority of the test drug over the reference drug.[193,197,198] One reason for this is that a one-sided statistical test is used for determining noninferiority, but a two-sided statistical test is needed for establishing superiority.[189] Once NI is established, superiority can be tested using the results for the primary outcome measure(s). According to guidance from the FDA, an NI study can be designed to first test noninferiority with a predetermined NI margin, and, if successful at proving noninferiority, the data can be analyzed for potential superiority of the test drug. Note the importance of the *sequential process* of first proving noninferiority, then analyzing for superiority. For instance, if the new antihypertensive NI trial discussed earlier provided results that showed the test drug to be noninferior, then an analysis of superiority would be appropriate and acceptable. This should be stated in the original NI trial protocol. Superiority can be tested prior to NI, even with a prespecified interim analysis, but the NI margin must be stated a priori to avoid potential manipulation of the margin.[185] Adjusting the NI margin to avoid the CI from crossing over would give a false NI result and is inappropriate. In addition, seeking the conclusion of NI from a failed superiority trial (one that shows no statistically significant difference between treatment groups) is inappropriate.[180,186] The only conclusion that can be made from this scenario is that the test drug is not superior to the reference drug. If a noninferiority conclusion is anticipated, an NI study design should be the initial choice.

Evaluation

Specific study design characteristics must be considered when evaluating the quality of an NI trial.[197,202,203] The determination of the NI margin is of great importance.[195,198] Correctly determining this margin is considered the greatest challenge in the design and interpretation of NI trials.[177] If noninferiority is established for the test drug, concluding that the test drug is efficacious can only be justified if the reference drug's efficacy has been confirmed with high-quality clinical trials against placebo. This is referred to as assay sensitivity.[177,194,196] The NI margin is set using historical placebo-controlled studies to determine the actual treatment effect of the reference drug. Two approaches to determine the NI margin are most frequently referenced: the fixed-margin approach and the synthesis approach. The fixed-margin approach is more conservative than the synthesis approach and is preferred by the FDA.[194]

Clarity of reporting which approach was used to establish the NI margin is important for literature evaluation and critique. For example, in a recent systematic review of NI studies published between 1966 and 2015, only 115 of 273 (42.1%) authors reported how the NI margin was determined in their study. Of the 115 NI studies, about 40% (47/115) used the fixed-margin or synthesis approaches to determine the NI margin. The description of how the NI margin was determined was reported significantly less frequently in journals with low-impact factors compared to those with high-impact factors (OR 0.20 95% CI 0.10–0.37, $p < 0.0001$).[199] There seems to be room for improvement with the reporting of how the NI margin was determined and the use of sound NI margin determination practices, thus underscoring the need for critical evaluation of this important NI study methodology.

In a noninferiority trial, it is key that the reference drug used is superior to placebo. The phrase historical evidence of sensitivity to drug effects (HESDE) has been used when past trials have been appropriately designed and conducted to confirm the superiority of the reference drug over placebo. Meta-analytic methods can be used to develop more precise estimates of reference drug effect when several studies are available. When multiple studies exist, all studies should be considered to avoid overestimating the reference drug's effect.[177] Only after a determination is made that these past studies are similar in design and conduct compared to the NI trial, regarding features that could alter the effect size, can the HESDE be used to select the NI margin. In other words, the historical studies and the new NI study should be as identical as possible regarding important characteristics. This is called the constancy assumption.[184,196] Note that establishing efficacy for the test drug using an NI trial design is seriously complicated by assay sensitivity and constancy assumptions that cannot be completely verified, leading to potentially inflated Type I error rate (see previous section in this chapter and Chapter 6).[186] In this instance, a Type I error occurs when noninferiority is established, but the true effect was inconclusive.

Another concern called **biocreep** or **placebo creep** potentially complicates using an active control to confirm efficacy, as is done with an NI trial.[184,199] Biocreep is the phenomenon where a somewhat inferior test drug is chosen as the reference drug for a future generation of NI trials. When this occurs with generation after generation of NI trials, the future reference drug eventually is no more efficacious than placebo.

As mentioned earlier, setting the NI margin post hoc can be interpreted as potential investigator manipulation to show desired results. For this reason, it is critical that the NI margin be set prospectively before the beginning of the trial. For all the aforementioned reasons, investigators should provide a detailed description of how the NI margin was determined.

The type of analysis used should also be determined prospectively. For the purposes of NI studies, a per-protocol (PP) analysis, where only the patients that completed the study are included in the analysis, is preferred over an intention-to-treat (ITT) analysis (see previous section in this chapter and Chapter 6).[197,198] The ITT analysis includes all patients that were randomized to treatment regardless of whether they completed the study duration, and smaller observed treatment effects may result since patients may not have stayed in the study long enough to see the maximum effect of the test drug. Using an ITT analysis with an NI trial can significantly increase the risk of falsely claiming noninferiority due to the potential of smaller observed treatment effects.[194] For this reason, a PP analysis is also used to cross-validate an ITT analysis.[177,205] Note that the PP analysis can be invalidated based on significant variation in dropout rates between treatment groups.[205] For example, a noninferiority study is completed, but there is an excessively large dropout rate due to safety and lack of return to the clinic visits. This provides a much smaller PP sample to be analyzed. If that PP sample is less than the required sample size to achieve statistical power, statistical significance ($p \geq 0.05$ if the alpha value is set at 0.05) may not be demonstrated. This lack of statistical significance shown could be real, and the test drug would fail to exhibit noninferiority (fail to reject the null hypothesis). However, since power was not met, the result could represent a Type II error (noninferiority is not demonstrated, but test drug is noninferior to reference) that invalidates the PP analysis (see a previous section of this chapter and Chapter 6 for explanation of Type II errors). The FDA and others suggest conducting and reporting both a PP and ITT analyses.[177,205,] Any differences in results between these two separate analyses should be examined closely by the reader.

NI trials have a larger sample size compared to superiority trials since the NI margin is frequently smaller than the treatment difference anticipated with superiority trials.[189,191,194] Sample size determination before the study is started can be difficult since variance of the estimated treatment effect and event rate may be unknown for the test drug at this point. When this issue is present for superiority studies, an **independent data monitoring committee (IDMC)** is formed to examine the blinded information during the trial (interim analysis). This committee looks for the occurrence of an unexpectedly low event rate so an upward adjustment in sample size can be proposed. This same approach to sample size reassessment and adjustment is applied to NI trials.[201,206] A clear explanation of how the blinded information was handled and how the IDMC was conducted should be provided in the article for evaluation.

One simple method that has been proposed to assist in remembering to evaluate some of the important characteristics of noninferiority trials uses the mnemonic "FACTS."[203] These five steps include the following:

1. Formulate a null hypothesis.
2. Assess the noninferiority margin.
3. Compare the intention-to-treat (ITT) and per-protocol (PP) analyses.
4. Translate CIs graphically (see Figure 4-5).
5. Summarize the clinical relevance of the results.

Although FACTS is helpful, this method does not cover all characteristics discussed in this section that should be evaluated to determine the quality of an NI trial.

Reporting NI trials in the literature remains inconsistent, and this is often the biggest issue when evaluating and interpreting trial results for quality.[183,207,208] The CONSORT statement was first published in 1996 and updated in 2010 to improve randomized controlled trial reporting in the medical literature.[9,209] An extension to the original CONSORT statement that specifically addressed reporting of NI and equivalence studies was first published in 2006, and the most recent update published in 2012 incorporates additional items to consider when reporting NI and equivalence studies beyond the items listed for traditional RCTs.[197] The updated CONSORT extension for NI and equivalence studies also provides guidance for what should be reported in the abstracts of NI and equivalence studies.[197] In addition to everything that should be reported in manuscripts about traditional RCTs, the authors suggest the following items to report in manuscripts about NI and equivalence studies:

- Identifying that the study is NI design in the title
- Four additional recommendations for reporting abstracts in NI studies:
  - Specific hypothesis concerning noninferiority and NI margin
  - All reported outcomes clearly marked as noninferiority or superiority
  - For primary outcome, its relation back to the NI margin
  - Conclusions related back to noninferiority and/or superiority hypotheses
- Rationale for using NI design

- Hypotheses regarding noninferiority including stating the NI margin and the reasoning for its choice
- Level of similarity between participants in the NI study and the studies that established the efficacy of the reference drug
- Level of similarity between the reference drug in the NI trial and the studies that established the efficacy of the reference drug
- Specifying the NI outcome(s) and whether hypotheses are noninferiority or superiority
- Level of similarity between the outcome(s) in the NI study and the studies that established the efficacy of the reference drug
- How sample size was calculated, specifically if calculated using an NI margin
- To which outcome(s) estimated sample size applies, specifically if related to an NI hypothesis
- Whether one- or two-sided CI(s) was/were used
- Recommendation to provide a figure showing CIs for NI outcomes(s) and the NI margin
- Interpretation of results in relation to the NI hypothesis and provide justification for concluding superiority from an NI design, if done

Case Study 4–3[200]

The TANGO I study was a phase 3, multicenter, randomized clinical trial that was conducted to evaluate the efficacy and safety of meropenem-vaborbactam (intervention) versus the piperacillin-tazobactam (control) in complicated urinary tract infections (UTIs). Eligible subjects were adults > 18 years old that had a complicated UTI or acute pyelonephritis. Investigators enrolled subjects over about 1.5 years in 60 sites across 17 countries in Asia, Europe, North and South America. Subjects were randomized 1:1 to receive either meropenem-vaborbactam or piperacillin-tazobactam for 10 days of total treatment, and those in the meropenem-vaborbactam group could have their dose blindly adjusted if they had a creatinine clearance <50 mL/min. The researchers had different primary efficacy endpoints to satisfy FDA and European Medicine Agency (EMA) criteria; however, this abbreviated abstract will only focus on the FDA endpoint, which was overall success, a composite outcome of clinical cure and microbial eradication at the end of IV treatment. The researchers set the noninferiority margin to 15%, so noninferiority could be concluded if the lower bound of the 95% CI of the difference in the primary efficacy endpoint was greater than −15%.

A total of 550 subjects were randomized; however, the final sample that comprised the microbiologic modified intention to treat (ITT) population was 374:192 in the treatment group and 182 in the control group. Baseline characteristics of the intervention and control groups were similar. The average study duration was 25 days. The overall success rate (i.e., primary efficacy endpoint) was 98.4% for the meropenem-vaborbactam group and 94.0% for the piperacillin-tazobactam group with a difference of 4.5%; 95% CI 0.7%–9.1%. According to the researchers' statistical plan, which had been established *a priori*, superiority of the interventions could be established over the control if the CI of the difference between the two treatments favored the intervention and did not include 0. Given the aforementioned results, the authors declared superiority of meropenem-vaborbactam with regard to overall success as compared to piperacillin-tazobactam.

1. Does this study need IRB approval?
2. What is the type of data being evaluated for the primary endpoint? What is a potential advantage of this data type?
3. Identify the null hypothesis and alternative hypothesis for this noninferiority study.
   a. Null hypothesis:
   b. Alternative hypothesis:
4. What is your conclusion if the 95% CI around the mean treatment difference for overall success, a composite of clinical cure and microbial eradication, does not include or cross over the established NI margin?
5. After showing noninferiority for the two drugs, the investigators performed a superiority analysis on the data. What is your reaction to this second analysis?

ADAPTIVE CLINICAL TRIALS

The FDA defines adaptive clinical trials as "a clinical trial design that allows for prospectively planned modifications to one or more aspects of the design based on accumulating data from subjects in the trial."[210] In simplest form, the ACT could be a well-designed randomized clinical trial with an interim analysis halfway through the study to identify if the original sample size determination is going to be adequate to meet the set power.[211] If this interim analysis shows the original sample size to be inadequate based on treatment effect, the response-adaptation of increasing the number of patients to be entered into the study will assure power is met by the end of the trial.

Classical clinical trial design is rigidly structured to investigate a set number of variables and prevent additional variables from being introduced that will confound the results. However, the disadvantage of such rigidity is the inability to make adjustments to the study as it progresses, and new information comes from those patients who have completed the trial. For example, if the investigators discover there is a specific patient group that responds to the treatment during the trial, adjustments to include only that patient population are not allowed. For that reason, a significant number of patients anticipated to not respond are exposed to a treatment that may cause severe side effects. ACT design provides flexibility to incorporate continuously emerging knowledge generated as a trial is carried out, such as limiting inclusion to only that specific patient population that responds.[212] The ACT study design provides the potential to save time and resources along with minimizing the exposure of subjects to possible dangerous therapies. Additional benefits include a more efficient developmental pathway for the drug, patients benefit from effective therapies earlier, and prescribers have more information on patients most likely to benefit from the drug. A review of ACT studies published between 2000 and 2014 revealed that ACT studies are increasing in numbers.[213] In addition, the ACT design is used most often in phase II clinical trials and in oncology research. Phase III ACT studies most often determine sample size once a statistically significant difference is noted during interim analyses instead of defining a sample size *a priori*.

Studies based on the ACT design are evaluated similarly to other randomized clinical trials; however, there are some specific factors to consider when assessing ACTs. First, the group responsible for identifying and initiating potential adaptations should not be included in the analysis of the results. All proposed adaptive changes should be based on evidence created by the continuous flow of information from the study along with clinical judgment.[214] In some cases, computer-generated adaptations using algorithms developed prior to the study may be used. Termination rules should already exist with specific criteria to take into consideration. In addition, it is very important that methods are incorporated to reduce the potential risk of bias. For example, the formation of an independent data and safety monitoring committee to conduct interim analyses on the information received from the ongoing study can alleviate the need for interactions with the company sponsoring the trial. Several types of bias have been identified that can have major effects on the results of a study. Table 4-11 presents several of these bias types in detail.

The benefits of ACT design encourage continued exploration for appropriate application to several therapeutic areas. Adaptations to study eligibility criteria, total sample size, randomization procedure, drug dose, schedule, treatment duration, concomitant treatments, patient evaluations for data collection, primary endpoint, secondary endpoints, and analytical methods to evaluate these endpoints can significantly improve the efficiency of drug development and overall patient care. However, readers should

TABLE 4–11. TYPES OF BIAS

Category of Bias	Name of Bias	Description	Methods of Control
Selection bias	Admission rate (Berkson) bias	Admission rates of exposed and unexposed cases and controls differ, resulting in a distortion of odds of exposure in hospital-based studies	*A priori* define inclusion and exclusion criteria All groups of subjects should have undergone identical diagnostic testing and there should be no difference in how exposure or disease status is determined
	Nonresponse bias	Nonrespondents may exhibit exposures or outcomes that differ from respondents, resulting in over- or underestimation of odds or risk	Match or adjust for confounding variables Use more than one control group
	Prevalence-incidence (Neyman) bias	Timing of exposure identification causes some cases to be missed	
	Unmasking bias	An innocent exposure causes a sign or symptom that precipitates search for a disease but does not itself cause the disease	
Information bias	Family history bias	Family members tend to share more information with family members who have similar diseases or exposures. Those family members without the disease or exposure may be unaware. Family historical information may vary widely depending on whether the person is a case or a control	Establish *a priori* explicit criteria for data collection methods on exposures and outcomes Blinded interviewer and subject to the hypotheses investigated Standardize data collection procedure, i.e., train observers, develop and refine survey questions and methods of recording answers
	Recall bias	Difference in how data collection occurs exists between cases and controls, or the exposed and unexposed, resulting in an abnormally high rate of recall of exposure or outcome in one group	Maintain aggressive contact with subjects to limit attrition (cohort designs) For surveys, obtain response rates ≥80% Assess for effects of potential confounders
	Exposure suspicion bias	Knowledge of a subject's disease status may influence both intensity and outcome of a search for exposure	

continued

TABLE 4–11. TYPES OF BIAS *(CONTINUED)*

Category of Bias	Name of Bias	Description	Methods of Control
Data analysis bias	*Post hoc* significance bias	When decisions regarding level of significance are selected a posteriori, conclusion may be biased	Establish *a priori* the statistical methods to be used to evaluate data Report how missing data are handled
	Data dredging bias	When data are reviewed for all possible associations without prior hypotheses, results are only suitable for hypothesis-forming activities	Assess associations between confounders and exposures and outcomes
	Significance bias	Confusing statistical significance with clinical significance	
	Correlation bias	Correlation do not equate with causation; concluding that correlation equating with causation can lead to serious errors	

Source: Adapted from Fletcher et al.[215]

be aware that the risk of bias in ACT studies is increased compared to standard clinical trial designs.

Conclusion

Practitioners of today are expected to have the skills, ability, and knowledge to problem solve, critically think, and formulate recommendations based upon published literature. Therefore, all practitioners, regardless of practice setting, need to learn how to efficiently locate, critically evaluate, and effectively formulate and communicate an evidence-based recommendation; incorporating these skills in daily practice is essential. A multitude of literature is published each year, and the quality varies significantly. Readers of the literature should not immediately accept the authors' conclusions; they should be able to assess the strengths and limitations of the source. The information within this chapter identifies and discusses many issues to consider while reading and analyzing controlled clinical trials. Although every clinical trial has limitations, those trials with appropriate design and well-presented results can be used to formulate recommendations in clinical practice. Using robust, validated techniques when evaluating clinical trials can allow practitioners to provide high-quality, evidence-based health care to our patients.

Self-Assessment Questions

Read the excerpt of the following clinical trial summary and answer questions 1 through 4.[216]

One single-center, double-blind, randomized controlled clinical trial assessed the effectiveness of oral glucosamine compared to placebo in patients with primary knee osteoarthritis. Subjects who met inclusion criteria were randomized in blocks of 4 to receive either 1500 mg of glucosamine or placebo once daily for 3 years. The primary endpoint was the change in radiographic joint space width which was assessed by two trained independent readers. Patient symptoms were also evaluated at each clinic visit, using the algo-functional severity index of Lequesne. The Lequesne index consists of five questions scored on a scale of 0–2, with 0 indicating no symptoms and 2 indicating severe symptoms.

Study investigators determined that 86 subjects per group were needed to have an 80% power to detect a difference of 0.33 mm between the groups. Results from all subjects were included in the final analyses, and a p value less than 0.05 was considered statistically significant.

After randomization, data from 101 patients in each group were available for the primary endpoint analysis. Subjects were distributed evenly across all treatment groups based upon predefined characteristics. After 3 years, the difference between the two groups was 0.36 mm (95% CI 0.13–0.59, $p < 0.01$) in the per-protocol group and 0.23 mm (95% CI 0.09–0.37, $p = 0.001$) in the intent-to treat population. The groups did not differ in the incidence of adverse events.

USE THE STUDY NARRATIVE TO ANSWER QUESTIONS 1–4

1. What type of endpoint is minimum joint space width?
   a. Composite
   b. Clinical
   c. Independent
   d. Surrogate

2. Regarding the per-protocol analysis, was the primary endpoint at year 3 statistically significant?
   a. Yes, because the 95% CI does not include 0.
   b. Yes, because the 95% CI does not include 1.
   c. No, because the p value is greater than alpha.
   d. No, because the 95% CI includes 1.

3. The authors used the algo-functional severity index of Lequesne to assess knee pain. What level of data is this?
   a. Continuous
   b. Nominal
   c. Ordinal

4. What was the most likely reason the study was designed to have two trained independent readers for all radiographs?
   a. To minimize bias, since radiograph readings can be subjective.
   b. To speed up reporting of the results.
   c. The IRB mandates at least two reviewers for all data.
   d. To increase power to find a difference.

5. Which of the following is true regarding surrogate endpoints?
   a. Prior to using surrogate endpoints in a trial, researchers should have evidence that the surrogate endpoints accurately predict clinical endpoints.
   b. Studying surrogate endpoints usually requires more money and time than studying clinical endpoints.
   c. Since surrogate endpoints are almost always comprised of other endpoints, clinicians should interpret surrogate endpoints with caution.
   d. Surrogate endpoints include events such as death, MI, or stroke.

6. A dual PPAR agonist, tesaglitazar, was compared to pioglitazone in a noninferiority study. The primary endpoint was percent change of HbA1c from baseline. The noninferiority margin was selected at 0.3%. When comparing the difference in the primary endpoint between tesaglitazar to pioglitazone, which of the following indicate(s) statistical noninferiority?
   a. −0.17 (95% CI −0.27, −0.06)
   b. 0.12 (95% CI 0.01, 0.22)
   c. 0.15 (95% CI −0.3, 0.26)
   d. a and b
   e. All of the above

7. A researcher is trying to determine an appropriate noninferiority margin for a comparative study between his company's new drug, fantastapril, and the standard treatment, enalapril. Numerous placebo-controlled studies indicate that enalapril reduces SBP (the primary endpoint) by 10% (95% CI 6–15%) compared to placebo. Which of the following would be the most appropriate noninferiority margin for a study comparing fantastapril and enalapril?
   a. 6%
   b. 10%
   c. 15%
   d. 30%

8. At the end of an 8-week trial, patients in the Fantastalol™ arm of the study had a mean SBP of 122 mmHg; patients in the Itsgreatalol™ arm had a mean SBP of 127 mmHg (p = 0.23). The prespecified alpha was 0.05. No sample size or power calculation was mentioned in the published research project. What can be concluded?

   a. The result was statistically significant and the chance of committing a Type II error was 23%.

   b. The result was not statistically significant; however, we cannot be sure that the study was powered appropriately.

   c. The result was not statistically significant; therefore, the medications have similar efficacy.

   d. The result was statistically significant; therefore, Fantastalol™ provides better blood pressure control than Itsgreatalol™.

9. Which term below accurately describes characteristics of a study or outside influences that may affect the true study results?

   a. Confounding variable

   b. Statistical significance

   c. Blinding

   d. Randomization

   e. Type I error

10. Which of the following statements about confounding variables is true?

   a. They represent the exposure of interest in a study.

   b. They improve our ability to determine the "true" effect.

   c. They are always evenly distributed between groups when using random selection.

   d. They represent a common limitation in clinical research.

11. An investigator would like to determine if a new weight-loss agent (Losealot®) causes subjects to lose *more weight* than another available weight-loss agent (ShredIt®). Given this, which of the following statements is the most appropriate *research/alternate* hypothesis?

   a. Subjects who take Losealot® will lose less weight than subjects who take ShredIt®.

   b. Subjects who take Losealot® will lose more weight than subjects who take ShredIt®.

   c. There will be a difference in weight loss between subjects who take Losealot® and subjects who take ShredIt®.

   d. There will be no difference in weight loss between subjects who take Losealot® and subjects who take ShredIt®.

12. Which of the following is true regarding data distribution?
    a. A normal distribution occurs when mean, median, and mode are numerically equal.
    b. 68% of data points are included within 2 standard deviations from the mean.
    c. 99% of data points are included within 1 standard deviation from the mean.
    d. 95% of data points are included within 3 standard deviations from the mean.
    e. Standard deviation and standard error of the mean are the same value.

13. Which of the following is true regarding Type I and Type II errors?
    a. Type II errors can occur when the H_0 is rejected.
    b. Type I errors can occur when the H_0 is accepted (fail to reject).
    c. Type I errors are associated with sample size.
    d. Type II errors are associated with statistically significant results.
    e. Type II can occur when the H_0 is accepted (fail to reject).

14. Which of the following is an example of a surrogate marker or endpoint?
    a. Death
    b. Stroke
    c. Myocardial infarction
    d. Hospital discharge
    e. Blood pressure

15. You are interested in assessing the degree to which a new antihypertensive (drug X) lowers blood pressure (BP) compared to an older medication (drug Y). You randomly assign an equal number of patients to the drug X group and the drug Y group for 12 weeks. You determine the mean change in BP from baseline to week 12 in both groups and compare the results. What would the null hypothesis (H_0) be for this study?
    a. Drug X will lower blood pressure more than drug Y.
    b. Drug Y will lower blood pressure more than drug X.
    c. There is no difference in blood pressure between drug X and drug Y.
    d. There is a difference in blood pressure between drug X and drug Y.

REFERENCES

1. Food and Drug Administration [Internet]. Silver Spring (MD). Drugs @ FDA: FDA-Approved Drugs. [cited 2020 Feb 20]. Available from: https://www.accessdata.fda.gov/scripts/cder/daf/index.cfm.
2. Johnson R, Watkinson A, Mabe M. The STM report. An overview of scientific and scholarly journal publishing. 5th ed. Published 2018 Sep [cited 2020 Feb 20]. Available from: https://www.stm-assoc.org/2018_10_04_STM_Report_2018.pdf.

3. Nathan JP. Drug information. The systematic approach: continuing education article. J Pharm Prac. 2013;26:78-84. doi:10.1177/0897190012474229.

4. US National Library of Medicine [Internet]. Bethesda (MD): PubMed tutorial. Building the search. [cited 2021 Jan 23]. Available from: https://www.nlm.nih.gov/bsd/disted/pubmedtutorial/020_010.html.

5. Nelson SJ, Schulman JL. Orthopaedic literature and MeSH. Clin Orthop Relat Res. 2010 Oct;468(10):2621-6. PMID: 20623263. PMCID: PMC3049625. doi:10.1007/s11999-010-1387-4.

6. U.S. Food and Drug Administration: how drugs are developed and approved [Internet]. Rockville (MD): U.S. Food and Drug Administration [updated 2019 Jan 07; cited 2021 Jan 23]. Available from: http://www.fda.gov/drugs/developmentapprovalprocess/how-drugsaredevelopedandapproved/default.htm.

7. Pihlstrom BL, Curran AE, Voelker HT, Kingman A. Randomized controlled trials: what are they and who needs them? Periodontol 2000. 2012;59(1):14-31. doi:10.1111/j.1600-0757.2011.00439.x.

8. Umscheid CA, Margolis DJ, Grossman CE. Key concepts of clinical trials: a narrative review. Postgrad Med. 2011;123(5):194-204.

9. Schulz KF, Altman DG, Moher D; CONSORT Group. CONSORT 2010 Statement: updated guidelines for reporting parallel group randomised trials. Ann Int Med. 2010;152(11):726-32. doi:10.7326/0003-4819-152-11-201006010-00232.

10. Strobe statement. Strengthening the reporting of observational studies in epidemiology. Version 4. [cited 2021 Jan 23]. Available from: http://www.strobe-statement.org.

11. Kendrach MG, Anderson HG. Fundamentals of controlled clinical trials. J Pharm Pract. 1998;XI(3):163-80. doi:10.1177/089719009801100308.

12. Friedman L, Furberg C, DeMets D. Fundamentals of clinical trials. 4th ed. New York: Springer; 2010.

13. Hershenberg R, Drabick DA, Vivian D. An opportunity to bridge the gap between clinical research and clinical practice: implications for clinical training. Psychotherapy (Chic). 2012;49(2):123-34. PMID: 22642520. PMCID: PMC3786339. doi:10.1037/a0027648.

14. Song F, Loke Y, Hooper L. Why are medical and health-related studies not being published? A systematic review of reasons given by investigators. In: Wicherts JM, editor. PLoS ONE. 2014;9(10):e110418. doi:10.1371/journal.pone.0110418.

15. Mathieu S, Boutron I, Moher D, Altman DG, Ravaud P. Comparison of registered and published primary outcomes in randomized controlled trials. JAMA. 2009;302(9):977-84. PMID: 19724045. doi:10.1001/jama.2009.1242.

16. Irwin RS. The role of conflict of interest in reporting of scientific information. Chest. 2009;136(1):253-9. PMID: 19584207. doi:10.1378/chest.09-0890.

17. International Committee of Medical Journal Editors: recommendations for the conduct, reporting, editing and publication of scholarly work in medical journals [Internet]. [place unknown] International Committee of Medical Journal Editors. [cited 2021 Jan 23]. Available from: http://www.icmje.org/icmje-recommendations.pdf.

18. Hayes A, Hunter J. Why is publication of negative clinical trial data important? Br J Pharmacol. 2012;167(7):1395-7.

19. Augustyn N, Welch SJ, Irwin RS. Managing information overload: the evolution of CHEST. Chest. 2012;142(1):1-5. PMID: 22796829. doi:10.1378/chest.12-1364.

20. Blumenthal D. Doctors and drug companies. N Engl J Med. 2004;351(18):1885-90. PMID: 15509823. doi:10.1056/NEJMhpr042734.

21. Harden RM, Lilley P. A fresh approach to publishing and reviewing papers in health professions education. Med Teach. 2013;35(1):1-3.

22. Weller A. Editorial peer-review. Its strengths and weaknesses. Medford (NJ): American Society for Information Science and Technology; 2001.

23. Rochon PA, Bero LA, Bay AM, et al. Comparison of review articles published in peer-reviewed and throwaway journals. JAMA. 2002;287(21):2853-6.

24. Rochon PA, Gurwitz JH, Cheung CM, Hayes JA, Chalmers TC. Evaluating the quality of articles published in journal supplements compared with the quality of those published in the parent journal. JAMA. 1994;272(2):108-13.

25. Schriger DL, Raffetto B, Drolen C, Cooper RJ. The effect of peer review on the quality of data graphs in Annals of Emergency Medicine. Ann Emerg Med. 2016. pii: S0196-0644(16)30366-3. doi:10.1016/j.annemergmed.2016.06.046. PubMed PMID: 27614587.

26. Wagner E, Middleton P. Effects of technical editing in biomedical journals: a systematic review. JAMA. 2002;287:2821-4.

27. Sharma M, Aarin A, Gupta P, Sachdeva S, Desai AV. Journal impact factor: its use, significance, and limitations. World J Nucl Med. 2014;13(2):146. PMCID: PMC4150161.

28. National Library of Medicine. Errata, retractions, and other linked citations in Pubmed [Internet]. [cited 2020 Nov 14]. Available from: https://www.nlm.nih.gov/bsd/policy/errata.html.

29. Lader EW, Cannon CP, Ohman EM, et al.; American College of Cardiology Foundation. The clinician as investigator: participating in clinical trials in the practice setting. Circulation. 2004;109(21):2672-9. PMID: 15173050. doi:10.1161/01.CIR.0000128702.16441.75.

30. International Committee of Medical Journal Editors. Recommendations for the conduct, reporting, editing, and publication of scholarly work in medical journals [Internet]. Available from: http://www.icmje.org/recommendations/.

31. Studdert DM, Mello MM, Brennan TA. Financial conflicts of interest in physicians' relationships with the pharmaceutical industry: self-regulation in the shadow of federal prosecution. N Engl J Med. 2004;351(18):1891-900. PMID: 15509824. doi:10.1056/NEJMlim042229.

32. Peat J, Elliott E, Baur L, Keena V. Scientific writing: easy when you know how. London: BMJ Books; 2002.

33. Iverson C, Christiansen S, editors. American Medical Association manual of style. A guide for authors and editors. 10th ed. New York: Oxford University Press; 2007.

34. Nelson HS, Bensch G, Pleskow WW, et al. Improved bronchodilation with levalbuterol compared with racemic albuterol in patients with asthma. J Allergy Clin Immunol. 1998;102(6 Pt 1):943-52. PMID: 9847435. doi:http://dx.doi.org/10.1016/S0091-6749(98)70332-X.

35. Socie G, de Gramont MA, Rio B, et al. Paroxysmal nocturnal haemoglobinuria: long-term follow-up and prognostic factors. French Society of Haematology. Lancet. 1996;348(9027):573-7. PMID: 8774569. doi:10.1016/s0140-6736(95)12360-1.

36. Hopewell S, Clarke M, Moher D, Wager E, Middleton P, Altman DG, Schulz KF; CONSORT Group. CONSORT for reporting randomized controlled trials in journal and conference abstracts: explanation and elaboration. PLoS Med. 2008;5(1):e20. PMID: 18215107. PMCID: PMC2211558. doi:10.1371/journal.pmed.0050020.

37. Harris AH, Standard S, Brunning JL, et al. The accuracy of abstracts in psychology journals. J Psychol. 2002;136(2):141-8. PMID: 12081089. doi:10.1080/00223980209604145.

38. Prasad S, Lee DJ, Yuan JC, Barao VA, Shyamsunder N, Sukotjo C. Discrepancies between Abstracts Presented at International Association for Dental Research. Annual Sessions from 2004 to 2005 and full-text publication. Int J Dent. 2012;2012:859561. doi:10.1155/2012/859561. Epub 2012 Feb 22. PubMed PMID: 22505912; PubMed Central PMCID: PMC3296196.

39. Kastelein JJ, Akdim F, Stroes ES, Zwinderman AH, Bots ML, Stalenhoef AF, Visseren FL, Sijbrands EJ, Trip MD, Stein EA, Gaudet D, Duivenvoorden R, Veltri EP, Marais AD, de Groot E; ENHANCE Investigators. Simvastatin with or without ezetimibe in familial hypercholesterolemia. N Engl J Med. 2008;358(14):1431-43. doi:10.1056/NEJMoa0800742.

40. Guimarães CA. Structured abstracts: narrative review. Acta Cir Bras. 2006;21(4):263-68. PMID: 16862349. doi:http://dx.doi.org/10.1590/S0102-86502006000400014.

41. Hartley J. Current findings from research on structured abstracts. J Med Libr Assoc. 2004;92(3):368-71. PMID: 15243644. PMCID: PMC442180.

42. Goldberg RJ, McManus DD, Allison J. Greater knowledge and appreciation of commonly-used research study designs. Am J Med. 2013;126(2):169.e1-8.

43. International Committee of Medical Journal Editors. Preparing a manuscript for submission to a medical journal. [cited 2020 Nov 14]. Available from: http://www.icmje.org/recommendations/browse/manuscript-preparation/preparing-for-submission.html#b.

44. Cuddy PG, Elenbaas RM, Elenbaas JK. Evaluating the medical literature. Part I: Abstract, introduction, methods. Ann Emerg Med. 1983;12(9):549-55. PMID: 6614609. doi:10.1016/S0196-0644(83)80296-0.

45. Cannon CP, Blazing MA, Giugliano RP, McCagg A, White JA, Theroux P, Darius H, Lewis BS, Ophuis TO, Jukema JW, De Ferrari GM, Ruzyllo W, De Lucca P, Im K, Bohula EA, Reist C, Wiviott SD, Tershakovec AM, Musliner TA, Braunwald E, Califf RM; IMPROVE-IT Investigators. Ezetimibe added to statin therapy after acute coronary syndromes. N Engl J Med. 2015;372(25):2387-97. doi:10.1056/NEJMoa1410489. Epub 2015 Jun 3. PubMed PMID: 26039521.

46. Veith FJ. How randomized controlled trials (RCTs) can be misleading: introduction. Semin Vasc Surg. 2011;24(3):143-5. PMID: 22153022. doi:10.1053/j.semvascsurg.2011.10.001.

47. Hulley SB, Cummings SR, Browner WS, Grady DG, Newman TB. Designing clinical research. 4th ed. Philadelphia (PA): Lippincott Williams & Wilkins; 2013.

48. Siddiqi AE, Sikorskii A, Given CW, Given B. Early participant attrition from clinical trials: role of trial design and logistics. Clin Trials. 2008;5(4):328-35. PMID: 18697847. PMCID: PMC2723836. doi:10.1177/1740774508094406.

49. Karalis DG, Ross AM, Vacari RM, Zarren H, Scott R. Comparison of efficacy and safety of atorvastatin and simvastatin in patients with dyslipidemia with and without coronary heart disease. Am J Cardiol. 2002;89(6):667-71.

50. Naylor CD, Guyatt GH, Bass E, et al. Users' guides to the medical literature. X. How to use an article reporting variations in the outcomes of health services. The Evidence-Based Medicine Working Group. JAMA. 1996;275(7):554-8. PMID: 8606478. doi:10.1001/jama.1996.03530310060034.

51. Tripepi G, Jager KJ, Dekker FW, Zoccali C. Selection bias and information bias in clinical research. Nephron Clin Pract. 2010;115(2):c94-9.

52. Sessler DI, Imrey PB. Clinical research methodology 3: randomized controlled trials. Anesth Analg. 2015;121(4):1052-64. doi:10.1213/ANE.0000000000000862.

53. Sankaré IC, Bross R, Brown AF, et al. Strategies to build trust and recruit African American and Latino community residents for health research: a cohort study. Clin Transl Sci. 2015;8(5):412-20. doi:10.1111/cts.12273.

54. Berger VW, Rezvani A, Makarewicz VA. Direct effect on validity of response run-in selection in clinical trials. Control Clin Trials. 2003;24(2):156-66. PMID: 12689737. doi:10.1016/S0197-2456(02)00316-1.

55. Wei SJ, Metz JM, Coyle C, et al. Recruitment of patients into an Internet-based clinical trials database: the experience of OncoLink and the National Colorectal Cancer Research Alliance. J Clin Oncol. 2004;22(23):4730-6. PMID: 15570073. doi:10.1200/JCO.2004.07.103.

56. Chan FK, Ching JY, Hung LC, et al. Clopidogrel versus aspirin and esomeprazole to prevent recurrent ulcer bleeding. N Engl J Med. 2005;352(3):238-44. PMID: 15659723. doi:10.1056/NEJMoa042087.

57. Department of Health and Human Services: Recruiting Human Subjects. Pressures in industry-sponsored clinical research [Internet]. Washington (DC): Department of Health and Human Services; [updated 2000 Jun; cited 2021 Jan 23]. Available from: http://oig.hhs.gov/oei/reports/oei-01-97-00195.pdf.

58. Hebert R. Newspaper advertising could distort research results. Nicotine Tob Res. 2000;2(4):317-8. PMID: 11197310. doi:10.1080/14622200020028038.

59. Refolo P, Sacchini D, Minacori R, Daloiso V, Spagnolo AG. E-recruitment based clinical research: notes for Research Ethics Committees/Institutional Review Boards. Eur Rev Med Pharmacol Sci. 2015;19(5):800-4.

60. Maiti R, Raghvendra M. Clinical trials in India. Pharmacol Res. 2007;56(1):1-10. PMID: 17391981. doi:10.1016/j.phrs.2007.02.004.

61. Nicholas J. Outsourcing clinical trials. J Natl Cancer Inst. 2012;104(14):1043-5. PMID: 22781429. doi:10.1093/jnci/djs323.

62. Guyatt GH, Sackett DL, Cook DJ. Users' guides to the medical literature. II. How to use an article about therapy or prevention. A. Are the results of the study valid? Evidence-Based

Medicine Working Group. JAMA. 1993;270(21):2598-601. PMID: 8230645. doi:10.1001/jama.1993.03510210084032.

63. Julious SA. Sample sizes for clinical trials with normal data. Stat Med. 2004;23(12):1921-86. PMID: 15195324. doi:10.1002/sim.1783.

64. Vickers AJ, de Craen AJ. Why use placebos in clinical trials? A narrative review of the methodological literature. J Clin Epidemiol. 2000;53(2):157-61. PMID: 10729687. doi:http://dx.doi.org/10.1016/S0895-4356(99)00139-0.

65. Yeh SS, DeGuzman B, Kramer T; M012 Study Group. Reversal of COPD-associated weight loss using the anabolic agent oxandrolone. Chest. 2002;122(2):421-8. PMID: 12171812. doi:http://dx.doi.org/10.1378/chest.122.2.421.

66. Baker SG, Lindeman KS. Rethinking historical controls. Biostatistics. 2001;2(4):383-96. PMID: 12933631. doi:10.1093/biostatistics/2.4.383.

67. Kunz R, Oxman AD. The unpredictability paradox: review of empirical comparisons of randomised and non-randomised clinical trials. BMJ. 1998;317(7167):1185-90. PMID: 9794851. PMCID: PMC28700. doi:http://dx.doi.org/10.1136/bmj.317.7167.1185.

68. Tramer MR, Reynolds DJ, Moore RA, McQuay HJ. When placebo controlled trials are essential and equivalence trials are inadequate. BMJ. 1998;317(7162):875-80. PMID: 9748192. PMCID: PMC1113953. doi:http://dx.doi.org/10.1136/bmj.317.7162.875.

69. Brodie MJ. Novel trial designs for monotherapy. Epileptic Disord. 2012;14(2):132-7. PMID: 22977899. doi:10.1684/epd.2012.0513.

70. Simons LA, Nestel PJ, Calvert GD, Jennings GL. Effects of MK-733 on plasma lipid and lipoprotein levels in subjects with hypercholesterolaemia. Med J Aust. 1987;147(2):65-8. PMID: 3299016.

71. Randomised trial of cholesterol lowering in 4444 patients with coronary heart disease: the Scandinavian Simvastatin Survival Study (4S). Lancet. 1994;344(8934):1383-9. PMID: 7968073. doi:10.1016/S0140-6736(94)90566-5.

72. Avenell A, Grant AM, McGee M, McPherson G, Campbell MK, McGee MA; RECORD Trial Management Group. The effects of an open design on trial participant recruitment, adherence, and retention: a randomized controlled trial comparison with a blinded, placebo-controlled design. Clin Trials. 2004;1(6):490-8. PMID: 16279289. doi:10.1191/1740774504cn053oa.

73. Montori VM, Jaeschke R, Schunemann HJ, Bhandari M, Brozek JL, Devereaux PJ, Guyatt GH. Users' guide to detecting misleading claims in clinical research reports. BMJ. 2004 Nov 6;329(7474):1093-6. PMID: 15528623. PMCID: PMC526126. doi:10.1136/bmj.329.7474.1093.

74. Gluud LL. Bias in clinical intervention research. Am J Epidemiol. 2006 Mar 15;163(6):493-50. PMID: 16443796. doi:10.1093/aje/kwj069.

75. Macklin R. The ethical problems with sham surgery in clinical research. N Engl J Med. 1999;341(13):992-6. PMID: 10498498. doi:10.1056/NEJM199909233411312.

76. Davidson M, Ma P, Stein EA, Gotto AM Jr, Raza A, Chitra R, Hutchinson H. Comparison of effects on low-density lipoprotein cholesterol and high-density lipoprotein cholesterol with rosuvastatin

versus atorvastatin in patients with Type IIa or IIb hypercholesterolemia. Am J Cardiol. 2002;89(3):268-75. PMID: 11809427. doi:http://dx.doi.org/10.1016/S0002-9149(01)02226-3.

77. Kendrach MG, Kelly-Freeman M. Approximate equivalent rosuvastatin doses for temporary statin interchange programs. Ann Pharmacother. 2004;38(7-8):1286-92. PMID: 15187217. doi:10.1345/aph.1D391.

78. Schwenzer KJ. Practical tips for working effectively with your institutional review board. Respir Care. 2008;53(10):1354-61. PMID: 18812000.

79. Enfield KB, Truwit JD. The purpose, composition, and function of an institutional review board: balancing priorities. Respir Care. 2008;53(10):1330-6. PMID: 18811996.

80. Schwenzer KJ. Protecting vulnerable subjects in clinical research: children, pregnant women, prisoners, and employees. Respir Care. 2008 Oct;53(10):1342-9. PMID: 18811998.

81. Dumville JC, Hahn S, Miles JN, Torgerson DJ. The use of unequal randomisation ratios in clinical trials: a review. Contemp Clin Trials. 2006;27(1):1-12.

82. Slobogean GP, Sprague S, Bhandari M. The tactics of large randomized trials. J Bone Joint Surg Am. 2012;94(Suppl 1):19-23.

83. Pitt B, Segal R, Martinez FA, et al. Randomised trial of losartan versus captopril in patients over 65 with heart failure (Evaluation of Losartan in the Elderly Study, ELITE). Lancet. 1997;349(9054):747-52.

84. Mertl SL. The fundamentals of Institutional Review Board operations. J Pharm Pract. 1996;IX:437-43. doi:10.1177/08971900960090060.

85. Horng S, Miller FG. Is placebo surgery unethical? N Engl J Med. 2002;347(2):137-9. PMID: 12110744. doi:10.1056/NEJMsb021025.

86. Collins R, MacMahon S. Reliable assessment of the effects of treatment on mortality and major morbidity, I: clinical trials. Lancet. 2001;357(9253):373-80. PMID: 11211013. doi:10.1016/S0140-6736(00)03651-5.

87. Roberts C, Torgerson D. Randomisation methods in controlled trials. BMJ. 1998;317(7168):1301. PMID: 9804722. PMCID: PMC1114206.

88. Kim J, Shin W. How to do random allocation (randomization). Clin Orthopedic Surg. 2014;6(1):103-9. doi:10.4055/cios.2014.6.1.103.

89. Dibao-Dina C, Caille A, Sautenet B, Chazelle E, Giraudeau B. Rationale for unequal randomization in clinical trials is rarely reported: a systematic review. J Clin Epidemiol. 2014;67(10):1070-5. doi:10.1016/j.jclinepi.2014.05.015.

90. Freemantle N, Calvert M, Wood J, Eastaugh J, Griffin C. Composite outcomes in randomized trials: greater precision but with greater uncertainty? JAMA. 2003;289(19):2554-9.

91. Egbewale BE. Random allocation in controlled clinical trials: a review. J Pharm Pharm Sci. 2014;17(2):248-53.

92. Bakal JA, Westerhout CM, Armstrong PW. Impact of weighted composite compared to traditional composite endpoints for the design of randomized controlled trials. Stat Methods Med Res. 2012 Jan 24. [Epub ahead of print]. 2015;24(6):980-8. PMID: 22275378. doi:10.1177/0962280211436004.

93. US Department of Health and Human Services. Guidance for clinical trial sponsors. [cited 2021 Jan 23]. Available from: https://www.fda.gov/downloads/RegulatoryInformation/Guidances/ucm127073.pdf.

94. Whitley E, Ball J. Statistics review 4: sample size calculations. Crit Care. 2002;6(4):335-41. PMID: 12225610. PMCID: PMC137461.

95. Guller U, DeLong ER. Interpreting statistics in medical literature: a vade mecum for surgeons. J Am Coll Surg. 2004;198(3):441-58. PMID: 14992748. doi:10.1016/j.jamcollsurg.2003.09.017.

96. Chan AW, Tetzlaff JM, Gøtzsche PC, Altman DG, Mann H, Berlin JA, Dickersin K, Hróbjartsson A, Schulz KF, Parulekar WR, Krleza-Jeric K, Laupacis A, Moher D. SPIRIT 2013 explanation and elaboration: guidance for protocols of clinical trials. BMJ. 2013;346:e7586. PMID: 23304. PMCID: PMC3541470. doi:10.1136/bmj.e7586.

97. Kaul S, Diamond GA. Trial and error: how to avoid commonly encountered limitations of published clinical trials. J Am Coll Cardiol. 2010;55(5):415-27. PMID: 20117454. doi:10.1016/j.jacc.2009.06.065.

98. Cohen M, Demers C, Gurfinkel EP, et al. A comparison of low-molecular-weight heparin with unfractionated heparin for unstable coronary artery disease: efficacy and safety of subcutaneous enoxaparin in Non-Q-Wave Coronary Events Study Group. N Engl J Med. 1997;337(7):447-52. PMID: 9250846. doi:10.1056/NEJM199708143370702.

99. Armstrong PW. Heparin in acute coronary disease: requiem for a heavyweight? N Engl J Med. 1997;337(7):492-4. PMID: 9250854. doi:10.1056/NEJM199708143370710.

100. Ohman EM. Enoxaparin reduced combined coronary events in unstable angina and non-Q-wave MI at 14 and 30 days [Comment]. ACP J Club. 1998;128:34. doi:10.7326/ACPJC-1998-128-2-034.

101. Expert Panel on Detection, Evaluation, and Treatment of High Blood Cholesterol in Adults. Executive summary of The Third Report of The National Cholesterol Education Program (NCEP) Expert Panel on detection, evaluation, and treatment of high blood cholesterol in adults (Adult Treatment Panel III). JAMA. 2001;285(19):2486-97. PMID: 11368702. doi:10.1001/jama.285.19.2486.

102. Frandsen CS, Dejgaard TF, Holst JJ, Andersen HU, Thorsteinsson B, Madsbad S. Twelve-week treatment with liraglutide as add-on to insulin in normal-weight patients with poorly controlled type 1 diabetes: a randomized, placebo-controlled, double-blind parallel study. Diabetes Care. 2015;38(12):2250-7. doi:10.2337/dc15-1037. Epub 2015 Oct 20. PubMed PMID: 26486191.

103. American Diabetes Association. Standards of medical care in diabetes-2017. Diabetes Care. 2017;40(1):S1. PMID: 28637892. doi:10.2337/dc17-0299.

104. Lader EW, Cannon CP, Ohman EM, Newby LK, Sulmasy DP, Barst RJ, Fair JM, Flather M, Freedman JE, Frye RL, Hand MM, Jesse RL, Van de Werf F, Costa F; American Heart Association. The clinician as investigator: participating in clinical trials in the practice setting: Appendix 2: statistical concepts in study design and analysis. Circulation. 2004;109:2672-9. PMID: 15173053. doi:http://dx.doi.org/10.1161/01.CIR.0000128702.16441.75.

105. Protocol for: Cannon CP, Blazing MA, Giugliano RP, McCagg A, White JA, Theroux P, Darius H, Lewis BS, Ophuis TO, Jukema JW, De Ferrari GM, Ruzyllo W, De Lucca P, Im K, Bohula EA, Reist C, Wiviott SD, Tershakovec AM, Musliner TA, Braunwald E, Califf RM; IMPROVE-IT Investigators. Ezetimibe added to statin therapy after acute coronary syndromes. N Engl J Med. 2015;372:2387-97. doi:10.1056/NEJMoa1410489.

106. Stone GW, McCullough PA, Tumlin JA, Lepor NE, Madyoon H, Murray P, Wang A, Chu AA, Schaer GL, Stevens M, Wilensky RL, O'Neill WW; CONTRAST Investigators. Fenoldopam mesylate for the prevention of contrast-induced nephropathy: a randomized controlled trial. JAMA. 2003;290(17):2284-91. PMID: 14600187. doi:10.1001/jama.290.17.2284.
107. Altman DG, Goodman SN, Schroter S. How statistical expertise is used in medical research. JAMA. 2002;287(21):2817-20. PMID: 12038922. doi:10.1001/jama.287.21.2817.
108. Whitley E, Ball J. Statistics review 3: hypothesis testing and P values. Crit Care. 2002;6(3):222-5. PMC137449. doi:10.1186/cc1493.
109. DeMuth JE. Overview of biostatistics used in clinical research. Am J Health-Syst Pharm. 2009;66(1):70-81. PMID: 19106347. doi:10.2146/ajhp070006.
110. Swinscow TDV. Statistics at square one. London: British Medical Association; 1983.
111. Kirby A, Gebski V, Keech AC. Determining the sample size in a clinical trial. Med J Aust. 2002;177(5):256-7. PMID: 12197821. doi:10.1.1.156.8676.
112. Tumlin JA, Wang A, Murray PT, Mathur VS. Fenoldopam mesylate blocks reductions in renal plasma flow after radiocontrast dye infusion: a pilot trial in the prevention of contrast nephropathy. Am Heart J. 2002 May;143(5):894-903. PMID: 12040355. doi:http://dx.doi.org/10.1067/mhj.2002.122118.
113. White IR, Carpenter J, Horton NJ. Including all individuals is not enough: lessons for intention-to-treat analysis. Clin Trials. 2012;9(4):396-407. PMID: 22752633. PMCID: PMC3428470. doi:10.1177/1740774512450098.
114. Ioannidis JPA, Evans JW, Gotzsche PC; CONSORT Group. Better reporting of harms in randomized trials: an extension of the CONSORT statement. Ann Intern Med. 2004;141(10):781-8. doi:10.7326/0003-4819-141-10-200411160-00009.
115. Guyatt G, Jaeschke R, Heddle N, Cook D, Shannon H, Walter S. Basic statistics for clinicians: 1. Hypothesis testing. CMAJ. 1995;152(1):27-32. PMID: 7804919. PMCID: PMC1337490.
116. Salkind NJ. Statistics for people who (think they) hate statistics. Thousand Oaks (CA): Sage Publications, Inc.; 2000.
117. Whitley E, Ball J. Statistics review 2: samples and populations. Crit Care. 2002;6(2):143-8. PMCID: PMC137296. doi:10.1186/cc1473.
118. Tu YK, Gilthorpe MS. Key statistical and analytical issues for evaluating treatment effects in periodontal research. Periodontol 2000. 2012;(1):75-88. PMID: 22507061. doi:10.1111/j.1600-0757.2011.00431.x.
119. Sun X, Briel M, Busse JW, You JJ, Akl EA, Mejza F, Bala MM, Bassler D, Metz D, Diaz-Granados N, Vandvik PO, Malaga G, Srinathan SK, Dahm P, Johnston BC, Alonso-Coello P, Hassouneh B, Walter SD Heels-Ansdell D, Bhatnagar N, Altman DG, Guyatt GH. Credibility of claims of subgroup effects in randomised controlled trials: systematic review. BMJ. 2012;344:e1553. PMID: 22422832. doi:http://dx.doi.org/10.1136/bmj.e1553.
120. Evans RB, O'Connor A. Statistics and evidence-based veterinary medicine: answers to 21 common statistical questions that arise from reading scientific manuscripts. Vet

Clin North Am Small Anim Pract. 2007;37(3):477-86. PMID: 17466751. doi:10.1016/j.cvsm.2007.01.006.

121. Glantz SA. Primer of biostatistics. 5th ed. New York: McGraw-Hill; 2002.

122. Ghert M, Petrisor B. Subgroup analyses: when should we believe them? J Bone Joint Surg Am. 2012;94(Suppl 1):61-4. PMID: 22810450. doi:10.2106/JBJS.L.00272.

123. Bucher HC, Guyatt GH, Cook DJ, Holbrook A, McAlister FA. Users' guides to the medical literature: XIX. Applying clinical trial results. A. How to use an article measuring the effect of an intervention on surrogate end points. Evidence-Based Medicine Working Group. JAMA. 1999;282(8):771-8. PMID: 10463714. doi:10.1001/jama.282.8.771.

124. Gorelick PB, Richardson D, Kelly M, Ruland S, Hung E, Harris Y, Kittner S, Leurgans S; African American Antiplatelet Stroke Prevention Study Investigators. Aspirin and ticlopidine for prevention of recurrent stroke in black patients: a randomized trial. JAMA. 2003;289(22):2947-57. PMID: 12799402. doi:10.1001/jama.289.22.2947.

125. Le Bars PL, Katz MM, Berman N, Itil TM, Freedman AM, Schatzberg AF. A placebo-controlled, double-blind, randomized trial of an extract of Ginkgo biloba for dementia. North American EGb Study Group. JAMA. 1997;278(16):1327-32. PMID: 9343463. doi:10.1001/jama.1997.03550160047037.

126. Postuma RB, Lang AE, Munhoz RP, Charland K, Pelletier A, Moscovich M, Filla L, Zanatta D, Rios Romenets S, Altman R, Chuang R, Shah B. Caffeine for treatment of Parkinson disease: a randomized controlled trial. Neurology. 2012;79(7):651-8. PMID: 22855866. PMCID: PMC3414662. doi:10.1212/WNL.0b013e318263570d.

127. Lee CM, Soin HK, Einarson TR. Statistics in the pharmacy literature. Ann Pharmacother. 2004;38(9):1412-8. PMID: 15199191. doi:10.1345/aph.1D493.

128. DeMets DL. Statistical issues in interpreting clinical trials. J Intern Med. 2004;255(5):529-37. PMID: 15078496. doi:10.1111/j.1365-2796.2004.01320.x.

129. Barter PJ, Caulfield M, Eriksson M, Grundy SM, Kastelein JJ, Komajda M, Lopez-Sendon J, Mosca L, Tardif JC, Waters DD, Shear CL, Revkin JH, Buhr KA, Fisher MR, Tall AR, Brewer B; ILLUMINATE Investigators. Effects of torcetrapib in patients at high risk for coronary events. N Engl J Med. 2007;357(21):2109-22. PMID: 17984165. doi:10.1056/NEJMoa0706628.

130. Lu T, Sheng H, Wu J, Cheng Y, Zhu J, Chen Y. Cinnamon extract improves fasting blood glucose and glycosylated hemoglobin level in Chinese patients with type 2 diabetes. Nutr Res. 2012;32(6):408-12. PMID: 22749176. doi:10.1016/j.nutres.2012.05.003.

131. Elenbaas JK, Cuddy PG, Elenbaas RM. Evaluating the medical literature, Part III: Results and discussion. Ann Emerg Med. 1983;12(11):679-86. PMID: 6356998. doi:10.1016/S0196-0644(83)80416-8.

132. Gupta S. Intention-to-treat concept: a review. Perspect Clin Res. 2011;2(3):109-12. PMID: 21897887. doi:10.4103/2229-3485.83221.

133. Ranstam J. Why the P-value culture is bad and confidence intervals a better alternative. Osteoarthr Cartil. 2012 Aug;20(8):805-8. PMID: 22503814. doi:10.1016/j.joca.2012.04.001.

134. Surrogate Endpoint Resources for Drug and Biologic Development. U.S. Food and Drug Administration. [cited 2021 23 Jan]. Available from: https://www.fda.gov/drugs/development-resources/surrogate-endpoint-resources-drug-and-biologic-development.

135. Pocock SJ, Ware JH. Translating statistical findings into plain English. Lancet. 2009;373(9679):1926-8. PMID: 19375158. doi:10.1016/S0140-6736(09)60499-2.

136. Sun X, Ioannidis JP, Agoritsas T, Alba AC, Guyatt G. How to use a subgroup analysis: user's guide to the medical literature. JAMA. 2014;311(4):405-11. PMID: 24449319. doi:10.1001/jama.2013.28506.

137. Sridharan L, Greenland P. Editorial policies and publication bias: the importance of negative studies. Arch Intern Med. 2009;169(11):1022-3.

138. Rothwell PM. External validity of randomised controlled trials: "to whom do the results of this trial apply?" Lancet. 2005;365(9453):82-93. PMID: 15639683. doi:10.1016/S0140-6736(04)17670-8.

139. Chobanian AV, Bakris GL, Black HR, Cushman WC, Green LA, Izzo JL Jr, Jones DW, Materson BJ, Oparil S, Wright JT Jr, Roccella EJ; National Heart, Lung, and Blood Institute Joint National Committee on Prevention, Detection, Evaluation, and Treatment of High Blood Pressure; National High Blood Pressure Education Program Coordinating Committee. The Seventh Report of the Joint National Committee on prevention, detection, evaluation, and treatment of high blood pressure: the JNC 7 report. JAMA. 2003;289(19):2560-72. PMID: 12748199. doi:10.1001/jama.289.19.2560.

140. Hass WK, Easton JD, Adams HP Jr, Pryse-Phillips W, Molony BA, Anderson S, Kamm B. A randomized trial comparing ticlopidine hydrochloride with aspirin for the prevention of stroke in high-risk patients. Ticlopidine Aspirin Stroke Study Group. N Engl J Med. 1989;321(8):501-7. PMID: 2761587. doi:10.1056/NEJM198908243210804.

141. Bhatt DL, Steg PG, Miller M, et al. Cardiovascular risk reduction with icosapent ethyl for hypertriglyceridemia. N Engl J Med. 2019;380(1):11-22. doi:10.1056/NEJMoa1812792.

142. Castell DO, Kahrilas PJ, Richter JE, Vakil NB, Johnson DA, Zuckerman S, Skammer W, Levine JG.. Esomeprazole (40 mg) compared with lansoprazole (30 mg) in the treatment of erosive esophagitis. Am J Gastroenterol. 2002 Mar;97(3):575-83. PMID: 11922549. doi:10.1111/j.1572-0241.2002.05532.x.

143. Whelton A, Fort JG, Puma JA, Normandin D, Bello AE, Verburg KM. Cyclooxygenase-2-specific inhibitors and cardiorenal function: a randomized, controlled trial of celecoxib and rofecoxib in older hypertensive osteoarthritis patients. Am J Ther. 2001;8(2):85-95. PMID: 11304662.

144. Guyatt G, Jaeschke R, Heddle N, Cook D, Shannon H, Walter S. Basic statistics for clinicians: 2. Interpreting study results: confidence intervals. CMAJ. 1995;152(2):169-73. PMID: 7820798. PMCID: PMC1337571.

145. Guyatt GH, Sackett DL, Cook DJ. Users' guides to the medical literature. II. How to use an article about therapy or prevention. B. What were the results and will they help me in caring for my patients? Evidence-Based Medicine Working Group. JAMA. 1994;271(1):59-63. PMID: 8258890. doi:10.1001/jama.1994.03510250075039.

146. Kendler DL, Marin F, Zerbini CAF, et al. Effects of teriparatide and risedronate on new fractures in post-menopausal women with severe osteoporosis (VERO): a multicentre, double-blind, double-dummy, randomised controlled trial [published correction

appears in Lancet. 2017 Nov 30 [published correction appears in Lancet. 2018 Dec 1;392(10162):2352]. Lancet. 2018;391(10117):230-40. doi:10.1016/S0140-6736(17)32137-2.

147. Jaeschke R, Guyatt G, Shannon H, Walter S, Cook D, Heddle N. Basic statistics for clinicians: 3. Assessing the effects of treatment: measures of association. CMAJ. 1995;152(3):351-7. PMID: 7828099. PMCID: PMC1337533.

148. Barratt A, Wyer PC, Hatala R, McGinn T, Dans AL, Keitz S, Moyer V, For GG; Evidence-Based Medicine Teaching Tips Working Group. Tips for learners of evidence-based medicine: 1. Relative risk reduction, absolute risk reduction and number needed to treat. CMAJ. 2004;171(4):353-8.

149. Colhoun HM, Betteridge DJ, Durrington PN, Hitman GA, Neil HA, Livingstone SJ, Thomason MJ, Mackness MI, Charlton-Menys V, Fuller JH, on behalf of the CARDS Investigators. Primary prevention of cardiovascular disease with atorvastatin in type 2 diabetes in the Collaborative Atorvastatin Diabetes Study (CARDS): multicentre randomised placebo-controlled trial. Lancet. 2004;364(9435):685-96. PMID: 15325833. doi:10.1016/S0140-6736(04)16895-5.

150. Kendrach MG, Covington TR, McCarthy MW, Harris CM. Calculating risks and number-needed-to-treat: a method of data interpretation. J Managed Care Pharm. 1997;3(2):179-83. doi:http://dx.doi.org/10.18553/jmcp.1997.3.2.179.

151. Feinstein AR. Principles of medical statistics. Boca Raton, FL: Chapman & Hall/CRC Press Co; 2002.

152. Manuscript Guidelines. Thousands Oak (CA): Sage Publications. Annals of Pharmacotherapy journal website. Manuscript Guidelines Web page. [cited 2021 Jan 23]. Available from: http://https://journals.sagepub.com/home/aop.

153. Clarke M, Alderson P, Chalmers I. Discussion sections in reports of controlled trials published in general medical journals. JAMA. 2002;287(21):2799-801. PMID: 12038916. doi:10.1001/jama.287.21.2799.

154. Mosdell KW. Literature evaluation I: controlled clinical trials. In: Malone PM, Mosdell KW, Kier KL, Stanovich JE, editors. Drug information: a guide for practitioners. 2nd ed. New York: McGraw-Hill; 2001. Chapter 6. p. 160.

155. Patrias K. Citing medicine: the NLM style guide for authors, editors, and publishers [Internet]. 2nd ed. Books and other individual titles on the internet. Wendling DL, technical editor. Bethesda (MD): National Library of Medicine (US); 2007 [updated 2018 May 18; cited 2021 Jan 23]. Chapter 22. Available from: http://nlm.nih.gov/citingmedicine.

156. Alhamoud HA, Dudum R, Young HA, Choi BG. Author self-disclosure compared with pharmaceutical company reporting of physician payments. Am J Med. 2016;129:59-63. http://dx.doi.org/10.1016/j.amjmed.2015.06.028.

157. Instructions to Authors. American Journal of Health-System Pharmacy website. [cited 2016 Oct 26]. Available from: https://academic.oup.com/ajhp/pages/General_Instructions.

158. Pharmaceutical Research and Manufacturers of America. 2016 Profile Biopharmaceutical Research Pharmaceutical Industry Profile 2016 [Internet]. Washington (DC): Pharmaceutical Research and Manufacturers of America. [updated 2016 Jul; cited 2021 Jan 23]. Available from: http://phrma.org/sites/default/files/pdf/biopharmaceutical-industry-profile.pdf.

159. Thompson DF. Understanding financial conflicts of interest. N Engl J Med. 1993;329(8):573-6. PMID: 8336759. doi:10.1056/NEJM199308193290812.

160. Wynia M, Boren D. Better regulation of industry-sponsored clinical trials is long overdue. J Law Med Ethics. 2009;37(3):395, 410-9, PMID: 19723252. doi:10.1111/j.1748-720X.2009.00402.x.

161. National Institutes of Health. Responsibility of applicants for promoting objectivity in research for which PHS funding is sought. [cited 2021 Jan 23]. Available from: http://grants.nih.gov/grants/policy/coi/coi_faqs.htm.

162. International Committee of Medical Journal Editors. Conflicts of Interest. [cited 2021 Jan 23]. Available from: http://www.icmje.org/conflicts-of-interest/.

163. Lievre M, Menard J, Bruckert E, Cogneau J, Delahaye F, Giral P, Leitersdorf E, Luc G, Masana L, Moulin P, Passa P, Pouchain D, Siest G. Premature discontinuation of clinical trial for reasons not related to efficacy, safety, or feasibility. BMJ. 2001;322(7286):603-5. PMID: 11238162. PMCID: PMC1119794. doi:http://dx.doi.org/10.1136/bmj.322.7286.603.

164. Gotzsche PC, Johansen HK. Meta-analysis of prophylactic or empirical antifungal treatment versus placebo or no treatment in patients with cancer complicated by neutropenia. BMJ. 1997;314(7089):1238-44. PMID: 9154027. PMCID: PMC2126615. doi:http://dx.doi.org/10.1136/bmj.314.7089.1238.

165. Rochon PA, Berger PB, Gordon M. The evolution of clinical trials: inclusion and representation. CMAJ. 1998;159(11):1373-4. PMID: 9861206. PMCID: PMC1229855.

166. Blumenthal D, Campbell EG, Anderson MS, Causino N, Louis KS. Withholding research results in academic life science: evidence from a national survey of faculty. JAMA. 1997;277(15):1224-8. PMID: 9103347. doi:10.1001/jama.1997.03540390054035.

167. Dickersin K, Min YI. Publication bias: the problem that won't go away. Ann N Y Acad Sci. 1993;703:135-46. PMID 8192291. doi:10.1111/j.1749-6632.1993.tb26343.x.

168. US National Institutes of Health [Internet]. Washington, DC: ClinicalTrials.gov. [cited 2021 Jan 23]. Available from: http://www.clinicaltrials.gov/.

169. US National Institutes of Health [Internet]. Washington, DC: FDAAA 801 Requirements Web page. [cited 2021 Jan 23]. Available from: http://www.clinicaltrials.gov/ct2/manage-recs/fdaaa.

170. Gotzsche PC. Lesson from and cautions about non-inferiority and equivalence randomized trials. JAMA. 2006; 295(10):11172-4.

171. Devereaux PJ, Manns BJ, Ghali WA, Quan H, Guyatt GH. Reviewing the reviewers: the quality of reporting in three secondary journals. CMAJ. 2001;164(11):1573-6. PMID: 11402795. PMCID: PMC81111.

172. ACP Journal Club [Internet]. [cited 2021 Jan 23]. Available from: https://www.acponline.org/clinical-information/journals-publications/acp-journal-club.

173. NEJM Journal Watch subscription Webpage [Internet]. [cited 2021 Jan 23]. Available from: https://www.secure.jwatch.org/subscribe.

174. Huitfeldt B, Hummel J. The draft FDA guideline on non-inferiority clinical trials: a critical review from European pharmaceutical industry statisticians. Pharmaceut Statist. 2011; 10:414-9.

175. De Muth JE. Basic statistics and pharmaceutical applications. 2nd ed. Boca Raton (FL): Chapman & Hall/CRC; 2006. 714 p.

176. Piaggio G, Elbourne DR, Altman DG, Pocock SJ, Evans SJ. Reporting of non-inferiority and equivalence randomized trials: an extension of the CONSORT statement. JAMA. 2006;295:1152-60.

177. U.S. Department of Health and Human Services, Food and Drug Administration, Center for Drug Evaluation and Research, and Center for Biologics Evaluation and Research. Guidance for industry non-inferiority clinical trials [Internet]. Silver Springs (MD); 2016 Nov [cited 2021 Jan 23] [63 p.]. Available from: https://www.fda.gov/downloads/Drugs/Guidances/UCM202140.pdf.

178. Suda KJ, Jurley AM, McKibbin T, Motl Moroney SE. Publication of non-inferiority clinical trials: changes over a 20-year interval. Pharmacotherapy. 2011; 31(9):833-9.

179. Head SJ, Kaul S, Bogers AJ, Kappetein AP. Non-inferiority study design: lessons to be learned from cardiovascular trials. Eur Heart J. 2012;33:1318-24.

180. Chiquette E, Posey LM, editors. Evidence-based pharmacotherapy. Washington, DC American Pharmaceutical Association; 2007. p. 211.

181. Wang SJ, Blume JD. An evidential approach to non-inferiority clinical trials. Pharmaceut Statis. 2011; 10:440-7.

182. Durkalski V, Silbergleit R, Lowenstein D. Challenges in the design and analysis of non-inferiority trials: a case study. Clin Trials. 2011; 8:601-8.

183. Wangge G, Klungel OH, Roes KCB, de Boer A, Hoes AW, Knol MJ. Room for improvement in conducting and reporting non-inferiority randomized controlled trials on drugs: a systematic review. PLoS ONE. 2010;5(10):e13550. doi:10.1371/journal.pone.0013550.

184. D'Agostino RB Sr, Massaro JM, Sullivan LM. Non-inferiority trials: design concepts and issues—the encounters of academic consultants in statistics. Statist Med. 2003;22:169-86.

185. Chen YHJ, Chen C. Testing superiority at interim analyses in a non-inferiority trial. Statist Med. 2012;31:1531-42.

186. Snapinn SM. Non-inferiority trials. Curr Control Trials Cardiovasc Med. 2000;1:19-21.

187. New drug approval: FDA's consideration of evidence from certain clinical trials—report to congressional requesters. Washington, DC: United States Government Accountability Office; 2010. p. 33. Report No.: GAO-10-798.

188. Turner JR, Durham TA. Must new drugs be superior to those already available? The role of noninferiority clinical trials. J Clin Hypertens. 2015; 17(4):319-21.

189. Kaji AH, Lewis RJ. Noninferiority trials: is a new treatment almost as effective as another? JAMA. 2015; 313(23):2371-2.

190. Guidelines on the choice of non-inferiority margin. London: European Medicines Agency (EMA); 2006.

191. Kaul S, Diamond G. Making sense of non-inferiority: a clinical and statistical perspective on its application to cardiovascular clinical trials. Prog Cardiovasc Dis. 2007; 49(4):284-99.

192. Musch DC, Gillespie BW. The state of being non-inferior. Ophthalmology. 2006; 113(1):1-2.

193. Pater C. Equivalence and non-inferiority trials—are they viable alternatives for registration of new drugs? (III). Curr Control Trials Cardiovasc Med [Internet]. 2004 Aug 17 [cited 2021 Jan 23]; 5(8): [7 p.] Available from: http://trialsjournal.biomedcentral.com/articles/10.1186/1468-6708-5-8.

194. Snapinn S, Jiang Q. Controlling the type 1 error rate in non-inferiority trials. Statis Med. 2008;27:371-81.

195. Hung JH, Wang SJ, Tsong Y, Lawrence J, O'Neil RT. Challenges and regulatory experiences with non-inferiority trial design without placebo arm. Biometrical J. 2009; 2:324-34.

196. Julious SA. The ABC of non-inferiority margin setting from indirect comparisons. Pharmaceut Statis. 2011;10:448-53.

197. Piaggio G, Elbourne DR, Altman DG, Pocock SJ, Evans S, for the CONSORT Group. Reporting of noninferiority and equivalence randomized trials: an extension of the CONSORT statement. JAMA. 2006;295(10):1152-61.

198. Norman GR, Streiner DL, editors. Biostatistics: the bare essentials. Shelton (CT): People's Medical Publishing House; 2008. p. 393.

199. Althunian TA, de Boer A, Klungel OH, et al. Methods of defining the non-inferiority margin in randomized, double-blind controlled trials: a systematic review. Trials. 2017;18:107. doi:10.1186/s13063-017-1859-x.

200. Kaye KS, Bhowmick T, Metallidis S, et al. Effect of meropenem-vaborbactam vs piperacillin-tazobactam on clinical cure or improvement and microbial eradication in complicated urinary tract infection: The TANGO I Randomized Clinical Trial. JAMA. 2018;319(8):788–99. doi:10.1001/jama.2018.0438.

201. Friede T, Kiser M. Blinded sample size reassessment in non-inferiority and equivalence trials. Statist Med. 2003;22:995-1007.

202. Bryant PJ, Pace HA, editors. The pharmacist's guide to evidence based medicine for clinical decision making. Bethesda (MD): American Society of Health-System Pharmacists; 2009. p. 198.

203. Thornby K-A, Johnson A, Ferrill MJ. Simplifying and interpreting the facts of noninferiority trials: a stepwise approach. Am J Health-Syst Pharm. 2014;71:1926-31.

204. Hung JH, Wang SJ, O'Neill R. A regulatory perspective on choice of margin and statistical inference issue in non-inferiority trials. Biometrical J. 2005;47:28-36.

205. Scott IA. Non-inferiority trials: determining whether alternative treatments are good enough. MJA. 2009;190:326-30.

206. Brown D, Volkers P, Day S. An introductory note to CHMP guidelines: choice of the non-inferiority margin and data monitoring committees. Statist Med. 2006; 25:1623-7.

207. Henanff AL, Giraudeau B, Baron G, Ravaud P. Quality of reporting of non-inferiority and equivalence randomized trials. JAMA. 2006; 295(10):1147-51.

208. Gopal AD, Desai NR, Tse T, Ross JS. Reporting of noninferiority trials in clinical trials. gov and corresponding publications. *JAMA*. 2015;313(11):1163-5.

209. Mohr D, Hopewell S, Schulz KF, Montori V, Gotzsche PC, Devereaux PH, et al. CONSORT 2010 explanation and elaboration: updated guidelines for reporting parallel group randomized trials. BMJ. 2010;340:c869.

210. Adaptive Design Clinical Trials for Drugs and Biologics. U.S. Food and Drug Administration. [cited 2021 23 Jan]. Available from: https://www.fda.gov/regulatory-information/search-fda-guidance-documents/adaptive-design-clinical-trials-drugs-and-biologics.

211. Mehta CR. Adaptive clinical trial designs with pre-specified rules for modifying the sample size: a different perspective. Statist Med. 2013;32:1276-9.

212. Bhatt DL, Mehta CR. Adaptive designs for clinical trials. N Engl J Med. 2016;375:65-74. doi:10.1056/NEJMra1510061.

213. Hatfield I, Allison A, Flight L, Julious S, Dimairo M. Adaptive designs undertaken in clinical research: a review of registered clinical trials. Trials. 2016;17:150.

214. Chow S. Adaptive clinical trial design. Annu Rev Med. 2014;65:405-15. doi:10.1146/annurev-med-092012-112310.

215. Fletcher RH, Wagner EH. Clinical epidemiology: the essentials. 3rd ed. Baltimore (MD): Williams & Wilkins; c1996. 283 p.

216. Pavelká K, Gatterová J, Olejarová M, Machacek S, Giacovelli G, Rovati LC. Glucosamine sulfate use and delay of progression of knee osteoarthritis. Arch Intern Med. 2002;162:2113-23. doi:10.1001/archinte.162.18.2113.

SUGGESTED READINGS

1. Schulz KF, Altman DG, Moher D; CONSORT Group. CONSORT 2010 Statement: updated guidelines for reporting parallel group randomised trials. Ann Intern Med. 2010;152(11):726-32. doi:10.7326/0003-4819-152-11-201006010-00232.

2. Stone GW, Pocock SJ. Randomized trials, statistics, and clinical inference. J Am Coll Cardiol. 2010;55(5):428-31. doi:10.1016/j.acc.2009.06.066.

3. Guyatt G, Rennie D, Meade MO, Cook DJ. User's guide to the medical literature: a manual for evidence-based clinical practice. 3rd ed. Columbus (OH): McGraw-Hill; 2015.

4. Kaul S, Diamond GA. Trial and error: how to avoid commonly encountered limitations of published clinical trials. J Am Coll Cardiol. 2010 Feb 2;55(5):415-27. doi:10.1016/j.jacc.2009.06.065.

5. Guller U, DeLong ER. Interpreting statistics in medical literature: a vade mecum for surgeons. J Am Coll Surg. 2004;198(3):441-58. doi:10.1016/j.jamcollsurg.2003.09.017.

6. Pihlstrom BL, Curran AE, Voelker HT, Kingman A. Randomized controlled trials: what are they and who needs them? Periodontol 2000. 2012;59(1):14-31. doi:10.1111/j.1600-0757.2011.00439.x.

7. Tu YK, Gilthorpe MS. Key statistical and analytical issues for evaluating treatment effects in periodontal research. Periodontol 2000. 2012;59(1):75-88. doi:10.1111/j.1600-0757.2011.00431.x.

8. DeMuth JE. Overview of biostatistics used in clinical research. Am J Health-Syst Pharm. 2009;66(1):70-81. doi:10.2146/sjhp070006.

9. Whitley E, Ball J. Statistics review 3: hypothesis testing and P values. Crit Care. 2002;6(3):222-5. doi:10.1186/cc1493.

10. Kendrach MG, Covington TR, McCarthy MW, Harris CM. Calculating risks and number-needed-to-treat: a method of data interpretation. J Managed Care Pharm. 1997;3(2):179-83.

11. Piaggio G, Elbourne DR, Pocock SJ, Evans SJW, Altman DG. Reporting of noninferiority and equivalence randomized trials. JAMA. 2012;308(24):2594-604. doi:10.1001/jama.2012.87802.

12. Askew JP. Journal club for the new practitioner: evaluation of a clinical trial. Am J Health-Syst Pharm. 2004;61(180):1885-7. doi:10.1093/ajhp/61.18.1885.

5

Chapter Five

Drug Literature Evaluation II: Beyond the Randomized Controlled Trial

Stacy L. Haber • Jason C. Cooper • Christopher S. Wisniewski • Cydney E. McQueen

Learning Objectives

After completing this chapter, the reader will be able to:

- Differentiate between four types of observational studies: case report/case series, cross-sectional study, case-control study, and cohort study (retrospective and prospective).
- Determine if the results of an observational study are valid based on a critical evaluation of its methods.
- Differentiate between three types of reviews: narrative (nonsystematic) review, qualitative systematic review, and quantitative systematic review (meta-analysis).
- Determine if the results of a systematic review are valid based on a critical evaluation of its methods.
- Differentiate between various other study designs: N-of-1 trials, health outcomes research, stability studies, bioequivalence studies, postmarketing studies, quality improvement research, survey research, and educational research.
- Evaluate the appropriateness of the methodology in various other study designs.
- Identify issues encountered in natural medicines medical literature that require special attention.

Key Concepts

1 The Strengthening the Reporting of Observational Studies in Epidemiology (STROBE) statement is a guidance document that describes the information that should be reported for a cross-sectional study, case-control study, or cohort study. Although developed to assist authors and reviewers/editors of journals, it can also serve as a tool to help readers identify important items for critical appraisal.

2 In the process of creating two or more groups of patients in observational studies, investigators may use a process called matching.

3 A confounding factor, or confounder, is something other than the independent variable that may affect the outcome in an observational study.

4 The Preferred Reporting Items for Systematic Reviews and Meta-analyses (PRISMA) statement is a guidance document that describes the information that should be reported for a systematic review. Although developed to assist authors and reviewers/editors of journals, it can also serve as a tool to help readers identify important items for critical appraisal.

5 Assessment of heterogeneity, the extent of dissimilarity in study results, is an important consideration for quantitative systematic reviews.

6 Failure to identify all relevant studies on a topic is a threat to the validity of a quantitative systematic review; thus, an assessment for publication bias should be performed.

7 Important research with which a health care professional should be familiar can be broadly organized by the reason the study or research is performed. These include studies conducted to help make therapeutic decisions, meet regulatory requirements, and examine and evaluate practice.

8 The principles and criteria used to analyze the quality of drug literature are used to analyze natural medicines medical literature; however, unique additional points such as standardization and purity must be considered.

Introduction

The randomized controlled trial is the strongest study design for clinical research, but several other designs, such as observational studies and reviews, are also commonly used. Each study design is useful for specific situations, has inherent strengths and weaknesses, and involves some unique methodologies. Because all relevant literature should be considered when practicing evidence-based medicine (EBM), it is vital to understand how to evaluate all study designs. The purpose of this chapter is to familiarize the health care practitioner with the uses, strengths, weaknesses, and unique methodologies for study designs beyond the randomized controlled trial.

The first section of this chapter covers observational studies. Observational studies typically (but not always [e.g., prospective cohort]) analyze data that already exist in large health care databases. Thus, they may be performed to evaluate events that are rare, to assess events that require a long period of time to develop, or to investigate the real-world effectiveness of a drug, which are often not possible to evaluate with randomized controlled trials. The second section addresses reviews. Reviews typically summarize data from studies that have been published previously. Because all relevant literature should be considered when practicing EBM, reviews are helpful to individual clinicians and often serve as the basis for the development of guidelines. In the third section, other types of literature are described; these include studies conducted to help make therapeutic decisions, meet regulatory requirements, and examine and evaluate practice. Lastly, some unique considerations for medical literature involving natural medicines are provided. Table 5-1 lists the study designs beyond the randomized controlled trial that are covered in this chapter.

TABLE 5–1. STUDY DESIGNS BEYOND THE RANDOMIZED CONTROLLED TRIAL

Study Design	Study Purpose
Case report/case series	Report observations in a single patient or a series of patients
Cross-sectional study	Identify prevalence of characteristics of diseases in populations
Case-control study	Determine association between disease states and previous exposure to risk factors
Cohort study	Determine association between risk factors and subsequent development of disease states
Narrative review (nonsystematic review)	Summarize data from multiple studies using nonsystematic, qualitative, and subjective methods
Qualitative systematic review	Summarize data from multiple studies using systematic, qualitative, and objective methods
Quantitative systematic review (meta-analysis)	Summarize data from multiple studies using systematic, quantitative, and objective methods
N-of-1 trial	Compare effects of drug to control during multiple observation periods in a single patient
Health outcomes research	Compare outcomes and costs of drug therapies or services
Stability study	Evaluate stability of drugs in various preparations (e.g., ophthalmologic, intravenous, topical, and oral)
Bioequivalence study	Assess whether products are similar in rate and extent of absorption
Postmarketing study	Examine efficacy and/or safety following approval of the drug by a regulatory authority
Quality improvement research	Determine the impact and/or economic value of systematic efforts
Survey research	Study the prevalence, distribution, and relationships of sociologic and psychologic variables through use of questionnaires applied to various populations
Educational research	Investigate aspects of education in order to further knowledge

Observational Studies

OVERVIEW

Outside of experimental trials, having a specific intervention within a defined patient sample, observational studies are used to determine associations between variables often involving a larger population.[1,2] Epidemiological studies are common examples of observational studies, as there is an overall interest in determining an association between exposures and outcomes. The Framingham Heart Study is an example of the first, large, prospective observational study to be performed in the United States.[3] Started in 1948, it is now in its third-generation cohort and has contributed considerable information and research to understanding cardiovascular disease risk factors (e.g., cholesterol levels, blood pressure, age) and how they affect the development of cardiovascular disease. Even though such cohorts can have thousands of patients and stretch over decades, all observational studies can only show associations in terms of risk factors or exposures and outcomes because there is no true intervention (i.e., independent variable) versus control group to analyze as in randomized controlled trials.[1,2] Despite the inability of observational studies to determine cause-and-effect, they offer many important contributions to the body of biomedical literature.

TYPES

● There are four main types of observational studies—a **case report/case series**, a **cross-sectional study**, a **case-control study**, and a **cohort study**. Case reports and case series are types of *descriptive* observational studies that do not involve a control group.[2,4] Cross-sectional, case-control, and cohort studies are types of *analytical* observational studies, which do involve control groups.[1,2] Because all observational studies involve human subjects, they need to be approved by an institutional review board (IRB).[5] The similarities and differences in these study types are discussed below. In addition, comparisons of analytical observational studies in terms of their relationships to time, exposures, and outcomes are provided in Table 5-2 and Figure 5-1. In the next section, a process for critically evaluating an analytical observational study design will be presented.

Case Report/Case Series

● A case report is a description of a clinical observation in a single patient, and a case series is a description of a clinical observation in a small group of patients.[2] Most would consider these to be the weakest type of evidence relating to EBM practices and research. However, case reports/case series can describe and recognize new diseases, report new or unusual side effects of medications, or detail rare clinical manifestations and presentations of currently

TABLE 5-2. CHARACTERISTICS OF OBSERVATIONAL STUDY DESIGNS

Observational Study Design	Concurrent Data Collection	Prospective Data Collection	Retrospective Data Collection	Exposure Known at Beginning of Study	Outcome Known at Beginning of Study	Study Determines Exposure Status	Study Determines Outcome Occurrence
Cross-sectional	X					X	X
Case-control			X		X	X	
Retrospective cohort			X	X			X
Prospective cohort		X		X			X

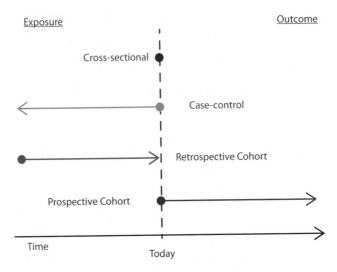

Figure 5–1. Graphical representation of observational study designs.
This figure represents four observational study designs in terms of exposures and outcomes, as well as in terms of time. Cross-sectional—Outcomes and exposures both occur at one point in time. Case-control—Outcomes are known (today); researchers use databases to go back in time to look at exposures. Retrospective cohort—Exposures occurred sometime in the past; through database manipulation and/or chart review, patients are followed over time to determine the outcome of the exposure. Prospective cohort—Exposures are known today within a particular cohort; the cohort is followed over time (i.e., in the future) to determine the outcome of the exposure.

known diseases. For example, in 1981 the Centers for Disease Control and Prevention (CDC) detailed the cases of five young men who were treated for *Pneumocystis carinii* pneumonia at three hospitals in Los Angeles, California.[6] These would be the first reports of human immunodeficiency virus and acquired immunodeficiency syndrome in the United States. Additionally, case reports/series can be the stimulus to remove a harmful medication from the market, as in the case of trovafloxacin, a previously available fluoroquinolone antibiotic. The first case reports related specifically to trovafloxacin-induced acute hepatitis were described in February 2000, although over 150 cases of general liver toxicity associated with trovafloxacin had been previously reported to the U.S. Food and Drug Administration (FDA) since December 1997 (initial FDA approval of trovafloxacin).[7] After further consideration of the totality of information related to liver dysfunction, the FDA subsequently removed trovafloxacin from the market in late 2000. Unfortunately, because case reports and case series describe a single patient or a small group of patients, and neither has a control group, observational statistics (e.g., prevalence, incidence) should not be applied (and often cannot be applied) to these publications.[2,4] Yet, case reports and case series can be used by clinicians and researchers to identify trends or generate hypotheses for future studies and larger clinical trials.

The Case Report (CARE) guidelines is a document that describes the information that should be reported for a case report.[8] The guidelines, which were published in 2013, are summarized with a 13-item checklist. An "explanation and elaboration" document with additional details was published in 2017.[9] Although the CARE guidelines were developed to assist authors and reviewers/editors of journals, they can also serve as a tool to help readers identify important items for critical appraisal. Appendix 5-1 contains a list of questions based on the CARE guidelines that can be used to evaluate the quality of case reports.[8]

Cross-Sectional Study

Cross-sectional studies are the "easiest" of the analytical observational studies to undertake, as they examine the prevalence of a risk factor or disease state within a population over a specific time period (e.g., how many people have the flu in November 2019 in Charleston County, Charleston, SC).[1,10,11] These are sometimes referred to as "point-in-time," "slice-in-time," or prevalence studies, as both exposures/risk factors and outcomes for these studies are collected at the same time. They are usually considered to be hypothesis-generating studies in which researchers can explore data sets for patterns and relationships and then propose a hypothesis for future examination in a larger study. Cross-sectional studies are usually structured as surveys or questionnaires; however, they can also be generated from electronic medical records or databases containing large amounts of epidemiologic data (e.g., state health department databases). For example, an electronic survey was sent to public health students of a large university in Southern California in May 2015 to determine what they knew or understood about vaccinations (e.g., beliefs, sources for health information, access to health care/insurance).[12] From the results of the survey, the authors ascertained how many students self-reported receiving the seasonal influenza vaccine in the previous 10 months. Although 88% of those who responded indicated that they had a good understanding of vaccinations and saw them as a positive for public health, only 43% reported getting vaccinated against influenza in the previous 10 months. However, in interpreting this cross-sectional study, one can only say that in May 2015 in Southern California within that sample of public health students, the prevalence of influenza vaccination (i.e., how many students were vaccinated) was less than 50% even though opinions and attitudes of vaccines/vaccinations were mostly positive. External validity of this study would be minimal, as the results could not be applied elsewhere (e.g., different students, different universities). Additionally, electronic medical records from the university would have been helpful to verify students' self-reporting of getting the vaccine.

Case-Control Study

Case-control studies are a step above cross-sectional studies in terms of level of evidence and study rigor, as more patients can be involved through the use of electronic medical records and large databases. Subsequently, more significant associations can be determined from the results due to the increased numbers of subjects, and because medical records and previously established databases are more dependable than surveys, observations may be considered more reliable. These types of studies examine a particular outcome of interest (e.g., adverse effect of a drug, disease/condition) and then go back in time (i.e., retrospective) to determine risk factors or exposures to what may have caused the particular outcome.[1,2] These studies are best to perform when a disease is rare (e.g., cystic fibrosis, sickle cell anemia) because more patients with the identified outcome of interest can be initially collected from a larger database or a smaller database over a longer period of time.[1,2,11] Once a database has been identified and patients with the outcome of interest have been selected, researchers can review patient health records to search for risk factors that may be associated with the development of disease and compare results with those who do not have the outcome of interest.

For example, researchers examined the association of acute pancreatitis with glucagonlike peptide 1 therapies, such as exenatide and sitagliptin.[13] Blue Cross Blue Shield databases identified patients with diabetes as well as acute pancreatitis (i.e., cases) and were paired with controls (i.e., patients with diabetes who did not have acute pancreatitis) in terms of similar age, sex, enrollment data, and complications. A pharmacy database was used to determine drug exposure to exenatide or sitagliptin. Researchers found that the odds for experiencing acute pancreatitis (i.e., the chances/probability of having the disease) were increased with current use of glucagonlike peptide 1 therapies (defined as use within 30 days), as well as recent use (defined as more than 30 days, but less than 2 years). Investigators searched patient charts retrospectively (all case-control studies are retrospective) to find pertinent data relating to the development of acute pancreatitis; however, the authors noted that they did not have access to all markers for acute pancreatitis, such as serum lipase, serum amylase, and radiographic imaging. Subsequently, not all risk factors for acute pancreatitis may have been identified if the data/database did not contain that information. This is an inherent disadvantage of such retrospective studies. Compliance via the pharmacy's database was also not able to be measured or guarantee that the medications were actually taken. Such missing or incomplete information could lead to decreased confidence in the association of glucagonlike peptide 1 therapies and acute pancreatitis. Although they did obtain a large group of acute pancreatic cases ($n = 1269$), larger, randomized controlled trials would be necessary, if possible, to prove cause-and-effect of experiencing acute pancreatitis after taking glucagonlike peptide 1 medications, as well as to reduce some of the limitations mentioned.

Of course, the limitations of a case-control study are just that. As it is retrospective in nature, researchers were restricted to the patient information which had already been collected in the database (i.e., all markers for acute pancreatitis, compliance/pill counts). In general, case-control studies are inexpensive to perform and can be completed in a relatively short amount of time as they are mostly performed via chart review using a small number of researchers/clinicians to collect the data.[1,2]

Cohort Study

Cohort studies, which can be either retrospective or prospective, are interested in what happens to patients (i.e., the outcome) after an exposure to a drug or risk factor.[10,11] These are sometimes referred to as "follow-up" studies. Cohort studies evaluate the relative risk of something occurring within a population over time (i.e., incidence rates). Prospective cohort studies are stronger than retrospective cohort studies and provide the highest level of evidence among all observational study designs.[2]

In general, a sample of the population is chosen without a particular disease or condition (e.g., chronic obstructive pulmonary disease).[1,2] Investigators usually start by evaluating one risk factor or exposure (e.g., smoking, environmental toxin) hypothesized to contribute to the disease and follow those patients over time to determine whether or not the disease occurs. Associations can then be made about whether certain risk factors or exposures are more likely to result in the development of a disease. Additional investigations can take place later to evaluate multiple risk factors associated with disease presentation, if desired. Traditional cohorts are two-armed, in that one group has been identified as having the risk factor or exposure of interest and the other group does not. Both groups are followed over time to determine if the development of disease is more common in one group than the other. Cohorts can also be single-arm studies (i.e., only one group has been exposed), but these can only show associations of disease development rates from the exposed group, as there is not another group available for comparison.

Retrospective cohort studies are cohort studies that go back in time via chart reviews with the help of large databases/electronic medical records and "follow" or observe patients having a particular exposure or risk factor of interest over time.[1,2] The retrospective nature of the cohort is that it has already been created or exists in a database, and researchers in the present can go back and utilize that data for whatever purpose they decide to study. This might sound similar to case-control studies, but in retrospective cohort studies (Table 5-2, Figure 5-1), only the exposure is the known item; the outcome of that exposure is unclear. However, the outcome has already occurred sometime in the past and can be "found" with the help of searching electronic medical records. For example, gastrointestinal clinicians may want to research whether taking pantoprazole leads to the development of rhabdomyolysis. In order for this to be a retrospective, two-armed cohort study, researchers could use the hospital's database today to identify patients who received pantoprazole during an inpatient admission within the past 6 months. These would be compared with a control group of similar patients who did not receive pantoprazole during that same time. The diagnosis of rhabdomyolysis would have been previously captured during the admission or at patient discharge through the electronic medical record. Researchers could then "follow" the patients over time and compare the rates of rhabdomyolysis between the cases and controls and determine the association of taking pantoprazole (exposure) in the development of rhabdomyolysis (outcome). Additionally, retrospective cohort studies may not necessarily be considered stronger in terms of evidence when compared with case-control studies, as the only difference is starting with the outcome (case-control) versus starting with a risk factor, exposure, or drug (retrospective cohort). Both are retrospective and must rely on previously established data.

As an example of a single-armed cohort study, 100,000 children in the United Kingdom born from 1988 to 1997 who received diphtheria-tetanus-whole-cell pertussis or diphtheria-tetanus vaccines within the first 6 months of life were evaluated for developmental disorders after exposure to thimerosal in infancy.[14] The two vaccines contained 50 µg of thimerosal (25 µg of mercury) and were routinely used in the United Kingdom. By 4 months of age, children could have received a total of up to 150-µg thimerosal (75-µg mercury) based on the accelerated 2/3/4 month vaccine schedule at that time. Researchers used the General Practice Research Database (established in 1987) to identify children who had received diphtheria-tetanus-whole-cell pertussis or diphtheria-tetanus vaccines (*exposure*). They further grouped patients by exposure to mercury/doses of vaccine at 3, 4, and 6 months; within the same database, researchers determined which patients had subsequently developed a neurological disorder (*outcome*) (e.g., tics, autism, attention-deficit disorder) later in life and compared rates among the three groups. Results showed an association of a higher risk of tics with increasing exposure to thimerosal/mercury, but a negative (i.e., protective) association in regards to developmental disorders/delay and attention-deficit disorder. For all other neurological disorders (e.g., autism), the researchers found no evidence of an association with exposure to thimerosal/mercury. However, rates of developmental disorders were not compared with children in the area who did not receive vaccinations (i.e., single-arm), making it possible only to show associations of disease development rates from the exposed group.

With prospective cohorts, subjects are followed from baseline or "now" until a time/point in the future.[1,2] Researchers can select single or multiple risk factors or exposures to track over time. These are different from retrospective cohorts, in that prospective cohorts evaluate a current exposure or risk factor present in a particular group of people (i.e., cohort). The cohort can be followed for months, years, or decades to determine how the known or chosen risk factor affects the progression of disease (e.g., diabetes, cardiovascular disease, Alzheimer's). So, the outcome is truly unknown at the start of the study. The Framingham Heart Study is a well-known example of a large, prospective observational study.[3]

As an example of a prospective cohort, infants and children of vitamin D–deficient mothers (less than 50 nmol/L) from the Avon Longitudinal Study of Parents and Children were evaluated for abnormal neurodevelopmental syndromes (*outcome*).[15] The Avon

Longitudinal Study of Parents and Children was originally designed in 1991 to follow children until 18 years of age for various health, social, and developmental outcomes.[16] Those children from vitamin D–deficient mothers were compared with infants and children from mothers having normal vitamin D levels based on maternal vitamin D intake (*exposure*) during pregnancy. The study by Darling and colleagues used pregnant women from the cohort with at least one serum 25-hydroxyvitamin D measurement during their pregnancy; their children were then evaluated prospectively (i.e., over a total of 18 years) for neurodevelopment markers (e.g., motor development, social skills, communication at 6–42 months; intelligence quotient at 8 years; reading ability at 9 years).[15] Results showed that children of mothers with a vitamin D deficiency were more likely to have lower scores in terms of motor development at 30 months and social development at 42 months when compared with children from mothers with a sufficient vitamin D level.

As one can probably guess from the above descriptions and examples, there are some inherent advantages and disadvantages to retrospective and prospective cohort studies.[1,2,10] The first advantage of retrospective cohorts, obviously, is time. It would be much quicker to search a previously established database for subjects exposed to a certain risk factor or medication and determine their outcomes (retrospective cohort) than it would be to set up a particular cohort now and follow them over the next 10 or 15 years (prospective cohort). In addition to time, prospective cohort studies are much more expensive to run/operate than retrospective cohort studies. However, with retrospective cohort studies, the researcher is bound by what data are available. Similar to case-control studies, if something was not recorded with the establishment of the database in the past (e.g., laboratory values, demographic information, intravenous infusion time), the data are not there. This is not true with prospective cohort studies, as researchers have the unique opportunity to make sure that all relevant values and information are recorded. Yet, in the case of prospective cohorts, it can be difficult to predict whether a new disease or condition might be prevalent in the future (e.g., 10 years from now) and might require a new set of data to be evaluated from the cohort. In general, cohort studies would not be used to evaluate rare diseases or outcomes because, especially with a prospective design, it might take decades to find enough patients with that rare disease in order to appropriately determine an association with a specific environmental factor, for example. Case-control studies would be better for evaluating risk factors and outcomes associated with rare diseases, because patients with the rare disease can be identified for inclusion as cases. Finally, it is important to remember that when compared with randomized controlled trials, cohort studies (retrospective and prospective) do not use a true intervention and cannot establish cause-and-effect.

Overall, in terms of observational studies, prospective cohorts would be the highest on the evidence-based medicine ladder due to their strength of design. They would be followed by retrospective cohorts, case-control studies, cross-sectional studies, and case reports/case series. However, one could argue that retrospective cohorts are equal to case-control studies in terms of strength of design due to their retrospective nature and reliance upon previously established databases and electronic medical records. Both are at similar risk for not having full data available for evaluation.

EVALUATION OF CROSS-SECTIONAL, CASE-CONTROL, AND COHORT STUDIES

In this section, a process for critically evaluating an analytical observational study will be presented. Most of the concepts apply to all designs, but the few that are unique to a particular type will be specified. The information will be addressed in the order that it commonly appears in publications, which is often driven by the Strengthening the Reporting of Observational Studies in Epidemiology (STROBE) statement.

❶ *The STROBE statement is a guidance document that describes the information that should be reported for a cross-sectional study, case-control study, or cohort study.*[17] *Although developed to assist authors and reviewers/editors of journals, it can also serve as a tool to help readers identify important items for critical appraisal.* The STROBE standards were released in 2007 and are summarized with a 22-item checklist. An "explanation and elaboration" document with additional details is also available.[18] The most common items found in the various sections of these observational studies are discussed below, and Appendix 5-1 contains a list of questions based on the STROBE statement that can be used to evaluate their quality.[17]

Title, Abstract, and Introduction

To begin, the design of the study should be appropriately described within the title or the abstract.[17] The title should be clear and descriptive, and the abstract should provide a complete summary of the results and conclusions of the study. If the abstract does not adequately state the overall methods and outcomes, there may be some biases on the part of the investigators or reasons why a balanced write-up was not performed. According to the STROBE statement, the abstract should provide a nonbiased and balanced summary of the outcomes. In the introduction, authors should describe the reasoning behind the current investigation and mention specific objectives of the study. There is also usually some discussion of previous knowledge, results, and/or hypotheses relating to the study at hand. Authors can then state their objectives and hypotheses, indicating what new information might come from the observational study being done. These should be supported by current literature. However, it is up to the reader to interpret the likelihood of the hypotheses, given what is already known about the disease state or area of research (e.g., are the investigators "reaching" for an association without adequate explanation).

Methods and Results

In the methods section of the article, authors should discuss the type of study design used (i.e., cross-sectional, case-control, cohort studies), as well as whether it is prospective or retrospective.[17] Evaluation of the study design should include the appropriateness of the study for assessing the outcome observed. For example, if the authors tried to set up a study to evaluate heart transplantations resulting from Barth syndrome (a rare autosomal recessive condition appearing in childhood that can result in neutropenia, decreased growth, and cardiomyopathy), a prospective cohort study might take years to complete in order to gather enough patients with that particular condition.[19] In that case, a retrospective cohort study would be a better methodology for research because Barth syndrome (exposure) is a rare condition which may lead to heart transplantation (outcome). Retrospective cohorts are helpful to evaluate rare risk factors or exposures over time and determine their outcome.

It is important to detail the setting of the study within the methods section.[5,17] This would include items such as the location (e.g., country, city) where the study took place and the patient recruitment sites (e.g., hospital, clinic). Dates of the study period should be listed in order to determine the applicability of the results to current therapy and practices. For instance, a retrospective cohort study about cardiovascular disease risk factors that was just published but examined cholesterol-related data from patients in 2010 might not be as applicable as the cholesterol guidelines have changed since then. A description of how data were collected would also be included in this section, as well as details about patient follow-up (e.g., seen in clinic every other month for 1 year, followed up via phone calls every week).

With all analytical observational studies, eligibility criteria, sources/methodology for selection of patients, and follow-up processes should be described.[17] Eligible patients in a study population are usually gathered via clinical or demographic information (e.g., condition/diagnosis or age/gender). These are presented as inclusion and exclusion criteria. Regarding the selection of patients, it is important to describe the population from which the groups were chosen (e.g., country, region). Both groups should be selected via chart review or from filtering data within the same database. It might be more difficult to interpret results from two different databases in two different regions of the country, for example, in addition to increasing the risk for biases. A description of follow-up procedures is necessary to determine whether adequate time was planned for outcomes or adverse events and also to detail which patients were lost to follow-up. A large number of recorded adverse events after 6 months might indicate that a medication may not be tolerable for certain patients. For example, if more elderly patients were found to experience significant renal failure after being exposed to a heart failure medication in a retrospective cohort design, the results may reveal an association of harm in patients greater than 65 years of age having been exposed to the medication for 6 months.

In terms of reporting results, the number of participants at each stage should be described (e.g., potentially eligible, examined for eligibility, confirmed and included in study, completed follow-up, analyzed in final results) and is usually presented as a flow chart/diagram or table within the results section.[17] Reasons for not including patient data or those lost to follow-up at each stage should also be available, as well as patient characteristics (e.g., demographic, clinical). Such information applies to the external validity (e.g., generalizability) of the study, as the results from the patients in the study may or may not be reflective or be representative of a particular patient population being treated (e.g., different country, region, area). For example, results from a Swedish retrospective cohort study of a Mediterranean diet on overall survival may not be applicable to patients in the United States because of factors related to the varying populations in those areas (e.g., genetics, activity level, lifestyle, food availability).[20] A summary of the follow-up time (e.g., average, total-person years of follow-up) is also necessary for prospective cohort studies.[17]

A good example of selecting appropriate patients and providing descriptions relating to eligibility criteria and follow-up would be the large case-control study by Yang and colleagues regarding long-term proton pump inhibitor therapy and the risk of hip fracture.[21] In selecting eligible subject for inclusion, researchers used the General Practice Research Database from the United Kingdom and searched for patients greater than 50 years of age who received at least one prescription for a proton pump inhibitor, patients who received at least one prescription for a histamine-2 receptor antagonist (but no proton pump inhibitor therapy), and patients having a documented acid suppression need but who did not use either therapy (acid suppression nonusers). Cases were those patients selected from the database with a hip fracture occurring at least 1 year after the planned follow-up for the study and were compared with controls (i.e., those without a hip fracture) found within the same database. In one part of the analysis, the authors identified 2722 hip fractures in 192,028 patients taking proton pump inhibitors for more than 1 year (1.41%) and 10,834 hip fractures in 1.4 million acid suppression nonusers (0.77%). These cases were then compared with 135,386 controls. After analysis, the researchers found an increased hip-fracture risk among long-term (i.e., greater than 1 year) proton pump inhibitor users.

❷ *In the process of creating two or more groups of patients in observational studies, investigators may use a process called* **matching**. Subjects that are in different treatment assignments can be paired or matched based on certain baseline characteristics (e.g., sex, age, race). Matching is often considered a strength of an observational study, as it minimizes baseline differences between groups.[22,23] Randomized controlled trials can avoid imbalanced groups by 1:1 randomization, but that option is not available for observational studies. Matching can be used to ensure that groups are similar, and by using more than one control per case (e.g., 2:1, 4:1), the sample size is increased and the precision of the results can be improved. However, it is sometimes difficult to determine which variables should be used to match groups in terms of characteristics (e.g., smoking status, date of admission, number of drinks/week). If matching is used, predisposition to the disease of interest should be similar in both groups, except for exposure to the risk factor under investigation. Matching may confound the interpretation of study results if groups are matched for a factor that is itself related to the exposure.[24] In studying lung cancer risks in a case-control study for example, this type of situation could exist if nonsmoking subjects (i.e., controls) had a family background of smokers. The exposure to second-hand smoke may muddle (i.e., confound) the effects of direct smoking on the case group because the nonsmokers have also been exposed to a factor that is itself related to the exposure. The result is both groups being exposed to indirect smoking in the past, which may have contributed to the development of lung cancer.

In observational studies, simplistic matching can only pair groups together on one or two characteristics. An advanced technique to better match groups is through **propensity scoring**, typically computed with logistic regression methods.[22] Propensity scoring is when each patient having the risk factor or exposure is assigned a score based on all observed baseline characteristics (e.g., sex, age, weight); they are then matched to patients without the risk factor or exposure having a similar baseline propensity score. This is different from matching cases and controls based on one or two characteristics, as the propensity score takes into account all traits. By observing all baseline characteristics through propensity scoring, this often leads to fewer statistically significant differences. In observational studies, matched propensity scoring between samples also allows investigators to have a more precise estimation of treatment response, approaching that of randomized controlled trials, by more closely matching groups based on these scores.

Weighting propensity scores is an alternative to matching and is useful to maximize precision, as well as to preserve larger portions of a study sample.[25] Additionally, weighting treatment and control groups allows them to be more representative of the specific population being studied. In one particular technique, the weighted average treatment effect approach, patients are weighted by the inverse of their propensity score. Subsequently, prognostic balance (i.e., similarity of variables having influence on developing the outcome) is improved by giving less weight to patients with higher propensity scores and more weight to those with lower scores.[22]

❸ *A confounding factor, or* **confounder***, is something other than the independent variable that may affect the outcome in an observational study.*[26] Confounders can be known or unknown; if known, they can be corrected for in the design of the study through matching or excluding those patients with the particular confounding variable. Issues related to confounding factors are common in observational studies because they are the product of not using a randomization schedule that evenly distributes the confounding factors between the study groups. For instance, in a cohort study evaluating the effects of sleep deprivation on pharmacy students during their schooling, sleep deprivation is a defined variable (exposure) and various outcomes associated with sleep deprivation, such as grades, interaction during lectures, and volunteer time provided to student organizations, are other defined variables. An example of a confounder would be age. If there were a greater number of older students in the exposure group, the outcomes could be poorer since older students have established lives with families and possibly other activities competing for their time. This confounding factor (age) could certainly have an effect on the outcome measures but have nothing to do with sleep deprivation. Confounding factors can mask actual associations or falsely demonstrate an apparent association that actually does not exist between variables in a study.[27] Whether the investigators have used a systematic process to identify known confounders should be identified within the methodology. In addition, careful consideration by the reader can sometimes identify confounders not mentioned by the authors. This would be considered a limitation and should raise caution about the reliability of the results.

It is also important to assess, correct, control, or adjust for confounding variables.[26,28] Methods to account for confounders relate to comparing baseline characteristics by stratification of characteristics. **Stratification** is when a particular sample is divided into subgroups based on characteristics that might have an effect on outcomes (e.g., stratifying smokers vs. nonsmokers in a lung cancer study). Another common statistical technique used to determine if confounders are related to the outcomes, as well as to increase confidence that confounding factors had no or minimal effects on the results, is with regression analysis.[29] For example, Florez and associates evaluated the relationship between rosiglitazone use and cardiovascular outcomes using case-control methods.[30] Individual cardiac events were separately analyzed from the composite cardiovascular outcome, death, myocardial infarction, and coronary revascularization. Risk ratios and confidence intervals (CIs) were reported as unadjusted, adjusted for baseline confounders, and adjusted for baseline and time-varying confounders (e.g., age, race, smoking status, education, duration of diabetes, previous cardiovascular event, blood pressure, total cholesterol, body mass index). The authors felt that it was important to adjust or control for such confounding factors, as they may be individually associated with diabetes, cardiovascular disease, or both.

In the methods section, patient exposures, outcomes, and any variables that might influence observational study results should be plainly defined, along with diagnostic criteria and definitions for chosen outcomes.[17] For each independent/dependent variable, methods for assessment and measurement need to be established.

Accurate measurement of patient exposures is essential to the validity of an observational study.[5] For example, the dose, strength, concentration, and duration of a medication would all be pertinent data to analyze and interpret. Such considerations might also involve the database from where the information was pulled (e.g., medical, pharmacy) and whether or not compliance, patient socioeconomic factors, and refills were assessed.

Similarly, accurate measurement of the outcomes is also essential.[31] For instance, a dual energy x-ray absorptiometry scan would produce more accurate measurement of bone mineral density than a peripheral qualitative ultrasound of the wrist. Sources for acquiring the outcome data can vary (e.g., VA database, private hospital database). When considering a particular source for a study, understand that different sources can affect the results as one database may be more sensitive than others. For example, the details provided regarding follow-up can be significantly different between provider notes, nursing notes, and radiology reports. Additionally, it is important to make similar efforts when measuring and validating outcomes between groups.[32,33] Finally, reliable and updated coding systems should be in place (e.g., International Classification of Diseases, 10th revision).

The outcomes evaluated in an observational study can be subjective (e.g., pain) versus objective (e.g., blood pressure).[5,11] Regardless of the type of outcome, standard definitions and protocols for collecting results relating to the outcome need to be defined a priori within the methods section. This would be especially important if a prospective cohort study were to use different centers or multiple investigators in reading a chest x-ray for diagnosis of pneumonia, for example. If available, standardized and validated tools (e.g., Hamilton Depression Rating Scale, visual analog scale) should be used to maintain uniformity in collecting and interpreting data.

When reporting outcomes in the results section, certain items need to be accounted for with each type of observational study.[17] Results from cross-sectional studies should contain only the outcomes for the particular timeframe measured. Case-control studies are best reported in terms of exposure category (e.g., hip fracture rates in patients taking proton pump inhibitors [cases] vs. patients taking proton pump inhibitors with no hip fractures [controls]). With retrospective or prospective cohort studies, the number of events which have occurred during the study should be reported for each outcome of interest, if more than one is identified. It could also be presented as events occurring over time by event rate per person-year of follow-up or a Kaplan-Meier plot/curve if the risk of the event changes over time. Readers should make sure that all results for the primary and secondary outcomes were included.

According to the STROBE statement, all statistical methods should be described a priori.[17] This would include methodology for controlling for confounders, examination of subgroups, and analysis of missing data. Things to detail for specific observational studies would be sampling and analytical methods for cross-sectional studies, matching of cases and controls for case-control studies if used, and loss to follow-up for prospective cohort studies.

In terms of statistical analysis, which is commonly found at the end of the methodology section just before the results, the three most common and important tests used in observational studies are the relative risk (RR), odds ratio (OR), and hazard ratio (HR).[1,34]

RR is also called the true risk and is used for prospective cohort studies. ORs, however, approximate RRs and are often found in cross-sectional, case-control, and retrospective cohort studies. RR ratios are more accurate of the true risk within a population because prospective cohort studies are better designed, are of better quality, and usually have more patients than cross-sectional, case-control, and retrospective cohort studies.[34] HRs often evaluate time-to-event data between groups and can be interpreted similarly to ORs. When using RR, ORs, or HRs to interpret data, if the result is greater than 1, then the risk of getting the outcome is associated more with the exposure or risk factor. For example, an RR of 3 would mean that there is three times the risk of getting an outcome from a particular exposure when compared with not being exposed. A result less than 1 would mean a protective effect from exposure (i.e., less likely of an association between the risk factor/exposure and outcome), whereas a result equal to 1 means no association. Confidence intervals are also recommended as estimates of precision involving RRs, ORs, and HRs. If CIs contain 1 as a value, then one can also say that there is no statistical significance or association between the risk factor/exposure and outcome. Confidence intervals can also describe the variability as to whether one particular risk factor or exposure is associated with development of an outcome. A wide or large CI should be questioned regarding the association of one risk factor causing the outcome, as other confounding factors may contribute. Varying statistical techniques (e.g., logistic regression analysis) are often used to adjust for confounders in order to minimize their effects in the overall analysis.

In general, the overall/main results should be listed as unadjusted and adjusted estimates (e.g., ORs, HRs) with precision measurements (e.g., p values, 95% CIs).[17] Adjusted measurements due to confounders should be included, if applicable, and why those particular confounding variables were adjusted. Thus, the measurements for unadjusted results can be compared with those adjusted for confounders to determine the magnitude and direction of change, as well as the statistical significance. Conclusions are based on adjusted results in order to limit confounders and get more precise estimates. In revisiting Florez and associates, both doses of rosiglitazone (4 and 8 mg) were associated with reduced myocardial infarction via unadjusted HRs (4 mg daily: HR = 0.604 [95% CI 0.388–0.939], $p < 0.05$; 8 mg daily: HR = 0.551 [95% CI 0.376–0.809], $p < 0.01$), but when the HRs were adjusted for baseline covariates and baseline/time-dependent covariates, both the 4-mg and 8-mg doses were not considered statistically significant for reduced myocardial infarction (4 mg daily: HR = 0.742 [95% CI 0.457–1.204], $p < 0.2$; 8 mg daily: HR = 0.749 [95% CI 0.473–1.184], $p < 0.4$).[30]

Any additional analyses (e.g., subgroup, sensitivity) should be stated within the methodology section. A sensitivity analysis is a statistical technique used to determine the strength of a particular analysis of a set of data by evaluating how results are affected by changes in methodology, unmeasured variables, and/or general assumptions.[35]

Sensitivity analyses often involve evaluating inclusion/exclusion criteria, outcome/exposure definitions, selection bias, confounding variables, and how to handle missing data.[17] An example would be with prescribing nonsteroidal anti-inflammatory drugs (NSAIDs) and the risk for gastrointestinal bleeds. Laporte and colleagues performed a multicenter case-control study that evaluated the risk of upper gastrointestinal bleeding associated with nonsteroidal anti-inflammatory drugs, including cyclooxygenase-2 inhibitors.[36] Cases were patients greater than 18 years of age who were admitted for an upper gastrointestinal bleed and were matched with controls (i.e., those without a gastrointestinal bleed). Medical records were reviewed for exposure to nonsteroidal anti-inflammatory drugs and/or other analgesics within the previous 21 days before admission. In order to reduce confounders by exposure to concomitant use of analgesics, a separate sensitivity analysis was done to assess the risk of gastrointestinal bleed from exposure to only one drug (e.g., rofecoxib). In looking at newer analgesics at the time (i.e., cyclooxygenase-2 inhibitors), initial results for rofecoxib showed an adjusted OR of 7.2 (95% CI 2.3–23.0). In comparison, the adjusted OR for ketorolac was highest at 24.7 (95% CI 8.0–77.0). The additional sensitivity analysis of patients being exposed to only one analgesic (i.e., rofecoxib only) indicated that estimates for risks were higher but did not change the overall ranking for medications associated with a greater risk of gastrointestinal bleed (i.e., ketorolac remained highest). The overall results of the study led the authors to conclude that cyclooxygenase-2 inhibitors did not result in decreased risk for gastrointestinal bleeds.

Finally, there are many types of biases that can be found in observational studies. Bias comes from errors in selecting, evaluating, or analyzing patients.[10] These known or unknown errors can ultimately skew the data and results. Appropriate steps should be taken by investigators to identify and address such biases. The reader should also interpret the results appropriately and determine what biases may apply. Table 5-3 lists common biases in observational studies and how to control for them.[37]

Discussion, Conclusion, and Funding

In any discussion section, it is important for the authors to summarize their results in terms of the primary outcome(s).[17] These should match with what is described in the abstract. Authors should also discuss the strengths and limitations of the study, including any known or perceived biases, problems with collecting data, or set up of the study (i.e., internal validity). Interpretations and potential conclusions of the results should be presented, considering limitations and generalizability to other patient populations (i.e., external validity). Other information, such as funding, authors' conflicts of interest, comparison to previous studies, and implications for future research are helpful in a robust discussion section.

TABLE 5–3. TYPES OF BIAS IN OBSERVATIONAL STUDY DESIGNS

Category of Bias	Name of Bias	Description	Methods of Control	Cross-Sectional	Case-Control	Cohort
Selection bias	Admission rate (Berkson) bias	Admission rates of exposed and unexposed cases and controls differ, resulting in a distortion of odds of exposure in hospital-based studies	A priori define inclusion and exclusion criteria. All groups of subjects should have undergone identical diagnostic testing and there should be no difference in how exposure or disease status is determined		X	
	Nonresponse bias	Nonrespondents may exhibit exposures or outcomes that differ from respondents, resulting in over- or underestimation of odds or risk	Match or adjust for confounding variables. Use more than one control group	X	X	X
	Prevalence-incidence (Neyman) bias	Timing of exposure identification causes some cases to be missed			X	X
	Unmasking bias	An innocent exposure causes a sign or symptom that precipitates search for a disease, but does not itself cause the disease		[a]	X	X
Information bias	Family history bias	Family members tend to share more information with family members who have similar diseases or exposures. Those family members without the disease or exposure may be unaware. Family historical information may vary widely depending on whether the person is a case or a control	Establish a priori explicit criteria for data collection methods on exposures and outcomes. Blinded interviewer and subject to the hypotheses investigated. Standardize data collection procedure, i.e., train observers, develop and refine survey questions and methods of recording answers	X	N/A	X

Bias	Description	Prevention			
Misclassification bias	Putting an individual, value, or characteristic into a category other than which it was originally assigned. This could lead to erroneous associations that are observed between different groups and the outcome of interest	Use accurate/ current measurements; carefully consider placement and categorization of subjects and values; and develop strict criteria/ definitions for conditions, groups, values.	X	X	X
Lag time bias	The time period before the enrollment or start date of the study, which was not taken into consideration before evaluating exposure	Define specific time periods for drug exposure	X	X	X
Confounding by indication	When an exposure seems to be associated with an outcome, but the outcome is actually caused by the indication for which the exposure was used/prescribed	Consider including a range of indications with varying risks associated with the outcome or stratify the results by different indications	X	X	X
Recall bias	Difference in how data collection occurs between cases and controls, or the exposed and unexposed, resulting in an abnormally high rate of recall of exposure or outcome in one group	Maintain aggressive contact with subjects to limit attrition (cohort designs) For surveys, obtain response rates ≥80%	X	N/A	X
Exposure suspicion bias	Knowledge of a subject's disease status may influence both intensity and outcome of a search for exposure	Assess for effects of potential confounders[a]		N/A	X

continued

TABLE 5–3. TYPES OF BIAS IN OBSERVATIONAL STUDY DESIGNS *(CONTINUED)*

Category of Bias	Name of Bias	Description	Methods of Control	Cross-Sectional	Case-Control	Cohort
	Surveillance bias	Increased possibility for a study outcome to be detected with more diagnostic tests or follow-up methods	Establish current guidelines specifying the frequency and description of testing processes			X
Data analysis bias	Post hoc significance bias	When decisions regarding level of significance are selected a posteriori, conclusion may be biased	Establish a priori the statistical methods to be used to evaluate data	X	X	X
			Report how missing data are handled			
	Data dredging bias	When data are reviewed for all possible associations without prior hypotheses, results are only suitable for hypothesis-forming activities	Assess associations between confounders and exposures and outcomes	X	X	X
	Significance bias	Confusing statistical significance with clinical significance		X	X	X
	Correlation bias	Correlation do not equate with causation; concluding that correlation equates with causation can lead to serious errors		X	X	X

aPotentially.
N/A = Not applicable.
Source: Adapted from Fletcher and Wagner.[37]

SUMMARY

Even though observational studies are not randomized controlled trials, they are still helpful in providing valuable information that can be used in practice. Observational studies can compile data on more subjects than randomized controlled trials, which can be very helpful in performing epidemiological studies that offer important data regarding public health or in learning more about rare adverse events and drug safety. For example, FDA Drug Safety Communications evaluate and include such studies and reports about adverse events when informing clinicians about postmarket safety. However, clinicians need to critically evaluate results from observational studies and appropriately apply them to their individual patients and practice. A main point to remember is that only associations between exposures and outcomes can be inferred from observational studies, as cause-and-effect analyses can be only obtained via randomized controlled trials. However, observational studies can still offer a great deal of information regarding the effectiveness of drugs once they are approved and prescribed for and used in the general public (e.g., real-word evidence).

Case Study 5–1: Observational Study

An observational study is published in Cancer Epidemiology, Biomarkers, and Prevention. It is a cohort study on the association between coffee consumption and risk of endometrial cancer. Coffee consumption was prospectively assessed in relation to endometrial cancer risk in the Nurses' Health Study with 67,470 females aged 34–59. The questionnaires collected the cumulative average coffee intake over a specific time period. Characteristics (e.g., age, diabetes, past oral contraceptive use, menopausal age) were compared between groups, but matching or propensity scoring was not utilized. Cox regression models calculated incidence rate ratios. Women who consumed four or more cups of coffee had a 25% lower risk of endometrial cancer than those who consumed less than one cup of coffee per day (multivariable RR 0.75; 95% CI 0.57–0.97; $p = 0.02$). The authors concluded that these results suggest four or more cups of coffee per day are associated with a lower risk of endometrial cancer in women.

- *What are some potential types of bias in this study?*
- *What are some potential confounders in this study?*
- *What are some ways to account for such confounders?*
- *If this study were quoted on the evening news, what important information would you want your patients to know?*

Reviews

OVERVIEW

The purpose of a review is to summarize existing literature on a topic. Reviews share the strength of being an efficient method for keeping up with the large amount of information presented to the health care professional every day. However, they become outdated once new data are published. In addition, they can be subject to author biases and inaccuracies due to limitations in their designs. Depending on the topic, they may involve a summary of randomized controlled trials, observational studies, or both. Thus, in order to critically evaluate reviews, readers must understand their unique methodologies as well as the strengths and limitations of the individual studies that they summarize.

TYPES

Reviews consist of three different entities—the **narrative review**, the qualitative **systematic review**, and the quantitative systematic review. The similarities and differences in these types are discussed below and summarized in Table 5-4. In the next section, a process for critically evaluating a systematic review will be presented.

TABLE 5–4. COMPARISON OF DIFFERENT TYPES OF REVIEWS

Feature	Narrative Review	Systematic Review	Meta-Analysis
Clinical question	Often broadly defined	Clearly defined and focused	Clearly defined and focused
Literature search	Methods not usually explicitly described	Predefined strategy, explicit and comprehensive	Predefined strategy, explicit and comprehensive
Studies included	Inclusion methods not usually described	Predefined inclusion and exclusion criteria	Predefined inclusion and exclusion criteria
Unpublished literature included	Not usually	Possibly	Possibly
Blinding of reviewers	No	Yes	Yes
Analysis of data— results of that analysis	Variable and subjective—**no new data produced**	Rigorous and objective— **no new data produced**	Rigorous and objective—**new data produced**
Results statistically evaluated	No	No	Yes
Type of results	Qualitative	Qualitative	Quantitative

Source: Reprinted with permission from Bryant PJ, Pace HA. The pharmacist's guide to evidence-based medicine for clinical decision making. Bethesda (MD): American Society of Health-System Pharmacists. ©2009. p. 123.

Narrative Review

A narrative (nonsystematic) review is a summary of previously conducted research that lacks systematic methods.[38] Narrative reviews may address broad rather than focused questions and generally do not apply methods such as formal criteria for selection of studies. In addition, they provide qualitative rather than quantitative information. Narrative reviews are useful in obtaining baseline knowledge on clinical topics that are unfamiliar to the reader. The authors, who may be experts on the topic, often provide interpretations of the selected evidence, which may be helpful in making clinical decisions. Narrative reviews provide information in much the same manner as found in textbooks, and because no new data are generated, they are classified as tertiary literature (see Chapter 3). Narrative reviews do not follow a universal structure so a standardized tool with items that should be reported has not been established; however, a list of questions that can be used to evaluate their quality is provided in Appendix 5-1.

Qualitative Systematic Review

A qualitative systematic review is a summary of previously conducted studies that uses specific criteria to address a question but does not statistically combine (i.e., pool) the data.[39] Unlike narrative reviews, a qualitative systematic review is designed to summarize all relevant studies on a focused clinical question by using specific inclusion and exclusion criteria. Thus, a qualitative systematic review may provide information that is more reliable than a narrative review that does not utilize such strict methodology. Because no new data are generated, a qualitative systematic review would also be classified as tertiary literature, although they are often used as secondary sources because they can lead readers to primary literature references. For some questions, a qualitative systematic review may have to be chosen by researchers over a quantitative systematic review because it is not possible to pool the data (e.g., questions for which the results of studies are fairly inconsistent). In such cases, the qualitative systematic review would typically report the range of values for outcomes, without calculating a single estimate of the effect. As an example, a qualitative systematic review that evaluates the effect of evolocumab on low-density lipoprotein (LDL) cholesterol concentrations as an outcome may report mean percent changes of -30.9% to -63.8% for the drug versus placebo groups among 10 included randomized controlled trials (in this case, the lowest and highest values are presented, as opposed to an average of the values, because the data were not pooled).

Quantitative Systematic Review

A quantitative systematic review, which may also be described as a meta-analysis, is a summary of previously conducted studies that uses specific criteria to address a question and statistically combines (i.e., pools) the data.[39] Because new data are generated, a quantitative systematic review would give information that is beyond that of a qualitative systematic review and would be classified as primary literature (see Chapter 3).

A meta-analysis would typically calculate a single estimate of effect for each endpoint. For example, a meta-analysis that evaluates the effect of evolocumab on LDL cholesterol concentrations as an outcome may report a pooled mean percent change of -54.6% (95% CI, -58.7% to -50.5%) for the drug versus placebo groups among 10 included randomized controlled trials (in this case, an average of the values is presented, as opposed to the lowest and highest values, because the data were pooled).

Meta-analyses are designed to provide greater insight into clinical dilemmas than individual clinical studies. They are especially useful when previous studies have been inconclusive or contradictory, or in situations where sample size may have been too small to detect a statistically significant difference between treatment and control groups (i.e., power was not met with required sample size). Meta-analyses assist in (1) supporting or refuting lesser quality evidence, (2) overcoming reduced statistical power of small studies, (3) assessing occurrence of rare events, (4) providing guidance with limited/conflicting data, (5) displaying sample sizes and treatment effects graphically, (6) assessing **heterogeneity** between studies and **publication bias**, (7) evaluating the natural history of disease, (8) improving estimates of effect size, and (9) answering new questions not posed at the start of individual trials.[40] The utility of such an analysis can be presented with a hypothetical situation regarding a new drug for smoking cessation. The drug may have only been analyzed in three phase III randomized controlled trials at the time it was approved by the FDA. In each of these trials, the percent of adverse cardiovascular events may be low but slightly higher (by an amount that is not statistically significant) in participants who received the drug compared to participants who received placebo. If the results from these three studies are pooled in a meta-analysis, the difference in the rates of adverse cardiovascular events between groups may become statistically significant. In this scenario, the meta-analysis, by evaluating a larger sample, is overcoming the limitation that most randomized controlled trials cannot accurately assess rare events due to their relatively small sample sizes.

Three different types of meta-analyses exist—a traditional meta-analysis, a meta-analysis of individual patient data, and a network meta-analysis. In the most common type, a traditional meta-analysis (also referred to as a pairwise analysis), aggregate data (study-level data, summary data) from studies are used to create pooled estimates that compare two groups.[39,41] Aggregate data are readily available to researchers but have limitations. Aggregate data are taken as summarized in published studies (and published studies may have handled some of the data slightly differently); thus, inconsistencies may be introduced into the meta-analysis.[42] For example, if each study defined its primary endpoint slightly differently, the primary endpoint of the meta-analysis will include these inconsistencies, which may contribute to heterogeneity in the results. In a meta-analysis of individual patient data (also referred to as individual participant data), data from each individual patient in each study (as opposed to aggregate data in each study) are used to create pooled estimates.[43] By using individual patient data, researchers can overcome the aforementioned limitation of traditional meta-analyses.[42] For example, when individual patient data are used, the primary endpoint of the meta-analysis can be defined in the same way for all data that are included, regardless of whether it was defined slightly differently in each study. In addition, a design of this type allows researchers to validate data, update data, and make statistical adjustments for the same variables across all included studies. Although gathering individual patient data for a meta-analysis is a much more extensive process, it is generally considered to be the ideal approach and is being utilized more frequently.[44] A limitation of traditional meta-analyses and meta-analyses of individual patient data involves the need for comparison of the same two groups in all included studies. In a network meta-analysis (also referred to as multiple treatment comparison meta-analysis or mixed treatment meta-analysis) multiple groups that may have not been investigated directly in head-to-head studies can be compared (e.g., if there are studies for drug A vs. placebo and drug B vs. placebo, a comparison of drug A vs. drug B can be made).[45] A design of this type may result in a greater understanding of the relative efficacy for all drugs in a class or all drugs used for a disease, but it will have the limitation of being derived from indirect evidence. In guidelines, indirect evidence may be rated down in quality by one to two levels depending on the extent of differences in patient populations, co-interventions, measurements of the outcome, and methods of the trials.[46] As with meta-analyses of individual patient data, network meta-analyses are growing within the medical literature.[47,48]

Cochrane Review

A Cochrane Review is a specific type of systematic review produced by Cochrane, an international organization of over 11,000 members and 68,000 supporters from more than 130 countries whose mission is "to promote evidence-informed health decision-making by producing high-quality, relevant, accessible systematic reviews and other synthesized research evidence."[49] Cochrane Reviews are subject to more stringent guidelines on their conduct and reporting than systematic reviews published in biomedical journals. The detailed process for development of a Cochrane Review of an intervention (e.g., planning a review, searching and selecting studies, collecting data, assessing risk of bias, analyzing data, interpreting results) is fully described in a handbook, part of which is available for free at https://training.cochrane.org/handbook.[50] To support the development of unbiased reviews, Cochrane does not accept commercial or conflicted sources of funding.[49] Finally, Cochrane Reviews are updated regularly to incorporate new research, unlike systematic reviews published in biomedical journals. For these reasons, Cochrane Reviews are viewed as an authoritative source and usually carry significant weight when considering the role of an intervention in the prevention or treatment of a disease. In total, more than 7700 Cochrane Reviews have been developed. Cochrane Reviews are published online in the Cochrane

Database of Systematic Reviews, which is a main component of the Cochrane Library and is accessible at https://www.cochrane.org, and they are also indexed in PubMed®. Since 2013, newly developed reviews are either immediately available for free or available for free 12 months after publication, depending on the access options chosen by the authors. Given the scientific rigor of a Cochrane Review, it is always advisable to determine if one has been produced on a topic, and if so, to consider any differences in the results compared to systematic reviews published in biomedical journals.

EVALUATION OF SYSTEMATIC REVIEWS (QUALITATIVE AND QUANTITATIVE)

In this section, a process for critically evaluating a qualitative or quantitative systematic review will be presented. Most of the concepts apply to both designs, but the few that are unique to quantitative systematic reviews will be specified. The information will be addressed in the order that it commonly appears in publications, which is often driven by the Preferred Reporting Items for Systematic Reviews and Meta-Analysis (PRISMA) statement.

❹ *The PRISMA statement is a guidance document that describes the information that should be reported for a systematic review.*[41,51] *Although developed to assist authors and reviewers/editors of journals, it can also serve as a tool to help readers identify important items for critical appraisal.* The PRISMA standards were released in 2009 and are summarized with a 27-item checklist and a four-phase flow diagram. An "explanation and elaboration" document with additional details is also available.[51,52] Shortly after release of the PRISMA standards, the International Prospective Register of Systematic Reviews (PROSPERO), a database of systematic reviews in the protocol stage, was launched to help avoid duplication of reviews and to enable comparisons of protocols with final reports.[53] In 2015, two PRIMSA extension documents were released with unique considerations for designs involving individual patient data (PRISMA-IPD) and network meta-analyses (PRISMA-NMA).[43,45] All of these sources are accessible for free at http://www.prisma-statement.org/.[54]

In addition to the PRISMA documents, an article on how to read a systematic review and apply the results to practice has been published in the Users' Guides to the Medical Literature.[39,51] The most common items found in the various sections of systematic reviews are discussed below, and Appendix 5-1 contains a list of questions based on the PRISMA Statement that can be used to evaluate their quality.[41] Other sources should be consulted for information on the unique aspects of more advanced designs (e.g., meta-analyses of individual patient data, network meta-analyses).

Title, Abstract, and Introduction

Considerations in the evaluation of the title, abstract, and introduction of a systematic review are similar to those for other study designs.[41,51] The title should address the type of review and not provide the result. The abstract should be an overview that includes the objective, data sources, eligibility criteria, synthesis methods, main results, and conclusion in a structured format. The introduction should summarize previously conducted research on the topic and provide the rationale for the review. Finally, the objective, which is often the last sentence of the introduction, should be clearly stated.

Methods and Results

The methods section of a systematic review often begins with a description of the search for studies. Inclusion of all relevant studies is vital to the validity of a review, so a comprehensive literature search is essential.[39,41,51] A comprehensive search typically involves the use of multiple databases, all of which should be listed with the date span covered.[41,51] For most systematic reviews, MEDLINE®, Embase®, and the Cochrane Central Register of Controlled Trials (CENTRAL) should be used at a minimum.[50,51] Depending on the topic, other databases may be consulted. For example, International Pharmaceutical Abstracts may index additional studies on the practice of pharmacy and PsycINFO® may index additional studies on the psychological sciences.[55,56] Within a database, the search terms used by the investigators should be chosen carefully and represent the key elements of the research question.[51] A well-constructed strategy will use various terms for a concept, which may involve acronyms, synonyms, and singular and plural forms of words. For example, in a meta-analysis on vitamin D supplementation to prevent acute respiratory tract infections, the following terms were used for the intervention: vitamin D, vitamin D2, vitamin D3, cholecalciferol, ergocalciferol, alphacalcidol, alfacalcidol, calcitriol, paricalcitol, and doxercalciferol.[57] Lastly, additional published and unpublished data may be identified by reviewing the bibliography of included studies, searching clinical trial registries (e.g., clinicaltrials.gov), contacting product manufacturers and study investigators, and seeking experts in the field.[39,51] "Grey literature" is a term that refers to data not formally published in standard sources such as journal articles (e.g., unpublished studies, conference abstracts).[50,58] Because published studies are more likely to show favorable results than unpublished studies, inclusion of grey literature is important for accuracy in a systematic review and is typically recommended. However, grey literature has not undergone rigorous peer-review and is more likely to have errors than published reports.

The eligibility criteria are typically provided next. Similar to how the inclusion and exclusion criteria of a randomized controlled trial determine which patients will be included, the inclusion and exclusion criteria of a systematic review determine which studies will be included. The criteria should address the participants, interventions, comparators, outcomes, and study designs (PICOS).[41,51] As an example, in a meta-analysis on aspirin for primary prevention of cardiovascular disease, the eligibility criteria required randomized trials (study design) of patients without preexisting cardiovascular disease (participants) which compared aspirin (intervention) to placebo or no treatment (comparators) and provided information on cardiovascular outcomes, bleeding outcomes, or cancer outcomes (outcomes).[59] The criteria may also address the length of follow-up, publication years, languages, and publication statuses of studies.[41,51] In the aforementioned meta-analysis of aspirin for prevention of cardiovascular disease, the trials were also required to have a follow-up of at least 12 months and be published in the English language.[59] The breadth of the eligibility criteria should be closely evaluated by readers.[39,51] Overly narrow criteria may lead to omission of relevant studies, whereas overly broad criteria may lead to inclusion of studies that are not adequately similar, and both of these scenarios may yield results that are not reliable.

The results of the search for studies will often be summarized with a figure and a table in the results section. As recommended in the PRISMA statement, a flow diagram summarizing the number of studies identified, screened, eligible, and included will often be provided.[41,51] The reasons for exclusions at each stage in the process should be shown. In addition, the first table in the results section is typically a summary of the key characteristics of the included studies. It often provides the sample size, groups, and study durations, as well as additional extracted data depending on the topic.

A process for assessing the quality (i.e., risk of bias) of the individual studies that are included in a systematic review is important.[39,41,51] Numerous scales and checklists exist for this purpose, but many are associated with significant limitations (e.g., rating a study as low quality due to lack of blinding, even if blinding was not possible). To overcome those limitations, the Cochrane risk-of-bias tool was developed and is recommended for systematic reviews of randomized controlled trials (systematic reviews of observational studies would require a different instrument).[50,51,60] It typically involves questions in six domains (randomization, allocation concealment, blinding, incomplete outcome data, selective outcome reporting, and other) to assess five types of bias (selection, performance, attrition, detection, and reporting) for each study. Each question is accompanied by criteria for making a judgment and phrased so that an answer of "yes" indicates a low risk of bias (desirable), "no" indicates a high risk (undesirable), and "unclear" indicates an uncertain risk. The process for how the ratings for each question are used to determine if the overall quality of a study is high (desirable) or low (undesirable) is not specified and thus may vary in systematic reviews.

The findings from the risk-of-bias assessments in a systematic review are often presented as tables or figures in the results section or the supplementary material.[39,51] Two common figures generated from the Cochrane risk-of-bias tool are provided in Figure 5-2. In the chart at the top, the researchers' judgments for each risk-of-bias item are presented as percentages across all included studies. For example, the results from assessments regarding blinding of participants and personnel indicate that 75% of included studies were at low risk of performance bias, 15% were at an unclear risk of performance bias, and 10% were at a high risk of performance bias. In the chart at the bottom, the researchers'

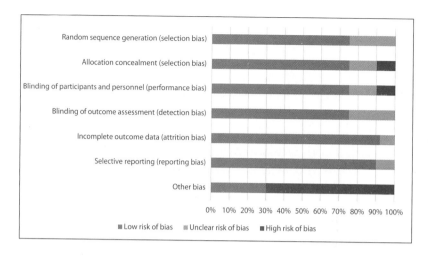

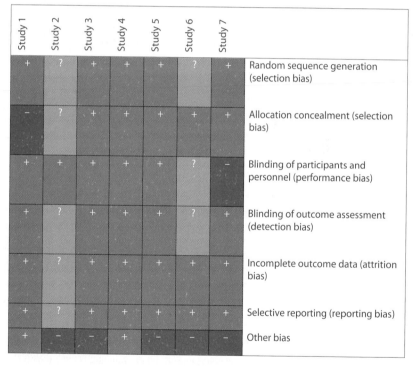

Figure 5–2. Assessment of study quality with the Cochrane risk-of-bias tool.

judgments for each risk-of-bias item are provided for each of the included studies. For instance, in Study 2, the risk of selection bias (from assessments regarding random sequence generation and allocation concealment), detection bias, attrition bias, and reporting bias were unclear, the risk of performance bias was low, and the risk of other bias was high. The amount of bias that is acceptable in a systematic review is not standardized and will vary depending on the topic. In general, the lower the risk of bias within individual studies (e.g., the higher the quality of individual studies), the more confidence one can place in the results.[39,51] In quantitative reviews, the effects of low-quality studies on the pooled result are frequently tested with a sensitivity analysis that excludes them.

Decisions in the aforementioned three procedures (performing the literature search, determining if studies meet the eligibility criteria, assessing the risk of bias) in addition to extracting the data from included studies may not always be clear.[39,41,51] Thus, having two or more investigators perform these tasks independently, with discrepancies resolved by another investigator or a consensus process, reduces the likelihood of errors and is considered a strength in the design. Although not always encountered, the extent of agreement among investigators for such tasks may be assessed with the κ statistic.[51,61] This statistic ranges from 0 to 1, where 0 indicates that the level of agreement does not exceed that expected by random chance and 1 indicates perfect agreement. On this scale, the values are commonly interpreted as follows: 0.01–0.20 as slight agreement, 0.21–0.40 as fair agreement, 0.41–0.60 as moderate agreement, 0.61–0.80 as substantial agreement, and 0.81–0.99 as almost perfect agreement. A threshold for an acceptable level of agreement in a systematic review has not been established, but higher values for the κ statistic are desirable and suggest that the criteria for making decisions in the procedures were clear and uniformly applied by all investigators.

In the methods section of a systematic review, the statistics will be described (refer to Chapter 6 for a more detailed description of the statistical terms and principles mentioned below). The statistic used to report an outcome of primary interest is commonly referred to as a principal summary measure.[39,41,51] If an outcome involves nominal data (i.e., data in categories that are not ranked), the principal summary measure will often be an RR, OR, or HR. For example, in a meta-analysis involving probiotics for irritable bowel syndrome, an RR was used as the principal summary measure for the effect on persistence of symptoms (the primary outcome, which involved nominal data).[62] If an outcome involves continuous data (i.e., data that are ranked with an equal distance between values), the principal summary measure will often be a difference in means. If individual studies in the review assessed the same outcome involving continuous data but measured it in different ways (e.g., all studies assessed depression, but measured it with different psychometric scales), the results may need to be converted to a uniform scale and reported as a standardized mean difference.[50] For instance, in the aforementioned meta-analysis involving probiotics, a standardized mean difference was used as the principal summary measure for the effect on global symptom or abdominal pain scores (a secondary outcome, which involved continuous data that was measured with different scales in individual studies).[62] Because of complex statistical challenges with combining ordinal data (i.e., data that are ranked without an equal distance between values), researchers will usually dichotomize it or handle it as continuous data in meta-analyses.[50] Lastly, as in individual studies, CIs, which are typically set at 95%, should be reported as an estimate of the precision of principal summary measures in systematic reviews.[39,41,51]

The results for the main analyses, using the chosen statistics, will typically be displayed with a **forest plot**.[39,41,51] Forest plots are extremely useful for quickly visualizing the results from many studies. As an example, a theoretical forest plot from a meta-analysis of 10 randomized controlled trials to determine if a drug increases the risk of fractures (as an adverse effect) is provided in Figure 5-3. On these plots, a solid vertical line is placed at the number that indicates no difference between the groups (1 for outcomes involving nominal data and 0 for outcomes involving continuous data).[39,51] In the example plot, the solid vertical line is placed at 1 (which represents no difference for the nominal endpoint of fractures), the RR values < 1 are labeled as favors drug (which indicates that the drug decreased the risk of fractures), and the RR values > 1 are labeled as favors placebo (which indicates that the drug increased the risk of fractures). The point estimate for the principal summary measure for each individual study is represented with a square on the forest plot, and its CI is represented with a horizontal line.[39,51] For the study by Richardson and colleagues in the example, the point estimate for the principal summary measure is an RR of 1.3, which is marked on the plot with a square; the horizontal line on the plot extends from 1.01, the lower limit of the CI, to 1.68, the upper limit of the CI. If the review is quantitative, the individual studies will be weighted differently in calculating the pooled result, and the weight will be reflected in the size of the square.[39,51] The weight is usually determined by the precision of the study relative to other studies in the review; studies that are more precise (i.e., have narrower CIs) will carry greater weight and thus have more influence on the pooled result than studies that are less precise (i.e., have wider CIs). In the example plot, the trial by Jacknowitz and colleagues had the narrowest CI and carried the most weight (16.06%, reflected on the plot with the largest square) in the analysis, and the trial by Frankel and colleagues had the widest CI and carried the lowest weight (0.78%, reflected on the plot with the smallest square). Lastly, if the review is quantitative, the pooled estimate will be depicted by a diamond (a dashed vertical line is sometimes centered on the estimate), with a width set by the lower and upper limits of the CI of the pooled estimate.[39,51] In the example, the pooled estimate was an RR of 1.06, depicted with a diamond on the plot (with a dashed vertical line that is centered on the estimate), and the CI ranged from 0.95 to 1.12, depicted by the width of the diamond; because the CI included 1, the authors of the meta-analysis would conclude that the drug was not associated with a significant increase in the risk of fractures (as an adverse effect) compared to placebo.

In order for a meta-analysis to produce valid results when the data are statistically combined, the individual studies must be adequately similar.[39,41,51] **❺** *Assessment of heterogeneity, the extent of dissimilarity of study results, is an important consideration for* *quantitative systematic reviews.* If there is a significant amount of dissimilarity of study results, the assumption is that the study designs (e.g., eligibility criteria, measurement of outcomes) may have differed significantly, and thus, the studies may not be adequately similar to statistically combine. To assess heterogeneity, two assessments are typically conducted: an assessment of the statistical significance of heterogeneity and an assessment of the magnitude of heterogeneity. The statistical tests and significance/acceptance levels used by the authors to perform these assessments should be described in the methods section. First, to determine the statistical significance of heterogeneity, the Q test, also known as the Cochran's Q test, is typically used. The Q test follows a chi-square distribution and is a yes-or-no test, with its result reported as a p value.[51,63,64] For this test, the null hypothesis is that the effect is the same in each study, so a nonstatistically significant p value means that random chance is likely to explain any heterogeneity and is the desirable result. Because the Q test has low sensitivity for heterogeneity, a liberal significance level of 10% has been proposed. Thus, a p value > 0.10 for a Q test would indicate that heterogeneity is not statistically significant (desirable), and a p value ≤ 0.10 for a Q test would indicate that heterogeneity is statistically significant (undesirable). Second, to determine the magnitude of heterogeneity, the I^2 statistic is frequently used. Values for this test range from 0% to 100%, with 0% indicating that all heterogeneity was due to random chance and being the perfect result. Thresholds for acceptable levels of heterogeneity have not been set with certainty, but the following estimates have been suggested: 0–40% as not important, 30–60% as moderate heterogeneity, 50–90% as substantial heterogeneity, and 75–100% as considerable heterogeneity.[50,51]

In addition to the results for the main analyses, the results for both assessments of heterogeneity will be provided on the forest plot of quantitative systematic reviews.[51] The statistical significance and magnitude of heterogeneity should be considered together and lead to similar conclusions. If heterogeneity is nonstatistically significant and lower in magnitude (p value ≥ 0.10 and lower I^2 values, often $< 50\%$), one should have increased confidence in the pooled result because the individual study results were reasonably similar. If heterogeneity is statistically significant and higher in magnitude (p value < 0.10 and higher I^2 values, often $> 50\%$), one should have decreased confidence in the pooled result because the individual study results were somewhat dissimilar. For example, on the theoretical forest plot in Figure 5-3, the p value for heterogeneity was 0.001 and the I^2 value was 73.1%. In this case, heterogeneity was statistically significant and high in magnitude (p value < 0.10 and I^2 value $> 50\%$) so one should have some concern about the validity of the pooled estimate as the individual study results were somewhat dissimilar. Because several factors may contribute to undesirable results for heterogeneity in meta-analyses (e.g., different doses, different populations), the strategies for addressing it are numerous and include not pooling the data or conducting additional analyses to investigate the reasons for it.[51,63] In the

Fractures

Study Name	RR	LCL	UCL	WGHT
Brown *et al.* 2000	1.36	0.79	2.32	5.51%
Richardson *et al.* 2001	1.3	1.01	1.68	11.68%
Sokol *et al.* 2003	0.91	0.43	1.4	4.85%
Wright *et al.* 2003	0.76	0.67	0.87	15.31%
Litchfield *et al.* 2006	1.36	1.07	1.72	12.19%
Grant *et al.* 2008	0.97	0.72	1.31	10.4%
Quan *et al.* 2011	0.91	0.7	1.19	11.36%
Frankel *et al.* 2014	1.14	0.21	6.27	0.78%
Jacknowitz *et al.* 2016	1	0.91	1.11	16.06%
Yang *et al.* 2018	1.3	1.01	1.66	11.86%
Overall: P=0.001, I²=73.1%	1.06	0.95	1.12	100%

Graph Generated by DistillerSR

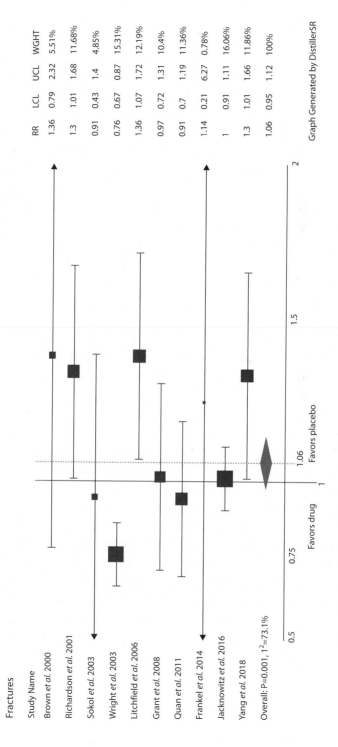

Figure 5–3. Summary of results with a forest plot. RR = Risk ratio; LCL = Lower confidence limit; UCL = Upper confidence limit; WGHT = Weight.

aforementioned forest plot, the trial by Wright and colleagues carried the second high-est weight in the analysis (15.31%) and was the only one with a statistically significant result that favored the drug (e.g., found that the drug significantly decreased the risk of fracture). Thus, it may be responsible for the undesirable results for heterogeneity (because of a difference in some aspect of its design), which could be assessed by per-forming a similar analysis in which it is not included as one of the trials.

The model for pooling data is another unique consideration for quantitative system-atic reviews.[41,51] Typically, data are combined statistically using a fixed-effect model or a random-effects model, which should be stated by the authors in the methods section. Fixed-effect models assume that the effect of an intervention is the same across studies and that the observed differences in results reflect random error (i.e., there is within-study variability but no between-study variability); they may be used when the heteroge-neity is zero.[51,52,63] Random-effects models assume that the effect of an intervention varies across studies and that the observed differences in results follow a particular distribution (i.e., there is within-study variability and between-study variability); they may be used when some heterogeneity is detected (i.e., heterogeneity is not zero). In the absence of any between-study heterogeneity, a fixed-effect model and a random-effects model will produce the same results. Because some heterogeneity is detected in most meta-analyses, random-effects models are encountered more frequently.

When critically evaluating the results of a quantitative systematic review, the effects of the model used to pool the data should be considered.[51] Generally, fixed-effect models produce CIs that are narrower (more likely to be statistically significant) than random-effects models, and the principal summary measures will be somewhat different.[51,63] For instance, in a meta-analysis on plant-based therapies for menopausal symptoms, pooled estimates were generated using both fixed-effect and random-effects models.[65] The fixed-effect model suggested a significant difference between red clover and placebo on the mean change in the number of daily hot flashes (mean difference −1.12, 95% CI −1.46 to −0.77), whereas the random-effects model suggested a nonsignificant difference (mean difference −1.84, 95% CI −3.87 to 0.19). Thus, it is important to confirm that the model used was appropriate for the amount of heterogeneity that was detected.[51] If some heterogeneity was detected and a random-effects model was used (the appropriate model when there is some heterogeneity), one can be reasonably confident in the pooled result. However, if some heterogeneity was detected and a fixed-effect model was used, one should have some concern in the pooled result (because it would be more likely to be sta-tistically significant than if the appropriate model was used). In the aforementioned meta-analysis involving red clover, more confidence should be placed in the results produced from the random-effects model because some heterogeneity was detected (heterogeneity for that analysis was statistically significant, with a p value < 0.001, and high in magnitude with an I^2 value = 97%).[65] Sometimes, if a random-effects model is chosen for the primary analysis, the fixed-effect model may be tested as a sensitivity analysis in order to assess the effects of heterogeneity on the outcome.

❻ *Failure to identify all relevant studies on a topic is a threat to the validity of a quantitative systematic review; thus, an assessment for publication bias should be performed.*[39,41,51] Publication bias is a situation that occurs when the decision to publish a study is based on the magnitude, direction, or statistical significance of the results. Because studies with positive results are more likely to be published than studies with negative results, publication bias can lead to inaccurate estimates of effect size when data are pooled.[51,66] The techniques for assessing publication bias should be described in the methods section, and the results of the assessments should be provided in the results section or the supplementary material.[39,51] Authors will most commonly utilize a **funnel plot**, which is a scatterplot that relates the estimate of effect size to the weight of each individual study (measured by precision), resulting in an inverted funnel.[39,51,63,67] Two hypothetical funnel plots are provided as examples in Figure 5-4. On these plots, a solid vertical line represents the pooled effect using a fixed-effects model, two diagonal lines represent pseudo CIs around the pooled effect for each standard error, and the circles represent individual studies; thus, in the absence of heterogeneity, 95% of studies should lie within the funnel.[39,51] Symmetry in an inverted funnel indicates that studies with smaller and larger effects than the pooled effect were included in the meta-analysis, which is the desirable result and suggests that publication bias is unlikely. For instance, in the funnel plot at the top of Figure 5-4, the individual studies are plotted symmetrically around the pooled treatment effect (six studies found a smaller treatment effect and are located on the left of the vertical line and seven studies found a larger treatment effect and are located on the right of the vertical line), which suggests that publication bias is unlikely. However, in the funnel plot at the bottom, the individual studies are not plotted symmetrically around the pooled treatment effect (eight studies found a smaller treatment effect and are located on the left of the vertical line and five studies found a larger treatment effect and are located on the right of the vertical line); the empty area in the funnel indicates that small studies that found a larger treatment effect may have been conducted but not published, which suggests that publication bias is likely.

Because visual inspection of funnel plots is subjective, statistical tests may also be conducted to aid in the assessment for publication bias.[39,51,63,67] Many tests exist for this purpose, but the Begg's test and Egger's test are common ones. With these tests, the null hypothesis is that symmetry exists in the funnel plot so a nonstatistically significant p value means that random chance is likely to explain any asymmetry and is the desirable result. Typically, a significance level of 5% is used. For example, if a Begg's test was used to assess the funnel plots in Figure 5-4, a p value of > 0.05 would be expected for the plot at the top, indicating that asymmetry was not statistically significant (desirable) and thus publication bias was unlikely; a p value of ≤ 0.05 would be expected for the plot

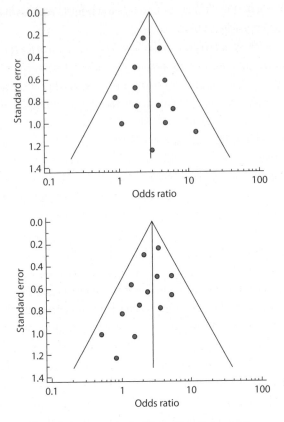

Figure 5–4. Assessment of publication bias with funnel plots.

at the bottom, indicating that asymmetry was statistically significant (undesirable) and thus publication bias was likely. In general, tests for funnel plot asymmetry should only be used for analyses that involve at least 10 studies because the power of the tests is inadequate to distinguish chance from real asymmetry when there are fewer studies.[50] In addition, it is important to note that many explanations exist for funnel plot asymmetry (e.g., heterogeneity); therefore, making decisions about the risk of publication bias with certainty is difficult.[51,63,67] However, because studies that are published are more likely to show favorable results, detection of potential publication bias in a meta-analysis could lead to an overestimation of a drug's benefit, and readers should lower their confidence in the findings.[39,51]

The last item to consider is the use of additional analyses.[41,51] Several types may be used in systematic reviews, with the most common being subgroup, sensitivity, and meta-regression analyses. The types and numbers of these analyses will vary based on the research question and the study design. The authors should describe the additional analyses that were planned a priori in the methods section. Results of additional analyses may be embedded within the forest plot for the main analyses or reported in separate tables or figures in the results section or supplementary material. Analyses that were performed post hoc should be interpreted with caution because the systematic review was not designed to assess them, though they may be useful in generating hypotheses for future studies.

The first type of additional analysis, a subgroup analysis, involves an evaluation of the result in subsets of the study sample (e.g., by gender, race, geographic location), with tests of interaction often used to determine if between-group differences are likely to be due to chance.[51,63] As an example, in the main analysis of a meta-analysis of randomized controlled trials for schizophrenia, augmentation with antidepressants was significantly more effective than placebo for depressive symptoms (standardized mean difference: −0.25, 95% CI −0.38 to −0.12).[68] In a subgroup analysis by type of patient, the following results were obtained: patients with treatment-resistant schizophrenia (standardized mean difference −0.61, 95% CI −0.96 to −0.26) and patients without treatment-resistant schizophrenia (standardized mean difference −0.23, 95% CI −0.36 to −0.09), with a p value of 0.04 for the test of interaction. From these data, augmentation with antidepressants appears to be beneficial for all patients (statistically significant benefits were detected in the overall group, in patients with treatment-resistant schizophrenia, and in patients without treatment-resistant schizophrenia) but may be significantly better in patients with treatment-resistant schizophrenia compared to patients without treatment-resistant schizophrenia (statistically significant test of interaction, with a greater standardized mean difference in patients with treatment-resistant schizophrenia).

The second type of analysis, a sensitivity analysis, is an assessment of the result under different conditions (e.g., using a different method of pooling data, removing low-quality studies, excluding an unusually large study).[51,63] They allow the reader to consider the robustness of the findings (data are considered robust if they do not change, or are insensitive to, small changes in the conditions). Generally, if the results are insensitive to small changes in the conditions, which may also be referred to as consistent with the primary analysis (in terms of favoring the drug or placebo and being statistically significant or not statistically significant), more confidence can be placed in the estimate of the treatment effect. For instance, in a sensitivity analysis in the aforementioned meta-analysis involving schizophrenia, an assessment of the result excluding trials that were not double-blinded yielded a statistically significant benefit for augmentation with antidepressants (standardized mean difference: −0.22, 95% CI −0.34 to −0.10), which was consistent with the statistically significant benefit for augmentation with antidepressants in the main analysis (standardized mean difference: −0.25, 95% CI −0.38 to −0.12).[68]

The last type of analysis, a meta-regression analysis (a term for multiple regression in a meta-analysis), is a statistical technique to evaluate the influence of certain covariates (e.g., drug dose, patient age, treatment duration) on the result and is typically reported as slope coefficients with CIs.[51,63] Because they often involve evaluation of dose-related and duration-related effects of a medication, they may add important information on a topic. In the example involving schizophrenia, a meta-regression analysis did not find a statistically significant influence on the result from the dose of antidepressant used for augmentation (slope coefficient: 0.0082, 95% CI −0.0033 to 0.0199).[68] In general, it is important to note that additional analyses, such as subgroup, sensitivity, and meta-regression analyses, will often involve fewer studies and fewer patients than the main analyses so their ability to detect statistically significant differences may be limited.[41,51]

Discussion, Conclusion, and Funding

As with other study designs, the final considerations in the evaluation of a systematic review involve the discussion, conclusion, and funding information.[51] In the discussion, the authors should summarize the main findings, compare the results to similar reviews, and provide theories for any differences.[41,51] Strengths and limitations of the review should be proposed. In addition, the authors may address the implications for clinical practice and suggest ideas for future research. The conclusion is typically provided as the last sentence of the discussion or in a separate section following the discussion. The conclusion should be clearly stated, based on the objective, and supported by the results. As with observational studies, the conclusions of a systematic review are generally limited to association versus causation, which is possible only with the methodological strength of randomized controlled trials. Information on funding, author contributions, and potential conflicts of interest are usually described at the end of a review. Although fewer systematic reviews than randomized controlled trials may involve industry sponsorship, it remains important to consider if any such relationships may have influenced the methods and conclusions.

SUMMARY

Reviews of all types are an essential part of the biomedical literature. Narrative reviews are helpful for obtaining a general overview on a particular topic.[39,51] Systematic reviews are often a critical first step in the development of guidelines and are more meaningful than an individual study when making clinical decisions for patients.[51,69] Although a universally accepted scale has not been established, systematic reviews, or multiple high-quality studies with consistent results, are typically considered the highest level of evidence.[51,70] Thus, as they continue to grow in numbers, it becomes increasingly important for health care professionals to understand how to critically evaluate them.

Case Study 5–2: Meta-Analysis

A meta-analysis was conducted to investigate whether statin therapy for patients with elevated LDL levels is associated with development of diabetes. PubMed®, Embase®, and the Cochrane Central Register of Controlled Trials from 2000 to 2015 were searched to identify relevant studies. Randomized, placebo-controlled trials that assessed statins for lipid-lowering effects and considered development of diabetes as an outcome were included. In addition, trials were required to involve at least 1000 patients and durations of at least 1 year. Two independent reviewers performed the data extraction and assessed study quality. ORs and 95% CIs were calculated using random-effects models. The primary outcome was development of diabetes measured by hemoglobin A1c levels. In total, 13 trials involving 88,132 participants were identified. Statin therapy was associated with an 8% increased risk for incident diabetes compared with placebo (OR 1.08; 95% CI 1.01–1.16; p value for heterogeneity = 0.32; I^2 = 11.7%). Meta-regression analyses showed that the result was consistent regardless of the statin dose or duration of statin use. A funnel plot was described as symmetrical with a p value of 0.67 from an Egger's test. The authors concluded that statin therapy was associated with a slightly increased risk of development of diabetes. Patients with moderate-to-high cardiovascular risk or existing cardiovascular disease should not discontinue statin therapy.

- *Inclusion of all relevant studies is vital to the validity of a systematic review. What are some terms that should be used to capture all studies involving statin therapy in a search of PubMed®?*
- *The eligibility criteria in a systematic review should address the PICOS. What are each of those elements and the additional criteria for this meta-analysis?*
- *Assessment of heterogeneity is an important consideration in a meta-analysis. What aspects of heterogeneity were assessed, were the results desirable, and how do the results impact your confidence in the findings?*
- *Assessment of publication bias is another important consideration in a meta-analysis. How was publication bias assessed, were the results desirable, and how do the results impact your confidence in the findings?*

Other Study Designs

When searching the literature, there are several types of research one might encounter that are not included in the traditional hierarchy of medical literature (observational studies, experimental studies, systematic reviews). ❼ *Important research with which a health care professional should be familiar can be broadly organized by the reason the study or research is performed. These include studies conducted to help make therapeutic decisions, meet regulatory requirements, and examine and evaluate practice.*

CONDUCTED TO HELP MAKE THERAPEUTIC DECISIONS

N-of-1 Trials

N-of-1 trials are controlled trials that often use gold-standard techniques, including randomization and blinding, conducted in a single patient in order to evaluate treatment effectiveness.[71-73] Because results from randomized controlled trials cannot predict effect in any one person, N-of-1 trials are useful to clinicians and patients, particularly for rare disease states, comorbid conditions, and patients using concurrent therapies. Because both study types involve a single patient, N-of-1 trials might be confused with case reports, but these two studies differ in several ways (Table 5-5), including that N-of-1 trials are controlled through repeated testing of the individual patient with both intervention and control, whereas case reports describe a single observation with no comparator.[74] While ethics board approval is not required for N-of-1 trials, should the primary interest of the research be to generalize the results for use in future patients, then the study should be treated as human subjects research and approved by an IRB.[71] Regardless, the patient should provide informed consent; consultation with a local IRB official may also be helpful in determining requirements for ethical approval.[72] The design and reporting of these studies has been established by the Consolidated Standards of Reporting Trials extension for reporting N-of-1 trials (CENT) 2015 Statement, which is available at http://www.consort-statement.org/extensions/overview/n-of-1.[73,75,76]

In N-of-1 trials, a patient serves as their own control for comparative purposes, making these studies a type of crossover trial. In order for an N-of-1 trial to be undertaken, the patient and clinician must first agree to assess a therapy.[71-73] Then, the patient is

TABLE 5–5. COMPARISON OF N-OF-1 TRIALS AND CASE STUDIES

	N-of-1 Trial	Case Study
Design	Prospective	Retrospective (most often)
Predefined methods	Yes	No
Clearly defined outcome measures	Yes	No
Randomization	Yes	No
Blinding	Yes	No
Multiple treatment periods	Yes	Not usually

Source: Adapted from Spilker.[74]

randomized to either the intervention or control, which could be placebo or active-control. Afterward, the patient receives the other agent (i.e., intervention or control) with the possibility of a washout period in between. A washout period is an amount of time between interventions to allow the drug to leave the participant's system so that effects from the first intervention do not cross into the next treatment interval. In this manner the patient is exposed in a challenge-withdrawal-challenge-withdrawal (i.e., "ABAB") sequence or the opposite sequence (i.e., "BABA"), depending on randomization.[71,73] Typically, the patient will repeat this sequence multiple times to increase the sample size and protect against random error caused by potential confounders.[71] Following the completion of each challenge, monitoring and quantitative assessment of effect should be documented. Repetitions of the paired treatment period should continue until the therapy is proven effective, ineffective, or dangerous; this typically requires a minimum of three paired exposures.[72]

Comparisons can then be made between the intervention and control once all data have been collected, either via data visualization or statistically. If inferential statistics are selected by the researchers, they should specify the number of treatment periods prior to starting the study.[72] Common statistical tests used include the sign test, paired t test, and Bayesian hierarchical models.

When conducting an N-of-1 trial, specific circumstances are required. First, there must be substantial doubt about whether the treatment will work for an individual patient. Patients must suffer from a chronic condition with documentable symptoms or established biomarkers (e.g., blood pressure). The treatment should have a fast onset of no more than a few days and termination of action of ideally hours to maintain the practicality and feasibility of conducting the study.[71,72] Because N-of-1 trials are easier to conduct when positive outcomes are revealed within a few days, giving consideration to how long it might take to see an effect of the therapy (i.e., the dosage and administration schedule is working as intended) is also important.[72] If the selected outcome is one that the researchers are trying to prevent, and thus occurs at an unknowable rate (e.g., asthma attack), the evaluation period should be long enough to see at least one occurrence of the event. In general, using three times the average number of days it takes to see one event provides 95% confidence that at least one event will be seen.

N-of-1 trials have several benefits. They provide flexibility in patient selection, allow patients to have a voice in their own care, control for patient-by-treatment interaction (patient characteristics are responsible for the response, not the treatment) and treatment-by-time interaction (chance that effects of treatments are variable over time), can reduce use of ineffective therapies, and can establish effectiveness directly in individuals.[71,73] Potential benefits that may be seen with an increase in the use of N-of-1 trials include cost savings, patient acceptance of the scientific method, clinician engagement with clinical research, and increased volume of data.

For N-of-1 trials to become more common, several barriers will need to be overcome.[71] Advocates of N-of-1 trials need to establish that this design has a concrete clinical and financial benefit for the entire health care community, including researchers, clinicians, and patients. Other areas that will require change in established practice include ethical standards, data analytics, and informatics.

Should one be exposed to an N-of-1 trial in practice, focusing on the established requirements for the appropriateness of conducting an N-of-1 trial is important. Consideration should be given to the acuity of the disease state, pharmacokinetics of the treatment, data collection procedures, and selection of outcomes. Furthermore, the design of the study should be evaluated, including whether gold-standard techniques like randomization and blinding are used, multiple sequences of the paired-treatment protocol are conducted, and analysis of the study results is suitable. Appendix 5-1 lists additional questions that one should utilize when reading an N-of-1 trial.

Health Outcomes Research

● **Health outcomes research** is defined as the effect clinicians and health care organizations have on improving patients' health.[77] This nebulous concept is much broader than systematic research conducted via observational and interventional trials used to identify or measure the benefit of a specific intervention on a specific disease state. Health outcomes research, which is used to complement clinical trial research by providing better information to inform patient, health provider, and health policy decisions, can focus on therapeutic, nontherapeutic, and economic concerns; the latter includes the subject of Chapter 7, pharmacoeconomics.[77,78] Regardless of the emphasis of any specific study, a generally accepted theme of health outcomes research is the evaluation of the patient experience, specifically outcomes that patients care about or that relate to how they feel, like ability to function, quality of life, or patient preference.[77–79]

The importance of patient-reported outcomes as a component of health outcomes research is illustrated by the emergence of patient-centered outcomes research, defined by the Agency for Healthcare Research and Quality (AHRQ) as the comparison of two or more interventions on health outcomes, including those important to patients.[79] Much of this research stems from the Patient-Centered Outcomes Research Institute (PCORI), an organization created in 2010, that is focused on identifying and answering critical research questions that help both patients and clinicians make better health care decisions via comparative effectiveness research. Given the focus on using outcomes important to patients, measuring how people feel, known as health-related quality of life (HR-QOL), is an essential part of conducting this type of outcomes research.[80]

When selecting therapies, patients and clinicians often focus on prolonging the life of the patient.[80] Assuming a patient accepts this as the goal and there is a therapy with proven efficacy, HR-QOL may be deemed less relevant; however, there are three situations when measuring HR-QOL becomes pertinent. First, should a life-prolonging treatment adversely affect HR-QOL, patients may feel a small increase in life expectancy is not worth the negative outcome. For example, chemotherapy often causes unbearable side effects and patients may not feel the additional time alive is worth the burden that the treatment has imposed on their life. Second, if the therapeutic goal is to improve life rather than prolong it, using assessments that measure HR-QOL is obvious. Lastly, when treating conditions that have known disease-oriented benefits measured by sur- rogate outcomes or physiologic parameters, it is possible that patient-oriented outcomes are not known or noticed; therefore, knowing that the physiologic benefit of the drug is also improving patient HR-QOL becomes important.

Assessments of HR-QOL have been organized into either general or specific mea- sures.[79,80] General measures are tools that capture physical and mental health on almost any adult and can be used across different disease states. A good example of a general HR-QOL measure that captures an individual's overall well-being is Short-Form 36, which is available at https://www.rand.org/health-care/surveys_tools/mos/36-item-short- form.html.[81] General measures can provide a direct comparison across various conditions but may produce superficial results and are less powerful than disease-specific tools.[80] Contrary to general measures, specific measures focus on an explicit disease, condi- tion, or symptom, and are more subject to change, but cannot be used across disease states. These measures, assuming appropriate development and vetting by researchers via a thorough survey of patients experiencing the condition, are beneficial because they can provide a comprehensive understanding of a particular disease state. Determining whether the overall or disease-specific quality of life is the focus for the patient will allow one to evaluate the tool selected by investigators when considering a therapy.

As an example, investigators could assess the overall health and quality of life of patients suffering from depression using the Short-Form 36 as a generic HR-QOL mea- sure. To focus on the disease of depression, the same researchers could assess the patients using the Hamilton Depression Rating Scale, a measure specific to that disease.[82] However, to compare the HR-QOL in patients with depression with those suffering from insomnia, researchers could not use the Hamilton Depression Rating Scale because it is specific to depression, but could use the Short-Form 36 to compare general HR-QOL.

When reading a study that has assessed HR-QOL, the first step is to look up the instrument that was used in the study.[80] After establishing the tool is current via a special- ized tertiary reference, utilizing a secondary database to find the original report of the tool can help provide context and ensure that the instrument has been properly investigated.

Furthermore, determining the measurement properties of any HR-QOL tool is impor- tant. Reliability, validity, and responsiveness are the three categories of measurement that will help establish use of the tool as appropriate.[80] Reliability allows one to accept that the results the tool produces will be consistent and reproducible across observers. If the results do not change a great deal over time but are different across patients based on the disease severity of each patient, then reliability of the assessment is high. Validity establishes that the assessment items are sensible and that the tool collects information that runs the gamut of issues important to patients. Finally, responsiveness of the tool is considered. Responsiveness is the ability of the tool to measure change over time within a specific patient.

In addition to giving consideration to these measurement properties before directly applying any results to a patient, it is important to determine if any evaluable aspect has been omitted.[80] Tools for HR-QOL first assess symptoms, then functional consequences of those symptoms, and lastly complex elements, like emotional function. While some tools include all three elements, this comprehensiveness may be unnecessary depending on a patient's desire; therefore, when looking at an HR-QOL assessment, ensure that the tool is not missing an element that a patient sees as a critical aspect of their care.

Finally, assessing the actual results of any study using HR-QOL requires some nuanced understanding of the disease state in addition to the tool itself. Looking at the minimally important difference, defined as the smallest change that would allow patients to derive a benefit, can help a reader decide whether or not the intervention would help a patient.[80] Other concepts to consider when evaluating a study that has used HR-QOL as an outcome assessment tool are included in Appendix 5-1.

CONDUCTED TO ACHIEVE REGULATORY CONSIDERATIONS

Stability Studies

Stability of a pharmaceutical product is defined by the United States Pharmacopeia (USP) as "extent to which a product retains, within specific limits and throughout its period of storage and use (that is, its shelf-life), the same properties and characteristics that it possessed at the time of its manufacture."[83] In order to ensure stability and thus establish the quality, safety, and efficacy of a product, stability testing must be performed. Stability testing includes a complex set of costly procedures requiring time and expertise.[84,85]

Stability studies establish the quality of an active pharmaceutical ingredient (API) or finished pharmaceutical product (FPP) when exposed to various environmental factors like temperature, light, and humidity.[85–87] Consideration must also be given to product-specific factors that could influence quality, such as interaction with excipients or packaging materials. The results of these tests, which reveal degradation attributable to exposure to thermal variances, moisture, and light, are used to determine the retest period for an API or the shelf life for an FPP. Stability studies are used to recommend storage conditions. The length of a stability study must be long enough and the range of exposures broad enough to address shipping as well as storage.

Because stability studies are conducted in order to meet regulatory standards, manufacturers rarely publish results in major medical journals, though manufacturers keep stability records and will usually provide this information upon request.[86] However, some testing to establish stability beyond manufacturers' recommendations, particularly for parenteral products, is conducted by health care professionals and published.

There are several international and national organizations responsible for overseeing the quality and stability testing of APIs and FPPs. The World Health Organization (WHO) published updated guidelines in 2018 outlining stability data requirements for registration of APIs and FPPs.[87] These guidelines are cross-referenced with the International Council for Harmonisation of Technical Requirements for Pharmaceuticals for Human Use, which also broadly address stability testing and evaluation.[88] Because the FDA is responsible for the quality of all drug products available in the United States, stability testing is also under the purview of this organization.[85] FDA guidance on stability testing is available on the government website and aligns with the International Council for Harmonisation guidelines.[85,88] Additional information on stability testing requirements to achieve current good manufacturing practice maintain that manufacturers must have a written testing program and that the results be used to determine storage conditions and expiration dates of products.[89] Finally, per the FDA, drug products marketed in the United States must adhere to USP and National Formulary standards.[83] The USP Guidelines include recommendations for preparation of pharmaceutical products via nonsterile and sterile compounding, beyond-use dating for pharmaceutical preparations that is based on stability and sterility data, and information on disposal of products that have reached their beyond-use date.

There is consistency across the above guidelines regarding expectations for stability study execution. When using stability studies supplied by the manufacturer, it can be helpful to review the guidelines to ensure that the study includes information required by regulators, including stress testing, selection of batches, specification, testing frequency, and storage conditions. For stability studies identified via literature searches, one should assess the applicability of the information to patient care, in a manner similar to reviewing other research, making sure that the study design has external validity to the specific circumstance. In addition to these considerations, the questions defined in Appendix 5-1 can help assess the value of the study.

Bioequivalence Studies

When manufacturers make generic drug products, they must prove that the new product is bioequivalent to the brand name or reference listed drug product in order to gain FDA approval.[90] To this end, **bioequivalence studies** are designed to show that the generic product has the same quality, safety, and efficacy of the reference product. Typically, this is achieved through crossover studies conducted within individual subjects using pharmacokinetic data. Assuming that the bioequivalence is established, the generic product can then be substituted for the branded drug per FDA regulations.[90,91] The FDA maintains the Orange Book (https://www.accessdata.fda.gov/scripts/cder/ob/index.cfm), a database that lists the reference drug and any approved generics that are considered bioequivalent.[92]

Demonstrating bioequivalence of the new generic product is a major component of the abbreviated new drug application.[91] The generic product is bioequivalent to the reference listed drug if "the rate and extent of absorption of the drug do not show a significant difference from the rate and extent of absorption of the listed drug when administered at the same molar dose of the therapeutic ingredient under similar experimental conditions in either a single dose or multiple doses." To establish comparative bioequivalence (i.e., not a significant difference), the current regulation used by the FDA requires that the entire 90% confidence interval of the geometric mean ratio of generic drug pharmacokinetic results falls within 80–125% of the reference drug.[90,91,93] The FDA allows for four study designs to establish bioequivalence, which are, in order of preference, pharmacokinetic, pharmacodynamic, clinical, and in vitro studies. In addition to subject data, the FDA recommends that manufacturers include the following pharmacokinetic data to establish bioequivalence: area under the blood concentration time-curve, peak drug concentration, and time-to-peak drug plasma concentration.

While it is possible that a health care provider would encounter a bioequivalence study, it is unlikely that the interpretation would affect patient care.[93] The appropriate regulating body will use the studies to determine if the generic product should be approved for use as a substitute for the reference product. Still, if one were to encounter bioequivalence research, certain criteria should be established in the methods section:

- Acceptable age and weight range for the subjects are defined.
- Clinical parameters used to characterize a normal, healthy adult (e.g., physical exam observations, hematological evaluations) are described.
- Subjects should be free of all drugs, including caffeine, nicotine, alcohol, and other recreational drugs for at least 2 weeks prior to testing because these factors can affect pharmacokinetic parameters.
- Subjects should be free of all dietary supplements (botanical and nonbotanical), as many of these products can interact with products under bioequivalence review.
- All subjects should receive the drug under the same conditions and all blood levels should be taken at the same intervals, which should be based on the half-life of the drug.
- The assay used to determine the blood levels should be validated.
- The same assay should be used for the test and reference drugs. Multiple assays are available to measure serum levels for some products. Results from the same assay for two drugs may demonstrate equivalence. However, if one assay type is used for the reference drug and another assay type is used for the test drug, the results may not demonstrate equivalence because the sensitivity and specificity of assays may be different.

- Bioequivalence testing may be performed in both fasting and fed states to assess the impact of food on bioavailability; however, food intake should be closely monitored and controlled.

In addition to considering these important components of bioequivalence study methodology, readers should be aware of cross-study evaluations, in which the blood concentration-time curve results of the same drug product, generated from separate studies, are compared. Because the same products may be tested with varying external factors, like subject populations, study conditions, and assay methodologies, differences in pharmacokinetic results can be seen despite the same drug being evaluated in these studies.[93] Should one encounter a bioequivalence study, assessing the methodology for appropriateness and reviewing the questions listed in Appendix 5-1 might prove useful.

Postmarketing Studies

Phase IV studies are designed to further research on a medication after approval by a regulating agency.[94] These studies help explain the way in which a medication is used in the real world, as they eliminate the strict inclusion and exclusion criteria typically used in preapproval studies. **Postmarketing studies**, a type of phase IV study, are mandated by a regulatory authority. These studies are needed because clinical trials prior to approval rarely include more than a few thousand patients and those seeking additional knowledge about medications cannot conduct scientific research prior to the drug becoming commercially available. Additionally, the FDA grants certain medications accelerated approval based on studies that demonstrate efficacy using surrogate markers; the FDA requires that these medications continue to be studied after approval in postmarketing studies focused on clinical efficacy.[95]

The real-world nature of postmarketing studies helps establish the **effectiveness** of an intervention, showing how a drug works once it has been made available to the entirety of the population.[94] This is opposed to the concept of **efficacy**, in which it is determined how well the medication works under ideal conditions. In addition to evaluating effectiveness, postmarketing studies can also be useful in establishing the safety of a medication by both identifying rare adverse effects and better defining adverse effect rates. They may show ways in which a medication could be used in an off-label manner, whether for use in diseases or populations not previously considered or via routes or schedules not yet established. Other ways that phase IV studies can be used include identifying drug-drug interactions, pharmacogenomic properties, and practice patterns; possibilities are limitless and ever-changing.

While postmarketing studies can be conducted voluntarily for research purposes by any investigator, the 1997 Food and Drug Administration Modernization Act (FDAMA) introduced the authority of the FDA to request postmarketing surveillance be conducted following approval of a medication.[96] These studies may include *requirements*, meaning that the FDA dictates some elements of the way the study is conducted, or *commitments*, in which the manufacturer has agreed to conduct the study but is not required to do so.[97] The FDA maintains a website that houses data, including the applicant, product, and status, on postmarketing requirements and commitments.[98]

Postmarketing studies can take many different forms, including cross-sectional, case-control, cohort, and randomized controlled trial; the general aspects of evaluating those studies apply to postmarketing investigations. Because postmarketing studies tend to focus on the safety of medications, there are specific components to consider. For example, reporting of adverse effects by subjects can vary and be inconsistent. Furthermore, while postmarketing studies help researchers identify rare events and further establish the prevalence and incidence of events, significant differences in safety outcomes may not be detected if the sample sizes are not sufficiently large. Referring to Appendix 5-1 for additional questions to ask when reading a postmarketing study is advised.

CONDUCTED TO EXAMINE AND EVALUATE PRACTICE

Quality Improvement Research

Quality improvement (QI) research (sometimes referred to as programmatic research) is conducted to determine whether systematic efforts, introduced under the belief that they will improve outcomes, are truly effective in producing those hypothesized benefits.[99] No matter how much an initiative makes sense or inductively should work, it is important for health care professionals to prove that practice is causing intended and likely better outcomes.[100] The overarching goal of QI research is to affect change in behavior, leading to improved outcomes through increased consistency, appropriateness, and efficiency via an applied initiative. As such, QI research does not assess the efficacy of any intervention, rather it determines whether clinicians adhere to changes developed to optimize health care. Put another way, the goal of QI is to do better, while the goal of research is to produce new knowledge; however, incorporating assessment of the new, seemingly better process is required to understand the nature and impact of the intervention.[99]

As an example, a QI study was designed to determine if introduced mechanisms were effective in reducing the high volume of vancomycin utilization in a neonatal intensive care unit.[101] Investigators established that while vancomycin is effective in reducing infant mortality from bacterial infection, overuse and adverse drug effects limit the use of the drug. They designed several initiatives to reduce the use of vancomycin in their neonatal intensive care unit, including the creation of an interdisciplinary team, a clinical-decision support tool to encourage pharmacist evaluation of antibiotic use at 48 hours, development of clinical pathways, and prospective antimicrobial stewardship review of orders for vancomycin. By evaluating the number of vancomycin days-of-therapy per

1000-patient days as the primary outcome, the researchers were able to demonstrate that the QI initiatives led to reduced vancomycin utilization through improved adherence and thus overall improvement of patient care.

Unlike randomized controlled trials, which establish the efficacy of an intervention through rigorous design intended to reduce bias, QI studies are conducted in a manner that can introduce high amounts of bias; therefore, researchers have developed a recommended design that focuses on how best to develop and report QI research.[99,100] The Standards for Quality Improvement Reporting Excellence (SQUIRE 2.0) guidelines, first published in 2008 and updated in 2016, were written to help standardize reporting of, and in turn improve the completeness, precision, and transparency of, QI research in health care.[99] SQUIRE 2.0 differs from other reporting standards described in this chapter (e.g., STROBE, PRISMA), in that it applies not to a specific study design but more broadly across the many various methods used in QI research.[102] More information and additional resources focused on the SQUIRE 2.0 initiative are available at http://squire-statement.org.

The designs utilized for QI research in health care range from single-center plan-do-study-act cycles of iterative changes to retrospective evaluation of large-scale programs to multicenter randomized trials.[99] Quasi-experimental designs are commonly utilized for QI research, including before-after studies and time series designs.[100] Before-after designs use historical controls, comparing results from a specified time prior to introducing the intervention with results during a similar timeframe after the intervention.[103] The design opens up the possibility of bias because other factors (e.g., changes in sample, changes in care) may influence the results during either of those two time periods. Time series studies collect data at multiple points in time from each subject, with an intervention being introduced in the middle of the observations. As such, data are collected on the subjects a number of times before the intervention and then a number of times after the intervention, allowing for the investigators to see a trend in impact of the intervention. These studies can be influenced by historical threats, as the effect of the intervention is difficult to establish without data from a control group.

Because QI research has no set study design, evaluation requires first determining the study design utilized by investigators. If it is one of the observational or interventional designs previously described, the study should be evaluated using tools from those sections. Another consideration that readers should assess is whether the QI research has been reviewed by an IRB. Ethics boards may consider QI research in a more lenient manner based on the fact that most studies are assessing common practices that do not put patients at an increased risk; while approval is not required, ideally the investigators should pursue local IRB review and report this in the publication.[104] In addition to asking questions pertinent to common study designs (e.g., were the results clinically important, was follow-up complete and long enough), questions listed in Appendix 5-1 can be used by readers when determining whether a particular QI report should be utilized to develop an initiative designed to improve patient outcomes. More information on QI in health care can be found in Chapter 18.

Survey Research

Survey research is the methodological collection of information from respondents including facts, opinions, knowledge, mindsets, and behaviors.[103] Typical characteristics that define survey research are large samples that include randomly selected participants, systematic instruments, and quantitative analysis (e.g., questionnaires with items rated numerically), although survey research can also be qualitative in nature or use a combination of both (i.e., mixed methods).[103,105] The use of an instrument that incorporates a systematic questionnaire or interview guide is an essential element of survey research. These instruments should be standardized for all participants. Surveys can be conducted during a single point in time, known as cross-sectional, or by repeating the survey across the same or similar sample more than once at different times, known as longitudinal.[103] Cross-sectional surveys are more common than longitudinal surveys.

Surveys are used frequently for various reasons. Because they collect information on human nature, surveys help researchers understand psychological and social behavior.[103,105] Surveys tend to be ubiquitous, not only in health research, but also in everyday life, making most people familiar with the concept of a survey, even if they are not involved in health research. Finally, surveys are great tools because they allow for a large amount of information to be collected from a potentially large pool of participants in a relatively short amount of time.

However, these characteristics also introduce the perception that surveys are easy to develop and use, which is not true.[105,106] As such, experts have developed survey research methodology to promote high-quality data that can be trusted.[106,107]

The first step is for researchers to develop a clearly defined research question.[103,106] In addition to selecting a topic of interest, investigators must review literature to see what is known about the topic and how the proposed research will fit into that knowledge, similar to any research project one might develop.

Once the research question is decided, a sample of interest, or sample frame, is to be defined.[105,106] As with other study designs, it is virtually impossible to collect data from every member of a population even with the range offered by survey research, though census surveys do attempt to collect information on every member of a population. Therefore, it is important that the sample is sufficient and represents the population of interest in terms and distribution of characteristics (e.g., demographics, socioeconomic status, disease severity and experience).[105] To do so, the population of interest must be clearly defined.[106] The manner in which participants are recruited is also important to consider because it can influence the ability of the research to achieve a representative sample. For example, a survey only using recruitment flyers posted at a local college would likely yield a younger sample than is representative of the population. Diverse recruitment strategies and probability sampling techniques, like simple random or stratified, will help researchers meet this goal.[105,106] For example, a survey of patients with type 2 diabetes in the United States would need to use strategies to include younger and older participants, those using and not using insulin, and those from both rural and urban settings in order to get as representative a sample as possible. When determining the number of participants to include in the survey research (i.e., sample size), researchers should consider the intent of the survey (descriptive vs. analytical) and likelihood of nonresponse.[106]

The most common methods for collecting survey research data are questionnaires and interviews.[103,105] While questionnaires can be administered by a professional, they are more likely to be self-administered via paper, email, or Internet-based programs (e.g., SurveyMonkey®). By combining paper and electronic methods (i.e., multimode), researchers may improve sample coverage and response rates since about 2% and 10% of Americans do not have telephone and Internet access, respectively.[107] Because this may introduce duplicative responses, this risk can be addressed via unique identification of indicators. While most multimode surveys do not make adjustments for effects of the survey methodology, there are techniques that can be used. Additionally, research has shown that improving the visual appeal with graphics and appropriate font size and logically ordering questionnaire items can enhance the response rate to electronic questionnaires.[105] Researchers should make sure to fully describe the questionnaire used in their report.[106]

When conducting interviews, phone, computer, or in-person interactions are standard.[105] Phone and computer surveys require less resources, but open up the potential for a low response rate. In-person interviews allow researchers to capture nonverbal communication of the participant, which may indicate that the interviewee does not understand the question and allow for clarification from the interviewer. While in-person interviews also offer the advantage of gathering more information than a questionnaire, the cost and time associated with this method are problems that can make them unreasonable to use, particularly for larger sample sizes.

Four types of error that are common in survey research have been reported in the literature, all of which negatively affect the generalizability of the results.[105] These include coverage error, sampling error, measurement error, and nonresponse error.[103,105] Coverage error occurs when individuals in the population are not given an opportunity to be included in the survey sample. Coverage error can be mitigated by using multiple methods of survey administration (e.g., Internet, telephone) to ensure that all individuals in the population have an opportunity to be contacted. Sampling error is when, by chance, the sample taken does not accurately represent all possible subjects of the population of interest. Using diverse recruitment strategies and large sample sizes can reduce the possibility of sampling error. Measurement error is a problem with how data are collected, either because questions do not coincide with the topic of interest or do not induce truthful answers from participants. Using valid and reliable survey tools, pretesting questions, and training interviewers can help reduce measurement bias in survey research.[105] Finally, nonresponse error occurs when individuals in a sample do not complete the survey; using attractive survey designs and following up with those not completing the survey are ways to mitigate this error.

The American Association for Public Opinion Research (AAPOR) has developed a framework for evaluating survey quality.[107] The guidance includes 17 questions across five domains; these were used to inform questions included in Appendix 5-1. As a reader of survey research, one should carefully consider whether researchers have used and described methodology that addresses each domain in order to accept the validity (i.e., the survey measures what it sought to measure) and reliability (i.e., the survey is capable of reproducing the results) of the survey research results.[106,107]

Researchers should be sure to describe the sample frame, a list of all members of the target population who may be sampled, in order for the reader to know how inclusive the sample is of the target population.[107] This is reliant upon the availability of resources that include most if not all of the target population. For example, should one want to survey the deans of all colleges of pharmacy in the United States, the American Association of Colleges of Pharmacy would have a complete list and the coverage of the target population by any sample taken would be full. However, if the target were international deans of colleges of pharmacy, that complete listing may not be as readily available and introduce the possibility of a coverage error. Should a full target population not be known or available, as is most likely the case, readers need to consider how respondents were identified and recruited, which should be reported by the researchers.

Consideration must be given to the manner in which the sample was selected, specifically whether a probability or nonprobability sampling methodology was used.[103,107] Probability sampling assigns a possibility of selection to each individual of the sample frame which allows for the use of inferential statistics, while nonprobability sampling does not involve the determination of how likely it is that each individual in the population be included in the sample. The latter, in the form of convenience sampling, is more likely to be used in survey research. Another consideration is how the researchers ensured that the sample was representative of the population and whether or not those methods were effective.[107] Using known characteristics (e.g., demographics, geographic location) of the target population to describe the sample so that distribution of these characteristics is similar between population and sample, including methods like quota and weighted sampling, is common. Comparing the sample and population distribution can be used to evaluate methodology for effectiveness. Finally, readers should assess whether the possibility of sampling error occurred during the study by considering recruitment strategies and sample size.

Clearly, attempting to survey individuals included in the sample without receiving a response from them causes issues in survey research. There are many reasons why those solicited to participate in a survey may not respond, so carefully considering how the methodology of the research may have introduced this likelihood is important. First and foremost, evaluating the response rate is an important factor in determining the value of the research results. Though there is no established standard for a "good" response rate, knowing the percentage of people who participated allows the reader to determine the potential for nonresponse bias, which is more likely if response rates are lower than 50–60%.[106–108] Other ways to potentially determine nonresponse error include contacting nonresponders to compare their characteristics with those of participants, comparing results with external data, assessing variation of internal data, and adjusting estimates after the survey is completed.[107,108]

From a reader perspective, it is important that researchers are transparent in their reporting of response. Including the flow of participants, from initial sample selection and contact through analysis, should be provided.[106,108] An item-by-item reporting of response rate may also be necessary should there be certain items that were answered by a small number of participants.

As mentioned, when discussing measurement error, it is important to consider the manner in which the survey was presented to the participant. How the survey was administered to the sample, the way the questions were written, the way the survey was organized, and the means by which truthfulness was determined are all aspects that researchers need to address to ensure reliable and valid survey results.[107] By describing the survey instrument, researchers allow the reader to make their own determination as to some of these evaluative points.[106]

Readers should be provided the amount of time the survey was in the field.[107] In general, the longer a survey is available to participants, the better because it offers more opportunity for response and can collect data differentiated by early and late responders. Despite this preference, there is no rule for how long a survey must be in the field.

Another consideration is whether or not participants were offered an incentive.[107] The type and value of any incentive might introduce bias. For example, low-income participants might be more likely to respond to the survey if they are offered a monetary incentive. Furthermore, some participants might not give full consideration to the survey in the interest of only participating to receive the incentive. While there are drawbacks to using incentives, there are also risks to not using them, mostly related to reducing response rates. Readers should know whether an incentive was offered and use that information to carefully consider how it might have affected the results of the research.

Survey research is a complex field, made more complicated by its overall prevalence and the ease with which it can be conducted (though not necessarily appropriately). Being equipped with the knowledge of methodology that conveys high-quality survey research will help readers make appropriate determinations about research they encounter. Using questions provided in Appendix 5-1 will also help readers evaluate survey research.

Educational Research

● **Educational research** has been defined as the "systematic and critical investigation of education that advances knowledge and benefits society by allowing people to live fuller lives."[109] The value of educational research is that it can help shape educational theory, assist with the development and management of conceptual frameworks, and influence future research, all pointing toward an ultimate goal of improving the quality of education. Educational research can take many forms; areas of evaluation include the scholarship of teaching and learning, enrollment and admissions processes, economic considerations like tuition and student debt, and faculty and student characteristics and perspectives.

Like much other research focused on a specific domain (e.g., QI research), educational research is not conducted via a particular study type, though using the traditional research method to determine the research question and choose the design that aligns with the goal of the research is necessary.[109] For example, should one want to know the prevalence of pharmacy students likely to seek postgraduate residency training, a cross-sectional study would be the most appropriate study design.

Approaches to research design that have been defined specific to educational research include quantitative, qualitative, mixed methods, and action research.[109] Quantitative research uses numbers and mathematics to define relationships, describe populations, and test hypotheses. Common ways to conduct quantitative educational research include surveys, performance assessments, and institutional and national databases. Pharmacy education studies commonly use surveys as quantitative tools, asking students to rate their experience on a Likert scale that asks their level of agreement or disagreement with a statement. Another example would be the use of quiz, exam, or course grades as quantitative outcomes specific to student performance. Qualitative research uses descriptive, nonnumerical data from surveys, focus groups, and documents to comprehend a specific population. In focus groups, students could be asked about their experience and they would be allowed to respond without a numerical designation or limitations. Qualitative research requires expertise in design and conduct of research because it necessitates more direct contact with participants and is more likely to introduce bias. The benefit of qualitative research is that it provides more direct and robust data because it allows for a closer interaction between researcher and participant and allows for more information regarding values, opinions, and behaviors of the participant. Mixed methods research combines quantitative and qualitative research in order to gain a complete understanding of an issue or population in a single study. For example, researchers in pharmacy education commonly conduct studies that include grades and numerical survey data as outcomes, then collect opinions via freeform questions or focus groups to better understand the quantitative results. Finally, action research is research conducted in a small setting by an investigator seeking to understand and solve a specific problem. These studies focus on a single, specific issue at the local level, commonly a single class, program, or school with the goal of improving outcomes or functionality. Action research relies on the willingness of educators to be self-aware of their own practice and performance, be able to critique their own performance, and be open to making changes based on the results of the action research they conduct. Investigators can use both quantitative and qualitative design during action research and, while valuable to the individual and potentially publishable, the results are unlikely to be generalizable because of the focused nature of the research.

Outcomes utilized in educational research should focus on the actual learning, rather than any perception of learning.[110] Using outcomes that allow students to subjectively answer how they feel they learned will produce poor data because learners tend to be poor evaluators of their own knowledge. Metacognition and motivation are two exceptions to this rule and allow researchers to use student confidence judgments (e.g., "I learned a lot," "I feel more confident") as outcomes. When the investigator wants to assess the metacognitive ability of students, which means whether students have improved their ability to understand what they do and do not know, researchers can evaluate how confident students are in relation to what they have learned. The second exception is when assessing student motivation, as perceived confidence can lead to improved self-efficacy and feed motivation (i.e., the better one thinks one is at learning, the more motivated one is to learn). Regardless of the exception, both metacognition and motivation assessments will be improved when tied to a measurement of learning.

Like all other research, reliability, validity, bias, and generalizability need to be considered when conducting and reading educational research.[109] Because ethical constraints limit the ability of educational research to be conducted via randomized controlled trials (i.e., it would be unethical to offer one group an educational intervention that was different than the way the control group was taught if the assessment affects the students' grades), much educational research consists of surveys, pre/post studies, and studies using historical controls.[110] Therefore, one should carefully consider the study design used and the inherent strengths and limitations of those designs when reading educational research. Additional questions that one might want to consider are listed in Appendix 5-1.[110,111]

Natural Medicines Medical Literature

OVERVIEW

Natural medicines (botanical and nonbotanical) information is a large and growing body of medical literature. As patients continue to use these products, despite some serious safety and quality issues, all health care practitioners must delve into the primary literature to be able to appropriately advise patients, even if only in the area of drug interactions. Effects on prescription medications can be both positive and negative, and drugs may also affect the efficacy or safety of the dietary supplements. As with standard drug literature, the ability to discern robust clinical evidence from weak clinical evidence is an essential skill that enables practitioners to make solid recommendations to patients and to other health care professionals. ❽ *The principles and criteria used to analyze the quality of drug literature are used to analyze natural medicines literature; however, unique additional points such as standardization and purity must be considered.*

Unfortunately, for most natural medicines, good clinical evidence is minimal. Without a body of large, controlled, methodologically sound clinical trials, practitioners must often make patient education decisions or recommendations based on safety and efficacy data from case reports, flawed trials, or information that is extrapolated from animal and/or in vitro studies. This can be appropriate, especially when the safety profile of the product is judged to be good, but decisions must include a very patient-specific risk-benefit analysis: weighing risks of occurrence of an interaction or side effect against possible benefits. Health literacy, the capacity to read, understand, and implement health information for appropriate decision-making and following of care instructions, is an important factor, as it is essential for the patient be able to accurately self-monitor for adverse effects or other problems. To further compound misinformation on natural medicines, often trials are mistakenly touted as supporting efficacy of a whole botanical natural medicine when they have actually been conducted using chemical extracts or combination products. Results from studies on such dissimilar products cannot be used to support efficacy or safety.

As with standard drug literature, well-considered meta-analyses or large well-designed, randomized, controlled clinical trials provide stronger clinical decision support than data from observational studies. The process to determine the quality and value of natural medicine medical literature is the same as standard medical literature. The criteria for analysis are the same, even when some aspects may be slightly different. For example, assessment of blinding strategy success should be performed in the same way by investigators. It could be argued that this assessment is even more critical because the blinding strategy may be more difficult due to the frequently distinctive or pungent tastes or odors of some natural medicines.

CONSIDERATIONS FOR NATURAL MEDICINES STUDIES

A few issues are unique to natural medicine studies, and certain types of methodological flaws are more common. In addition to standard literature evaluation criteria, specifics to consider include the following:

- Standardization of chemical components
- Quality and purity of product formulations

- Adequate trial duration and sample size
- Location of natural medicine literature—international literature inclusion

Standardization of the chemical components is very important. Plant-derived products contain many different chemical entities that fluctuate with the growing and harvesting conditions, the plant's age, and which part of the plant is used. One or more chemical entities could be considered active constituents, that is, responsible for desired pharmacologic action, which may or may not be accurately identified. Other components may be marker compounds, compounds that allow estimation of levels of other, less easily assayed chemicals. Natural medicines are standardized by controlling the amount of one chemical entity, either an active constituent (if known) or a marker compound. For example, St. John's wort extracts can be standardized to either hypericin or hyperforin content, both of which have pharmacologic activity and are used as marker compounds.[112] Using a standardized chemical concentration allows for comparisons between study products and marketed products as well as between various brands of one product. It is vital to assess standardization methods used by investigators when evaluating a trial. Investigators should discuss and document the plant or chemical substance(s) as well as the strength or salt form utilized. This is an essential consideration for grouping trials appropriately to make "apples-to-apples" comparisons of results, whether reading individual trials or analyzing the appropriateness of trial inclusion into a meta-analysis.

Plant parts are also important to consider. If a trial evaluated use of a herb's root, but the product about which a practitioner is searching for information contains the herb's leaves and flowers, the results cannot be extrapolated. The "apples-to-apples" concept also applies to nonbotanical natural medicines, generally in terms of differences in salt forms. For example, glucosamine sulfate monotherapy has more evidence of benefit in osteoarthritis patients, while glucosamine hydrochloride monotherapy has little supportive evidence.[113,114]

The quality of products used in trials of natural medicines is always a matter of concern. Natural medicines can be adulterated with heavy metals, synthesis byproducts, or prescription medications. Although U.S. dietary supplement manufacturers of all sizes are now legally required to follow FDA and USP good manufacturing practice, the reality is that many small companies do not; many poor-quality natural medicines and other supplements are on the market, as evidenced by frequent recalls.[115] Some manufacturers voluntarily participate in the USP's Dietary Supplement Verification Program (http://www.quality-supplements.org/), and products must meet USP monograph standards.[116] Available USP Verified supplements are primarily vitamins, minerals, and a few nonbotanical supplements such as fish oil and melatonin. Although USP has more than 50 monographs for botanical supplements available, currently only three marketed turmeric or curcumin products meet USP standards. This is especially concerning considering that botanicals, or products derived from them, often have chemical constituents that are volatile; possible degradation must be considered when interpreting results of a trial.[117] Investigators should take active steps to verify that products used in studies are stable throughout the duration of a clinical trial and discuss this in study reports. The extension of the Consolidated Standards of Reporting Trials checklist for trials of herbal medicines offers extensive examples of appropriate reporting of standardization, plant part, and quality issues and is accessible for free at http://www.consort-statement.org/extensions/overview/herbal-medicinal/interventions.[118–120]

Sufficient study samples and appropriate duration of therapy are essential for accurate assessment of both efficacy and safety, yet inadequacies in both are common flaws in natural medicine trials. This may be a function of lack of knowledge of appropriate trial design or lack of sufficient funding. Small groups may not have adequate statistical power to detect a potential difference between a treatment and a placebo. Adverse reactions or drug interactions can be overlooked in smaller groups versus larger ones, and a small study sample decreases generalizability to broader patient populations. Dependent upon the mechanism of action, some natural medicines may take several weeks to months before patients experience full, or even noticeable, benefit. If study duration is too short, natural medicines may appear less efficacious than they actually are. On the other hand, when true effect sizes are only small to moderate, a short trial may tend to overestimate responses. Patients will often exhibit greater responses in the beginning of clinical trials, perhaps because of contributing placebo effect, which may attenuate as the trial proceeds. And, just as with standard drug trials, shorter study periods cannot predict outcomes or safety issues associated with long-term use.

A majority of natural medicine trials are conducted in Europe and Asia. Most health professionals are familiar with the MEDLINE® database, whether searched through PubMed® or another platform. Unfortunately, studies of natural medicines published in international journals cannot be found when only searching the MEDLINE® database. Embase® is another index of abstracts from a wider variety of international journals, many of which are published in English.

No matter which databases are searched, use of adequate keywords or indexing terms is important. This is especially true for botanical medicines—plants have multiple common names and different spellings (e.g., ginkgo, gingko, ginko), disparate plants share common names, and official botanical taxonomy changes frustratingly frequently. Any database search should include multiple search terms in order to ensure thoroughness. Additionally, searching the references of obtained articles (i.e., bibliographic searches) is useful to identify citations of trials.

With the increased use of general online searching to identify scientific literature, the use of misleading or outright fraudulent "publications" by natural medicine manufacturers is on the increase as well. These will often be full-text articles that appear to be from reputable scientific journals; they may be used as a citation of "clinically proven" on a sales website. However, investigation will reveal that the journal does not actually exist or was created to serve as a "home base" for non-peer-reviewed articles. Any studies located by a general Internet search must be verified as authentic before use.

CONSIDERATIONS FOR CANNABIS AND CANNABINOID STUDIES

With the number of states that have legalized medicinal cannabis or other cannabinoid medicines such as extracts and cannabidiol (CBD) oil, health care providers must be prepared for increasing questions from patients concerning these natural medicines. Yet, because of the federal classification of cannabis that limits research, clinical data are extremely limited, and published trials are rarely robust in size or design; this situation is slowly changing as more research is being allowed. An exception is for Epidiolex®, a cannabis extract of CBD, which was first approved in 2018 for treatment of two severe seizure disorders.[121] To gain approval, this particular CBD product had to meet all requirements necessary for any prescription drug. Research on Epidiolex® cannot be used to support decisions about efficacy or safety of any other CBD products.

When examining the existing literature for cannabis and cannabinoid medicines, all of the considerations for natural medicines studies generally apply, but with the addition of "Dosage form and route of administration." These considerations, with changes pertinent to cannabis and cannabinoid trials, are as follows:

- Standardization of chemical components
  - ○ The same concept of standardization for extracts applies, but whole plant extracts of cannabis are not as commonly used. An exception might be hemp or cannabis extracts specifically for CBD, where the aim is to exclude or limit any delta-9-tetrahydrocannabinol (THC).
  - ○ Standardization of whole plant cannabis, often administered via vaping or smoking, is rarely able to be accomplished beyond comparisons of CBD or THC amounts. This is problematic because other cannabinoids and other chemical components with pharmacologic effects, such as terpenes, can vastly differ between strains of cannabis or even between harvests, if grown in the outdoors.
- Quality and purity of product formulations
  - ○ No U.S. standards exist for quality and purity of non-FDA-approved natural cannabis medicinal products. Researchers must take steps to analyze the quality of the products used in clinical trials, and trial reports must include sufficient detail regarding the formulations to be able to appropriately compare results of trials.

- Adequate trial duration and sample size
  - Cannabis trials are often of short duration, which may have a variable impact on interpretation of results, depending upon the disease state under study.
  - Small sample size, often due to limitations in funding, restricts both generalization of results and the ability to uncover clinically significant differences between treatment groups.
- Location of literature—international literature inclusion
  - Because cannabis is (as of this writing) still a Schedule I controlled substance at the federal level, very few U.S. studies exist; therefore, searches must include international literature.
  - Searches using the term "cannabinoid" will return results that include studies of the synthetic drugs dronabinol and nabilone. As these are usually not applicable to clinical decisions regarding whole cannabis or extract use, they must be specifically withdrawn or extracted from the search. This must be done carefully and it may be necessary to do this manually, rather than electronically, as using a logical operator (e.g., filter) in a search that excludes something may inadvertently exclude articles that primarily cover the topic of interest simply because there is a brief mention of the aspect that is not of interest.
- Dosage form and route of administration
  - Both whole cannabis plant material and various extracts can be used by more than one route of administration, with differing onset of action, effects, and adverse events. The same amount of the same batch of whole plant cannabis will have different results and adverse effects when administration is via smoking, vaping, or oral ingestion.

SUMMARY

Natural medicine use continues to be prevalent despite fluctuations in ages or ethnicities choosing to use supplements and changes in the popularity of specific products.[122] Pharmacists must serve as reliable and approachable information resources for natural medicine information, just as they do for other medications. In community settings, supplements are often placed with over-the-counter products near the pharmacy, so that pharmacists are easily accessible for consumer questions and patient education. The ability to effectively evaluate natural medicine literature is essential to making informed recommendations and appropriately counseling patients who have natural medicine questions.

As previously mentioned, natural medicine clinical trials should be evaluated for quality with the same criteria as used for FDA-approved medications. The difference lies in greater emphasis upon certain aspects that are known to often be problematic in natural medicine trials. See Appendix 5-1 for a list of specific questions to aid in the analysis of natural medicine trials.

Case Study 5–3: Study Testing a Natural Medicine

You are evaluating a trial examining effects of a proline-rich polypeptide (PRP) complex derived from ovine colostrum, Colostrinin®. Animal studies demonstrated immune-modulating effects. Human blood studies found that the complex induced cytokines, including interferon γ, and human subjects experienced enhanced immunomodulatory activity and psychotropic activity described as mood elevation and cognitive stimulation. This randomized, double-blinded trial of 46 subjects with Alzheimer's disease in Poland compared 100 μg of Colostrinin® ($n = 15$) to 100-μg selenium ($n = 15$) and to placebo ($n = 16$) for a year. Treatments were given every other day for 3 weeks, followed by a 2-week rest. This cycle was repeated a total of 10 times. The primary outcome measure to determine efficacy was the Mini Mental State Examination (MMSE), which was administered five times during the course of the study. Subjective evaluations of daily functioning and mood were provided by caregivers to the assessing psychiatrists. Power was not addressed, and statistical analysis utilized the Student's t test. The three subject groups were subdivided into three strata according to disease severity as determined by baseline Mini Mental State Examination scores: mild (17–24), moderate (12–16), and severe (≤ 11). Study results demonstrated improvement in the Mini Mental State Examination scores in the Colostrinin® group, 19.5–24.3, 14.3–16.7, and 11.0–12.0, respectively, in the mild, moderate, and severe strata, though only the change in the mild strata was statistically significant ($p = 0.02$). Mini Mental State Examination scores worsened in all strata, though not significantly, in the selenium group and worsened significantly ($p = 0.005$ to $p = 0.03$) in all strata in the placebo group. Researchers remarked on the improvement of memory demonstrated, but no data were presented. All reported adverse effects were mild and transient, though most were in the Colostrinin® group, occurring at the beginning of the first treatment cycle. Approximately 30% of the Colostrinin® group experienced speech flow disturbances, insomnia, and/or anxiety.

- *You are evaluating this trial because a caregiver for patient with Alzheimer's disease has asked about a colostrum product currently being heavily promoted by a local natural foods store. This product is concentrated bovine colostrum that has been dried and encapsulated. How could the formulation of the product used in this study be a problem to extrapolating the study results to the patient under consideration?*

- *Like this trial, many natural medicine trials are conducted outside the United States. Why should you take this into consideration?*
- *What is your opinion regarding the patient numbers for this trial?*

Conclusion

This chapter provides important information on study designs beyond the randomized controlled trial. For example, observational studies are limited to determining associations, as opposed to causation, due to their inherent weaknesses, but provide an important strength of involving large numbers of patients. Quantitative systematic reviews can improve estimates of effect size by combining data from multiple studies, but the literature search must be comprehensive, heterogeneity must be minimal, and individual studies must be of high quality in order for the results to be valid. Other types of studies, including N-of-1 trials, health outcomes research, stability studies, bioequivalence studies, postmarketing studies, QI research, survey research, and educational research, will also need to be critically evaluated in practice. Additionally, for the growing body of literature on natural medicines, special considerations such as standardization and purity are required. Thus, by understanding the principles presented in this chapter for evaluating study designs beyond the randomized controlled trial, health care practitioners can enhance their ability to practice EBM.

Self-Assessment Questions

For each of the following questions, please select the *best* answer:

Study #1: It is hypothesized that hormone replacement therapy in postmenopausal women may play a beneficial role in preventing osteoporosis. A group of patients receiving hormone replacement therapy and a group of patients not receiving hormone replacement therapy are followed over a 20-year period. The development of osteoporosis as assessed by bone mineral density in each group is compared and the RR associated with the use of hormone replacement therapy and the development of osteoporosis is calculated.

Study #2: There is a concern that the use of hormone replacement therapy in postmenopausal women may cause an increased risk of breast cancer. A study is conducted to test this hypothesis. Medical charts from a group of patients previously admitted to the hospital with the diagnosis of breast cancer is compared to medical charts from a group of patients previously admitted to the hospital without breast cancer. The groups are matched by age, sex, date of admission, and other confounding factors such as alcohol use. Use of hormone replacement therapy in each group is assessed and compared. An OR for the risk of breast cancer related to use of hormone replacement therapy is calculated.

Study #3: An investigator identifies a study sample of women aged 20–45 years. During a single office visit, the investigator measures bone mass in the women. He also questions them about their past and present exercise habits. The investigator determines that women involved with rigorous exercise before the onset of menses have a greater bone mass.

1. Which listing of observational designs is in the correct order for the studies described above?
   a. Cohort, case-control, cross-sectional
   b. Cross-sectional, case-control, cohort
   c. Case-control, cohort, case series
   d. Cohort, cross-sectional, case-control

2. Which ranking of observational study designs is in order of decreasing rigor?
   a. Retrospective cohort > case series > case-control
   b. Cross-sectional > case-control > retrospective cohort
   c. Case-control > case report > prospective cohort
   d. Prospective cohort > case-control > case series

3. Which observational study design involves a control group and retrospective data collection?
   a. Case series
   b. Cross-sectional
   c. Case-control
   d. Prospective cohort

4. Which technique is used to produce groups that are similar at baseline in observational studies?
   a. Adjustment of odds ratios
   b. Propensity score matching
   c. Randomization
   d. Sensitivity analyses

5. Which of the following is a confounding variable in an observational study to evaluate whether medications used to treat attention-deficit/hyperactivity disorder are associated with cardiovascular events?
   a. Methylphenidate
   b. Myocardial infarction
   c. Smoking
   d. Sudden cardiac death

6. Which characteristic is unique to quantitative systematic reviews?
   a. Focused clinical question
   b. Comprehensive literature search
   c. Specific inclusion and exclusion criteria
   d. Method for pooling data

7. What does the Cochrane risk-of-bias tool assess in a systematic review?
   a. Likelihood of publication bias
   b. Quality of individual studies that are included
   c. Statistical significance of the results for the main analysis
   d. Consistency among reviewers in determining if studies meet the eligibility criteria

8. In a meta-analysis on feverfew for migraines, the p value for heterogeneity was 0.00001 and the I^2 value was 72% for the pooled analysis of the primary outcome. Which of the following is an accurate interpretation of the heterogeneity?
   a. Low in extent
   b. Not assessed adequately
   c. Not statistically significant
   d. Undesirable

9. In a meta-analysis on medications to treat alcohol dependence, the pooled result using a random-effects model for the primary outcome of return to drinking was RR 0.89 (95% CI, 0.67–0.99). Which trial would have carried the most weight in the analysis?
   a. N=25; RR 1.08 (95% CI, 0.91–1.27)
   b. N=68; RR 0.85 (95% CI, 0.79–0.99)
   c. N=104; RR 0.94 (95% CI, 0.87–1.01)
   d. N=212; RR 0.58 (95% CI, 0.31–1.10)

10. Which results are desirable for publication bias evaluated with a funnel plot in a quantitative systematic review?
   a. Symmetry; $p = 0.65$
   b. Symmetry; $p = 0.04$

    c. Asymmetry; $p = 0.01$

    d. Asymmetry; $p = 0.15$

11. Which type of study is typically conducted after a medication has been approved and is necessary to meet regulatory requirements?

    a. Stability

    b. Bioequivalence

    c. Postmarketing

    d. Quality improvement

12. Which type of research is affiliated with a specific study design?

    a. N-of-1

    b. Health outcomes

    c. Quality improvement

    d. Educational

13. Which element is essential in survey research?

    a. Systematic questionnaire

    b. Convenient population of interest

    c. Simple recruitment strategy

    d. Well-intentioned research question

14. Which characteristic is important to identify in a botanical natural medicine study?

    a. Duration, because these studies are often long

    b. Number of participants, because these studies are often large

    c. Legal status, because the FDA must approve plant-derived medicines

    d. Standardization, because plant-derived products often contain many different chemical entities

15. Your hospital is considering a request to allow the use of powdered ginger root capsules for prevention and treatment of postoperative nausea and vomiting. Which literature would be appropriate to include in your analysis to make a final decision?

    a. Two retrospective analyses of powdered ginger root capsules in 3845 women for prevention of pregnancy-associated nausea and vomiting

    b. A randomized, single-blind, placebo-controlled trial of powdered ginger root capsules in 80 patients with previous severe postoperative nausea and vomiting

    c. A randomized, double-blind, placebo-controlled trial of dried standardized ginger leaf extract in 372 patients with previous moderate postoperative nausea and vomiting

    d. Two randomized controlled trials of ginger root extract added to standard antiemetic therapy in 423 patients receiving chemotherapy for gynecological malignancies

REFERENCES

1. Mann CJ. Observational research methods. Research design II: cohort, cross sectional, and case-control studies. Emerg Med J. 2003;20(1):54-60.

2. DiPietro NA. Methods in epidemiology: observational study designs. Pharmacotherapy. 2010;30(10):973-84. doi:10.1592/phco.30.10.973.

3. Tsao CW, Vasan RS. Cohort profile: the Framingham Heart Study (FHS): overview of milestones in cardiovascular epidemiology. Int J Epidemiol. 2015;44(6):1800-13. doi:10.1093/ije/dyv337.

4. Vandenbroucke JP. In defense of case reports and case series. Ann Intern Med. 2001;134(4):330-4. doi:10.7326/0003-4819-134-4-200102200-00017.

5. Shields KM, DiPietro NA, Kier KL. Principles of drug literature evaluation for observational study designs. Pharmacotherapy. 2011;31(2):115-27. doi:10.1592/phco.31.2.115.

6. Gottlieb MS, Schroff R, Schanker HM, Weisman JD, Fan PT, Wolf RA, Saxon A. *Pneumocystis carinii* pneumonia and mucosal candidiasis in previously healthy homosexual men: evidence of a new acquired cellular immunodeficiency. N Engl J Med. 1981;305(24):1425-31. doi:10.1056/nejm198112103052401.

7. Lucena MI, Andrade RJ, Rodrigo L, Rodrigo L,Salmeron J,Alvarez A,Lopez-Garrido MJ,Camargo R, Alcantara R. Trovafloxacin-induced acute hepatitis. Clin Infect Dis. 2000;30(2):400-1. doi:10.1086/313680.

8. Gagnier JJ, Kienle G, Altman DG, Moher D, Sox H, Riley D. The CARE guidelines: consensus-based clinical case reporting guideline development. BMJ Case Rep. 2013. doi:10.1136/bcr-2013-201554.

9. Riley DS, Barber MS, Kienle GS, Aronson JK, von Schoen-Angerer T, Tugwell P, Kiene H, Helfand M, Altman DG, Sox H, Werthmann PG, Moher D, Rison RA, Shamseer L, Koch CA, Sun GH, Hanaway P, Sudak NL, Kaszkin-Bettag M, Carpenter JE, Gagnier JJ. CARE guidelines for case reports: explanation and elaboration document. J Clin Epidemiol. 2017;89:218-35. doi:10.1016/j.jclinepi.2017.04.026.

10. Chenghui L. Principles of research design and drug literature evaluation. Burlington (MA): Jones & Bartlett Learning; c2015. Chapter 19, Evaluating observational studies; p. 307-22.

11. Goldwire M, Babby J. The clinical practice of drug information. Burlington (MA): Jones & Bartlett Learning; c2016. Chapter 14, Evidence-based medicine; p. 253-90.

12. Rogers CJ, Bahr KO, Benjamin SM. Attitudes and barriers associated with seasonal influenza vaccination uptake among public health students; a cross-sectional study. BMC Public Health. 2018;18(1):1131. doi:10.1186/s12889-018-6041-1.

13. Singh S, Chang HY, Richards TM, Weiner JP, Clark JM, Segal JB. Glucagonlike peptide 1-based therapies and risk of hospitalization for acute pancreatitis in type 2 diabetes mellitus: a population-based matched case-control study. JAMA Intern Med. 2013;173(7):534-9. doi:10.1001/jamainternmed.2013.2720.

14. Andrews N, Miller E, Grant A, Stowe J, Osborne V, Taylor B. Thimerosal exposure in infants and developmental disorders: a retrospective cohort study in the United kingdom does not support a causal association. Pediatrics. 2004;114(3):584-91. doi:10.1542/peds.2003-1177-L.

15. Darling AL, Rayman MP, Steer CD, Golding J, Lanham-New SA, Bath SC. Association between maternal vitamin D status in pregnancy and neurodevelopmental outcomes in childhood: results from the Avon Longitudinal Study of Parents and Children (ALSPAC). Br J Nutr. 2017;117(12):1682-92. doi:10.1017/S0007114517001398.

16. Boyd A, Golding J, Macleod J, Lawlor DA, Fraser A, Henderson J, Molloy L, Ness A, Ring S, Smith GD. Cohort profile: the "children of the 90s"–the index offspring of the Avon Longitudinal Study of Parents and Children. Int J Epidemiol. 2013;42(1):111-27. doi:10.1093/ije/dys064.

17. von Elm E, Altman DG, Egger M, Pocock SJ, Gotzsche PC, Vandenbroucke JP. The Strengthening the Reporting of Observational Studies in Epidemiology (STROBE) statement: guidelines for reporting observational studies. Ann Intern Med. 2007; 147(8):573-7.

18. Vandenbroucke JP, von Elm E, Altman DG, Gøtzsche PC, Mulrow CD, Pocock SJ, Poole C, Schlesselman JJ, Egger M. Strengthening the Reporting of Observational Studies in Epidemiology (STROBE): explanation and elaboration. Ann Intern Med. 2007;147(8):W163-94. doi:10.7326/0003-4819-147-8-200710160-00010-w1.

19. Aprikyan AA, Khuchua Z. Advances in the understanding of Barth syndrome. Br J Haematol. 2013;161(3):330-8. doi:10.1111/bjh.12271.

20. Bellavia A, Tektonidis TG, Orsini N, Wolk A, Larsson SC. Quantifying the benefits of Mediterranean diet in terms of survival. Eur J Epidemiol. 2016;31(5):527-30. doi:10.1007/s10654-016-0127-9.

21. Yang YX, Lewis JD, Epstein S, Metz DC. Long-term proton pump inhibitor therapy and risk of hip fracture. JAMA. 2016;296(24):2947-53. doi:10.1001/jama.296.24.2947.

22. Agoritsas T, Merglen A, Shah ND, O'Donnell M, Guyatt GH. Adjusted analyses in studies addressing therapy and harm: users' guides to the medical literature. JAMA. 2017;317(7):748-59. doi:10.1001/jama.2016.20029.

23. Song JW, Chung KC. Observational studies: cohort and case-control studies. Plast Reconstr Surg. 2010;126(6):2234-42. doi:10.1097/PRS.0b013e3181f44abc.

24. Aschengrau A, Seage GR. Essentials of epidemiology in public health. 2nd ed. Sudbury (MA): Jones & Bartlett Publishers; c2008. 479 p.

25. Desai RJ, Franklin JM. Alternative approaches for confounding adjustment in observational studies using weighting based on the propensity score: a primer for practitioners. BMJ. 2019;367:l5657. doi:10.1136/bmj.l5657.

26. Normand SL, Sykora K, Li P, Mamdani M, Rochon PA, Anderson GM. Readers guide to critical appraisal of cohort studies: 3. Analytical strategies to reduce confounding. BMJ. 2005;330(7498):1021-3. doi:10.1136/bmj.330.7498.1021.

27. Rochon PA, Gurwitz JH, Sykora K, Mamdani M, Streiner DL, Garfinkel S, Normand ST, Anderson GM. Reader's guide to critical appraisal of cohort studies: 1. Role and design. BMJ. 2005;330(7496):895-7. doi:10.1136/bmj.330.7496.895.

28. Mamdani M, Sykora K, Li P, Normand S-LT, Streiner DL, Austin PC, Rochon PA, Anderson GM. Reader's guide to critical appraisal of cohort studies: 2. Assessing potential for confounding. BMJ. 2005;330(7497):960-2. doi:10.1136/bmj.330.7497.960.

29. Hayden GF, Kramer MS, Horwitz RI. The case-control study: a practical review for the clinician. JAMA. 1982;247(3):326-31.

30. Florez H, Reaven PD, Bahn G, Moritz T, Warren S, Marks J, Reda D, Duckworth W, Abraira C, Hayward R, Emanuele N. VADT Research Group. Rosiglitazone treatment and cardiovascular disease in the Veterans Affairs Diabetes Trial. Diabetes Obes Metab. 2015;17(10):949-55. doi:10.1111/dom.12487.

31. Greenhalgh T. How to read a paper: the basics of evidence-based medicine. 5th ed. Hoboken (NJ): Wiley-Blackwell Publishing Ltd; c2014. 253 p.

32. Grimes DA, Schulz KF. Cohort studies: marching towards outcomes. Lancet. 2002;359(9303):341-5. doi:10.1016/S0140-6736(02)07500-1.

33. Matthews DE, Farewell VT. Using and understanding medical statistics. 4th ed. Basel (NY): Karger; c2007. 345 p.

34. Kier KL. Biostatistical applications in epidemiology. Pharmacotherapy. 2011;31(1):9-22. doi:10.1592/phco.31.1.9.

35. Schneeweiss S. Sensitivity analysis and external adjustment for unmeasured confounders in epidemiologic database studies of therapeutics. Pharmacoepidemiol Drug Saf. 2006;15(5):291-303. doi:10.1002/pds.1200.

36. Laporte J, Ibáñez L, Vidal X, Vendrell L, Leone R. Upper gastrointestinal bleeding associated with the use of NSAIDs: newer versus older agents. Drug Saf. 2004;27(6):411-20. doi:10.2165/00002018-200427060-00005.

37. Fletcher RH, Wagner EH. Clinical epidemiology: the essentials. 3rd ed. Baltimore (MD): Williams & Wilkins; c1996. 283 p.

38. Green BN, Johnson CD, Adams A. Writing narrative literature reviews for peer-reviewed journals: secrets of the trade. J Chiropr Med. 2006;5(3):101-17. doi:10.1016/s0899-3467(07)60142-6.

39. Murad MH, Montori VM, Ioannidis JP, Jaeschke R, Devereaux PJ, Prasad K, Neumann I, Carrasco-Labra A, Agoritsas T, Hatala R, Meade MO, Wyer P, Cook DJ, Guyatt G. How to read a systematic review and meta-analysis and apply the results to patient care: users' guides to the medical literature. JAMA. 2014;312(2):171-9. doi:10.1001/jama.2014.5559.

40. Crowther M, Lim W, Crowther MA. Systematic review and meta-analysis methodology. Blood. 2010;116(17):3140-6. doi:10.1182/blood-2010-05-280883.

41. Moher D, Liberati A, Tetzlaff J, Altman DG. Preferred reporting items for systematic reviews and meta-analyses: the PRISMA statement. Ann Intern Med. 2009;151(4):264-9.

42. Lyman GH, Kuderer NM. The strengths and limitations of meta-analyses based on aggregate data. BMC Med Res Methodol. 2005;5:14. doi:10.1186/1471-2288-5-14.

43. Stewart LA, Clarke M, Rovers M, Riley RD, Simmonds M, Stewart G, Tierney JF. PRISMA-IPD Development Group, Preferred reporting items for systematic review and meta-analyses of individual participant data: the PRISMA-IPD statement. JAMA. 2015;313(16):1657-65. doi:10.1001/jama.2015.3656.

44. Riley RD, Lambert PC, Abo-Zaid G. Meta-analysis of individual participant data: rationale, conduct, and reporting. BMJ. 2010;340:c221. doi:10.1136/bmj.c221.

45. Hutton B, Salanti G, Caldwell DM, Chaimani A, Schmid CH, Cameron C, Ioannidis JPA, Straus S, Thorlund K, Jansen JP, Mulrow C, Catalá-López F, Gøtzsche PC, Dickersin K, Boutron I, Altman DG, Moher D. The PRISMA extension statement for reporting of systematic reviews incorporating network meta-analyses of health care interventions: checklist and explanations. Ann Intern Med. 2015;162(11):777-84. doi:10.7326/m14-2385.

46. Guyatt GH, Oxman AD, Kunz R, Woodcock J, Brozek J, Helfand M, Alonso-Coello P, Falck-Ytter Y, Jaeschke R, Vist G, Akl EA, Post PN, Norris S, Meerpohl J, Shukla VK, Nasser M, Schünemann HJ GRADE Working Group GRADE guidelines: 8. Rating the quality of evidence-indirectness. J Clin Epidemiol. 2011;64(12):1303-10. doi:10.1016/j.jclinepi.2011.04.014.

47. Lee AW. Review of mixed treatment comparisons in published systematic reviews shows marked increase since 2009. J Clin Epidemiol. 2014;67(2):138-43. doi:10.1016/j.jclinepi.2013.07.014.

48. Nikolakopoulou A, Chaimani A, Veroniki AA, Vasiliadis HS, Schmid CH, Salanti G. Characteristics of networks of interventions: a description of a database of 186 published networks. PLoS One. 2014;9(1):e86754. doi:10.1371/journal.pone.0086754.

49. Cochrane [Internet]. London: Cochrane; c2019 [cited 2020 Jan 2]. Available from: https://www.cochrane.org

50. Higgins JPT, Thomas J, Chandler J, Cumpston M, Li T, Page MJ, Welch VA, editors. Cochrane handbook for systematic reviews of interventions [Internet]. Version 6.0. London: Cochrane; 2019 [updated 2019 Jul; cited 2020 Jan 2]. 1 p. Available from: https://training.cochrane.org/handbook

51. Haber SL, Fairman KA, Sclar DA. Principles in the evaluation of systematic reviews. Pharmacotherapy. 2015;35(11):1077-87. doi:10.1002/phar.1657.

52. Liberati A, Altman DG, Tetzlaff J, Mulrow C, Gøtzsche PC, Ioannidis JPA, Clarke M, Devereaux PJ, Kleijnen J, Moher D. The PRISMA statement for reporting systematic reviews and meta-analyses of studies that evaluate health care interventions: explanation and elaboration. Ann Intern Med. 2009;151(4):W65-94.

53. Booth A, Clarke M, Dooley G, Ghersi D, Moher D, Petticrew M, Stewart L. The nuts and bolts of PROSPERO: an international prospective register of systematic reviews. Syst Rev. 2012;1:2. doi:10.1186/2046-4053-1-2.

54. PRISMA: transparent reporting of systematic reviews and meta-analyses [Internet]. Oxford: PRISMA; c2015 [cited 2020 Jan 2]. Available from: http://www.prisma-statement.org/.

55. International Pharmaceutical Abstracts: user guide [Internet]. Boston (MA): Clarivate Analytics; c2019 [cited 2020 Jan 2]. [1 screen]. Available from: https://support.clarivate.com/ScientificandAcademicResearch/s/article/International-Pharmaceutical-Abstracts-User-guide?language=en_US

56. American Psychological Association. PsycINFO [Internet]. Washington (DC): American Psychological Association; c2019 [cited 2020 Jan 2]. [1 screen]. Available from: https://www.apa.org/pubs/databases/psycinfo/

57. Martineau AR, Jolliffe DA, Hooper RL, Greenberg L, Aloia JF, Bergman P, Dubnov-Raz G, Esposito S, Ganmaa D, Ginde AA, Goodall EC, Grant CC, Janssens W, Jensen ME, Kerley

CP, Laaksi I, Manaseki-Holland S, Mauger D, Murdoch DR, Neale R, Rees JR, Simpson S, Stelmach I, Kumar GT, Urashima M, Camargo CA, Griffiths CJ. Vitamin D supplementation to prevent acute respiratory tract infections: systematic review and meta-analysis of individual participant data. BMJ. 2017;356:i6583. doi:10.1136/bmj.i6583.

58. Hopewell S, McDonald S, Clarke M, Egger M. Grey literature in meta-analyses of randomized trials of health care interventions. Cochrane Database Syst Rev. 2007;2:Mr000010. doi:10.1002/14651858.MR000010.pub3.

59. Zheng SL, Roddick AJ. Association of aspirin use for primary prevention with cardiovascular events and bleeding events: a systematic review and meta-analysis. JAMA. 2019;321(3):277-87. doi:10.1001/jama.2018.20578.

60. Higgins JP, Altman DG, Gotzsche PC, Jüni P, David Moher D, Oxman AD, Savovic J, Schulz KF, Weeks L, Sterne JAC Cochrane Bias Methods Group; Cochrane Statistical Methods Group. The Cochrane Collaboration's tool for assessing risk of bias in randomised trials. BMJ. 2011;343:d5928. doi:10.1136/bmj.d5928.

61. Viera AJ, Garrett JM. Understanding interobserver agreement: the kappa statistic. Fam Med. 2005;37(5):360-3.

62. Ford AC, Quigley EM, Lacy BE, Lembo AJ, Saito YA, Schiller LR, Soffer EE, Spiegel BM, Moayyedi P. Efficacy of prebiotics, probiotics, and synbiotics in irritable bowel syndrome and chronic idiopathic constipation: systematic review and meta-analysis. Am J Gastroenterol. 2014;109(10):1547-61. doi:10.1038/ajg.2014.202.

63. Lau J, Ioannidis JP, Schmid CH. Quantitative synthesis in systematic reviews. Ann Intern Med. 1997;127(9):820-6.

64. Huedo-Medina TB, Sanchez-Meca J, Marin-Martinez F, Botella J. Assessing heterogeneity in meta-analysis: Q statistic or I2 index? Psychol Methods. 2006;11(2):193-206. doi:10.1037/1082-989x.11.2.193.

65. Franco OH, Chowdhury R, Troup J, Voortman T, Kunutsor S, Kavousi M, Oliver-Williams J C, Muka T. Use of plant-based therapies and menopausal symptoms: a systematic review and meta-analysis. JAMA. 2016;315(23):2554-63. doi:10.1001/jama.2016.8012.

66. Hopewell S, Loudon K, Clarke MJ, Oxman AD, Dickersin K. Publication bias in clinical trials due to statistical significance or direction of trial results. Cochrane Database Syst Rev. 2009;1:Mr000006. doi:10.1002/14651858.MR000006.pub3.

67. Jin Z, Zhou X, He J. Statistical methods for dealing with publication bias. Stat Med. 2015;34(2):343-60. doi:10.1002/sim.6342.

68. Helfer B, Samara MT, Huhn M, Klupp E, Leucht C, Zhu Y, Engel RR, Leucht S. Efficacy and safety of antidepressants added to antipsychotics for schizophrenia: a systematic review and meta-analysis. Am J Psychiatry. 2016;173(9):876-86. doi:10.1176/appi.ajp.2016.15081035.

69. Guyatt GH, Oxman AD, Schunemann HJ, Tugwell P, Knottnerus A. GRADE guidelines: a new series of articles in the Journal of Clinical Epidemiology. J Clin Epidemiol. 2011;64(4):380-2. doi:10.1016/j.jclinepi.2010.09.011.

70. Balshem H, Helfand M, Schunemann HJ, Oxman AD, Kunz R, Brozek J, Vist GE, Falck-Ytter Y, Meerpohl J, Norris S, Guyatt GH. GRADE guidelines: 3. Rating the quality of evidence. J Clin Epidemiol. 2011;64(4):401-6. doi:10.1016/j.jclinepi.2010.07.015.

71. Kravitz RL, Duan N, editors, and the DEcIDE Methods Center N-of-1 Guidance Panel (Duan N, Eslick I, Gabler NB, Kaplan HC, Kravitz RL, Larson EB, Pace WD, Schmid CH, Sim I, Vohra S). Design and implementation of N-of-1 trials: a user's guide [Internet]. AHRQ Publication No. 13(14)-EHC122-EF. Rockville (MD): Agency for Healthcare Research and Quality; 2014 Jan [cited 2020 Jan 3]. 88 p. Available from: https://effectivehealthcare.ahrq.gov/sites/default/files/pdf/n-1-trials_research-2014-5.pdf

72. Guyatt G, Zhang Y, Jaeschke R, McGinn T. N-of-1 randomized clinical trials. In: Guyatt G, Rennie D, Meade MO, Cook DJ, editors. Users' guides to the medical literature: a manual for evidence-based clinical practice. 3rd ed. New York: McGraw-Hill; c2015. p. 151-62.

73. Vohra S, Shamseer L, Sampson M, Bukutu C, Schmid CH, Tate R, Nikles J, Zucker DR, Kravitz R, Guyatt G, Altman DG, Moher D. CONSORT extension for reporting N-of-1 trials (CENT) 2015 statement. BMJ. 2015;350:h1738. doi:10.1136/bmj.h1738.

74. Spilker B. Single-patient clinical trials. In: Spilker B, editor. Guide to clinical trials. New York: Raven Press; c1991. p. 277-82.

75. Shamseer L, Sampson M, Bukutu C, Schmid CH, Nikles J, Tate R, Johnston BC, Zucker D, Shadish WR, Kravitz R, Guyatt GC, Altman DG, Moher D, Vohra S. CONSORT extension for reporting N-of-1 trials (CENT) 2015: explanation and elaboration. BMJ. 2015;350:h1793. doi:10.1136/bmj.h1793.

76. CONSORT: transparent reporting of trials [Internet]. Ottawa: The CONSORT Group; c2019 [cited 2020 Jan 2]. N-of-1 trials; [1 screen]. Available from: http://www.consort-statement.org/extensions/overview/n-of-1

77. Gidron Y. Health outcomes research. In: Gellman MD, Turner JR, editors. Encyclopedia of behavioral medicine. New York: Springer; 2013:924-5.

78. Jefford M, Stockler MR, Tattersall MH. Outcomes research: what is it and why does it matter? Intern Med J. 2003;33(3):110-8.

79. Patient-Centered Outcomes Research (PCOR) at AHRQ. Dissemination of PCOR [Internet]. Rockville (MD): Agency for Healthcare Research and Quality; c2010-2019 [reviewed 2016 Oct; cited 2019 Aug 10]. [about 2 screens]. Available from: https://www.ahrq.gov/pcor/dissemination-of-pcor/index.html

80. Furukawa TA, Scott IA, Guyatt G. Measuring patients' experience. In: Guyatt G, Rennie D, Meade MO, Cook DJ, editors. Users' guides to the medical literature: a manual for evidence-based clinical practice. 3rd ed. New York: McGraw-Hill; c2015. p. 219-34.

81. 36-Item Short Form Survey (SF-36) [Internet]. Santa Monica (CA): RAND Health Care; c1994-2020 [cited 2020 Jan 6]. Available from: https://www.rand.org/health-care/surveys_tools/mos/36-item-short-form.html

82. Hamilton M. A rating scale for depression. J Neurol Neurosurg Psychiatry. 1960;23:56-62.

83. USP-NF [Internet]. Rockville (MD): United States Pharmacopeia, Inc.; c2019 [cited 2019 Nov 22]. Available from: https://online.uspnf.com/uspnf

84. Bajaj S, Singla D, Sakhuja N. Stability testing of pharmaceutical products. J Appl Pharm Sci. 2012;2(3):129-38.

85. U.S. Food and Drug Administration. Guidance for industry: Q1A(R2) stability testing of new drug substances and products [Internet]. Rockville (MD): U.S. Food and Drug

Administration; 2003 Nov [cited 2019 Aug 10]. 25 p. Available from: https://www.fda.gov/media/71707/download

86. Bing CD, Nowobliski-Vasillos A. Extended stability for parenteral drugs. 6th ed. Bethesda (MD): American Society of Health-System Pharmacy; 2017:340.

87. WHO Expert Committee of Specifications for Pharmaceutical Preparations. Stability testing of active pharmaceutical ingredients and finished pharmaceutical products [Internet]. Geneva (Switzerland): World Health Organization; 2018 Jun 7 [cited 2019 Aug 10]. 44 p. Available from: https://extranet.who.int/prequal/sites/default/files/documents/TRS1010_Annex10.pdf

88. ICH: harmonisation for better health. Evaluation for stability data: QE1. ICH harmonised tripartite guidelines [Internet]. International Conference on Harmonisation of Technical Requirements for Registration of Pharmaceuticals for Human Use. Geneva (Switzerland): The International Council for Harmonisation of Technical Requirements for Registration of Pharmaceuticals for Human Use; 2003 Feb 6 [cited 2019 Aug 10]. 19 p. Available from: https://database.ich.org/sites/default/files/Q1E_Guideline.pdf

89. U.S. Food and Drug Administration. Current good manufacturing practice for finished pharmaceuticals [Internet]. Rockville (MD): U.S. Food and Drug Administration; 2019 Apr 1 [cited 2019 Aug 10]. [1 screen]. Available from: https://www.accessdata.fda.gov/scripts/cdrh/cfdocs/cfcfr/CFRSearch.cfm?fr=211.166

90. Chow SC. Bioavailability and bioequivalence in drug development. Wiley Interdiscip Rev Comput Stat. 2014;6(4):304-12. doi:10.1002/wics.1310.

91. U.S. Food and Drug Administration. Guidance for industry: bioequivalence studies with pharmacokinetic endpoints for drugs submitted under an ANDA. Draft guidance [Internet]. Rockville (MD): U.S. Food and Drug Administration; 2013 Dec [cited 2019 Aug 10]. Available from: http://www.fda.gov/ucm/groups/fdagov-public/@fdagov-drugs-gen/documents/document/ucm377465.pdf

92. U.S. Food and Drug Administration. Orange book: approved drug products with therapeutic equivalence evaluations [Internet]. Rockville (MD): U.S. Food and Drug Administration; 2019 Nov [cited 2019 Nov 22]. Available from: https://www.accessdata.fda.gov/scripts/cder/ob/index.cfm

93. Johnson SB. Bioavailability and bioequivalence testing. In: Allen LV, Lawson LA, Adejare A, Desselle SP, Felton LA, Moffat AC, Perrie Y, Popovich NG, Shermock KM, Wall DS, editors. Remington: the science and practice of pharmacy. 22nd ed. Philadelphia (PA): Pharmaceutical Press; 2013:349-59.

94. Suvarna V. Phase IV of drug development. Perspect Clin Res. 2010;1(2):57-60.

95. Naci H, Smalley KR, Kesselheim AS. Characteristics of preapproval and postapproval studies for drugs granted accelerated approval by the U.S. Food and Drug Administration. JAMA. 2017;318(7):626-36. doi:10.1001/jama.2017.9415.

96. U.S. Food and Drug Administration. Guidance for industry: Reports on the Status of Postmarketing Study Commitments. Implementation of Section 130 of the Food and Drug Administration Modernization Act of 1997 [Internet]. Rockville (MD): U.S. Food and Drug Administration; 2006 Feb [cited 2019 Aug 10]. Available from: https://www.fda.gov/media/72535/download

97. U.S. Food and Drug Administration. Postmarketing requirement and commitments: introduction [Internet]. Rockville (MD): U.S. Food and Drug Administration; 2016 Jan 12 [cited 2019 Aug 10]. Available from: https://www.fda.gov/drugs/guidance-compliance-regulatory-information/postmarket-requirements-and-commitments

98. U.S. Food and Drug Administration. Postmarketing requirement and commitments. Rockville (MD): U.S. Food and Drug Administration; 2019 Jul 24 [cited 2019 Aug 10]. Available from: https://www.accessdata.fda.gov/Scripts/cder/pmc/index.cfm

99. Ogrinc G, Davies L, Goodman D, Batalden P, Davidoff F, Stevens D. SQUIRE 2.0 (Standards for Quality Improvement Reporting Excellence): revised publication guidelines from a detailed consensus process. BMJ Qual Saf. 2016;25(12):986-92. doi:10.1136/bmjqs-2015-004411.

100. Fan E, Laupacis A, Pronovost PJ, Guyatt G, Needham DM. How to use an article about quality improvement. In: Guyatt G, Rennie D, Meade MO, Cook DJ, editors. Users' guides to the medical literature: a manual for evidence-based clinical practice. 3rd ed. New York: McGraw-Hill; c2015. p. 175-88.

101. Hamdy RF, Bhattarai S, Basu SK, Hahn A, Stone B, Sadler ED, Hammer BM, Galiote J, MD,b,d, Slomkowski J, Casto AM, Korzuch KP, Chase H, Nzegwu N, Greenberg I, Ortiz N, Blake C, Chang J, James E, Bost JE, Payne AS, RK, Soghier L. Reducing vancomycin use in a level IV NICU. Pediatrics. 2020;146(2):e20192963. doi:10.1542/peds.2019-2963.

102. SQUIRE: promoting excellence in healthcare improvement reporting [Internet]. SQUIRE; c2017 [cited 2019 Aug 10]. Available from: http://squire-statement.org

103. Shi L. Health services research methods. 2nd ed. Clinton Park (NY): International Thomson Publishing; 2008. 481 p.

104. Casarett D, Karlawish JH, Sugarman J. Determining when quality improvement initiatives should be considered research: proposed criteria and potential implications. JAMA. 2000;283(17):2275-80. doi:10.1001/jama.283.17.2275.

105. Ponto J. Understanding and evaluating survey research. J Adv Pract Oncol. 2015;6(2):168-71.

106. Draugalis JR, Coons SJ, Plaza CM. Best practices for survey research reports: a synopsis for authors and reviewers. Am J Pharm Educ. 2008;72(1):11. doi:10.5688/aj720111.

107. AAPOR: American Association for Public Opinion Research. Evaluating survey quality in today's complex environment [Internet]. Oakbrook Terrace (IL): American Association for Public Opinion Research; c2019 [cited 2019 Aug 10]. Available from: https://www.aapor.org/Education-Resources/Reports/Evaluating-Survey-Quality.aspx

108. Draugalis JR, Plaza CM. Best practices for survey research reports revisited: implications of target population, probability sampling, and response rate. Am J Pharm Educ. 2009;73(8):142. doi:10.5688/aj7308142.

109. McLaughlin JE, Dean MJ, Mumper RJ, Blouin RA, Roth MT. A roadmap for educational research in pharmacy. Am J Pharm Educ. 2013;77(10):218. doi:10.5688/ajpe7710218.

110. Persky AM, Romanelli F. Insights, pearls, and guidance on successfully producing and publishing educational research. Am J Pharm Educ. 2016;80(5):75. doi:10.5688/ajpe80575.

111. A closer look at scientifically based research: how to evaluate educational research. The Journal. 2004;31:24.

112. Zirak N, Shafiee M, Soltani G, Mirzaei M, Shebkar A. *Hypericum perforatum* in the treatment of psychiatric and neurodegenerative disorders: current evidence and potential mechanisms of action. J Cell Physiol. 2019;234(6):8496-508. doi:10.1002/jcp.27781.

113. Ogata T, Ideno Y, Akai M, Seichi A, Hagino H, Iwaya T, Doi T, Yamada K, Chen A-Z, Li Y, Hayashi K. Effects of glucosamine in patients with osteoarthritis of the knee: a systematic review and meta-analysis. Clin Rheumatol. 2018;37(9):2479-87. doi:10.1007/s10067-018-4106-2.

114. Towheed TE, Maxwell L, Anastassiades TP, Shea B, Houpt J, Robinson V, Hochberg MC, Wells G. Glucosamine therapy for treating osteoarthritis. Cochrane Database Syst Rev. 2005;2:CD002946. doi:10.1002/14651858.CD002946.pub2.

115. U.S. Food and Drug Administration. Recalls, market withdrawals, and safety alerts: dietary supplements [Internet]. Rockville: U.S. Food and Drug Administration; c2020 [cited 2020 May 1]. [1 screen]. Available from: https://www.fda.gov/safety/recalls-market-withdrawals-safety-alerts

116. QualitySupplements [Internet]. The United States Pharmacopeial Convention; c2020 [cited 2020 Jan 2]. Available from: https://www.quality-supplements.org/

117. Stoney CM, Coates P, Briggs JP. Integrity of active components of botanical products used in complementary and alternative medicine. JAMA. 2008;300(17):1995. doi:10.1001/jama.2008.557.

118. CONSORT: Transparent Reporting of Trials. Herbal medicinal interventions [Internet]. Ottawa: The CONSORT Group; c2019 [cited 2020 Jan 2]. [1 screen]. Available from: http://www.consort-statement.org/extensions/overview/herbal-medicinal/interventions

119. Gagnier JJ, Boon H, Rochon P, Moher D, Barnes J, Bombardier C. Reporting randomized, controlled trials of herbal interventions: an elaborated CONSORT statement. Ann Intern Med. 2006;144(5):364-7. doi:10.7326/0003-4819-144-5-200603070-00013.

120. Gagnier JJ, Boon H, Rochon P, Moher D, Barnes J, Bombardier C. Recommendations for reporting randomized controlled trials of herbal interventions: explanation and elaboration. J Clin Epidemiol. 2006;59(11):1134-49. doi:10.1016/j.jclinepi.2005.12.020.

121. Epidiolex (Cannabidiol) Oral Solution. Carlsbad (CA): Greenwich Biosciences, Inc.; 2020. Package insert.

122. Dickinson A, Blatman J, El-Dash N, Franco JC. Consumer usage and reasons for using dietary supplements: report of a series of surveys. J Am Coll Nutr. 2014;33(2):176-82. doi:10.1080/07315724.2013.875423.

SUGGESTED READINGS

1. von Elm E, Altman DG, Egger M, Pocock SJ, Gotzsche PC, Vandenbroucke JP; STROBE Initiative. The Strengthening the Reporting of Observational Studies in Epidemiology (STROBE) statement: guidelines for reporting observational studies. Ann Intern Med. 2007;147(8):573-7.

2. DiPietro NA. Methods in epidemiology: observational study designs. Pharmacotherapy. 2010;30(10):973-84. doi:10.1592/phco.30.10.973.

3. Kier KL. Biostatistical applications in epidemiology. Pharmacotherapy. 2011;31(1):9-22. doi:10.1592/phco.31.1.9.

4. Shields KM, DiPietro NA, Kier KL. Principles of drug literature evaluation for observational study designs. Pharmacotherapy. 2011;31(2):115-27. doi:10.1592/phco.31.2.115.

5. Moher D, Liberati A, Tetzlaff J, Altman DG; PRISMA Group. Preferred reporting items for systematic reviews and meta-analyses: the PRISMA statement. Ann Intern Med. 2009;151(4):264-9.

6. Murad MH, Montori VM, Ioannidis JP, Jaeschke R, Devereaux PJ, Prasad K, Neumann I, Carrasco-Labra A, Agoritsas T, Hatala R, Meade MO, Wyer P, Cooke DJ, Guyatt G. How to read a systematic review and meta-analysis and apply the results to patient care: users' guides to the medical literature. JAMA. 2014;312(2):171-9. doi:10.1001/jama.2014.5559.

7. Haber SL, Fairman KA, Sclar DA. Principles in the evaluation of systematic reviews. Pharmacotherapy. 2015;35(11):1077-87. doi:10.1002/phar.1657.

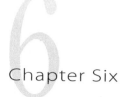

Chapter Six

The Application of Statistical Analysis in the Biomedical Sciences

Ryan W. Walters

Learning Objectives

After completing this chapter, the reader will be able to:

- Define the population being studied and describe the method most appropriate to sample a given population.
- Identify and describe the dependent and independent variables and indicate whether any covariates were included in analysis.
- Identify and define the four scales of variable measurement.
- Describe the difference between descriptive and inferential statistics.
- Describe the mean, median, variance, and standard deviation and why they are important to statistical analysis.
- Describe the properties of the normal distribution and when an alternative distribution should be, or should have been, used.
- Describe several common epidemiological statistics.
- Identify and describe the difference between parametric and nonparametric statistical tests and when their use is most appropriate.
- Determine whether the appropriate statistical test has been performed when evaluating a study.

Key Concepts

❶ There are four scales of variable measurement consisting of nominal, ordinal, interval, and ratio scales that are critically important to consider when determining the appropriateness of a statistical test.

❷ Measures of central tendency are useful to quantify the distribution of a variable's data numerically. The most common measures of central tendency are the mean, median, and mode, with the most appropriate measure of central tendency dictated by the variable's scale of measurement.

❸ Variance is a key element inherent in all statistical analyses, but standard deviation is presented more often. Variance and standard deviation are related mathematically.

❹ The last observation carried forward (LOCF) technique used often with the data from clinical trials introduces significant bias into the results of statistical tests.

❺ The central limit theorem states when equally sized samples are drawn from a non-normal distribution, the plotted mean values from each sample will approximate a normal distribution as long as the non-normality was not due to outliers.

❻ There are numerous misconceptions about p values and it is important to know how to interpret them correctly.

❼ Clinical significance is far more important than statistical significance. Clinical significance can be quantified by using various measures of effect size.

❽ The selection of the appropriate statistical test is based on several factors including the specific research question, the measurement scale of the dependent variable (DV), distributional assumptions, the number of DV measurements, as well as the number and measurement scale of independent variables (IVs) and covariates, among others.

Introduction

Knowledge of statistics and statistical analyses is essential to constructively evaluate literature in the biomedical sciences. This chapter provides a general overview of both descriptive and inferential statistics that will enhance the ability of the student or practitioner to interpret results of empirical literature within the biomedical sciences by evaluating the appropriateness of statistical tests employed, the conclusions drawn by the authors, and the overall quality of the study.

Alongside Chapters 4 and 5, diligent study of the material presented in this chapter is an important first step to critically analyze the often-avoided methods or results sections of published biomedical literature. Be aware, however, that this chapter cannot substitute for more formal didactic training in statistics, as the material presented here is not exhaustive with regard to either statistical concepts or available statistical tests. Thus, when reading a journal article, if doubt emerges about whether a method or statistical test was used and interpreted appropriately, do not hesitate to consult appropriate references or an individual who has more formal statistical training. This is especially true if the empirical evidence is being considered for implementation in practice. Asking questions is the key to obtaining knowledge!

For didactic purposes, this chapter can be divided into two sections. The first section presents a general overview of the processes underlying most statistical tests used in the biomedical sciences. It is recommended that all readers take the time required to thoroughly study these concepts. The second section, beginning with the section entitled "Selecting the Appropriate Statistical Test," presents descriptions, assumptions, examples, and results of numerous statistical tests commonly used in the biomedical sciences. This section does not present the mathematical underpinnings, calculation, or programming of any specific statistical test. It is recommended that this section serve as a reference to be used concurrently alongside a given journal article to determine the appropriateness of a statistical test or to gain further insight into why a specific statistical test was employed.

Populations and Sampling

When investigating a particular research question or hypothesis, researchers must first define the population to be studied. A population refers to any set of objects in the universe, while a sample is a fraction of the population chosen to be representative of the specific population of interest. Thus, samples are chosen to make specific generalizations about the population of interest. Researchers typically do not attempt to study the entire population because data cannot be collected for everyone within a population. This is why a sample should ideally be chosen at random. That is, each member of the population must have an equal probability of being included in the sample.

For example, consider a study to evaluate the effect a calcium channel blocker (CCB) has on blood glucose levels in Type 1 diabetes mellitus (DM) patients. In this case, all Type 1 DM patients would constitute the study population; however, because data could never be collected from all Type 1 DM patients, a sample that is representative of the Type 1 DM population would be selected. There are numerous sampling strategies, many beyond the scope of this text. Although only a few are discussed here, interested readers are urged to consult the list of suggested readings at the end of this chapter for further information.

A random sample does not imply that the sample is drawn haphazardly or in an unplanned fashion, and there are several approaches to selecting a random sample. The most common method employs a random number table. A random number table theoretically contains all integers between 1 and infinity that have been selected without any trends or patterns. For example, consider the hypothetical process of selecting a random sample of Type 1 DM patients from the population. First, each patient in the population is assigned a number; say 1 to N, where N is the total number of Type 1 DM patients in the population. From this population, a sample of 200 patients is requested. The random number table would randomly select 200 patients from the population of size N. There are numerous free random number tables and generators available online; simply search for "random number table" or "random number generator" in any search engine.

Depending on the study design, a completely random sample may not be most appropriate when selecting a representative sample. On occasion, it may be necessary to separate the population into mutually exclusive groups called strata, where a specific factor (e.g., race, gender) will create separate strata to aid in analysis. In this case, the random sample is drawn within each stratum individually. This process is termed "stratified random sampling." For example, consider a situation where the race of the patient was an important variable in the Type 1 DM study. To ensure the proportion of each race in the population is represented accurately, the researcher stratifies by race and randomly selects patients within each stratum to achieve a representative study sample.

Another method of randomly sampling a population is known as cluster sampling. Cluster sampling is appropriate when there are natural groupings within the population of interest. For example, consider a researcher interested in the patient counseling practices of pharmacists across the United States. It would be impossible to collect data from all pharmacists across the United States. However, the researcher has read literature suggesting regional differences within various pharmacy practices, not necessarily including counseling practices. Thus, he or she may decide to randomly sample within the four regions of the United States defined by the U.S. Census Bureau (i.e., West, Midwest, South, and Northeast) to assess for differences in patient counseling practices across regions.[1]

Another sampling method is known as systematic sampling. This method is used when information about the population is provided in list format, such as in the telephone book, election records, class lists, or licensure records, among others. Systematic sampling uses an equal-probability method where one individual is selected initially at random and every nth individual is then selected thereafter. For example, the researchers may decide to take every 10th individual listed after the first individual is chosen.

Finally, researchers often use convenience sampling to select participants based on the convenience of the researcher. That is, no attempt is made to ensure the sample is representative of the population. However, within the convenience sample, participants may be selected randomly. This type of sampling is often used in educational research. For example, consider a researcher evaluating a new classroom instructional method to increase exam scores. This type of study will use the convenience sample of the students in their own class or university. Obviously, significant weaknesses are apparent when using this type of sampling, most notably, limited generalization.

Variables and the Measurement of Data

A variable is the characteristic that is being observed or measured. Data are the measured values assigned to the variable for each individual member of the population. For example, a variable would be the participant's biological sex, while the data is whether the participant is male or female.

In statistics, there are three types of variables: dependent (DV), independent (IV), and confounding or nuisance. The DV is the response or outcome variable for a study, while an IV is a variable that is manipulated. A confounding variable (often referred to as covariate) is any variable that has an effect on the DV over and above the effect of the IV, but is not of specific research interest. Putting these definitions together, consider a study to evaluate the effect a new oral hypoglycemic medication has on glycosylated hemoglobin (HbA1c) compared to placebo. Here, the DV consists of the HbA1c data for each participant, and the IV is treatment group with two levels (i.e., treatment vs. placebo). Initially, results may suggest the medication is very effective across the entire sample; however, previous literature has suggested participant race may affect the effectiveness of this type of medication. Thus, participant race is a confounding variable and would need to be included in the statistical analysis. After statistically controlling for participant race, the results may indicate that the medication was significantly more effective in the treatment group.

SCALES OF MEASUREMENT

❶ *There are four scales of variable measurement consisting of nominal, ordinal, interval, and ratio scales that are critically important to consider when determining the appropriateness of a statistical test.*[2] Think of these four scales as relatively fluid; that is, as the data progress from nominal to ratio, the information about each variable being measured is increased. The scale of measurement of DVs, IVs, and confounding variables is an important consideration when determining whether the appropriate statistical test was used to answer the research question and hypothesis.

A **nominal scale** consists of categories that have no implied rank or order. Examples of nominal variables include gender (e.g., male vs. female), race (e.g., Caucasian vs. African American vs. Hispanic), or disease state (e.g., absence vs. presence). It is important to note that, with nominal data, the participant is categorized into one, and only one, category. That is, the categories are mutually exclusive.

An **ordinal scale** has all of the characteristics of a nominal variable with the addition of rank ordering. It is important to note the distance between rank-ordered categories cannot be considered equal; that is, the data points can be ranked but the distance between them may differ greatly. For example, in medicine a commonly used pain scale is the Wong-Baker Faces Pain Rating Scale.[3] Here, the participant ranks pain on a 0–10 scale by selecting a face that conveys their degree of pain; however, while it is known that a rating of 8 indicates the participant is in more pain than a rating of 4, there is no indication that a rating of 8 hurts twice as much as a rating of 4.

An **interval scale** has all of the characteristics of an ordinal scale with the addition that the distance between two values is now constant and meaningful. However, it is important to note that interval scales do not have an absolute zero point. For example, temperature on a Celsius scale is measured on an interval scale (i.e., the difference between $10°C$ and $5°C$ is equivalent to the difference between $20°C$ and $15°C$). However, $20°C/10°C$ cannot be quantified as twice as hot because there is no absolute zero (i.e., the Celsius scale does not have an index of "no temperature").

Finally, a **ratio scale** has all of the characteristics of an interval scale, but ratio scales have an absolute zero point. The classic example of a ratio scale is temperature measured on the Kelvin scale, where 0 K represents the absence of molecular motion. Theoretically, researchers should not confuse absolute and arbitrary zero points. However, the difference between interval and ratio scales is generally trivial as these data are analyzed by identical statistical procedures and are both numerical.

CONTINUOUS VERSUS CATEGORICAL VARIABLES

Continuous variables generally consist of data measured on interval or ratio scales. However, if the number of ordinal categories is large (e.g., seven or more), they may be considered continuous.[4] Be aware that continuous variables may also be referred to as quantitative in the literature. Examples of continuous variables include age, body mass index (BMI), or uncategorized systolic or diastolic blood pressure values.

Categorical variables consist of data measured on nominal or ordinal scales because these scales of measurement have naturally distinct categories. Examples of categorical variables include gender, race, or blood pressure status (e.g., hypotensive, normotensive, prehypertensive, hypertensive). In the literature, categorical variables are often termed "discrete" or if a variable is measured on a nominal scale with only two distinct categories it may be termed "binary" or "**dichotomous**."

Note that it is common in the biomedical literature for researchers to categorize continuous variables. Although not wholly incorrect, categorizing a continuous variable will always result in loss of information about the variable. For example, consider the role that participant age has on the probability of experiencing a cardiac event. Although age is a continuous variable, younger individuals typically have much a lower probability compared to older individuals. Thus, the research may divide age into four discrete categories: <30, 31–50, 51–70, and 70+. Note that assigning category cutoffs is generally an arbitrary process. In this example, information is lost by categorizing age because after categorization, the exact age of the participant is unknown. That is, an individual's age is defined only by their age category. For example, a 50-year-old individual is considered identical to a 31-year-old individual because they are in the same age category and qualitatively different from a 51-year-old individual given they are in different categories.

Descriptive Statistics

There are two types of statistics—descriptive and inferential. Descriptive statistics present, organize, and summarize a variable's data by providing information regarding the appearance of the data and distributional characteristics. Examples of descriptive statistics include measures of central tendency, variability, shape, histograms, boxplots, and scatterplots. These descriptive measures are the focus of this section.

Inferential statistics indicate whether a difference exists between groups of participants or whether an association exists between variables. Inferential statistics are used to determine whether the difference or association is real or whether it is due to some random process. Examples of inferential statistics are the statistics produced by each statistical test described later in the chapter. For example, the t statistic produced by a t test.

MEASURES OF CENTRAL TENDENCY

❷ *Measures of central tendency are useful to quantify the distribution of a variable's data numerically. The most common measures of central tendency are the mean, median, and mode, with the most appropriate measure of central tendency dictated by the variable's scale of measurement.*

The **mean** (indicated as M in the literature) is the most common and appropriate measure of central tendency for normally distributed data (see the "Common Probability Distributions" section later in the chapter) measured on an interval or ratio scale. The mean is the arithmetic average of a variable's data. Thus, the mean is calculated by summing a variable's data and dividing by the total number of participants with data for the specific variable. It is important to note that data points that are severely disconnected from the other data points can significantly influence the mean. These extreme data points are termed "outliers."

The **median** is most appropriate measure of central tendency for data measured on an ordinal scale. The median is the absolute middle value in the data; therefore, exactly half of the data is above the median and exactly half of the data is below the median. The median is also known as the 50th percentile. Note that the median can also be presented for continuous variables with skewed distributions (see the "Measures of Distribution Shape" section later in the chapter) and for continuous variables with outliers. A direct comparison of a variable's mean and median can give insight into how much influence outliers had on the mean.

Finally, the **mode** is the most appropriate measure of central tendency for nominal data. The mode is a variable's most frequently occurring data point or category. Note that it is possible for a variable to have multiple modes; a variable with two or three modes is referred to as bimodal and trimodal, respectively.

MEASURES OF VARIABILITY

Measures of variability are useful in indicating the spread of a variable's data. The most common measures of variability are the range, interquartile range, variance, and standard deviation. These measures are also useful when considered with appropriate measures of central tendency to assess how the data are scattered around the mean or median. For example, consider the two histograms in Figure 6-1. Both histograms present data for 100 participants that have identical mean body weight of 185 pounds. However, notice the variability (or dispersion) of the data is much greater for Group 2. If the means for both groups were simply taken at face value, the participants in these two groups would be considered similar; however, assessing the variability or spread of data within each group illustrates an entirely different picture. This concept is critically important to the application of any inferential statistical test because the test results are heavily influenced by the amount of variability.

The simplest measure of variability is the range, which can be used to describe data measured on an ordinal, interval, or ratio scale. The range is a crude measure of variability calculated by subtracting a variable's minimum data point from its maximum data point. For example, in Figure 6-1 the range for Group 1 is 30 (i.e., 200 – 170), whereas the range from Group 2 is 90 (i.e., 230 – 140).

The interquartile range (indicated as IQR in the literature) is another measure of dispersion used to describe data measured on an ordinal scale; as such, the IQR is usually presented alongside the median. The IQR is the difference between the 75th and 25th percentile. Therefore, because the median represents the 50th percentile, the IQR presents the middle 50% of the data and always includes the median.

The final two measures of variability described are the variance and standard deviation. These measures are appropriate for normally distributed continuous variables

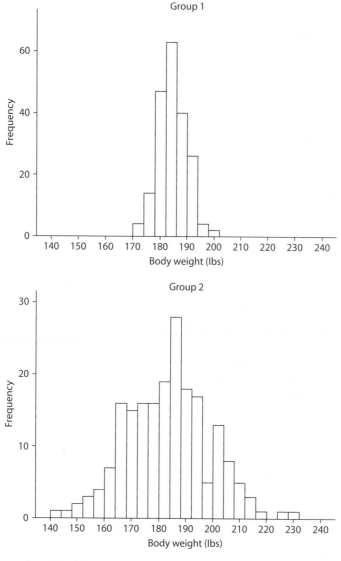

Figure 6–1. Differences in variability between two groups with identical means.

measured on interval or ratio scales. ❸ *Variance is a key element inherent in all statistical analyses, but standard deviation is presented more often. Variance and standard deviation are related mathematically.* Variance is the average squared deviation from the mean for all data points within a specific variable. For example, consider Figure 6-1 where the mean for both Groups 1 and 2 was 185 pounds. Say a specific participant in Group 1 had a body weight of 190 pounds. The squared deviation from the mean for this participant would be equal to 25 pounds. That is, $190 - 185 = 5$ and $5^2 = 25$). To calculate variance, the squared deviations are calculated for all data points. These square deviations are then summed across participants and then divided by the total number of data points (i.e., N) to obtain the average squared deviation. Some readers may be asking why the deviations from the mean are squared. This is a great question! The reason is that summing unsquared deviations across participants would equal 0. That is, deviations resulting from values above and below the mean would cancel each other out. While the calculation of variance may seem esoteric, conceptually all that is required to understand variance is that larger variance values indicate greater variability. For example, the variances of Groups 1 and 2 in Figure 6-1 were 25 and 225, respectively. While the histograms did not present these numbers explicitly, the greater variability in Group 2 can be observed clearly. The importance of variance cannot be overstated. It is the primary parameter used in all parametric statistical analyses, and this is why it was presented in such detail here. With that said, variance is rarely presented as a descriptive statistic in the literature. Instead, variance is converted into a standard deviation as described in the next paragraph.

As a descriptive statistic, the standard deviation (indicated as SD in the literature) is often preferred over variance because it indicates the average deviation from the mean presented on the same scale as the original variable. Variance presented the average deviation in squared units. It is important to note that the standard deviation and variance are directly related mathematically, with standard deviation equal to the square root of the variance (i.e., $SD = \sqrt{variance}$). Thus, if the standard deviation is known, the variance can be calculated directly, and vice versa. When comparing variability between groups of participants, the standard deviation can provide insight into the dispersion of scores around the mean, and, similar to variance, larger standard deviations indicate greater variability in the data. For example, from Figure 6-1, Group 1 had a standard deviation of 5 (i.e., $\sqrt{25}$) and Group 2 had a standard deviation of 15 (i.e., $\sqrt{225}$). Again, the greater variability within Group 2 is evident.

MEASURES OF DISTRIBUTION SHAPE

Skewness and kurtosis are appropriate measures of shape for variables measured on interval or ratio scales, and indicate asymmetry and peakedness of a distribution, respectively. They are typically used by researchers to evaluate the distributional assumptions of a parametric statistical analysis.

Skewness indicates the asymmetry of distribution of data points and can be either positive or negative. Positive (or right) skewness occurs when the mode and median are less than the mean, whereas negative (or left) skewness occurs when mode and median are greater than the mean. As stated previously, the mean is sensitive to extremely disconnected data points termed "outliers"; thus, it is important to know the difference between true skewness and skewness due to outliers. True skewness is indicated by a steady decrease in data points toward the tails (i.e., ends) of the distribution. Skewness due to outliers is indicated when the mean is heavily influenced by data points that are extremely disconnected from the rest of the distribution. For example, consider the histogram in Figure 6-2. The data for Group 1 provides an example of true-positive skewness, whereas the data for Group 2 provides an example of negative skewness due to outliers.

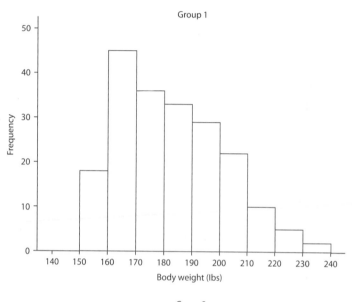

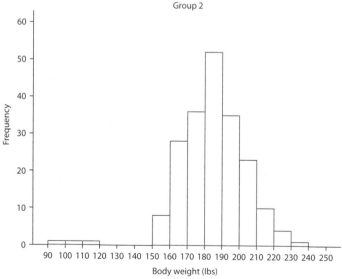

Figure 6–2. True-positive skewness and negative skewness due to outliers.

Kurtosis indicates the peakedness of the distribution of data points and can be either positive or negative. Plotted data with a narrow, peaked distribution and a positive kurtosis value is termed "leptokurtic." A leptokurtic distribution has small range, variance, and standard deviation with the majority of data points near the mean. In contrast, plotted data with a wide, flat distribution and a negative kurtosis value is referred to as platykurtic. A platykurtic distribution is an indicator of great variability, with large range, variance, and standard deviation. Examples of leptokurtic and platykurtic data distributions are presented for Groups 1 and 2, respectively, in Figure 6-2.

GRAPHICAL REPRESENTATIONS OF DATA

Graphical representations of data are incredibly useful, especially when sample sizes are large, as they allow researchers to inspect the distribution of individual variables. There are typically three graphical representations presented in the literature—histograms, boxplots, and scatterplots. Note that graphical representations are typically used for continuous variables measured on ordinal, interval, or ratio scales. By contrast, nominal, dichotomous, or categorical variables are best presented as count data, which are typically reported in the literature as frequency and percentage.

A histogram presents data as frequency counts over some interval; that is, the x-axis presents the values of the data points, whether individual data points or intervals, while the y-axis presents the number of times the data point or interval occurs in the variable (i.e., frequency). Figures 6-1 and 6-2 provide examples of histograms. When data are plotted, it is easy to observe skewness, kurtosis, or outlier issues. For example, reconsider the distribution of body weight for Group 2 in Figure 6-2, where each vertical bar represents the number of participants having body weight within 10-unit intervals. The distribution of data has negative skewness due to outliers, with outliers being participants weighing between 90 and 120 pounds.

A boxplot, also known as a box-and-whisker plot, provides the reader with five descriptive statistics.[5] Consider the boxplot in Figure 6-3, which presents the same data as the Group 2 histogram in Figure 6-2. The thin-lined box in a boxplot indicates the IQR, which contains the 25th to 75th percentiles of the data. Within this thin-lined box is a thick, bold line depicting the median, or 50th percentile. From both ends of the thin-lined box extends a tail, or whisker, depicting the minimum and maximum data points up to 1.5 IQRs beyond the median. Beyond the whiskers, outliers and extreme outliers are identified with circles and asterisks, respectively. Note that other symbols may be used to identify outliers depending on the statistical software used. Outliers are defined as data points 1.5–3.0 IQRs beyond the median, whereas extreme outliers are defined as data points greater than 3.0 IQRs beyond the median. The boxplot corroborates the information provided by the histogram in Figure 6-2 as participants weighing between 90 and 120 pounds are defined as outliers.

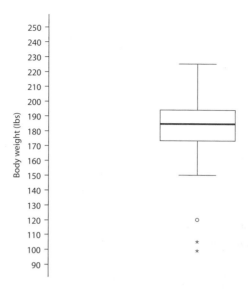

Figure 6–3. Boxplot of body weight with outliers. Circles represent values 1.5–3.0 IQRs, Asterisks represent values > 3.0 IQRs.

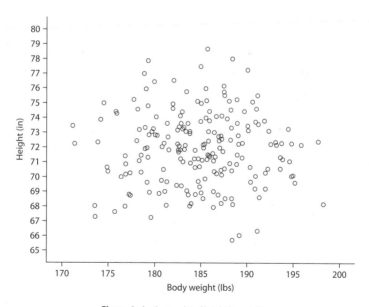

Figure 6–4. Scatterplot of height by weight.

Finally, a scatterplot presents data for two variables both measured on a continuous scale. That is, the *x*-axis contains the range of data for one variable, whereas the *y*-axis contains the range of data for a second variable. In general, the axis choice for a given variable is arbitrary. Data are plotted in a similar fashion to plotting data on a coordinate plane during an introductory geometry class. Figure 6-4 presents a scatterplot of height in inches and body weight in pounds. The individual circles in the scatterplot are a participant's height in relation to their weight. Because the plot is bivariate (i.e., there are two variables), participants must have data for both variables in order to be plotted. Scatterplots are useful in visually assessing the association between two variables as well as assessing assumptions of various statistical tests such as linearity and absence of outliers.

Common Probability Distributions

Up to this point, data distributions have been discussed using very general terminology. There are numerous distributions available to researchers; far too many to provide a complete listing, but all that needs to be known about these available distributions is that each has different characteristics to fit the unique requirements of the data. Globally, these distributions are termed "probability distributions," and they are incredibly important to every statistical analysis conducted. Thus, the choice of distribution used in a given statistical analysis is nontrivial as the use of an improper distribution can lead to incorrect statistical inference. Of the distributions available, the normal and binomial distributions are used most frequently in the biomedical literature; therefore, these are discussed in detail. To provide the reader with a broader listing of available distributions, this section also presents brief information about other common distributions used in the biomedical literature and when they are appropriately used in statistical analyses.

THE NORMAL DISTRIBUTION

The normal distribution, also called Gaussian distribution, is the most commonly used distribution in statistics and one that occurs frequently in nature. It is used only for continuous variables measured on interval or ratio scales. The normal distribution has several easily identifiable properties based on the numerical measures of central tendency, variability, and shape. Specifically, this includes the following characteristics:

1. The primary shape is bell-shaped.
2. The mean, median, and mode are equal.
3. The distribution has one mode, is symmetric, and reflects itself perfectly when folded at the mean.
4. The skewness and kurtosis are 0.
5. The area under a normal distribution is, by definition, equal to 1.

It should be noted that these five properties are considered the gold standard. In practice, however, each of these properties will be approximated; namely, the curve will

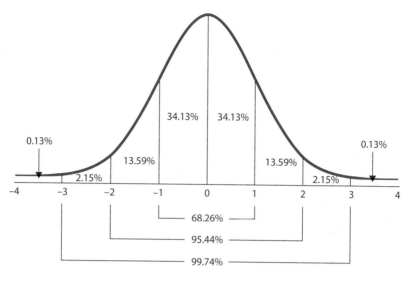

Figure 6–5. The standard normal distribution.

be roughly bell-shaped, the mean, median, and mode will be roughly equal, and skewness and kurtosis may be evident but not greatly exaggerated. For example, the distribution of data for Group 2 in Figure 6-1 is approximately normal.

Several additional properties of the normal distribution are important; consider Figure 6-5. First, the distribution is completely defined by the mean and standard deviation. Consequently, there are an infinite number of possible normal distributions because there are an infinite number of mean and standard deviation combinations. In the literature, this property is often stated as the mean and standard deviation being sufficient statistics for describing the normal distribution. Second, the mean can always be identified as the peak (or mode) of the distribution. Third, the standard deviation will always dictate the spread of the distribution. That is, as the standard deviation increases, the distribution becomes wider. Finally, roughly 68% of the data will occur within one standard deviation above and below the mean, roughly 95% within two standard deviations, and roughly 99% within three standard deviations.

THE STANDARD NORMAL DISTRIBUTION

Among the infinite number of potential normal distributions, only the standard normal distribution can be used to compare all normal distributions. Although this may seem confusing on the surface, a clearer understanding of the standard normal distribution is made possible by considering the standard deviation. Initially, when converting a normal distribution to a standard normal distribution, the data must be converted into standardized scores referred to as *z* **scores**. A *z* score converts the units of the original data into standard deviation units. That is, a *z* score indicates how many standard deviations a data point is from the mean. When converted to *z* scores, the new standard normal distribution will always have a mean of 0 and a standard deviation of 1. The standard normal distribution is presented in Figure 6-5.

It is a common misconception that converting data into *z* scores creates a standard normal distribution from data that was not normally distributed. This is never true. A standardized distribution will always have the same characteristics of distribution from which it originated. That is, if the original distribution was skewed, the standardized distribution will also be skewed.

The key benefit to using the standard normal distribution is that converting the original data to *z* scores allows researchers to compare different variables regardless of the original scale. Remember, a standardized variable will always be expressed in standard deviation units with a mean of 0 and standard deviation of 1. Therefore, differences between variables may be more easily detected and understood. For example, it is possible to compare standardized variables across studies. It should go without stating that the only requirement is that both variables measure the same construct. After *z* score standardization, the age of two groups of participants from two different studies can be compared directly.

THE BINOMIAL DISTRIBUTION

Many discrete variables can be dichotomized into one of two mutually exclusive groups, outcomes, or events (e.g., dead vs. alive). Using the binomial distribution, a researcher can calculate the exact probability of experiencing either binary outcome. In clinical trials, the binomial distribution is used often to evaluate binary outcomes and can be used when an experiment assumes the four characteristics listed below:

1. The trial occurs a specified number of times (analogous to sample size, *n*).
2. Each trial has only two mutually exclusive outcomes (success vs. failure in a generic sense, *x*). Also, be aware that a single trial with only two outcomes is known as a Bernoulli trial, a term that may be encountered in the literature.
3. Each trial is independent, meaning that one outcome has no effect on the other.
4. The probability of success remains constant throughout the trial.

An example may assist with the understanding of these characteristics. The binomial distribution consists of the number of successes and failures during a given study period. When all trials have been run, the probability of achieving exactly *x* successes (or failures) in *n* trials can be calculated. Consider flipping a fair coin. The coin is flipped for a set number of trials (i.e., *n*), there are only two possible outcomes (i.e., heads or tails), each trial is not affected by the outcome of the last, and the probability of flipping heads or tails remains constant throughout the trial (i.e., 0.50).

By definition, the mean for the binomial distribution is equal to the number of successes in a given trial. That is, if a fair coin is flipped 10 times and heads turns up on six flips, the mean is 0.60 (i.e., 6/10). Further, the variance of the binomial distribution is fixed by the mean. While the equation for the variance is not presented, know that the variance is largest at a mean of 0.50, decreases as the mean diverges from 0.50, and is symmetric (e.g., the variance for a mean of 0.10 is equal to the variance for a mean of 0.90). Therefore, because variance is fixed by the mean, the mean is the sufficient statistic for the binomial distribution.

In reality, the probability of experiencing an outcome is rarely 0.50. For example, biomedical studies often use all-cause mortality as an outcome variable, and the probability of dying during the study period is generally lower than staying alive. At the end of the trial, participants can experience only one of the outcomes—dead or alive. Say a study sample consists of 1000 participants, of which 150 die. The binomial distribution allows for the calculation of the exact probability of having 150 participants die in a sample of 1000 participants.

OTHER COMMON PROBABILITY DISTRIBUTIONS

As mentioned in the introduction to this section, there are numerous probability distributions available to researchers, with their use determined by the scale of measurement of the DV as well as the shape (e.g., skewness) of the distribution. When reading journal articles, it is important to know whether the appropriate distribution has been used for statistical analysis as inappropriate use of any distribution can lead to inaccurate statistical inference.

Table 6-1 provides a short list of the several commonly used distributions in the biomedical literature. Of note here is that alternative distributions are available when statistically analyzing non-normally distributed continuous data or data that cannot be normalized such as categorical data. The take away message here is that non-normal continuous data does not need to be forced to conform to a normal distribution.

The only DV scale presented in Table 6-1 that has not been discussed thus far is count data. An example of count data would be a count of the number of hospitalizations during a 5-year study period. It is clear from the example that count data cannot take on negative values. That is, a participant cannot have a negative number of hospitalizations. Both the Poisson and negative binomial distributions are used when analyzing count data. The Poisson distribution assumes the mean and the variance of the data are identical. However, in situations where the mean and variance are not equal, the negative binomial distribution allows the variance of the distribution to increase or decrease as needed. As

TABLE 6–1. COMMON PROBABILITY DISTRIBUTIONS AND WHEN THEY ARE APPROPRIATE TO USE

Distribution Name	DV Scale	Distribution Characteristics	Comments
Normal	Continuous		
Gamma	Continuous	Positive skew	
Inverse Gaussian	Continuous	Positive skew	
Exponential	Continuous	Positive skew	Data has to be > 0
Log-normal[a]	Continuous	Positive skew	Data has to be > 0
Weibull	Continuous	Positive or negative skew	
Gompertz	Continuous	Positive or negative skew	
Poisson	Count	Mean = variance	Data ≥ 0
Negative Binomial	Count	Mean ≠ variance	Data ≥ 0
Bernoulli	Binary		One trial; 2 categories
Binomial	Binary		Repeated Bernoulli trials; 2 categories
Categorical	Categorical		One trial; > 2 categories
Multinomial	Categorical		Repeated trials; > 2 categories

[a]DV = dependent variable. Log = natural log or ln.

a point of possible confusion, the negative binomial distribution does not allow negative values. The negative in negative binomial is a result of using a negative exponent in its mathematical formula.

TRANSFORMATION OF NON-NORMAL DISTRIBUTIONS

Transformations are usually employed by researchers to force a non-normal distribution into a distribution that is approximately normal. Although on the surface this may appear reasonable, data transformation is an archaic technique. As such, transformation is not recommended for the three reasons provided below.

First, although parametric statistical analyses assume normality, the distribution of the actual DV data is not required to be normally distributed. As stated in the previous section, and highlighted in Table 6-1, if non-normality is observed, alternative distributions exist allowing proper statistical analysis of non-normal data without transformation. For this reason alone, transformation is rarely necessary.

Second, transforming the DV data potentially prevents effects of an IV from being observed. As an overly simplistic example, consider the distribution of body weight data presented in Figure 6-6. Say the body weight data were collected from a sample of men and women. Obviously, the data in Figure 6-6 is bimodal and not normally distributed. In this situation, a researcher may attempt to transform the data, but transformation would

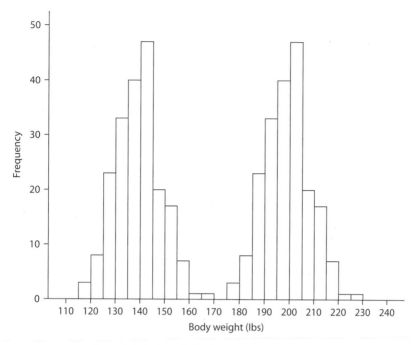

Figure 6–6. Body weight data for a group of men and women.

obscure the effects of an obvious IV—gender. That is, women tend to be lighter compared to men, and this is observed in these data, with women being grouped in the left distribution and men grouped in the right distribution. If transformation were performed successfully, inherent differences between men and women would be erased.

Third, although data transformation will not affect the rank order of the data, it can significantly cloud interpretation of statistical analyses. That is, after transformation all results must be interpreted in the transformed metric, which can become convoluted quickly, making it difficult to apply results to the untransformed data used in the real world. Thus, when reading a journal article where the authors employed any transformation, be aware that the results are in the transformed metric and ensure that the authors' interpretations remain consistent with this metric.

Although transformation is not recommended, it can be used appropriately, and it will inevitably be encountered when reading the literature, especially for skewed distributions. Therefore, it is useful to become familiar with several of the techniques used to transform data. Transformations for positive skewness differ from those suggested for negative skewness. Mild positive skewness is typically remedied by a square root transformation. Here, the square root of all data is calculated and this square root data is used in analysis. When positive skewness is severe, a natural log transformation is used. When data are skewed negatively, researchers may choose to reflect their data to make it positively skewed and apply the transformations for positive skewness described above. To reflect data, a 1 is added to the absolute value of the highest data point and all data points are subtracted from this new value. For example, if the highest value in the data is 10, a 1 is added to create 11, and then all data points are subtracted from 11 (e.g., $11 - 10 = 1, 11 - 1 = 10$). In this manner, the highest values become the lowest and the lowest become the highest. It should be clear that this process considerably convolutes data interpretation!

Epidemiological Statistics

The field of epidemiology investigates how diseases are distributed in the population and the various factors (or exposures) influencing this distribution.[6] Epidemiological statistics are not unique to the field of epidemiology, as much of the literature in the biomedical sciences incorporates some form of these statistics, such as odds ratios. Thus, it is important to have at least a basic level of understanding of these statistics. In this section, the most commonly used epidemiological statistics are discussed briefly, including ratios, proportions, rates, incidence and prevalence, relative risk and odds ratios as well as sensitivity, specificity, and predictive values.

RATIO, PROPORTIONS, AND RATES

Ratios, proportions, and rates are terms used interchangeably in the medical literature without regard for the actual mathematical definitions. Further, there are a considerable number of proportions and rates available to researchers, each providing unique information. Thus, it is important to be aware of how each of these measures is defined and calculated.[7]

- A ratio expresses the relationship between two numbers. For example, consider the ratio of men to women diagnosed with multiple sclerosis (MS). If, in a sample consisting of only MS patients, 100 men and 50 women are diagnosed, the ratio of men to women is 100 to 50, or 100:50, or 2:1. Remember that the order in which the ratio is presented is vitally important; that is, 100:50 is not the same as 50:100.

- A proportion is a specific type of ratio indicating the probability or percentage of the total sample that experienced an outcome or event without respect to time. Here, the numerator of the proportion, representing patients with the disease, is included in the denominator, representing all individuals at risk. For example, say 850 non-MS patients are added to the sample of 150 MS patients from the example above to create a total sample of 1000 patients. Thus, the proportion of patients with MS is 0.15 or 15% (i.e., 150/1000).

A rate is a special form of a proportion that includes a specific study period, typically used to assess the speed at which the event or outcome is developing.[8] A rate is equal to the number of events in a specified time period divided by the length of the time period. For example, say over a 1-year study period, 50 new cases of MS were diagnosed out of the 850 previously undiagnosed individuals. Thus, the rate of new cases of MS within this sample is 50 per year.

INCIDENCE AND PREVALENCE

Incidence quantifies the occurrence of an event or outcome over a specific study period within a specific population of individuals. The incidence rate is calculated by dividing the number of new events by the population at risk, with the population at risk defined as the total number of people who have not experienced the outcome. For example, consider the 50 new cases of MS that developed from the example above from the 850 originally undiagnosed individuals. The incidence rate is approximately 0.06 (i.e., 50/850). Note the denominator did not include the 150 patients already diagnosed with MS because these individuals could longer be in the population at risk.

Prevalence quantifies the number of people who have already experienced the event or outcome at a specific time point. Prevalence is calculated by dividing the total number of people experiencing the event by the total number of individuals in the population. Note that the denominator is everyone in the population, not just individuals in the population at risk. For example, the diagnosed MS cases (i.e., 50 + 150 = 200) would be divided by the population that includes them. That is, the prevalence of MS in this sample is 0.20 (i.e., 200/1000).

Finally, it is important to consider both incidence and prevalence when describing events or outcomes. This is because prevalence varies directly with incidence and the duration of the sickness or disease. For example, consider influenza where the duration of the sickness is relatively short. Thus, while incidence of new influenza cases may be high, the overall prevalence may be low because most individuals recover quickly. By contrast, consider individuals diagnosed with asthma. Because asthma is incurable, the prevalence of the disease may be high, whereas the incidence may be low depending on the total number of new cases diagnosed throughout the year.

RELATIVE RISK AND ODDS RATIO

Relative risk is defined as the ratio (or probability) of the incidence of an event occurring in individuals exposed to a stimulus compared to the incidence of the event in those not exposed to the stimulus. Relative risk can be calculated directly from the cohort study design (see Chapter 5). Briefly, this design is typically a prospective observational design

	Event	No Event	
Exposed	A	B	A+B
Unexposed	C	D	C+D
	A+C	B+D	A+B+C+D

Figure 6–7. Example of a 2 × 2 contingency table.

comparing the incidence of experiencing an event in cohorts of exposed and unexposed individuals over time.

Relative risk is used when comparing the probability of an event occurring to all possible events considered in a study. For example, consider the risk of developing lung cancer in those who are exposed and unexposed to secondhand smoke over a 10-year study period. Upon study conclusion, the 2 × 2 contingency table, shown in Figure 6-7, is created containing frequency counts of events for two groups exposed and unexposed to the secondhand smoke stimulus. This table provides all data necessary to calculate the incidence of the event for both exposed and unexposed individuals. Relative risk is calculated by dividing the proportion of individuals who suffered the event in the exposed group (i.e., A/A+B) by the proportion of individuals who suffered the event in the unexposed group (i.e., C/C+D). Relative risk provides a single number ranging from 0 to infinity, and there are three resulting interpretations provided below.[6]

1. If relative risk equals 1, the risk of experiencing the event is equal within the exposed and unexposed groups. Thus, there is no association between being exposed to the stimulus and experiencing the event.
2. If relative risk is greater than 1, the exposed group has a greater risk of experiencing the event compared to the unexposed group. Thus, there is a positive association or detrimental effect (risk factor) of being exposed to the stimulus.
3. If relative risk is less than 1, the exposed group has a lower risk of experiencing the event compared to the unexposed group. Thus, there is a negative association or protective effect of being exposed to the stimulus.

When relative risk is inappropriate to use, such as in a case-control study (see Chapter 5), researchers will often present an odds ratio. Odds are calculated by dividing the proportion of people experiencing an event by the proportion of people not experiencing an event. Thus, an odds ratio is a ratio of two odds; one for individuals exposed to the stimulus and the other for those not exposed to the stimulus. Odds ratios range from 0 to infinity. They have three interpretations identical to those presented above for relative risk, simply substitute the odds ratio for relative risk. Odds ratios can be calculated for both cohort and case-control designs. A case-control study compares cases that have experienced the event and controls who have not, and then assesses whether each individual was exposed to a stimulus or not. Thus, a case-control study is retrospective.

Odds ratios are used when comparing events to nonevents with its calculation depending on the study design. For example, consider comparing a group of individuals who developed measles to those who did not and then determining whether they received all recommended vaccinations. In a cohort study, the odds ratio is calculated by dividing the odds of experiencing the event in the exposed group (i.e., A/B) by the odds the unexposed group who experienced the event (i.e., C/D). In a case-control study, the odds ratio is calculated by dividing the odds that cases were exposed to the risk (i.e., A/C) by the odds that the controls were exposed (i.e., B/D).

Relative risk and odds ratios are comparable in magnitude only when the outcome under study is rare (e.g., some cancers). It is important to consider that odds ratios consistently overestimate risk when the outcome is more common (e.g., hyperlipidemia). As a result, relative risk should be used if possible and caution should be exhibited when interpreting odds ratios.

SENSITIVITY, SPECIFICITY, AND PREDICTIVE VALUES

Sensitivity, specificity, and positive and negative predictive values indicate the ability of a test to identify correctly those experiencing the event and those who did not. For example, consider the rapid flu test. Four outcomes result from this test that are required for the calculation of sensitivity, specificity, and the predictive values:

1. True positives (TP) have the flu and have a positive rapid flu test result.
2. False positives (FP) do not have the flu, but have a positive rapid flu test result.
3. True negatives (TN) do not have the flu and have a negative rapid flu test result.
4. False negatives (FN) have the flu, but have a negative rapid flu test result.

Sensitivity is the probability a diseased individual will have a positive test result and is the true-positive rate of the test. It is calculated by dividing true positives by all individuals who actually have the disease (i.e., TP/TP+FN). **Specificity** is the probability that a disease-free individual will have a negative test result and is the true-negative rate of the screening test. It is calculated by dividing true negatives by all disease-free individuals (i.e., TN/TN+FP).

Positive and negative predictive values are calculated to measure the accuracy of the screening test. Both predictive values are directly related to disease prevalence; that is, the higher the prevalence, the higher the predictive value.[6] Positive predictive value provides the proportion of individuals who test positive for the disease and actually have the disease. It is calculated by dividing true positives by all individuals with a positive test result (i.e., TP/TP+FP). Negative predictive value provides the proportion of individuals who test negative and are actually disease-free. It is calculated by dividing true negatives by all individuals with a negative test result (i.e., TN/TN+FN).

It is important to identify the implications all four values have to new and existing research. When designing a study involving a screening test, researchers must indicate a standard cutoff score for their screening. That is, qualify who is to be considered diseased and who will be considered disease-free. This decision clearly reflects the repercussions of classifying individuals as false negatives or false positives. For example, consider a screening tool for early stage breast cancer, where there are considerable consequences for both false positives and false negatives. On the one hand, a patient with a false positive may be referred for unnecessary testing that is painful and expensive, not to mention emotionally taxing. On the other hand, a false negative has more serious implications, since the patient may not receive any treatment until the disease has progressed.

Types of Study Design

The distinction between experimental, quasi-experimental, and nonexperimental research is important, both from a study design perspective and when evaluating literature. Although experimental designs are considered the gold standard by many, do not discount research conducted using quasi-experimental and nonexperimental designs, as long as the limitations are considered. Each of these types of designs will be discussed below.

EXPERIMENTAL DESIGNS

In the biomedical sciences, experimental designs are typically referred to as a randomized controlled trial (RCT). A full treatment of experimental design is presented in Chapters 4 and 5, so the discussion provided here will only touch the tip of the iceberg on experimental designs. Interested readers are encouraged to consult the suggested readings provided at the end of this chapter for more information.

First, experimental designs always allow the researcher to manipulate levels of an IV. For example, consider a drug trial assessing the effectiveness of a new cancer medication. For this trial, four groups of participants are randomly assigned to a different dose of a medication. Thus, there are four levels of the IV. The researcher, within ethical and theoretical constraints, can manipulate the size of the dose, if the participants will be measured multiple times, and the length of the study period.

Second, in experimental design, participants are randomly assigned to levels of the IV. Thus, any participant has a chance of being placed in any single group, which theoretically provides initial equivalence of participants across study groups. There are many different methods and theories of randomization and the chance of being in one group versus another does not necessarily have to be equal. For example, consider a study that has two treatment groups and one placebo group where the researcher is interested in the difference between the treatment groups. Because the difference in the DV between the placebo and either treatment group will usually be larger than the difference in the DV between the treatment groups, the researcher may randomize more participants to the treatment groups to increase statistical power to detect the difference between treatments. Note that the concept of statistical power is discussed in the "Statistical Inference" section in this chapter as well as in Chapter 4. Often a 2:1 or 3:1 randomization schedule will be used with two or three times as many participants, respectively, being randomized to treatment as opposed to placebo.

Third, causality can be determined with proper experimental control of error. For example, the effectiveness of a cancer drug can be better explained by reducing sources of error due to the participant (e.g., age, health status), setting (e.g., prescriber's office), or diagnostic tests (e.g., measurement accuracy).

Finally, it should be noted RCTs have limitations. The primary limitation is cost, as RCTs are extremely costly requiring many considerations including space, personnel, and participants. RCTs also may have limited **external validity** and generalizability due to extreme control over experimental conditions that do not necessarily translate to real world situations. For example, RCTs generally use very strict inclusion and exclusion criteria to control all factors that could influence the effect of the drug under study; however, after approval, the patients who are prescribed the drug might not map closely onto those inclusion and exclusion criteria from the RCT (e.g., a patient with multiple comorbid conditions may have been excluded from the RCT, but is prescribed the drug after approval). Third, it is difficult, if not impossible, to study rare events with an RCT due to ethical concerns (e.g., a patient being denied treatment by being randomized to a control group) and the considerable sample size required.

QUASI-EXPERIMENTAL DESIGNS

Quasi-experimental designs are used more often in the social sciences but can be observed in the biomedical literature. On the surface, these types of designs appear to be experimental; however, they lack one key aspect, random assignment.

For example, consider examining the effectiveness of a new dialysis treatment. Most dialysis patients are already in the care of a nephrologist at a specific clinic. Because nephrologists typically see numerous patients, randomizing patients to specific levels of treatment (i.e., the IV) within a group that is under the care of the same nephrologist may be infeasible logistically or may lead to medication errors. Thus, the entire clinic must be randomized. That is, all patients within a specific clinic will receive one treatment.

Advantages of quasi-experimental designs include reduced cost and a quicker time-line compared to RCTs with the addition of possible increases in external validity due to conditions being more consistent with the real world. The disadvantages, however, are considerable. This is most notable with the lack of random assignment. Nonrandom assignment may create dissimilar groups based on any number of characteristics that are potentially related to the success of the treatment. For example, consistent differences in patient demographics (e.g., sickness) may result from a dialysis clinic in the suburbs being compared to a dialysis clinic in a more urban setting. Further, causation cannot be implied and statistical analysis can potentially be rendered uninformative.[9]

NONEXPERIMENTAL DESIGNS

Nonexperimental designs have several advantages over RCTs, primarily lower cost, a quicker timeline to publication, and a broader range of participants.[10] The advantages of nonexperimental studies over RCTs have prompted their widespread use in the biomedi-cal sciences. Overall, these studies tend to be nonrandomized, retrospective, and cor-relational in nature and are distinct because the researcher cannot manipulate the IV(s).

For example, consider a 5-year retrospective study assessing the effectiveness of statin therapy on preventing cardiac events. The researcher has knowledge of which patients ini-tiated statin therapy, but has no control over the drug, dose, adherence, etc. Although the researcher may assign patients to groups based on different doses, the researcher cannot randomly assign patients to a specific drug nor can they manipulate the dose. In addition, nonexperimental research often fails to indicate causality, which is due to lack of experi-mental control and randomization as well as inability to identify all confounding variables. Finally, it is important to note that while nonexperimental designs are ubiquitous in the biomedical sciences, treatment effects may be different when compared to RCTs.[11]

Case Study 6–1

Consider a single-institution study to evaluate a new patient-centered intervention that focused on reducing 30- and 90-day all-cause hospital readmissions in patients with a pri-mary discharge diagnosis of ST-segment elevation acute myocardial infarction (STEMI). The total length of enrollment was 12 months and individual patients were followed for 90 days. The patient-centered intervention included disease education from the discharg-ing physician and medication education from a hospital pharmacist that focused on adherence, interactions, and side effects. Further, postdischarge case management was conducted by a nurse practitioner who focused on the patient's needs while at home and coordinated subsequent care. At the end of the study, patients receiving the intervention are compared to a group of patients who had routine discharges.

Please answer the following questions:

1. Describe the population of interest.
2. What type of sampling strategy is most appropriate? Why?
3. What is the DV for this study? How many levels does the DV have? What is the scale of measurement?
4. What is the appropriate measure of central tendency for this DV? Why? How should this data be presented in an article?
5. What is the IV for this study? How many levels does the IV have? What is the scale of measurement?
6. What are some confounding variables?
7. Was the control group adequate for comparison? Why or why not? How could you improve the quality of the control group?
8. What distribution will be used in data analysis? Why?
9. What epidemiological statistic(s) is most appropriate? Why?

The Design and Analysis of Clinical Trials

The U.S. National Institutes of Health (NIH) defines clinical trials into two types: interventional and observational studies.[12] In this chapter, two specific types of interventional clinical trials are discussed—the randomized controlled trial (RCT) and adaptive clinical trial (ACT). The experimental design of RCTs and ACTs are discussed at length in Chapters 4 and 5, so the descriptions provided in this chapter are minimal. Briefly, RCTs and ACTs are both protocol-based, meaning that every step of the study from design to analysis is identified **a priori**. They are prospective studies where participants are followed over time using strict experimental control to indicate reliably the causality between the DV and manipulated IV.

THE DESIGN OF CLINICAL TRIALS

Parallel-Groups Design

The most common RCT is a parallel-groups design where the IV typically involves participants randomized into fixed levels of treatment, also known as treatment arms, with each arm indicating a different treatment or comparison.[13-16] That is, participants are randomly assigned to one, and only one, treatment arm. As stated in the previous section, the sample size within each group does not have to be equal and can vary depending on estimated statistical power to detect treatment effects.

There are two parallel-groups designs frequently used in the biomedical sciences—group comparison and matched pairs.[15] Briefly, a group comparison design simultaneously compares at least two groups of participants after each group is randomized to a different level of the IV. In a matched pairs design, participants are matched based on one or more characteristics (e.g., age, race) and then randomized to levels of the IV.

Crossover Design

The second most common RCT is a crossover design. A crossover design has the primary advantage of each participant serving as his or her own control.[13,15] The primary advantage of a crossover design is that it requires fewer participants in comparison to a parallel-groups design due to the fact that at the end of the study all participants will have been in all treatment arms. A disadvantage is that a crossover design cannot be used in a study where the first drug may cure the participant (e.g., an antibiotic given for an infection), since there would be no reason for the participant to crossover to the other agent.

For example, consider a 1-month study that includes two treatment arms. For a parallel-groups design, say 20 participants are required; that is, 10 participants are randomized to each treatment arm. By contrast, in a crossover design, only 10 subjects are required because each participant receives both treatments—10 participants receive the first treatment and the same 10 participants receive the second treatment. While both designs have two total measurements, in the parallel-groups design, two individual groups of participants provide one measurement each, whereas in the crossover design the same group of participants provides both measurements.

At this point, a common question is whether the effect of the first treatment carries over to influence the effect of the second treatment. This is a considerable concern in crossover designs and is dealt with by including a washout period between treatments. While the maximum duration of the washout period is arbitrary, it must be long enough that the effect of the first treatment is absent prior to beginning the second treatment, but not be so long that participant attrition becomes a concern.

Adaptive Design

A more recent advancement to the RCT is the adaptive design or ACT. Although an ACT is possibly cheaper and more ethical than an RCT, this design is much more complex to both implement and analyze. Briefly, ACTs implement changes or adaptations in the design of the study based on the results of a predetermined set of interim statistical analyses.

Interim analyses can be based on blinded or unblinded data, with the resulting adaptations aimed at establishing a more efficient, safer, and informative trial that is more likely to demonstrate treatment effects.[17]

For example, consider a 3-year study examining the effect of three different large doses of vitamin D on parathyroid hormone. Because implementing large doses of vitamin D is controversial, ethical considerations require this study to be adaptive. Here, the interim analyses would provide important information regarding the effectiveness and safety of the doses. Say, for example, that the ACT has interim analyses scheduled quarterly. Further, say that at the end of the second quarter of the first year the interim analyses indicated that the group receiving the highest dose of vitamin D had twice the risk of developing kidney stones compared to the other two groups. Thus, the group receiving the highest dose of vitamin D could have their dose reduced or the group could be dropped from the study completely. After these adaptations are implemented, the study continues as designed.

THE ANALYSIS OF CLINICAL TRIALS

The analysis of clinical trials typically involves evaluating repeated-measures data where participants are followed prospectively over time or conducting an endpoint analysis using only the last observation or measurement. Regardless of the study design, the choice of the appropriate statistical test to analyze these data is based primarily on the scale of measurement of the DV, but other factors should also be considered (see the "Selecting the Appropriate Statistical Test" section later in the chapter).

Because an endpoint analysis is straightforward conceptually, a brief discussion of repeated-measures design and analysis considerations is presented. Using a repeated-measures design allows researchers to study the treatment effects over time in a smaller sample of participants due to the increased statistical power. Briefly, a repeated-measures design increases statistical power by removing the error variance due to the participant. That is, each participant serves as their own control. Removing error variance is important because it results in larger test statistics and an increased probability of achieving statistical significance. However, a repeated-measures design has limitations relevant to clinical trials, primarily participant attrition and nonadherence.

Attrition and nonadherence can assume many forms in a clinical trial. For example, participants may drop out of the study, fail to complete all required measurements, receive incorrect treatment or doses, or a myriad of other possible protocol violations. Thus, the first part of this section will discuss how the analysis of clinical trials typically handles missing data due to attrition and nonadherence. The final sections discuss the analysis of parallel-group, crossover, and adaptive designs.

Intent-to-Treat and Per-Protocol Approaches

Two analytical approaches exist for clinical trials—intent-to-treat (ITT) and per-protocol (PP). The ITT approach is often employed in the presence of violations to protocol or patients being lost to follow-up. ITT is the approach most often used in the biomedical literature. ITT requires the analysis to include all participants in the arm to which they were randomized originally. That is, treatment effects are best evaluated by the planned treatment protocol rather than the actual treatment given.[18]

For example, consider a participant randomized to receive treatment A but who instead receives treatment B. For analysis, this participant would be considered as receiving treatment A. It should be noted that if a large number of protocol violations of this nature occur, the study would be discontinued; thus, these occurrences are relatively rare. It is important to note that the ITT approach has considerable weaknesses. Most notably, for ITT to be unbiased, attrition and nonadherence are considered to occur completely at random.[14] However, this is an untestable hypothesis. Further, the ITT approach can dilute treatment effects simply by including nonadherent participants by employing the last observation carried forward (LOCF) technique discussed later in this section.

By comparison, the PP approach evaluates only compliant participants with complete data. Although this analysis is straightforward analytically and allows researchers to evaluate a more accurate treatment effect, it has substantial limitations, primarily, reduced statistical power compared to an ITT approach, because participants with incomplete data are not considered in analysis.[18]

Because the ITT approach considers all participants with at least one measurement, an imputation or replacement method is often employed for missing measurements. The LOCF technique is one of the most commonly used imputation methods. This method uses the last recorded measurement for a participant for every missing measurement. For example, consider a study measuring HbA1c measured on four occasions over a 1-year study period. If a participant had only the first two measurements, the second (i.e., last) measurement would be imputed for measurements three and four. ❹ *From this example, it is clear the LOCF technique not only dilutes treatment effects by assuming that the measurement is constant, but also introduces significant bias into the results of statistical tests.* Therefore, be cautious when evaluating a study that has employed the LOCF technique. As a result of these limitations, better imputation approaches have been suggested including multiple imputation and the use of maximum likelihood estimation. These techniques are beyond the scope of this chapter, but are valid and produce unbiased estimates if data are considered missing at random.[19,20]

Analyzing Parallel-Groups Designs

When analyzing a parallel-groups design, the traditional approach is to conduct an endpoint analysis using only the final measurement. If the DV is continuous, analysis will typically require an independent-samples t test for two groups, one-way analysis of variance (ANOVA) for more than two groups, or analysis of covariance (ANCOVA) for two or more groups, statistically controlling for a baseline DV measurement. If the DV is categorical, an endpoint analysis will typically require a chi-square test or logistic regression analysis. Note that these analyses are discussed in detail in the in the sections addressing statistical tests later in the chapter.

For example, consider a study designed to assess the effect of lubiprostone compared to placebo in treating chronic constipation associated with Parkinson disease. Following randomization, this 1-month study will assess constipation symptoms twice—at the end of the second and fourth weeks. An endpoint analysis would only consider the treatment effect at the end of week 4, ignoring the measurement at the end of week 2. Thus, it is clear that this type of analysis does not consider the repeated measures, and, as a result, does not consider the changes occurring over time. Further, an endpoint analysis does not take full advantage of statistical power increases from a longitudinal design as discussed in the "Analysis of Clinical Trials" section.

By contrast, to assess for change over time using repeated measures for a continuous DV, researchers often employ a mixed between-within ANOVA or mixed-effects linear regression. Briefly, these analyses assess differences between treatment groups as well as changes over time within treatment groups. The major benefit of these analyses is provided by the interaction effect, which evaluates whether the change over time was different between the two treatment arms (see Figure 6-8). To evaluate group differences in change over time for a categorical DV, researchers are required to employ a mixed-effects logistic regression. This analysis allows the researcher to evaluate group differences and interaction effects. In general, mixed-effects analyses are extremely complex and even a brief overview of this analysis is well beyond the scope of this chapter. With that said, when these analyses are most appropriate is provided in the "Selecting the Appropriate Statistical Tests" section later in the chapter. Interested readers are encouraged to consult the suggested readings at the end of the chapter for a treatment of this analysis.

As an example of analyzing a parallel-groups design, reconsider the lubiprostone example that evaluated chronic constipation associated with Parkinson disease using a 1-month study during which constipation symptoms were assessed at the end of the second and fourth weeks. The results are presented graphically in Figure 6-8. Notice that two groups experience drastically different change in constipation symptoms between the end of week 2 and the end of week 4. The between-group difference in constipation symptoms over time is the interaction effect. Because a lower number of symptoms are indicative of treatment success, Figure 6-8 shows that the effect of lubiprostone is more effective compared to placebo over the study period.

Following a statistically significant interaction effect, researchers can conduct follow-up or post hoc tests to determine where the significant difference occurred. In Figure 6-8,

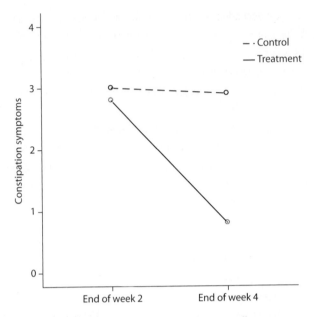

Figure 6–8. Statistically significant interaction effect.

there is likely no statistically significant difference in constipation symptoms between groups at the end of week 2, but there is a likely statistically significant difference at the end of week 4. Therefore, post hoc tests can assist researchers in identifying the shortest treatment time or minimum effective dose by indicating where treatment effects diminish (e.g., the slope plateaus) or indicating when differences between doses converge and are no longer statistically significant.

Analyzing Crossover Designs

The purpose of the crossover design is to study treatment effects using the participant as his or her own control. Remember, in a crossover design each participant receives all treatment arms, with an adequate washout period occurring between arms to prevent the carryover of treatment effects. For example, consider the lubiprostone example described in the "Analyzing Parallel-Groups Designs" section. Instead of having two treatment arms as in a parallel-groups design, the crossover design would randomize participants into a different treatment order. That is, Group A would receive lubiprostone and Group B would receive placebo for the first 2 weeks. At the end of the 2-week study period, constipation symptoms are assessed. Next, all participants are required to have a 3-week washout period purported to effectively eliminate any carryover effects of the lubiprostone. Note that during the washout period the placebo is not given either. After the washout period, Group A would receive placebo and Group B would receive lubiprostone for 2 weeks. At the end of this second 2-week study period, constipation symptoms are assessed again.

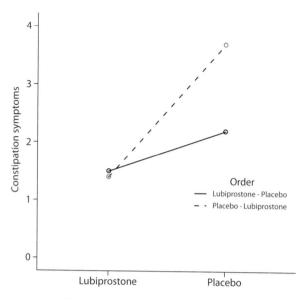

Figure 6–9. Statistically significant order effect.

Statistically, a crossover design requires an initial test for order effects. If the DV is continuous, order effects are assessed by evaluating the interaction effect between order of treatment and the IV using a mixed between-within ANOVA or a mixed-effects linear regression. These analyses are described in detail in the "Selecting the Appropriate Statistical Test" section later in the chapter, but for now consider both analyses useful when evaluating interaction effects. When testing for order effects, a statistically significant interaction indicates that the order in which the treatments were received influenced the treatment effect. For example, say that receiving lubiprostone prior to placebo had a different treatment effect than receiving placebo prior to lubiprostone. A clear order effect is presented in Figure 6-9. Notice the effect of placebo differs depending on the order in which it was received. The presence of a statistically significant order effect can have multiple explanations. Considering the example and Figure 6-9, it is clear the washout period may not have been long enough, as the effectiveness of lubiprostone carried over to measurement of the placebo. In addition, the groups may have been initially different following randomization. Whenever a statistically significant order effect is identified, no further analysis is conducted as any subsequent analyses are biased by this order effect. However, if the interaction is nonsignificant and the DV is continuous, an endpoint analysis is typically evaluated via paired-samples *t* test (also explained in detail in the "Selecting the Appropriate Statistical Test" section later in the chapter). That is, treatment differences between lubiprostone and placebo are assessed without respect to the order in which the treatments were received.

Analyzing Adaptive Designs

The statistical analyses and considerations used when analyzing adaptive designs are similar to parallel-groups and crossover designs. If the DV is continuous, statistical tests used during the interim analyses or on the study endpoint typically include an independent-samples t test for comparing two groups, one-way ANOVA for comparing more than two groups, or ANCOVA for statistically controlling baseline DV measurement. Note that the DV for the interim analyses is the most recent measurement. If the DV is categorical, an interim analysis will typically require a chi-square test or logistic regression analysis. All of the analyses mentioned are discussed in detail in the "Statistical Tests" section later in the chapter.

Several important considerations are required when analyzing and interpreting the results from adaptive designs.[17] First, all interim and endpoint analyses suffer the potential risk of inflated Type I errors. Briefly, a Type I error can be thought of as a false positive. That is, the statistical test could indicate a statistically significant result when the result is actually not significant. Type I error has been discussed in Chapter 4 and is discussed in the "Statistical Inference" section later in the chapter. With this definition in mind, as the number of interim analyses increases, the probability of finding a false positive might increase as well. To adjust for this possibility, researchers will often make the criteria for achieving statistical significance more conservative by adjusting alpha (see the "Statistical Inference" section later in the chapter for a full description of alpha). Note that adjusting alpha is not a ubiquitous practice and there is no universal recommendation for doing so. Just be aware that inflated Type I errors may be an issue in an ACT.

Second, estimates of population parameters may be biased. That is, any adaptation can reduce the generalizability to the original population sampled, produce underestimated or overestimated parameter estimates, and produce misleading confidence intervals. Researchers must carefully document and provide rationale for adaptations resulting from interim analysis. Failure to do so will indicate that results should be viewed with extreme caution.

Finally, when all adaptations are considered, the overall results of the endpoint analyses may actually be invalid, providing inaccurate support for treatment effects. Consumers of research are urged strongly to consider these factors when interpreting and evaluating research using adaptive designs.

Statistical Inference

Inferential statistics provide the probability that a difference or association is actually observed in the population based on the analysis of sample data. Inferential statistics allow researchers to make rational decisions in the presence of random processes and variation. This section presents several requirements that need to be considered prior to conducting and evaluating the result of a statistical test. First, the sampling distribution and application of the **Central Limit Theorem** are discussed, followed by hypothesis testing, as well as Type I and Type II errors and statistical power. Then, the difference between statistical and clinical significance is presented. Finally, the appropriate uses of parametric and nonparametric statistical tests are provided as well as a brief description of degrees of freedom.

SAMPLING DISTRIBUTIONS AND THE CENTRAL LIMIT THEOREM

Statistical inference uses sampled data to make conclusions about a specific population. Because quality samples are chosen randomly, the means produced from these samples are also random.[21] Given this information, it is important to remember that the mean may not be exactly representative of the population and will vary from sample to sample. However, the law of large numbers states that as the size of the sample increases, the sample mean will move closer to the population mean. Further, as the number of samples increases, the mean of the sample means will begin to approximate the population mean.

❺ *The central limit theorem states when equally sized samples are drawn from a non-normal distribution, the plotted mean values from each sample will approximate a normal distribution as long as the non-normality was not due to outliers.*

A distribution of the sampled means calculated from repeated samples is termed the "distribution of sampling means." For example, consider a study to analyze the mean value of blood urea nitrogen (BUN) in the general, healthy population, where the researcher selects 100 random samples of ten healthy participants. Each sample of ten will provide a mean BUN value. Although mean BUN will vary from sample to sample, when the 100 sample means are plotted in a histogram, this distribution of sampling means will begin to approximate the actual population distribution.

The Central Limit Theorem states that sufficiently large samples should approximate a normal distribution of sampling means as long as the data do not contain outliers. A sufficiently large sample is generally considered to consist of 30 or more participants or a situation where the degrees of freedom for the statistical test are greater than 20.[22] Note that degrees of freedom are discussed later in this section. In addition, researchers must be careful not to confuse the issue of having a large enough sample to achieve statistical significance and a large enough sample to be representative of the population.

As with any normal distribution, the standard deviation of the distribution of sampling means can be calculated. This is termed the "standard error of the mean (SEM)." The SEM is equal to the standard deviation divided by the square root of the sample size and reflects variability within the sample means. That is, how precisely the sample mean was estimated. Further, standard error is used in the majority of statistical tests. It is important when evaluating the literature to understand the relationship between the standard deviation and the SEM. Researchers often present the SEM to show variability or noise in their data but the SEM (variability of the mean estimate) will always be smaller than the standard deviation (variability in the observed data); thus, the use of SEM will suggest the data is less variable and often more appealing.

HYPOTHESIS TESTING

A hypothesis indicates a theory about the population regarding an outcome the researcher is interested in studying. The statistical analyses discussed in this chapter evaluate two types of hypotheses: the null hypothesis and the alternative or research hypothesis. That is, the analyses discussed employ procedures generally known as null hypothesis significance testing (NHST). The **null hypothesis** (H_0) assumes no difference or association between the different study groups or variables, whereas the **alternative hypothesis** (H_A or H_1) states that there is a difference or association between the different study groups or variables. A representative, ideally random, sample is then drawn from the population of interest to estimate the difference or relationship and test whether this difference or relationship rejects or fails to reject the null hypothesis. It is important to note that failing to reject the null hypothesis does not indicate the null hypothesis is true. This is a common misconception observed frequently in the literature. There are often many other reasons for failing to reject the null hypothesis including inadequate experimental design, inadequate control over extraneous variables, and inadequate sample size to detect the effect of interest, among others.

When testing a specific hypothesis, a researcher is required to determine whether their hypothesis is directional or not. A directional hypothesis requires a **one-tailed** hypothesis test, whereas a nondirectional hypothesis requires a **two-tailed** hypothesis test. For example, consider a hypothesis which states that initiating statin therapy will lower low-density lipoproteins (LDL). Note that use of the term "lower" implies directionality and requires a one-tailed test. If, however, the researchers were looking for any effect of statin therapy, whether lowering or raising LDL, the hypothesis is nondirectional and would require a two-tailed test. In the literature, it is generally more acceptable to use a two-tailed test, even if the hypothesis is directional because a two-tailed test is more conservative statistically, thereby reducing the probability of a spurious statistical significance.

ERROR AND STATISTICAL POWER

It is essential that researchers establish how much error they are willing to accept before initiating a study. NHST can only result in four possible outcomes, which can be observed

TABLE 6-2. FOUR POSSIBLE OUTCOMES OF NULL HYPOTHESIS SIGNIFICANCE TESTING (NHST)

Decision	Truth	
	False H_0	True H_0
Reject H_0	Correctly Reject H_0	Type I Error
Fail to Reject H_0	Type II Error	Correctly Fail to Reject H_0

in Table 6-2. Type I and Type II have been discussed at length in Chapter 4, but briefly, a **Type I error** occurs when a statistical test rejects the null hypothesis by indicating a statistically significant difference when, in fact, the null hypothesis is true (i.e., false positive). A **Type II error** occurs when the researcher fails to reject the null hypothesis by not indicating a statistically significant difference when, in fact, the null hypothesis is false (i.e., false negative). Type I and Type II errors are interconnected; that is, as the probability of one error increases the other decreases. Researchers must consider these two errors carefully when designing studies, weighing whether a false positive is more or less concerning than a false negative.

Statistical power was developed as a method allowing researchers to calculate the probability of finding a statistically significant result, when, in fact, one actually exists. This topic has been discussed in Chapter 4. Essentially, increasing statistical power reduces the probability of committing a Type II error; however, it can also increase the probability of committing a Type I error as described in the previous paragraph. Statistical power is influenced by four factors: alpha defined as the probability value at which the null hypothesis is rejected, effect size defined as the size of the treatment effect (discussed later), error variance defined as the precision of the measurement instrument, and the sample size. Statistical power can be increased by increasing alpha, effect size, or sample size as well as by decreasing error variance. Note that statistical power of 0.8 has been defined as adequate.[23] However, some researchers use 0.9 or higher in the biomedical sciences, indicating that a false negative is more detrimental than a false positive, such as when evaluating the effectiveness of a novel breast cancer treatment.

STATISTICAL VERSUS CLINICAL SIGNIFICANCE

Alpha and *p* Values

The next step in the research process is to employ a statistical test to assess whether a difference or relationship is due to random variation. The researcher is interested in determining whether the observed difference or relationship rejects or fails to reject the null hypothesis. **Alpha** (α) is the conventionally designated decision criterion for rejecting the null hypothesis and ranges from 0 to 1. Alpha is defined as the theoretical probability of rejecting the null hypothesis conditional on the null hypothesis being true. Alpha does not represent the exact Type I error rate; instead, alpha is the upper bound of the Type I error rate. Although most studies set alpha at 0.05, this value is arbitrary. A more conservative (i.e., $\alpha = 0.01$) or liberal ($\alpha = 0.10$) alpha may be used in an attempt to show greater support for rejecting or retaining the null hypothesis, respectively. As an example, conservative alpha levels are often used to protect against Type I errors, whereas liberal alpha values are often used in drug equivalency trials where researchers are using data to show nonsignificant differences between the drugs.

Conceptually related to alpha is the probability value (i.e., *p* **value**). Statistical tests produce p values that range from 0 to 1. The formal definition of a p value is the probability of obtaining a test statistic as large as or larger than the one obtained, conditional on the null hypothesis being true. Graphically, a p value is directly indicative of the area under the probability distribution used by the statistical test. Note that the area under any proper probability distribution is 1. A quick glance at the appendices of any introductory statistics textbook will provide area under the curve values for various distributions. In more general terms, $p = 0.05$ indicates 5% of the distribution's area is to the left or right of the associated test statistic depending on whether it is positive or negative. For example, consider a one-tailed statistical test with a positive test statistic and reconsider Figure 6-5. A z score of 1.645 leaves approximately 5% of the distribution to the right of this value. This example highlights how a p value less than 0.05 indicates that less than 5% of the values (or area) lies beyond a specific test statistic value. As an alternative example, consider a two-tailed (i.e., nondirectional) statistical test. A z score of 1.96 leaves approximately 2.5% of the distribution to the right of this value, whereas a z score of -1.96 leaves approximately 2.5% of the distribution to the left of this value. Thus, a two-tailed test also leaves 5% of the area under the distribution when the two parts are aggregated. Regardless of whether a one- or two-tailed test was used, in general, if a p value is less than the specified alpha, the researcher rejects the null hypothesis and the difference or relationship is considered statistically significant. Alternatively, if the p value is equal to or greater than alpha, the researcher has failed to reject the null hypothesis and the difference or relationship is not considered statistically significant.

❻ *There are numerous misconceptions about p values and it is important to know how to interpret them correctly.* Be aware that there is continuing difficulty when interpreting p values, even among statisticians.[24] Therefore, it is important to be cognizant of several misconceptions about p values that are stated commonly in the literature. First, a p value is not the exact probability of committing a Type I error. Second, the p value is not the probability that the null hypothesis is true, nor is $1 - p$ the probability that the alternative hypothesis is true. Third, a small p value is not evidence that the results will replicate nor can p values be compared directly across studies. Fourth, a p value indicates nothing about the magnitude of a difference or relationship. For example, a small p value (e.g., $p = 0.00001$) does not indicate a larger treatment effect than a larger p value (e.g., $p = .049$). Finally, for better or worse, alpha in NHST is treated like a cliff. For example, if alpha is set at 0.05 and a p value of 0.051 is obtained, a researcher will often state that a p value of 0.051 was trending toward significance or that the p value indicated marginal or moderate significance. These statements are often wholly incorrect! Thinking back to the discussion of one-tailed versus two-tailed significance tests provided in the "Hypothesis Testing" section, trending can only occur if the hypothesis is directional using a one-tailed test and the result obtained was in the hypothesized direction. Results can never be trending toward significance if the hypothesis was nondirectional using a two-tailed test because the alternative claim that the result was trending away from significance cannot be challenged.

Confidence Intervals

Statistical significance can also be established by calculating a confidence interval around the estimated population parameters (e.g., sample means, slopes) or test statistics (e.g., t). A confidence interval provides a range of scores likely to contain the unknown population parameter, and generally, a confidence interval is reported using a 95% confidence level. The calculation of confidence intervals includes both sample size and variability where smaller confidence intervals indicate less variability in the data. A 95% confidence interval is calculated by multiplying 1.96 by the SEM and adding or subtracting this value from the estimated parameter to find the upper and lower confidence limits, respectively. A 95% confidence interval indicates that if repeated random sampling occurs within the population of interest under consistent conditions (e.g., sample size), the true population parameter would be included in the interval 95% of the time (i.e., the interval is random and the population parameter is fixed).

Confidence intervals can be used to indicate statistical significance without the use of statistical tests. This process varies according to whether the researcher is examining population parameters or test statistics. For example, consider Figures 6-10, 6-11, and 6-12. In each figure, HbA1c values are being compared for a treatment and placebo group. Further, mean HbA1c for each group is presented as the circle, while the 95% confidence intervals are the whiskers extending above and below the means. The overlap of the confidence intervals between groups is directly related to p values; that is, less overlap is indicative of larger differences resulting in smaller p values. In Figure 6-10, notice that the confidence intervals do not overlap; thus, this difference can be assumed statistically significant at least at $p < 0.05$. Statistical significance can also be indicated when the confidence intervals overlap as long as the overlap is less than approximately 50% of a whisker, as in Figure 6-11.[25] That is, if the lower whisker of the confidence interval for one group (Placebo in Figure 6-11) shares less than 50% overlap with the upper whisker of the other group's confidence interval (Treatment in Figure 6-11). Finally, as shown in Figure 6-12,

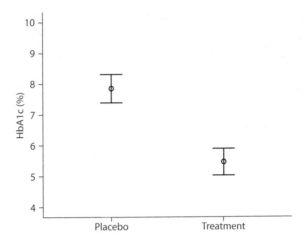

Figure 6–10. Statistically significant result indicated by nonoverlapping 95% confidence intervals.

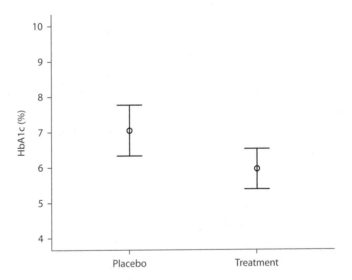

Figure 6–11. Statistically significant result indicated by overlapping 95% confidence intervals.

substantial overlap in confidence intervals indicates a nonstatistically significant difference (i.e., $p > 0.05$).

Determining statistical significance using confidence intervals around test statistics (e.g., t) uses procedures that vary based on the statistical test employed. For most parametric tests of group differences and correlation, a 95% confidence interval around the test statistic containing 0 is not considered statistically significant at an alpha of 0.05. That is, statistical significance for these types of analyses are essentially testing that the

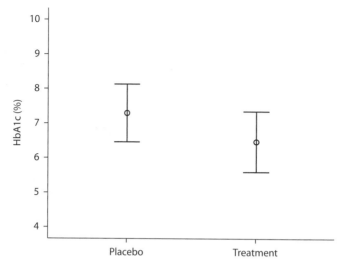

Figure 6–12. Overlapping 95% confidence interval indicating a nonsignificant result.

difference or relationship is different from 0 (i.e., $H_0 = 0$). Thus, a 95% confidence interval containing 0 essentially indicates that it is plausible the true population difference or relationship could be 0.[26] For example, consider the commonly used independent-samples t test to evaluate for a difference between two group means (this statistical test is discussed later in the chapter). Say that the test statistic produced was 2, but the confidence interval ranged from −0.5 to 4.5. Based on this sample, the difference would not be considered statistically significant because it is plausible that in 95% of samples of the same size, the true population parameter could in fact be 0.

Alternatively, the 95% confidence interval for test statistics based on ratios (e.g., odds ratios) that contain 1 are not considered statistically significant at an alpha of 0.05. Remember from the "Epidemiological Statistics" section that an odds ratio or relative risk of 1 indicates no difference. Thus, a 95% confidence interval for a relative risk or an odds ratio that contains 1 indicates that it is plausible the true population parameter could in fact be an odds ratio or relative risk of 1. For example, say the result of a logistic regression analysis produced an odds ratio of 2.5 (this statistical test is discussed later in the chapter). This value is greater than 1 indicating an increase in odds of experiencing the event. However, say the 95% confidence interval ranged from 0.50 to 15.0. Because the confidence interval contains 1, the odds ratio of 2.5 is not statistically significant using an alpha of 0.05.

Clinical Significance and Effect Size

❼ *Clinical significance is far more important than statistical significance. Clinical significance can be quantified by using various measures of effect size.* When evaluating the significance of the finding, statistical significance (e.g., $p < 0.05$) does not indicate clinical significance. Statistical significance can be manipulated in several ways, most easily by increasing sample size drastically. A sample size increase may artificially reduce error variance, which in turn reduces the standard error on which the test statistic is based. Reducing the standard error increases the value of the test statistic necessarily resulting in a smaller p value.

As an example, using a sample of 10,000 patients, researchers may find a CCB reduced blood glucose significantly in Type I DM patients. However, on examining the estimated parameters, the statistically significant difference in blood glucose was only 2 mg/dL, a decrease considered clinically insignificant.

This example highlights the importance of identifying and interpreting the clinical significance or effect size of all studies. While a complete discussion of effect size is beyond the scope of this chapter, larger effect size values are always preferred. Briefly, two different types of effect sizes exist. First, standardized difference effect sizes indicate a standardized difference between groups in standard deviation units. Examples commonly seen in the literature include Cohen's **d**, Glass' Δ, and Hedges' **g**. As indicated by their name, standardized difference effect sizes are used when evaluating mean differences between groups. Further, because the effect sizes are standardized, it may be easier to think of them as z scores described previously. Second, effect size may also be reported as the proportion of variance explained. That is, how much of the reason a participant had a specific value of the DV is due to the IV. Examples commonly observed in the literature include R^2, ω^2, and η^2.

Given this information, it is important to remember that the definition of clinical significance varies by substantive area; thus, the definition of clinical significance to a bench researcher may be qualitatively different from an evidence-based practitioner. Finally, not all studies will provide an effect-size estimate, especially in the biomedical sciences. Thus, research must be viewed with warranted skepticism until it can be determined whether the statistically significant difference or relationship is clinically meaningful.

PARAMETRIC VERSUS NONPARAMETRIC STATISTICAL TESTS

The primary difference between parametric and nonparametric statistical tests is that parametric tests make assumptions regarding the descriptive characteristics of the normal distribution (i.e., mean, variance, skewness, and kurtosis). Nonparametric tests make a few or no distributional assumptions. In general, **parametric tests** are used only for interval and ratio scales, whereas **nonparametric tests** can be employed for any scale of measurement. Regardless, if the DV is measured on a continuous scale, the decision of which statistical test to employ typically begins with parametric tests. Because they assume a normal distribution, all parametric tests have several conservative and easily violated assumptions. These assumptions are testable, but vary depending on the statistical test employed. Therefore, in the sections that follow, all assumptions are described for each statistical test. It is important to know that employing a parametric test in the presence of a nondefined distribution will lead to inaccurate, biased, and unreliable parameter estimates. Therefore, when reading a journal article, if the authors neglect to provide information regarding assumption testing, caution should be exercised as it is unknown how much bias exists in their results.

Some assumption violations challenge the robustness of parametric tests greater than others. **Robustness** is defined as the ability of the statistical test to produce correct inferences in the presence of assumption violations. In most situations, any assumption violation requires the researcher to employ a nonparametric test, and most parametric tests have a widely used nonparametric alternative. Most, but not all, nonparametric statistical tests are distribution free, meaning they do not make inferences based on a defined probability distribution. Further, additional strengths of nonparametric tests include the ability to assess small sample sizes and the ability to assess data from several different populations.[27] However, it must be noted if the assumptions of a parametric test are tenable, parametric tests have greater statistical power to detect real effects compared to their nonparametric alternative(s).[28]

DEGREES OF FREEDOM

Degrees of freedom (df) are a vital component of all statistical tests, as most probability distributions, and statistical significance are based on them. Degrees of freedom are provided for all statistical tests and are a useful indicator of adequate sample size in the presence of assumption violations. For example, recall that the Central Limit Theorem states the distribution of sampling means is approximately normal with degrees of freedom greater than 20. Thus, the Central Limit Theorem operates independently of the distribution of the actual raw data. Therefore, if a researcher indicates that degrees of freedom for the statistical test is greater than 20, the results can typically be viewed as robust.

The definition of degrees of freedom is obscure and beyond the scope of this chapter; however, a brief description is provided. Degrees of freedom are conceptually defined as the number data points that are free to vary. Not all data is free to vary because values may have to be fixed by a specific sample parameter, such as the group mean. For example, consider a group of three participants who have a mean age of 50 years. Because the mean is 50, two of the participants can be of almost any age greater than 0. The third participant, however, must be the age that creates the mean of 50. Thus, if participant A is 40 and participant B is 45, participant C must be 65. That is, $[40+45+65]/3 = 50$. If instead, participant A is 75 and participant B is 40, then participant C must be 35. Therefore, because the age of two of the three participants could be just about any age greater than 0, there are two degrees of freedom (i.e., 2 df).

Calculating degrees of freedom becomes increasingly complex in accordance with the complexity of the statistical test. That is, degrees of freedom for bivariate tests, such as those evaluating the difference between two group means, are easier to calculate and conceptualize than multivariate tests with multiple DVs. For the analyses described later in the chapter, calculation of degrees of freedom is not explained explicitly, but it is important to note the distribution, probability, and statistical significance of all statistical tests are based on degrees of freedom. Further, degrees of freedom will usually be subscripted next to the test statistic for all parametric tests as well as for some nonparametric tests, such as the chi-square test. Subscripted degrees of freedom should be provided in the brief results section for all statistical tests described.

Selecting the Appropriate Statistical Test

While the information presented in this chapter has outlined the underlying processes of most statistical tests used in the biomedical sciences, the remainder of the chapter uses all previous information as a base to begin integrating more directly useful information. This section presents decision trees that allow for determination of whether the appropriate statistical test was used in a journal article.

❽ *The selection of the appropriate statistical test is based on several factors including the specific research question, the measurement scale of the DV, distributional assumptions, the number of DV measurements, as well as the number and measurement scale of IVs and covariates, among others.* Tables 6-3 and 6-4 provide decision trees to identify the most appropriate statistical test based on the unique set of factors for statistical tests of group differences and statistical tests of association, respectively.

FACTOR 1: THE RESEARCH QUESTION

The first factor that needs to be addressed when selecting the most appropriate statistical test is whether the research question is phrased to evaluate differences or associations. In general, the last paragraph of the Introduction to any journal article should explicitly state the research questions, so give close attention to the phrasing of these questions. This may seem mundane, but it is important to note that all parametric tests of group differences are mathematically equivalent to parametric tests of association. Therefore, various parametric statistical tests can often be used interchangeably to answer the same research question. This can be seen in Tables 6-3 and 6-4 where one-way ANOVA can be used in the same situations as simple linear regression analysis. The overall statistical inference would be identical. This can be an overwhelmingly confusing concept for those

TABLE 6–3. CHOOSING THE MOST APPROPRIATE STATISTICAL TEST OF GROUP DIFFERENCES

	DV Scale	Distributional Assumptions Met	Repeated DV Measurements	Number of DV Measurements	Number of IVs	IV Levels	Covariates Allowed	Appropriate Statistical Test
Differences from Known Population	Continuous	Yes	No	1	0		No	One-sample z test
	Continuous	Yes	No	1	0		No	One-sample t test
	Dichotomous		No	1	0		No	Binomial test
	Continuous		No	1	0		No	Kolmogorov-Smirnov test
Between-Group Differences	Continuous	Yes	No	1	1	2	No	Independent-samples t test
	Ordinal or higher	No	No	1	1	2	No	Mann-Whitney test
	Ordinal or higher	No	No	1	1	2	No	Median test
	Continuous	Yes	No	1	1	≥2	No	One-way ANOVA
	Ordinal or higher	No	No	1	1	≥2	No	Kruskal-Wallis test
	Continuous	Yes	No	1	1	≥2	Yes	ANCOVA
	Continuous	Yes	No	1	≥2	≥2	No	Factorial ANOVA
Within-Group Differences	Continuous	Yes	Yes	2	0		No	Paired-samples t test
	Ordinal or higher	No	Yes	2	0		No	Signed-rank test
	Ordinal or higher	No	Yes	2	0		No	Sign test
	Continuous	Yes	Yes	≥2	0		No	One-way RM-ANOVA
	Ordinal or higher	No	Yes	≥2	0		No	Friedman test
	Continuous	Yes	Yes	≥2	1	≥2	No	Mixed BW-ANOVA
	Dichotomous		Yes	2	0		No	McNemar test
	Dichotomous		Yes	≥2	0		No	Cochran Q test

TABLE 6-4. CHOOSING THE MOST APPROPRIATE STATISTICAL TEST OF ASSOCIATION

	DV Scale	Distributional Assumptions Met	Number of IVs	IV cale	Covariates Allowed	Appropriate Statistical Test
One Sample Association	Categorical		1	Categorical	No	Chi-square test
	Categorical		1	Categorical	No	Fisher's exact test
	Categorical		1	Categorical	Yes	Mantel-Haenszel test
Correlation and Regression	Continuous	Yes	1	Continuous	No	Pearson's correlation
	Continuous	No	1	Continuous	No	Spearman's rank-order correlation
	Continuous	Yes	1	Any	No	Simple linear regression
	Continuous	Yes	≥ 2	Any	Yes	Multivariable linear regression
	Dichotomous		1	Any	No	Simple logistic regression
	Dichotomous		≥ 2	Any	Yes	Multivariable logistic regression
Within-Group Regression	Continuous	Yes	≥ 0	Any	Yes	Mixed-effects linear regression[a]
	Dichotomous		≥ 0	Any	Yes	Mixed-effects logistic regression[a]
Time-to-Event	Continuous	Yes	≥ 2		Yes	Cox proportional-hazards model
Reliability	Nominal		0		No	Kappa

[a]Mixed-effects linear and logistic regression models are complex analyses beyond the scope of this chapter. However, be aware that these analyses are available. Also, note that there is varying terminology used among researchers when describing these types of models; thus, in the literature mixed-effects models may be termed multilevel, hierarchical, nested, random effects, random coefficient, or random parameter models. The actual procedure for conducting the analyses remains identical regardless of the label attached to them.

with more novice statistical backgrounds. However, in general, when a research question is phrased to evaluate group differences (e.g., to determine whether two different dose regimens of dapagliflozin result in different mean A1c levels compared to placebo) follow the decision tree provided in Table 6-3, and when a research question is phrased to evaluate associations between variables (e.g., to determine whether a comorbidity such as diabetes is associated with receipt of an antihypertensive prescription), follow Table 6-4.

FACTOR 2: SCALE OF MEASUREMENT

• The second factor to consider is the measurement scale of the DV. This is a much more concrete concept, but requires a thorough understanding of the four scales of variable measurement. Remember, nominal and ordinal scales are roughly classified as discrete or categorical, whereas interval and ratio scales are classified as continuous. Although it is often inappropriate, continuous variables may be also categorized into discrete variables. For example, categorization often occurs in the biomedical sciences with variables such as blood pressure, where exact systolic or diastolic blood pressure values are combined and categorized into low, normal, or high blood pressure.

FACTOR 3: DISTRIBUTIONAL ASSUMPTIONS

• The distributional assumptions of a statistical test involve complex explanations beyond the scope of this chapter. However, there are a few concepts to remember regarding distributions, most of which have been described in the "Common Probability Distributions" section. First, distributional assumptions are required for all statistical tests using a continuous DV. Remember, the search for the most appropriate statistical test usually begins with parametric options, and all parametric statistical tests require a normal distribution (or application of the Central Limit Theorem). Second, the distribution of the actual DV data is never considered when assessing distributional assumptions. Distributional assumptions are based on residual values, which represent the difference between the outcome predicted by the statistical model and the actual, observed outcome. Residuals are discussed in detail later in the simple linear regression analysis section. Third, if the distributional assumptions are violated, two options are generally available. First, the researcher could use a more appropriate distribution (see Table 6-1) or, second, they could employ a nonparametric statistical test. It is also common to see data transformation to attempt to force a normal distribution, but the considerable downside of this archaic technique was discussed previously in the "Transformation of Non-Normal Distributions" section. It is more common in the biomedical literature to see a nonparametric test used, but be aware more statistically savvy researchers will use alternative distributions if the distributional assumption is violated.

FACTOR 4: REPEATED MEASURES

• The number of DV measurements is critically important to determine whether an appropriate statistical test was used. Note that studies using one DV measurement are known as **cross-sectional**, whereas studies using two or more DV measurements are known as **longitudinal**. If the DV was measured on multiple occasions, there is inherent association or correlation across DV measurements. That is, DV values from the same person inherently have a higher correlation compared to DV values from different people. Therefore, if a statistical test does not account for this correlation, the standard errors will be biased and improper statistical inference will occur.

FACTOR 5: INCLUSION OF COVARIATES

• It is also critically important to consider the number of IVs and covariates, their scale of measurement, the number of categorical IV levels, and whether the IVs and/or covariates interact. Note that the distribution of the IV or covariate is never considered in the statistical analysis. With that said, the scale of measurement for each IV and covariate is important when deciding which statistical test to employ. In general, ANOVA will usually be employed for categorical IVs, whereas regression analysis is required for continuous IVs. Note that the wording of the last sentence was chosen specifically. That is, although it was stated earlier that ANOVA and regression are mathematically equivalent, ANOVA cannot be used with continuous IVs. However, regression analysis can be used with any combination of IVs and covariates measured on any scale. This can be a confusing distinction.

• Another important concept is the number of levels for each categorical IV. Remember, a level can be thought of as the number of groups being studied and evaluated. When testing group differences, researchers will typically employ a t test for two levels and ANOVA for three or more groups. Determining the number of levels is important because with three or more groups, the statistical test is an **omnibus test**. That is, an overall test result will be provided indicating a difference between at least two of the groups, but the test will not indicate specifically which groups differ. The concept of an omnibus test is discussed throughout the "Statistical Tests" section later in the chapter. Finally, whether an IV interacts with another IV or covariate is critically important. It is important to note that ANOVA can handle interactions between categorical IVs. Remember, an interaction indicates that the value of one IV is dependent on the value of another IV. For example, treatment group differences may be smaller in older patients (i.e., a treatment group-by-age interaction). However, if there is an interaction between a categorical IV and a continuous covariate, an ANOVA-type analysis, such as ANCOVA, cannot be used and a form of regression analysis must be used instead. Whether an interaction exists is an empirical question that is testable and described in the "Analysis of Covariance" section later in the chapter.

FACTOR 6: CLUSTERING

Finally, other factors exist when determining whether the appropriate statistical test was used, but many are beyond the scope of this chapter. One key factor worth considering, however, is based on the concept of clustering (also known as nesting). Classic examples of clustering include children nested within the same classroom or patients nested within the same doctor. Clustering creates statistical issues that are similar to using a cross-sectional analysis on longitudinal data. That is, DV measurements from children nested within the same classroom have greater associations compared to DV measurements from children in different classrooms. Failing to account for clustering will result in biased standard errors and incorrect statistical inference. Although a description of the statistical analysis for clustered data is too complex for this chapter, recognizing when an analysis should account for (or should have accounted for) clustering is relatively easy, and the number of clustering levels can get as complex as the researcher desires. For example, patients could be nested within a doctor, the doctor could be nested within a clinic, the clinic could be nested within a hospital system, the hospital system could be nested within a city, and so on. When reading a journal article, take time to consider whether clustering should have been considered by the researchers. Do not be disheartened by the possibility of seeing an exorbitant number of clustering levels in any journal article. If clustering is considered, most studies in the biomedical sciences will only use two or three clustering units. The takeaway message is that careful thought must be undertaken when evaluating a study, especially when considering clustering. If clustering levels were not considered, but should have been, interpret all results with caution.

As an example of how to use Tables 6-3 and 6-4, say a researcher wanted to examine the effect a new statin medication had on the number of low-density lipoproteins (LDL) using a sample of 200 healthy patients. Although LDL has received a bad reputation, research has shown that the size of the LDL particles carrying the cholesterol is more predictive of future cardiovascular problems than the absolute LDL value measured in mg/dL.[29] More specifically, cholesterol carried by large, buoyant LDLs (i.e., Pattern A) has little association with cardiovascular problems, whereas cholesterol carried by small, dense LDLs (i.e., Pattern B) has been associated with a myriad of cardiovascular problems.[30] Therefore, a statin that only targets cholesterol carried by small, dense LDL is needed. Based on lipoprotein particle profile (LPP) testing, patients were placed into one of two groups based on LDL particle size (i.e., the IV: Pattern A vs. Pattern B). The outcome for the study was LDL measured in mg/dL. Baseline measurements and demographic data were used as covariates and included categorized age (i.e., 40–49, 50–59, etc.), race, socioeconomic status indicated by whether the patient's mother graduated from high school, comorbid conditions, concurrent medications, and baseline LDL. The researchers hypothesized that the statin should reduce LDL significantly more in

Pattern A patients compared to Pattern B patients. The analysis was completed at the end of a 6-month study period. In the method section, the researchers stated that baseline characteristics and demographic data were compared between the two groups of patients. Due to the presence of outliers, Mann-Whitney tests were used for all continuous variables and chi-square tests were used for categorical variables. For the primary analysis, multiple linear regression was used. No assumption violations were indicated.

The example above contains similar information to what is typically provided in the overwhelming majority of published literature. Thus, using the example information above, Tables 6-3 and 6-4 can be used to determine whether the statistical tests employed were appropriate. Note that all three of these tests are described in detail later in the chapter. For the baseline and demographic data, using Table 6-3, the Mann-Whitney test was used because the DV scale was continuous, distributional assumptions were not met due to outliers, the DV was only measured on one occasion, there was one IV with two levels, and no covariates were considered. Further, using Table 6-4, chi-square tests were used because both the DV and IV were categorical and no covariates were considered. For the primary analysis, using Table 6-4, multiple linear regression analysis was used because the scale of the DV was continuous, the distributional assumptions were met, there was one IV with two levels, covariates were considered measured on both categorical and continuous scales, and although the DV was measured twice, the baseline measurement was used only as an additional covariate. Based on this information, all three statistical tests were used appropriately.

Case Study 6–2

Consider an RCT designed to evaluate the effect of clopidogrel as an inhibitor of adenosine diphosphate (ADP)–induced platelet aggregation. Platelet aggregation was measured via impedance aggregometry, which is more representative of physiological conditions as it uses whole blood. Upon consent, blood was drawn to quantify baseline percent inhibition of platelet aggregation, after which participants were randomized to either a 75 mg/day or 150 mg/day dose of clopidogrel to be taken for 14 days. On study day 15, blood was drawn to assess platelet aggregation inhibition. Beginning at study day 15, the patients were instructed to hold their clopidogrel dose through study day 28, on which blood was drawn to assess platelet aggregation inhibition. On study day 29, participants received the clopidogrel dose to which they were not randomized initially (e.g., if randomized initially to a 75 mg/day dose, they would now receive the 150 mg/day dose) to be taken for an additional 14 days. On study day 42, blood was drawn to assess platelet aggregation inhibition. Beginning on study day 43, patients were instructed to hold their clopidogrel dose. The primary outcome was impedance change across measurements. Prior to study initiation, it was estimated that 160 participants would be required per group to achieve 90% statistical power to detect an impedance change difference of 15% using a one-tailed alpha of 0.05.

Please answer the following questions:

1. Is the design parallel-groups, crossover, or adaptive? How do you know?
2. What was the length of the wash-out period?
3. What does it mean to say that the estimated sample size achieved 90% power?
4. Is a one-tailed hypothesis test appropriate? Why or why not?
5. At the end of the first study year, data from 60 participants were collected. If the researched analyzed the data on these 60 participants, when the study was powered for 160 participants, what type of analysis is this?
6. At the end of the second study year, data from 120 participants were collected. If these data are also analyzed, what limitations must be considered when evaluating the results?
7. At the end of the third study year, data from 160 patients is collected. Results indicated that the difference in platelet inhibition between the two clopidogrel doses was statistically significant as $p < 0.000001$. Does this p value indicate a large difference? Does this p value indicate a clinically meaningful difference? Does this p value indicate that this result is likely to replicate if the study was conducted again? What associated statistical information should the surgeon present to provide the clinical significance of this study?

Introduction to Common Statistical Tests

The remainder of this chapter describes the application and assumptions of numerous parametric and nonparametric statistical tests commonly used in the biomedical sciences. Note that this section only covers statistical tests applicable to study designs with one measured DV. A description and list of assumptions are provided for each statistical test as well as an example with an associated results section as it would likely appear in the literature. It is important to take careful note of the assumptions for each statistical test, as these assumptions are vital in determining whether correct statistical inference can be inferred from the statistical test results. The discussion of statistical tests begins with tests for nominal and categorical data, followed by statistical tests for evaluating group differences and associations. Finally, a brief discussion of a Bayesian framework and its estimation methods is provided.

TESTS FOR NOMINAL AND CATEGORICAL DATA

Nonparametric Tests

Pearson's Chi-Square Test

Pearson's chi-square test (or simply the chi-square test) is one of the most common statistical tests used in the biomedical sciences. It is used to assess for significant differences between two or more mutually exclusive groups for two variables measured on a nominal scale. Note that the data may also be ordinal if the number of rank-ordered categories is small (e.g., 3 or 5); however, the test does not consider rank order. The chi-square test assesses for differences between actual or observed frequency counts and the frequency count that would be expected if there actually were no differences in the data.

As an example, consider a study to determine whether a significant difference in gender exists between three treatment groups. In most journal articles, a 2×3 (i.e., gender by treatment group) contingency containing the observed frequency counts within each cell will typically be presented. This table would appear similar to Figure 6-7 but with another row or column. The expected frequencies are rarely presented in the literature. Next, a chi-square (χ^2) statistic should be presented with appropriate degrees of freedom subscripted next to the chi-square symbol (e.g., χ^2_2 for two degrees of freedom). As stated above, the number of degrees of freedom will vary based on the analysis. If the probability of the difference is below alpha; that is, if the observed frequencies are different from the expected frequencies, the test is considered statistically significant indicating a significant gender difference between the groups. The results of a statistically significant gender difference are presented as follows:

The results of the chi-square test indicated a statistically significant gender difference between treatment groups ($\chi^2_2 = 11.59$, $p < 0.05$).

When the chi-square test is based on a contingency table larger than 2×2, the test is considered an omnibus test. That is, in the example above for the 2×3 table, the chi-square test indicated that a statistically significant gender difference existed between at least two treatment groups, but failed to indicate specifically which treatment groups differed. In these situations, post hoc chi-square tests (or Fisher's exact tests if expected frequencies are low, see the next section) are used to determine where statistically significant differences occurred. For example, in the 2×3 chi square above, three 2×2 post hoc chi-square tests are required. Specifically, gender compared between groups A and B, gender compared between groups A and C, and gender compared between groups B and C. A sample results section including the post hoc chi-square test results is presented below:

Statistically significant gender differences were indicated across the three treatment groups ($\chi^2_2 = 11.59$, $p < 0.05$). Post hoc chi-square tests indicated statistically significant gender differences between groups A and B ($\chi^2_1 = 6.54$, $p < 0.05$) and between groups B and C ($\chi^2_1 = 10.26$, $p < 0.05$), with group B including significantly more males compared *to both groups A and C. Further, no statistically significant gender difference was indicated between groups A and C.*

The assumptions of the chi-square test include:

1. Data for both variables being compared must be categorical.
   a. Note that continuous data can be categorized; however, information will be lost via categorization.
2. The categories must be mutually exclusive.
   a. That is, each individual can fall into one, and only one, category.
3. The total sample size must be large.
   a. The expected frequencies in each cell must not be too small. For chi-square tests with degrees of freedom greater than 1 (i.e., when the number of columns and/or rows are greater than 2), no more than 20% of the cells should have expected frequencies less than 5. Further, no cell should have an expected frequency less than 1.[31] This is a difficult assumption to verify from the literature, outside of calculating the expected frequencies by hand. However, if an article fails to indicate this assumption was tested, view results with caution.

Fisher's Exact Test

Fisher's exact test is ubiquitous in the biomedical literature. The test can only be applied to 2×2 contingency tables and is most useful when the sample size is small. As such, it is often used when the adequacy of expected frequencies assumption of the chi-square test is violated. Conceptually, Fisher's exact test is identical to the chi-square test, in that the two variables being compared must be nominal and have mutually exclusive categories.

For example, consider a study assessing for differences in cardiac events in dialysis patients who initiated β-blocker therapy compared to patients who did not initiate therapy. Note, both variables are dichotomous (i.e., event vs. no event; β-blocker vs. no β-blocker). Fisher's exact test provides the exact probability of observing this particular set of frequencies within each cell of the contingency table. Results of a statistically significant Fisher's exact test are presented below. Notice only a *p* value is provided:

The results of a Fisher's exact test indicated patients initiating β-blocker therapy had significantly fewer cardiac events compared to patients failing to initiate therapy ($p < 0.05$).

The assumptions of Fisher's exact test include:

1. Data for both variables being compared must be dichotomous.
   a. Note that continuous data can be dichotomized; however, information will be lost via categorization.
2. The dichotomous categories must be mutually exclusive.
   a. That is, each individual can fall into one, and only one, category.

Mantel-Haenszel Chi-Square Test

The Mantel-Haenszel chi-square test (aka, Cochran-Mantel-Haenszel test or Mantel-Haenszel test) measures the association of three discrete variables, which usually consist of two dichotomous IVs and one categorical confounding variable or covariate used as a stratification variable.

For example, consider a study assessing the presence or absence of lung cancer in smokers and nonsmokers (the IVs) after stratifying for frequent exposure to secondhand smoke (the dichotomous covariate; exposure vs. no exposure). A 2×2 contingency table is created at each level of secondhand smoke. That is, a contingency table for exposure and another for no exposure. This test produces a chi-square statistic (χ^2_{MH}), with a statistically significant result indicating a significant difference in the presence of lung cancer for smokers and nonsmokers across the levels of the covariate (i.e., exposed vs. unexposed). A statistically significant result is presented as follows:

The results of a Mantel-Haenszel chi-square test indicated the proportion of nonsmokers developing lung cancer was significantly greater for those exposed to secondhand smoke $(\chi^2_{MH} = 29.67, 1 df, p < 0.05)$.

The assumptions of the Mantel-Haenszel chi-square test include:

1. Data of the IVs must be dichotomous.
   a. Note that continuous data can be dichotomized; however, information will be lost via categorization.
2. The dichotomous categories must be mutually exclusive.
   a. That is, each individual can fall into one, and only one, category.
3. Data of the covariate must be categorical.
   a. Again, note that continuous data can be dichotomized; however, information will be lost via categorization.

The Kappa Statistic

The kappa statistic (aka, Cohen's kappa or κ) is a measure of inter-rater reliability or agreement for a categorical variable measured on a nominal scale. That is, kappa indicates how often individual raters using the same measurement scale indicate identical scores. Kappa provides the proportion of agreement corrected for chance and ranges from 0 indicating no agreement to 1 indicating perfect agreement.

Because this statistic corrects for chance agreement, it is more appropriate than simply calculating overall percent agreement.[32] In fact, percent agreement should rarely be used and published results using percent agreement should be viewed with caution. Kappa can be applied to a variable with any number of categories, with the understanding that as the number of categories increase, overall agreement will undoubtedly decrease. That is, the more choices two raters have, the less likely they are to agree.

As an example, consider 100 professional school applicants, who each interview with two faculty members. After the interview is complete, each faculty member rates the applicant as accept, deny, or waitlist. Kappa is then used to calculate the agreement between faculty members. Results using the kappa statistic are presented as follows:

Cohen's kappa was employed to measure the agreement between faculty members in determining whether applicants should be accepted, denied, or waitlisted. Results indicated moderate agreement between faculty members ($\kappa = 0.75$).

The assumptions of the kappa statistic include:

1. Each object (e.g., the applicant in the example above) is rated only one time.
2. The outcome variable is nominal with mutually exclusive categories.
   a. That is, each individual can fall into one, and only one, category.
3. There are at least two independent raters.
   a. That is, each rater provides one, and only one, response for each applicant.

TESTING FOR DIFFERENCES FROM THE POPULATION

Parametric Tests

One-Sample z Test

The one-sample z test is used to assess for a difference between the mean of the study sample and a known population mean using a continuous DV.

For example, consider data collected from a random sample of 1000 patients with borderline high cholesterol who were not taking cholesterol-lowering medications and did not have diabetes, for which their mean serum total cholesterol was 210 mg/dL. The researcher is interested in determining whether the total cholesterol of this sample is significantly higher than the mean total cholesterol of nondiabetics who were not taking cholesterol-lowering medications within the general population for whom the mean total cholesterol level was 200 mg/dL with a standard deviation of 28.[33] A one-sample z test provides a z score indicating how many standard errors the sample mean is from the known population mean and if this difference is large enough to be considered statistically significant based on specific degrees of freedom. Note that degrees of freedom will be subscripted next to the z score (e.g., z_{999}). Results of a statistically significant one-sample z test with no assumption violations are provided as follows:

Results of a one-sample z test indicated a statistically significant difference in total cholesterol between the study sample and population ($z_{999} = 11.3, p < 0.05$), with the study sample having significantly higher total cholesterol compared to the general population (210.01 vs. 186.67 mg/dL, respectively).

Assumptions of the one-sample z test include:

1. The DV is measured on an interval or ratio scale.

2. The sampling distribution of means for the DV is normal.
   a. This can be assured by applying the Central Limit Theorem.
3. The population mean and standard deviation are known.
4. The observations are independent.
   a. That is, each participant provides one, and only one, observation (i.e., data or response).

One-Sample *t* Test

Only in rare cases is the population standard deviation known; thus, test statistics often must be based on sample data (i.e., standard deviation and sample size). The one-sample *t* test is used in situations where only the population mean is known, or can at least be estimated by very large amounts of data. It is used only for a continuous DV.

For example, consider a study to compare the mean total cholesterol of a random sample of 1000 adults aged 20 years of age or older with high cholesterol (e.g., mean: 220 mg/dL, SD: 20 mg/dL) to the mean total cholesterol of the general population. In 2016, the National Center for Health Statistics (NCHS) determined that the mean serum total cholesterol for adults in the United States aged 20 years and older was 191 mg/dL.[34] Notice, no population standard deviation is available; thus, a one-sample *t* test is required. Note that this test produces a *t* statistic, which can be considered similar to a *z* score when samples are large. In general, a *t* test will approximate a *z* test with a sample size of around 30. The result of a statistically significant one-sample *t* test with no assumption violations is presented as follows:

Results of a one-sample t test indicated a statistically significant difference in total cholesterol between the study sample and population ($t_{999} = 45.9$, p < 0.05), with the study sample having significantly higher total cholesterol compared to individuals aged 20 or older in the general population (210 mg/dL vs. 191 mg/dL, respectively)

Assumptions of the one-sample *t* test include:

1. The DV is measured on an interval or ratio scale.
2. The sampling distribution of means for the DV is normal.
   a. This can be assured by applying the Central Limit Theorem.
3. The population mean is known.
4. The observations are independent.
   a. That is, each participant provides one, and only one, observation (i.e., data or response).

Nonparametric Tests

Binomial Test

The binomial test is used when the DV is dichotomous and all of the possible data or outcomes fall into one, and only one, of the two categories. The binomial test uses the binomial distribution to test the exact probability of whether the sample proportion differs from the population proportion. Further, the binomial test is often used in the literature when sample sizes are small and violate the assumptions of the chi-square test, specifically low expected frequencies.[27]

For example, say a fair coin is flipped 10 times, and lands on heads six of the 10 flips. The expected population proportion is 0.50; that is, if the coin is fair, as the number of flips increases the coin should land on heads 50% of the time. Because the coin landed on heads six of the 10 flips, the statistical test is whether this proportion (i.e., 6/10 or 0.60) is statistically different from the expected proportion (i.e., 0.50). In this case, the binomial test indicates the difference between these proportions is not significant and results are presented as follows:

Results of the binomial test indicated the probability of flipping six heads in 10 flips was not statistically different from the expected population proportion of 0.50 (p > 0.05).

The assumptions of the binomial test include:

1. Data for both variables being compared must be dichotomous.
   a. Note that continuous data can be dichotomized; however, information will be lost via categorization.
2. The dichotomous categories must be mutually exclusive.
   a. That is, each individual can fall into one, and only one, category.
3. The population proportion is known.
4. The observations are independent.
   a. That is, each participant provides one, and only one, observation (i.e., data or response).

Kolmogorov-Smirnov One-Sample Test

The Kolmogorov-Smirnov one-sample test is a goodness-of-fit test used to determine the degree of agreement between the distribution of a researcher's sample data and a theoretical population distribution.[27] That is, it allows researchers to compare the distribution of their sample data against a given probability distribution for a continuous DV (see Table 6-1).

For example, consider a study where HbA1c data were collected for a random sample of 100 patients with diabetes. The researcher is interested in determining whether the distribution of HbA1c data was sampled from a population of patients with an underlying normal distribution. That is, the researcher is interested in whether the sample data is normally distributed. A nonsignificant Kolmogorov-Smirnov test indicates the sample distribution and the hypothesized normal distribution are not statistically different; that is, the distribution of sample data can be considered normally distributed. Results of the Kolmogorov-Smirnov test are presented as follows:

Results of the Kolmogorov-Smirnov test indicated HbA1c variable had a nonsignificant departure from normality (p > 0.05); thus, the data are considered to result from a normal distribution.

The assumptions of the Kolmogorov-Smirnov one-sample test include:

1. The DV is measured on an interval or ratio scale.
2. The underlying population distribution is theorized or known.
   a. That is, the researcher must specify the correct probability distribution to test the sample data against. If the distribution is unknown, the test is inappropriate.
3. The observations are independent.
   a. That is, each participant provides one, and only one, observation (i.e., data or response).

TESTING FOR DIFFERENCES BETWEEN GROUPS

Parametric Tests

Independent-Samples t Test

The independent-samples t test (aka, Student's t test) is used to assess for a statistically significant difference between the means of two independent, mutually exclusive groups using a continuous DV.

For example, consider testing for a mean difference in a methacholine challenge at the end of an 8-week study period in two groups of asthma patients receiving either fluticasone or placebo. Methacholine challenge was measured by a 20% decrease in forced expiratory volume in one second (FEV1; PC20). The independent-sample t test provides the t statistic and probability of obtaining a difference of this size or larger based on specific degrees of freedom, which are usually subscripted (e.g., t_{31}). Results of a statistically significant independent-samples t test with no assumption violations are presented as follows:

The results of an independent-samples t test indicated a statistically significant difference between groups (t_{31} = 9.654, p < 0.05), with asthma patients receiving fluticasone displaying significantly better lung function compared to placebo (mean PC20 = 10.7 vs. 3.8 mg/mL, respectively).

The assumptions of the independent-samples t test include:

1. The DV is measured on an interval or ratio scale.
2. The sampling distribution of means for the DV within each level of the IV (i.e., group) is normal.
   a. This can be assured by applying the central limit theorem.
3. The IV is dichotomous.
   a. Note that continuous data can be dichotomized; however, information will be lost via categorization.
4. The IV categories are mutually exclusive.
   a. That is, each individual can fall into one, and only one, category.

5. Homogeneity of variance is assured.

   a. That is, the variance within each group is similar. A crude indicator of a violation of this assumption (i.e., heterogeneity) is the ratio of the largest variance to smallest variance being greater than 10:1.[22] For example, most studies do not provide the variance for each variable; however, the standard deviation is reported consistently. Remember, variance is simply the standard deviation squared. Thus, consider two variables with standard deviations of 5 and 10. The homogeneity of variance assumption can be tested by squaring the standard deviations (i.e., $5^2 = 25$ and $10^2 = 100$, respectively) and finding their ratio (i.e., $100/25 = 4$). In this case, the ratio is less than 10:1; thus, the assumption is not violated.

6. The observations are independent.

   a. That is, each participant provides one, and only one, observation (i.e., data or response).

One-Way Between-Groups Analysis of Variance

A one-way between-groups analysis of variance (ANOVA) is an extension of the independent-samples t test to situations where researchers want to assess for mean differences between three or more mutually exclusive groups using a continuous DV.

For example, consider the fluticasone example from the "Independent-Samples t Test" section earlier in the chapter, but in addition to the placebo group, include two groups receiving different doses of fluticasone (e.g., 113 or 232μg). The use of three independent-samples t tests to test for mean differences between groups (i.e., 113 μg vs. placebo, 232 μg vs. placebo, 113 μg vs. 232 μg) is inappropriate due to a possible increase in Type I error. Instead, one-way ANOVA is used to partition the variance between and within groups to determine if a statistically significant group difference exists. This partitioning can be observed in the two numbers presented for degrees of freedom (i.e., $F_{2,27}$ indicates 2 between-group degrees of freedom and 27 within-group degrees of freedom). The result of a statistically significant one-way ANOVA with no assumption violations is presented as follows:

Results of a one-way ANOVA indicated a statistically significant difference between groups ($F_{2,27} = 6.89$, $p < 0.05$).

ANOVA provides an omnibus F test; that is, an overall test assessing the statistical significance between the three or more group means. A statistically significant omnibus F test indicates a statistically significant difference between at least two group means. To determine which groups differ specifically, a series of post hoc tests are conducted. Post hoc tests are simply tests comparing individual groups to one another; thus, post hoc tests can be viewed as a series of independent-samples t tests. That is, two-group comparisons. Because post hoc tests increase the number of statistical tests used, they often use a more conservative alpha to control for potential Type I errors. With this in mind, the significant one-way ANOVA in the example above would require three adjusted post hoc tests. That is, 113 µg vs. placebo, 232 µg vs. placebo, and 113 µg vs. 232 µg. The most commonly used post hoc tests in the literature include the Tukey and Scheffé tests. Be aware that the Scheffé test is the most conservative post hoc test available and some methodologists argue that the test may be too conservative, increasing the probability of committing a Type II error. A suitable alternative is the Tukey test, which is conservative, but to a lesser degree. In most cases, the two tests will indicate similar results and both are viewed as acceptable.

The results of a statistically significant one-way ANOVA including post hoc tests are presented as follows:

Results of a one-way ANOVA indicated a statistically significant difference between groups ($F_{2,27}$ = 6.89, $p < 0.05$). Post hoc Tukey tests indicated statistically significant differences (at $p < 0.05$) between placebo (3.8 mg/mL) and 113 µg dose of fluticasone (10.7 mg/mL) as well as between placebo and the 232 µg dose of fluticasone (12.2 mg/mL). No statistically significant differences were indicated between the 113 µg and 232 µg doses of fluticasone.

The assumptions for one-way ANOVA include:

1. The DV is measured on an interval or ratio scale.
2. The sampling distribution of means for the DV within each level of the IV is normal.
   a. This can be assured by applying the Central Limit Theorem.
3. The levels of the IV are mutually exclusive.
   a. That is, each individual can fall into one, and only one, category.
4. Homogeneity of variance is assured.
   a. That is, the variance within each group is similar. A crude indicator of a violation of this assumption (i.e., heterogeneity) is the ratio of the largest variance to smallest variance being greater than 10:1.[22] For example, most studies do not provide the variance for each variable; however, the standard deviation is reported consistently. Remember, variance is simply the standard deviation squared. Thus, consider two variables with standard deviations of 5 and 10. The homogeneity of variance assumption can be tested by squaring the standard deviations (i.e., $5^2 = 25$ and $10^2 = 100$, respectively) and finding their ratio (i.e., $100/25 = 4$). In this case, the ratio is less than 10:1; thus, the assumption is not violated.
5. The observations are independent.
   a. That is, each participant provides one, and only one, observation (i.e., data or response).

Factorial Between-Groups Analysis of Variance

A factorial between-groups analysis of variance (aka, factorial ANOVA) is an extension of the one-way between-groups ANOVA to a study with more than one IV using a continuous DV.

For example, consider a study to evaluate for differences in heart rate measured by beats per minute (bpm) between men and women following either a 30-mg dose of pseudoephedrine or placebo. In the literature, this may be described as a 2 × 2 factorial design indicating two IVs (i.e., gender and treatment) each with two levels (i.e., male vs. female; pseudoephedrine vs. placebo). This type of design produces two main effects—one for gender and one for treatment—and an interaction effect between gender and treatment. Thus, three separate F tests are provided, one for each effect, with statistical significance determined separately for each effect.

It is extremely important to note that if the interaction effect is statistically significant, the results of the main effects cannot be interpreted directly, as the IVs are dependent on each other. From the example, a statistically significant interaction effect indicates treatment effects differ depending on the gender of the participant. That is, pseudoephedrine had a different effect for males than it did for females. However, if the interaction effect is not significant, main effects can and should be interpreted. When interpreting the main effect of an IV, the levels of the other IV are averaged or marginalized. That is, interpreting the main effect of gender is done irrespective of whether the participants received pseudoephedrine or placebo. Likewise, interpreting the main effect of treatment is done irrespective of the participant's gender.

Similar to one-way, between-groups ANOVA, following a statistically significant main effect or interaction, post hoc tests may be required to identify where statistically significant differences occurred. There are a number of post hoc tests available depending on whether the interaction or main effects are statistically significant including the Tukey and Scheffé tests.[35] Each post hoc test adjusts alpha more or less conservatively to reduce potential Type I errors. Post hoc tests for factorial ANOVA used in the literature are often termed "simple comparisons," "simple contrasts," "simple main effects," or "interaction contrasts." While each uses a slightly different procedure, they are used to accomplish the same goal—identify group differences.

In the biomedical sciences, the results of a nonsignificant interaction effect for a 2 × 2 factorial between-groups ANOVA with no assumption violations are presented as follows:

Results of a 2 (Gender; male vs. female) × 2 (Treatment; pseudoephedrine vs. placebo) factorial between-groups ANOVA indicated a nonsignificant interaction effect between gender and treatment ($p > 0.05$). However, the main effect for gender was statistically significant ($F_{1,26} = 21.36$, $p < 0.05$), with males having significantly higher heart rates than females (91.6 vs. 84.3 bpm, respectively). Further, the main effect of treatment was also statistically *significant (F$_{1,26}$ = 15.24, p < 0.05), with pseudoephedrine resulting in a significantly higher heart rate compared to placebo (70.3 vs. 65.2 bpm, respectively).*

The results of a 2 × 2 factorial between-groups ANOVA with a statistically significant interaction and no assumption violations are presented as follows:

Results of a 2 (gender; male vs. female) × 2 (treatment; pseudoephedrine vs. placebo) factorial between-groups ANOVA indicated a statistically significant interaction effect between gender and treatment (F$_{1,26}$ = 15.42, p < 0.05). Simple main effects were assessed to identify at which treatment level gender differed. Results indicated pseudoephedrine increased heart rate significantly higher for males compared to females (90.5 vs. 82.4 bpm, respectively). No statistically significant gender difference in heart rate was indicated for the placebo group.

The assumptions of factorial between-groups ANOVA include:

1. The DV is measured on an interval or ratio scale.
2. The sampling distribution of means for the DV within each level of the IV is normal.
   a. This can be assured by applying the Central Limit Theorem.
3. The levels of the IVs are mutually exclusive.
   a. That is, each individual can fall into one, and only one, category.
4. Homogeneity of variance is assured.
   a. That is, the variance within each group is similar. A crude indicator of a violation of this assumption (i.e., heterogeneity) is the ratio of the largest variance to smallest variance being greater than 10:1.[22] For example, most studies do not provide the variance for each variable; however, the standard deviation is reported consistently. Remember, variance is simply the standard deviation squared. Thus, consider two variables with standard deviations of 5 and 10. The homogeneity of variance assumption can be tested by squaring the standard deviations (i.e., $5^2 = 25$ and $10^2 = 100$, respectively) and finding their ratio (i.e., 100/25 = 4). In this case, the ratio is less than 10:1; thus, the assumption is not violated.
5. The observations are independent.
   a. That is, each participant provides one, and only one, observation (i.e., data or response).

Analysis of Covariance

Analysis of covariance (ANCOVA) is an extension of both one-way between-groups ANOVA and factorial between-groups ANOVA. ANCOVA evaluates main effects and interactions using a continuous DV after statistically adjusting for one or more continuous confounding variables. That is, ANCOVA adjusts all group means to create the situation as if all participants scored identically on the covariate.[22]

For example, consider a study comparing atenolol to placebo (IV) and assessing their effects on systolic blood pressure (DV). The researchers note, however, that previous research has shown systolic blood pressure and BMI to be highly correlated.[36] Thus, the analysis will include BMI as a covariate assessing the effect of atenolol on systolic blood pressure over and above the effect of BMI on systolic blood pressure. If the atenolol group has greater BMI values compared to the placebo group, ANCOVA will adjust the systolic blood pressure within both groups to account for this initial difference in BMI.

In ANCOVA, covariates are continuous, measured before the DV, and correlated with the DV. It should be noted that ANCOVA is closely related to linear regression. Thus, although not completely necessary, it may be useful to revisit this section after reading the Simple Linear Regression and Multivariable Linear Regression sections presented later in the chapter. In ANCOVA, group means are statistically adjusted by the magnitude of the association (i.e., slope) between the DV and covariate.[39] That is, the greater the association, the more useful the covariate and better the adjustment. Thus, the goal of the covariate is to reduce error variance thereby increasing the statistical power of the test. From the example, mean systolic blood pressure for the atenolol and placebo groups are adjusted by the association between BMI and systolic blood pressure. Because previous research has shown the association between systolic blood pressure and BMI to be considerable, the statistical power of this test will undoubtedly be increased.

When presenting the results of ANCOVA, researchers should provide adjusted means; that is, the mean of the DV at each level of the IV after adjusting for the covariate. Published research that does not present adjusted means should be viewed with caution. Further, the effect of the covariate must also be presented which provides information regarding the effectiveness of the covariate in adjusting group means. Finally, it should be noted that ANCOVA is more suited for experimental design in which participants are randomized to groups, as opposed to nonexperimental designs without randomization. Remember, ANCOVA is used to adjust group means as if all participants had identical covariate values. However, in nonexperimental research, important covariates may have been missed and causality is difficult to infer—a characteristic intrinsic to all nonexperimental work. Thus, the limitations may be significant when applying ANCOVA to nonexperimental designs and results must be viewed cautiously.[9]

In the biomedical sciences, the results of a statistically significant ANCOVA with no assumption violations are presented as follows:

Results of a one-way ANCOVA indicated a statistically significant group differences in systolic blood pressure after adjusting for BMI ($F_{1,17} = 7.98$, $p < 0.05$), with patients receiving atenolol having significantly lower systolic blood pressure compared to placebo (adjusted means = 118 vs. 141 mmHg, respectively). The relationship between systolic blood pressure and BMI was also statistically significant after adjusting for group ($F_{1,17} = 39.85$, $p < 0.05$) with a pooled within-group correlation of 0.61.

The assumptions of ANCOVA include:

1. The DV is measured on an interval or ratio scale.
2. The sampling distribution of means for the DV and covariate(s) within each level of the IV is normal.
   a. This can be assured by applying the Central Limit Theorem.
3. The levels of the IV are mutually exclusive.
   a. That is, each individual can fall into one, and only one, category.
4. Homogeneity of variance is assured.
   a. That is, the variance within each group is similar. A crude indicator of a violation of this assumption (i.e., heterogeneity) is the ratio of the largest variance to smallest variance being greater than 10:1.[22] For example, most studies do not provide the variance for each variable; however, the standard deviation is reported consistently. Remember, variance is simply the standard deviation squared. Thus, consider two variables with standard deviations of 5 and 10. The homogeneity of variance assumption can be tested by squaring the standard deviations (i.e., $5^2 = 25$ and $10^2 = 100$, respectively) and finding their ratio (i.e., $100/25 = 4$). In this case, the ratio is less than 10:1; thus, the assumption is not violated.
5. Homogeneity of regression is assured.
   a. This assumption requires the association between the DV and covariate to be the same within each level of the IV. A violation of this assumption renders ANCOVA inappropriate, and the authors should use linear regression instead. However, violation is difficult to detect from the literature, as most authors fail to provide the appropriate information in the narrative. Thus, when reading a journal article employing ANCOVA, if the author fails to indicate whether this assumption was tested, results must be viewed with caution.
6. The covariate(s) is measured reliably and without error.
7. The observations are independent.
   a. That is, each participant provides one, and only one, observation (i.e., data or response).

Nonparametric Tests

Mann-Whitney Test

The Mann-Whitney test (aka, Mann-Whitney U test, Wilcoxon rank-sum test) is the nonparametric alternative to the independent-samples t test and is one of the most powerful nonparametric tests.[27] It is used when the distributional assumptions for the parametric test are violated or when the DV is measured on an ordinal scale. The Mann-Whitney test is based on ranked data. That is, instead of using the actual values of the DV, as an independent-samples t test does, each participant's DV value is ranked with the highest value receiving the highest rank and the lowest value receiving the lowest rank. The ranks within each group are then summed and the test assesses whether the difference in ranked sums between groups is statistically significant.

For example, consider a performance improvement study assessing gender differences in patient satisfaction of hospital stay following total hip replacement surgery. The measurement instrument uses a Likert-type scale with four possible responses anchored from Strongly Disagree to Strongly Agree. A statistically significant Mann-Whitney test indicates gender differences in patient satisfaction, with the group with the highest ranked sums indicating higher satisfaction. The results of the Mann-Whitney test are presented as follows:

The results of a Mann-Whitney test indicate a statistically significant gender difference in patient satisfaction following total hip replacement surgery (z = 2.65, p < 0.05), with males indicating higher satisfaction scores compared to females.

The assumptions of the Mann-Whitney test include:

1. The DV is measured on an ordinal, interval, or ratio scale.
2. The IV is dichotomous.
   a. Note that continuous data can be categorized into a dichotomous variable; however, information will be lost.
3. The levels of the IV are mutually exclusive.
   a. That is, each individual can fall into one, and only one category.
4. The observations are independent.
   a. That is, each participant provides one, and only one, observation (i.e., data or response).

Median Test

The median test is used to assess whether two mutually exclusive groups have different medians. There is no parametric alternative to the median test; however, the nonparametric Mann-Whitney test can be used as an adequate alternative. The test calculates the medians within each group and then classifies the data within each group as either above or below the respective group median. Further, because the test is based on the median, it can be used appropriately for skewed distributions or data containing outliers.

For example, consider a study designed to evaluate staff knowledge of infection control between a rural and urban hospital that each had high prevalence of hospital-acquired infections.[37] A 15-item questionnaire was developed to assess knowledge in which each question was scored 0 or 1 and then summed across all items. The median for each group (i.e., hospital) served as the appropriate descriptive statistic as the data were left skewed. As such, the median test was used to determine whether statistically significant knowledge differences existed between hospitals. The results of a statistically significant median test are presented as follows:

The results of the median test indicated no statistically significant differences in knowledge between the rural and urban hospital (median = 11.8 vs. 12.0, respectively; p > 0.05).

Assumptions of the median test include:

1. The DV is measured on an ordinal, interval, or ratio scale.
2. Samples sizes are sufficiently large.
    a. If sample sizes are small, say less than 5 in each group, Fisher's exact test should be used instead. From the example, this means using a 2 (Group; male vs. female) × 2 (Median; above vs. below) contingency table.
3. The observations are independent.
    a. That is, each participant provides one, and only one, observation (i.e., data or response).

Kruskal-Wallis One-Way ANOVA by Ranks

The Kruskal-Wallis one-way ANOVA by ranks (or simply, the Kruskal-Wallis test) is the nonparametric alternative to the one-way between-groups ANOVA. The test is an extension of the Mann-Whitney test to assess group differences between three or more mutually exclusive groups. The Kruskal-Wallis test is typically used when distributional assumptions are violated or when the DV is measured on an ordinal scale. Further, the Kruskal-Wallis test is based on rank sums similar to the Mann-Whitney test. The DV scores are ranked from highest to lowest, summed, and statistically significant of group differences are evaluated based these rank sums.

For example, consider a study evaluating regional differences in whether volunteer preceptors believe they have adequate time available to dedicate to their experiential pharmacy students.[38] In this study, the DV was measured on an ordinal 4-point Likert-type scale; thus, the Kruskal-Wallis test was used in lieu of one-way between-groups ANOVA. The results of the statistically significant Kruskal-Wallis test are presented as follows:

Results of the Kruskal-Wallis test indicated regional differences regarding whether volunteer preceptors believe they have adequate time to dedicate to experiential students $(\chi^2_6 = 33.07, p < 0.05)$.

Similar to a one-way between-groups ANOVA, the Kruskal-Wallis test is an omnibus test. That is, the test will determine whether an overall statistically significant difference exists between groups, but will not indicate specifically which groups differed statistically. Thus, post hoc tests are required. In this situation, the Mann-Whitney test is used to compare all two-group combinations. From the example, post hoc tests would include West vs. Midwest, West vs. South, West vs. Northeast, and so on for a total of six post hoc tests. The results of the Kruskal-Wallis test including Mann-Whitney post hoc tests are presented as follows:

Results of the Kruskal-Wallis test indicated regional differences regarding whether volunteer preceptors believe they have adequate time to dedicate to experiential students ($\chi^2_6 = 33.07$, $p < 0.05$). Post hoc Mann-Whitney tests indicated preceptors in the West disagreed more compared to preceptors located in the Midwest ($p < 0.05$) and agreed less with preceptors in the South ($p < 0.05$). No other statistically significant group differences were indicated.

The assumptions of the Kruskal-Wallis test include:

1. The DV is measured on an ordinal, interval, or ratio scale.
2. The IV is categorical.
    a. Note that continuous data can be categorized; however, information will be lost.
3. The levels of the IV are mutually exclusive.
    a. That is, each individual can fall into one, and only one category.
4. Each group has approximately the same distribution.
    a. Although the Kruskal-Wallis test does not assume data are distributed normally, if the distribution for one level of the IV is skewed negatively and the other levels are skewed positively, the results produced by the test may be inaccurate.
5. The data do not include a large number of ties.
    a. Tied values are given average ranks. Typically, if less than 25% of the data are ties, the test is unaffected.[27]
6. The observations are independent.
    a. That is, each participant provides one, and only one, observation (i.e., data or response).

TESTING FOR WITHIN-GROUP CHANGE

Parametric Tests

Paired-Samples t Test

The paired-samples t test (aka, matched t test or nested t test) is used when one group of participants in measured twice or two groups of participants are matched on specific characteristics. In both cases, the assumption of independence, or mutually exclusive groups, is violated. This statistical test is only appropriate using a continuous DV.

When one group of participants is measured twice, it is known as a repeated-measures design. Repeatedly measuring participants is a valid method for reducing error and increasing statistical power, which requires fewer participants. The simplest repeated-measures design is termed "a pretest-posttest design." For example, consider measuring the therapeutic knowledge of 20 fourth year pharmacy (P4) students prior to clinical rotations (i.e., pretest) and following rotations (i.e., posttest) to assess for increases in therapeutic knowledge. Therapeutic knowledge was measured using a discriminating

20-question test. The paired-samples t test assesses for a statistically significant change in correct responses from pretest to posttest.

When two groups of participants are matched on specific characteristics, it is called a matched design. For example, when studying the effects of a new statin medication on hyperlipidemia, researchers would identify a group of patients to receive the statin and then identify a matched control group by matching individuals based on age, race, gender, BMI, and years with diagnosis. Note that the matched control group does not receive any medication. Matching participants serves the same purpose as repeated measures—reduce error variance—but is often more difficult because as the number of matching criteria increases the probability of finding a suitable match decreases.

Results of a statistically significant paired-samples t test with no assumption violations using the pretest-posttest design example above is presented as follows:

The results of a paired-samples t test indicated a statistically significant difference in therapeutic knowledge between pretest and posttest scores ($t_{19} = 3.25$, $p < 0.05$). Therapeutic knowledge increased significantly following clinical rotations (mean = 10.4 correct responses at pretest vs. a mean of 16.5 at posttest).

The assumptions of the paired-samples t test include:

1. The DV is measured on an interval or ratio scale.
2. The two DV measurements are associated.
3. The sampling distribution of means for both DV measurements is normal.
    a. This can be assured by applying the Central Limit Theorem.
4. Homogeneity of variance for both DV measurements is assured.
    a. That is, the variance within each group is similar. A crude indicator of a violation of this assumption (i.e., heterogeneity) is the ratio of the largest variance to smallest variance being greater than 10:1.[22] For example, most studies do not provide the variance for each variable; however, the standard deviation is reported consistently. Remember, variance is simply the standard deviation squared. Thus, consider two variables with standard deviations of 5 and 10. The homogeneity of variance assumption can be tested by squaring the standard deviations (i.e., $5^2 = 25$ and $10^2 = 100$, respectively) and finding their ratio (i.e., $100/25 = 4$). In this case, the ratio is less than 10:1; thus, the assumption is not violated.

One-Way Repeated-Measures Analysis of Variance

A one-way repeated-measures ANOVA (aka, repeated-measures ANOVA) is an extension of the paired-samples t test to situations where the continuous DV is measured three or more times. Again, this can occur when the same participants are measured repeatedly or when three or more matched groups are measured once. A repeated-measures ANOVA is used to indicate whether a statistically significant change occurred between the repeated measurements.

For example, reconsider the pretest-posttest design described in the Paired-Samples *t* test section early in the chapter. Briefly, a researcher is interested in testing whether therapeutic knowledge of 20 pharmacy students in their last year of college changes before and after clinical rotations. To be applicable to repeated-measures ANOVA, students would be tested on a third occasion 6 months after posttest to assess knowledge retention. That is, the design measures therapeutic knowledge at pretest, posttest, and 6-month follow-up. The repeated-measures ANOVA is then used to test whether a statistically significance change occurred between the repeated measurements.

Some researchers prefer to use repeated-measures ANOVA over paired-samples *t* tests when participants are only measured twice. This is an appropriate use of repeated-measures ANOVA as repeated-measures ANOVA can be used in any situation when a paired-samples *t* test is appropriate. The results would be identical. However, the test statistic from the repeated-measures ANOVA will be an *F* value instead of a *t* value produced by the paired-samples *t* test. This is a nonissue, though, as the *F* value in this situation is simply t^2.

In most cases, repeated-measures ANOVA has more statistical power than a paired-samples *t* test. This has been alluded to in the "Analysis of Clinical Trials" and "Paired-Samples *t* Test" sections earlier in the chapter. In general, increasing the number of repeated measures further reduces error, which allows for more precise measurement and decreases the overall probability of committing a Type I error. With that said, increasing the number of repeated measurements has diminishing returns in statistical power. That is, for most studies, statistical power will increase drastically by adding a few additional repeated measurements, but the magnitude of this increase weakens rapidly between four and six measurements, with little to no increases in statistical power beyond the seventh measurement.[39] Finally, if a study has more than 10 repeated measurements, a time series analysis may be more appropriate than repeated-measures ANOVA.

In addition, a brief discussion of the key assumption of repeated-measures ANOVA is useful as a basic understanding of this assumption will assist in determining whether the test statistics produced from the analysis are correct. This key assumption, known as sphericity, states that the variances of the differences between repeated measurements are equal. For example, consider a study with three repeated measurements. For the sphericity assumption to be satisfied, the variance of the difference between the first and second measurements must be similar to the variance of the difference between the first and third and second and third. This assumption tends to be restrictive, as most differences closer in time tend to have less variability compared to measurements further apart in time. Sphericity is a testable assumption using Mauchly's test, and a violation can severely bias the statistical inference. Therefore, when reading a journal article, if the authors fail to provide information regarding the assurance or violation of the sphericity assumption, results and interpretations must be viewed with caution.

Briefly reconsider the example provided above where 20 pharmacy students in their final year have therapeutic knowledge measured before clinical rotations (i.e., pretest), once immediately after rotations (i.e., posttest), and at a 6-month follow-up. That is, therapeutic knowledge is measured on three separate occasions. A statistically significant repeated-measures ANOVA with no assumption violations will be presented as follows:

The results of a one-way repeated-measures ANOVA indicated a statistically significant difference in therapeutic knowledge between pretest, posttest, and 6-month follow-up $(F_{2,38} = 9.87, p < 0.05)$.

With more than two repeated measurements the one-way repeated-measures ANOVA is an omnibus test. That is, the F test will identify whether a statistically significant difference exists between repeated measures, but will not indicate specifically which repeated measurements differ. Thus, *post hoc* tests, known as pairwise comparisons, are required. Similar to other analysis requiring *post hoc* tests, there are numerous adjusted pairwise comparisons available. Each type of pairwise comparison adjusts alpha differently, with some being more conservative. It may be simpler to think of these comparisons as a series of paired-samples t tests with adjusted alpha values. That is, adjusted paired-samples t tests comparing the first and second repeated measurements, the first and third, the second and third, and so on. The additional information required to present results of a statistically significant one-way repeated-measures ANOVA with no assumption violations are presented as follows:

The results of a one-way repeated-measures ANOVA indicated a statistically significant difference in therapeutic knowledge between pretest, posttest, and 6-month follow-up $(F_{2,38} = 9.87, p < 0.05)$. *Results of the pairwise comparisons indicated a statistically significant increase in therapeutic knowledge from pretest to posttest (mean = 5.50 vs. 15.90, respectively, p < 0.05). Further, no statistically significant difference was indicated from posttest to 6-month follow-up (mean = 15.90 vs. 15.50, respectively) indicating therapeutic knowledge was retained 6 months following clinical rotations.*

The assumptions of the one-way repeated-measures ANOVA include:

1. The DV is measured on an interval or ratio scale.
2. All DV measurements are associated.
3. The sampling distribution of means for all DV measurements is normal.
   a. This can be assured by applying the Central Limit Theorem.
4. Homogeneity of variance for all DV measurements is assured.
   a. That is, the variance within each group is similar. A crude indicator of a violation of this assumption (i.e., heterogeneity) is the ratio of the largest variance to smallest variance being greater than 10:1.[22] For example, most studies do not provide the variance for each variable; however, the standard deviation is reported consistently. Remember, variance is simply the standard deviation

squared. Thus, consider two variables with standard deviations of 5 and 10. The homogeneity of variance assumption can be tested by squaring the standard deviations (i.e., $5^2 = 25$ and $10^2 = 100$, respectively) and finding their ratio (i.e., $100/25 = 4$). In this case, the ratio is less than 10:1; thus, the assumption is not violated.

5. Sphericity is assured for designs with three or more repeated measurements.

   a. This is a complex assumption discussed above. In general, sphericity is violated when the variance of the differences between measurements are not similar.

Mixed Between-Within Analysis of Variance

A mixed between-within analysis of variance (aka, factorial ANOVA with repeated measures or split-plot ANOVA) is a combination of factorial between-groups ANOVA and repeated-measures ANOVA. The mixed terminology highlights this combination, and indicates that the design considers two or more levels of the IV when a continuous DV is measured repeatedly. It is important to note that a mixed between-within ANOVA is qualitatively different from a mixed-effects analysis involving random effects (see Table 6-4). The simplest case is a 2×2 pretest-posttest design, using two mutually exclusive treatment groups measured on two separate occasions. The primary advantage of this analysis is that it allows researchers to assess the interaction effect evaluating whether two groups changed differently over time in addition to between-subjects main effect indicating the overall effect irrespective of measurement and within-subjects main effect indicating the overall effect irrespective of group.

As an example, consider a study examining the effectiveness of vilazodone (a selective serotonin reuptake inhibitor [SSRI] and serotonin agonist) compared to repeated-dose intravenous ketamine over a 12-week study period. The researcher hypothesizes that vilazodone is more effective than ketamine in reducing symptoms of clinical depression. Prior to initiating treatment, 20 patients with diagnosed clinical depression are measured on the Beck Depression Inventory II (BDI-II).[40] Following this pretest or baseline measurement, each patient is randomized to receive one of two treatment options, the vilazodone or ketamine, with ten patients in each group. Patients then initiate the prescribed medication therapy and at the end of the 12-week study period BDI-II scores are measured again. A mixed between-within ANOVA provides researchers with a separate F tests for the interaction effect, between-groups main effect, and within-groups main effect each evaluated with specific degrees of freedom. Within this example, the primary effect of interest is the interaction effect, evaluating whether BDI-II scores changed differently within the vilazodone group compared to the ketamine group from pretest to posttest.

Similar to factorial ANOVA discussed above, only if the interaction effect is nonsignificant can the researcher evaluate the statistical significance of overall group mean difference or between-group main effect and the overall change in BDI-II scores or within-group main effect. That is, a statistically significant interaction effect indicates that the change in BDI-II scores from pretest to posttest changed differently in the group receiving vilazo- done compared to the group receiving ketamine or vice versa. Stated another way, the reduction in symptoms from pretest to posttest was dependent on whether the patient received vilazodone or ketamine. In this example, the researcher's hypothesis would be supported by a statistically significant interaction effect; that is, vilazodone was more effec- tive at reducing the symptoms associated with clinical depression compared to ketamine.

Although the example above was for a 2 (Group: vilazodone vs. intravenous ket- amine) × 2 (Measurement: pretest vs. posttest) design, a mixed between-within ANOVA can be used for a design with any number of IVs with any number of levels or repeated measures. This is often seen in the literature. For example, consider the pretest-posttest study evaluating the effectiveness of three treatment groups (e.g., vilazodone , intra- venous ketamine, and a dopamine reuptake inhibitor such as bupropion) in reducing symptoms of clinical depression. This would be considered a 3 × 2 design. Or, con- sider the same study evaluating for additional gender differences within these three treatments. This would be considered a 3 × 2 × 2 design. It must be noted that as the number and levels of the IVs increase so does the complexity of interpreting results. Thus, extreme care must be taken when interpreting results and implementing sugges- tions supported by these types of designs. Consultation with an individual well versed in research methodology and statistical analysis is advised prior to implementing findings into an evidence-based practice.

Because a mixed between-within ANOVA is an extension of factorial between-groups ANOVA and repeated-measures ANOVA, post hoc tests or pairwise comparisons may be required for any IV with three or more levels. That is, when there are more than three lev- els of the between-groups IV (e.g., vilazodone, intravenous ketamine, and bupropion), the between-groups main effect is an omnibus test. A statistically significant between-groups main effect indicates that a statistically significant difference in BDI-II scores exists, but does not indicate specifically which groups differ significantly. Further, with three or more repeated measures, a statistically significant within-groups main effect indicates a differ- ence between repeated measures, but fails to indicate specifically which measurements differ significantly. The post hoc tests and pairwise comparisons for factorial between- groups ANOVA and repeated-measures ANOVA, respectively, are also appropriate for a mixed between-within ANOVA.

The results of a 2 × 2 mixed between-within ANOVA with no assumption violations for a nonsignificant interaction effect and statistically significant between- and within- groups main effects is presented as follows:

The results of a 2 (Group: vilazodone vs ketamine) × 2 (Measurements: pretest vs. post- test) mixed between-within ANOVA failed to indicate a statistically significant interaction

($F_{1,18} = 1.215$, p > 0.05). However, both main effects were statistically significant. Overall, patients receiving the vilazodone *had lower BDI-II scores compared to patients receiving intravenous ketamine ($F_{1,18} = 27.97$, p < 0.05; mean = 29.41 vs. 47.50, respectively). Further, an overall decrease in depressive symptoms was indicated from pretest to posttest ($F_{1,18} = 24.74$, p < 0.05; mean = 49.86 vs. 35.72, respectively).*

With a statistically significant interaction effect, results of the mixed between-within ANOVA with no assumption violations are presented as follows:

The results of a 2 (Group: vilazodone vs. intravenous ketamine) × 2 (Measurements: pretest vs. posttest) mixed between-within ANOVA indicated a statistically significant interaction effect ($F_{1,18} = 10.37$, p < 0.05). Simple main effects were assessed to identify statistically significant treatment differences at pretest and posttest individually. Results indicated no statistically significant difference between the vilazodone and ketamine at pretest (mean = 48.53 vs. 50.23, respectively). However, at posttest, a statistically significant difference was indicated, with the vilazodone group having significantly lower BDI-II scores compared to the ketamine group (mean = 24.63 vs. 47.53, respectively).

The assumptions of a mixed between-within ANOVA include:

1. The DV is measured on an interval or ratio scale.
2. All DV measurements are associated.
3. The sampling distribution of means at each level of the IV(s), collapsed across the repeated DV measurements, is normal.
   a. This can be assured by applying the Central Limit Theorem.
4. Homogeneity of variance for all DV measurements within each level of the IV(s) is assured.
   a. That is, the variance within each group is similar. A crude indicator of a violation of this assumption (i.e., heterogeneity) is the ratio of the largest variance to smallest variance being greater than 10:1.[22] For example, most studies do not provide the variance for each variable; however, the standard deviation is reported consistently. Remember, variance is simply the standard deviation squared. Thus, consider two variables with standard deviations of 5 and 10. The homogeneity of variance assumption can be tested by squaring the standard deviations (i.e., $5^2 = 25$ and $10^2 = 100$, respectively) and finding their ratio (i.e., $100/25 = 4$). In this case, the ratio is less than 10:1; thus, the assumption is not violated.
5. Sphericity is assured for designs with three or more repeated measurements.
   a. This is a complex assumption discussed briefly above for one-way repeated-measures ANOVA. In general, sphericity is violated when the variance of the differences between measurements are not similar.

Nonparametric Tests

Wilcoxon Signed-Rank Test

The Wilcoxon signed-rank test (aka, signed-rank test) is the nonparametric alternative to a paired-samples t test. Note that this is a different test from the Wilcoxon rank-sum test discussed above. The test is used typically to assess for differences between two repeated measurements or two matched groups when distributional assumptions are violated or when the DV is measured on an ordinal scale. The signed-rank test is based on ranked difference scores (e.g., difference between pretest and posttest), with the highest difference score receiving the highest rank and the lowest difference score receiving the lowest rank.

For example, consider single group pretest-posttest study evaluating the secondary effect of weight loss in pounds while on exenatide therapy in a sample of 20 Type I DM patients. Prior to initiating exenatide therapy, all patients are weighed (i.e., pretest). At the end of a 1-year study period, patients are weighed again (i.e., posttest). For this study, the DV has numerous outliers; thus, the signed-rank test is used in lieu of paired-samples t test to assess for a change in patient weight from pretest to posttest. The result of a statistically significant signed-rank test is presented as follows:

The results of the signed-rank tests indicated a statistically significant decrease in body weight from pretest to posttest ($z = 2.32$, $p < 0.05$).

The assumptions of the signed-rank test include:

1. The DV measured repeatedly on an ordinal, interval, or ratio scale.
2. The two DV measurements are associated.
3. The two measurements come from populations with the same median.
4. There should not be a large number of difference scores equal to 0.
5. That is, the number of participants having no change (i.e., difference score of 0) should be low.

Friedman Two-Way ANOVA by Ranks

The Friedman two-way ANOVA by ranks test (aka, Friedman's test) is the nonparametric alternative to the one-way repeated-measures ANOVA and is an extension of the signed-rank test to a situation with three or more repeated measurements. Similar to the other nonparametric tests, it is most often used when distributional assumptions are violated or the DV is measured on an ordinal scale. The Friedman test is based on ranked data, with higher scores receiving higher ranks, and is used to assess for statistically significant differences between repeated measurements.

For example, reconsider the exenatide example described in the "Wilcoxon Signed-Rank Test" section above. Briefly, the example consisted of a onetime pretest-posttest study evaluating the secondary effect of weight loss in pounds while on exenatide therapy in a sample of 20 Type I DM patients. To extend this design to be applicable to Friedman's test, consider a study where patients are weighed prior to initiating exenatide therapy, 6 months after initiation, and 1 year after initiation. Thus, each patient is weighed on three occasions. Because the distribution of weight has numerous outliers, Friedman's test is employed. The results of a statistically significant Friedman's test are presented as follows:

The results of Friedman's test indicated statistically significant differences in body weight between the three repeated measurements ($\chi^2_2 = 15.21$, p < 0.05).

Similar to the one-way repeated-measures ANOVA, Friedman's test is an omnibus test. That is, it assesses whether a statistically significant difference exists between the repeated measurements, but does not indicate specifically which measurements differ significantly. Thus, a series of post hoc tests are required. For the example above, three signed ranks tests are required to test for differences between measurements: pretest vs. 6 months, pretest vs. 1 year, and 6 months vs. 1 year. The results of a statistically significant Friedman's test including the additional post hoc tests are presented as follows:

The results of Friedman's test indicated statistically significant differences between the three repeated measurements ($\chi^2_2 = 15.21$, p < 0.05). Post hoc signed-rank tests indicated a statistically significant decrease in body weight from pretest to 6-month follow-up (z = 2.65, p < 0.05), with no statistically significant difference between the 6-month and 1-year follow-up (z = 0.51, p > 0.05). Thus, results suggest weight loss occurred rapidly, within 6 months of initiating exenatide therapy, and was sustained through 1 year of therapy.

The assumptions of the Friedman test include:

1. The DV is measured repeatedly on an ordinal, interval, or ratio scale.
2. All DV measurements are associated.
3. The DV measurements come from populations with the same median.

The Sign Test

The sign test is another nonparametric alternative to the paired-samples *t* test. Similar to the signed-rank test, the sign test is used typically when distributional assumptions are violated or when the DV is measured on an ordinal scale. The sign test is used to assess for differences between two repeated measurements or two matched groups. The sign test is typically less powerful than the signed-rank test as the signed-rank test uses more information from the data to calculate the test statistic. Nevertheless, the sign test is presented here because it is seen in the literature; however, in most situations, the signed-rank test should have been used.

For example, consider a pretest-posttest study to evaluate change in BMI following a physical activity intervention in a sample of 20 third-grade students. In this study, BMI was measured at the beginning of the school year (i.e., pretest) and again after the school year was complete (i.e., posttest). The sign test assesses whether statistically significant change occurred between the two measurements. The results of a statistically significant sign test are presented below. Notice that no test statistic is presented, only a p value.

The results of the sign test indicated a statistically significant decrease in BMI from pretest to posttest ($p < 0.05$).

The assumptions of the sign test include:

1. The DV is measured repeatedly on an ordinal, interval, or ratio scale.
2. The two DV measurements are associated.

The McNemar Test of Change

The McNemar test of change (aka, McNemar's test) is an extension of the chi-square and Fisher's exact test when participants are measured on two separate occasions and assesses the statistical significance of observed changes between the two repeated measurements. McNemar's test is only applicable to a DV measured on a nominal scale; however, continuous variables can be artificially dichotomized, with the understanding that information will be lost.[27,41]

McNemar's test is often used for pretest-posttest studies to assess change following an intervention or treatment. For example, consider a study to determine the effectiveness of an influenza vaccination across two consecutive flu seasons. At the beginning of the first flu season, 20 participants are randomized to receive either vaccination or placebo with ten in each group. At the end of the first flu season, participants are asked whether they were diagnosed with the flu or not (i.e., yes vs. no). Then, at the beginning of the second flu season, participants who received the vaccination originally will receive placebo and those who received placebo originally will receive the vaccination. At the end of the second flu season, participants are asked again whether they were diagnosed with flu. McNemar's test is used in this study to statistically test whether the flu vaccination was effective, where participants diagnosed with flu while taking placebo should not have developed flu with the vaccination. That is, the participant's outcome changed depending on the treatment received.

A critically important caveat is that McNemar's test only considers participants who changed between the two repeated measurements, with participants who did not change removed from analysis. Thus, if a researcher believes that change will be rare, the McNemar test may be inappropriate because the statistical power of this test may be extremely reduced due to the sample size decrease from removing participants who did not change.

Based on the example above, the results of a statistically significant McNemar test are presented below. Notice that no test statistic is provided, only the p value.

The results of a statistically significant McNemar's test indicated a statistically signifi-cant change between treatment and placebo ($p < 0.05$), with the vaccination significantly reducing influenza diagnoses compared to placebo.

The assumptions of the McNemar test include:

1. The DV is measured repeatedly on a dichotomous scale.
2. The two DV measurements are associated.

The Cochran Q Test

The Cochran Q test (aka, Cochran's Q) is an extension of McNemar's test to situations where participants are measured repeatedly on three or more separate occasions.[27] Similar to McNemar's test, the DV must be measured repeatedly on a nominal scale.

In the biomedical literature, Cochran's Q is often used to assess stability of a treat-ment over time or to compare the effectiveness of several treatments. In meta-analysis, it is also used to assess heterogeneity (i.e., instability, inconsistency) of effects reported between included studies. For example, consider a study evaluating the effectiveness of the combination treatment sildenafil and psychotherapy in reducing symptoms of erectile dysfunction (ED).[42] Eight patients with psychogenic ED attended weekly psychotherapy sessions and ingested 50 mg of sildenafil citrate orally as needed over a 6-month period. Symptoms of ED were assessed at baseline, 6 months (i.e., end of treatment), and at a 3-month posttreatment follow-up. For this study, Cochran's Q was used to evaluate a change in the stage of remission for patients dichotomized into ED vs. no ED. A statisti-cally significant finding indicated change from baseline and the possibility of sustaining effects at posttreatment follow-up. That is, all patients were diagnosed with ED at base-line; thus, a statistically significant change indicates patients indicated remission of ED symptoms at some point.

In the literature, the results of the Cochran Q test may be presented with a χ^2 statistic and a p value; however, in other studies, the results may only present a p value. Although failing to include the test statistic provides less information, it does not necessarily dam-age the integrity of results. The result of a statistically significant Cochran's Q for the example above is presented as follows:

The results of Cochran's Q indicated a statistically significant change in psychogenic ED symptoms from baseline ($p < 0.05$) suggesting a combination of psychotherapy and 50-mg sildenafil are effective in reducing ED symptoms.

Because Cochran's Q is used to assess change over three or more repeated mea-sures, it is an omnibus test. That is, the test will determine whether a statistically signifi-cant change occurred between the repeated measurements, but will not indicate where the change occurred. Thus, post hoc tests are required. For Cochran's Q, a series of McNemar tests comparing each repeated measurement serve as post hoc tests. In this example, three separate McNemar tests are required comparing baseline vs. 6 months, baseline vs. posttreatment follow-up, and 6 months vs. posttreatment follow-up. The results of a statistically significant Cochran's Q including results of post hoc McNemar tests are presented as follows:

The results of the Cochran Q test indicated a statistically significant change in psychogenic ED symptoms from baseline ($p < 0.05$). Post hoc McNemar tests indicated statistically significant changes from baseline at 6 months as well as at posttreatment follow-up (all $p < 0.05$). These results suggest the combination of psychotherapy and sildenafil is effective in reducing ED symptoms and this effect continued to reduce ED symptoms up to 3 months following treatment completion.

The assumptions of the Cochran test include:

1. The DV measured repeatedly on a dichotomous scale.
2. All DV measurements are associated.

TESTING FOR RELATIONSHIPS OR ASSOCIATIONS

When exploring the association or relationship between two or more variables, two specific types of analyses are employed—correlation or regression. These analyses are applied to determine the magnitude and direction of an association or relationship. Correlation analysis indicates the co-relationship of two variables. That is, correlation describes how one variable changes in relation to another. It is critically important to note that correlation cannot imply causation.

For example, consider the positive association between serum creatinine and BUN concentrations. In most cases, as creatinine increases so does BUN, but increasing creatinine does not cause BUN to increase or vice versa. Instead, the cause of the BUN and creatinine increase might be due to renal failure.

Regression analysis is a type of correlational analysis used to predict the value of one variable from the value of another variable. In this type of analysis, researchers attempt to determine the amount of variance in the DV that is explained by the IVs or covariates. Note that regression analysis can also permit multiple IVs and/or covariates measured on any scale. With the inclusion of multiple IVs or covariates this type of analysis is often referred to as multivariable regression analysis. While the definition of an IV and covariate is not always concrete, it is easier to think of an IV as the primary variable of interest and a covariate as a variable correlated with the DV, but not of specific interest.

For example, consider a multivariable analysis assessing the effect statin use (IV) had on all-cause mortality due to heart failure (DV) during a 5-year study period after statistically controlling for age, gender, race, comorbid conditions, and concurrent medications (covariates). The covariates may explain the reason a patient died, but are not of specific research interest.

This section begins by discussing bivariate, or two-variable, techniques followed by multivariable techniques. The discussion in this section will progress in a similar fashion to the statistical tests already presented where parametric tests will be discussed first, followed by the nonparametric alternatives.

Parametric Tests

Pearson's Product-Moment Correlation

Pearson's product-moment correlation (aka, Pearson's correlation or Pearson's r) is one of the most commonly used correlation measures. It measures the direction and strength of a linear relationship between two continuous variables. Pearson's r ranges from -1 and $+1$, with r of 0 indicating no relationship. That is, the correlation is stronger as it approaches -1 or 1. A positive correlation (e.g., 0.3 or 0.99) indicates that as the values of one variable increase so do the values of the other variable, while a negative correlation (e.g., -0.5 or -0.8) indicates that as the values of one variable increase, the values of the other variable decrease. Pearson's r tests whether the correlation of two variables is different from 0 (i.e., no relationship); thus, a statistically significant r indicates the slope of the linear relationship is not horizontal.

For example, research has shown a moderate, but statistically significant, positive correlation ($r = 0.25$) between weight in kilograms and platelet count in men aged 20–55.[43] Thus, in men, as weight increases, so does platelet count. However, the magnitude of this increase varies from person to person. That is, for any individual man, a 1-kg increase in body weight may indicate an increase in platelet count that is different from the platelet count increase for another man. It should be noted the value of r is dimensionless because it is based on standardized scores. That is, measuring weight in pounds or kilograms in the example above will not change the value of the correlation. Finally, be aware that r is substantially affected by outliers, so researchers must identify and remove them from analysis or use the nonparametric Spearman's rho discussed below.

The relationship between two variables can be assessed visually by plotting the data on a scatterplot. In fact, this practice is highly recommended.[5] The magnitude of the correlation is directly related to the strength of the linear relationship. Take a moment to consider Figures 6-13 and 6-14. In Figure 6-13, the value of Pearson's r is approximately 1 indicating a near perfect relationship between the two variables. Notice the dots on the scatterplot lay near the best-fit line and that the slope of this line is fairly steep. The positive correlation coefficient indicates that as the values of Continuous Variable 1 increase so do the values of Continuous Variable 2. In Figure 6-14, Pearson's r is approximately 0. Here, notice the dots are scattered all over the plot with no real direction, and the best-fit line is almost perfectly horizontal, which indicates no relationship between the two continuous variables.

To highlight the substantial effect outliers have on Pearson's r, take a moment to draw an outlier on Figure 6-13, say, a value of 45 for Continuous Variable 1 and a value

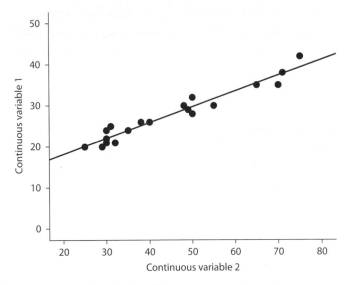

Figure 6–13. Scatterplot showing a positive correlation.

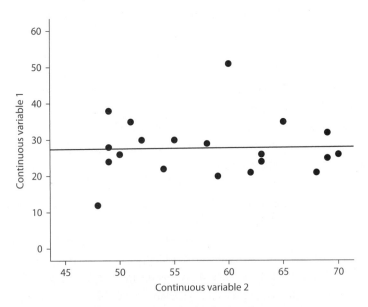

Figure 6–14. Scatterplot showing no correlation.

of 25 for Continuous Variable 2. Visualize what effect this outlier has on the previously strong positive correlation and how it would pull the best-fit line toward horizontal significantly weakening the correlation.

The result of a statistically significant Pearson's product-moment correlation with no assumption violations using the example above is presented as follows:

The results of a Pearson's product-moment correlation indicate a statistically significant moderate relationship between body weight in kilograms and platelet count ($r_{81} = 0.252, p < 0.05$) indicating body weight increased in concordance with platelet count.

Assumptions of the Pearson's product-moment correlation include:

1. Both variables are measured on an interval or ratio scale.
2. There are no outliers.
3. The relationship between the variables is linear.
4. **Homoscedasticity** is assured.
   a. The assumption states that the variability around the best-fit line of the linear relationship is the same for all data. A violation of this assumption can be seen within a scatterplot. For example, consider a scatterplot where the lower values for a variable fall near the best-fit line and higher values for this same variable fall far from the best-fit line. In this situation, the variability around the line is not constant. The tenability of this assumption is difficult to ascertain in a journal article; thus, ensure the authors noted that it was tested.
5. The observations are independent.
   a. That is, each participant provides one, and only one, observation (i.e., data or response) for each variable.

Simple Linear Regression

As stated in the previous section, the magnitude or size of the correlation is directly related to the strength of the linear relationship. The pattern of this linear relationship is typically indicated by the regression line, which is another name for the best-fit line presented in Figures 6-13 and 6-14. The regression line is a best-fit line describing how the continuous DV changes as values of the IV change. Similar to Pearson's *r*, the statistical test in simple linear regression is whether the slope of the regression line is statistically different from 0, or, stated another way, whether the regression line has no slope or is horizontal. Simple linear regression, however, takes Pearson's *r* one step further, where the regression line is used to predict values of the DV for a given value of the IV.[21] This is incredibly useful to evidence-based practitioners looking to implement findings into their practice.

The algebraic linear regression equation is: $\hat{y} = a + bx$. Here, *a* is the intercept of the regression line with the *y*-axis, *b* is the slope of the regression line, *x* is the value of the IV, and $\hat{y}$ (pronounced *y*-hat) is the predicted value of the DV. The intercept is interpreted as the predicted value of the DV when the value of the IV is 0. The slope is interpreted as the overall change in the DV for a one-unit increase in the IV. Further, it is important to note that the value of Pearson's correlation between the DV and IV is incorporated into the mathematical equation for the slope.

As an example, consider the association between systolic blood pressure measured in millimeters of mercury (mmHg) and height in centimeters for 100 children aged 5–7 years.[44] The results of this study indicated a positive Pearson correlation between height and systolic blood pressure of 0.33. Moving beyond basic correlation, the researchers used a simple linear regression analysis to predict a child's systolic blood pressure from their height. Results indicated an intercept value of 46.28 mmHg and a slope of 0.48. Using these values, the linear regression equation would be: $\hat{y} = 46.28 + (0.48*\text{Height})$. Using the interpretation of the intercept and slope provided above, the intercept value of 46.28 is the predicted systolic blood pressure for a child 0 cm tall, whereas the slope indicates that a 1-cm increase in height increases systolic blood pressure by 0.48 mmHg. From this interpretation, it is obvious that a child with a height of 0 cm is impossible. This is a prime example of the awareness readers must have when interpreting the intercept. That is, unless it makes theoretical sense to have a meaningful zero point for the IV, the interpretation of the intercept is never useful. This situation, however, should not suggest the intercept is meaningless to prediction. Instead, the intercept is simply a starting point for predicting the outcome. For example, say we want to predict systolic blood pressure for a child that is 115 cm tall; the linear regression equation becomes: $\hat{y} = 46.28 + (0.48*115)$, which equals 101.48 mmHg.

It is important to note that the predicted values of the DV are rarely identical to the actual observed values. That is, a child 115 cm tall in this sample may actually have a systolic blood pressure of 105 mmHg, but have a predicted value of 101.48 mmHg. The difference between the actual and predicted scores is referred to as a **residual value** or residual error. For the example child above, the residual value is 3.52 mmHg (i.e., $105 - 101.48$). Residual values are always calculated for all participants included in the regression analysis, and one of the assumptions of linear regression is that the residual values follow a normal distribution; this is where the assumption of normality originates for all parametric statistical tests. The tenability of this assumption is a key indicator of the reliability of the results. Therefore, if a researcher fails to describe the distribution of residuals alongside their results, the study should be read and interpreted with caution.

In addition, the interpretation of slope used in the above example is only appropriate for IVs measured on a continuous scale. If instead the IV is categorical, interpretation is slightly different. For example, consider replacing height in the example above with the dichotomous IV gender. In this situation, the researcher must specify which level of gender will serve as the reference or comparison category that is coded 0 for analysis. That is, specify which level of the IV the calculated slope represents. Note that every published study should indicate which group served as the reference category, and if the authors fail to provide a reference category, interpretation becomes impossible. Continuing, if females are specified as the reference category, the slope for gender provides the overall difference in predicted systolic blood pressure for males compared to females. Interpretation follows this logic. For example, using an example similar to the above, say a simple linear regression analysis indicated the intercept was 115.54 and the slope for gender was 15.20 with females considered the reference category. The new linear regression equation would be: $\hat{y} = 115.54 + 15.20*\text{Male}$. Thus, the intercept value of 115.54 now represents the average systolic blood pressure for a woman (i.e., when Male = 0) and the slope indicates that the predicted value of systolic blood pressure will be 15.20 mmHg higher for a man (i.e., when Male = 1) compared to a woman. Admittedly, these interpretations can be confusing, but understanding this concept is critically important to proper interpretation of study results.

The primary test used in simple linear regression is an omnibus between-groups ANOVA. It may seem esoteric, but linear regression and ANOVA are mathematically equivalent. The omnibus ANOVA provides an F test indicating whether the IV explains a statistically significant amount of variance in the DV. Stated another way, the omnibus test determines whether the IV reliably predicts the DV. Only if the ANOVA is statistically significant is the slope of the individual IV interpreted. Most research studies will provide the results of the ANOVA prior to presenting the slope of the IV. Further, the ANOVA results presented in simple linear regression will be presented identically to the one-way between-groups ANOVA examples discussed above. The statistical significance of the IV will most often be presented with the regression slope and potentially an associated t value. The slope is critical to proper interpretation of any regression analysis; thus, if the slope is not presented in the narrative portion or in a table, complete interpretation of the regression analysis is impossible and the study is essentially useless.

Finally, the amount of variance in the DV explained by the IV must also be considered. That is, how much of the reason why a participant has a particular value on the DV is attributable to their IV value. As a side note, the word "explained" should not and does not imply causality, as causality in correlational studies is extremely difficult to determine. The amount of variance explained in simple linear regression is quantified by an effect size estimate termed the "coefficient of determination." This coefficient is calculated by squaring the Pearson's r between the IV and DV (i.e., r^2 or R^2). The coefficient will often be presented as a proportion, ranging from 0 to 1, with higher values indicating more reliable prediction. From the example above, remember the correlation between a child's height and systolic blood pressure was 0.33. Thus, approximately 0.11 (i.e., 0.33^2) of the child's measured systolic blood pressure can be explained by the child's height. Said another way, approximately 11% of the reason a child has a particular systolic blood pressure value is explained by his or her height.

In the literature, the result of a statistically significant simple linear regression analysis with no assumption violations will be presented as follows:

The results of a simple linear regression analysis indicated a child's height significantly predicts systolic blood pressure ($F_{1,98}$ = 12.03, p < 0.05, r^2 = 0.11), with a 1-cm increase in height resulting in a 0.48-mmHg increase in systolic blood pressure.

The assumptions of simple linear regression include:

1. The DV is measured on an interval or ratio scale.
2. There are no outliers.
3. The relationship between the DV and IV is linear.
4. Homoscedasticity is assured.
   a. The assumption states that the variability around the regression line is the same for all data. A violation of this assumption can be seen within a scatterplot. For example, consider a scatterplot where the lower values for a variable fall near the regression line and higher values for this same variable fall far from the regression line. In this situation, the variability around the regression line is not constant. The tenability of this assumption is difficult to ascertain in a journal article; thus, ensure the authors noted that it was tested.
5. Residuals are distributed normally.
   a. Residuals are the difference between the actual and predicted values. Authors will need to state that they tested this assumption.
6. The observations are independent.
   a. That is, each participant provides one, and only one, observation (i.e., data or response) for each variable.

Multivariable Linear Regression

Multivariable linear regression (aka, multiple linear regression) is an extension of simple linear regression for designs with one continuous DV and multiple IVs or covariates measured on any scale. Remember, an IV is defined as an explanatory variable of specific research interest, while a covariate is a nuisance variable that is significantly associated with the DV, but not of specific research interest. That is, covariates are typically included because they are related to the DV or because previous research has indicated they are important. In multiple linear regression, IVs can be any combination of continuous or discrete variables (e.g., height, gender). Further, this analysis is often a better option than simple linear regression because the inclusion of additional IVs often explains a higher percentage of variance in the DV. That is, multiple linear regression produces higher R^2 values.

For example, previous research has shown a statistically significant negative Pearson's correlation between serum 25-hydroxyvitamin D (i.e., 25(OH)D; ng/mL) and serum parathyroid hormone (PTH; pg/mL) of −0.28.[45] Based on this correlation, the percentage of variance in serum PTH explained by serum 25(OH)D is 8% (i.e., -0.28^2). That is, 8% of the reason a participant has a predicted serum PTH value is associated with their serum 25(OH)D level. In an effort to increase this percentage of variance explained, a new study is designed to determine the effect serum 25(OH)D has on serum PTH after statistically adjusting for age, BMI, total calcium intake, and serum creatinine. Thus, a multiple linear regression analysis will be used to determine whether there is an effect of serum 25(OH)D on serum PTH over and above the effect of the covariates. That is, multiple linear regression assesses the unique correlation between 25(OH)D and serum PTH after removing the effects already accounted for by age, BMI, total calcium intake, and serum creatinine.

The percentage of variance explained in multiple linear regression is always referred to as R^2, where the R indicates the multiple correlation. That is, R is the multivariate extension of Pearson's r and is defined as the combined or total correlation between all IVs and the DV. Similar to Pearson's r, R ranges from -1 to 1, with 0 indicating no relationship. Thus, as R approaches -1 or 1, the association between the IVs and DV becomes stronger. In addition, most studies will also present an adjusted R^2 value, sometimes labeled R^2_{adj} in the literature. Adjusted R^2 is interpreted exactly the same as R^2, but it is adjusted for the sample size used in the study. When reading a study, comparing R^2 and adjusted R^2 is incredibly useful to interpretation, as large differences between the two indicates significant issues with the analysis, such as inadequate sample size, which essentially render the regression model useless and not generalizable to the population. Finally, it should be noted a multiple linear regression model will never explain 100% of the variance in the DV. However, do not disregard studies reporting low values of R^2 because the definition of what constitutes a large R^2 value varies by research arena. That is, lower R^2 values are expected when using human participants because measurement error is usually high. For example, consider a study using participant self-reported daily calorie intake. Large R^2 values are expected for bench research studies because in well-conducted bench research measurement error is typically not an issue. For example, think about a biomedical research study using analytic chemistry.

In general, the results of a multiple linear regression model are interpreted in an almost identical fashion to simple linear regression. As a result, please reconsider the section on simple linear regression if necessary. Similar to simple linear regression, multiple regression produces a regression equation allowing for prediction of DV values based on the y-intercept and the slope of the regression line for each IV or covariate. Briefly, the intercept is the predicted value of the DV when all values of the IVs and covariates are 0, while the slope quantifies the change in the predicted DV with a one-unit increase in the IV or covariates. Again, the regression equation is incredibly useful to evidence-based practitioners looking to implement findings into their practice. For example, consider the multiple regression example above, where serum PTH was predicted from 25(OH)D and a set of covariates. Based on the regression equation from this study, the practitioner can provide the patient with empirical evidence regarding which variables (i.e., age, BMI, total calcium intake, serum creatinine, and serum 25(OH)D) to increase or decrease, if possible, in an effort to optimize serum PTH levels and increase bone production.

The overall test of the multiple linear regression model is an omnibus between-groups ANOVA, which indicates at least one of the IVs or covariates significantly predicts the DV. However, this omnibus test fails to indicate which IVs or covariates significantly predict the DV. Thus, the statistical test for each IV or covariate is considered. Each of the statistical tests for the IVs and covariates can be considered similar to a post hoc test; however, unlike the post hoc tests discussed for ANOVA-type models above, alpha remains unadjusted. In most studies, the results of the individual IVs or covariates are presented as regression slope or t values. Note that regardless of which result an author presents, the p values will be identical. Further, interpretation of the slopes for the individual coefficients is also slightly different compared to simple linear regression. In multiple linear regression, interpretation of a particular IV or covariate is statistically adjusted for all other IVs and covariates in the regression model similar to ANCOVA.

An example may help clarify this information. Consider a situation where the result of a statistically significant multiple linear regression analysis based on the example above indicates 25(OH)D has a statistically significant slope of -1.5 pg/mL. Because the analysis is multivariable, this slope must be interpreted considering all covariates included in the model. Thus, the slope of -1.5 pg/mL indicates that after adjusting for age, BMI, total calcium intake, and serum creatinine, a one-ng/mL increase in 25(OH)D decreases predicted serum PTH 1.5 pg/mL.

Based on the example, the results of a statistically significant multiple linear regression analysis with no assumption violations are presented below. Notice the effects of statistically significant covariates (i.e., BMI and serum creatinine) are also described; however, authors will vary on which covariates, if any, they choose to interpret.

The results of a multivariable linear regression analysis indicated age, BMI, total calcium intake, serum creatinine, and 25(OH)D significantly predicted serum PTH ($F_{5,472} = 21.82$, $p < 0.05$, adjusted $R^2 = 0.18$). After adjusting for covariates, 25(OH)D significantly predicted serum PTH (slope $= -1.5$, $p < 0.05$). That is, with all else held constant, a 1 ng/mL increase in serum 25(OH)D resulted in a 1.5 pg/mL decrease in serum PTH. Regarding the individual covariates, after adjustment, increases in BMI and serum creatinine (slope $= 0.75$ and 2.12, respectively, both $p < 0.05$) resulted in higher serum PTH levels. Finally, after adjustment, age and total calcium intake were not associated with serum PTH.

The assumptions of multiple linear regression include:

1. The DV is measured on an interval or ratio scale.
2. Absence of **multicollinearity** is assured.

a. That is, no Pearson's r between any IVs and covariates should be greater than 0.90, as correlations this high indicate the variables are redundant. That is, high correlations indicate the variables may be measuring the same construct. Including redundant variables will significantly bias results. Most published studies provide Pearson correlations between the DV, IVs, and covariates; thus, a violation of this assumption is easy to identify.

3. There are no outliers.

4. The relationship between the DV and IVs and between the DV and covariates is linear.

5. Homoscedasticity is assured.

a. The assumption states that the variability around the regression line is the same for all data. A violation of this assumption can be seen within a scatterplot. For example, consider a scatterplot where the lower values for a variable fall near the regression line and higher values for this same variable fall far from the regression line. In this situation, the variability around the regression line is not constant. The tenability of this assumption is difficult to ascertain in a journal article; thus, ensure the authors noted that it was tested.

6. Residuals are distributed normally.

a. Residuals are the difference between the actual and predicted values.

7. The observations are independent.

a. That is, each participant provides one, and only one, observation (i.e., data or response) for each variable.

Nonparametric Tests

Spearman Rank-Order Correlation Coefficient

The Spearman rank-order correlation coefficient (r_s), also known as Spearman's rho (ρ), is the nonparametric alternative to Pearson's r. This correlation is used when two continuous variables have outliers, when the variables are measured on an ordinal scale, or when the relationship is nonlinear. Similar to the other nonparametric statistical tests discussed previously, this correlation is based on rank-ordered data as opposed to the actual values. The value of r_s ranges between -1 and 1, with 0 indicating no association. Thus, as r_s approaches -1 or 1, the association between the two variables becomes stronger. A statistically significant r_s indicates that the association is significantly different from 0.

As an example, consider a study to assess the effect of long-chain omega-3 fatty acid supplementation on psychosocial functioning in depressed heart failure patients.[46] Spearman's rank-order correlation was used in this study due to skewed distributions and outliers. The study found a statistically significant negative r_s of -0.40, suggesting that a 2000-mg daily dose of pure eicosapentaenoic acid (EPA) taken for 12 weeks was associated with lower depression symptoms compared to baseline.

Based on the example above, the result of a statistically significant Spearman rank-order correlation coefficient is presented as follows:

The Spearman rank-order correlation analysis was employed in lieu of Pearson's correlation due to skewed distribution and the presence of outliers. Results indicated a statistically significant negative association between baseline and 12-week depression scores for participants who received a 2000-mg daily dose of EPA ($r_s = -0.40, p < 0.05$).

The assumptions of the Spearman rank-order correlation coefficient include:

1. The two variables are measured on an ordinal, interval, or ratio scale.
2. The relationship between the two rank-ordered variables is linear.
   a. Although the relationship between the two variables based on their actual values may be nonlinear, the relationship based on rank-ordered data must be linear. This assumption typically cannot be tested by what the authors provide in the narrative. Thus, when authors fail to indicate whether the assumption was tested results should be viewed with caution.
3. The observations are independent.
   a. That is, each participant provides one, and only one, observation (i.e., data or response) for each variable.

Logistic Regression

The interpretation of a logistic regression analysis is similar to linear regression; thus, a basic understanding of the interpretation of simple and multiple linear regression is extremely useful. Please reconsider reading the sections discussing simple and multivariable linear regression as much of the material discussed here is simply an extension of the material described in detail previously.

Logistic regression is used when the DV is measured on a dichotomous scale and the relationship between the DV and IV is nonlinear. This analysis is ubiquitous in the biomedical sciences. It is important to note that in any logistic regression analysis, the measurement scale of the DV is always considered unordered. That is, the dichotomous DV is always considered to be measured on a nominal scale. While the logistic regression analyses discussed here are only for a dichotomous DV, an extension of logistic regression is available for a categorical DV with three or more categories. This analysis is termed "multinomial logistic regression," with the definition of multinomial being multiple nominal categories. Interpretation of results from this analysis is similar to the analyses discussed in this section and interested readers are encouraged to consider the suggested readings at the end of the chapter.

As an example of a design requiring a simple logistic regression analysis, consider a 5-year study designed to assess the effect that the duration of statin use measured as percentage of time on any statin during the study period has on all-cause mortality in a sample of Veterans Administration patients previously experiencing congestive heart failure. Note that the DV is dichotomous (i.e., dead vs. alive). Further, a simple logistic regression analysis can always be extended to a multivariable analysis by including additional IVs and covariates in an effort to explain more of the reason why patients experienced the outcome of interest. For example, consider a multivariable extension to the study above where the effect duration of statin use has on all-cause mortality is assessed after controlling for age, race, gender, concurrent medications, and comorbid conditions.

For all logistic regression models, researchers must choose a reference category for the DV. When identified, the reference category is used as a comparison group for the primary outcome of interest. In most situations, the reference category is typically the category determined by the researcher to be of less specific interest. For example, consider all-cause mortality, a dichotomous DV (i.e., dead vs. alive). Most studies are interested in the individuals who died; essentially the researcher wants to identify the primary reasons for death. Thus, with patients alive at the end of the study period considered the reference category, all regression slopes are calculated for patients who died compared to patients who lived. Thus, the first step in properly interpreting the results of logistic regression analysis is to identify the primary outcome of interest and the reference category within the DV. It should be noted that most authors will not explicitly identify the primary outcome of interest or the reference category; however, this information can be obtained easily as all results and interpretations are typically written in relation to the primary outcome of interest.

Similar to linear regression, a logistic regression analysis provides a regression equation that can be used to predict the probability of experiencing primary outcome of interest. Briefly, the regression equation contains a y-intercept and slope values for all IVs included in the analysis. This equation is interpreted slightly different from linear regression because the association between the DV and IV is nonlinear. That is, because probability is bounded between 0 and 1, the slope must essentially shut off at these bounds. However, the usefulness of the equation is the same. That is, the equation can be used to assist evidence-based practitioners in instructing patients regarding what changes need to be made to optimize or prevent a specific outcome.

The primary statistical test in logistic regression determines whether the logistic model including all IVs or covariates better predicts the probability of experiencing the outcome of interest compared to the model with no IVs or covariates. That is, a logistic regression analysis determines whether the IVs significantly predict the primary outcome of interest. Similar to linear regression, this overall test is an omnibus chi-square test. If this omnibus chi-square test is statistically significant, the statistical significance of each IV or covariate is assessed and interpreted. These tests of individual predictors can be thought of as post hoc tests, and typically no adjustment is made to alpha. When interpreting the results for individual predictors, authors typically provide two values, the slope and odds ratio.

The slope is interpreted similar to linear regression; however, slopes in logistic regression indicate changes in the **log-odds** (aka, **logits**) of experiencing the outcome of interest. That is, a one-unit increase in the IV indicates a change in the predicted log-odds of experiencing the primary outcome of interest. While a full description of log-odds or logits is beyond the scope of this chapter, they can be thought of simply as a linear transformation of probability. That is, after transformation, log-odds or logits are linear; thus, their values can be interpreted similarly to slopes in linear regression. For example, reconsider the 5-year study assessing the effect duration of statin use, measured as percentage of time on any statin during the study period, has on all-cause mortality. Say, the slope for statin use is −0.25. With death considered the primary outcome of interest and alive serving as the reference category, this slope suggests that a 1% increase in statin use during the study period resulted in a 0.25-unit decrease in the log-odds of dying. Note this was a decrease because the slope was negative. Based on this interpretation, a common question is, what does a 0.25-unit decrease in log-odds mean? While the slope is integral in producing the regression equation, the interpretation in log-odds can be fairly convoluted. Thus, logistic regression provides an alternative value that some individuals find easier to interpret—the odds ratio.

The odds ratio produced by a logistic regression analysis is calculated and interpreted similarly to the odds ratios discussed in the "Epidemiological Statistics" section earlier in the chapter. Briefly, odds ratios range from 0 to infinity, with 1 indicating no association. Therefore, an odds ratio above 1 indicates an increase in the odds of experiencing the primary outcome of interest, whereas an odds ratio below 1 indicates a decrease in the odds of experiencing the primary outcome of interest. For example, reconsider the example above with a slope of −0.25. The associated odds ratio for this slope is 0.78. Because the odds ratio is below 1, a 1% increase in statin use is associated with a 22% (i.e., 1 − 0.78) decrease in the odds of dying during the study period.

It is important to be aware that authors will vary the information they present in journal articles, as one article may only provide slopes as log-odds and another article may provide odds ratios. This is not an issue, however, because there is a direct mathematical relationship between slopes and odds ratios. That is, the slope is the natural log of the odds ratio (i.e., ln 0.78 = −0.25) and the odds ratio is simply the exponentiated slope (i.e., $e^{-0.25} = 0.78$). It should become clear that this mathematical relationship is where the definition of log-odds originates; they are literally the log of the odds. Given this relationship, if an author provides log-odds, the odds ratio can be easily calculated to ease interpretation. Also, note that regardless of which value the authors present, the associated p value will be identical. That is, a statistically significant slope will have a statistically significant odds ratio, and vice versa.

Finally, similar to linear regression, the primary reason a researcher includes additional IVs and covariates in a multivariable logistic regression model are to increase the amount of variance explained in the primary outcome of interest. However, unlike R^2 in linear regression, there is no accepted measure for quantifying explained variance in logistic regression, although several R^2 values exist, with the most common including the Nagelkerke R^2 and the Cox and Snell R^2. These pseudo-R^2 values are used to approximate R^2 from linear regression and are interpreted in similar fashion.

Based on the example described above, the result of a simple logistic regression analysis is presented as follows:

The results of a simple logistic regression analysis indicated a statistically significant association between duration of statin use and all-cause mortality. ($\chi^2_1 = 13.65$, $p < 0.05$) where a 1% increase in duration of statin use resulted in a 22% decrease in the odds of dying during the study period.

An example of a multivariable logistic regression analysis, with the addition of age, race, gender, concurrent medications, and comorbid conditions as covariates is presented below. Notice in this example, the researcher is not interested in the individual effects of the covariates, as they are not interpreted.

The results of a multivariable logistic regression analysis indicated a statistically significant overall association between the variables as a set and all-cause mortality ($\chi^2_1 = 156.02$, $p < 0.05$). After controlling for age, race, gender, concurrent medications, and comorbid conditions, duration of statin use significantly predicted all-cause mortality (OR = 0.62, $p < 0.05$). Thus, holding all variables constant, a 1% increase in statin use resulted in a 38% decrease in all-cause mortality.

The assumptions of logistic regression include:

1. The DV is discrete with mutually exclusive categories.
2. The sample size is large.
   a. A very rudimentary rule is to have at least 50 participants per variable included in the model. A large sample is required so that the parameters (e.g., slopes, standard errors) are estimated accurately.[47] Using this rule, a model with 10 IVs or covariates requires a minimum of 500 participants (i.e., 10*50 = 500).
3. Adequacy of expected frequencies is assured.
   a. This assumption applies only to categorical IVs and is the same assumption as the chi-square test. That is, no more than 20% of cells can have expected frequencies less than 5. This is a difficult assumption to verify, outside of calculating the expected frequencies by hand. Thus, if an article fails to indicate this assumption was tested, view results with caution. However, most studies using logistic regression will have large sample sizes and this assumption is rarely violated.
4. Linearity in the logit is assured.
   a. Remember, logit and log-odds are synonyms. This is a convoluted assumption, and difficult to explain without getting into mathematical detail. However, the

logit is defined as the linear transformation of probability. This assumption is tested by determining whether the relationship between continuous IVs or covariates and the DV is linear. This is a key assumption, and a violation severely biases results. Thus, if authors do not mention the assumption was assured in the methods or results sections, view results with caution.

5. Absence of multicollinearity assured.

   a. That is, no Pearson's r between any continuous IVs and covariates should be greater than 0.90, as correlations this high indicate the variables are redundant. That is, high correlations indicate the variables may be measuring the same facet. Including redundant variables will significantly bias results.

6. There are no outliers.

7. The observations are independent.

   a. That is, each participant provides one, and only one, observation (i.e., data or response) for each variable.

Survival Analysis

Survival analysis (or failure analysis) consists of three of the most commonly used statistical techniques in the biomedical sciences—life tables, the Kaplan-Meier method, and Cox proportional-hazards model or Cox regression. Survival analysis is concerned with time-to-event data; that is, the time to experience an outcome of interest. For example, consider a study designed to examine whether a new immunotherapy, in comparison to chemotherapy, prolongs remission in women previously diagnosed with breast cancer over a 20-week study period.

In survival analysis, participants who do not experience the outcome of interest are considered to survive, while those who experience the event are considered to fail. Although this is fairly grim terminology, survival and failure do not necessarily imply living or dying. For example, in the example above, failure was defined as breast cancer recurrence, not death. In survival analysis, the outcome will typically be dichotomous, patients do not need to enter the study at the same time because enrollment can be continuous, and patients are followed until the study ends which is known as end of follow-up.

Patients who do not experience the event by the end of follow-up, who are lost to follow-up, or who drop out of the study are termed "censored." The key advantage survival analysis has over the analyses presented above, particularly logistic regression, is that it can handle censored data, which is essentially incomplete data. That is, censored data are considered incomplete because the researcher does not know when or if participants experienced the event. Survival analysis can handle censored data because the DV is time, which is a continuous variable allowed to vary for each participant. Thus, as long as a participant has a survival time indicated, they are included in analysis. The key point here is that survival time for a censored participant is the time until they were censored, whether that is end of follow-up or whether they left the study for reasons other than suffering the event. Thus, all participants who entered the study are included in analysis regardless of whether they experienced the event or are censored, because the analysis only considers the time they were in the study.

Life Tables

Life tables present time-to-event data in table format. That is, a life table tabulates the time that has elapsed until an event is experienced. Life tables are used to indicate the proportion of individuals surviving or not experiencing the event based on fixed or varying time intervals.

For example, reconsider the example above evaluating the effectiveness of the new immunotherapy in preventing recurrence of breast cancer. A life table allows the researcher to tabulate the cumulative proportion of women who do not have a recurrence of breast cancer at any interval, whether it is 6 months, 1 year, or 3 years.

As stated in the introduction to this section, life tables can be based on fixed or varying time intervals. Life tables based on fixed time intervals have a significant weakness, as they do not consider the exact time within the specified interval when the patient experienced the event. Thus, depending on the length of the time interval, a great amount of information could be lost regarding the exact time the event was experienced. That is, the longer the time interval, the less precise a researcher can be regarding the exact moment the event occurred. Thankfully, better methods have emerged, particularly the Kaplan-Meier method.

The Kaplan-Meier Method

The Kaplan-Meier method is the most widely used estimator of survival time in the biomedical sciences.[48] The Kaplan-Meier method is an extension of the life table using varying time intervals. Using this method, the cumulative proportion surviving is recalculated every time an event occurs.[49]

As an example, instead of assessing the total number of women who have a breast cancer recurrence at fixed intervals of 6 months, the Kaplan-Meier method recalculates the proportion of women surviving every time a woman in the study has a recurrence. In most studies, Kaplan-Meier data is presented as a graph of the cumulative survival over the study period known as a Kaplan-Meier curve. The Kaplan-Meier curve presents either a survival or hazard function, where the survival function is the cumulative frequency of participants not experiencing the event, whereas the hazard function is the cumulative frequency of participants experiencing the event. A Kaplan-Meier curve is provided in the vast majority of published literature using survival analysis and will appear similar to the survival curve presented in Figure 6-15. Note that for ease of interpretation, the curve in Figure 6-15 only presents data for the sample of women initiating the new immunotherapy and does not include

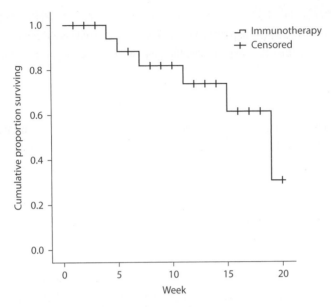

Figure 6-15. Kaplan-Meier curve.

data for women initiating chemotherapy. Notice that the *y*-axis indicates the cumulative proportion of women surviving, while the *x*-axis indicates the total number of weeks of the study. The solid line represents the survival function. That is, the cumulative proportion of women not experiencing the event at any given time. The survival function indicates when a woman experienced the event when the function steps down. For example, by week 5, two women have experienced the event, indicated by the two steps in the survival function. Further, notice the vertical dashes throughout the survival function. These dashes indicate individual women who were censored. That is, women dropped out of the study for reasons other than experiencing the event such as side effects or they simply were lost to follow-up by moving out of the area. Few studies provide explicit information regarding censored participants on the Kaplan-Meier curve because most survival analyses involve large samples. Thus, the dashes in Figure 6-15 are usually omitted from the curve; however, frequency counts of censored participants are always provided within the narrative or in table format.

The Kaplan-Meier curve can also be presented for multiple groups. For example, consider the overall survival of women initiating immunotherapy compared to women initiating chemotherapy. Figure 6-16 presents a Kaplan-Meier curve where the survival functions for both treatment groups are presented simultaneously. Interpretation of these survival functions is identical to the methods described above for Figure 6-15. However, with two or more treatment groups, a statistical test must be conducted to assess for a statistically significant group difference in survival rate. The most common test in the biomedical literature is the log-rank test (aka, the Mantel-Cox test).[49] A statistically

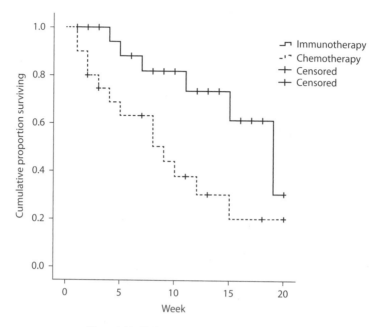

Figure 6-16. Kaplan-Meier curve—comparing groups.

significant log-rank test indicates there is a significant difference in survival rate between the groups. However, it is important to note that a Kaplan-Meier curve and associated log-rank test have no way of indicating why the breast cancer recurred beyond the possibility of the therapy being ineffective.

Based on the survival functions presented in Figure 6-16, the results of a statistically significant log-rank test are presented as follows:

Based on Kaplan-Meier curves, the results of the log-rank test indicated a statistically significant difference in duration of breast cancer remission between immunotherapy and chemotherapy groups $(\chi^2_1 = 5.68, p < 0.05)$, with women initiating the immunotherapy experiencing significantly longer breast cancer remission.

It should be noted that when more than two treatment groups are being compared the log-rank test is an omnibus test. That is, with three or more groups, a statistically significant log-rank test will indicate that a statistically significant difference exists between groups, but will not indicate specifically which groups differ. Thus, post hoc log-rank tests are required to determine where a significant difference in survival occurred.

For example, consider the addition of another treatment group to the breast cancer example, say, women who do not want to initiate any therapy. Following a statistically significant omnibus log-rank test, three post hoc log-rank tests would be required to determine whether statistically significant differences in survival rate occurred between immunotherapy vs. chemotherapy, immunotherapy vs. no therapy, and chemotherapy vs. no therapy.

The results of statistically significant post hoc tests are presented as follows:

Based on Kaplan-Meier curves, the results of the log-rank test indicated a statistically significant difference in breast cancer recurrence between the three treatment groups ($\chi^2_2 = 9.76$, p < 0.05). Post hoc log-rank tests indicated women initiating immunotherapy experienced significantly longer breast cancer remission compared to women receiving chemotherapy or women choosing not to receive therapy (both p < 0.05). No statistically significant difference was indicated between women initiating chemotherapy and women receiving no therapy.

Cox Proportional Hazards Model

Although the Kaplan-Meier method is effective in assessing for overall differences in survival, the analysis is unable to identify the association between covariates and survival. That is, the Kaplan-Meier method cannot identify whether the IV significantly predicts survival, and for many studies, prediction is a far more important consideration. Thus, a form of regression analysis is required. The Cox proportional hazards model (aka, Cox regression) is a semiparametric method used to predict the risk of experiencing an event of interest. Note that the DV is a dichotomous variable and the analysis is considered semiparametric because it includes both parametric and nonparametric components. In addition, all predictor variables in a Cox regression are termed "covariates." That is, in the literature, authors will not identify a distinction between IVs and covariates. Finally, it should also be noted that most published studies progress from Kaplan-Meier curves and log-rank tests to Cox regression analysis. That is, the Kaplan-Meier curve will first present the survival functions for the covariate of interest as well as associated log-rank tests and then authors will present the results of a Cox regression assessing for the relationship between covariates and the event of interest.

The interpretation of Cox regression can be considered a combination of linear and logistic regression; however, the primary difference is that in Cox regression results are considered time dependent. That is, Cox regression is concerned with the time-dependent risk of experiencing the event instead of the overall occurrence of events as in logistic regression. Remember, the DV is time. For example, consider a study designed to assess the effect duration of statin use, measured as percentage of time in any statin during the study period, has on all-cause mortality in a sample of Veterans Administration patients previously experiencing congestive heart failure. If the researchers were interested in the effect duration of statin use had on prolonging the time until death during the study period, a Cox regression analysis is the analysis of choice. Again, the primary consideration in Cox regression is the risk of experiencing the event, not in the overall probability of the event as in logistic regression.

Similar to linear and logistic regression, Cox regression can be simple or multivariable. For example, in the example above a simple Cox regression analysis was required because only duration of statin use was used to predict the risk of death. However, if the study was extended to statistically control for age, gender, race, comorbid conditions, and concurrent medications, a multivariable Cox regression is appropriate. That is, assess the effects duration of statin use had on the risk of death over and above the effects of the other covariates.

Similar to logistic regression analysis, within the DV the researcher must choose the primary event of interest and the associated reference category. When identified, the reference category is used as a comparison group for the event of interest. In most situations, the reference category is typically the category determined by the researcher to be of less specific interest. For example, consider all-cause mortality, a dichotomous outcome variable, in which most studies are interested in the individuals who died. Thus, patients who lived are usually considered the reference category and all regression slopes are calculated for patients who died compared to patients who lived. Therefore, the first step in properly interpreting the results of a Cox regression analysis is to identify the event and the reference category. If an author does not explicitly state the reference category, this information can be obtained easily as all results and interpretations are typically written in relation to the primary event of interest.

It is critically important to note that in the literature, authors will report using one of two different Cox regression analyses—with or without time-varying covariates. The decision of which model to use is based on whether the proportionality of hazards assumption was violated. This assumption typically applies to all categorical covariates and states that, although events can begin to occur at any time during the study period, when events do begin, the rate at which events occur between levels of a categorical covariate must remain constant over time. That is, when events begin to occur, the survival functions for the groups must be the same or roughly parallel.

For example, reconsider Figure 6-16. Here, the proportionality of hazards assumption is not violated because events occur at approximately the same rate in each group. Notice women initiating the new immunotherapy did not begin experiencing breast cancer recurrence until week 4, as indicated by no steps in the curve until week 4, whereas women in the chemotherapy group began experiencing the recurrence at week 1, steps occurred immediately. However, when events began to occur in either group, they occurred at approximately the same rate. That is, the slopes of the survival functions are roughly parallel. Thus, the proportionality of hazards assumption is not violated and the treatment group covariate is assumed to have constant survival rates over time. More specifically, in this situation a Cox regression without time-varying covariates is appropriate.

By contrast, a violation of the proportionality assumption is provided in Figure 6-17. Notice that in this figure, events began occurring at roughly around weeks 3 and 4 within both treatment groups. However, the survival functions are drastically different, and in fact intersect twice. In general, any time survival functions intersect, the proportionality of

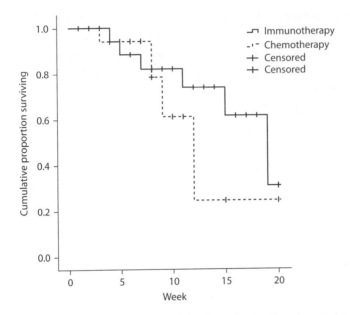

Figure 6–17. Kaplan-Meier curve showing violation of proportionality of hazards assumption.

hazards assumption can be considered violated, because the rate of survival within each group varies across time. In this situation, Cox regression with time-varying covariates would be required.

In conclusion, when reading a journal article, take careful notice of the Kaplan-Meier curves presented prior to the Cox regression analysis. A violation of this assumption is likely any time survival functions intersect. If a violation is observed, identify whether the appropriate Cox regression analysis was employed. That is, if a violation is indicated, Cox regression with time-varying covariates must be used. If Cox regression without time-varying covariates was used in the presence of a violation, results and interpretations are biased to some unknown extent.

Similar to the other forms of regression discussed, Cox regression allows research-ers to produce a regression equation useful in determining the overall risk score for a patient based on specific characteristics. The primary difference in Cox regression, how-ever, is that there is no y-intercept representing the baseline hazard function. Thus, overall risk is calculated simply by using the slopes for the covariates. Even without the intercept, however, this regression equation remains useful for evidence-based practitioners when consulting their patients on changes required for decreasing the risk of experiencing an unfavorable event.

Identical to logistic regression, the overall statistical test in Cox regression is whether the model including the covariates predicts the risk of experiencing the event significantly better than the model with no covariates. That is, a Cox regression analysis determines whether the covariates significantly predict the risk of experiencing the primary event of interest. This overall test is an omnibus chi-square test. Only if this omnibus chi-square test is statistically significant does the researcher evaluate the statistical significance of each covariate. The tests of individual predictors are usually more important and these will be presented in all studies using a Cox regression model. Tests of individual predictors will be presented by regression slopes and/or hazard ratios.

In Cox regression, slopes are interpreted similar to logistic regression. However, for this analysis, a one-unit increase in a covariate results in an increase or decrease in the log-hazard or log-risk of experiencing the event. Although a full description of log-risk is beyond the scope of this chapter, they can be thought of simply as a linear transformation of probability of experiencing the event. That is, after transformation, log-risks are linear and their values can be interpreted similarly to slopes in linear regression. For example, say the slope for women initiating the new immunotherapy was -0.65. That is, women initiating chemotherapy served as the reference or comparison group. Thus, the slope represents a 0.65-unit decrease in the log-risk of breast cancer recurrence for immunotherapy compared to chemotherapy. A 0.65-unit decrease in log-hazard is difficult to explain and beyond the scope of this chapter; thus, the presentation and interpretation of hazard ratios are often a useful alternative.

The hazard ratio produced by a Cox regression analysis is calculated and interpreted similarly to the relative risk discussed in the "Epidemiological Statistics" section earlier in the chapter. It is important to note that a hazard ratio will approximate a relative risk only when the proportionality of hazards assumption is satisfied and censoring is minimal. Briefly, hazard ratios range from 0 to infinity, with 1 indicating no association. Therefore, a hazard ratio above 1 indicates an increase in the risk of experiencing the event, whereas a hazard ratio below 1 indicates a decrease in the risk of experiencing the event. For example, reconsider the example above where the slope for the new immunotherapy was -0.65. The associated hazard ratio for this slope is 0.52. Because the hazard ratio is below 1, initiating immunotherapy resulted in a 48% (i.e., $1 - 0.52$) decrease in the risk of breast cancer recurrence compared to chemotherapy.

It is important to consider that authors may vary the information they present in journal articles, as one study may only provide slopes and another study may only provide hazard ratios. This is not an issue because there is a direct mathematical relationship between slopes and hazard ratios. That is, the slope is simply the natural log of the hazard ratio (i.e., $\ln 0.52 = -0.65$), whereas the hazard ratio is simply the exponentiated slope (i.e., $e^{-0.65} = 0.52$). It should become clear that this mathematical relationship is where the definition of log-risk originates; they are literally the log of the risk. Thus, if an author only provides slopes, the hazard ratio can be easily calculated to ease interpretation. Also, note that regardless of which value the authors present, the associated p value will be identical. That is, a statistically significant slope will have a statistically significant hazard ratio, and vice versa.

Finally, similar to logistic regression, no commonly accepted R^2 exists for Cox regression to indicate proportion of variance explained by the predictor variables, although several have been suggested.[48] Thus, when reading a journal article, do not be discouraged by authors failing to provide this information.

Based on the breast cancer example above, a statistically significant multivariable Cox regression analysis is presented below. Note that this Results section will typically be presented in addition to the results of the Kaplan-Meier analysis above.

No violation of the proportionality of hazards assumption was indicated; thus, a Cox regression without time dependent covariates was conducted to assess the effectiveness of immunotherapy compared to chemotherapy in preventing breast cancer recurrence after adjusting for age, concurrent medications, and comorbid conditions. Results indicated the covariates, as a set, significantly predicted risk of breast cancer recurrence ($\chi^2_8 = 63.12$, $p < 0.05$). Holding age, concurrent medications, and comorbid conditions constant, women initiating immunotherapy experienced a 48% decrease in the risk of breast cancer recurrence compared to women initiating chemotherapy.

The assumptions of Cox regression include:

1. Time is measured on an interval or ratio scale.
2. Sample size must be large.
    a. A very rudimentary rule is to have at least 50 participants per variable included in the model. A large sample is required so that the parameters (e.g., slopes, standard errors) are estimated accurately.[47] Using this rule, a model with 10 IVs and covariates requires a minimum of 500 participants (i.e., 10*50 = 500).
3. Proportionality of hazards is assured.
    a. The survival functions for all categorical covariates must be similar.
4. No differences between withdrawn and remaining cases exist.
    a. Because Cox regression can handle censored data, participants who are lost to follow-up must not differ from those whose outcome is known. That is, participants who dropped out of the study must not be different from those who completed it. For example, women who dropped out of immunotherapy group because they are experiencing unbearable side effects that do not occur in the chemotherapy group.
5. Absence of multicollinearity is assured.
    a. That is, no Pearson's r between any continuous covariates should be greater than 0.90, as correlations this high indicate the variables are redundant. High correlations indicate the variables may be measuring the same facet. Including redundant variables will significantly bias results.
6. There are no outliers.

7. Observations are independent.
   a. That is, each participant provides one, and only one, observation (i.e., data or response) for each variable.

Case Study 6–3

Although warfarin is inexpensive and effective in treating deep vein thrombosis (DVT), pulmonary embolism (PE), and atrial fibrillation (AF), it requires close monitoring of international normalized ratio (INR) due to its narrow therapeutic index, interpatient dosing variability, and drug and food interactions. Therefore, appropriate management in an inpatient setting is essential. A 2-year retrospective study was conducted using medical records of patients admitted for DVT, PE, and/or AF who were on warfarin during their hospital stay to identify whether the patients were actively managed by either a hospital pharmacist or physician and then compare whether patients achieved therapeutic INR. A total of 150 patient charts were identified with 115 (76.7%) patients being pharmacist-managed and 35 (23.3%) being physician-managed.

Please answer the following questions:

1. What is the DV for this study? What is its scale of measurement?
2. What is the IV for this study? How many levels does the IV have?
3. Say the researchers used the chi-square test for the outcome. What research question would this statistical test answer?
4. Say the researchers instead used logistic regression. What research question would this statistical test answer?
5. Say the researchers instead used the Kaplan-Meier method. What research question would this statistical test answer? What additional information would be required to conduct this statistical test?
6. Say the researchers used Cox proportional-hazards model. What research question would this statistical test answer? What additional information would be required to conduct this statistical test?
7. Failing to achieve therapeutic INR by day 5 has been shown to influence the duration of parenteral therapy bridging as well as hospital length of stay. Say that the researchers classified patients as achieving therapeutic INR within 5 days or not. Results of the chi-square test indicated no statistically significant difference between those who were pharmacist- or physician managed (43.5% vs. 42.9%, respectively, $p = .948$).

However, when considering patients who achieved therapeutic INR after inpatient day 5 as censored, results of the Kaplan-Meier method indicated a statistically significant difference favoring the patients who were pharmacist-managed. How could these apparently conflicting statistical test results be possible?

Conclusion

A thorough understanding of statistical methods is integral to effectively evaluating medical literature. Being cognizant of the effect study design has on results, interpretation, and generalization is incredibly important to implementing evidence-based practice. Statistical analyses are simply a piece of the puzzle when evaluating literature, since the study design and research question determine the appropriate analyses. It must be noted that simply because a study is published does not define it as a quality study. Further, all research has flaws, some trivial, others significant. A reader's task is to determine whether these flaws prevent the research from being credible.[50] Thus, when reviewing an empirical study, the following steps must be considered carefully:

1. Thoughtfully consider the study design (see Chapters 4 and 5). This includes, but is not limited to, the theory, specific research question(s), randomization, sample characteristics, data collection methods, variables, and outcomes. A poor design will lead to inaccurate or biased estimates, leading to an inferior study.
2. Evaluate the statistical test. Is it appropriate for the research question? Did the author test for assumption violations? If no assumption tests are stated, can violations be determined from the descriptive statistics provided? Was the test interpreted properly? Were effect size (i.e., clinical significance) measures provided?
3. Evaluate the discussion section. Are the results interpreted within the context of the sample and population? Are generalizations accurate? What were the limitations? How does the study lend itself to future research?

Finally, to reiterate, this chapter is by no means exhaustive of all statistical tests, nor does it provide a complete overview of statistical tests. Interested readers are encouraged to consult any of the suggested readings below for a more thorough treatment of the topics discussed.

Self-Assessment Questions

1. Consider a randomized controlled trial in which patients were randomized to a treatment or control condition using a 1:1 allocation ratio (i.e., equal group sizes). The randomization schedule was designed to ensure that an equal number of males and females are enrolled, and also that within each biological sex, the allocation ratio was maintained at 1:1. What type of sampling design is this?
   a. Convenience sample
   b. Cluster sample
   c. Stratified random sample
   d. Multistage sample

2. The independent variable in question 1 has which measurement scale?
   a. Nominal
   b. Ordinal
   c. Interval
   d. Ratio

3. Say a continuous variable, such as board scores from the North American Pharmacist Licensure Examination (NAPLEX) are categorized into pass vs. not pass, where ≥ 75 is determined to be the cutoff for passing. If this new categorical variable were included in a statistical analysis, pharmacists who passed the NAPLEX with a score of 75 would be considered qualitatively superior from individuals who did not pass with a score of 74.
   a. True
   b. False

4. The most appropriate measure of central tendency for continuous, non-normally distributed data is:
   a. Mean
   b. Median
   c. Mode
   d. Range

5. Variance is an incredibly important statistic that is used in all statistical analyses. Although, most journal articles will only report the standard deviation, it is easy to translate between standard deviation and variance. For example, say the standard deviation of a continuous variable is reported to be 4. What is the variance?
   a. 2
   b. 8

c. 16

d. 4

6. What does the width of the box in a boxplot represent?

   a. The interquartile range

   b. The range of data up to 1.5 interquartile ranges from the median

   c. Outliers

   d. Extreme outliers

7. A z score of -1 indicates that a specific data point is what?

   a. The data point is 1 standard deviation above variable's mean.

   b. The data point is 1 interquartile range from the variable's median.

   c. The variable has a range of 1.

   d. The data point is 1 standard deviation below the variable's mean.

8. An odds ratio of 1.25 indicates that:

   a. There is a 25% decrease in the odds of experiencing some outcome.

   b. There is a 75% increase in the odds of experiencing some outcome.

   c. One group is 25% less likely to experience the outcome compared to another group.

   d. There is a 25% increase in the odds of experiencing some outcome.

9. A study in which clinics are randomized to treatment vs. control would be an example of which study design?

   a. Nonexperimental

   b. Experimental

   c. Quasi-experimental

   d. None of the above

10. A 2-year study in which participants receive one, and only one, of two treatments without planned interim analyses or modifications is an example of what type of study design?

    a. A crossover design

    b. A randomized controlled trial

    c. A parallel-groups design

    d. An adaptive design

11. A statistical test is used to evaluate for differences between two treatment groups. Alpha is set at 0.05. The statistical test indicates $p = 0.0001$, which is statistically significant. This small p value indicates a clinically significant difference.

    a. True

    b. False

12. Statistical power of 0.95 (or 95%) indicates that:
    a. The statistical test result was not statistically significant when in fact the result does exist in the population.
    b. The probability of finding a statistically significant effect when one exists in the population.
    c. The statistical test result is significant when in fact the result does not exist in the population.
    d. The result of the statistical test will be true in the population.

13. The 95% confidence interval indicates that:
    a. There is a 95% probability that the true population parameter is within the interval.
    b. If repeated random sampling occurred from the population of interest using identical sample sizes, the true population parameter would be included in the 95% of 95% confidence intervals.
    c. There is 95% certainty that the parameter estimate is correct.
    d. None of the above.

14. A nonparametric test is most appropriate when:
    a. The distributional assumptions of a parametric statistical test is violated.
    b. There are larger numbers of outliers.
    c. The sample size is small.
    d. All of the above.

15. A drug safety trial is designed to evaluate the proportion of patients who suffered congestive heart failure (i.e., yes vs. no) after taking a new drug compared to placebo. Patients were followed for 2 years. The analysis will control for a variety of patient characteristics (e.g., age, biological sex, comorbidities). Which analysis is appropriate given the research question?
    a. A multivariable logistic regression model
    b. The multivariable Cox proportional-hazards model
    c. Pearson's chi-square test
    d. Mantel-Haenszel chi-square test

REFERENCES

1. United States Census Bureau. Census regions and divisions of the United States [Internet]. [Cited 2010 Jun 24.] Available from: http://www.census.gov/geo/www/us_regdiv.pdf
2. Stevens SS. On the theory of scales of measurement. Science. 1946;103(2684):677-80.
3. Hockenberry MJ, Wilson D. Wong's essentials for pediatric nursing. 8th ed. St. Louis (MO): Mosby; 2009.

4. Tabachnick BG, Fidell LS. Using multivariate statistics. 5th ed. Boston (MA): Pearson Education Inc.;2007.

5. Tukey JW. Exploratory data analysis. Reading (MA): Addison-Wesley; 1977.

6. Gordis L. Epidemiology. Philadelphia (PA): Saunders Elsevier; 2009.

7. Hennekens CH, Buring JE. Epidemiology in medicine. In: Mayrent SL, editor. Philadelphia (PA): Lippincott, Williams, and Wilkins; 1987.

8. Friis RH. Epidemiology 101. Sudbury (MA): Jones and Bartlett Publishers; 2010.

9. Campbell DT, Stanley JC. Experimental and quasi-experimental designs for research. Chicago (IL): Rand McNally & Company; 1963.

10. Feinstein AR. Epidemiologic analyses of causation: the unlearned scientific lessons of randomized trials. J Clin Epidemiol. 1989;42(6):481-9.

11. Ioannidis JP, Haidich AB, Pappa M, Pantazis N, Kokori SI, Tektonidou MG, Contopoulos-Ioannidis DG, Lau J. Comparison of evidence of treatment effects in randomized and non-randomized studies. JAMA. 2001;286(7):821-30.

12. United States National Institutes of Health. Understanding Clinical Trials [Internet]. [Cited 2010 Jun 25]. Available from: http://clinicaltrials.gov/ct2/info/understand#Q18

13. Hopewell S, Dutton S, Yu L-M, Chan A-W, Altman DG. The quality of reports of randomized trials in 2000 and 2006: comparative study of articles indexed in PubMed. BMJ. 2010;340(c723):1-8.

14. Everitt BS, Pickles A. Statistical aspects of the design and analysis of clinical trials. 2nd ed. River Edge (NJ): Imperial College Press; 2004.

15. Chow S, Liu J. Design and analysis of clinical trials: concepts and methodologies. 2nd ed. Hoboken (NJ): John Wiley & Sons; 2004.

16. International Conference on Harmonisation of Technical Requirements for Registration of Pharmaceuticals for Human Use (ICH). Statistical Principles for Clinical Trials E9 [Internet]. [Cited 2010 Jun 26]. Available from: http://www.ich.org/LOB/media/MEDIA485.pdf

17. United States Department of Health and Human Services. Guidance for industry: Adaptive design clinical trials for drugs and biologics [Internet]. [Cited 2010 Jun 18]. Available from: http://www.fda.gov/downloads/Drugs/GuidanceComplianceRegulatoryInformation/Guidances/UCM201790.pdf

18. Lachin JM. Statistical considerations in the intent-to-treat principle. Control Clin Trials. 2000;21(3):167-89.

19. Enders CK. A primer on the use of modern missing-data methods in psychosomatic medicine research. Psychosom Med. 2006;68(3):427-36.

20. Rubin DB. Inference and missing data. Biometrika. 1976;63(3):581-92.

21. Moore DS. The basic practice of statistics. 2nd ed. New York: W. H. Freeman and Company; 2000.

22. Tabachnick BG, Fidell LS. Experimental design using ANOVA. Belmont (CA): Duxbury Press; 2007.

23. Cohen J. Statistical power analysis for the behavioral sciences. 2nd ed. Hillsdale (NJ): Lawrence Erlbaum Associates Inc.; 1988.

24. Nickerson RS. Null hypothesis significance testing: a review of an old and continuing controversy. Psychol Methods. 2000;5(2):241-301.

25. Cumming G, Finch S. Inference by eye: confidence intervals and how to read pictures of data. Am Psychol. 2005;60(2):170-80.

26. Cumming G, Finch, S. A primer on the understanding, use, and calculation of confidence intervals that are based on central and noncentral distributions. Educ Psychol Meas. 2001;61(4):532-74.

27. Siegel S, Castellan NJ. Nonparametric statistics for the behavioral sciences. 2nd ed. New York: McGraw-Hill Inc.; 1988.

28. Sheskin DJ. Handbook of parametric and nonparametric statistical procedures. 3rd ed. Boca Raton (FL): CRC Press; 2000.

29. Krauss RM, Burke DJ. Identification of multiple subclasses of plasma low density lipoproteins in normal humans. J Lipid Res. 1982;23(1):97-104.

30. Austin MA, King MC, Vranizan KM, Krauss RM. Atherogenic lipoprotein phenotype: a proposed genetic marker for coronary heart disease risk. Circ. 1990;82:495-506.

31. Cochran WG. Some methods for strengthening the common χ^2 tests. Biometrics. 1954;10(4):417−51.

32. Cohen J. A coefficient of agreement for nominal scales. Educ Psychol Meas. 1960;20(1):37-46.

33. Mercado CI, Gregg E, Gillespie C, Loustalot F. Trends in lipid profiles and descriptive characteristics of US adults with and without diabetes and cholesterol-lowering medication use—National Health and Nutrition Examination Survey, 2003-2012, United States. PLOS ONE. 2018;13(3):e0193756.

34. United States Center for Disease Control and Prevention. National Center for Health Statistics. Cholesterol [Internet]. [Cited 2020 Apr 21]. Available from: https://www.cdc.gov/nchs/data/hus/2018/023.pdf

35. Keppel G, Wickens TD. Design and analysis: a researcher's handbook. 4th ed. Upper Saddle River (NJ): Prentice Hall; 2004.

36. Hardy R, Kuh D, Langenberg C, Wadsworth ME. Birthweight, childhood social class, and change in adult blood pressure in the 1946 British birth cohort. Lancet. 2003362(9391):1178-83.

37. Lien LTQ, Chuc NTK, Hoa NQ, Lan PT, Thoa NTM, Riggi E, Tamhankar AJ, Lundborg C. Knowledge and self-reported practices of infection control among various occupational groups in a rural and an urban hospital in Vietnam. Sci Rep. 2018;8:5119.

38. Skrabal MZ, Jones RM, Walters, RW, Nemire RE, Soltis DA, Kahaleh AA, Hritcko PM, Boyle CJ, Assemi M, Turner P. National volunteer preceptor survey of experiential student loads, quality of time issues, and compensation: differences in responses based on region, type of practice setting, and population density. J Pharm Prac. 2010;23(3):265-72.

39. Vickers AJ. How many repeated measures in repeated measure designs? Statistical issues for comparative trials. Br Med Res Methodol. 2003;3(22):1-9.

40. Beck AT, Steer RA, Brown GK. Manual for Beck Depression Inventory-II. San Antonio (TX): Psychological Corporation; 1996.

41. Jekel JF. Epidemiology, biostatistics, and preventative medicine. 3rd ed. Philadelphia (PA): Asunders Elseiver; 2007.

42. Melnik T, Abdo CHN. Psychogenic erectile dysfunction: comparative study of three therapeutic approaches. J Sex Marital Ther. 2005;31(3):246-55.

43. Siebers RWL, Carter JM, Wakem PJ, Maling TJB. Interrelationship between platelet count, red cell count, white cell count and weight in men. Clin Lab Hematol. 1990;12(3);257-62.

44. Petrie A, Sabin C. Medical statistics at a glance. 2nd ed. Malden (MA): Blackwell Publishing Ltd.; 2005.

45. Need AG, Horowitz M, Morris HA, Nordin BEC. Vitamin D status: effects of parathyroid hormone and 1,25-dihydroxyvitamin D in post menopausal women. Am J Clin Nutr. 2000; 71(6):1577-81.

46. Jiang W, Whellan DJ, Adams KF, Babyak MA, Boyle SH, Wilson JL, Patel CB, Rogers JG, Harris WS, O'Connor CM. Long-chain omega-3 fatty acid supplements in depressed heart failure patients: results of the OCEAN trial. JACC Heart Fail. 2018;6(10):833-43.

47. Aldrich JH, Nelson FD. Linear probability, logit, and probit models. Sage University paper series on quantitative applications in the social sciences, series no. 07-045. Newbury Park (CA): Sage Publications, Inc.; 1984.

48. Allison PD. Survival analysis using the SAS system: a practical guide. 2nd ed. Cary (NC): SAS Institute Inc.; 2010.

49. Kleinbaum DG, Klein M. Survival analysis: a self learning text. 2nd ed. New York: Springer; 2005.

50. Simon SD. Is the randomized clinical trial the gold standard of research? J Androl. 2001;22(6):938-43.

SUGGESTED READINGS

The suggested readings below are for interested readers to gain further insight into some of the topics covered in this chapter. Note that most of the information provided in the first half of this chapter can be obtained in any introductory statistics textbook.

EPIDEMIOLOGICAL STATISTICS

1. Gordis L. Epidemiology. Philadelphia (PA): Saunders Elsevier; 2009.

CLINICAL SIGNIFICANCE AND EFFECT SIZE

2. Cohen J. Statistical power analysis for the behavioral sciences. 2nd ed. Hillsdale (NJ): Lawrence Erlbaum Associates Inc.; 1988.

STUDY DESIGN AND RANDOMIZED CONTROLLED TRIALS

3. Campbell DT, Stanley JC. Experimental and quasi-experimental designs for research. Boston (MA): Houghton Mifflin Company; 1966.

4. Chow S, Liu J. Design and analysis of clinical trials: concepts and methodologies. 2nd ed. Hoboken (NJ): John Wiley & Sons; 2004.

NONPARAMETRIC STATISTICAL TESTS
5. Siegel S ,Castellan NJ. Nonparametric statistics for the behavioral sciences. 2nd ed. New York: McGraw-Hill, Inc.; 1988.

ANOVA DESIGNS
6. Keppel G, Wickens TD. Design and analysis: a researcher's handbook. 4th ed. Upper Saddle River NJ: Prentice Hall; 2004.

LINEAR REGRESSION, LOGISTIC REGRESSION, SURVIVAL ANALYSIS
7. Tabachnick BG, Fidell LS. Using multivariate statistics. 5th ed. Boston (MA): Pearson Education Inc.; 2007.
8. Stevens J. Applied multivariate statistics for the social sciences. 4th ed. Mahwah (NJ): Lawrence Erlbaum Associates, Inc.; 2002.
9. Cohen P, Cohen J, West SG, Aiken LS. Applied multiple regression/correlation analysis for the behavioral sciences. 3rd ed. Mahwah (NJ): Lawrence Erlbaum Associates Inc.; 2003.
10. Hosmer DW, Lemeshow S. Applied logistic regression. 3nd ed. New York: John Wiley and Sons; 2013.
11. Kleinbaum DG, Klein M. Survival analysis: a self-learning text. 2nd ed. New York: Springer; 2005.

CLUSTERING AND NESTING
12. Snijders TAB, Bosker RJ. Multilevel analysis: an introduction to basic & advanced multilevel modeling. 2nd ed. Thousand Oaks (CA): Sage Publications; 2011.
13. Hox J. Multilevel analysis: techniques and applications. 2nd ed. New York: Routledge; 2010.
14. Raudenbush SW, Bryk AS. Hierarchical linear models: applications and data analysis methods. 2nd ed. Newbury Park (CA): Sage Publications; 2002.

STATISTICAL ANALYSIS IN THE BAYESIAN FRAMEWORK
15. Gelman A, Hill J. Data analysis using regression and multilevel/hierarchical models. New York: Cambridge University Press; 2007.
16. Kruschke JK. Doing Bayesian data analysis: a tutorial with R, JAGS, and Stan. 2nd ed. Waltham (MA): Academic Press; 2015.
17. Gelman A, Carlin JB, Stern HS, Dunson DB, Vehtari A, Rubin DB. Bayesian data analysis. 3rd ed. Boca Raton (FL): CRC Press; 2013.

7
Chapter Seven

Pharmacoeconomics

James P. Wilson • Karen L. Rascati

Learning Objectives

After completing this chapter, the reader will be able to:

- Describe the four types of pharmacoeconomic analysis: cost-minimization analysis (CMA), cost-benefit analysis (CBA), cost-effectiveness analysis (CEA), and cost-utility analysis (CUA).
- Describe the advantages and disadvantages of the different types of pharmacoeconomic analyses.
- List and explain the 10 steps that should be found in a well-conducted pharmacoeconomic study.
- List the six steps in a decision analysis.
- Give examples of the application of the pharmacoeconomic evaluation techniques to the formulary decision process, including decision analysis.
- Apply a systematic approach to the evaluation of the pharmacoeconomic literature.

Key Concepts

❶ Pharmacoeconomics identifies, measures, and compares the costs and consequences of pharmaceutical products and services.

❷ Pharmacoeconomic studies categorize costs into four types: direct medical, direct non-medical, indirect, and intangible.

❸ Perspective is a pharmacoeconomic term that describes whose costs are relevant based on the purpose of the study.

❹ There are four ways to measure outcomes, and each type of outcome measurement is associated with a different type of pharmacoeconomic analysis: cost-minimization analysis (CMA), cost-benefit analysis (CBA), cost-effectiveness analysis (CEA), and cost-utility analysis (CUA).

❺ There are two common methods that economists use to estimate a value for health-related consequences, the human capital approach and the willingness-to-pay approach.

❻ A CUA takes patient preferences, also referred to as utilities, into account when measuring health consequences.

❼ All four types of analyses described (CMA, CBA, CEA, and CUA) should follow 10 general steps.

❽ A sensitivity analysis allows one to determine how the results of an analysis would change when these best guesses or assumptions are varied over a relevant range of values.

❾ Decision analysis is the application of an analytical method for systematically comparing different decision options. Decision analysis graphically displays choices and performs the calculations needed to compare these options.

Introduction

The introduction of new, high cost, technologies, including new drugs, has received increased attention. During 2019, 48 novel drugs were approved by the Food and Drug Administration (FDA).[1] Media has brought the high costs of medication to the attention to the general public. For example, Luxturna (for blindness) is priced at $850,000 and Zolgensma (for spinal muscular atrophy) is priced at $2.1 million.[2,3]

The increase in the number of new drugs combined with the increase in costs of established drugs provides a great challenge for all health care. The new organizations created by the Affordable Care Act (ACA) to provide access to health care insurance for Americans, in addition to existing managed care organizations (MCOs), all desire to deliver quality care while minimizing costs.[4,5]

Pharmacy and therapeutics (P&T) committees are responsible for evaluating these new drugs and determining their potential value to organizations. Evaluating drugs for formulary inclusion can often be an overwhelming task. The application of pharmacoeconomic methods to the evaluation process may help streamline formulary decisions.

This chapter presents an overview of the practical application of pharmacoeconomic principles. Students and health professionals are often asked to gather and evaluate literature to support the decision process.

Pharmacoeconomics: What Is It and Why Do It?

❶ *Pharmacoeconomics identifies, measures, and compares the costs and consequences of pharmaceutical products and services.*[6] Decision-makers can use these methods to evaluate and compare the total costs of treatment options and the outcomes associated with these options. To show this graphically, think of two sides of an equation: (1) the inputs (costs) used to procure and use the drug and (2) the health-related outcomes (see Figure 7-1).

The center of the equation, the drug product, is symbolized by Rx. If only the left-hand side of the equation is measured without regard for outcomes, this is a cost analysis (or a partial economic analysis). If only the right-hand side of the equation is measured without regard to costs, this is a clinical or outcome study (not an economic analysis). In order to be a true pharmacoeconomic analysis, both sides of the equation must be considered and compared.

Relationships of Pharmacoeconomics to Outcomes Research

Outcomes research is defined as an attempt to identify, measure, and evaluate the end results of health care services. It may include not only clinical and economic consequences, but also outcomes, such as patient health status and satisfaction with their health care.[7] Pharmacoeconomics is a type of outcomes research, but not all outcomes research is pharmacoeconomic research.[8] The ECHO model—assessing the Economic, Clinical, and Humanistic Outcomes of health care interventions—was first introduced in the early 1990s.

Models of Pharmacoeconomic Analysis

The four types of pharmacoeconomic analysis all follow the diagram shown in Figure 7-1; they measure costs or inputs in dollars and assess the outcomes associated with these costs. Pharmacoeconomic analyses are categorized by the method used to assess outcomes. If the outcomes are assumed to be equivalent, the study is called a **cost-minimization analysis** (CMA); if the outcomes are measured in dollars, the study is called a **cost-benefit analysis** (CBA);

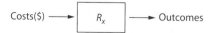

Figure 7–1. The pharmacoeconomic equation.

TABLE 7–1. FOUR TYPES OF PHARMACOECONOMIC ANALYSIS

Methodology	Cost Measurement Unit	Outcome Measurement Unit
Cost-minimization analysis	Dollars	Assumed to be equivalent in comparable groups analysis
Cost-benefit analysis	Dollars	Dollars
Cost-effectiveness analysis	Dollars	Natural units (life years gained, mmHg blood analysis [CEA] pressure, mmol/L blood glucose)
Cost-utility analysis	Dollars	Quality-adjusted life year (QALY) or other utilities

if the costs are measured in natural units (e.g., cures, years of life, blood pressure), the study is called a **cost-effectiveness analysis** (CEA); if the outcomes take into account patient preferences (or utilities), the study is called a **cost-utility analysis** (CUA) (Table 7-1). Each type of analysis includes a measurement of costs in dollars.

Assessment of Costs

First, the assessment of costs (the left-hand side of the equation) will be discussed. A discussion of the four types of costs and timing adjustments for costs follows.

TYPES OF COSTS

Costs are calculated to estimate the resources (or inputs) that are used in the production of an outcome. ❷ *Pharmacoeconomic studies categorize costs into four types.* **Direct medical costs** are the most obvious costs to measure. These are the medically related inputs used directly in providing the treatment. Examples of direct medical costs would include costs associated with pharmaceutical products, physician visits, emergency room visits, and hospitalizations. **Direct nonmedical costs** are costs directly associated with treatment, but are not medical in nature. Examples include the cost of traveling to and from the physician's office or hospital, babysitting for the children of a patient, and food and lodging required for patients and their families during out-of-town treatment. **Indirect costs** involve costs that result from the loss of productivity due to illness or death. Please note that the accounting term "indirect costs," which is used to assign overhead, is different from the economic term, which refers to a loss of productivity of the patient or the patient's family due to illness. **Intangible costs** include the costs of pain, suffering, anxiety, or fatigue that occur because of an illness or the treatment of an illness. It is difficult to measure or assign values to intangible costs.

Treatment of an illness may include all four types of costs. For example, the cost of surgery would include the direct medical costs of the surgery (medication, room charges, laboratory tests, and physician services), direct nonmedical costs (travel and lodging for the preoperative day), indirect costs (due to the patient missing work during the surgery and recuperative period), and intangible costs (due to pain and anxiety). Most studies only report the direct medical costs. This may be appropriate depending on the objective of the study or the perspective of the study. For example, if the objective is to measure the costs to the hospital for two surgical procedures that differ in direct medical costs (for example, using high-dose versus low-dose aprotinin in cardiac bypass surgery), but that are expected to have similar nonmedical, indirect, and intangible costs, measuring all four types of costs may not be warranted.

In order to determine what costs are important to measure, the perspective of the study must be determined. ❸ *Perspective is a pharmacoeconomic term that describes whose costs are relevant based on the purpose of the study.* Economic theory suggests that the most appropriate perspective is that of society. Societal costs would include all categories of costs, including costs to the insurance company, costs to the patient, intangible costs, and indirect costs due to the loss of productivity. Although this may be the most appropriate perspective according to economic theory, it is rarely seen in the pharmacoeconomic literature. The most common perspectives used in pharmacoeconomic studies are the perspective of the institution or the perspective of the payer. The payer perspective may include the costs to the third-party plan, the patient, or a combination of the patient copay and the third-party plan costs.

TIMING ADJUSTMENTS FOR COSTS

When costs are estimated from information collected for more than a year before the study or for more than a year into the future, adjustment of costs is needed. If retrospective data are used to assess resources used over a number of years, these costs should be adjusted to the present year. For example, if the objective of the study is to estimate the difference in the costs of antibiotic A versus antibiotic B in the treatment of a specific type of infection, information on the past utilization of these two antibiotics might be collected from a review of medical records. If the retrospective review of these medical records dates back for more than a year, it may be necessary to adjust the cost of both medications by calculating the number of units (doses) used per case and multiplying this number by the current unit cost for each medication. Sometimes past costs are adjusted to current costs using the medical consumer price index (MCPI) which is used to multiply past costs by each year's MCPI inflation rate.[9] Bringing past costs forward to the same year is sometimes referred to as annuitization.

If costs are estimated based on dollars spent or saved in future years, another type of adjustment, called discounting, is needed. There is a time value associated with money. Most people (and businesses) prefer to receive money today, rather than later. Therefore, a dollar received today is worth more than a dollar received next year—the time value of money. Discount rate, a term from finance, approximates the cost of capital by considering the projected inflation rate and the interest rates of borrowed money and then estimates the time value of money. From this parameter, the present value (PV) of future expenditures and savings can be calculated. The discount factor is equal to $1/(1 + r)^n$, where r is the discount rate and n is the year in which the cost or savings occur. For example, if the costs of a new pharmaceutical care program are $5000 per year for the next 3 years, and the discount rate is 5%, the present value (PV) of these costs is $14,297 ($5000 year 1 + $5,000/1.05 year 2 + $5,000/[1.05]^4 year 3) (note that discounting does not start until year 2). The most common discount rates currently seen in the literature are 3–5%, the approximate cost of borrowing money today.

Assessment of Outcomes

The methods associated with measuring outcomes (the right-hand side of the equation) will be discussed in this section. ❹ *As shown in Table 7-1, there are four ways to measure outcomes: CMA, CBA, CEA, and CUA.* Each type of outcome measurement is associated with a different type of pharmacoeconomic analysis. The advantages and disadvantages of each type of analysis will be discussed in this section.

COST-MINIMIZATION ANALYSIS

For a CMA, costs are measured in dollars, and outcomes are assumed to be equivalent. One example of a CMA is the measurement and comparison of costs for two therapeutically equivalent products, like glipizide and glyburide.[10] Another example is the measurement and comparison of using prostaglandin E2 on an inpatient versus an outpatient basis.[11] In both cases, all the outcomes (e.g., efficacy, incidence of adverse drug interactions) are expected to be equal, but the costs are not. Some researchers contend that a CMA is not a true pharmacoeconomic study, because costs are measured, but outcomes are not. Others say that the strength of a CMA depends on the evidence that the outcomes are the same.[12] This evidence can be based on previous studies, publications, FDA data, or expert opinion. The advantage of this type of study is that it is relatively simple compared to the other types of analyses because outcomes need not be measured. The disadvantage of this type of analysis is that it can only be used when outcomes are assumed to be identical.

Examples

A hospital needs to decide if it should add a new intravenous antibiotic to the formulary, which is therapeutically equivalent to the current antibiotic used in the institution and has the same adverse event profile. The advantage of the new antibiotic is that it only must be administered once per day versus three times a day for the comparison antibiotic. Because the outcomes are expected to be nearly identical, and the objective is to assess the costs to the hospital (e.g., the hospital perspective), only direct medical costs need to be estimated and compared. The direct medical costs include the daily costs of each medication, the pharmacy personnel time used in the preparation of each dose, and the nursing personnel time used in the administration of each dose. Even if the cost of the new medication is a little higher than the cost of the current antibiotic, the lower cost of preparing and administering the new drug (once a day vs. three times per day) may offset this difference. Direct nonmedical, indirect, and intangible costs are not expected to differ between these two alternatives, and they need not be included if the perspective is that of the hospital, so these costs are not included in the comparison.

Mithani and Brown[13] examined once-daily intravenous administration of an aminoglycoside versus the conventional every 8-hour administration (Table 7-2). The drug acquisition cost was in Canadian dollars ($Can) 43.70 for every 8 hours dosing, and $Can 55.39 for the single-dose administration. Not including laboratory drug-level measurements, the costs of the intravenous bag ($Can 29.32), preparation ($Can 13.81), and administration ($Can 67.63) were $Can 110.76 for the three-times daily administration versus $Can 42.23 (intravenous bag $Can 10.90, preparation $Can 6.20, and administration $Can 25.13) for the single daily dose. With essentially equivalent clinical outcomes, the once-daily administration of the aminoglycoside minimized hospital costs ($Can 97.62 vs. $Can 154.46).

COST-BENEFIT ANALYSIS

A CBA measures both inputs and outcomes in monetary terms. One advantage to using a CBA is that alternatives with different outcomes can be compared, because each outcome

TABLE 7–2. EXAMPLE OF COST MINIMIZATION

Type of Cost	Every 8 Hours	Once Daily
Drug acquisition cost	$43.70	$55.39
Minibag cost	$29.32	$10.90
Preparation cost	$13.81	$6.20
Administration costs	$67.63	$25.13
Total cost	$154.46	$97.62

is converted to the same unit (dollars). For example, the costs (inputs) of providing a pharmacokinetic service versus a diabetes clinic can be compared with the cost savings (outcomes) associated with each service, even though different types of outcomes are expected for each alternative. Many CBAs are performed to determine how institutions can best spend their resources to produce monetary benefits. For example, a study conducted at Walter Reed Army Medical Center looked at costs and savings associated with the addition of a pharmacist to its medical teams.[14] Discounting of both the costs of the treatment or services and the benefits or cost savings is needed if they extend for more than a year. Comparing costs and benefits (outcomes in monetary terms) is accomplished by using one of two methods. One method divides the estimated benefits by the estimated costs to produce a benefit-to-cost ratio. If this ratio is more than 1, the choice is cost beneficial. The other method is to subtract the costs from the benefits to produce a net benefit calculation. If this difference is positive, the choice is cost beneficial. The example at the end of this section will use both methods for illustrative purposes.

Another more complex use of CBA consists of measuring clinical outcomes (e.g., avoidance of death, reduction of blood pressure, and reduction of pain) and placing a dollar value on these clinical outcomes. This type of CBA is not often seen in the pharmacy literature, but will be discussed here briefly. This use of the method still offers the advantage that alternatives with different types of outcomes can be assessed, but a disadvantage is that it is difficult to put a monetary value on pain, suffering, and human life. ❺ *There are two common methods that economists use to estimate a value for these health-related consequences, the human capital (HC) approach and the willingness-to-pay (WTP) approach.* The HC approach assumes that the values of health benefits are equal to the economic productivity that they permit. The cost of disease is the cost of the lost productivity due to the disease. A person's expected income before taxes and/or an inputted value for nonmarket activities (e.g., housework and childcare) is used as an estimate of the value of any health benefits for that person. The HC approach was used when calculating the costs and benefits of administering a meningococcal vaccine to college students. The value of the future productivity of a college student was estimated at $1 million in this study.[15] There are disadvantages to using this method. People's earnings may not reflect their true value to society, and this method lacks a solid literature of research to back this notion. The WTP method estimates the value of health benefits by estimating how much people would pay to reduce their chance of an adverse health outcome. For example, if a group of people is willing to pay, on average, $100 to reduce their chance of dying from 1:1000 to 1:2000, theoretically a life would be worth $200,000 [$100/(0.001−0.0005)]. Problems with this method include the issue that what people say they are willing to pay may not correspond to what they actually would pay, and it is debatable if people can meaningfully answer questions about a 0.0005 reduction in outcomes.

Example

An independent pharmacy owner is considering the provision of a new clinical pharmacy service. The objective of the analysis is to estimate the costs and monetary benefits of two possible services over the next 3 years (Table 7-3). Clinical Service A would cost $50,000 in start-up and operating costs during the first year, and $20,000 in years 2 and 3. Clinical Service A would provide an added revenue of $40,000 each of the 3 years, Clinical Service B would cost $40,000 in start-up and operating costs the first year, and $30,000 for years 2 and 3. Clinical Service B would provide added revenue of $45,000 for each of the 3 years. Table 7-3 illustrates the comparison of both options using the perspective of the independent pharmacy with no discounting and when a discount rate of 5% is used. Although both services are estimated to be cost beneficial, Clinical Service B has both a higher benefit-to-cost ratio and a higher net benefit when compared to Clinical Service A.

COST-EFFECTIVENESS ANALYSIS

This is the most common type of pharmacoeconomic analysis found in the pharmacy literature. A CEA measures costs in dollars and outcomes in natural health units such as cures, lives saved, or blood pressure. An advantage of using a CEA is that health units are common outcomes practitioners can readily understand and these outcomes do not need to be converted to monetary values. On the other hand, the alternatives used in the comparison must have outcomes that are measured in the same units, such as lives saved with each of two treatments. If more than one natural unit outcome is important when conducting the comparison, a cost-effectiveness ratio should be calculated for each type of outcome. Outcomes cannot be collapsed into one unit measure in CEAs as they can with CBAs (outcome = dollars) or CUAs (outcome = **quality-adjusted life years [QALYs]**). Because CEAs are the most common type of pharmacoeconomic study in the pharmacy literature, many examples are available. Bloom and others[16] compared two medical treatments for gastroesophageal reflux disease (GERD), using both healed ulcers confirmed by endoscopy and symptom-free days as the outcomes measured. Law and others[17] assessed two antidiabetic medications by comparing the percentage of patients who achieved good glycemic control as the outcome measure.

A cost-effectiveness grid (Table 7-4) can be used to illustrate the definition of cost-effectiveness. In order to determine if a therapy or service is cost-effective, both the costs and effectiveness must be considered. Think of comparing a new drug with the current standard treatment. If the new treatment is (1) both more effective and less costly (cell G), (2) more effective at the same price (cell H), or (3) has the same effectiveness at a lower price (cell D), the new therapy is considered cost-effective. On the other hand, if the new drug is (1) less effective and more costly (cell C), (2) has the same effectiveness

TABLE 7–3. CBA EXAMPLE CALCULATIONS

	Year 1 Dollars (No Discounting in Year 1)	Year 2 Dollars (Discounted Dollars)	Year 3 Dollars (Discounted Dollars)	Total Dollars (Discounted Dollars)	Benefit-to-Cost Ratio (Discounted Dollars)	Net Benefit Dollars (Discounted Dollars)
Costs of A	$50,000 ($50,000)	$20,000 ($19,048)	$20,000 ($18,140)	$90,000 ($87,188)	$120,000/$90,000 = 1.33:1 ($114,376/87,188 = 1.31:1)	$120,000 − $90,000 = $30,000 ($114,376 − 87,188 = 27,188)
Benefits of A	$40,000 ($40,000)	$40,000 ($38,095)	$40,000 ($36,281)	$120,000 ($114,376)		
Costs of B	$40,000 ($40,000)	$30,000 ($28,571)	$30,000 ($27,211)	$100,000 ($95,782)	$135,000/100,000 = 1.35:1 ($128,673/95,782 = 1.34:1)	$135,000 − 100,000 = 35,000 ($128,673 − 95,782 = 32,891)
Benefits of B	$45,000 ($45,000)	$45,000 ($42,857)	$45,000 ($40,816)	$135,000 ($128,673)		

TABLE 7-4. COST-EFFECTIVENESS GRID

Cost-Effectiveness	Lower Cost	Same Cost	Higher Cost
Lower effectiveness	A	B	C
Same effectiveness	D	E	F
Higher effectiveness	G	H	I

but costs more (cell F), or (3) has lower effectiveness for the same costs (cell B), then the new product is *not* cost-effective. There are three other possibilities: (1) the new drug is more expensive and more effective (cell I)—a very common finding, (2) less expensive but less effective (cell A), or (3) has the same price and the same effectiveness as the standard product (cell E). For the middle cell E, other factors may be considered to determine which medication might be best. For the other two cells, an incremental cost-effectiveness ratio (ICER) is calculated to determine the extra cost for each extra unit of outcome. It is left up to the readers to determine if they think the new product is cost-effective, based on a value judgment. The underlying subjectivity as to whether the added benefit is worth the added cost is a disadvantage of CEA.

Example

An MCO is trying to decide whether to add a new cholesterol-lowering agent to its preferred formulary. The new product has a greater effect on lowering cholesterol than the current preferred agent, but a daily dose of the new medication is also more expensive. Using the perspective of the MCO (e.g., direct medical costs of the product to the MCO), the results will be presented in three ways in Tables 7-5–7-7 to illustrate the various ways that costs and effectiveness are presented in the literature. Table 7-5 presents the simple listing of the costs and outcomes of the two alternatives. Sometimes for each alternative, the costs and various outcomes are listed but no ratios are conducted—this is termed a cost-consequence analysis (CCA).

The second method of presenting results includes calculating the average cost-effectiveness ratio (ACER) for each alternative. Table 7-6 shows the cost-effectiveness ratio for the two alternatives. The ACER is the ratio of resources used per unit of clinical benefit, and implies that this calculation has been made in relation to doing nothing or no treatment. In this case, the current medication costs $40 for every 1 mg/dL decrease in LDL while the new medication under consideration costs $50 for the same decrease.

In clinical practice, the question is infrequently "Should we treat the patient or not?" or "What are the costs and outcomes of this intervention versus no intervention?" More often the question is "How does one treatment compare with another treatment in costs and outcomes?" To answer this more common question, an ICER is calculated. The ICER is the ratio of the difference in costs divided by the difference in outcomes.

TABLE 7-5. LISTING OF COSTS AND OUTCOMES

Alternative	Costs for 12 Months of Medication	Lowering of LDL in 12 Months (mg/dL)
Current preferred medication	$1,000	25
New medication	$1,500	30

LDL = low-density lipoprotein.

TABLE 7-6. COST-EFFECTIVENESS RATIOS

Alternative	Costs for 12 Months of Medication	Lowering of LDL in 12 Months	Average Cost per Reduction in LDL
Current preferred medication	$1,000	25 mg/dL	$40 per mg/dL
New medication	$1,500	30 mg/dL	$50 per mg/dL

LDL = low-density lipoprotein.

Most economists agree that an ICER (the extra cost for each added unit of benefit) is the more appropriate way to present CEA results. Table 7-7 shows the incremental cost-effectiveness (the extra cost of producing one extra unit) of the new medication compared to the current medication. For the new medication, it costs an additional $100 for every additional decrease in LDL of 1 mg/dL. The formulary committee would need to decide if this increase in cost is worth the increase in outcomes. In this example, the costs and benefits of the medications are estimated for only 1 year; discounting is not needed. If incremental calculations produce negative numbers, this indicates that one treatment is both more effective and less expensive, or dominant, compared to the other option. The magnitude of the negative ratio is difficult to interpret, so it is suggested that authors instead indicate which treatment is the dominant one. As mentioned before, when one of the alternatives is both more expensive and more effective than another, the ICER is used to determine the magnitude of added cost for each unit in health improvement (see CEA grid, cell I, Table 7-4).

Clinicians must then wrestle with this type of information—it becomes a clinical call. Many economists will argue that this uncertainty is why cost-effectiveness may not be the preferred method of pharmacoeconomic analysis.

COST-UTILITY ANALYSIS

❻ *A CUA takes patient preferences, also referred to as utilities, into account when measuring health consequences.*[18] The most common unit used in conducting CUAs is

TABLE 7–7. INCREMENTAL COST-EFFECTIVENESS RATIO

Alternative	Costs for 12 Months of Medication	Lowering of LDL in 12 Months	Incremental Cost per Marginal Reduction in LDL
Current preferred medication	$1,000	25 mg/dL	($1,500 − $1,000)/(30 mg/dL − 25 mg/dL) = $100 per mg/dL
New medication	$1,500	30 mg/dL	

LDL = low-density lipoprotein.

QALYs (Quality Adjusted Life Year(s)). A QALY is a health utility measure combining quality and quantity of life, as determined by some valuations process. The advantage of using this method is that different types of health outcomes can be compared using one common unit (QALYs) without placing a monetary value on these health outcomes (like CBA). The disadvantage of this method is that it is difficult to determine an accurate QALY value. This is an outcome measure that is not well understood or embraced by many providers and decision-makers. Therefore, this method is not commonly seen in the pharmacy literature. One reason researchers are working to establish methods for measuring QALYs is the belief that one year of life (a natural unit outcome that can be used in CEAs) in one health state should not be given the same weight as one year of life in another health state. For example, if two treatments both add 10 years of life, but one provides an added 10 years of being in a healthy state and the other adds 10 years of being in a disabled health state, the outcomes of the two treatments should not be considered equal. Adjusting for the quality of those extra years is warranted. When calculating QALYs, one year of life in perfect health has a score of 1 QALY. If health-related **quality of life** (HR-QOL) is diminished by disease or treatment, one year of life in this state is less than 1 QALY. This unit allows comparisons of morbidity and mortality. By convention, perfect health is assigned 1 per year and death is assigned 0 per year. How are scores between these two determined? Different techniques for determining scales of measurement for QALY are discussed below.

There are three common methods for determining QALY scores: rating scales (RS), standard gamble (SG), and time trade-off (TTO). A rating scale consists of a line on a page, somewhat like a thermometer, with perfect health at the top (100) and death at bottom (0). Different disease states are described to subjects, and they are asked to place the different disease states somewhere on the scale indicating preferences relative to all diseases described. As an example, if they place a disease state at 70 on the scale, the disease state is given a score of 0.7 QALYs.

The second method for determining patient preference (or utility) scores is the standard gamble method. For this method, each subject is offered two alternatives. Alternative one is treatment with two possible outcomes resulting in either the return to normal health or immediate death. Alternative two is the certain outcome of a chronic disease state for life. The probability (p) of dying is varied until the subject is indifferent between alternative one and alternative two. As an example, a person considers two options: a kidney transplant with a 20% probability of dying during the operation (alternative one) or dialysis for the rest of his life (alternative two). If this percent is his or her point of indifference (he or she would not have the operation if the chances of dying during the operation were any higher than 20%), the QALY is calculated as $1 - p$ or 0.8 QALY.

The third technique for measuring health preferences is the TTO method. Again, the subject is offered two alternatives. Alternative one is a certain disease state for a specific length of time t, the life expectancy for a person with the disease, then death. Alternative two is being healthy for time x, which is less than t. Time x is varied until the respondent is indifferent between the two alternatives. The proportion of the number of years of life a person is willing to give up ($t - x$) to have his or her remaining years (x) of life in a healthy state is used to assess his or her QALY estimate. For example, a person with a life expectancy of 50 years is given two options: being blind for 50 years or being completely healthy (including being able to see) for 25 years. If the person is indifferent between these two options (he or she would rather be blind than give up any more years of life), the QALY for this disease state (blindness) would be 0.5. Table 7-8 contains examples of disease states and QALY estimates for each disease state listed.

As one might surmise, QALY measurement is not regarded as being as precise or scientific as natural health unit measurements (like blood pressure and cholesterol levels) used in CEAs. Some issues in the measurement of QALYs are debated in the literature. One issue concerns whose viewpoint is the most valid. An advantage of having patients with the disease of interest determine health state scores is that these patients may understand the effects of the disease better than the general population, whereas some believe these patients would provide a biased view of their disease compared with other diseases they have not experienced. Some contend that health care professionals could provide good estimates because they understand various diseases, but others argue that these professionals may not rate discomfort and disability as seriously as patients or the general population.

Another issue that has been addressed regarding patient preference or utility-score measures is the debate over which is the best measure. Utility scores calculated using one method might differ from those using another. Finally, utility measures have been criticized for not being sensitive to small, but clinically meaningful, changes in health status.

Example

An article by Kennedy and associates[19] assessed the costs and utilities associated with two common chemotherapy regimens (vindesine and cisplatin [VP], and cyclophosphamide, doxorubicin, and cisplatin [CAP]) and compared the results with the costs and

TABLE 7–8. SELECTED QALY ESTIMATES

Disease State	QALY Estimate
Complete health	1.00
Moderate angina	0.83
Breast cancer: removed breast, unconcerned	0.80
Severe angina	0.53
Cancer spread, constant pain, tired, not expected to live long	0.16
Death	0.00

utilities of using best supportive care (BSC) in patients with non–small cell lung cancer. The perspective was that of the health care system or the payer. Using the TTO method, treatment utility scores were estimated by personnel of the oncology ward. Although the chemotherapy regimens provide a longer survival (VP = 214 days, CAP = 165 days) than BSC (112 days), the quality of life TTO score was higher for BSC (0.61) compared with the chemotherapy regimens (0.34). When survival time is multiplied by the TTO scores, the use of BSC results in an estimated 0.19 QALYs, which is similar to VP (0.19 QALYs), but higher than CAP (0.15 QALY). The costs to the health care system for the three options are about $5000 for BSC, $10,000 for VF, and $7000 for CAP (the authors reported median costs instead of average costs due to the abnormality of the cost data). Cost-utility ratios are calculated similarly to cost-effectiveness ratios, except that the out-come unit is QALYs. Therefore, the cost-utility ratio is about $26,000/QALY for BSC and about $44,000–$52,000/QALY for the chemotherapy regimens. Because BSC is at least as effective, as measured by QALYs, and is less expensive than the other two options, a marginal (or incremental) cost-utility ratio does not need to be calculated. Marginal cost-utility ratios only need to be calculated to estimate the added cost for an added benefit, not when the added benefit comes at a lower cost.

Performing an Economic Analysis

Conducting a pharmacoeconomic analysis can be challenging. Resources (time, exper-tise, data, and money) are limited. Data used to construct a model may be impossible to obtain due to lack of computer automation. Comparative studies of drug treatments may not be available or poorly designed. Results of clinical trials may not apply at the institu-tion performing the analysis due to lack of resources.

Methods for conducting a pharmacoeconomic analysis have been described above. **❼** *All four types of analyses described (CMA, CBA, CEA, and CUA) should follow 10 general steps.*

See Table 7-9. A modified practical approach to these steps based on the work developed by Jolicoeur and others[20] will be reviewed.

STEP 1: DEFINE THE PROBLEM

This step is self-explanatory. What is the question or objective that is the focus of the analysis? An example might be, "The objective of the analysis is to determine what medications for the treatment of urinary tract infections (UTIs) should be included on formulary." Perhaps one of the drugs being evaluated is a new drug recently approved by the FDA. Should the new drug be added to the drug formulary? The important thing to remember with this step is to be specific.

STEP 2: DETERMINE THE STUDY'S PERSPECTIVE

It is important to identify from whose perspective the analysis will be conducted. As mentioned in the "Assessment of Costs" section, this will determine the costs to be evaluated. Is the analysis being conducted from the perspective of the patient or from that of the health system, clinic, accountable care organization, or society? Depending on the perspective assigned to the analysis, different results and recommendations based on those results may be identified. If deciding on whether to add a new antibiotic to a formulary for treating UTIs, the perspective of the institution or payer would probably be used.

STEP 3: DETERMINE SPECIFIC TREATMENT ALTERNATIVES AND OUTCOMES

In this step, all treatment alternatives to be compared in the analysis should be identified. This selection should include the best clinical options and/or the options that are used most often in that setting at the time of the study. If a new treatment option

TABLE 7–9.   STEPS IN PERFORMING AN ECONOMIC ANALYSIS

Step 1	Define the problem
Step 2	Determine the study's perspective
Step 3	Determine specific treatment alternatives and outcomes
Step 4	Select the appropriate pharmacoeconomic method or model
Step 5	Measure inputs and outcomes
Step 6	Identify the resources necessary to conduct the analysis
Step 7	Establish the probabilities for the outcomes of the treatment alternatives
Step 8	Construct a decision tree
Step 9	Conduct a sensitivity analysis
Step 10	Present the results

is being considered, comparing it with an outdated treatment or a treatment with low efficacy rates is a waste of time and money. This new treatment should be compared with the next best alternative or the alternative it may replace. Keep in mind that alternatives may include drug treatments and nonpharmacologic treatments. For the UTI example, a new antibiotic would probably be compared with fluoroquinolones or sulfa drugs, or even the use of cranberry juice—old or gold standard therapy—but still the usual and most commonly used therapy. Today's expensive new chemical entities are very unlikely to cost less than standard therapy, and because of this, newer drugs are sometimes compared to the most recent, more expensive drugs used as alternative therapy.

The outcomes of those alternatives should include all anticipated positive and negative consequences or events that can be measured. Remember, outcomes may be measured in a variety of ways: lives saved, emergency room visits, hospitalizations, adverse drug reactions, dollars saved, QALYs, and so forth. For the UTI example, cure rates would be the most important outcome.

STEP 4: SELECT THE APPROPRIATE PHARMACOECONOMIC METHOD OR MODEL

The pharmacoeconomic method selected will depend on how the outcomes are measured (see Table 7-1). Costs (inputs) for all four types of analyses are measured in dollars. When all outcomes for each alternative are expected to be the same, a CMA is used. If all outcomes for each alternative considered are measured in monetary units, a CBA is used. When outcomes of each treatment alternative are measured in the same nonmonetary (i.e., clinical or humanistic) units, a CEA is used. When patient preferences for alternative treatments are being considered, a CUA is used. For the UTI example, cure rates are a natural clinical unit measure, so a CEA would be conducted.

STEP 5: MEASURE INPUTS AND OUTCOMES

All resources consumed by each alternative should be identified and measured in monetary value. The cost for each alternative should be listed and estimated (see "Assessment of Costs" section). The types of costs that will be measured will depend on the perspective chosen in Step 2. When evaluating alternatives over a long period of time (e.g., greater than 1 year), the concept of adjusting for time through annuitization or discounting or both should be applied. For the UTI example, if the perspective is that of an acute care hospital, only inpatient costs of treatment are measured. If the perspective is that of the third-party payer, all direct medical costs for the treatment are included whether they are provided on an inpatient or outpatient basis.

Measuring outcomes can be relatively simple (e.g., cure rates) or relatively difficult (e.g., QALYs). Outcomes may be measured prospectively or retrospectively. Prospective measurements tend to be more accurate and complete, but may take considerably more time and resources than retrospective data retrieval. Prospectively it is possible to define exactly what data to capture, but because it is necessary to wait for the patients to complete therapy, these types of studies may take months to years to complete. A data set on the shelf (computer) can be available now, but may or may not have all the data fields of interest. For the UTI example, cure rates attributed to the new product may be estimated from previous clinical trials, expert opinion, or measured prospectively in the population of interest.

STEP 6: IDENTIFY THE RESOURCES NECESSARY TO CONDUCT THE ANALYSIS

The availability of resources to conduct the study is an important consideration. Lack of access to important data can severely limit the validity of an analysis, as can the accuracy of the data itself. Data may be obtained from a variety of sources, including clinical trials, medical literature, medical records, prescription profiles, or computer databases. Before proceeding with the project, evaluate whether reliable sources of data are accessible or the data can be collected within the timeframe and budget allocated for the project.

STEP 7: ESTABLISH THE PROBABILITIES FOR THE OUTCOMES OF THE TREATMENT ALTERNATIVES

Probabilities for the outcomes identified in Step 3 should be determined. This may include the probability of treatment failures or success, or adverse reactions to a given treatment or alternative. Data for these can be obtained from the medical literature, clinical trials, medical records, expert opinion, prescription databases, as well as institutional databases. For the UTI example, probabilities of a cure rate for the new medication can be found in clinical trials or obtained from the FDA-approved labeling information. See Table 7-10. Probabilities of cure rates for the previous treatments (e.g., sulfonylureas) can also be found in clinical trials or by accessing medical records. If prospective data collection is conducted, the probabilities of all alternatives will be directly measured instead of estimated.

STEP 8: CONSTRUCT A DECISION TREE

Decision analysis can be a very useful tool when conducting a pharmacoeconomic analysis (see the "Steps in Decision Analysis" section for a step-by-step review). Constructing a

TABLE 7–10. STEPS IN DECISION ANALYSIS

Step 1	Identify the specific decision (therapeutic or medical problem)
Step 2	Specify alternatives
Step 3	Specify possible outcomes and probabilities
Step 4	Draw the decision analysis structure
Step 5	Perform calculations
Step 6	Conduct a sensitivity analysis (vary cost estimates)

decision tree creates a graphic display of the outcomes of each treatment alternative and the probability of their occurrence. Costs associated with each treatment alternative can be determined and the respective cost ratios derived. An example using a decision tree is provided in Figure 7-2.

STEP 9: CONDUCT A SENSITIVITY ANALYSIS

Whenever estimates are used, there is a possibility that these estimates are not precise. These estimates may be referred to as assumptions. For example, if the researcher assumes the discount rate is 5%, or assumes the efficacy rate found in clinical trials will be the same as the efficacy rate in the general population, this is a best guess used to conduct the calculations. ❽ *A sensitivity analysis allows one to determine how the results of an analysis would change when these best guesses or assumptions are varied over a relevant range of values.* For example, if the researcher assumes that the appropriate discount rate is 5%, this estimate should be varied from 0% to 10% to determine if the same alternative would still be chosen within this range. In order to vary many assumptions at one time, a probabilistic sensitivity analysis (changing each variable at random and recalculating) can be conducted that simulates many patients randomly being processed through the decision model using a range of estimates chosen for the analysis.[21]

STEP 10: PRESENT THE RESULTS

The results of the analysis should be presented to the appropriate audience, such as P&T committees, medical staff, or third-party payers. The steps outlined in this section should be employed when presenting the results. State the problem, identify the perspective, and so on. It is imperative to acknowledge or clarify any assumptions.

Although none of the models presented above are perfect, their utility may lead to better decision-making when faced with the difficult task of evaluating new drugs or technology for health care systems.

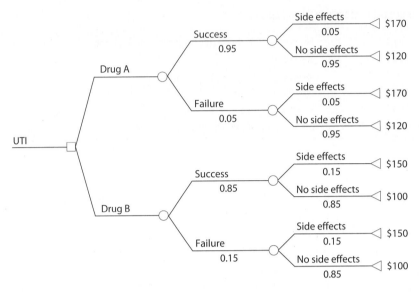

Figure 7–2. Decision tree for UTI example.

What is Decision Analysis?

Decision analysis is a tool that can help visualize a pharmacoeconomic analysis. ❾ *It is the application of an analytical method for systematically comparing different decision options. Decision analysis graphically displays choices and performs the calculations needed to compare these options.* It assists with selecting the best or most cost-effective alternative. Decision analysis is a tool that has been utilized for years in many fields, but has been applied to medical decision-making more frequently in the last 10 years. This method of analysis assists in making decisions when the decision is complex and there is uncertainty about some of the information.

Discussions of the medical uses of decision analysis have been included in collections of pharmacoeconomic bibliographies,[22–26] and in such specific topic areas as CEAs,[27] CUAs,[28] CBAs,[29] CMAs,[30] policies,[31] formulary processes,[32] pharmacy practices,[33] and drug product development.[34]

STEPS IN DECISION ANALYSIS

The steps in the decision process are enumerated in greater detail in several articles,[35–39] and are relatively straightforward, especially with the availability of computer programs that greatly simplify the calculations.[39] Articles reporting a decision analysis should include a picture of the decision tree, including the costs and probabilities utilized. The steps in a decision analysis will be outlined using the UTI example. The six steps involved in performing a decision analysis are provided below, and in Table 7-10.

Step 1: Identify the Specific Decision

Clearly define the specific decision to be evaluated (what is the objective of the study?). Over what period of time will the analysis be conducted (e.g., the episode of care, a year)? Will the perspective be that of the ill patient, the medical care plan, an institution/organization, or society? Specifying who will be responsible for the costs of the treatment will determine how costs are measured. For the UTI example, the decision was whether to add a new antibiotic to the formulary to treat UTIs. The perspective was that of the institution and the time period was 2 weeks.

Step 2: Specify Alternatives

Ideally, the two most effective treatments or alternatives should be compared. In pharmacotherapy evaluations, makers of innovative new products may compare or measure themselves against a standard (older or well-established) therapy. This is most often the case with new chemical entities. For pharmaceutical products, dosage and duration of therapy should be included. When analyzing costs and outcomes of pharmaceutical services, these services should be described in detail. For the UTI example, the use of the new medication (drug A) will be compared with that of a sulfa drug (drug B).

Step 3: Specify Possible Outcomes and Probabilities

For each potential outcome, an estimated probability must be determined (e.g., 95% probability of a cure or a 7% incidence of adverse events). Probability values should be selected or collected from the best designed and least biased sources that are relevant to the question and population under study: including well-conducted randomized, controlled trials (RCTs); observational data, including cohort, case-control, and cross-sectional studies; uncontrolled experiments; descriptive series; and expert opinion.[40]

Table 7-11 shows the outcomes and probabilities for the UTI example. The probabilities represent the chances or likelihood of treatment success or adverse events, and the costs associated with them.

Step 4: Draw the Decision Analysis Structure

A **decision tree** is a *decision support* tool that uses a *tree-like model* of decisions and their possible consequences, including *chance* event outcomes, resource costs, and *utility*. Lines are drawn to joint decision points (branches or arms of a decision tree), represented either as choice nodes, chance nodes, or final outcomes. Nodes are places in the decision tree where decisions are allowed; a branching becomes possible at this point. There are three types of nodes: (1) a choice node is where a choice is allowed (as between two drugs or two treatments), (2) a chance node is a place where chance (natural occurrence) may influence the

TABLE 7–11. OUTCOMES AND PROBABILITIES, UTI EXAMPLE

	Drug A	Drug B
Effectiveness probability	0.95	0.85
Side effect probability	0.05	0.15
Cost of medication	$120	$100
Cost of side effects	$50	$50

decision or outcome expressed as a probability, and (3) a terminal node is the final outcome of interest for that decision. Probabilities are assigned for each possible outcome, and the sum of the probabilities must add up to 1. Most computer-aided software programs utilize a square box to represent a choice node, a circle to represent a chance node, and a triangle for a terminal branch or final outcome. Figure 7-2 illustrates the decision tree for the UTI example.

Step 5: Perform Calculations

The first consideration should be the present value, or cost, of resources If the study is over a period of less than 1 year, actual costs are utilized in the calculations. If the study period is greater than 1 year, then costs should be discounted or standardized (converted to PV). For each branch of the tree, costs are totaled and multiplied by the probability of that arm of the tree. These numbers (costs × probabilities) calculated for each arm of the option are added for each alternative. Example calculations are given in Tables 7-12, 7-13, and 7-14. The UTI example would be a cost-effectiveness type of study, so the difference in the cost for each arm would be divided by the difference in effectiveness for each arm to produce an ICER (see Table 7-14).

Step 6: Conduct a Sensitivity Analysis (Vary Cost Estimates)

Because these decision trees or models are constructed with best guesses, a sensitivity analysis is conducted. The highest and lowest estimates of costs and probabilities are inserted into the equations, to determine the best case and worse case answers. These estimates should be sufficiently varied to reflect all possible true variations in values. For the UTI example, the new drug (drug A) would be added to the formulary if the committee thought the added cost ($150) was worth the added benefit (one more successful treatment) (see Table 7-12). Some might not agree with the probability of the adverse events of drug A; because the therapy is new, they may believe 5% may be an underestimate. If the estimate is increased to a 10% adverse event rate for the new drug and the marginal cost-effectiveness ratio is recalculated, the recalculated ratio would be $175 per added treatment success. Again, the committee would have to decide if the added cost is worth the added benefit.

TABLE 7–12. DECISION ANALYSIS CALCULATIONS FOR DRUG A

	Cost	Probability	Probability × Cost ($)
Outcome 1	$120 + $50 = $170	0.95 × 0.05 = 0.0475	8.08
Outcome 2	$120	0.95 × 0.95 = 0.9025	108.30
Outcome 3	$120 + $50 = $170	0.05 × 0.05 = 0.0025	0.42
Outcome 4	$120	0.05 × 0.95 = 0.0475	5.70
Total		1	122.5

TABLE 7–13. DECISION ANALYSIS CALCULATIONS FOR DRUG B

	Cost	Probability	Probability × Cost ($)
Outcome 1	$100 + $50 = $150	0.85 × 0.15 = 0.1275	19.12
Outcome 2	$100	0.85 × 0.85 = 0.7225	72.25
Outcome 3	$100 + $50 = $150	0.15 × 0.15 = 0.0225	3.38
Outcome 4	$100	0.15 × 0.85 = 0.1275	12.75
Total		1	107.50

TABLE 7–14. INCREMENTAL COST-EFFECTIVENESS RATIO

	Alternative Costs of Drug and Treating Side Effects ($)	Effectiveness in Treating UTI (%)	Incremental Cost per Treatment Success
Drug A	$122.50	95	($122.50 − $107.50)/ (0.95 − 0.85) = $150
Drug B	$107.50	85	

Decision analysis is being used more commonly in pharmacoeconomic evaluations. The use and availability of computer programs[34] to assist with the multiple calculations makes it fairly easy for someone to automate their evaluations. Examples of software available for this purpose include TreeAge Pro (http://www.treeage.com), DPL (http://www.syncopation.com), and DecisionPro® (http://www.decisionpro.biz). The prices for these software packages range from less than $100 for student versions to over $1000 for professional versions. Decision analyses can also be conducted using Microsoft Excel (http://office.microsoft.com/en-us/excel).

Example

An article by Botteman and others[41] used a decision-tree analysis to model the cost-effectiveness of enoxaparin compared to warfarin for the prevention of complications (deep vein thrombosis, venous thromboembolisms, and postthrombotic syndromes) due

to hip replacement surgery. Data for this model were obtained through published literature and expert opinion. The model was created to assess both short-term (immediately
after surgery) and long-term (followed until death or 100 years old) costs and consequences. The perspective was that of the payer, and a discount rate of 3% was used for
the long-term analysis. Results: for the short-term model, therapy with enoxaparin was
more expensive (+$133 per patient), but had a better outcome (+0.04 QALY per patient).
For the long-term model, therapy with enoxaparin saved money (−$89 per patient) and
had a better outcome (+0.16 QALY per patient), and was therefore the dominant (saves
money and has a better outcome) choice. Both univariate (one item varied) and probabilistic (multiple items varied) sensitivity analyses were conducted and indicated that the
results were robust.

Steps in Reviewing Published Literature

It is more likely that a practicing pharmacist will be asked to evaluate published literature on the topic of pharmacoeconomics, rather than conduct a study. When evaluating
the pharmacoeconomics literature for making a formulary decision, or selecting the best
product for an institution, a systematic approach to evaluating the pharmacoeconomics
literature can make the task easier.

Several authors[16,42–48] cite methodology to assist in systematically reviewing the
pharmacoeconomic literature. If a study is carefully reviewed to ensure that the author(s)
included all meaningful components of an economic evaluation, the likelihood of finding
valid and useful results is high. The steps for evaluating studies are similar to the steps
for conducting studies, because the readers determine whether the proper steps were followed when the researcher conducted the study. When evaluating a pharmacoeconomic
study, at least the following 10 questions should be considered.

1. Was a well-defined question posed in an answerable form? The specific questions
   and hypotheses should be clearly stated at the beginning of the article.
2. Is the perspective of the study addressed? The perspective should be explicitly
   stated, not implied.
3. Were the appropriate alternatives considered? Head-to-head comparisons of the
   best alternatives provide more information than comparing a new product or service with an outdated or ineffective alternative.
4. Was a comprehensive description of the competing alternatives given? If products are compared, dosage and length of therapy should be included. If services
   are compared, explicit details of the services make the paper more useful. Could
   another researcher replicate the study based on the information given?

5. What type of analysis was conducted? The paper should address if a CMA, CEA, CBA, or CUA was conducted. Some studies may conduct more than one type of analysis (i.e., a combination of a CEA and a CUA). Some studies, especially older published studies, incorrectly placed the terms "benefit" or "effectiveness analysis" in the title of the article, when many were actually CMA studies.

6. Were all the important and relevant costs and outcomes included? Check to see that all pertinent costs and consequences were mentioned. Depending on the specific objectives and perspective, different costs and outcomes measures may be important.

7. Was there justification for any important costs or consequences that were not included? Sometimes, the authors will admit that although certain costs or consequences are important, they were impractical (or impossible) to measure in their study. It is better that the authors state these limitations, than to ignore them.

8. Was annuitization needed? If so, was it conducted? Was discounting appropriate? If so, was it conducted? If the treatment cost or outcomes are extracted more than one year back or extrapolated for more than one year in the future, the time value of money must be incorporated into the cost estimates.

9. Are all assumptions stated? Were sensitivity analyses conducted for these assumptions? Many of the values used in pharmacoeconomic studies are based on assumptions. For example, authors may assume the adverse event rate is 5%, or that adherence with a regimen will be 80%. These types of assumptions should be stated explicitly. For important assumptions, was the estimate varied within a reasonable range of values?

10. Was an unbiased summary of the results presented? Sometimes, the conclusions seem to overstate or exaggerate the data presented in the results section. Did the authors use unbiased reasonable estimates when determining the results? In general, are the study results believable?

Case Study 7–1

Title: Cost-Utility Analysis of Best Supportive Care versus Oncoplatin and Oncotaxel in the Treatment of Recurrent Metastatic Breast Cancer

Background: For patients diagnosed with recurrent metastatic breast cancer, the prognosis is grim. Two agents, Oncoplatin and Oncotaxel, have been used to help prolong the lives of these patients (authors would cite clinical literature here for real pharmaceutical products). As with other chemotherapy treatments, the toxic effects of the medications can be severe and vastly decrease the patient's quality of life. Some would argue that the small increase in life expectancy from these agents might not be worth the trade-off in suffering from the adverse effects of the agents during the treatment period. Instead of chemotherapy, palliative treatments, such as best supportive care (BSC), have been suggested as an option. BSC includes measures to keep the patient comfortable. These may include medications to alleviate pain, antibiotics, or radiotherapy to reduce tumor size. The objective of this study was to compare the costs and utility of two chemotherapy treatments, Oncoplatin and Oncotaxel, with those of BSC in patients with recurrent metastatic breast cancer.

Methods: The practice sites for data collection included three oncology clinics that are part of a multihospital, multiclinic health care system. Utility scores were collected via the **time trade-off** (TTO) method. A panel of experts helped create descriptions of the health states of patients undergoing the different treatment options. Based on these descriptions, utility scores were elicited from two sources: oncology nurses at the three clinics and a random sample of patients from general (nononcology) clinics associated with the health care system.

Data on treatment and survival time were collected for the past 3 years from a retrospective analysis of charts at three oncology clinics. Medical services and procedures associated with these treatment options were recorded. Treatment data included medications and their administration, as well as laboratory, radiology, and various types of medical visits (physician, clinic, emergency room, and hospital). Charges listed by the health care system in 2013 were used to estimate current costs for each service or procedure.

Results: Table 7-1A lists the costs and survival times found by the review of charts. Although the chemotherapy regimens provided a longer survival (Oncoplatin, 200 days; Oncotaxel, 160 days) than BSC (130 days), the utility score was higher for BSC (0.60–0.61) compared with the chemotherapy regimens (0.32–0.35). Oncology nurses gave similar estimates compared with the group of nononcology patients.

If the difference in quality of life is not incorporated into the analysis, cost-effectiveness calculations based on survival time alone (life years saved [LYS]) indicate that chemotherapy is more effective but at a higher cost (Table 7-1B). When survival time is adjusted for the differences in utilities (preferences) for treatment, the use of BSC is dominant over both chemotherapy treatments because of its lower cost and higher QALY estimate.

Sensitivity analyses were conducted by reducing cost estimates using the clinic's cost-to-charge ratio of 0.83:1 and by varying the days of survival by their 95% confidence intervals. As with the comparison of oncology nurses versus patient utility estimates, the results were robust.

Conclusion: There are some limitations to this study. The data were collected from a small sample of patients. Although data were collected from three clinics, these clinics were all part of the same health care system. Oncology treatment in other clinics may vary in both costs and outcomes. Although utility scores were collected from health care professionals and general patients, they were not collected from patients with metastatic breast cancer. We believed that administering the instrument to these women might have placed an undue burden on patients with a poor prognosis. Actual cost data were not available, so charge data were used as a proxy, and a sensitivity analysis was conducted on this variable.

As with previous research, using BSC was found to be less expensive than using chemotherapy agents to treat advanced cancer. Although BSC may not be as effective as chemotherapy in traditional measures of effectiveness (e.g., survival time, progression-free survival time), when preferences for a less toxic treatment are factored into the decision, BSC may become the preferred treatment, and it should be considered as an option (Tables 7-15 and 7-16).

■ CRITIQUE OF CUA ARTICLE

1. Complete title: The title identified the type of study (CUA), the treatments that were being compared (BSC, Oncoplatin, and Oncotaxel), and the disease state (metastatic breast cancer).

2. Clear objective: The objective of this study was "to compare the costs and utility of two chemotherapy treatments, Oncoplatin and Oncotaxel, with those of best supportive care." This was clear.

3. Appropriate alternatives: The three alternatives were BSC, Oncoplatin, and Oncotaxel. A case was made that BSC is sometimes overlooked as a valid option. Based on the clinical literature cited, the readers would determine if the two chemotherapy options were appropriate.

4. Alternatives described: Chemotherapy dosing is very individualized, and data were collected from three clinics; average doses of agents were not included. BSC was defined as keeping the patient comfortable, including providing pain medications, antibiotics, and radiotherapy, if needed.

5. Perspective stated: The perspective of the study was not explicitly stated. Because the researchers only report measuring direct medical costs, the perspective could have been that of the payer or that of the health care system that included the three oncology clinics. Charges were measured, so the perspective is still unclear. If actual costs to the health system were estimated, the perspective could have been the health care system. If reimbursed costs were used, the perspective could have been that of the average third-party payer.

6. Type of study: The study was correctly identified as a CUA because outcomes were valued in QALYs. For comparison purposes, incremental cost-effectiveness ratios were also calculated based on length of survival for the three options, so the answer could be that both a CUA and a CEA were conducted.

TABLE 7–15. COMPOSITE ARTICLE DATA

	BSC	Oncoplatin	Oncotaxel
	(N = 29)	(N = 36)	(N = 35)
Treatment Charges			
Mean	$5,000	$10,000	$7,000
(SD)	($1,000)	($2,000)	($2,000)
Survival (days)			
Mean	130 days	200 days	160 days
Range	110–140 days	180–215 days	110–190 days
Utility Scores			
Oncology Nurses	0.60	0.35	0.35
Utility Scores			
Nononcology Patients	0.61	0.32	0.32

TABLE 7–16. COMPOSITE ARTICLE CALCULATIONS

	BSC	Oncoplatin	Oncotaxel
	(N = 29)	(N = 36)	(N = 35)
Cost-Effectiveness Cost per LYS = (cost/days) * 365 days/year	$14,038	$18,250	$15,969
Incremental Cost per LYS = [Δ Costs/Δ days] * 365 days/year		Oncoplatin vs. BSC = $26,071 per additional LYS	Oncotaxel vs. BSC = $24,333 per additional LYS
Cost Utility $QALY = \dfrac{days \times utility}{365\ days/year}$	O = 0.21 QALY P = 0.22 QALY	O = 0.19 QALY P = 0.17 QALY]	O = 0.15 QALY P = 0.14 QALY
Average Cost per QALY Cost/QALY	O = $23,809 P = $22,727	O = $52,631 P = $58,823	O = $46,667 P = $50,000
Incremental Cost per QALY = [Δ Costs/Δ QALYs]	Both Oncoplatin and Oncotaxel dominated by BSC For both O and P estimates	Oncoplatin vs. Oncotaxel O = $75,000 per additional QALY P = $100,000 per additional QALY	

BSC = Best supportive care; LYS = Life-years saved; QALY = Quality-adjusted life-year; O = based on utility scores from oncology nurses; P = based on utility scores from nononcology patients.

7. Relevant costs: Because we are unsure of the perspective of the study, it is difficult to determine if relevant costs were measured. It seems as if all relevant direct medical costs were measured. Patient costs, such as time traveling to and from the clinic, might be different for BSC than for chemotherapy, but these costs were not measured.

8. Relevant outcomes: Outcomes of the treatment were measured by determining the length of life from chart reviews and utilities via two groups, oncology nurses and general patients. The TTO technique was used to elicit utility scores. A description of the health states used in eliciting these responses would have been a helpful addition to the article.

9. Adjustment or discounting: Data were collected from charts that spanned a 3-year period. To adjust for this, units of service were multiplied by current charges for each service. Discounting was not needed because neither costs nor outcomes were extrapolated into the future.

10. Reasonable assumptions: One assumption was that utility scores from the oncology staff would be accurate. To test this assumption, scores were also obtained from another group (a random sample of nononcology patients). Another assumption was that charges were a valid substitute for actual costs.

11. Sensitivity analyses: Sensitivity analyses were conducted. Utility scores from two groups were compared, and costs and survival time were varied. Although the authors indicated that results were insensitive to these analyses, a table with the numbers based on these new calculations would have been useful.

12. Limitations addressed: The authors did address some of their limitations at the beginning of the conclusion section. One limitation that was not addressed is that patients were not randomized to the three treatment options. It is possible that patients who received BSC were different from those who received chemotherapy. They may have been older or may have been in a more advanced stage of the disease.

13. Generalizations appropriate: Because data on both costs and outcomes were collected from only one health care system (albeit from three clinics within the system), caution should be used when extrapolating to other populations who are treated in other settings.

14. Unbiased conclusions: The authors state that when survival is adjusted for patient preferences, BSC is a valid option for treating patients with recurrent metastatic breast cancer. BSC costs less than chemotherapy treatments and provides a higher QALY score. Sensitivity analyses found the results to be robust (i.e., not sensitive to changes in estimates).

Many articles, several journals, and numerous texts have been devoted to pharmacoeconomics. Research and further development and refinement of the analysis tools are ongoing. It can be expected that the literature on pharmacoeconomics will continue to expand rapidly, not only for use in proving the value of new therapies, but for invalidating the worth of standard therapies. Grutters,[42] Husereau,[43] Duran,[44] Chiou,[45] Ofman,[46] Edwards,[47] among others, cite references to assist readers in understanding and assessing economic analyses of health care as well as providing checklists (with examples and explanations) to evaluate published articles.

Selected Pharmacoeconomic Websites

Articles that provide an overview of the field of pharmacoeconomics, its changing methodologies, and recent advances can often be found readily at Internet sites devoted to this area of specialization. These sites usually highlight articles that are not necessarily drug or therapy specific. Many present an overview or validation of methodologies. Several pharmacoeconomic websites are included as references. They were selected because they all have multiple links to other pharmacoeconomic-related sites.

Conclusion

Many health care organizations continue to be challenged with managing costs of pharmacotherapy. With the proliferation of health care programs under the Affordable Care Act, each entity will be building pharmacoeconomic models that can be useful tools for evaluating the costs of pharmaceuticals in these plans. The ability to objectively measure and compare costs may also produce better decisions about the choice of pharmaceuticals for a formulary. Decision analysis is one of the many tools finding increased utilization in the field of medicine, and pharmacoeconomics specifically. As the science of pharmacoeconomics becomes more standardized, rigorous comparisons among several papers on the same topic will be possible (and necessary). For a more in-depth review of the principles and concepts of pharmacoeconomics, please see textbooks devoted to the topic, such as Essentials of Pharmacoeconomics[49] or Methods for the Economic Evaluation of Health Care Programmes.[50,51]

Self-Assessment Questions

1. A patient has a nurse come to their home to administer an IV antibiotic—this can be categorized as what type of cost?
   a. Direct medical cost
   b. Direct nonmedical cost
   c. Indirect cost
   d. Intangible cost

2. A parent staying home from work because they have a mild case of the COVID virus can be categorized as what type of cost?
   a. Direct medical cost
   b. Direct nonmedical cost
   c. Indirect cost
   d. Intangible cost

3. For which of the following would Alternative A be considered cost-effective when compared to the standard Alternate B.
   a. Alternative A costs less than Alternative B.
   b. Alternative A is more effective than Alternative B.
   c. Alternative A is more effective than Alternative B, and Alternative A costs less than Alternative B.
   d. Alternative A is less effective than Alternative B, but Alternative A costs more than Alternative B.

4. When an article states that the results of an analysis are *sensitive* to a particular variable this means:
   a. The results vary depending on the range of that variable, thereby strengthening your confidence in the study results.
   b. The results vary depending on the range of that variable, thereby weakening your confidence in the study results.
   c. The results do not vary depending on the range of that variable, thereby strengthening your confidence in the study results.
   d. The results do not vary depending on the range of that variable, thereby weakening your confidence in the study results.

5. If Project A costs $30,000 this year, $40,000 in year 2, and $50,000 in year 3, what are the total 3-year costs in present value (PV) terms using a 5% discount rate. Do not begin discounting until year 2. Round to the nearest $1000.
   a. $100,000
   b. $113,000

c. $120,000
d. $127,000

6. If a researcher evaluates cost per life year saved (LYS), what type of study is being conducted?
   a. CEA
   b. CBA
   c. CMA
   d. CUA

7. Most economists agree that the most appropriate way to present cost-effectiveness data is using:
   a. An incremental cost-effectiveness ratio.
   b. A simple cost-effectiveness ratio.
   c. A net benefit ratio.
   d. A benefit-to-cost ratio.

8. In order to estimate utilities, researchers use:
   a. Rating scale methods.
   b. Time trade-off methods.
   c. Standard gamble methods.
   d. Any of the above methods may be used.

9. A disadvantage of using the human capital method to value health is:
   a. The value estimated depends on a person's earning potential.
   b. People may not pay what they indicate they are willing to pay.
   c. Both of the above.
   d. None of the above.

10. Drug A costs $3000 and saves $6000. What is the benefit-to-cost ratio for Drug A?
    a. 0.50:1
    b. 0.80:1
    c. 1.67:1
    d. 2:1

11. Drug B cost $5000 and saves $7500. What is the benefit-to-cost ratio for Drug B?
    a. 0.75:1
    b. 0.80:1
    c. 1.5:1
    d. 1.33:1

12. Based on these results from questions 10 and 11 which option would you choose?
    a. Drug A is the more cost-beneficial option.
    b. Drug B is the more cost-beneficial option.
    c. They are equally cost-beneficial.
    d. Not able to calculate based on information given.

For questions 13–15 use the following abstract:

Title: Cost-utility of asthmazolimide (fictitious drug) in the treatment of severe persistent asthma.

Background: Some patients with severe persistent asthma are not controlled with standard treatment (defined in this study as a combination of long-acting beta agonists [LABAs] and inhaled corticosteroids [ICS]). Clinical trials have shown improved outcomes for these patients if asthmazolimide is added to their regimen.

Objective: The objective of this study was to estimate the cost per quality-adjusted life year (QALY) of the addition of asthmazolimide to standard treatment for patients enrolled in a randomized controlled trial. The perspective of the study was the third-party payer.

Methods: Patients with severe persistent asthma in a health plan were enrolled in the study using a pre-post study design. The index date for each patient was his or her date of enrollment. Two years of preindex utilization and costs of medical services were recorded using retrospective data collection, and patients were followed prospectively for 1 year after their index date. For the first 12 months after enrollment, patients recorded their use of any asthma-related medical services and prescriptions and kept a daily symptom diary. Then patients had asthmazolimide added to their regimen for the next 12-month period and again kept tract of their asthma-related medical services and prescriptions and a diary of daily symptoms. Costs of preindex services were adjusted to 2019 costs to the health plan. QALYs were calculated using utility weights for various asthma-related symptoms that were estimated from a previous study using the time trade-off (TTO) method.

Results: A total of 216 patients were enrolled in and completed the study. Asthma-related health plan costs increased after the addition of asthmazolimide (mostly from an increase in prescription costs) by an average of $800 per year. Fewer symptoms and less severe symptoms were reported after the addition of the new drug, resulting in an average increase of 0.1 QALY, for an incremental cost per QALY ratio of (*for calculating the answer, see question 13, below*).

Conclusion: For these 216 patients, the addition of asthmazolimide to their medication regimen resulted in a reduction of symptoms at a reasonable cost to the health plan.

13. What number should be included in the blank in the abstract?
    a. $800
    b. $8000
    c. $80
    d. $80,000

14. In the abstract, was discounting needed? Was it conducted?
    a. Not needed, not conducted
    b. Needed, not conducted
    c. Needed, conducted
    d. Not needed, conducted

15. In the abstract, was adjustment needed? Was it conducted?
    a. Not needed, not conducted
    b. Needed, not conducted
    c. Needed, conducted
    d. Not needed, conducted

REFERENCES

1. Novel drug approvals for 2019 [Internet]. Bethesda (MD): U.S. Food and Drug Administration; 2019 [cited 2020 Apr 1]. 6 p. Available from: https://www.fda.gov/drugs/new-drugs-fda-cders-new-molecular-entities-and-new-therapeutic-biological-products/novel-drug-approvals-2019

2. Luxturna gene therapy for blindness to cost $850,000 [Internet]. New York: NBC News; 2018 Jan 3 [updated 2018 Jan 4; cited 2020 Mar 29]. 3 p. Available from: https://www.nbc-news.com/health/health-news/luxturna-gene-therapy-blindness-cost-850-000-n834261

3. At $2.1 million, new gene therapy is the most expensive drug ever [Internet]. New York: National Public Radio; 2019 May 24 [cited 2020 Mar 29]. 3 p. Available from: https://www.npr.org/sections/health-shots/2019/05/24/725404168/at-2-125-million-new-gene-therapy-is-the-most-expensive-drug-ever

4. Wang Z, Salmon JW, Walton SM. Cost effectiveness analysis and the formulary decision-making process. J Manag Care Pharm. 2004;10(10):48-59.

5. Chernew, ME, Conway PH, Frakt AB. Transforming Medicare's payment systems: progress shaped by the ACA. Health Affairs. 2020;39(3):413–20.

6. Bootman JL, Townsend RJ, McGhan WF. Introduction to pharmacoeconomics. In: Bootman JL, Townsend RJ, McGhan WF, editors. Principles of pharmacoeconomics. 2nd ed. Cincinnati (OH): Harvey Whitney Books; 1996. p. 5-11.

7. Kozma CM, Reeder CE, Schulz RM. Economic, clinical, and humanistic outcomes: a planning model for pharmacoeconomic research. Clin Ther. 1993;15(6):1121-32.

8. Rascati KL. Essentials of pharmacoeconomics. Philadelphia (PA): Wolters Kluwer/ Lippincott Williams & Wilkins; 2009. p. 3.

9. Measuring price change in the CPI: medical care [Internet]. Washington (DC): U.S. Bureau of Labor Statistics; 2020 Mar 20 [cited 2020 May 15]. Available from: https://www.bls.gov/cpi/factsheets/medical-care.htm

10. Nadel HL. Formulary conversion from glipizide to glyburide: a cost-minimization analysis. Hosp Pharm. 1995;30(6):467-9, 472-4.

11. Farmer KC, Schwartz WJ, Rayburn WF, Turnball G. A cost-minimization analysis of intracervical Prostaglandin E2 for cervical ripening in an outpatient versus inpatient setting. Clin Ther. 1996;18(4):747-56.

12. Newby, D., Hill, S. Use of pharmacoeconomics in prescribing research. Part 2: cost-minimization analysis—when are two therapies equal? J Clin Pharm Ther. 2003;28(2):145-50.

13. Mithani H, Brown G. The economic impact of once-daily versus conventional administration of gentamicin and tobramycin. PharmacoEconom. 1996;10(5):494-503.

14. Bjornson DC, Hiner WO, Potyk RP, Nelson BA, Lombardo FA, Morton TA, Larson LV, Martin BP, Sikora RG, Cammarata FA. Effects of pharmacists on health care outcomes in hospitalized patients. Am J Hosp Pharm. 1993;50:1875-84.

15. Jackson LA, Schuchat A, Gorsky RD, Wenger JD. Should college students be vaccinated against meningococcal disease? A cost-benefit analysis. Am J Public Health. 1995;85(6):843-5.

16. Bloom BS, Hillman AL, LaMont B, Liss C, Schwartz JS, Stever GJ. Omeprazole or ranitidine plus metoclopramide for patients with severe erosive oesophagitis. PharmacoEconom. 1995;8(4):343-9.

17. Law AV, Pathak DS, Segraves AM, Weinstein CR, Arneson WH. Cost-effectiveness analysis of the conversion of patients with non-insulin-dependent diabetes mellitus from glipizide to glyburide and of the accompanying pharmacy follow-up clinic. Clin Ther. 1995;17(5):977-87.

18. Kaplan RM. Utility assessment for estimating quality-adjusted life years. In: Sloan FA, editor. Valuing health care: costs, benefits, and effectiveness of pharmaceuticals and other medical technologies. Cambridge (NY): Cambridge University Press; 1995.

19. Kennedy W, Reinharz D, Tessier G, Contandriopoulos AP, Trabut I, Champagne F, Ayoub J. Cost-utility analysis of chemotherapy and best supportive care in non-small cell lung cancer. PharmacoEconom. 1995;8(4):316-23.

20. Jolicoeur LM, Jones-Grizzle AJ, Boyer JG. Guidelines for performing a pharmacoeconomic analysis. Am J Hosp Pharm. 1992;49:1741-7.

21. Shaw JW, Zachry WM. Application of probabilistic sensitivity analysis in decision analytic modeling. Formulary (USA). 2002;37:32-34, 37-40.

22. McGhan WF, Lewis NJW. Basic bibliographies: pharmacoeconomics. Hosp Pharm. 1992;27:547-8.

23. Wanke LA, Huber SL. Basic bibliographies: cancer therapy pharmacoeconomics. Hosp Pharm. 1994;29:402.

24. Skaer TL, Williams LM. Basic bibliographies: biotechnology pharmacoeconomics I. Hosp Pharm. 1994;29:1053-4.

25. Skaer TL, Williams LM. Basic bibliographies: biotechnology pharmacoeconomics II. Hosp Pharm. 1994;29:1136.

26. McGhan WF. Basic bibliographies: pharmacoeconomics. Hosp Pharm. 1998;33:1270, 1273.

27. Duggan AE, Tolley K, Hawkey CJ, Logan RF. Varying efficacy of Helicobacter pylori eradication regimens: cost effectiveness study using a decision analysis model. BMJ. 1998;316:1648-54.

28. Messori A, Trippoli S, Becagli P, Cincotta M, Labbate MG, Zaccara G. Adjunctive lamotrigine therapy in patients with refractor y seizures: a lifetime cost-utility analysis. Eur J Clin Pharmacol. 1998;53(6):421-7.

29. Ginsberg G, Shani S, Lev B. Cost benefit analysis of risperidone and clozapine in the treatment of schizophrenia in Israel. PharmacoEconom. 1998 Feb;13:231-41.

30. Sesti AM, Armitstead JA, Hall KN, Jang R, Milne S. Cost-minimization analysis of hand held nebulizer LC vs UC metered dose inhaler protocol for management of acute asthma exacerbations in the emergency department. ASHP Midyear Clinical Meeting; 32: MCS-7: 1997 Dec 8–12; New Orleans, Louisiana.

31. Hinman AR, Koplan JP, Orenstein WA, Brink EW. Decision analysis and polio immunization policy. Am J Pub Health. 1988;78:301-3.

32. Kessler JM. Decision analysis in the formulary process. Am J Health Syst Pharm. 1997;54:S5-S8.

33. Einarson TR, McGhan WF, Bootman JL. Decision analysis applied to pharmacy practice. Am J Hosp Pharm. 1985;42:364-71.

34. Walking D, Appino JP. Decision analysis in drug product development. Drug Cosmet Ind. 1973;112:39-41.

35. Rascati KL. Decision analysis techniques practical aspects of using personal computers for decision analytic modeling. Drug Benefit Trends. 1998 July;33-36.

36. Richardson WS, Detsky AS. Users' guides to the medical literature. Part 7. How to use a clinical decision analysis. Part A. Are the results of the study valid? JAMA. 1995;273:1292-5.

37. Richardson WS, Detsky AS. Users' guides to the medical literature. Part 7. How to use a clinical decision analysis. Part B. What are the results and will they help me in caring for my patients? JAMA. 1995;273:1610-3.

38. Baskin LE. Practical pharmacoeconomics. Cleveland (OH): Advanstar Communications; 1998.

39. Sacristán JA, Soto J, Galende I. Evaluation of pharmacoeconomic studies: utilization of a checklist. Ann Pharmacother. 1993;27:1126-32.

40. Mandelblatt JS, Fryback DG, Weinstein MC, Russell LB, Gold MR. Assessing the effectiveness of health interventions for cost-effectiveness analysis. Panel on Cost-Effectiveness in Health and Medicine. J Gen Intern Med. 1997;12(9):551–8. doi. org/10.1046/j.1525-1497.1997.07107.x.

41. Botteman MF, Caprini J, Stephens JM, Nadipelli V, Bell CF, Pashos CL, Cohen AT. Results of an economic model to assess cost-effectiveness of enoxaparin, a low-molecular-weight heparin, versus warfarin for the prophylaxis of DVT and associated long-term complications in total hip replacement surgery in the United States. Clin Ther. 2002:24(11):1960-86.

42. Grutters J, Seferina S, Tjan-Heijnen V, van Kampen R, Goettsch W, Joore M. Bridging trial and decision: a checklist to frame health technology assessments for resource allocation decisions. J Int Soc Pharmacoecon Outcomes Res. 2011 July;14(5):777-84.
43. Husereau D, Drummond M, Petrou S, Carswell C, Moher D, Greenberg D, Augustovski F, Briggs AH, Mauskopf J, Loder E. Consolidated Health Economic Evaluation Reporting Standards (CHEERS) statement. BMJ. 2013;346:f1049.
44. Doran C. Critique of an economic evaluation using the Drummond checklist. Appl Health Econ Health Pol. 2010;8(6):357-9.
45. Chiou C, Hay J, Ofman J, Bloom BS, Neumann PJ, Sullivan SD, Yu H-T, Keeler EB, Henning JM, Ofman JJ, Development and validation of a grading system for the quality of cost-effectiveness studies. Medical Care [serial online]. 2003 January;41(1):32-44.
46. Ofman J, Sullivan S, Neumann PJ, Chiou CF, Henning JM, Wade SW, Hay J. Examining the value and quality of health economic analyses: implications of utilizing the QHES. J Managed Care Pharmacy: JMCP [serial online]. 2003 January;9(1):53-61.
47. Edwards R, Charles J, Lloyd-Williams H. Public health economics: a systematic review of guidance for the economic evaluation of public health interventions and discussion of key methodological issues. BMC Public Health [serial online]. 2013 October 24;13(1):1001.
48. Mullins CD, Flowers LR. Evaluating economic outcomes literature. In: Grauer DW, Lee J, Odom TD, editors. Pharmacoeconomics and outcomes: applications for patient care. 2nd ed. Kansas City (MO): American College of Clinical Pharmacy; 2003.
49. Rascati, KL. Essentials of pharmacoeconomics. 2nd ed. Philadelphia (PA): Wolters Kluwer/Lippincott Williams & Wilkins; 2013.
50. Drummond MF, Sculpher MJ, Torrance GW, O'Brien BJ, Stoddart GL. Methods for the economic evaluation of health care programmes. 3rd ed. Oxford, New York: Oxford University Press; 2005.
51. Neumann PJ, Sanders GD, Russell LB, Siegel JE, Ganiats TG, editors. Cost-effectiveness in health and medicine. 2nd ed. New York: Oxford University Press; 2016.

SUGGESTED READINGS

1. Health care costs, quality, and outcomes ISPOR book of terms. Lawrenceville (NJ): International Society for Pharmacoeconomics and Outcomes Research; 2020 Edition in Press.
2. Husereau D, Drummond M, Petrou S, Carswell C, Moher D, Greenberg D, Augustovski F, Briggs AH, Mauskopf J, Loder E. Consolidated Health Economic Evaluation Reporting Standards (CHEERS) statement. Value Health. 2013 Mar;16(2):e1-e5.
3. Rascati, KL. Essentials of pharmacoeconomics. 3rd ed. Philadelphia: Wolters Kluwer/Lippincott Williams & Wilkins; 2021.
4. Drummond MF, Sculpher MJ, Claxton K, Stoddart GL, Torrance, GW. Methods for the economic evaluation of health care programmes. 4th ed. Oxford, New York: Oxford University Press; 2015.
5. Neumann PJ, Sanders GD, Russell LB, Siegel JE, Ganiats TG, editors. Cost-effectiveness in health and medicine. 2nd ed. New York: Oxford University Press; 2016.

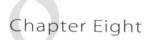

Chapter Eight

Evidence-Based Clinical Practice Guidelines

Jeanine P. Abrons • Pavnit Kukreja

Learning Objectives

After completing this chapter, the reader will be able to:

- Define clinical practice guideline.
- Define evidence-based medicine (EBM).
- Discuss collaboration and roles of health care professionals and pharmacists in the development and use of evidence-based clinical practice guidelines.
- Describe how guidelines influence health care delivery.
- Discuss appropriate use of the GRADE (Grading of Recommendations, Assessment, Development, and Evaluation) system for grading the quality of evidence and the strength of recommendations.
- Describe methods of evaluating clinical practice guidelines.
- Identify the key issues involved in the implementation and use of clinical practice guidelines.
- Identify sources of published clinical practice guidelines.

Key Concepts

❶ Clinical practice guidelines or "guidelines" are recommendations for providing optimal patient care. The development of evidence-based guidelines incorporates a systematic review of the available evidence, often relying heavily on randomized controlled trials (RCTs) for guidance on best practices in treatment and interventions. For screening and diagnosis, guidelines commonly use evidence from other study designs. Each guideline may also use different study types/levels and expert knowledge to assess the benefits and harms of interventions for topics or disease states.

❷ EBM is the conscientious, explicit, and judicious development and use of current best evidence in making decisions about the care of individual patients.

❸ Evaluation of the appropriateness of guideline use in various settings should include the consideration of the strength, quality, and applicability of the guideline to the practice setting.

❹ Formulation and articulation of clinical questions to be addressed by a guideline provide direction for subsequent steps in the development of a guideline.

❺ Evaluation of evidence quality, which is the basis for recommendations, is a crucial aspect for the interpretation and use of a guideline.

❻ The GRADE system presents all evidence considered in the creation of a guideline and weighs the strength of the criteria. Judgments made are transparent. Summarized tables of evidence and findings are created.

❼ Before selecting a clinical practice guideline for use in any practice setting, the health care professional needs to evaluate the quality of published guidelines. The Appraisal of Guidelines for Research Evaluation (AGREE) Enterprise created a useful tool for evaluating clinical practice guidelines.

❽ An optimal method for the use of guidelines to improve the quality of patient care does not exist.

❾ ECRI developed a website called ECRI Guidelines Trust® that serves as a respository of clinical practice guidelines.

Introduction

● USE OF CLINICAL PRACTICE GUIDELINES TO OPTIMIZE PATIENT CARE

❶ *Clinical practice guidelines or "guidelines" are recommendations for providing optimal patient care. Evidence-based guidelines are developed through a systematic review of the available evidence, often relying heavily on RCTs for guidance on best practices in treatment and interventions.[1] For screening and diagnosis, guidelines commonly use evidence from other study designs. Each guideline may also use different study types/levels of evidence and expert knowledge to assess the benefits and harms of interventions for topics or disease states.*

What is the General Purpose of a Guideline?

A clinical practice guideline is a set of statements or recommendations, ideally based on a systematic review of evidence. Intentions of these recommendations include improving quality of care while decreasing the cost of care and improving patient safety. Guidelines review the potential risks and benefits of various management strategies (e.g., screening, diagnosis, and/or intervention) for a practice specialty or a specific setting for clinical care and provide recommendations for or against use. Interventions include medication use or other types of therapy (e.g., radiation, surgery, physical therapy).[2] Governments, professional associations, managed care and quality assurance organizations, third-party payers, and utilization review groups develop guidelines. The purpose of a guideline, the methods used to develop each guideline, the format of the recommendations, and the strategies suggested for their use and implementation vary widely. Guidelines have the potential to influence many decisions about health-related interventions, including reimbursement for therapies or services. Examples include the establishment of formularies and compensation or coverage of medications or other interventions. As such, it is vital for health care professionals must become familiar with guidelines and evaluate the criteria used to assess their validity.

What are the Considerations in Developing a Guideline?

The development of clinical practice guidelines includes the use of systematic approaches and problem solving to assess the relevance and completeness of information available to formulate recommendations. In interpreting a guideline, a health care practitioner should be able to describe the answers to clinical questions that the guideline addresses. Completion of a literature search identifies new studies to ensure the guideline includes current practices and scientific findings. Clinical expertise, epidemiology, and biostatistics principles should be used to evaluate the rigor of the studies identified by the literature search. This review of the existing literature can be used to determine whether the guideline is complete and accurate.

What Should You Know about Evidence Included in Guidelines?—The Challenge of Staying Up-to-Date

Limitations do exist with the use of guidelines. For example, the available information and technologies used in health care rapidly evolve, and information may become quickly outdated. Therefore, health care providers should remember that interventions described are limited to a given point in time (typically up to the time of guideline publication).

The challenge of keeping guidelines up-to-date is further affected by the significant time lag that occurs between the actual translation of research into clinical practice and the use of guidelines in practice. Delay in the sharing of knowledge of well-studied, efficacious treatments has resulted in underutilization of appropriate interventions and continued use of interventions proven to be ineffective.[3] The development of accurate, complete, and transparent guidelines with continued updates may facilitate the more rapid adoption of available evidence into clinical practice. Preferably, guidelines should be updated whenever new information becomes available, which can occur multiple times per year, if and when significant revisions are warranted (as are done with some guidelines). However, most guidelines are updated annually, or sometimes less frequently.

Despite this limitation, guidelines can assist with the identification of indicators for care quality. Appropriately developed guidelines provide health care practitioners with concise summaries of relevant, high-quality evidence to differentiate between efficacious and nonefficacious interventions. They assist with clinical decision-making and facilitate the discussion of available care options. Guidelines may establish a common ground to coordinate care, especially when patient care decisions involve multiple health care practitioners and when transitions of care between settings occur.[4]

How can Guidelines Improve the Quality of Care?

Critical issues in reforming the U.S. health care system include access to care, cost, and quality. Quality and safety were a significant focus as highlighted in reports published by the National Academy of Medicine, formerly known as the Institute of Medicine (IOM), on quality of care problems in the United States, and recommendations to improve patient safety, and to reduce preventable medical errors.[5-8] The central concepts in these reports relate to the use of the best available evidence, the use of decision support tools and informatics, and including patients in health care decisions. The National Academies of Sciences, Engineering, and Medicine reports explicitly dealt with standards for clinical practice guidelines, systematic reviews of comparative effectiveness research, and providing care at a lower cost.[1,9,10] These documents and standards highlighted improvements in technology, quality of access to electronic records, and more exceptional ability to use the data from processes of care to provide valuable information to learn what works best. These concepts are central to improving the validity and usefulness of clinical practice guidelines.

This chapter will present a review of clinical practice guidelines and the related concept of EBM; review evidence-based methods for guideline development, evaluation, and use; and provide directions to locate sources of guidelines.

Evidence-Based Medicine and Clinical Practice Guidelines

❷ *EBM is the conscientious, explicit, and judicious development and use of current best evidence in making decisions about the care of individual patients.*[11]

The practice of EBM integrates individual clinical knowledge with published clinical evidence from systematic research. EBM is often mistaken for, or reduced to, one of its several components, critical appraisal of the literature. However, EBM requires both clinical expertise and knowledge of individual patient's circumstances, beliefs, priorities, and values to be useful. External evidence must inform, but not replace, clinical expertise. It is clinical expertise that determines if and how the external evidence applies to the individual patient. The development and use of clinical practice guidelines are among the tools used in EBM. The first published use of the term "evidence-based" was in the context of clinical guidelines.[12] An understanding of EBM is necessary to understand the purpose of guidelines. The Center for Evidence-Based Medicine (CEBM) is an important and respected world resource on EBM.[13]

WHERE DID THE TERM "EVIDENCE-BASED MEDICINE" COME FROM?

Physicians, led by the founding father of EBM, David Sackett, at McMaster University in Hamilton, Ontario were the first to use the term "evidence-based medicine." These physicians, known as the Evidence-Based Medicine Working Group, published a description of what they considered a new paradigm for medical practice and teaching.[14] The group articulated views on changes that were occurring in medical practice related to the use of medical literature to more effectively guide decision-making. They stated that the foundation for the paradigm shift rested in advances in clinical research, such as the development of RCTs and meta-analyses.

WHAT ARE THE SPECIFIC STEPS USED IN EBM?

The practice of EBM has focused on five linked steps: (1) the conversion of information need into a clearly defined answerable clinical question, (2) the search for the best available evidence for a problem, (3) appraisal of the validity, impact, and applicability of the evidence, (4) the incorporation of clinical expertise and knowledge of the patient's unique characteristics within this appraisal, and (5) evaluation of the first four activities and identification of ways to improve them.[15] These activities are similar to the systematic approach to drug information requests of Watanabe and colleagues[16] developed in 1975, which continue to be used today.

After the original paper on EBM was published by the Evidence-Based Medicine Working Group,[14] a description of appropriate training methods on evidence-based care was written to enable practitioners to locate, evaluate, and apply the best evidence.[17] The report recognized that not all practitioners have the time or interest to use primary literature and noted the potential use of sources of appropriately preappraised evidenced. Examples include clinical practice guidelines and systematic reviews produced with evidence-based methods. However, the authors note that practitioners should interpret medical literature individually to judge the quality of preappraised resources. This step would enable health care practitioners to know when recommendations provided are applicable, and to determine when to use the original literature.[17]

HOW ARE EBM AND GUIDELINES RELATED?

A review of the EBM philosophy, published by Eddy in 2005,[18] describes an approach that is similar to that of the Evidence-Based Medicine Working Group. In this review, guidelines are a second approach to EBM. The approach has four important features: (1) small, specially trained groups analyze evidence and develop the guideline, (2) an explicit, rigorous process is used, (3) the guideline is not specific to an individual patient but rather should be applicable to a class or group of patients, and (4) the guideline should indirectly help, guide, or motivate health care providers to deliver certain types of care to people, not directly determine the care for a specific patient.[18]

Health care professionals face the complicated reality of a continually changing and increasing body of medical information. To practice effective, high-quality medicine, memorization of vast amounts of information is not always reasonable. As a result, it is necessary to develop skills to acquire and critically assess knowledge rapidly in order to make clinical decisions.[19] These abilities align with the decision-making process of EBM and use of clinical practice guidelines.

Guideline Development Methods and Evaluation

An understanding of the clinical practice guideline development process is essential to health care practitioners. Although relatively few practitioners will participate in guideline development, they should be able to determine on their own whether a guideline is credible based on the methodology used to create it, and whether or not it applies to their practice setting.

❸ *Evaluation of guideline quality, applicability, and appropriateness of use in a given practice setting depends primarily on the ability to distinguish methods that minimize potential biases in development.* A lack of understanding of the process for guideline development could lead to inappropriate interpretations of guideline recommendations, which could lead to the use of ineffective or harmful therapy.

WHO CREATES GUIDELINES?

Many organizations develop clinical practice guidelines. Examples of organizations include, but are not limited to, professional societies (e.g., American Academy of Neurology [AAN],[20] American College of Chest Physicians [CHEST],[21] Infectious Disease

Society of America [IDSA][22]) and government agencies (e.g., Advisory Committee on Immunization Practices [ACIP],[23] Centers for Disease Control and Prevention [CDC],[24] National Institutes of Health [NIH],[25] and the United States Preventative Services Task Force [USPSTF][26]). Although there are currently no universally endorsed standards for guideline development, progress has been made through the collaboration of key organizations and individuals to improve standardization.

HOW DOES ONE ENSURE THAT THE INFORMATION INCLUDED IN A GUIDELINE IS VALID?

The recommendations included in guidelines must come from high-quality research. The following sections describe organizations that help ensure the availability of high-quality research.

The EQUATOR Network (Enhancing the Quality and Transparency of Health Research) brings together researchers, journal editors, peer reviewers, reporting guideline developers, research funding bodies, and other collaborators.[27] The EQUATOR network intends to "improve the quality of research publications and of research itself." Such organizations maintain a comprehensive collection of reporting guidelines for main study types (e.g., CONSORT guidelines to evaluate/interpret randomized trials,[28] STROBE guidelines for evaluation of observational studies[29]). The EQUATOR network promotes the use of reporting guidelines to ensure consistency in processes and an ability to evaluate the strength of literature.[27] Many endorsed standards for research can be located on the EQUATOR network website and can be applied to ensure that the literature used in clinical practice guidelines is sound.

The CONSORT statement was developed through a collaboration of epidemiologists, methodologists, statisticians, researchers, and journal editors to improve the quality of the reporting results of randomized trials.[28] This statement guides improvement in the completeness and adequacy of randomized controlled trial research reported. The goal is to describe the systematic approach used, the findings, and the meaning of results. CONSORT establishes a checklist of items for the reporting of randomized trials.[28]

Many endorsed standards for research can be located on the EQUATOR Network website and can be applied to ensure the literature used in clinical practice guidelines is sound. In 2008, the IOM developed and promoted standards for systematic reviews of comparative effectiveness research and evidence-based clinical practice guidelines.[1] The Committee on Standards for Systematic Reviews of Comparative Effectiveness Research and the Committee on Standards for Developing Trustworthy Clinical Practice Guidelines were formed. In 2011, the committees published standards for systematic reviews of comparative effectiveness research and for developing rigorous, trustworthy clinical practice guidelines.[1,9]

The IOM was another source of standards to ensure the development of useful guidelines. The IOM proposed eight standards (Table 8-1) for developing evidence-based

TABLE 8–1. STANDARDS FOR DEVELOPING TRUSTWORTHY CLINICAL PRACTICE GUIDELINES[1]

1. Establishing Transparency
   1.1 The processes by which clinical practice guidelines are developed and funded should be detailed explicitly and publicly accessible.

2. Management of Conflict of Interest (COI)
   2.1 Prior to selection of the guideline development group (GDG), individuals considered for membership should declare all interests and activities potentially resulting in COI with guideline development, by written disclosure to those convening the GDG:
      - Disclosure should reflect all current and planned commercial (including services from which a clinician derives a substantial proportion of income), noncommercial, intellectual, institutional, and patient–public activities pertinent to the potential scope of the clinical practice guideline.

   2.2 Disclosure of COIs within GDG:
      - All COI of each GDG member should be reported and discussed by the prospective development group prior to the onset of his or her work.
      - Each panel member should explain how his or her COI could influence the clinical practice guideline development process or specific recommendations.

   2.3 Divestment
      - Members of the GDG should divest themselves of financial investments in which they or their family members have, and not participate in marketing activities or advisory boards of entities whose interests could be affected by clinical practice guideline recommendations.

   2.4 Exclusions
      - Whenever possible, GDG members should not have COI.
      - In some circumstances, a GDG may not be able to perform its work without members who have COIs, such as relevant clinical specialists who receive a substantial portion of their incomes from services pertinent to the clinical practice guideline.
      - Members with COIs should represent no more than a minority of the GDG.
      - The chair or cochairs of a guideline should not have COIs.
      - Funders should have no role in clinical practice guideline development.

3. Guideline Development Group Composition
   3.1 The GDG should be multidisciplinary and balanced, comprising a variety of methodological experts and clinicians, and populations to be affected by the clinical practice guideline.
   3.2 Patient and public involvement should be facilitated by including (at least at the time of clinical question formulation and draft clinical practice guideline review) a current or former patient, and a patient advocate or patient/consumer organization representative in the GDG.
   3.3 Strategies to increase effective participation of patient and consumer representatives, including training in appraisal of evidence, should be adopted by GDGs.

4. Clinical Practice Guideline—Systematic Review Intersection
   4.1 Clinical practice guideline developers should use systematic reviews that meet standards set by the Institute of Medicine's Committee on Standards for Systematic Reviews of Comparative Effectiveness Research.
   4.2 When systematic reviews are conducted specifically to inform particular guidelines, the GDG and systematic review team should interact regarding the scope, approach, and output of both processes.

continued

TABLE 8–1. STANDARDS FOR DEVELOPING TRUSTWORTHY CLINICAL PRACTICE GUIDELINES[1] *(CONTINUED)*

5. Establishing Evidence Foundations for and Rating Strength of Recommendations

   5.1 For each recommendation, the following should be provided:
   - An explanation of the reasoning underlying the recommendation, including:
     - a clear description of potential benefits and harms;
     - a summary of relevant available evidence (and evidentiary gaps), description of the quality (including applicability), quantity (including completeness), and consistency of the aggregate available evidence;
     - an explanation of the part played by values, opinion, theory, and clinical experience in deriving the recommendation.
   - A rating of the level of confidence in (certainty regarding) the evidence underpinning the recommendation.
   - A rating of the strength of the recommendation in light of the preceding bullets.
   - A description and explanation of any differences of opinion regarding the recommendation.

6. Articulation of Recommendations

   6.1 Recommendations should be articulated in a standardized form detailing precisely what the recommended action is, and under what circumstances it should be performed.

   6.2 Strong recommendations should be worded so that compliance with the recommendation(s) can be evaluated.

7. External Review

   7.1 External reviewers should comprise a full spectrum of relevant stakeholders, including scientific and clinical experts, organizations (e.g., health care, specialty societies), agencies (e.g., federal government), patients, and representatives of the public.

   7.2 The authorship of external reviews submitted by individuals and/or organizations should be kept confidential unless that protection has been waived by the reviewer(s).

   7.3 The GDG should consider all external reviewer comments and keep a written record of the rationale for modifying or not modifying a clinical practice guideline in response to reviewers' comments.

   7.4 A draft of the clinical practice guideline at the external review stage or immediately following it (i.e., prior to the final draft) should be made available to the general public for comment. Reasonable notice of impending publication should be provided to interested public stakeholders.

8. Updating Guidelines

   8.1 The date of clinical practice guideline publication, date of pertinent systematic evidence review, and proposed date for future clinical practice guideline review should be documented in the clinical practice guideline.

   8.2 Literature should be monitored regularly following clinical practice guideline publication to identify the emergence of new, potentially relevant evidence and to evaluate the continued validity of the clinical practice guideline.

   8.3 Clinical practice guidelines should be updated when new evidence suggests the need for modification of clinically important recommendations. For example, a clinical practice guideline should be updated if new evidence shows that a recommended intervention causes previously unknown substantial harm; that a new intervention is significantly superior to a previously recommended intervention from an efficacy or harms perspective; or that a recommendation can be applied to new populations.

clinical practice guidelines. When reviewing a guideline for potential use or implementation at a practice setting, these steps can be used as a checklist for the health care practitioner to consider in reviewing the guideline. The major steps in their proposed standards include[1]:

- Establishing transparency
- Management of conflict of interest
- Guideline development group composition
- Clinical practice guideline and systematic review intersection
- Establishing evidence foundations for and rating strength of recommendations
- Articulation of recommendations
- Conduct an external review
- Establishment of a plan for guideline updates

Each of these steps is discussed separately below.

ESTABLISHING TRANSPARENCY

The processes of developing a guideline should be shared with the intended audience. Additionally, sources of funding for the guideline should be transparent. Specifically, this information should be explicitly detailed and publicly available. This transparency helps users to understand the basis of recommendations, who developed them, as well as other considerations for their interpretation. The clinical experience of the guideline development group members and potential **conflicts of interest (COIs)** are stated as well to ensure members are knowledgeable on the topic area and free of important COIs.[1]

MANAGEMENT OF CONFLICTS OF INTEREST

This step is essential in both the creation and interpretation of guidelines to clarify potential COIs by members of the guideline development group. Conflicts of interest include not only financial conflicts of interest, but also include intellectual disputes that may occur as a result of previous research published by the individual, institutional COI, and patient-public activities.[1] Individuals considered for membership on a guideline panel should declare potential COIs. Individuals with potential COIs may still be considered for participation on a panel depending on the type and degree of conflict, and with appropriate management and disclosure.[30] The exclusion of any individuals with possible conflicts could result in the elimination of the majority of individuals with the critical expertise needed.[31] Controversies over the sponsorship of guideline development and publication exist,[32] and potential COIs by panel members[33] are sometimes present. In general, guideline development groups should limit potential conflicts of interest as much as possible, and health care practitioners should assess whether conflicts exist or appear to have influenced recommendations.

CHEST, for example, is a prominent guideline-development group that emphasizes management of COIs in their guideline development process.[34] A methodologist with no COIs is the primary author of each guideline. Panel members who have conflicts are "approved with management," meaning that they are subject to oversight and may have limited participation in discussions and final decisions on the direction or strength of a recommendation.[35]

● ESTABLISHMENT OF MULTIDISCIPLINARY GUIDELINE DEVELOPMENT GROUPS

A step in the guideline development process that is important to consider during evaluation of a guideline is the establishment of a well-rounded guideline development group. The composition of the team involved in the clinical practice guideline development should be multidisciplinary. Guidelines ideally include all groups that have a stake in the development and use of a guideline. Team members for each guideline include specialized physicians; providers involved in the treatment of patients; representatives of other disciplines involved in providing care (e.g., pharmacy, physical therapy, respiratory therapy, nursing, occupational therapy, social work, dentistry); experts with knowledge of the applicable research methods; individuals with expertise in systematically searching for evidence; and patient representatives or caregivers. Patient involvement is essential in formulating and prioritizing the questions to be addressed by the guideline.[1]

Case Study 8-1

You have been selected to review the literature as part of a committee to choose a clinical practice guideline for use within your health system. As you evaluate the available guidelines, what are the first four steps that you want to take to ensure that the approach is valid and provides a summary of high-quality evidence for your institution?

CLINICAL PRACTICE GUIDELINE AND SYSTEMATIC REVIEW INTERSECTION

Clinical practice guidelines and systematic reviews are concepts that overlap. (See Chapter 5 for more information on systematic reviews.) Systematic reviews synthesize evidence that guideline development groups can use when forming recommendations based on available evidence.[1] It is recommended that clinical practice guideline developers conduct systematic reviews that meet the IOM standards for systematic reviews of comparative effectiveness research. The standards include the following steps (these are described in more detail below):[9]

- An appropriate topic for the creation of a guideline was selected.
- The clinical questions to be addressed were defined.
- The study screening selection criteria were determined and described.
- A systematic search for evidence was conducted.
- Individual studies were critically appraised.
- The body of evidence was synthesized.

Select an Appropriate Topic for Creation of a Guideline

Health care practitioners can compare the process of selecting a topic for guideline development to the selection of topics for a medication use evaluation, or for any quality improvement program (see Chapter 18). Guidelines improve the quality and outcomes of care. As with any clinical management decision, assessments of the potential benefits of guideline development and implementation are made. Characteristics of disease states with the maximum potential to benefit from guideline development include:

- High prevalence
- High frequency and severity of associated morbidity or mortality
- Available high-quality evidence for the efficacy of treatments that may reduce morbidity or mortality
- Feasible implementation of the treatment based on expertise and resources required
- Potential cost-effectiveness
- Evidence that current practice is not optimal
- Evidence of practice variation (i.e., patients with similar characteristics are provided different services or a substantially different frequency of services in different geographic locations)
- Available personnel, expertise, and resources to develop and implement the practice guideline

As an example, the American Heart Association (AHA) identified reasons for developing evidence-based guidelines for cardiovascular disease prevention in women, which includes the incidence of heart disease-related morbidity and mortality in women.[36] The organization believed that it was essential to identify and prevent the incidence of coronary heart disease (CHD) in women as a separate population and recognized that patient characteristics could differ between clinical trials and practice.[36]

Define the Clinical Questions to be Addressed

In addition to the selection of a topic, the issues that recommendations in the guideline address should be defined. How does the transparency of decision-making or action steps improve the recommendations for screening, confirmation, diagnosis, treatment, and surveillance of disease? Decision-making points are expressed as clinical questions.

❹ *Formulation and articulation of clinical questions to be addressed by a guideline provide direction for subsequent steps in the development of a guideline.* The clinical questions provide direction for the systematic review of the literature, and the outline for recommendations in the guideline. The question should be clearly defined first to enable a literature review to look for relevant studies and evidence and support the development of useful and valid conclusions.

Health care practitioners should review guidelines to determine if a clear description of the questions addressed were provided and should consider if the issues are useful in practice. Depending on the overall goals of a guideline, questions may include: What is the best diagnostic test or method of screening? What forms of treatment or prevention are most effective? What is the quantification of the potential harms of treatment? What comorbidities change recommendations? What costs are associated with different management strategies?

To allow health care professionals to easily assess whether clinical questions addressed in a guideline are relevant to their practice setting, many guideline development groups have carefully framed the questions using the Patients-Interventions-Comparison-Outcomes (PICO) model, which includes the following parts[37,38]:

- Patients: Which patients did the guideline consider? How were they described? Did any subgroups require special consideration? This step is similar to the statement of the inclusion and exclusion criteria in a clinical study, but usually not as restrictive.
- Interventions: Which interventions or treatments did the guideline consider?
- Comparison: What other interventions or treatments were compared with the interventions considered?
- Outcome: What measurement was most important to the patient (e.g., mortality, morbidity, treatment complications, rates of relapse, physical function, quality of life, costs)?

The clinical questions define the relevant patient population, the management strategies considered, and the outcomes of care that the guideline intends to achieve. Questions are analyzed for different clinical scenarios and practice settings to ensure that guidelines are of sufficient scope to avoid significant gaps in decision-making. There is no standard for the number of questions required. However, if the number of questions becomes substantial, it may be necessary to break the guideline into subtopics. Subtopics may be determined to construct a guideline for making recommendations for screening or diagnosis in one guideline and recommendations for treatment in another. Subtopics may be based on differentiation of populations or severities of disease (e.g., New York Heart Association classes of heart failure) or based on other demographic factors that might impact patient care recommendations.

Determine the Methods and Criteria for Study Selection

Guidelines should specify the types of published or unpublished research analyzed to ensure the inclusion of appropriate literature. Keywords from the focused clinical questions addressed by a recommendation should be defined to indicate the types of patients, interventions, comparators, and outcomes of studies. The evidence considered, including the types of studies (e.g., observational studies, diagnostic studies, economic studies, and qualitative studies), should be described.

The inclusion of additional studies may again be revisited at a later stage of guideline development. It is possible and common that based on an initial review of the evidence, initial questions are modified or new questions are formed. Often the scope of articles included is expanded. Guideline creators should share the reasons for changing search criteria to enable the clinician to understand the reasons for the changes.

Once the keywords and criteria are defined, evidence-based guidelines require that relevant evidence was found and appraised. A first step in identifying this material is through an extensive literature search. In most cases, more than one person is involved in searching for evidence and selecting studies. Clear criteria ensure consistency in the methods used to select the studies. Inconsistent retrieval of evidence between evaluators adds a potential for bias in the guideline.

Many guideline development groups first search to identify prior guidelines or systematic reviews of similar or closely related questions. Available bibliographic resources such as MEDLINE®, Current Contents®, Embase®, Science Citation Index, The Cochrane Library, International Pharmaceutical Abstracts, and Cumulative Index to Nursing and Allied Health Literature (CINAHL) are searched. Evidence may also be obtained from citations listed in published bibliographies and textbooks, and literature identified by researchers and content experts. Recording of keywords and other search criteria (e.g., Medical Subject Headings [MeSH] terms from MEDLINE®, limits by publication year, language, and study types) allow duplication of the process. Retrieved articles are then considered for relevance and fit with the criteria for inclusion as predetermined by the panel. Guideline developers keep a log of excluded studies and the rationale for their exclusion.

An extensive review of search strategies (e.g., word-phrasing and refinement of search terms) is beyond the scope of this chapter. Most guideline development groups use highly trained methodologists, librarians, or drug information specialists to perform searches. A carefully planned and executed search is necessary to maximize search efficiency and avoid missing relevant evidence.

Critically Appraise Individual Studies

Health care practitioners should appraise individual studies to identify relevant literature to apply to practice and to assess the basis of guidelines. Review each included study using checklists to evaluate the strength of the article (e.g., CONSORT guidelines). Study design problems or biases can be identified by this step. Considerations include the type of study (i.e., randomized controlled clinical trial, cohort study, or case-control study), the sample size or population used, and the statistical power to support or identify the effects of the intervention. Next, a review to assess the representativeness of the total population in the inclusion and exclusion criteria and whether the control group adequately removes factors that complicate findings.

Additionally, a well-structured article or study should provide for the health care practitioner with the randomization methods, group composition, definitions of interventions and outcome measures, attrition rates, methods of data collection and statistical analysis, unique characteristics of the study population, and blinding. Consider whether the results of different trials are consistent or if there is significant heterogeneity. An analysis of the safety of treatments includes the amount of evidence, the number of participants evaluated, and the length of time. Potential adverse events that occur infrequently may not be identified if studies do not have a sufficient sample size or if sample populations are narrowly defined or are not representative of the entire population impacted by the condition. See Chapters 4 and 5 for information on literature evaluation, along with Chapter 6, for evaluating statistical tests used in studies. Chapter 7 provides additional details on cost considerations.

Synthesize the Body of Evidence

Guidelines often have effectively summarized key themes from included studies. Whether using a guideline or summarizing its contents, it is essential to present information clearly to highlight characteristics, quality of individual studies, the scope of evidence, and potential benefits and risks of intervention. If available, guidelines use a meta-analysis as a statistical way to summarize or estimate the treatment effect size. See Chapter 5 for information on meta-analyses.

Case Study 8–2

Building on Case 8-1, you are asked to summarize the guideline that was selected for the pharmacy and therapeutics (P&T) committee at your hospital. You must describe the clinical questions defined. Based on the guidelines, you are asked to recommend what treatments or medications should be covered or excluded under your health system's plan. Using the PICO format, frame the clinical questions addressed by the guideline and the potential usefulness of the guideline to your health system.

ESTABLISHMENT OF THE FOUNDATIONS OF EVIDENCE AND RATING RECOMMENDATION STRENGTH

Rating the quality of the evidence and strength of recommendations within the guideline is the next step.

The National Comprehensive Cancer Network (NCCN) is an excellent example of an organization with established foundations of evidence and rating recommendation strength. Four categories for recommendations used are:[39]

- Category 1: Based on high-level evidence with the uniform consensus that the intervention is appropriate
- Category 2A: Based on lower-level evidence with a uniform consensus that the intervention is appropriate
- Category 2B: Based on lower-level evidence consensus that the intervention is appropriate
- Category 3: Based on any level of evidence and with disagreement that the intervention is appropriate

The organization further defines when to use various interventions as preferred interventions (based on superior efficacy, safety, evidence, and affordability), other recommendations (less efficacious, more safety concerns, less data, and less affordability), and usefulness in certain circumstances (or populations). This additional classification provides additional clarity between the quality of the evidence and the level of information.[39]

The Grading of Recommendation, Assessment, Development, and Evaluation (GRADE) Working Group has developed the most accepted system for determining the strength of recommendations and rating quality of evidence.[40] The **GRADE system** is a system used by CHEST[41] and by many other developers of high-quality guidelines. More details on the GRADE system are provided below. By rating the quality of evidence, the guideline creators establish the level of confidence in the estimates of the effects.

GRADE System of Grading Quality of Evidence and Strength of Recommendations

The GRADE Working Group began in 2000 as an informal collaboration of people who recognized the shortcomings of the systems available at that time to clarify the strength of recommendations. The group sought to offer recommendations for improvement. This section will begin with the history of the guidelines and proceed into how the guidelines assess the quality and strength of recommendations in greater detail.[42]

The GRADE Working Group first published a standardized grading method for determining the quality of the evidence and the strength of clinical practice recommendations in 2004.[43] The group believed that a grading system would provide consistent and transparent judgments on the evidence quality and recommendation strength. Ultimately, the group felt that the GRADE system supported more informed choices in health care.[44] The GRADE criteria were last updated in 2016.[45] Since the publishing of the original criteria in 2004, the GRADE Working Group has issued over 70 publications related to the methodology located on the GRADE website.[44]

⑤ *Evidence quality and the basis for recommendations should be evaluated in the interpretation and use of a practice guideline.*

How is the balance between benefits and risks communicated?

Health care practitioners consider the balance between benefits and risks with a treatment or intervention before deciding to implement a guideline. Health care practitioners also attempt to determine whether the findings have external validity. The strength of the recommendation and the balance of benefit to harm for the patient is communicated.[44]

The GRADE system established definitions of evidence quality and the strength of recommendations. The quality of evidence describes the amount of confidence that an estimate of effect is correct.[43] The GRADE system also assesses the validity of the results of the individual studies for outcomes and judgments evaluated by the health care practitioner. The assessment of evidence quality across studies for each outcome includes the following:[44]

- Outcomes that were critical to the recommendations
- The overall evidence quality provided across outcomes
- The balance between benefits and harms to patients
- The strength of the recommendations

The GRADE system defines clinical questions using the PICO model to consider all outcomes that are important to patients.[45] Outcomes are classified as critical; important, but not critical; or of limited importance. Guideline developers may use a nine-point scale with seven to nine representing critical outcomes, four to six representing important outcomes, and one to three representing outcomes of limited importance. Critical outcomes are given more weight in the final recommendations. The GRADE system additionally considers outcomes related to possible harms of therapy.[45]

The evidence quality and study strength inform the recommendation. Randomized trials are considered higher quality evidence and observational studies to be lower quality evidence with the GRADE system.[46] Ratings are increased or decreased based on five reasons (Table 8-2): risk of bias, inconsistency, indirectness, imprecision, publication bias. The level of confidence similarly can be increased based on three reasons: large effect sizes, dose response, and all plausible confounding.[46]

TABLE 8–2. GRADE SYSTEM TO RATING CONFIDENCE IN EFFECT ESTIMATES[28]

1. Establish Initial Level of Confidence		2. Consider Lowering or Raising Level of Confidence		3. Final Level of Confidence Rating
Study Design	**Initial Confidence in an Estimate of Effect**	Reasons for Considering Lowering or Raising Confidence		**Confidence in an Estimate of Effect Across those Considerations**
		↓ Lower if	**↑ Higher if**	
Randomized trials →	High confidence	Risk of Bias	Large effect	High
		− 1 Serious	+ 1 Large	⊕⊕⊕⊕
		− 2 Very serious	+ 2 Very large	Moderate
		Inconsistency	Dose response	⊕⊕⊕
		− 1 Serious	+ 1 gradient found	Low
		− 2 Very serious	All plausible residual confounding and bias	⊕⊕
		Indirectness	+ 1 Would reduce a demonstrated effect or	Very low
		− 1 Serious	+ 1 Would suggest a spurious effect if no effect was observed	⊕
		− 2 Very serious		
Observational studies	Low confidence	Imprecision		
		− 1 Serious		
		− 2 Very serious		
		Publication bias		
		− 1 Likely		
		− 2 Very Likely		

GRADE = Grading of Recommendations Assessment, Development, and Evaluation.

Health care practitioners should use the GRADE system in combination with clinical judgments to inform recommendations for individual patients. An assessment of bias that could impact the strength of the recommendations is available to the health care practitioner based upon several factors.[47] When correctly completed, randomized study designs have tremendous power to reduce the potential for biased results. However, health care practitioners should recognize limits to randomized controlled trials, including the applicability to real-world populations due to potentially restrictive inclusion criteria. Other study types, such as observational studies (e.g., cohort, case-control) with strong methods, provide additional high-quality evidence. The quality of each study should be assessed based on the adequacy of the concealment of allocation of subjects when randomizing patients, the type of blinding used, presence or absence of a follow-up, the reported outcomes, whether or not the trial stopped early, presence or absence of a validated outcome measure, and whether other design or execution errors were found.[48] Refer to Chapters 4 and 5 for additional discussion on interpretation of data from different study types.

In 2016, the 21st Century Cures Act placed additional focus on the use of real-world data (RWD) and real-world evidence (RWE) and the importance of these factors in the formation of health care decisions. The Food and Drug Administration (FDA) uses RWD and RWE to monitor for postmarking safety and adverse events that may impact regulatory decisions. These data are also used by health care practitioners to support decisions of coverage that may be made, based on guidelines. RWD can support the expansion of approved indications for drugs. RWD and RWE may harness data from sources such as mobile devices, wearables, and biosensors, and have answered questions previously presumed infeasible to answer.[49] The use of RWD and RWE has partially addressed the challenge of ensuring that studies are representative of the patients who will use the treatments. One limitation with RWD, however, is the ability to replicate findings of clinical trials. For example, RWD derived from claims databases may be missing information like compliance, the indication for the use of the drug, or the endpoint evaluated (if the endpoint are not in the electronic health record). One recent study found that only 15% of studies evaluating RWD replicated clinical trial results. As the opportunity to use RWD/RWE grows, designing systems or even observational studies to capture relevant RWD should be considered.[50]

Another challenge in the interpretation of studies and guidelines is how results are evaluated and presented. Inconsistency of results between different studies can reduce confidence that the results are valid. The quality of evidence is rated higher if included studies find consistent results. When the point estimates of results vary widely across studies, confidence intervals show overlap, or statistical tests for heterogeneity are significant, and there is a lack of explanation of differences, the quality of evidence is lower.[51]

The GRADE criteria further address considerations of consistency by examining subject inclusion criteria. The "directness of results" is the extent subjects, interventions, and outcomes of a study are similar to the target population for a recommendation.[52] Ideally, the study subjects are similar to the target population in informing clinicians of the safety and efficacy of an intervention. When the subjects differ from the patients typically treated for the condition, confidence in the ability to achieve the same response is lost, and the evidence quality is lower. Common examples of factors that may differ in subjects have consisted of age, gender, race, other comorbidities, or severity of illness.

Another factor considered in the interpretation of guidelines is the type of outcome used. When studies use **surrogate endpoints** or intermediate outcomes, consider whether the desired benefits are reliably estimated. Surrogate endpoints are laboratory values or physical assessments that predict the actual clinical events and are imperfect predictors of the actual outcomes. For example, the time from the presentation of surrogate endpoints to the achievement of the ultimate clinical outcome may differ. Surrogate endpoints and indirect evidence are necessary when no studies are available to compare different interventions directly, which is common with new drugs. Lack of studies comparing different interventions is a common situation with new drugs studied on a limited basis, such as those only compared to placebo or lacking a control group altogether. When data comparing treatments are lacking, it is difficult to determine which treatment is more effective and to estimate the size of a potential treatment difference.[52]

Confidence intervals are often used to assess the measure of precision in study results (see Chapter 6).[52] When using a 95% confidence interval, the treatment is not proven effective if the 95% confidence interval crosses the boundary of benefit versus harm. For example, when the relative risk of a clinical event is 0.8, but the 95% confidence interval is from 0.5 to 1.1, the result is generally not considered to be statistically significant. The confidence interval does not exclude the possibility of a reduction or increase in the risk of the event. Also, if the confidence interval extends into a point where the size of the clinical benefit is no longer greater than the potential adverse effects, the burden of treatment, and costs, the level of evidence is lower, and the treatment may not be beneficial to use. Other statistical concepts considered in studies and guidelines is the absolute risk difference or number needed to treat (NNT).[52–54] Absolute risk differences take into consideration the baseline risk or the risk of the event with no treatment. The NNT calculates the number of subjects that need to receive treatment in order for one subject to achieve a significant outcome. These measures are more meaningful values to represent the size of a potential treatment benefit than relative values.

The presence of publication bias can impact evidence quality and should be assessed. Risk of publication bias can be present with new therapies or in situations when there are relatively few studies published and particularly when the sample size is small.[47] Many factors may contribute to publication bias. One example that may contribute to publication bias is the preference to publish positive results versus negative results. In 2015, the

World Health Organization (WHO) provided mandatory guidance to publish any results from trials on clinical trial registry sites within 12 months of study completion. Although the results may be available on sites like clinicaltrials.gov, researchers may delay publishing the results in journals, which may lead to issues in identifying the results in literature searches. Therefore, guideline creators should review clinical trial registries when formulating guidelines.

The GRADE system can provide health care practitioners with an examination of confidence of the evidence.[55–57] Decreases in confidence levels occur due to study limitations, the inconsistency of results, imprecision, and reporting bias.[56] In general, the absence of factors for rating the evidence lower results in the decision to place the confidence in evidence at a higher level.

The GRADE system assigns a grade of evidence to express the confidence that the true effect is close to the estimate of the impact. This grade is based on the components discussed above. Grades or levels of evidence include[47]:

- High = very confident
- Moderate = moderately confident
- Low = limited confidence
- Very low: very little confidence

Many guidelines collapse the low and very low confidence grades into a single grade.

Grades are assigned in the same manner for both the evidence for harm and benefits. This continuity creates a challenge if the evidence of quality for harms differs from that of the benefits. Treatment recommendations rely on both the magnitude and desirability of benefits and harms and care should be taken to demonstrate how evidence translates into specific clinical situations. Clinicians should consider treatment alterations to individualize care. The GRADE working group recommends the following definitions to categorize the trade-off between benefits and harms[44]:

- *Net benefits:* The intervention clearly does greater good than harm.
- *Trade-offs:* There are important trade-offs between the benefits and harms.
- *Uncertain trade-offs:* It is not clear whether the intervention does greater good than harm.
- *No net benefits:* The intervention clearly does not do more good than harm.

Categorizing benefits and risks is based on estimated size and confidence intervals of the effect of the main outcomes, the quality of evidence, ability to extrapolate evidence to different patients or settings, and uncertainty of the baseline risk of disease events in the population of interest.[45]

Finally, the GRADE system assigns categories of recommendations for whether to use an intervention. The categories include a strong or weak recommendation in support of the use of an intervention, and a strong or weak recommendation against the use of an intervention.[44] These recommendations are based on the balance of benefits to risk, the quality rating of the evidence, value variability, differences between patients and circumstances, and resource use implications. Implications on resource use are often the most difficult to make because they can change substantially over time and in different settings.[44]

❻ *The GRADE system attempts to ensure that all evidence that is important to making a decision has been judged with explicit criteria. Judgments made are transparent. Evidence profiles and tables summarizing findings are created to facilitate the best use of evidence.*

Although the GRADE system may appear complicated, it provides a balance of the needs for simplicity and for full consideration of issues impacting clinical decision-making. It has assisted in providing the rationale for recommendations. The evidence profile[57] and summary of findings tables[56–59] produced with the GRADE process are useful for explaining judgments that lead to recommendations in the clinical use of the guideline. See Appendix 8-1 for an example of an evidence profile.

ARTICULATION OF RECOMMENDATIONS

When reading and interpreting guidelines, health care practitioners should look for the strength of a recommendation in the phrasing. When using the GRADE system, a strong recommendation is introduced by terms such as "We recommend" or "Clinicians should," and a weak recommendation begins with the terms "We suggest," "Clinicians might," or "Clinicians may."

Health care practitioners may be more able to process the potential impact of guidelines after an in-depth read by referring to quick reference guides or executive summaries, which give overviews of the recommendations. These summaries are convenient to use in patient care.

When reading guidelines, health care practitioners should recognize that the GRADE system helps clarify what is being recommended. Clear clinical practice recommendations are often difficult to reach. Data may not be adequate to form absolute recommendations for every patient and scenario in the creation of guidelines. Many uncertainties exist about the benefits and harms of interventions based on patient differences. Responses to a treatment may vary, and patient preferences are not considered in the determination of the desirability of outcomes and aversion to risk. Rigid language and absolute recommendations can be dangerous, mainly when presented in a simplistic manner because clinical decision-making is complex, and individual judgment is necessary. By describing uncertainty and providing broad boundaries for appropriate practice, differences of opinion are allowed. Rigid guidelines, based on data that is not conclusive may be worse than having no written guidelines.

Clinical guidelines influence the different elements of practice. Recommendations for future research to further strengthen knowledge on a topic often are included. The process of developing clinical guidelines often calls attention to gaps in scientific information. This generation of new data increases our understanding of a disease process or treatment.

CONDUCT AN EXTERNAL REVIEW

Health care practitioners should consider whether guidelines have undergone an external review. When using an external review, categories of stakeholders and participants review a draft of the guideline and give comments.[1] Based on feedback from the review, revisions may be incorporated and documented.

ESTABLISHMENT OF A PLAN FOR GUIDELINE UPDATES

When guidelines are released, they have the potential to quickly become outdated with the emergence of new evidence or research findings. Regular review of the literature to identify new technology or new evidence that may impact the guideline, and a specific plan for updating or expiration of a guideline should be created to ensure that the information provided is timely and current.[1] The duration of the review interval is dependent upon the topic and knowledge of ongoing studies.

Case Study 8–3

Adoption and adherence to the guidelines that have been recommended for internal use within your health care system is reviewed. You know that the use and adoption of the guideline by health care providers within the system varies. How can you identify and address barriers to the use of the guidelines by providers in your health system? Describe approaches to addressing these barriers based upon the articles presented from this chapter.

Guideline Evaluation Tools

❼ *Before selecting a clinical practice guideline for use in any practice setting, the health care professional needs to evaluate the quality of published guidelines. The Appraisal of Guidelines for Research and Evaluation (AGREE) Enterprise created a useful tool for evaluating clinical practice guidelines.* The AGREE Enterprise is an international group of researchers and policymakers. This collaboration has produced a series of tools, used for appraisal of clinical practice guidelines.[60] One of these tools is the **AGREE II instrument**, which is summarized in Table 8-3.[61-63] Another tool is the AGREE Global Rating Scale (GRS), which is a short-item tool to evaluate the quality and reporting of practice guidelines.[64] The CheckUp tool[65] evaluates the completeness of reporting in updated guidelines, and the GUIDE-M model helps to optimize the implementation of practice guidelines. These tools are used to evaluate guideline quality before considering the adoption of the guideline.

TABLE 8–3. AGREE II DOMAINS AND ITEMS FOR ASSESSMENT[42]

Domain 1. Scope and Purpose

1. The overall objective(s) of the guideline is (are) specifically described.

2. The health question(s) covered by the guideline is (are) specifically described.

3. The population (patients, public, etc.) to whom the guideline is meant to apply is specifically described.

Domain 2. Stakeholder Involvement

4. The guideline development group includes individuals from all the relevant professional groups.

5. The views and preferences of the target population (patients, public, etc.) have been sought.

6. The target users of the guideline are clearly defined.

Domain 3. Rigor of Development

7. Systematic methods were used to search for evidence.

8. The criteria for selecting the evidence are clearly described.

9. The strengths and limitations of the body of evidence are clearly described.

10. The methods for formulating the recommendations are clearly described.

11. The health benefits, side effects, and risks have been considered in formulating the recommendations.

12. There is an explicit link between the recommendations and the supporting evidence.

13. The guideline has been externally reviewed by experts prior to its publication.

14. A procedure for updating the guideline is provided.

Domain 4. Clarity of Presentation

15. The recommendations are specific and unambiguous.

16. The different options for management of the condition or health issue are clearly presented.

17. Key recommendations are easily identifiable.

Domain 5. Applicability

18. The guideline describes facilitators and barriers to its application.

19. The guideline provides advice and/or tools on how the recommendations can be put into practice.

20. The potential resource implications of applying the recommendations have been considered.

21. The guideline presents monitoring and/or auditing criteria.

Domain 6. Editorial Independence

22. The views of the funding body have not influenced the content of the guideline.

23. Competing interests of guideline development group members have been recorded and addressed.

Overall Guideline Assessment

Rate the overall quality of the guideline: 1 lowest possible quality—2,3,4,5,6—7 highest possible quality

I would recommend this guideline for use: Yes, Yes with modifications, No

AGREE = Appraisal of Guidelines for Research and Evaluation.

Use of Clinical Practice Guidelines

❽ *The most effective methods for the use of guidelines to achieve an improved quality of care have not been determined.* Institutional, organizational, local practice, political, and even individual practitioner characteristics influence the choice of a guideline for use in clinical practice. In a review of clinical practice guideline adoption, the variables that affected the success of implementation or use of a guideline included guideline-related factors, health care practitioner personal factors, practice setting characteristics, incentives, regulation, and patient factors.[66] Personal factors related to physician attitudes included lack of agreement with the recommendations, the requirement of learning new skills or changing practice routine, self-efficacy, outcome expectancy, and motivation. Guideline-related factors include complexity, accessibility, and applicability. External factors included organizational constraints on the use of the guideline. For example, the consideration of the local context of a guideline is essential to successful implementation as well as the buy-in of local consensus groups or opinion leaders. Strategies to improve guideline use may consider workflow interventions (e.g., clinical reminders, decision support systems, and standing orders) and provider-focused interventions (e.g., education and training, clinical outreach visits, marketing to opinion leaders).[67]

Despite a prior belief that using multiple strategies to improve guidelines was more effective, one extensive review of guideline implementation strategies concluded that imperfect evidence exists to support decisions about which combination of strategies is best.[67] The most common strategies used to promote guideline use in the systematic review were the use of reminders, educational materials, audit and feedback, and patient-directed interventions. The most frequent strategies used in multifaceted interventions were educational materials, educational meetings, reminders, audits, feedback, and patient-directed interventions.[67] The local policy-leader should consider these strategies in promoting the use of guidelines by the clinical practitioner. The guideline development group also must consider these strategies in providing resources to assist with guideline dissemination and use. The number of anticipated effects with the use of the intervention also must be considered.[67]

How an intervention will impact whether a guideline is adopted can be examined with analyses of the impact to patient care measures. Examples of the process of care measures include frequency of prescribing a specific therapy, providing patient education, or ordering laboratory tests in accordance with a guideline. Overall, 86% of interventions tested achieved positive improvements in the process of care measures. Most interventions from guidelines produced modest to moderate improvements in care.[67] Further research is required to estimate the efficacy and efficiency of strategies to implement guidelines into practice. Health care practitioners should consider other local factors such as characteristics of patients, professionals, and the environment as potential facilitators and barriers to implementation.[68]

Cabana and colleagues[69] conducted a systematic review of the literature regarding barriers to physician adherence to guidelines. A barrier is any factor that limits or restricts complete physician adherence to a guideline. Seven general categories of barriers were identified; examples or a description of each are provided (Table 8-4). The importance of each barrier varies depending on the characteristics of the specific guideline and the local health system characteristics.[69] Knowledge of these potential barriers in the use of guidelines will facilitate successful implementation. Considerations may include changes required, values and routines, resources required, the specificity of advice, and perceived consequences to health care practitioners.[70] In consideration of values, facilitating the individual practitioners must not only value but also understand the methodology of the guidelines. He or she must view the source as being credible to be willing to use the guideline's recommendations.[71] A systematic approach to that engages clinicians in the process of addressing these values and other considerations such as is important to overcome these barriers to guideline use.[72]

CLINICAL DECISION SUPPORT SYSTEMS

One manner of addressing barriers to implementation and use of a guideline is to provide support systems and resources to assist with the translation of knowledge and evidence into feasible practices. **Clinical decision support (CDS) systems** "provide clinicians, staff, patients or other individuals with knowledge and person-specific information, intelligently filtered or presented at appropriate times, to enhance health and health care."[73] These systems can be used to facilitate guideline implementation. Jia and colleagues[74] analyzed recent systematic reviews of trials assessing the effects of CDS systems that combined clinical knowledge with patient characteristics and provided basic or advanced guides to participants using the systems. The review found that CDS systems reduce medication errors by impacting the process of care but may inconsistently improve patient outcomes.[74]

Despite this inconsistency of outcomes, CDS systems remain a standard process by which many health systems implement approved guidelines. Specifically, the systems address challenges to guideline use. The challenges addressed can include competing for demands on health care practitioner time, and limits to "accurate, timely and accessible patient data in user-friendly formats." Electronic health records (EHRs) are CDS systems that provide performance monitoring and feedback to the health care practitioner, sometimes tying financial incentives into their performance.[75]

CDS systems also have limitations or challenges. Wright and colleagues used a method to summarize expert opinions on malfunctions with alerts in CDS systems called the Delphi method.[75] In the review of evidence related to CDS, the authors summarize the benefits such as improved quality and safety while also describing the challenges of

TABLE 8–4. SEVEN CATEGORIES OF BARRIERS[45]

Barrier Category	Examples of Barriers Identified or Description of Barrier
Lack of awareness	Did not know the guideline existed
Lack of familiarity	Could not correctly answer questions about guideline content or self-reported lack of familiarity
Lack of agreement	Difference in interpretation of the evidence
	Benefits not worth patient risk, discomfort, or cost
	Not applicable to patient population in their practice
	Credibility of authors questioned
	Oversimplified cookbook
	Reduces autonomy
	Decreases flexibility
	Decreases physician self-respect
	Not practical
	Makes patient-physician relationship impersonal
Lack of self-efficacy	Did not believe that they could actually perform the behavior or activity recommended by the guideline, e.g., nutrition or exercise counseling
Lack of outcome expectancy	Did not believe intended outcome would occur even if the practice was followed, e.g., counseling to stop smoking
Inertia of previous practice	This barrier relates primarily to motivation to change practice, whether the motivation is professional, personal, or social. It was also noted that guidelines that recommend eliminating a behavior are more difficult to implement than guidelines that recommend adding a new behavior
External barriers	Patient resistance/nonadherence
	Patient does not perceive need
	Perceived to be offensive to patient
	Causes patient embarrassment
	Lack of reminder system
	Not easy to use, inconvenient, cumbersome, confusing
	Lack of educational materials
	Cost to patient
	Insufficient staff, consultant support, or other resources
	Lack of time
	Lack of reimbursement
	Increased malpractice liability
	Not compatible with practice setting

maintaining the systems (e.g., cost, time, and complexity). CDS systems have reliability limits, and available resources constrain best practices for their design and implementation (e.g., knowledge, vendors, tools, finances).[75]

Designers of the best CDS systems work to create more intuitive systems and tools. CDS systems may be more user-friendly if they include considerations such as the ability to be customized to new needs/interventions; methods to improve the effectiveness of the tool; improvements to the human-computer interface (e.g., how does the tool work within the current workflow; are alerts and reminders appropriate or excessive); means of summarizing and prioritizing patient information, as well as prioritizing and filtering other information.[76]

ACADEMIC DETAILING

Academic detailing is a process traditionally used to educate health care practitioners on evidence-based practice, which may include the use of guidelines.[76-78] This educational technique summarizes a clinical issue with the goal of improving the quality and safety of patient outcomes. However, the effectiveness of this technique in influencing health care practitioners has varied. A study by Yeh and colleagues used a Delphi exercise to establish expert consensus on what approaches were most effective in producing change.[77] The experts suggest providing support when using academic detailing to the health care practitioners for clinical decision-making, including educational support. When delivering information, the message should be tailored to the individual health care practitioner and should include feasible strategies with suggestions on how to approach challenging situations or cases. Finally, the importance of developing specific skills (i.e., overcoming barriers to change in individual health care practitioners) was encouraged.[77] Additional information on academic detailing is available in Chapter 25.

EFFECT OF GUIDELINES ON QUALITY OF CARE AND PATIENT OUTCOMES

Grimshaw and Russell published one of the first systematic literature reviews and evaluations of the effect of practice guidelines.[79] They conducted an extensive literature search and identified 59 studies that evaluated the impact of guidelines on physician behavior or patient outcomes. All but four of the studies showed some benefit from the guidelines. However, the magnitude of the benefits and the significant impact on patient care were not impressive in all cases.

Guidelines should contain all necessary elements of routine care for most individuals with a specific condition. However, sometimes guidelines do not adequately address all comorbidity or polypharmacy issues. Additionally, they may or may not include all patient situations.[80] As a result, guidelines should prompt consideration of what specific characteristics of an individual patient might warrant departures from the guidance provided. Guidelines are not perfect; therefore, construction of systems that apply evidence can address patient and system-specific factors, just as the guidelines indicate where care delivery can be improved.[19]

CHALLENGES WITH GUIDELINE IMPLEMENTATION

Even with improvements in clinical practice guideline development, several difficulties remain with the implementation, utilization, evaluation, and revision of guidelines.[81] As pressures on drug prices, sustainability, and provider performance increase, guidelines often establish value for money spent. Usually, public and private health plans begin by defining coverage for a treatment or service, and exclusion of coverage initially by the use of guidelines. However, the difficulty of applying guidelines to complex patients and situations creates a need for ways to deviate from these guidelines. Cost-effectiveness evaluations can appraise medications or treatments individually to determine coverage or inclusion and to provide a wider range of available options.[82,83]

Cost-effectiveness evaluations combat the inability of guidelines to address all patient considerations due to the complexities of patients. Guidelines should direct clinical decision-making, but the health care practitioner should recognize that they may not apply to all situations.[82-85] Additionally, harm may result from following recommendations from multiple individual guidelines for patients with numerous medical conditions. Treatments may become overly complicated, costly, and interact with each other.[85] Although not yet proven, it might be possible to adapt guidelines to facilitate decisions in the presence of multimorbidity.[86,87]

Another challenge when using guidelines is recognizing which guideline is the most relevant or which organization is the most recognized authority for the guideline content. When different groups develop guidelines on the same topic, they can arrive at different recommendations. Packer describes just such a problem with previously developed heart failure guidelines.[87] He reviewed areas of differences in the guidelines that were developed by the European Society of Cardiology in comparison with those by the American College of Cardiology/American Heart Association/Heart Failure Society of America. Examples of the differences involved details of the indications for one medication, or class of drugs, compared to alternatives, and variations in recommended doses. Issues with recommendations of therapy in patients with diabetes in addition to heart failure also were mentioned. The differing recommendations most likely occurred due to differences in judgment and gaps or shortcomings in the evidence.

FUTURE METHODS

The GRADE Working Group continues to evaluate improved methods for presenting recommendations in guidelines that will be more adaptable and feasible for use by clinicians, as well as more readily implementable.[88,89] One focused effort is the evaluation of new ways of formatting and using explanatory footnotes in evidence tables to improve understanding of the certainty of evidence.[90-92] Members of the group have published resources to educate health professionals on how to interpret and use recommendations in guidelines developed with the GRADE approach.[93] For pharmacists or other health professionals charged with the implementation of clinical practice guidelines, further review of these references would be useful.

TOOLS FOR IMPLEMENTATION

Additional tools are available for those who are developing, implementing, or using guidelines. The Guideline International Network (GIN)—McMaster Guideline Development Checklist is a checklist used by guideline developers to plan and track the process of guideline development.[81,94,95] Additionally, McMaster University created a web-based application called GRADEpro to support the guideline development process. GRADEpro provides guidance ranging from the composition of a guideline team to the identification of the subject of the guideline. It also covers guideline dissemination.[96] Video tutorials regarding multiple aspects of guideline development are available from this organization.[97]

Case Study 8-4

Referring to Case Study 8-1, you implemented a new clinical practice guideline within your health care system but need to consider updates to literature. Describe a process of locating updates to clinical practice literature between guideline updates.

Sources of Clinical Practice Guidelines

❾ The Agency for Healthcare Research and Quality (AHRQ) previously funded a site called the National Guideline Clearinghouse, which provided a listing of numerous guidelines. Following the defunding of AHRQ, the need for a similar site existed. *ECRI developed a website called ECRI Guidelines Trust® that serves as a respository of clinical practice guidelines.*[98] Determining where guidelines exist and what is a comprehensive review of the literature is critical to identifying an appropriate guideline for use in patient care. Systematic reviews can help develop or assess specific practice guidelines. These reviews historically have been produced by organizations such as the Cochrane Library, in addition to other websites that collect and provide health care–related information designed to support evidence-based medicine.

There are several mechanisms to locate current clinical practice guidelines or systematic reviews. Websites such as the National Institutes of Health's National Center for Complementary and Integrative Health consolidate a list of clinical practice guidelines and to further assist health care practitioners in identifying relevant guidelines.[99] PubMed also publishes many guidelines published in the peer-reviewed medical literature.[100] One method of searching for guidelines in PubMed is to do an advanced search. First, enter *"practice guideline"* in the publication type field of the record, or use the MeSH filter term *"practice guideline* or *clinical guideline"* in conjunction with other terms for the specific disease or therapy of interest. Search additional publication types by including the following terms: consensus development conference, guideline, and meta-analysis.[100] going directly to the guideline-writing organizations' websites may be a mechanism to identify when a guideline was most recently updated. Additionally, apps are also available which serve as guideline repositories.[100–102]

Systematic review articles are useful in augmenting findings of clinical practice guidelines. These reviews begin with the statement of focused clinical questions. They involve comprehensive searches of evidence and use uniformly applied, and criterion-based selection of evidence in the reviews. Systematic reviews perform rigorous critical appraisal of studies chosen and sometimes provide a quantitative summary of the evidence (i.e., meta-analysis).[103] Published literature search strategies assist with locating systematic reviews.[104,105] Additional information on systematic reviews is presented in Chapter 5.

Multiple professional organizations, academic centers, independent research centers, and government agencies are involved in the development of clinical practice guideline activities. These organizations offer updated information, and many provide access to guidelines on their websites. Of note, the U.S. Preventive Services Task Force provides health care practitioners tools to guide to clinical preventive services and related evidence syntheses.[106] AHRQ continues to offer consolidated evidence reports and summaries, comparative effectiveness reviews, technical reviews and summaries, publications and reports of the Surgeon General, and other resources available from their websites.[107] The GIN Library provides access to the International Guideline Library, development and training resources, relevant literature, a health topic collection, relevant links, and other tools.[95] Some of the resources from this website require membership for access.[95] Finally, the Cochrane Collaboration has a list of databases offering online access to medical evidence.[108]

Conclusion

Clinical practice guidelines are used in health care to facilitate the use of evidence in clinical practice to improve the quality of care, patient safety, and assess cost-effectiveness. Guidelines can assist clinical decision-making and may enhance quality of care and patient outcomes and are used by organizations to direct the efficient use of resources. Guideline methodology exists to enhance the validity and transparency of guideline development and use. The active involvement of practitioners in the preparation and implementation of evidence-based clinical practice guidelines is vital. An understanding of evidence-based methodology will prepare health care practitioners to participate in this process as well as to understand how to use these guidelines in practice effectively. Training in drug information is valuable in the preparation and implementation of evidence-based clinical practice guidelines.

Self-Assessment Questions

1. Which groups or organization types are commonly involved in guideline development?
   a. Federal and state governments
   b. Professional societies and associations
   c. Managed care organizations
   d. Third-party payers
   e. All of the above

2. Which characteristic is common between guideline development and drug information practices?
   a. Decision-making and recommendations based on individual experience
   b. Assurance of cost savings
   c. A clear specific definition of clinical questions
   d. Lack of interdisciplinary participation

3. Clinical practice guidelines are essential to getting research findings into practice because:
   a. Well-studied new treatments proven effective are substantially underutilized.
   b. Interventions found to be ineffective or harmful continue to be provided.
   c. Research information is not readily available for implementation into practice.
   d. a and b only are essential.
   e. b and c only are important.

4. Recommendations for optimizing patient care that are developed by systematically reviewing the evidence and assessing the benefits and harms of health care interventions is the definition for:
   a. Strengths of recommendations
   b. Evidence-based medicine

   c. Clinical practice guidelines

   d. Systematic reviews

5. Which of the following is among the five core competencies for health professionals as recommended in a landmark Institute of Medicine report?

   a. Deliver patient-centered care.

   b. Participate in interdisciplinary teams.

   c. Utilize informatics.

   d. All of the above.

6. The first step in the Institute of Medicine's proposed standards for developing evidence-based clinical practice guidelines is:

   a. Conduct a systematic review for qualifying evidence.

   b. Establish an interdisciplinary guideline development group.

   c. Establish transparency.

   d. Manage conflict of interest.

7. Development of a clinical practice guideline should:

   a. Include a hospital administrator

   b. Be an interdisciplinary process

   c. Be made up of panel members without any conflicts of interest

   d. Have a pharmacist leading the effort

8. Which of the following characteristics associated with a disease would suggest that it would be a good topic for the development and implementation of a practice guideline?

   a. Evidence that current practice is optimal

   b. Evidence of little variation in current practice

   c. Availability of high-quality evidence for the efficacy of treatments that reduce morbidity or mortality

   d. Low frequency and/or severity of morbidity or mortality

9. In the PICO model for framing clinical questions, the C represents:

   a. Collaboration

   b. Comparison

   c. Clinical

   d. Control

10. When using the GRADE system, which of the following information should be incorporated with guideline recommendations?

   a. Quality of evidence across studies for each critical outcome

   b. Strength of the recommendations

    c. The balance between benefits and harms

    d. a and b only

11. When using the GRADE system, all of the following are reasons for lowering the level of confidence rating *except*:

    a. Publication bias

    b. Imprecision

    c. Indirectness

    d. Consistency

12. When using the GRADE system, which of the following is a reason for rating the level of confidence higher?

    a. Dose-response relationship

    b. Large effect size

    c. b and c only

    d. a, b, and c

13. All of the following are true regarding the AGREE II instrument for guideline evaluation *except*:

    a. Created by an international group of researchers and policymakers

    b. Provides a framework to assess the quality of guidelines

    c. Assesses the quality of the clinical content

    d. Provides a methodological strategy for the development of guidelines

14. External barriers to clinical practice guideline implementation include all of the following *except*:

    a. Cost to patient

    b. Increased malpractice liability

    c. Insufficient staff, consultant support, or other resources

    d. Lack of reimbursement

15. All of the following statements about clinical practice guidelines are true *except*:

    a. Clinical practice guidelines should contain all necessary elements of routine care for most individuals with a specific condition.

    b. Clinical practice guidelines should not prompt consideration of the specific characteristics of an individual patient that might warrant departures from the guideline.

    c. Clinical practice guidelines represent an application of decision support systems to facilitate providing quality clinical care.

    d. Clinical practice guidelines should be part of the continuous improvement of systems of care.

REFERENCES

1. Institute of Medicine, Committee on Standards for Developing Trustworthy Clinical Practice Guidelines. Clinical practice guidelines we can trust [Internet]. Washington (DC): National Academies Press; 2011 [cited 2016 Sep]. Available from: http://nationalacademies.org/HMD/Reports/2011/Clinical-Practice-Guidelines-We-Can-Trust.aspx

2. American Academy of Family Physicians. Clinical practice guideline manual [Internet]. 2017 Dec [cited 2020 May 5]. Available from: https://www.aafp.org/patient-care/clinical-recommendations/cpg-manual.html

3. President's Advisory Commission on Consumer Protection and Quality in the Health Care Industry. Quality first: better health care for all Americans [Internet]. Agency for Healthcare Research and Quality; 1998 Jul 18 [cited 2020 May 5]. Available from: http://archive.ahrq.gov/hcqual/final/

4. Jones RH, Ritchie JL, Fleming BB, Hammermeister KE, Leape LL. 28th Bethesda Conference. Task Force 1: clinical practice guideline development, dissemination, and computerization. J Am Coll Cardiol. 1997;29:1133-41.

5. Institute of Medicine, Committee on Quality Health Care in America. Crossing the quality chasm: a new health system for the 21st century [Internet]. Washington (DC): National Academy Press; 2001 [cited 2020 May 5]. Available from: https://www.ncbi.nlm.nih.gov/books/NBK222274/

6. Institute of Medicine, Committee on Data Standards for Patient Safety. Patient safety: achieving a new standard for care [Internet]. Aspden P, Corrigan JM, Wolcott J, Erikson SM, editors. Washington (DC): National Academies Press; 2004 [cited 2020 May 5]. Available from: https://www.nap.edu/read/10863/chapter/1

7. Institute of Medicine, Committee on Quality of Health Care in America. To err is human: building a safer health system [Internet]. Kohn LT, Corrigan JM, Donaldson MS, editors. Washington (DC): National Academy Press; 2000 [cited 2020 May 5]. Available from: https://www.nap.edu/read/9728/chapter/1#ix

8. Institute of Medicine, Committee on Identifying and Preventing Medication Errors. Preventing medication errors [Internet]. Aspden P, Wolcott J, Bootman JL, Cronenwett LR, editors. Washington (DC): National Academies Press; 2007 [cited 2020 May 5]. Available from: https://www.nap.edu/read/11623/chapter/1

9. Institute of Medicine, Committee on Standards for Systematic Reviews of Comparative Effectiveness Research. Finding what works in health care: standards for systematic reviews [Internet]. Eden J, Levit L, Berg A, Morton S, editors. Washington (DC): National Academies Press; 2011 [cited 2020 May 5]. Available from: https://www.nap.edu/catalog/13059/finding-what-works-in-health-care-standards-for-systematic-reviews

10. Institute of Medicine, Committee on the Learning Health Care System in America. Best care at lower cost: the path to continuously learning health care in America [Internet]. Smith M, Saunders R, Stuckhardt L, McGinnis JM, editors. Washington (DC): National Academies Press; 2012 [cited 2020 May 5]. Available from: http://www.nationalacademies.org/hmd/Reports/2012/Best-Care-at-Lower-Cost-The-Path-to-Continuously-Learning-Health-Care-in-America.aspx

11. Centre for Evidence-Based Medicine. Evidence-based medicine: what's in a name? [Internet]. 2015 Dec 15 [cited 2020 May 5]. Available from: https://www.cebm.net/2015/12/evidence-based-medicine-whats-in-a-name/.

12. Sackett DL, Rosenberg WM, Gray JA, Haynes RB, Richardson WS. Evidence-based medicine: what it is and what it isn't. BMJ. 1996;312:71-72.

13. Centre for Evidence-Based Medicine [Internet]. University of Oxford [cited 2020 May 5]. Available from: https://www.cebm.net/.

14. Evidence-Based Medicine Working Group. Evidence-based medicine: a new approach to teaching the practice of medicine. JAMA. 1992;268:2420-5.

15. Straus SE, Glasziou P, Richardson WS, Haynes RB. Evidence-based medicine: how to practice & teach it. 4th ed. New York: Churchill Livingstone; 2011.

16. Watanabe AS, McCart G, Shimomura S, Kayser S. Systematic approach to drug information requests. Am J Hosp Pharm. 1975; 32:1282-5.

17. Guyatt GH, Meade MO, Jaeschke RZ, Cook DJ, Haynes RB. Practitioners of evidence-based care: not all clinicians need to appraise evidence from scratch, but all need some skills. BMJ. 2000;320:954-5.

18. Eddy DM. Evidence-based medicine: a unified approach. Health Aff. 2005;24:9-17.

19. Chassin MR. Is health care ready for Six Sigma quality?. Milbank Q. 1998;76:565-91, 510.

20. American Academy of Neurology. Policy and guidelines [Internet]. [Cited 2020 May 5]. Available from: https://www.aan.com/policy-and-guidelines/guidelines/

21. American College of Chest Physicians. CHEST guidelines and resources [Internet]. [Cited 2020 May 5]. Available from: https://www.chestnet.org/Guidelines-and-Resources

22. Infectious Diseases Society of America (IDSA). IDSA practice guidelines [Internet]. Arlington (VA) [cited 2020 May 5]. Available from: https://www.idsociety.org/practice-guideline/practice-guidelines/#/date_na_dt/DESC/0/+/

23. Advisory Committee on Immunization Practices. Vaccine recommendations and guidelines of the ACIP [Internet]. Centers for Disease Control and Prevention [cited 2020 May 5]. Available from: https://www.cdc.gov/vaccines/hcp/acip-recs/index.html

24. Centers for Disease Control and Prevention (CDC). Viral hepatitis: surveillance guidelines and forms [Internet]. 2018 Apr 18 [cited 2020 May 5]. Available from: https://www.cdc.gov/hepatitis/statistics/GuidelinesAndForms.htm

25. National Institutes of Health (NIH). NIH guidelines [Internet]. Office of Science Policy [cited 2020 May 5]. Available from: https://osp.od.nih.gov/biotechnology/nih-guidelines/

26. U.S. Preventative Services Task Force. Recommendations [Internet]. Rockville (MD) [cited 2020 May 5]. Available from: https://www.uspreventiveservicestaskforce.org/uspstf/topic_search_results?topic_status=P

27. EQUATOR Network. Enhancing the quality and transparency of health research [Internet]. UK EQUATOR Centre [cited 2020 May 5]. Available from: http://www.equator-network.org/about-us/equator-network-what-we-do-and-how-we-are-organised/

28. Consolidated Standards of Reporting Trials (CONSORT). CONSORT 2010 statement [Internet]. [Cited 2020 May 5]. Available from: http://www.consort-statement.org/consort-2010

29. Strengthening the Reporting of Observational Studies in Epidemiology (STROBE). STROBE statement: guidelines for reporting observational studies [Internet]. UK EQUATOR Centre [cited 2020 May 5]. Available from: https://www.equator-network.org/reporting-guidelines/strobe/.

30. Fye WB. The power of clinical trials and guidelines and the challenge of conflicts of interest. J Am Coll. Cardiol. 2003;41:1237-42.

31. Choudhry NK, Stelfox HT, Detsky AS. Relationships between authors of clinical practice guidelines and the pharmaceutical industry. JAMA. 2002;287:612-7.

32. Curtiss FR. Consensus panel, national guidelines, and other potentially misleading terms. J Manag Care Pharm. 2003;9:574-5.

33. Van der Weyden MB. Clinical practice guidelines: time to move the debate from the how to the who. Med J Aust. 2002;176:304-5.

34. American College of Chest Physicians. CHEST guideline development [Internet]. [Cited 2020 May 5]. Available from: http://www.chestnet.org/Guidelines-and-Resources/About-CHEST-Guidelines/Guideline-Development

35. American College of Chest Physicians. Evidence-based clinical practice guidelines: leadership conflict-of-interest (COI) policy [Internet]. 2010 Oct 29 [updated 2019 Mar; cited 2020 May 5]. Available from: http://www.chestnet.org/-/media/chesnetorg/About-ACCP/Documents/GovernanceLeadershipCOIPolicy_UploadedJune2019.ashx?la=en&hash=4003DECFDE7075D468A5B3DAFAAE40163445E19F

36. Mosca L, Appel LJ, Benjamin EJ, Berra K, Chandra-Strobos N, Fabunmi RP, Grady D, Haan CK, Hayes SN, Judelson DR, Keenan NL, McBride P, Oparil S, Ouyang P, C Oz M, Mendelsohn ME, Pasternak RC, Pinn VW, Robertson RM, Schenck-Gustafsson K, Sila CA, Smith SC Jr, Sopko G, Taylor AL, Walsh BW, Wenger NK, Williams CL. Evidence-based guidelines for cardiovascular disease prevention in women. J Am Coll Cardiol. 2004;43:900-21.

37. Schardt C, Adams MB, Owens T, Keitz S, Fontelo P. Utilization of the PICO framework to improve searching PubMed for clinical questions. BMC Med Inform Decis Mak. 2007 Dec 1;7(1):16.

38. Richardson WS, Wilson MC, Nishikawa J, Hayward RS. The well-built clinical question: a key to evidence-based decisions. ACP J Club. 1995;123:A12-A13.

39. National Comprehensive Cancer Network (NCCN). Levels of evidence and consensus of recommendations [Internet]. Plymouth Meeting (PA) [cited 2020 May 5]. Available from: https://www.nccn.org/professionals/development.aspx

40. Guyatt GH, Oxman AD, Schunemann HJ, Tugwell P, Knottnerus A. GRADE guidelines: a new series of articles in the Journal of Clinical Epidemiology. J Clin Epidemiol. 2011;64:380-2.

41. Diekemper RL, Patel S, Mette SA, Ornelas J, Ouellette DR, Casey KR. Making the GRADE: CHEST updates its methodology. Chest. 2018;153(3):756-9.

42. The GRADE Working Group. What is GRADE? [Internet]. [Cited 2020 May 5]. Available from: https://www.gradeworkinggroup.org/

43. Atkins D, Best D, Briss PA, Eccles M, Falck-Ytter Y, Flottorp S, Guyatt GH, Harbour RT, Haugh MC, Henry D, Hill S, Jaeschke R, Leng G, Liberati A, Magrini N, Mason J,

Middleton P, Mrukowicz J, O'Connell D, Oxman AD, Phillips B, Schünemann HJ, Edejer TT-T, Varonen H, Vist GE, Williams JW Jr, Zaza S. GRADE Working Group. Grading quality of evidence and strength of recommendations. BMJ. 2004;328:1490.

44. The GRADE Working Group. Criteria for applying or using GRADE [Internet]. [Updated and approved 2016; cited 2020 May 5]. Available from: http://www.gradeworkinggroup.org/docs/Criteria_for_using_GRADE_2016-04-05.pdf

45. The GRADE Working Group. Publications [Internet]. [Cited 2020 May 5]. Available from: http://www.gradeworkinggroup.org/

46. Balshem H, Helfand M, Schunemann HJ, Oxman AD, Kunz R, Brozek J, Vist GE, Falck-Ytter Y, Meerpohl J, Norris S, Guyatt GH. GRADE guidelines: 3. Rating the quality of evidence. J Clin Epidemiol. 2011;64:401-6.

47. Guyatt GH, Oxman AD, Vist G, Kunz R, Brozek J, Alfonso-Coello P, Montori V, Akl EA, Djulbegovic B, Falck-Ytter Y, Norris SL, Williams JW JR, Atkins D, Meerpohl J, Schünemann HJ. GRADE guidelines: 4. Rating the quality of evidence-study limitations (risk of bias). J Clin Epidemiol. 2011;64:407-15.

48. U.S. Food and Drug Administration (FDA). Real-world evidence [Internet]. [Updated 2020 March 23; cited 2020 May 5]. Available from: https://www.fda.gov/science-research/science-and-research-special-topics/real-world-evidence?utm_campaign=Public%20Meeting%20on%20Pediatric%20Medical%20Device%20Development&utm_medium=email&utm_source=Eloqua&elqTrackId=EDDF399A3ABC271ED83669580AA5E3C1&elq=3924857ada5c44328e2e56862f4b020d&elqaid=4216&elqat=1&elqCampaignId=3315

49. Bartlett VL, Dhruva SS, Shah ND, Ryan P, Ross JS. Feasibility of using real-world data to replicate clinical trial evidence. JAMA Network Open. 2019;2(10):e1912869

50. Guyatt GH, Oxman AD, Kunz R, Woodcock J, Brozek J, Helfand M, Alonso-Coello P, Glaszious P, Jaeschke R, Akl EA, Norris S, Vist G, Dahm P, Shukla VK, Higgins J, Falck-Ytter Y, Schünemann HJ. GRADE Working Group. GRADE guidelines: 7. Rating the quality of evidence--inconsistency. J Clin Epidemiol. 2011;64:1294-1302.

51. Guyatt GH, Oxman AD, Kunz R, Woodcock J, Brozek J, Helfand M, Alonso-Coello P, Falck-Ytter Y, Jaeschke R, Vist G, Alk EA, Post PN, Norris S, Meerpohl J, Shukla VK, Nasser M, Schünemann HJ, GRADE Working Group. GRADE guidelines: 8. Rating the quality of evidence-indirectness. J Clin Epidemiol. 2011;64:1303-10.

52. Guyatt GH, Oxman AD, Kunz R, Brozek J, Alfonso-Coello P, Rind D, Devereaux PJ, Montori VM, Freyschuss B, Vist G, Jaeschke R, Filliams JR JW, Murad MH, Snclair D, Falck-Ytter Y, Meerpohl , Whittington C, Thorlund K, Andrews J, Schünemann HJ, GRADE guidelines 6. Rating the quality of evidence-imprecision. J Clin Epidemiol. 2011;64:1283-93.

53. Guyatt GH, Oxman AD, Sultan S, Glasziou P, Akl EA, Alfonso-Coello P, Atkins D, Kunz R, Brozek J, Montori V, Jaeschke R, Rind D, Dahm P, Meerpohl M, Vist G, Berliner E, Norris S, Falck-Ytter Y, Murad MH, Schünemann HJ, GRADE Working Group. GRADE guidelines: 9. Rating up the quality of evidence. J Clin Epidemiol. 2011;64:1311-16.

54. Schünemann HJ, Oxman AD, Brozek J, Glasziou P, Jaeschke R, Vist GE, Williams JW Jr, Kunz R, Craig J, Montori VM, Bossuyt P. Rating quality of evidence and strength of recommendations: GRADE: grading quality of evidence and strength of recommendations for diagnostic tests and strategies. BMJ. 2008;336(7653):1106.

55. Hill AB. The environment and disease: association or causation? Proc R Soc Med. 1965;58:295-300.

56. Guyatt G, Oxman AD, Akl EA, Kunz R, Vist G, Brozek J, Norris S, Falck-Ytter Y, Glasziou P, DeBeer H, Jaeschke R, Rind D, Meerpohl J, Schünemann HJ. GRADE guidelines: 1. Introduction-GRADE evidence profiles and summary of findings tables. J Clin Epidemiol. 2011;64:383-94.

57. Guyatt GH, Oxman AD, Santesso N, Helfand M, Vist G, Kunz R, Brozek J, Norris S, Meerpohl J, Djulbegovic B, Alonso-Coello P, Post PN, Busse JW, Glasziou P, Christensen R, Schünemann HJ. GRADE guidelines: 12. Preparing a summary of findings tables-binary outcomes. J Clin Epidemiol. 2013;66:158-72.

58. Guyatt GH, Thorlund K, Oxman AD, Walter SD, Patrick D, Furukawa TA, Johnston BC, Karanicolas P, Akl EA, Kunz R, Brozek J, Kupper LL, Martin SL, Meerpohl JJ, Alonso-Coello P, Christensen R, Schunemann HJ. GRADE guidelines: 13. Preparing summary of findings tables and evidence profiles-continuous outcomes. J Clin Epidemiol. 2013;66:173-83.

59. AGREE Enterprise. AGREE tools [Internet]. The AGREE Research Trust [cited 2020 May 5]. Available from: https://www.agreetrust.org/resource-centre/

60. Seto K, Matsumoto K, Kitazawa T, Fujita S, Hanaoka S, Hasegawa T. Evaluation of clinical practice guidelines using the AGREE instrument: comparison between data obtained from AGREE I and AGREE II. BMC Res Notes. 2017;10(1):716.

61. Brouwers MC, Kho ME, Browman GP, Burgers JS, Cluzeau F, Feder G, Fervers B, Graham ID, Grimshaw J, Hanna SE, Littlejohns P, Makarski J, Zitzelsberger L. AGREE II: advancing guideline development, reporting, and evaluation in health care. CMAJ. 2010;182:E839-E842.

62. AGREE Enterprise. Appraisal of Guidelines for Research & Evaluation (AGREE) II Instrument [Internet]. The AGREE Research Trust [cited 2020 May 5]. Available from: https://www.agreetrust.org/resource-centre/agree-ii/

63. AGREE Enterprise. AGREE global rating scale (GRS) [Internet]. The AGREE Research Trust [cited 2020 May 5]. Available from: https://www.agreetrust.org/resource-centre/agree-ii-grs-instrument/

64. AGREE Enterprise. CheckUp [Internet]. The AGREE Research Trust [cited 2020 May 5]. Available from: https://www.agreetrust.org/resource-centre/checkup/

65. AGREE Enterprise. Guide-M Publications [Internet]. The AGREE Research Trust [cited 2020 May 5]. Available from: https://www.agreetrust.org/resource-centre/guide-m/guideline-implementability-for-decision-excellence-model-guide-m/

66. Fischer F, Lange K, Klose K, Greiner W, Kraemer A. Barriers and strategies in guideline implementation—a scoping review. Healthcare. 2016;4(3):36.

67. Grimshaw JM, Thomas RE, MacLennan G, Fraser C, Ramsay CR, Vale L, Whitty P, Eccles MP, Matowe L, Shirran L, Wensing M, Dijkstra R, Donaldson C. Effectiveness and efficiency of guideline dissemination and implementation strategies. Health Technol Assess. 2004;8:3-72.

68. Francke AL, Smit MC, de Veer AJ, Mistiaen P. Factors influencing the implementation of clinical guidelines for health care professionals: a systematic meta-review. BMC Med Inform Decision Mak. 2008;8(1):38.

69. Cabana MD, Rand CS, Powe NR, Wu AW, Wilson MH, Abboud PA, Rubin HR. Why don't physicians follow clinical practice guidelines?: A framework for improvement. JAMA. 1999;282(15):1458-65.

70. Grol R, Dalhuijsen J, Thomas S, Veld C, Rutten G, Mokkink H. Attributes of clinical guidelines that influence use of guidelines in general practice: observational study. BMJ. 1998;317:858-61.

71. Beauchemin M, Cohn E, Shelton RC. Implementation of clinical practice guidelines in the healthcare setting: a concept analysis. Adv Nursing Sci. 2019;42(4):307-24.

72. Doherty JA, Crelia SJ, Smith MW, Rosenblum SF, Rumsey EM, Mabry-Hernandez IR, Ngo-Metzger Q. Large health "systems" prevention guideline implementation: a qualitative study. Am J Prevent Med. 2018;54(1):S88-S94.

73. Health IT.gov. What is clinical decision support? [Internet]. The Office of the National Coordinator for Health Information Technology (ONC) [cited 2020 May 5]. Available from: https://www.healthit.gov/topic/safety/clinical-decision-support

74. Jia P, Zhang L, Chen J, Zhao P, Zhang M. The effects of clinical decision support systems on medication safety: an overview. PloS One. 2016 Dec 15;11(12):e0167683.

75. Wright A, Ash JS, Ai A, Hickman TT, Wiesen JF, Galanter W, McCoy AB, Schreiber R, Longhurst CA, Sittig DF. Best practices for preventing malfunctions in rule-based clinical decision support alerts and reminders: results of a Delphi study. Int J Med Inform. 2018;1(118):78-85.

76. Sittig DF, Wright A, Osheroff JA, Middleton B, Teich JM, Ash JS, Campbell E, Bates DW. Grand challenges in clinical decision support. J Biomed Inform. 2018;41(2):387-92.

77. Yeh JS, Van Hoof TJ, Fischer MA. Key features of academic detailing: development of an expert consensus using the Delphi method. Am Health Drug Benefits. 2016 Feb;9(1):42.

78. Horowitz CR, Goldberg HI, Martin DP, Wagner EH, Fihn SD, Christensen DB, Cheadle AD. Conducting a randomized controlled trial of CQI and academic detailing to implement clinical guidelines. Jt Comm J Qual Improv. 1996;22:734-50.

79. Grimshaw JM, Russell IT. Effect of clinical guidelines on medical practice: a systematic review of rigorous evaluations. Lancet. 1993;342:1317-22.

80. Nobili A, Garattini S, Mannucci PM. Multiple diseases and polypharmacy in the elderly: challenges for the internist of the third millennium. J Comorb. 2011;1(1):28-44.

81. Kredo T, Bernhardsson S, Machingaidze S, Young T, Louw Q, Ochodo E, Grimmer K. Guide to clinical practice guidelines: the current state of play. Int J Qual Health Care. 2016;28:122-28.

82. Garrison LP.Jr Cost-effectiveness and clinical practice guidelines: have we reached a tipping point?—An overview. Value Health. 2016 Jul 1;19(5):512-15.

83. McCauley JL. Guidelines and value-based decision making an evolving role for payers. North Carolina Med J. 2015 Sep 1;76(4):243-46.

84. Gagliardi AR, Brouwers MC, Palda VA, Lemieux-Charles L, Grimshaw JM. How can we improve guideline use? A conceptual framework of implementability. Implement Sci. 2011 Dec;6(1):26.

85. Boyd CM, Darer J, Boult C, Fried LP, Boult L, Wu AW. Clinical practice guidelines and quality of care for older patients with multiple comorbid diseases: implications for pay for performance. JAMA. 2005;294:716-24.

86. Guthrie B, Payne K, Alderson P, McMurdo ME, Mercer SW. Adapting clinical guidelines to take account of multimorbidity. BMJ. 2012;345:e6341.

87. Packer M. The room where it happens: a skeptic's analysis of the new heart failure guidelines. J Card Fail. 2016;22:726-30.

88. Alonso-Coello P, Schünemann HJ, Moberg J, Brignardello-Petersen R, Akl EA, Davoli M, Treweek S, Mustafa RA, Rada G, Rosenbaum S, Morelli A, Guyatt GH, Oxman AD. GRADE Working Group. GRADE Working Group. GRADE Evidence to Decision (EtD) frameworks: a systematic and transparent approach to making well-informed healthcare choices. 1: Introduction. BMJ. 2016;353:i2016.

89. Alonso-Coello P, Oxman AD, Moberg J, Brignardello-Petersen R, Akl EA, Davoli M, Treweek S, Mustafa RA, Rada G, Rosenbaum S, Morelli A, Guyatt GH, Oxman AD. GRADE Working Group. GRADE Evidence to Decision (EtD) frameworks: a systematic and transparent approach to making well-informed healthcare choices. 2: Clinical practice guidelines. BMJ. 2016;353:i2089.

90. Carrasco-Labra A, Brignardello-Petersen R, Santesso N, Neumann I, Mustafa RA, Mbuagbaw L, Ikobaltzeta IE, DeStio C, McCullagh LJ, Alonso-Coello P, Meerpohl JJ, Vandvik PO, Brozek JL, Akl EA, Bossuyt P, Churchill R, Glenton C, Rosenbaum S, Tugwell P, Welch V, Garner P, Guyatt G, Schünemann HJ. Improving GRADE evidence tables part 1: a randomized trial shows improved understanding of content in the summary of findings tables with a new format. J Clin Epidemiol. 2016;74:7-18.

91. Langendam M, Carrasco-Labra A, Santesso N, Mustafa RA, Brignardello-Petersen R, Ventresca M, Heus P, Lasserson T, Moustgaard R, Brozek J, Schünemann HJ. Improving GRADE evidence tables part 2: a systematic survey of explanatory notes shows more guidance is needed. J Clin Epidemiol. 2016;74:19-27.

92. Santesso N, Carrasco-Labra A, Langendam M, Brignardello-Petersen R, Mustafa RA, Heus P, Lasserson T, Opiyo N, Kunnamo I, Sinclair D, Garner P, Treweek S, Tovey D, Akl EA, Tugwell P, Brozek JL, Guyatt G, Schünemann HJ. Improving GRADE evidence tables part 3: detailed guidance for explanatory footnotes supports creating and understanding GRADE certainty in the evidence judgments. J Clin Epidemiol. 2016;74:28-39.

93. Neumann I, Santesso N, Akl EA, Rind DM, Vandvik PO, Alonso-Coello P, Agoritsas T, Mustafa RA, Alexander PE, Schünemann HJ, Guyatt GH. A guide for health professionals to interpret and use recommendations in guidelines developed with the GRADE approach. J Clin Epidemiol. 2016;72:45-55.

94. Guidelines International Network (GIN) and McMaster University. GIN-McMaster Guideline Development Checklist[Internet]. McMaster University [cited 2020 May 5]. Available from: https://cebgrade.mcmaster.ca/guidecheck.html

95. Guidelines International Network (G-I-N) [Internet]. 2020 May 1 [cited 2020 May 5]. Available from: http://www.g-i-n.net

96. McMaster University. GRADEpro [Internet]. [Cited 2020 May 5]. Available from: https://cebgrade.mcmaster.ca/gradepro.html

97. McMaster University. GRADEpro Tutorials [Internet]. [Cited 2020 May 5]. Available from: https://gradepro.org/guidelines-development#develop-tuts

98. ECRI. Guidelines Trust [Internet]. [Cited 2020 May 5]. Available from: https://guidelines.ecri.org/

99. National Center from Complementary and Integrative Health. Clinical practice guidelines [Internet]. National Institutes of Health [cited 2020 May 5]. Available from: https://nccih.nih.gov/health/providers/clinicalpractice.htm

100. National Library of Medicine. PubMed [Internet]. National center for biotechnology information [cited 2020 May 5]. Available from: https://www.ncbi.nlm.nih.gov/pubmed/

101. Guideline central [Internet]. [Cited 2020 May 5]. Available from: https://www.guidelinecentral.com/

102. Alliance for the implementation of clinical guidelines [Internet]. [Cited 2020 May 5]. Available from: https://aicpg.org

103. Cook DJ, Mulrow CD, Haynes RB. Systematic reviews: synthesis of best evidence for clinical decisions. Ann Intern Med. 1997;126:376-80.

104. Hunt DL, McKibbon KA. Locating and appraising systematic reviews. Ann Intern Med. 1997;126:532-38.

105. Montori VM, Wilczynski NL, Morgan D, Haynes RB. Optimal search strategies for retrieving systematic reviews from Medline: analytical survey. BMJ. 2005;330:368.

106. U.S. Preventative Services Task Force [Internet]. 2017 Sep [cited 2020 May 5]. Available from: https://www.uspreventiveservicestaskforce.org/

107. Agency for Health Quality Research (AHRQ). Research findings [Internet]. [Updated 2020 March; cited 2020 May 5]. Available from: https://www.ahrq.gov/research/findings/index.html

108. The Cochrane Collaboration. Evidence-based health care [Internet]. [Cited 2020 May 5]. Available from: http://www.cochrane.org/about-us/evidence-based-health-care/webliography/databases

SUGGESTED READINGS

1. AGREE Next Steps Consortium. Appraisal of Guidelines for Research & Evaluation (AGREE) II instrument. Available from: http://www.agreetrust.org/wp-content/uploads/2013/10/AGREE-II-Users-Manual-and-23-item-Instrument_2009_UPDATE_2013.pdf

2. Guyatt GH, Oxman AD, Schunemann HJ, Tugwell P, Knottnerus A. GRADE guidelines: a new series of articles in the Journal of Clinical Epidemiology. J Clin Epidemiol. 2011;64:380-2.

3. Institute of Medicine Committee on Standards for Developing Trustworthy Clinical Practice Guidelines. Clinical practice guidelines we can trust. Available from: http://nationalacademies.org/HMD/Reports/2011/Clinical-Practice-Guidelines-We-Can-Trust.aspx

4. Institute of Medicine Committee on Standards for Systematic Reviews of Comparative Effectiveness Research. Finding what works in health care: standards for systematic reviews. Available from: https://www.nap.edu/catalog/13059/finding-what-works-in-health-care-standards-for-systematic-reviews

Chapter Nine

Journal Clubs

Benjamin A. Witt • Brian S. Hoffmaster

Learning Objectives

After completing this chapter, the reader will be able to:

- Describe the process of developing a journal club presentation.
- Discuss the benefits of journal club participation.
- Apply the concepts of literature evaluation to a journal club presentation.
- Describe effective strategies to increase interest and engagement in journal clubs.
- Describe techniques to add clinical relevance to journal club presentations.

Key Concepts

❶ There is no standard method for implementing a journal club. Journal clubs are flexible in order to meet the needs of the participants.

❷ A journal club can often target articles specific to their area of practice, and practitioners use the journal club as a way to stay current with new developments and clinical evidence in one's specialty area.

❸ As teaching tools, journal clubs are an active-learning method used to enhance knowledge of clinical trial design, biostatistics, and literature evaluation.

❹ Case reports, letters, and nonsystematic reviews should not be the focus of a journal club discussion.

❺ Journal club presenters should draw original conclusions related to the findings of the study that they are presenting. Presenters should share evidence to support this critique with the group.

❻ Discussion among journal club participants can serve as an outlet for providing diverse clinical insight and perspectives.

Introduction

Journal clubs have become a staple in the professional development and continuing education of health care practitioners across many disciplines. ❶ *However, there is no standard method for implementing a journal club. Journal club design and execution are flexible in order to meet the needs of the participants.* The purpose of this chapter is to provide general guidance and suggestions that can be used to design a successful journal club that will meet the needs of the reader.

Journal clubs are groups of individuals who meet regularly to discuss and critically evaluate the biomedical literature.[1,2] Documentation of journal clubs dates back to the 1800s, at which time they served the purpose of sharing educational resources to keep current with new findings published in the medical literature.[1,2] As postgraduate education and training of health care practitioners continue to evolve, so does the journal club. Today, journal clubs are widely used by health care professionals in many disciplines.[3]

Due to the sheer volume of the present-day literature, it is impractical to expect to be able to read every piece of original research that is published. Journal clubs are one solution to keep current with literature in one's area of practice. Members of a particular journal club often have similar professional interests and practice areas. ❷ *Thus, a journal club can often target articles specific to an area of practice, and practitioners use the journal club as a way to stay current with new developments and clinical evidence in one's specialty area.* Additional aims of journal clubs include teaching and practicing **critical appraisal** skills, improving understanding of statistical methods and research design, and fostering the development of evidence-based practice.[2,4-6] Journal club participation can also help presenters hone their public speaking and meeting facilitation skills, improve professionalism and ethics, and serve as an outlet for socialization among peers.[7] Journal club presentations have become a mainstay of literature-evaluation education in the training of health care professionals in the United States.[8] ❸ *As teaching tools, journal clubs are an active-learning method used to enhance knowledge of clinical trial design, biostatistics, and literature evaluation.*[9] Journal clubs are also used in practice to help answer clinical questions, with the intent of applying the knowledge gained to current or anticipated treatment decisions. Journal clubs can also choose to focus on nonclinical topics, such as management and leadership, depending on the need of the participants.[10,11] No matter the intent, journal clubs are a great way to learn about new drug therapies, apply literature evaluation techniques, and apply clinical reasoning skills.

Conducting Journal Clubs

There are numerous considerations when implementing a journal club, and there is no one right design for proper execution. The method of delivery and setting can vary considerably to meet the needs of the participants and achieve the intended purpose. The main factor in holding a successful journal club is to define the expectations of participants and presenters clearly. See Table 9-1 for common considerations when starting a journal club.

EXPECTATIONS OF PARTICIPANTS

Journal clubs facilitators are commonly practitioners or academicians.[12] The facilitator handles the logistics of the journal club, including designating the presenter or presenters for each session, inviting participants, securing the meeting space, and communicating the logistics of the journal club to all the participants.[12] The facilitator may also select the journal article; however, the presenter(s) may take more ownership if they are allowed to choose their article.[13] If not selected by the facilitator, articles should still be screened and approved by the facilitator to assure relevance to practice and suitability for presentation. Once selected, the article should be announced to or shared with all the participants before the presentation date, via an agreed method, so that they may be prepared for a meaningful discussion at the journal club.

Journal clubs have at least one designated presenter who is responsible for providing an overview and critique of the selected article. The presenter is also responsible for engaging other participants by steering the conversation with carefully constructed and

TABLE 9−1. CONSIDERATIONS WHEN PREPARING A JOURNAL CLUB

Who will be invited to attend?	How often will the journal club meet?
Who will facilitate the meetings?	How long will each session last?
How will articles be selected?	Which journal club format will be used?
Is a handout or slide set required?	Will food be provided or permitted?
Will attendance be mandatory?	What technology or resources will be available?
Where will the presentation be held?	Will an evaluation or feedback form be used?

thought-provoking questions. Either the facilitator or presenter should assume the role of keeping the discussion on track and focused, making sure that the discussion starts and ends on time, and that participants are meaningfully contributing to the dialogue.

Ideally, a content expert will be present to participate in the discussion. In clinical practice, a content expert is typically a practitioner with expertise in the area that is the focus of discussion. Having a content expert provides practical insight into how the intervention being discussed applies to real practice. Additionally, including a drug information specialist or clinician with advanced training in clinical investigation can help add depth to the discussion of research methods, study design, and biostatistics.

JOURNAL CLUB SETTING

Journal clubs can take place in many settings and may depend on the structure. Journal clubs that are integrated into coursework will typically take place in the classroom setting, a familiar space often rich in technology that can help aid in discussion. Commonly, this setting is more structured than a practice setting and follows a format designed by the faculty. However, journal clubs can take place in more informal settings, such as in a home or a public place; such an environment may make newer participants more comfortable and likely to engage in discussion. Journal clubs taking place at work may also be held on patient units, or in an office or conference room setting. While the content of the discussion should not change, knowing the environment will help the presenter best prepare based on the knowledge of available resources. For example, if presenting a journal club formally by using a set of PowerPoint® slides, the facilitator or presenter needs to ensure that the venue includes a way to display them. If necessary, physical copies of slides may need printed and brought in, or electronic copies disseminated in advance for use on tablets or laptop computers. Keeping a recurring schedule and meeting place may help increase attendance.[12] Additionally, providing food has been shown to increase journal club turnout when attendance is not mandatory.[14] No matter the setting, it is essential for a presenter to be aware of the given environment and prepared to maximize the learning opportunity of a journal club.

JOURNAL CLUB FORMAT

Journal clubs can be conducted in different formats. First is a presentation-based journal club, in which the presenter will present an overview of a study, along with their critique (as discussed in Chapters 4 through 6). This format is commonly used for student presenters, as it is the easiest to evaluate and assess their critique and evaluation of the article. This format is often integrated into health sciences curricula as a method to develop, apply, and evaluate the principles of literature evaluation and biostatistics, in addition to developing public-speaking skills. The creation of a slide set or a handout often accompanies this format. The presentation-based journal club should allow time for questions and discussion.

The second style of journal club is a discussion-based journal club, which is often the more prevalent style of journal club outside of the classroom setting. In this format, attendees generally read and critique the selected article in advance and are expected to participate in active discussion. In this capacity, the presenter may be expected to provide enough background to set the stage for the article, including any relevant treatment guidelines, related therapies, and more information about the disease state in question. The presenter should also be prepared to keep the discussion focused and on track with the use of guiding questions. Typically, this format of journal club is used to evaluate current literature for new and emerging therapies but is also a great time to practice the critical evaluation skills that were presented in Chapters 4 through 6. Slide sets and handouts are less common in this setting, but the facilitator may choose to use them. Appendices 4-1 and 5-1 provide suggestions of questions and other items for discussion.

Lastly, this age of ever-expanding technologies has paved the way for online journal clubs, also referred to as **virtual journal clubs**. Using video-conferencing software (e.g., Apple FaceTime®, Google Hangouts™, Skype®, Zoom), clinicians from various locations can meet together to help increase access and attendance to the journal club. This synchronous format is particularly attractive for multisite health systems in which a commute may be a deterrent to participation, and may also be used among nonaffiliated sites wishing to hold interactive journal clubs focused on specialty topics.[15,16] In this format, the journal club may also promote socializing and professional networking by increasing communication among practitioners of similar interests and training, such as among postgraduate residents and fellows within specialty tracks. Asynchronous online journal clubs, which allow each participant to post at their availability, are also an option and may increase participation due to increased convenience.[17]

Online journal clubs hosted on popular microblogging websites such as Twitter® are an emerging concept.[18] These journal clubs can include either asynchronous or synchronous discussions about primary literature. Despite a limited length of posts using such a system, several Twitter®-based journal clubs have a successful online presence.[19] Data regarding participation in these online journal clubs are generally descriptive in nature, including numbers of participants, tweets or posts, followers, and uses of hashtags. As with other virtual journal clubs, the primary advantage of this format includes the ability to reach a wide number of participants without geographical limitations. This format can help practitioners within a certain specialty keep up-to-date with new literature in their area by connecting experts in that specialty area. Potential drawbacks to using this format of journal club can include a lack of familiarity with the platform being used, as well as a hesitancy of participants to share their thoughts in a public forum.[20]

Case Study 9–1

A residency preceptor has established a journal club and has made it a required rotation activity for pharmacy students and residents at the site. This activity has been required of residents and students for several years now, but interest from pharmacy staff appears low, and turnout is now less than it has been in past years.

• *What measures can be taken to increase participation from staff members?*

Preparing the Presentation

SELECTING ARTICLES

Articles can be selected in a variety of fashions. Typically, high-quality primary literature from reputable journals and **landmark trials** are selected for student presentations in the classroom. One way to gauge the prominence of a journal is by its **impact factor**, a measure of the average number of citations received by recent articles in a journal. Alternately, an instructor may pick articles that appear in familiar news sources (e.g., television, newspaper, electronic media), which allows students to understand the significant limitations of what may be learned from such sources (e.g., was the clinical significance of a finding of a study overstated or outright embellished?). For practicing clinicians, the focus is typically on analyzing a new article to keep abreast of medical literature, evaluating a piece of original research to help answer a clinical question, or for teaching purposes related to a recent case. One way for clinicians to stay up-to-date with new literature is to identify key journals relevant to one's practice and monitor the table of contents of each new issue for articles that appear useful to one's practice. Articles surrounding clinical controversies are particularly well-suited for journal clubs because participants may have different insights and evidence to provide to the discussion. Ideas may also be solicited from participants in advance of the meeting to gather ideas for therapies or disease states to target as the topic of discussion. This allows participants to offer suggestions of topics that they believe to be timely or clinically relevant and may help to spur interest and subsequent turnout and participation. Note that articles do not need to produce positive results to be the topic of discussion. Drotrecogin alfa (activated; Xigris®) was most likely the topic of countless journal clubs following the publication of the PROWESS-SHOCK trial; this medication was used for years for the prevention of death in patients with severe sepsis at high risk for death until being withdrawn from the market when it was determined to be no better than placebo.[21] While the randomized controlled trial is a mainstay of the journal club, it is important to review other study designs that were discussed in Chapters 4 and 5; this is an opportune time to consider different study designs such as cohort studies, noninferiority studies, and meta-analyses, including their individual strengths and weaknesses. ❹ *Case reports, letters, and nonsystematic reviews should not be the focus of a journal club discussion.*

CONSIDERATIONS FOR PREPARATION

When evaluating the article, the reader should collect enough background information to obtain an adequate perspective. The onus of providing enough background to set the stage for discussion is typically on the presenter, who should address any pertinent treatment guidelines, comparable therapies and the place in therapy of the agent being studied, and any relevant disease-state-specific information such as epidemiological information. The reader should always review any supplements or appendices to selected articles when these are available. Ideally, each participant should be supplied with the article for discussion well in advance, to allow time for thoughtful critique. If the presenter uses a handout, it should be brief; remember that each participant should have already read the article. Slide sets are often not necessary for discussion-based journal clubs and may inadvertently distract from the discussion. As previously described, the presenter should come prepared with questions aimed at generating discussion. Questions should be open-ended to gather as many opinions as possible and to allow participants to expand upon their ideas. Participants may also be provided with questions to answer or a checklist to complete before attending the journal club, if desired, which may help new participants feel more prepared and likely to participate actively during the discussion.

DELIVERING THE PRESENTATION

Presenters should always set the stage for the discussion by first communicating the reason for choosing the selected article and providing any pertinent background for the study. The audience, nature of the article, and the article's background discussion will guide the amount of detail provided. For instance, if the research being discussed is the **pivotal trial** for a new medication with a novel mechanism of action, it is worth dedicating extra time to discussing the pharmacology of the new therapy. Pertinent background about related articles (e.g., a letter to the editor, commentaries) and previous trials with the same therapy should be included. The introduction should let participants know why they should care about the study being discussed.

After setting the stage, stating the purpose of the study, and providing pertinent background information, the study methods should be discussed. How were patients recruited? Were the selected outcome variables appropriate for what was being studied? Was the trial of adequate length? This is also a great time to incorporate statistics into the discussion. Were statistical methods described? If so, were they appropriate? If the presenter disagrees with the methods, this is an opportunity to state what should ideally have been done. If the presenter had to review the statistical tests or concepts used, others could likely benefit from this knowledge as well. As a general rule, if it was necessary to look it up, consider including it in the discussion! These are just a few of the most common items discussed from the methods section; see Appendices 4-1 and 5-1 for more comprehensive examples that can also be used to prepare a checklist for presenters to consider.

Next, the results and conclusions of the study are discussed. Are the results well described? Are results presented for each specified endpoint? How many patients were lost to follow up? It is crucial to address the strengths and limitations of the study during the discussion, keeping in mind the internal and external validities of the results. The participants may discuss additional strengths and limitations beyond those included in the article. The authors' conclusions should be clearly stated. **❺** *Journal club presenters should draw original conclusions related to the findings of the study that they are presenting. Evidence to support this critique should be shared with the group.*

Case Study 9–2

The pharmacist in Case Study 9-1 has been able to increase turnout to their monthly journal club discussion. However, there is often debate on whether or not certain aspects of the study are valid, which often leads to disagreement among members.

- *What is a reasonable approach to help address these issues?*

ADDING CLINICAL RELEVANCE

After presenting and critiquing the article, the findings of the article need to be put into perspective. How does the article compare to other literature available on the topic? How should this new information be used in practice? If the study is investigating a new medication, how should it be recommended or used? If the presenter would use or recommend it, in what specific patient population or clinical scenario would the therapy be most appropriate? The discussion creates an opportune time to present a case vignette of how this therapy might be used in a real-life situation. **❻** *Discussion among journal club participants can serve as an outlet for providing diverse clinical insight and perspectives.*

Other essential items to consider when presenting a journal club include practical issues and its external validity, which may not be thoroughly discussed by the study's investigators. For instance, is the new agent significantly more expensive than the comparator or standard of care? Is the medication available only via a restricted access program, such as a Risk Evaluation Mitigation Strategy (REMS)? Is there a significant dose burden or complex dosage regimen that may be a barrier to adherence? Answering these questions can help tie the results of the study to clinical practice. Keep in mind that the external validity of the study's findings cannot exist if the internal validity of the study (i.e., how well the research was conducted) was not established.

After critical appraisal and journal club discussion of a recently published article, participants may choose to write a **letter to the editor** to describe their analysis of the study.[5,22] Authoring a letter to the editor for publication is a method for reinforcing critical appraisal skills, and many participants will find the group format less intimidating than pursuing this scholarly activity alone. Well-constructed and thoughtful letters should be considered for submission to the journal in which the article was published.[16] Many journals will outline their requirements for submission of a letter. The possibility of a potential publication may serve as an outlet for stimulating interest in journal club attendance and participation.

Case Study 9–3

The pharmacist from Case Studies 9-1 and 9-2 has seen great success with the changes in the journal club program. There is increased interest from the other health-system hospitals, and the second- and third-shift pharmacy staff are also hoping to find a way to participate.

- *What options could you suggest?*

Conclusion

The focus and execution of journal clubs can vary greatly and should be tailored to meet the specific need of the group. Careful and critical analysis of study design and statistical methods should be included when discussing original research. The use of a checklist or template will help guide participants through the literature evaluation process. Presenters should aim to maximize practical information and clinical relevance in their presentation to increase the benefit to other participants. The use of technology may be considered to increase the reach and participation in journal clubs.

Self-Assessment Questions

1. Which one of the following is **NOT** a primary goal of journal club participation?
   a. Practice critical appraisal skills
   b. Become a content expert in a therapeutic discipline
   c. Keep current with newly published literature
   d. Improve understanding of statistical methods and research design

2. Journal club presenter(s) should:
   a. Avoid discussing the author's conclusions.
   b. Provide their own original conclusions.
   c. Avoid discussing the rationale for selecting the study.
   d. Adopt the author's conclusions as their own.

3. Critical appraisal is the process of systematically and critically evaluating scientific research for relevance and value within a specific context.
   a. True
   b. False

4. Discussions of clinical controversies should be avoided during a journal club.
   a. True
   b. False

5. Which of the following is a potential benefit of journal club participation?
   a. Gain comfort with public speaking.
   b. Increase critical appraisal skills.
   c. Keep abreast of new medical literature.
   d. All of the above.

6. Which of the following is least likely to help promote participation in the discussion?
   a. Use of a presentation-style format and slide set
   b. Use of open-ended questions
   c. Sending participants a literature review checklist
   d. Sending participants the selected article in advance

7. Journal clubs are an active-learning method used to enhance knowledge of clinical trial design, biostatistics, and literature evaluation.
   a. True
   b. False

8. Which of the following statements best describe journal clubs? Journal clubs:
   a. Do not allow participants to apply literature evaluation techniques.
   b. Have no standard method for implementation.
   c. Do not allow participants to apply clinical reasoning skills.
   d. Have no facilitator or discussion leader.

9. Only trials with positive results are suitable for journal club discussion.
   a. True
   b. False

10. Attendance and participation in journal clubs can be increased by:
    a. Hosting the session in a virtual journal club format
    b. Providing food or snacks to those in attendance
    c. Gathering ideas from staff for journal club topics
    d. All of the above

11. An impact factor is an objective way to gauge the relative prestige of a scientific journal.
    a. True
    b. False

12. The discussion format of virtual journal clubs can be:
    a. Asynchronous
    b. Synchronous
    c. Asynchronous or synchronous

13. Monitoring the table of contents of several journals can help you identify articles related to your practice.
    a. True
    b. False

14. One potential advantage of a virtual journal club is the ability to include participants from multiple practice sites without the need for travel.
    a. True
    b. False

15. One potential drawback of a virtual journal club is the hesitancy of participants to share their thoughts online.
    a. True
    b. False

REFERENCES

1. Linzer M. The journal club and medical education: over one hundred years of unrecorded history. Postgrad Med J. 1987;63(740):475-8.
2. Lizarondo LM, Grimmer-Somers K, Kumar S. Exploring the perspectives of allied health practitioners toward the use of journal clubs as a medium for promoting evidence-based practice: a qualitative study. BMC Med Educ. 2011;11:66.
3. Deenadayalan Y, Grimmer-Somers K, Prior M, Kumar S. How to run an effective journal club: a systematic review. J Eval Clin Pract. 2008;14(5):898-911.
4. Matthews DC. Journal clubs most effective if tailored to learner needs. Evid Based Dent. 2011;12(3):92-3.
5. Stallings A, Borja-Hart N, Fass J. New practitioners forum: strategies for reinventing journal club. Am J Health-Syst Pharm. 2011;68(1):14-6.
6. Mezgebe M, Chesson MM, Thurston MM. Pharmacy student perceptions regarding understanding of and confidence in literature evaluation following a student-led journal club. Curr Pharm Teach Learn. 2019;11(6):557-64.
7. Cave MT, Clandinin DJ. Revisiting the journal club. Med Teach. 2007;29(4):365-70.
8. O'Sullivan TA, Phillips J, Demaris K. Medical literature evaluation education at US schools of pharmacy. Am J Pharm Educ. 2016;80(1):5.
9. Arif SA, Gim S, Nogid A, Shah B. Journal clubs during advanced pharmacy practice experiences to teach literature evaluation skills. Am J Pharm Ed. 2012;76(5):article 88, 1-8
10. Flarey DL. Journal club: a tool for health care management and development. Health Care Superv. 1993;11(3):53-8.
11. Wombwell E, Murray C, Davis SJ, Palmer K, Nayar M, Konkol J. Leadership journal club. Am J Health-Syst Pharm. 2011;68(21):2026-7.
12. Hattoy SL, Childress B, Jett A, Motney J. Enhancing experiential education: implementing and improving the journal club experience. Curr Pharm Teach Learn. 2015;7:389-94.
13. Al Achkar M. Redesigning journal club in residency. Adv Med Educ Pract. 2016;7:317-20.
14. Lee AG, Boldt HC, Golnik KC, Arnold AC, Oetting TA, Beaver HA, Olson RJ, Carter K. Using the Journal Club to teach and assess competence in practice-based learning and improvement: a literature review and recommendation for implementation. Surv Ophthalmol. 2005;50(6):542-8.
15. Miller Quidley A, LeClaire A, Glick Frasiolas J, Berger K, Gonzales JP, Oyen L. Implementation of a national, Web-based critical care pharmacy journal club. Am J Health-Syst Pharm. 2015;72(15):1260-2.
16. Devabhakthuni S, Reed BN, Watson K. Interactive Web-based regional journal club for postgraduate year 2 pharmacy residents in cardiology. Am J Health-Syst Pharm. 2016;73(17):1300.

17. Lizarondo L, Kumar S, Grimmer-Somers K. Online journal clubs: an innovative approach to achieving evidence-based practice. J Allied Health. 2010;39(1):e17-22.
18. Roberts MJ, Perera M, Lawrentschuk N, Romanic D, Papa N, Bolton D. Globalization of continuing professional development by journal clubs via microblogging: a systematic review. J Med Internet Res. 2015;17(4):e103.
19. Bolderston A, Watson J, Woznitza N, Westerink A, Di Prospero L, Currie G, Beardmore C, Hewis J. Twitter journal clubs and continuing professional development: An analysis of a #MedRadJClub tweet chat. Radiography (Lond). 2018;24(1):3-8.
20. Lin M, Joshi N, Hayes BD, Chan TM. Accelerating knowledge translation: reflections from the online ALiEM-Annals global emergency medicine journal club experience. Ann Emerg Med. 2017;69(4):469-74.
21. Ranieri VM, Thompson BT, Barie PS, Dhainaut JF, Douglas IS, Finfer S, Gardlund B, Marshall JC, Rhodes A, Artigas A, Payen D, Tenhunen J, Al-Khalidi HR, Thompson V, Janes J, Macias WL, Vangerow B, Williams Md, PROWESS-SHOCK Study Group. Drotrecogin alfa (activated) in adults with septic shock. N Engl J Med. 2012;366(22):2055-64.
22. Green BN, Johnson CD. Use of a modified journal club and letters to editors to teach critical appraisal skills. J Allied Health. 2007;36(1):47-51.

SUGGESTED READINGS

1. Deenadayalan Y, Grimmer-Somers K, Prior M, Kumar S. How to run an effective journal club: a systematic review. J Eval Clin Pract. 2008;14(5):898-911.
2. Green BN, Johnson CD. Use of a modified journal club and letters to editors to teach critical appraisal skills. J Allied Health. 2007;36(1):47-51.
3. Lizarondo L, Kumar S, Grimmer-Somers K. Online journal clubs: an innovative approach to achieving evidence-based practice. J Allied Health. 2010;39(1):e17-22.
4. McLeod P, Steinert Y, Boudreau D, Snell L, Wiseman J. Twelve tips for conducting a medical education journal club. Med Teach. 2010;32(5):368-370.
5. Miller Quidley A, LeClaire A, Glick Frasiolas J, Berger K, Gonzales JP, Oyen L. Implementation of a national, web-based critical care pharmacy journal club. Am J Health-Syst Pharm. 2015;72(15):1260, 1262.
6. Stallings A, Borja-Hart N, Fass J. New practitioners forum: strategies for reinventing journal club. Am J Health-Syst Pharm. 2011;68(1):14-6.
7. Stapleton JJ. The successful journal club. Clin Podiatr Med Surg. 2007;24(1):51-5.

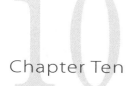

Chapter Ten

Peer Review

David M. Peterson

Learning Objectives

After completing this chapter, the reader will be able to:

- Explain the purpose and role of peer review in biomedical publishing.
- Provide an overview of the peer review process.
- Describe reasons to participate in peer review.
- List three ways to identify peer review opportunities.
- Describe the potential contents of a peer review resource file.
- List three reasons to decline a peer review invitation.
- Describe the elements of a three-read approach to performing peer review.
- Discuss the most important aspects of a manuscript to assess during peer review.
- Describe attributes of a manuscript that would support a publishing recommendation of accept, accept with revisions, and reject.
- Describe the process for involving a learner in a peer review assignment.

Key Concepts

❶ The peer review process helps to ensure that published articles fill a gap in the current literature, meet the aims and quality standards of the respective journal, and ethically report valid results based upon sound methodology.

❷ Despite its importance, the majority of health care professionals are never formally trained in performing peer review.

❸ Peer review is a critical evaluation of a manuscript that has been submitted for publication, performed by a content expert who serves as a neutral party between the publisher and manuscript author.

❹ Unless specifically requested by the editor, peer reviewers should not focus upon grammar, spelling, and punctuation, except if these aspects of the manuscript significantly interfere with comprehension of the manuscript.

❺ Insufficient knowledge of the manuscript topic is an important reason to consider declining a peer review invitation.

❻ A conflict of interest occurs in peer review when the reviewer's private interests (i.e., competing interests) diverge from their responsibilities as a reviewer and either affect or could appear to affect their assessment of the manuscript.

❼ One of the most important things a reviewer can do is to assess whether the manuscript fills a needed gap in the body of literature, and advances knowledge in this area.

❽ When submitting comments to the author, it is important to maintain a constructive and professional tone. Comments should be objective, constructive, and actionable. The reviewer should also seek balance in comments, addressing positive aspects of the manuscript as well as areas for improvement.

❾ Many skilled practitioners with exceptional literature evaluation skills never participate in peer review because they lack an understanding of the process and fear that they are inadequate to participate in the process.

Introduction

Peer review is an important aspect of the publication process for biomedical journals. ❶ *The peer review process helps to ensure that published articles fill a gap in the current literature, meet the aims and quality standards of the respective journal, and ethically report valid results based upon sound methodology.*[1-3] Peer review also helps to refine and improve the manuscript prior to publication.[1] Article submissions to biomedical journals far exceed publishing capacity, and the work of peer reviewers can assist in determining which submissions are most appropriate for publication.[2,3]

❷ *Despite its importance, most health care professionals are never formally trained in performing peer review.*[4,5] Most journals offer guidelines or instructions for peer reviewers, but no additional training. Generally, peer reviewers do not receive feedback from editors addressing ways that they can improve future reviews. The quality of peer reviews is not consistent between reviewers, and a decline in review quality has been noted in recent years.[6] Guidance on navigating the peer review process, and instructions on performing a thorough review, may make peer review more accessible to new reviewers, improve the quality of peer reviews, and in turn help to improve the quality of the published literature.[5] The goal of this chapter is to provide information and instruction on the peer review process. This chapter will begin by providing a general overview of peer review, its value, and role. The remainder of the chapter provides practical tools to help the reader participate in peer review and involve learners in the process.

What Is Peer Review?

❸ *Peer review is a critical evaluation of a manuscript that has been submitted for publication, performed by a content expert who serves as a neutral party between the publisher and manuscript author.*[3,4] The peer reviewer will submit comments and a publishing recommendation to the editor based upon their evaluation. The peer reviewer may be selected for expertise related to the main topic of the manuscript being reviewed (e.g., diabetes management, medication reconciliation, staffing models) or they may be selected for expertise related to the methodology or statistical analyses described in the manuscript (e.g., Bayesian statistical analysis, adaptive trial design, guideline development models).[2,5] Although the peer reviewer is usually vetted by the publisher, the reviewer should neither be an employee of the publisher nor be affiliated with the manuscript author(s).[7] The peer reviewer usually serves as a volunteer, and does not receive financial compensation for performing a review.[4,8] The peer review process is most commonly referred to in the context of peer-reviewed journals, but book chapters, online publications, grant proposals, and informational databases may also undergo a peer review process.[4]

The details and specifics of the peer review process differ from journal to journal, but there are also many similarities between journals. No single type of peer review (e.g., blinded vs. **open peer review**) is clearly better than the others.[12,15,16] A detailed account of all the different types of peer review is beyond the scope of this chapter. Instead, the chapter will focus on the most common forms of peer review for biomedical journals and highlight a few variations where possible. The number of peer reviewers assigned to evaluate a manuscript varies, ranging from one to several, with two or three reviewers being fairly common.[2,9] In terms of journal article publication, peer review is generally performed after the manuscript is submitted to the journal editor, but prior to final copyediting and publication. The exact timing of peer review can vary somewhat. On one extreme, some journals request feedback from peer reviewers immediately upon receiving a manuscript submission, while other journals perform an initial evaluation of the manuscript prior to enlisting the help of peer reviewers. However, copyediting occurs after peer review, so that time is not wasted copyediting a manuscript that will not ultimately be published in that journal. Editors of peer-reviewed journals are not obligated to obtain peer review for a manuscript prior to rejection, and most editors will screen for major flaws and to ensure the manuscript fits within the scope of the journal prior to sending the manuscript to peer reviewers.[2] The comments and recommendations of peer reviewers carry different weights with different journals and editors, but regardless of the journal, the decision to publish a manuscript or not ultimately rests upon the editor, not the peer reviewer.[3] The peer reviewer is sometimes described as a **referee**, and peer-reviewed publications may be described as **refereed publications**. However, because the decisions of a referee in most contexts (e.g., sports) are considered final, some consider this terminology misapplied in the peer review setting, where the editor makes the final publication decision.

There is no objective measure for what constitutes a "good" peer review.[6] A high-quality review will be based upon thoughtful consideration of the manuscript and its scientific merit, will present a balanced and organized assessment of the strengths and limitations of the manuscript, and will be written in a courteous tone.[2,4,6] Other important attributes of a peer review are addressed in more detail in the Performing Peer Review section of this chapter. ❹ *Unless specifically requested by the editor, peer reviewers should not focus upon grammar, spelling, and punctuation, except if these aspects of the manuscript significantly interfere with comprehension of the manuscript.*[6] These aspects of the manuscript will be addressed by the journal's copyeditors, allowing the peer reviewer to focus efforts upon the other aspects of the manuscript.[2]

Criticisms and Variations of Peer Review

The true value of peer review is a topic that has been heavily debated.[1,3] While some sources consider peer review an essential part of the publication process, others argue that it delays publication, increases expenses for the journal, and offers limited benefits.[10–12] Although peer review is an imperfect process, it is still considered the gold standard for biomedical journal publications.[3,13] Two innovations that are frequently described as possible ways to improve the peer review process include open review and postpublication review.[12,14,15]

BLINDED VS. OPEN REVIEW

Traditionally, biomedical peer review has been a blinded process, where the reviewer's name and affiliation are withheld from the author.[16] The two subtypes of blinded peer review include **single-blind peer review**, in which the reviewer is aware of the author's information, and **double-blind peer review**, in which the author's information is withheld from the reviewer.[17] The purpose of blinded review is to elicit an unbiased evaluation of the manuscript by a reviewer who feels comfortable sharing honest opinions because their identity is concealed. The reviewer whose identity is not known may be less susceptible to outside influences, such as pressure from the author or others within the field of practice. Concealing the identity of the author (double-blind review) is used to reduce bias during the review process that could be attributed to recognition of the author or their affiliations. For instance, in an unblinded setting, a manuscript submitted by a professor at an Ivy League university is probably much more likely to receive a favorable review than a comparable manuscript submitted by a professor at a community college. Even when journal editors attempt to initiate a double-blind review, details within the manuscript, or the reviewer's familiarity with the work of others within their field, often unintentionally results in author identification.[1,15,18]

Blinded review formats may have unintended consequences such as a lack of transparency, a lack of accountability for the reviewer, and overexpression of negative comments by the reviewer.[1,15,18] Open review is an alternative to blinded review where the identity of the author and reviewer are not withheld from each other.[17] The British Medical Journal (BMJ) and some of the journals of BioMed Central (BMC; e.g., Head & Face Medicine, Journal of Cardiothoracic Surgery) are examples of publications that utilize an open review process.[14,19] Proposed advantages of open review include increasing accountability of reviewers, placing authors and reviewers on equal footing, reducing time spent by editorial staff to remove identifiers from manuscripts, and promoting a transparent scientific dialogue between authors and reviewers.[14,15,18] Open review makes it easier to acknowledge reviewers, because their identity does not need to be concealed. An open review format may prompt some reviewers to perform a more thorough evaluation of the manuscript than they would in a blinded setting. It may also help ensure that reviewers complete their peer review assignments in a timely manner. Reviewers may also be less likely to include personal attacks or acrimonious comments in reviews if their identity is not hidden. Open peer review is perceived as being fairer by authors due to greater reviewer accountability, but studies comparing open and blinded review have not identified significant differences in the quality of the reviews yielded through the different processes.[1,15]

There are some potential drawbacks to an open review format. Open review could bias the results of the review by inhibiting the reviewer's comments and producing more or less favorable reviews based upon the nature of the relationship between the author and reviewer (e.g., mentor/mentee relationship, competing institutions). Some peer reviewers may be less willing to participate in an open review process due to fear of repercussion from a displeased author, particularly if the author is a senior authority within the field.[1,17]

PREPUBLICATION VS. POSTPUBLICATION PEER REVIEW

Prepublication peer review has long been the standard review format for biomedical journals. With increased ease of access to publications and easier worldwide communication between the members of a biomedical community due to online access, some argue that prepublication review is an antiquated system that should be replaced by postpublication review.[12] In postpublication peer review, once an article is published online, anyone who is interested can post a review in a forum-like setting. Whereas the prepublication peer review process includes only a small number of reviewers, usually two or three, the number of potential reviewers in an online postpublication setting is unlimited. Proponents of postpublication review assert that eliminating prepublication review will result in faster publication times, lower editor workload, and the larger pool of reviewers to provide a more thorough review.[12] In contrast to a prepublication peer review process, which examines the manuscript at only one point in time, postpublication peer review could result in a much more dynamic type of article that is updated and corrected as reviews are posted.[15]

Some elements of postpublication peer review have been adopted, in the sense that many journals provide content online, and subscribers are able to post comments and critiques for the articles where others can see. However, movement to a fully postpublication peer review process, in place of prepublication peer review, is uncommon. One drawback to postpublication review is that less popular article topics may never undergo a thorough review, while more popular topics may undergo rigorous and continual evaluation and updating. Without the responsibility associated with a formal assignment, postpublication peer reviewers may be less likely to expend the time and energy that is typically dedicated to a prepublication peer review assignment, and thus some details may never be examined. Another challenge of postpublication peer review centers on the uncertainty it creates when citing an article undergoing this process, because the article may change in significant ways after the citation has already been made.[9] Rather than replacing prepublication peer review, the role of postpublication review may instead function to complement the more traditional peer review format.[20]

Reasons to Participate in Peer Review

Performing peer review generally offers no tangible rewards, and often little or no acknowledgment. Due to a shortage of experienced reviewers,[2,21] many journals and organizations are experimenting with methods to provide acknowledgment and benefits to reviewers.[14,21] The BMJ now offers continuing medical education credits when reviewers submit peer reviews that meet quality standards.[14] Some journals publish an annual list of reviewers who have contributed during the past year, and some even offer financial perks to reviewers, such as free or discounted books or journal subscriptions.[1,19,22] To address the lack of formal recognition for peer reviewers, a peer review registry entitled Publons (**https://publons.com/about/home/**) was created,[8,23] but use of this website has not been universally adopted.

Many peer reviewers see participation in the peer review process as a professional responsibility, especially if they have published themselves.[10,24] Upon submitting a manuscript to a peer-reviewed journal, an author has engaged the services of a peer reviewer, and participating as a peer reviewer is a way of returning the favor.[24] Peer review is a manner of contributing to the body of available literature that requires a lesser investment of time than authoring a manuscript. Participation in peer review may be a necessary step toward promotion for some professionals.[24] It can be added to a curriculum vitae to demonstrate active participation in the research community. Some peer reviewers may be invited to participate in the editorial board for a journal.[27] Peer review also provides the reviewer with an opportunity to stay current in areas of expertise and to exercise literature evaluation skills.[27]

Locating Peer Review Opportunities

There is no set pathway for becoming a peer reviewer. Many journals identify peer reviewers from the pool of prior authors who have published articles with them.[1] However, there are also other methods for locating peer review opportunities that do not require authorship in the journal. Some journals include an electronic peer review application on the journal's website that can be completed to request consideration as a peer reviewer (e.g., American Journal of Health-System Pharmacy [AJHP]).[2] Online peer review applications commonly ask for background and contact information, credentials, and areas of expertise or interest.

Even if the journal's website does not include an electronic application, it is still a great place to start when looking for peer review opportunities. The website will usually address the role of peer review at that specific journal and may provide instructions for requesting a peer review appointment. If no instructions are available, the website should include contact information for the editor. In that case, the prospective reviewer can send a professional email request to the editor with a curriculum vitae attached, requesting consideration as a peer reviewer. For more information on writing a formal request, please refer to Chapter 13.

Journals will often host exhibitor booths at national society meetings (e.g., ASHP Midyear Clinical Meeting). Stopping by the journal's booth is a good way to collect more information about their peer review process and their manner for selecting peer reviewers.

At times, one or more members of the editorial staff may be at the booth, offering the prospective peer reviewer an opportunity for a face-to-face conversation.

Finally, peer review opportunities can be identified via colleague referral. When journals send manuscript review invitations to established peer reviewers, they often ask the reviewers to recommend colleagues with expertise on that topic who may also serve as reviewers. Establishing good rapport with colleagues and letting them know of interests in becoming a peer reviewer, as well as areas of expertise, can result in peer review opportunities through referral.

In the case of referral, the journal already has an article for which they are seeking a reviewer, so the prospective peer reviewer may get an immediate invitation to review the article. In most other instances, the reviewer will need to wait patiently, to see when the first review request arrives. Often, the prospective reviewer may not even know if they were accepted by the journal as a reviewer until the first review invitation arrives, which may take several months. The first review invitation will usually include information on how to access the journal's publication management software, where the article can be accessed, the review can be submitted, and the reviewer can update contact information and add or refine areas of expertise.

Preparing for Peer Review

In addition to this book chapter, several review articles have been published that discuss the peer review process and address the elements of a high-quality review (see "Suggested Readings"). Studying these articles will provide the reviewer with the knowledge base necessary to perform peer review. Many of these articles include lists of specific attributes to look for when reviewing a manuscript. Even after studying a few instructional articles, the first time reviewing a manuscript can be a bit intimidating. Without any prior experience to measure the review against, it can be difficult for the first-time reviewer to determine if they have done a good job or not. If possible, performing the first review with a colleague who has peer review experience can be extremely helpful. For additional information on the mentor-mentee relationship when reviewing an article, refer to the "Involving Learners in Peer Review" section of this chapter.

CREATING A PEER REVIEW RESOURCE FILE

After studying instructional articles about performing peer review, avoid the temptation to place these articles in a virtual or actual recycling bin. Keeping helpful articles accessible in a peer review resource file can be extremely helpful. The resource file could be a physical or electronic file depending on the preferences of the reviewer, as long as it is easily accessible. When a peer review invitation arrives, the reviewer need not spend time searching for hints and pointers, and instead can quickly review the materials already collected in the resource file. Other contents of the resource file could include the reviewer's notes and submissions from prior reviews, and peer review instructions from the journals with which the reviewer frequently works. The actual manuscripts provided by journals during the peer review process remain property of the author, and all print or electronic copies of the manuscript must be destroyed upon completion of the peer review assignment.[3] However, the review notes and comments remain the property of the reviewer and can be useful to reflect upon to spark the thought process during subsequent reviews.

Reporting criteria for different publication types, such as the Consolidated Standards of Reporting Trials (CONSORT)[25] or Preferred Reporting Items for Systematic Reviews and Meta-Analyses (PRISMA),[26] are also useful items to include in the resources file.

Even experienced reviewers can benefit from maintaining a peer review resource file. Because many reviewers only perform a review once every few months, a quick refresher on the most important items and aspects to assess in a manuscript will help to ensure that the reviewer is both thorough and efficient. Maintaining a peer review resource file will allow the reviewer the benefits of a quick refresher without wasting time hunting down resources.

Case Study 10–1

You have recently finished a PGY1 residency and would like to participate in peer review, but you're not sure where to start. A number of your colleagues already participate in peer review, but you feel a little embarrassed that you do not really understand the peer review process.

- *What are some things you can do to prepare to participate in peer review?*
- *How might you locate an opportunity to participate in peer review?*

Reasons to Decline a Peer Review Invitation

Before considering the methods and details of performing peer review, it is important to note that not every review invitation will be a good fit, and the reviewer will need to carefully consider each invitation to decide whether to accept it or not. There are several valid and important reasons to consider declining the review of a specific manuscript. Common reasons for declining an opportunity include lack of time, lack of expertise, and conflicts of interest.[3] See below for a discussion on each of these reasons. Accepting a peer review invitation that is not a good fit is a disservice to the editor and author, and reflects poorly upon the reviewer. If a reviewer has concerns about their ability to adequately review a given manuscript, an email or call to the editor to discuss concerns is often helpful. The editor will generally be grateful for the reviewer's honest and thoughtful consideration of their peer review responsibilities. Whether the reviewer plans to accept or decline the peer review invitation, it is important to let the editor know as soon as possible. Time waiting for a peer reviewer to respond to an invitation slows the publication process, and in the case of a declined invitation, delays locating an alternate reviewer.[2]

When assessing whether to accept a peer review invitation or not, the reviewer should consider their history of reviewing for this journal. If a reviewer consistently declines peer review invitations, the editor may reduce or withhold future review opportunities, opting to send these opportunities to peer reviewers who are more likely to accept the invitation. Again, if a manuscript is not a good fit for the reviewer, it is in the best interest of the reviewer to decline, even considering the potential risk of receiving fewer review invitations in the future. A peer reviewer who serves multiple journals and finds that they receive more invitations than are possible to fulfill may want to consider limiting their reviews only to the journals that are most aligned with their interests or scope of practice. Most journals maintain an electronic profile for each peer reviewer where the reviewer can indicate areas of expertise, and this can also be used to manage the number of invitations received. Reducing the number of areas of expertise selected in the profile to those where the reviewer has the greatest aptitude will both reduce the number of review invitations received and help to ensure that review invitations fall within the reviewer's greatest areas of expertise. The online peer reviewer profiles on many journals' sites offer other features that can help manage review invitations, such as indicating when the peer reviewer will be on vacation or otherwise unavailable, and selecting approximately how many review invitations are desired per year.[9,27]

LACK OF TIME

One of the most common reasons to decline a peer review invitation is lack of time. Each review request will indicate the due date for the review. When deciding whether to accept a review, it is important to realistically consider any projects and commitments that may interfere with meeting this deadline. It is also important to consider the amount of time that will need to be dedicated to the review. Experienced reviewers should plan to spend 3 hours or more reviewing a manuscript. A study of reviewers for the BMJ determined that review quality improved with increasing time spent on the review up to 3 hours, but not beyond 3 hours.[28] However, many experts suggest that several hours may be needed to perform a thorough and accurate review.[6,29,30] Inexperienced reviewers will generally need more time than those with experience.

Delays in peer review submissions can interfere with a journal's publication timeline. If meeting the review deadline will pose a challenge, it is better to decline the invitation than to submit the review late or to submit an incomplete or hurried attempt at a review. If a few extra days may make the difference between accepting or declining a review assignment, a conversation with the editor is warranted. Some editors are willing to slightly extend the deadline on the review in these circumstances. Likewise, after accepting a review invitation, any unexpected circumstances that will interfere with your ability to meet the review deadline should prompt a communication with the editor.[2]

LACK OF EXPERTISE

❺ *Insufficient knowledge of the manuscript topic is an important reason to consider declining a peer review invitation.* The reviewer must have a working knowledge of the specific manuscript topic as well as familiarity with how that topic fits into the wider body of literature.[4] In a study of pharmacy journal editors, knowledge in the content area of the review was the peer reviewer characteristic that was rated as most important to enhancing manuscript quality.[31] If the reviewer is not confident that they have the expertise to properly review a manuscript, it is best to decline the invitation.[6] If the lack of expertise is discovered after accepting the invitation, a discussion with the editor is warranted.

CONFLICT OF INTEREST

❻ *A conflict of interest occurs in peer review when the reviewer's private interests (i.e., competing interests) diverge from their responsibilities as a reviewer and either affect or could appear to affect their assessment of the manuscript.* Conflicts of interest can be difficult to define because everyone has some private interests that could potentially influence their judgment. One measure for determining if a conflict of interest exists is to assess whether a reasonable unblinded observer would wonder if the peer reviewer's competing interests motivated their assessment of the manuscript. If a potential conflict of interest exists, the reviewer should notify the editor as soon as possible to determine a course of action. In this scenario, the editor serves as the unblinded observer to help assess the significance of the potential conflict of interest. There are several types of conflict of interest and each type is composed of an unlimited number of different scenarios, situations, and examples. A few of the important types of conflicts of interest include financial ties, personal relationships, academic pursuits, and institutional affiliations.[7] Examples of these conflicts of interest are included in Table 10-1.

TABLE 10–1. CONFLICT OF INTEREST EXAMPLES[7]

- Financial ties—A clinician who has received speaker fees from a drug manufacturer now receives a peer review invitation for a manuscript describing a clinical trial for an investigational medication owned by the same drug manufacturer (note: this would also be a conflict of interest if the investigational drug was owned by a competing manufacturer).
- Personal relationships—A provider is reading a manuscript for a peer review assignment and deduces that the manuscript was written by a beloved mentor (note: this would also be a conflict of interest if the manuscript was written by his arch rival).
- Academic pursuits—A professor has been working tirelessly for several weeks to complete a systematic review comparing the different pharmacologic weight loss medications she will soon be submitting for publication, when a peer review invitation arrives describing a very similar manuscript.
- Institutional affiliations—A health plan director receives a peer review request for a manuscript submitted by a local competitor.

Case Study 10–2

You have accepted an invitation to review a manuscript. During your first reading of the manuscript, you realize that the manuscript was submitted by someone at your institution, with whom you closely work.

- *How should you respond to this situation?*

Performing Peer Review

Performing peer review can be a daunting process. The author of a manuscript has spent numerous hours preparing their work, hoping that it will be published, and now the reviewer is asked to judge whether the manuscript is worthy of publication or not. This is a weighty responsibility that should not be taken lightly, but if the reviewer is qualified and applies a stepwise approach to reviewing the manuscript, it will be a manageable and rewarding experience. The sections that follow provide a suggested overall approach to performing peer review, specific details to look for and assess during peer review, and considerations when constructing the review that will ultimately be submitted to the editor.

A THREE-READ APPROACH

Peer review invitations usually arrive as an email. The email will include a brief description or abstract of the article, the due date, and instructions for accepting or declining the invitation (see "Reasons to Decline a Peer Review Invitation"). Upon accepting the invitation, the reviewer will usually be provided with an internet link to the full manuscript, the journal's guidelines for reviewers, and an electronic form used when submitting the review. The reviewer will usually have about 2 or 3 weeks to perform and submit the review, depending on the timeline defined by the editor. Over the course of the process, the reviewer will likely need to read the article at least two or three times.[6,30] This chapter will outline a three-read approach, but some reviewers may find two reads of the manuscript sufficient, and others may require four or more reads to complete the assignment. There is no objective "right" way to perform peer review, so the reader should adapt this material to match their strengths and preferences.

Before beginning the review, it is important to be familiar with the journal's instructions for reviewers. These instructions will provide the reviewer with helpful guidance on performing the review and will clarify expectations and submission requirements of the publisher. It is also a good idea to examine the journal's review submission form prior to starting the review. A review submission form that poses very specific questions for the reviewer to address might prompt attention to different aspects of the manuscript than one that is composed of a free-text field where the reviewer can place any comments that seem important and appropriate.

Perform the first read of the article as soon as possible after accepting the review invitation. The goal of the first read is to get a general sense of the article topic, to assess whether it makes sense and is understandable, and to identify any major flaws in the methodology that might make further review unnecessary. As thoughts or questions emerge about the manuscript during this first read, make a quick note of them to refer to later, and keep moving on through the manuscript. The first read of the manuscript should not take much longer than it would take to read any other journal article, because the goal is not to fully critique the article, but to merely try to understand it and start generating notes and ideas that can be further investigated during subsequent reads of the manuscript. Performing the first read early on allows the reader time to ponder and process thoughts about the manuscript before proceeding to the second read.[30] New and important insights about a manuscript often come while performing unrelated tasks, such as driving to work, mowing the lawn, or washing dishes. Allowing time between readings provides an opportunity for these thoughts to surface.

This first read also allows the reviewer to quickly ensure that the monograph falls within their scope of expertise and to scan for any potential conflicts of interest. Although the information in the review invitation is usually enough to determine the appropriateness of serving as a peer reviewer for the manuscript, sometimes additional details from the full manuscript reveal unforeseen conflicts of interest or limitations to reviewer's expertise. The reviewer should notify the editor as soon as possible if problems related to expertise or a conflict of interest are identified. This permits the editor to identify a substitute reviewer, if needed, without further delay.[6]

The second read of the manuscript will ideally occur within a few days of the first read. Waiting a day or so to read the article the second time will help the reviewer to approach the article with new vision and insight. Inconsistencies and nuances that were not apparent during the first read will almost magically appear on the second pass. Points that were confusing or unclear during the first read may become understandable during the second read. The second read of the manuscript will be the most thorough and time consuming of the three, likely requiring a larger time commitment than the first and third readings combined.[30] Having a list of assessment questions present alongside the manuscript, an example of which is shared in Table 10-2, can be very helpful in maintaining focus during this voyage through the manuscript.[32] Most of the reviewer's notes and comments on the article will be generated during the second read.[30] Because editors usually require the review to be submitted electronically, using a word processing program to document notes as thoughts arise can help with organization and reduce the time needed to create the review submission later on. When the review is complete, the notes will already be in a format that can easily be edited and polished, and then copied from the word processing program and pasted into the appropriate fields of the submission form.

The third read of a manuscript serves as a final scan to look for any missed details or inconsistencies, and resolve any pending concerns or questions.[6] Taking the time to review notes from the first and second reads before launching into the third read will help orient the reviewer to the task at hand. If any portions of the manuscript were unclear or confusing during the first two reads, the third read provides an opportunity to circle back to these sections for reassessment. If they remain unclear or confusing after the third read, it is very likely that the casual reader would also struggle with them, and it is worth pointing these out so that they can be clarified.[30] Any new items or issues identified in this final read will be added to the notes from earlier reads of the manuscript. The compiled notes from the three readings of the manuscript will provide the content for the review submission.

Case Study 10–3

You have just received your first peer review invitation.

- *What should you do before accepting this invitation?*
- *Once you've accepted the invitation, what should you do next?*

KEY THINGS TO LOOK FOR WHEN PERFORMING PEER REVIEW

Having some things in mind to look for when reviewing a manuscript will generally be more productive than casually reading the manuscript from beginning to end. Some of the key items to look for will differ depending on the type of manuscript (e.g., narrative review vs. clinical trial), but others apply to any type of manuscript. This section will summarize some fundamental items to look for in all manuscripts, followed by some specific questions to ask about the manuscript during the review process. For additional ideas of things to look for in specific types of manuscript types (e.g., randomized controlled trials), please refer to Chapters 4 and 5 of this book, addressing literature evaluation skills, and Chapter 6, which addresses statistics.

Role of the Manuscript in the Complete Body of Literature

❼ *One of the most important things a reviewer can do is to assess whether the manuscript fills a needed gap in the body of literature, and advances knowledge in this area.* Reviewers should be experts in the areas in which they volunteer to review, which will make it much easier to assess the importance of a submitted manuscript. Despite the reviewer's expertise with the topic, a search of the medical literature using PubMed, Embase, or another database of publications specific to the topic is often necessary.[32] For instance, if the submitted manuscript is a narrative review of medications used for weight loss, and several other narrative reviews on this topic have already been published in the past few years, the manuscript may not have much to add to the current body of literature. However, if the manuscript addresses the topic from a unique perspective, such as the perspective of the ambulatory care pharmacist, it still may fill a knowledge gap that makes it a welcome and useful publication. Likewise, if a few new medications have recently been approved for this indication, and prior reviews did not include information on the newer medications, it could also fill a gap, despite the initial impression of the reviewer that this area of publication is already saturated.

Appropriateness for Publication in the Specific Journal

Does the manuscript match the scope of the journal and the interests of the journal's readership? An in-depth analysis of new methods for diagnosing dermatologic diseases would be more appropriate for a dermatologic journal than a pulmonology journal. Even within the fairly narrow scope of pharmacy journals, some focus heavily on pharmaceutics, while others focus on clinical practice, and still others are more focused on pharmacy reimbursement models and pharmacy logistics. A quick visit to the journal's website will reveal the goals and scope of the publication, as well as the different categories of articles that are published in the journal. A well-written manuscript addressing a valid gap in the body of literature may be worthy of publication, but still may not be the best fit for this specific journal.

Comprehension

● Does the manuscript make sense? After an initial read of the manuscript, the reviewer should be able to understand the article, including its goal, methods, and findings. In the case of a study, the manuscript should provide sufficient detail that the reader, provided appropriate resources, could replicate the study.[30] As stated earlier, assessment of grammar does not fall within the scope of peer review. However, if a manuscript is so poorly written that it is incomprehensible, it is not appropriate for publication; at least not yet.[2,6,30]

Methodology

● Was the methodology appropriate to address the stated goals of the manuscript? The most perfectly worded manuscript may not be appropriate for publication if it is lacking in methodologic rigor. Assessing the methodology used in a trial is a great opportunity to exercise literature evaluation skills. A manuscript with severely flawed methodology is unlikely to result in a useful publication, even if changes to the manuscript are made. Flawed methodology is a reason to recommend rejection of the manuscript, because simple fixes are not enough to make up for methodologic deficits; it is likely that the study will need to be repeated using appropriate methodology and resubmitted at a later date. Reporting criteria, such as the CONSORT or PRISMA statements, are useful references when assessing the methodology and reporting of results.[5]

Specific Questions for the Reviewer to Consider

Having a list of questions to refer to can be very helpful when reviewing a manuscript. Table 10-2 provides some examples of questions to consider during peer review. Additional examples are available in Appendices 4-1 and 5-1.

THINGS TO AVOID WHEN REVIEWING AN ARTICLE

● One of the most common errors of peer reviewers is excessive focus on grammar and style.[6] Unless specifically requested by the editor, peer review does not include editing or proofreading. The peer reviewer should generally avoid editing for grammar, punctuation, or spelling unless these aspects of the manuscript significantly impact the meaning and comprehension of the manuscript. This allows the reviewer to focus on other aspects of the manuscript. If the grammatical aspects of the manuscript greatly interfere with the readability or understanding of the manuscript, this should be brought to the attention of the author and editor.[2,6,32]

The reviewer should also avoid recommending changes to the manuscript based purely upon personal preference.[30] It is very rare to review a manuscript that is worded exactly how the reviewer would have worded it if the roles of author and reviewer were reversed. In this sense, the reviewer must take the rather subjective assignment of peer

TABLE 10–2. SAMPLE QUESTIONS TO CONSIDER WHEN REVIEWING A MANUSCRIPT[4,6,32,33]

- Is the title succinct and descriptive of the actual manuscript?
- Does the abstract follow conventions of the journal and reflect the content of the full manuscript?
- Is the rationale clearly stated?
- Does the introduction include a summary of the body of literature up to this point?
- Does the manuscript fill a gap in the current body of literature?
- Are the objectives clearly stated?
- Are the objectives supported and adequately addressed in the body of the manuscript?
- Was institutional review board approval obtained, if applicable?
- Were inclusion and exclusion criteria described?
- Is the methodology equipped to adequately address the objectives?
- Are the methods reproducible?
- Are primary and secondary endpoints defined?
- Are statistical tests used appropriately?
- Are data reported clearly and without errors or inconsistencies?
- Are all patients accounted for in the results?
- Are tables and figures labeled appropriately so that they can stand alone?
- Do included tables and figures supplement and improve the manuscript without repeating unnecessary details?
- Are there things addressed in the text that could more clearly be represented by a table or figure?
- Are the conclusions appropriate based upon the methods and results?
- Are strengths and limitations of the manuscript described?
- Are potential sources of bias addressed?
- Were conflicts of interest addressed?
- Are the bibliographic citations current and pertinent?
- Are there any signs of duplicate publication, plagiarism, or other ethical concerns?
- Are reporting conventions followed (e.g., CONSORT, PRISMA)?

review and make it as objective as possible. If a change to the manuscript would greatly improve objective clarity, then it is worth mentioning, but if the change is only a matter of writing style, it is best left unstated during peer review.

CONSTRUCTING THE REVIEW SUBMISSION

Once the reviewer has thoroughly evaluated the manuscript and documented comprehensive notes on their findings, it is time to submit the review to the editor. In most cases the review will be submitted to the editor electronically through the journal's website or a third-party portal. Formats for the final review vary between different journals. The simplest format consists of three items: a publishing recommendation, comments to the author, and comments to the editor. In place of general comments to the author, some journals have a more guided format for the review, requesting separate comments on each section of the manuscript (e.g., title, abstract, introduction, conclusion) or addressing different qualities of the manuscript (e.g., methodology, place in current body of literature). Other journals pose specific questions for the reviewer to address in the review (e.g., How original is the research described in this manuscript?). The simple format of a publishing recommendation, comments to the author, and comments to the editor will be described in additional detail below.

Making a Publishing Recommendation

In most instances the peer reviewer will be asked to submit an overall publishing recommendation for the manuscript. In a blinded review setting, this recommendation is seen by the editor, but not the author. The reviewer's recommendation will be considered by the editor, but the editor is under no obligation to follow the recommendation. Options for the publishing recommendation vary between journals, but the most basic format includes the following three options: accept, accept with revisions, and reject. Other journals may offer additional options such as accept with minor revisions, accept with major revisions, or reject and resubmit. A recommendation to accept (i.e., publish) a manuscript should be made if the manuscript fills a needed gap in the body of literature and the reviewer's assessment does not identify any deficiencies related to content, methodology, clarity, conclusions, or ethical standards. A manuscript rated as accept may still include some minor revision recommendations in the reviewer's comments, but by marking accept the reviewer suggests to the editor that these changes are recommended, but optional. Reviewers often have a challenge determining whether a manuscript should be rated as accept with revisions or reject. When facing this challenge, the reviewer should consider whether there are any **fatal flaws** in the manuscript, such as inappropriate methodology, that render the results unimportant or unbelievable. Major flaws in the methods of a study cannot be overcome by proper grammar and nice flow, and rejection should be recommended. Regardless of how well-written the manuscript is, a study question based upon erroneous assumptions cannot be fixed through editing and requires restarting the study from the beginning. In contrast, a study with sound methodology but exaggerated conclusions could be corrected and published without repeating the study, and thus could be marked as accept with revisions. Other examples of manuscripts that should be marked for rejection include manuscripts that clearly fall outside of the journal's scope, manuscripts with ethical problems (e.g., lack of consent, plagiarism), manuscripts that do not fill an important role in the body of literature, and manuscripts that are so poorly written that they are incomprehensible.[6]

Comments to the Author

Comments to the author are also visible to the editor. Most of the comments made by the peer reviewer will be submitted in this section. This section will usually be free-text, and the electronic notes created by the reviewer during the three-read approach will provide most of the material. Comments should be orderly so that they are easily followed by the author and editor. Follow any specific format and organization instructions provided by the journal. If the journal does not specify a preferred format for these comments, the reviewer can organize the comments in the way that seems most logical.[6,30,32]

Usually it is best to start the comments to the author with an overall assessment of the document, followed by a section-by-section breakdown of the manuscript. The overall assessment should address the summative impression of the manuscript, its place in the full body of literature, how well it fits within the scope of the journal, and any major methodologic deficiencies or fatal flaws. The overall assessment should support the publishing recommendation, especially if rejection is recommended. The section-by-section assessment will provide feedback on each section of the manuscript (e.g., title, abstract, introduction, methods) in the same order as the manuscript. Many of the notes formulated during the three-read approach can simply be copied and pasted into this section of the review submission, but first they should be proofread for grammar or spelling mistakes, reviewed and edited for clarity, and organized into a sequence appropriate for submission. Use of headings for each section, and a bulleted or numbered list within each section, will help keep the comments organized and make them easier for the author and editor to interpret. When referring to a specific part of the manuscript, include the page, paragraph, and line number to ensure the author and editor know exactly which part of the manuscript is being addressed (e.g., "The last sentence of paragraph 2 on page 4 states...."). The section-by-section assessment should also be supportive of the publishing recommendation, and should include both positive and constructive comments. Comments to the author should be balanced, fair, and objective.[4,6,30,32]

A Word about Tone

8 *When submitting comments to the author, it is important to maintain a constructive and professional tone. Comments should be objective, constructive, and actionable. The reviewer should also seek balance in comments, addressing positive aspects of the manuscript as well as areas for improvement.*[2,4,6,12,30,32] However, the peer reviewer's primary responsibility is to critically evaluate the manuscript, not to praise the author.[30] The nature of the comments should be consistent with the overall recommendation submitted to the editor. A manuscript marked for acceptance will primarily have positive comments with minor critiques or ideas for improvements. In contrast, if rejection is recommended, the comments should include sufficient detail to support that recommendation. Acrimonious, sarcastic, or destructive comments have no place in peer review.[2,4,6,12,30,32]

Comments to the Editor

Comments made to the editor are confidential and not available to the author. Comments to the editor should generally be limited, because the majority of the comments will be addressed to the author, and thus will also be visible to the editor. Comments to the editor should include a short explanation of the reasons for the publication recommendation (e.g., accept, accept with revisions, reject) made by the reviewer. The comments to the editor should also be used to describe any sensitive topics that are important to bring to the editor's attention. For instance, if the reviewer identifies clear examples of plagiarism in the manuscript, this needs to be addressed in the comments to the author as well as the comments to the editor, though the tone and message will be different between the two comments. The comments to the author may state "several of the passages are worded almost identically to the wording in the cited sources, such as lines 3–7 on page 2, the second paragraph on page 3, and the third paragraph on page 5. This will need to be addressed." In contrast, the comments to the editor may state "I am concerned about plagiarism in the manuscript. During my review I identified several passages that are almost identical to the source documents (see Comments to Author), and I fear that there may be others that I did not have time to detect." Both of these comments address the concern of plagiarism, but are tailored for their respective audiences.[6,30,32]

If the reviewer is not able to evaluate a specific part of the manuscript due to lack of expertise, this should also be addressed in the comments to the editor.[4,12] An example of this could be unfamiliarity with the statistical methods described. Ideally any lack of expertise was already brought to the attention of the editor either prior to accepting the peer review invitation or after the first reading of the manuscript.[2] Even if a lack of expertise was already pointed out, the comments to the editor is a fitting place to remind the editor of this potential gap in the review. Lastly, if a learner or colleague helped with the review, their name and affiliation should be included in this section (see the "Involving Learners in Peer Review" section).[2,30,32]

THE IMPORTANCE OF CONFIDENTIALITY

During peer review, the reviewer will have access to prepublication manuscripts and data. These materials remain the property of the author and must be treated with confidentiality. The reviewer should never disclose the content of the manuscript or any details about it. The author must also avoid using any information from the prepublication manuscript to further their own personal publications. If a peer reviewer wishes to involve a colleague or a learner on a review, permission should be secured from the editor prior to sharing the manuscript. Upon completing the review submission, the peer reviewer must destroy all print and electronic copies of the prepublication manuscript.[3]

Involving Learners in Peer Review

Students of the health sciences quickly learn to refer to respected journals as peer-reviewed journals, but often lack a full understanding of the peer review process or even the definition of peer review. As noted earlier, there is usually no formal training for health care professionals on developing the peer review skills. Involving learners in the peer review process early can help them develop skills that they might otherwise never obtain.[4,5] ❾ *Many skilled practitioners with exceptional literature evaluation skills never participate in peer review because they lack an understanding of the process and fear that they are inadequate to participate in the process.* Today's learners represent the future of peer review, and their development as reviewers is essential to sustaining this process in years to come.[2] Peer review offers learners the opportunity to apply many of the skills they obtain during their education in a real-world setting that offers the opportunity to use their skills to provide a valuable contribution to the body of published literature. Involving learners not only benefits the learners themselves, but often results in a more robust review because the review is a product of multiple perspectives rather than just one. Just as there is no single "right way" to review an article submission, there is no single way to involve learners in this process. This section will outline a process that can be molded to the preferences and situations of a specific mentor and learner.

OBTAINING PERMISSION FROM THE EDITOR

Because of the confidential nature of peer review assignments, the first step in involving a learner in the process should always be to obtain permission from the editor.[6] Most editors are happy to allow learners to participate in the process, because they recognize learners as a resource for future reviewers.[2] Still, it is important to always request this permission to avoid a breach of confidentiality.[4] Some editors may request that learners sign agreements similar to those signed by the peer reviewer, while others may just indicate that their approval.

FIRST MEETING WITH THE LEARNER

The first meeting between the mentor and the learner will be used to provide an overview of the peer review process, establish ground rules and expectations, and provide the learner with a copy of the manuscript. Providing the learner with information about the peer review process will help the learner understand why peer review is important and help them visualize their role in this process. This chapter and other resources (see "Suggested Readings") can be used to help the learner gain this necessary foundation. The learner should be provided with reading materials that they can look at after this meeting to expand their understanding of this process. These materials are indispensable for the learner, and they will provide a detailed listing of important things that the learner should look for or consider when performing the review of the article. Before providing the learner with a copy of the manuscript, it is important to discuss the need for confidentiality as it applies to this process.[4] Upon addressing the role of peer review and the need for confidentiality, the learner can be provided with a copy of the manuscript.

During this first meeting it is also important to discuss the specific reviewer instructions provided by the journal and provide the learner with a copy of these instructions to refer back to during their actual review. The reviewer and learner should examine the submission form for the journal, which will help them understand the format of the final review. For instance, does the journal provide the opportunity to provide confidential comments to the editor, or just comments that are shared between the editor and author. The publishing recommendation field is also important to identify (e.g., accept, accept with revisions, reject), so that both parties can carefully consider the recommendation they will need to provide to summarize their publishing recommendation for the manuscript.

In addition to the expectations of the journal, the mentor should also address their personal expectations of the learner. For instance, is the learner expected to provide electronic notes or will written notes suffice? To make the submission process as easy as possible for the mentor, electronic notes created in word processing software will generally be the most efficient format, allowing the mentor to pool the comments of the learner and the reviewer together for final submission. Providing the learner with sample notes from prior reviews performed by the mentor can greatly aid the learner in understanding the amount and type of comments that are typical for a review. Help the learner to understand the amount of time that should be dedicated to perform a review—this will help avoid a situation where the learner dedicates insufficient time to construct a comprehensive review, or on the other extreme dedicates numerous hours to a review. An experienced reviewer should plan to spend at least 3 hours reviewing a manuscript; the first-time reviewer should probably plan to spend more than that.[6,28-30]

Lastly, the mentor should establish a date for the second meeting so that both parties have a deadline for completion of the review. Ideally, this second meeting should take place a few days before the review is due to the editor, allowing the mentor time to synthesize the two reviews prior to submission.

SECOND MEETING WITH THE LEARNER

The second meeting with the learner is an opportunity to compare notes and share observations. As the mentor, avoid starting this session by lecturing and instructing the learner on the things that they should have noticed about the article. Instead, allow the learner to guide the initial discussion in this session. Start the session by encouraging the learner to share their overall observations about the manuscript, their initial thoughts on a publishing recommendation for the manuscript, and what they learned through this process. Often, the learner's comments and observations will differ from those of the mentor. This is part of the beauty of this process. Reassure the learner that even if two experienced reviewers participated in this process together, their observations would likely be quite different. Neither one is wrong—different people will notice different things, and combining the observations of two reviewers will result in a more comprehensive and useful review. Indeed, this is one reason that most journals engage multiple reviewers to examine a single manuscript prior to making a publishing decision.[2,16] As the learner shares their thoughts and observations, encourage them by emphasizing their accurate observations and constructively discuss any observations that may be misguided. Compare the overall observations and recommendation of the learner with those of the those of the mentor. The learner often takes great satisfaction in learning that they made important observations that the mentor may have missed.

After discussing major observations, the learner and mentor can systematically move through the manuscript, discussing specific observations for the different sections of the manuscript (e.g., title, abstract, methods). After a thorough discussion of the manuscript, the mentor and learner can circle back to the publishing recommendation to see if their discussion has altered their feelings about the publishing recommendation. Often, the learner's initial recommendations may lean toward a more favorable publishing recommendation, but with additional discussion, it may become apparent that the best recommendation is to reject the manuscript. Learners may be quite hesitant to make a recommendation to reject a manuscript initially. Discussing publications rates for the specific journal may help the learner feel more comfortable making a recommendation to reject. For instance, knowing that a journal only publishes about 20% of manuscript submissions can help the learner understand that not all manuscript submissions can receive a recommendation for publication. Once the mentor and learner have come to a consensus on their recommendation for the article, most of the hard work is done. If the learner has created an electronic summary of the manuscript, make sure to get a copy of the document to simplify synthesis of the final review.

The second meeting with the learner is also a good time to provide the learner with feedback on their review. Clear feedback that addresses the insights and oversights of the learner will help the learner develop as a reviewer. This is also a good time to discuss with the learner how to get involved in the process of peer review (see the "Locating Peer Review Opportunities" section). If the learner is near the completion of their training, it may be appropriate to ask the learner if they would like the mentor to refer peer review invitations to them in the future that fit their scope of interest.

FINALIZING THE REVIEW AND PROVIDING FOLLOW-UP

If the learner has provided the mentor with an electronic copy of the review, synthesizing comments should be a quick and easy process. Ultimately, the mentor is the one who is signing off on the review, so the mentor will only want to incorporate comments from the learner with which they agree. Most journals will not notify the reviewer of whether the manuscript will be published or not, but by watching the table of contents for the journal, the reviewer will learn if it was published. Many journals will provide the reviewer with a summary of comments by other peer reviewers. This can be a valuable piece of feedback for the reviewer as well as the learner. By sharing this correspondence with the learner, the learner will have additional examples to refer to from a variety of different perspectives. It will become apparent that some reviewers may not dedicate much time to review, while others may provide comprehensive comments that suggest a very thorough review.

Conclusion

Peer review is a gold standard for biomedical publications. Peer review assists journal editors in deciding which manuscripts to publish and helps improve the quality of manuscripts prior to publication. Although most health care professionals receive no formal training in peer review, resources are available to help obtain the necessary skills and knowledge to participate in peer review. Involving learners in peer review will help them develop skills necessary to contribute to the body of literature and help to sustain the future of peer review.

Self-Assessment Questions

1. Which of the following is *not* a *main purpose* of peer review?
   a. Improve the manuscript prior to publishing.
   b. Assist the editor in determining if a manuscript should be published.
   c. Edit for grammar and spelling errors.
   d. Determine if the manuscript fills a gap in the medical literature.
   e. Critically evaluate the methodology described in the manuscript.

2. Most journals provide formal training for peer reviewers.
   a. True
   b. False

3. When does peer review of a manuscript usually occur?
   a. Before the manuscript is submitted to a journal
   b. After the manuscript is submitted to a journal, but prior to copyediting and publication
   c. After the manuscript has undergone final copyediting but before publication
   d. After publication
   e. None of the above

4. Peer review is considered a gold standard for biomedical publications.
   a. True
   b. False

5. Which of the following is *not* a potential advantage of using an open review format instead of a blinded review format?
   a. Improved transparency
   b. Ease of acknowledging reviewers
   c. Increased accountability of reviewers
   d. Reduced risk of author retaliation following manuscript rejection
   e. All of the above are potential advantages of open review

6. Which of the following is an appropriate reason to participate in peer review?
   a. Professional responsibility
   b. Way of contributing to the medical literature
   c. Professional advancement
   d. All of the above
   e. Only b and c

7. Which of the following is a way to identify a peer review opportunity?
   a. Referral by a colleague
   b. Visit booths for journals at national conferences
   c. Sign up on the journal's website
   d. All of the above are valid options
   e. None of the above are valid options

8. Which of the following should *not* be kept in a peer review resource file?
   a. Review articles about peer review
   b. Your notes from a prior peer review
   c. The manuscript from a prior peer review
   d. Peer review guidelines from a journal you review for
   e. Reporting criteria such as CONSORT or PRISMA

9. Which of the following is a valid reason to decline a peer review invitation?
   a. Lack of time
   b. Lack of expertise
   c. Conflict of interest
   d. Personal relationship with the author
   e. All of the above are valid reasons to decline a peer review invitation

10. Which of the following statements about peer review is correct?
   a. Time spent reviewing a manuscript, up to 3 hours, results in a review of higher quality.
   b. Time spent reviewing a manuscript does not correlate with the quality of the review.
   c. Several sources suggest that completing a high-quality review can require several hours.

    d. Both a and c are correct.

    e. None of the above are correct.

11. If a peer reviewer designates that a manuscript should be rejected, the editor is ethically bound to reject the manuscript.

    a. True

    b. False

12. A publishing recommendation of "reject" is most appropriate in which scenario?

    a. Substantial plagiarism is identified in the manuscript.

    b. The methodology of an experimental trial contains major flaws.

    c. Patients were not consented prior to an experimental trial.

    d. All of the above.

    e. Both a and b.

13. Which of the following is true about submitting written comments during peer review?

    a. Written comments are not necessary as long as a publishing recommendation is made.

    b. It is more important that comments are courteous than that they are true.

    c. Most of the comments should be directed to the author.

    d. Most of the comments should be directed to the editor.

    e. None of the above are true.

14. It is necessary to obtain permission from the editor prior to sharing a manuscript with a student who will assist you on peer review of the manuscript.

    a. True

    b. False

15. Which statement is true about involving learners in peer review?

    a. Most journals are hesitant to allow learners to participate in the process.

    b. Comments and ideas generated by the learner should not be incorporated into the mentor's review submission.

    c. The first meeting with a learner is used to set expectations.

    d. The learner will generally need to dedicate less time to reviewing the manu-script than the mentor.

    e. Learners are often more likely than mentors to recommend rejection for a manuscript.

ACKNOWLEDGMENTS

The author wishes to gratefully acknowledge Rachael Freeman, PharmD, BCPS for her ideas and contributions related to involving learners in the peer review process, which was originally developed as a Pharmacy Grand Rounds presentation at University of Utah Health, Salt Lake City, Utah.

REFERENCES

1. Riley BJ, Jones R. Peer review: acknowledging its value and recognising the reviewers. Br J Gen Pract. 2016;66(653):629-30.
2. Hasegawa GR. An editor's perspective on peer review. Am J Health-Syst Pharm. 2017;74(24):2090-4.
3. International Committee of Medical Journal Editors. Recommendations for the conduct, reporting, editing, and publication of scholarly work in medical journals [Internet]. c2018 [updated 2018 Dec; cited 2019 Sep 4]. Available from: http://www.icmje.org/recommendations/
4. Benos DJ, Kirk KL, Hall JE. How to review a paper. Adv Physiol Educ. 2003;27(2):47-52.
5. Alam S, Patel J. Peer review: tips from field experts for junior reviewers. BMC Med. 2015;13:269.
6. DiDomenico RJ, Baker WL, Haines ST. Improving peer review: what reviewers can do. Am J Health-Syst Pharm. 2017;74(24):2080-4.
7. World Association of Medical Editors. Conflict of interest in peer-reviewed medical journals [Internet]. c2016 [updated 2009 Jul 25; cited 2019 Sep 4]. Available from: http://wame.org/conflict-of-interest-in-peer-reviewed-medical-journals
8. Rajpert-De Meyts E, Losito S, Carrell DT. Rewarding peer-review work: the Publons initiative. Andrology. 2016;4(6):985-6.
9. Berquist TH. Peer review: is the process broken? AJR Am J Roentgenol. 2017;209(1):1-2.
10. Gannon F. The essential role of peer review. EMBO Rep. 2001;2(9):743.
11. Manchikanti L, Kaye AD, Boswell MV, Hirsch JA. Medical journal peer review: process and bias. Pain Physician. 2015;18(1):E1-E14.
12. Kelly J, Sadeghieh T, Adeli K. Peer review in scientific publications: benefits, critiques, & a survival guide. EJIFCC. 2014;25(3):227-43.
13. Haines ST, Baker WL, DiDomenico RJ. Improving peer review: what journals can do. Am J Health-Syst Pharm. 2017;74(24):2086-9.
14. The BMJ. Resources for reviewers [Internet]. c2019 [cited 2019 Sep 4]. Available from: https://www.bmj.com/about-bmj/resources-reviewers
15. Resnik DB, Elmore SA. Ensuring the quality, fairness, and integrity of journal peer review: a possible role of editors. Sci Eng Ethics. 2016;22(1):169-88.
16. Napolitani F, Petrini C, Garattini S. Ethics of reviewing scientific publications. Eur J Intern Med. 2017;40:22-5.
17. Faggion CM Jr. Improving the peer-review process from the perspective of an author and reviewer. Br Dent J. 2016;220(4):167-8.
18. Smith R. Peer review: reform or revolution? BMJ. 1997;315(7111):759-60.
19. BioMed Central. Advancing peer review at BMC [Internet]. c2019 [cited 2019 Oct 10]. Available from: https://www.biomedcentral.com/about/advancing-peer-review

20. Luo L, Rubens FD. Traditional peer review and post-publication peer review. Perfusion. 2016;31(6):443-4.

21. Keating NL, Mohile SG. Increasing engagement in peer review. J Geriatr Oncol. 2019;10(4):526-7.

22. Sage Publishing. Reviewer Rewards [Internet]. c2019 [cited 2019 Sep 4]. Available from: https://us.sagepub.com/en-us/nam/reviewer-rewards

23. Publons [Internet]. [cited 2019 Sep 4]. Available from: https://publons.com/.

24. Hak DJ, Giannoudis P, Mauffrey C. Increasing challenges for an effective peer-review process. Eur J Orthop Surg Traumatol. 2016;26(2):117-8.

25. Schulz KF, Altman DG, Moher D. CONSORT 2010 statement: updated guidelines for reporting parallel group randomized trials. Ann Intern Med. 2010;152(11):726-32.

26. Moher D, Liberati A, Tetzlaff J, Altman DG. Preferred reporting items for systematic reviews and meta-analyses: the PRISMA statement. Ann Intern Med. 2009;151(4):264-9, W264.

27. Pytynia KB. Why participate in peer review as a journal manuscript reviewer: what's in it for you? Otolaryngol Head Neck Surg. 2017;156(6):976-7.

28. Black N, van Rooyen S, Godlee F, Smith R, Evans S. What makes a good reviewer and a good review for a general medical journal? JAMA. 1998;280(3):231-3.

29. Blockeel C, Drakopoulos P, Polyzos NP, Tournaye H, Garcia-Velasco JA. Review the "peer review". Reprod Biomed Online. 2017;35(6):747-9.

30. Hoppin FG Jr. How I review an original scientific article. Am J Respir Crit Care Med. 2002;166(8):1019-23.

31. Janke KK, Bzowyckyj AS, Traynor AP. Editors' perspectives on enhancing manuscript quality and editorial decisions through peer review and reviewer development. Am J Pharm Educ. 2017;81(4):73.

32. Smith DV, Stokes LB, Marx K, Aitken SL. Navigating manuscript assessment: the new practitioner's guide to primary literature peer review. J Oncol Pharm Pract. 2019;25(1):94-100.

33. Zellmer WA. What editors expect of reviewers. Am J Hosp Pharm. 1977;34(8):819.

SUGGESTED READINGS

1. Hasegawa GR. An editor's perspective on peer review. Am J Health-Syst Pharm. 2017;74(24):2090-4.

2. DiDomenico RJ, Baker WL, Haines ST. Improving peer review: what reviewers can do. Am J Health-Syst Pharm. 2017;74(24):2080-4.

3. Hoppin FG Jr. How I review an original scientific article. Am J Respir Crit Care Med. 2002;166(8):1019-23.

4. Smith DV, Stokes LB, Marx K, Aitken SL. Navigating manuscript assessment: the new practitioner's guide to primary literature peer review. J Oncol Pharm Pract. 2019;25(1):94-100.

11

Chapter Eleven

Legal Aspects of Drug Information

Martha M. Rumore

Learning Objectives

● *After completing this chapter, the reader will be able to:*

- Describe the legal issues related to the provision of drug information (DI).
- Apply various legal theories that impose liability on pharmacists providing DI.
- Describe how pharmacists can help protect themselves from malpractice claims resulting from the provision of DI.
- Explain the Doctrine of Drug Overpromotion as it pertains to the 1997 Food and Drug Administration Modernization Act (FDAMA).
- Identify the liability concerns inherent with off-label drug use and informed consent.
- Describe U.S. copyright law as it pertains to the provision of DI.
- Identify copyright, liability, and privacy issues arising from the Internet and Social Media.
- Describe the legal and ethical challenges emerging in telemedicine and cybermedicine.
- Describe the DI plan that addresses the Health Insurance Portability and Accountability Act (HIPAA) of 1996.
- Explain the legal issues involved with industry support for pharmaceutical educational activities.

Key Concepts

❶ Currently, most litigation concerning pharmacists involves negligence.
❷ There are a number of ways in which tort liability can relate to the provision of DI: incomplete information, inappropriate quality information, outdated information, inappropriate analysis, or dissemination of information.

❸ There are at least three key areas of labeling and advertising liability: the learned inter-mediary rule, which is a defense to failure to warn actions; the doctrine of overpromo-tion, under which adequate warning is alleged to have been diluted by communications failing to adequately convey the full impact of the warning; and promotion of off-label use or Food and Drug Administration (FDA) unapproved indications.

❹ DI is currently being obtained from a number of Internet/social media and mobile apps and there is the possibility of DI liability for information obtained from these sources.

❺ Pharmacists providing DI must have a working knowledge of copyright law both to avoid liability and to protect their own literary works.

❻ HIPAA Privacy Rule is not intended to disrupt or discourage adverse event reporting or DI in any way.

❼ The FDA, the American Council for Continuing Medical Education (ACCME), and the Pharmaceutical Research and Manufacturers of America (PhRMA) have established educational policies, guidelines, or guidances, which allow communication between industry and the continuing medical education (CME) providers.

Introduction

An understanding of the legal aspects of drug information (DI) can help a practitioner in day-to-day practice, as well as provide some possible ways to protect himself or herself in the legal system. This chapter is intended to examine legal issues and should not be considered legal advice.

There are a myriad of legal issues confronting the various facets of DI. These legal issues cross over a number of traditional legal specialties, including computer law, adver-tising law, privacy law, intellectual property law, telecommunications law, and tort law. This chapter provides an overview and discussion of the key legal issues involving intel-lectual property rights, **torts**, privacy, and advertising and promotion that may arise in the provision of DI.

Decades after the genesis of drug information services, the legal duties of pharma-cists providing DI are still evolving. Today, most pharmacy curriculums, board certifica-tions, and postgraduate year one (PGY1) residencies include DI, realizing that whether a student specializes in DI or not, it is an integral part of pharmacist-supervised patient care. Pharmacists can and will be held liable for their conduct relating to DI. This chapter begins with an examination of the expanded liability of the DI specialist, which is defined as those pharmacists who either work in DI centers or who spend the majority of their working day providing DI (e.g., clinical managers, drug information specialists, and PGY1 and postgraduate year two [PGY2] residents). The liability inherent in the provisions of DI to patients as an integral component of pharmacist-supervised patient care will be covered as will recommendations for prevention and mitigation of liability. The chapter then explores copyright, privacy, legal issues pertaining to Internet/social media, direct-to-consumer-advertising, **off-label** use, as well as industry support for educational activities.

Tort Law

Pharmacists' functions such as online searching, monitoring or recommending drug therapy, preparing drug alerts and pharmacy bulletins, participating in pharmacy and therapeutics (P&T) committees, conducting medication use evaluations (MUE), writing and revising medication policies, training residents, pharmacy students, and pharmacy staff, and identifying adverse drug events entail legal obligations of proper performance.

Minimal practice standards for clinicians have been put forth to delineate functions and activities that may be considered essential to the provision of DI services. Position papers and standards of the American Society of Health-System Pharmacists (ASHP) and The Joint Commission (TJC), as well as Accreditation Council for Pharmacy Education (ACPE) curriculum standards, and literature regarding appropriate management of DI requests remove any doubt about the level of expertise needed.[1-3] Minimal standards of performance and a consistent level of competence must be assured by clinicians promoting or offering DI regardless of the practice site. Although there are no standards to accredit DI centers, professional standards of performance may be used by courts as an objective measuring tool for the standard of care.

The pharmacy profession is assuming an increased legal responsibility to provide DI in accordance with the Pharmacist's Patient Care Process adopted by the Joint Commission of Pharmacy Practitioners.[4] The physician has been considered the learned intermediary responsible for communicating the manufacturer's warnings to the patient. However, cases in which pharmacists failed to counsel or warn patients are showing a trend in pharmacist liability.[5] Although most cases still maintain that the pharmacist has no duty to warn, a minority of cases in various jurisdictions demonstrate that the pharmacist's duty to warn of foreseeable complications of drug therapy is becoming a recognized part of the expanded legal responsibility of pharmacists. Courts have been more willing to apply a duty to warn where the pharmacist voluntarily assumes the duty, or has special knowledge about a patient, or the prescription is dangerous as written.[6]

Where the patient is at higher risk than the general population, the courts have uniformly found liability. Today, pharmacists providing DI may be more likely to be held to the same standards as physicians when determining standard of care.

❶ *Currently, most litigation concerning pharmacists involves negligence.* Traditionally, physicians remain responsible for their patients and must exert **due care**; that is, a physician who knows or should have known that the information provided was improper may be held liable for negligence. Therefore, it is safe to assume that a legal cause of action pertaining to the provision of DI will be founded on the theory of negligence as the direct or **proximate cause** of personal injury or death. Malpractice liability based on negligence refers to failure to exercise the degree of care that a prudent (reasonable) person would exercise under the same circumstances. Elements of negligence include the four Ds: (1) duty breached, (2) damages, (3) direct causation, and (4) defenses absent. To establish a negligent failure, actual conduct must be compared with what is considered standard professional conduct. Typically, this is accomplished by introducing evidence of the relevant professional standards or testimony from expert witnesses such as college of pharmacy faculty or other DI practitioners. Once the duty of care is established, the plaintiff would need a preponderance of evidence to prove that: (1) the information provided was materially deficient, (2) the deficient information was a proximate cause of injury suffered (or at least a substantial contributing factor), (3) the recipient reasonably relied on the information provided, (4) the information deficiency was due to failure to exercise reasonable care, and (5) the pharmacist knew or should have known that the safety or health of another may have depended on the accuracy of the information provided.

Expanding on the first element of negligence, duty breached, it is important to be aware of the fact that the duty must be a legal duty, not a moral or ethical duty. Although there are many ethical dilemmas pertaining to the provision of DI by pharmacists and they can sometimes give rise to a cause of action, an ethical breach is not necessarily a legal breach. Similarly, conduct that is considered unprofessional in the broad sense (e.g., rudeness) is distinct from legal duty.

In a study of DI requests, those from consumers rather than health professionals raised more ethical issues.[7] For example, should a pharmacist respond to a drug identification request for someone else's medication? Is the situation different if the medication is a drug of abuse and the inquiry is from a parent, relative, teacher, or police officer? Current law provides little guidance for disclosure of DI for questionable purposes; therefore, pharmacists must exercise independent professional judgment and assume legal responsibility for that judgment when exercised.

Case Study 11–1

The anticoagulation pharmacist receives an order for enoxaparin in a patient who is receiving warfarin. The patient's current INR is 5.2. The anticoagulation pharmacist is a board certified ambulatory care pharmacist (BCACP). The pharmacist dispenses the enoxaparin and the patient is harmed.

- *What factors favor finding the pharmacist liable for negligence?*
- *Is the prescription dangerous as written?*
- *Is the specialist more liable than the generalist?*
- *Who may be liable in this situation—the pharmacist, the physician, or the clinic?*

Suppose a patient develops a reaction that is believed to be caused by a drug, and the pharmacist is consulted to find any case reports of this drug causing the reaction. If the case is available online, but not in print, and the pharmacist had access to online databases, but did not consult them, was the pharmacist required to do so? Did the pharmacist exert reasonable care? Reasonable care (i.e., that which is considered acceptable and responsible) is the standard applied for negligence. What if the pharmacist searched MEDLINE® but not Embase® databases, or vice versa, and thereby failed to retrieve the case? Should the pharmacist have searched both? There are no clear answers here. Who can say what a reasonable search might have been on a given day? However, using outdated references would more likely constitute an inadequate search. In a German case, a court held a business and patent information service to be responsible for not having used updated materials.[8]

In a highly publicized case involving a clinical trial being conducted at Johns Hopkins University, a researcher conduced an incomplete PubMed® search only back to 1966 regarding lung damage from hexamethonium.[9] Although articles published in the 1950s and other sources such as TOXLINE® and IBM Micromedex® warned of such dangers, the researcher had not consulted these references resulting in a patient's death.

Cases against pharmacists have held that pharmacists who gain information about the unique susceptibility of a patient are liable for failure to warn of the risks. In Dooley v. Everett, the court held the pharmacist liable for failing to warn a patient of the interaction of theophylline with erythromycin that produced seizures and consequent brain damage.[10] Similarly, in Hand v. Krakowski, the pharmacist failed to alert either the patient or physician of the drug interaction between the patient's psychotropic drug and alcohol.[11] The fact that the medication profile indicated that the patient was an alcoholic created a foreseeable risk of injury and, therefore, a duty to warn on the part of the pharmacist.

Recently, this liability applied to DI advice the pharmacist provided on a nonprescription (over-the-counter [OTC]) product. Pharmacists can be sued for malpractice and negligence for inaccurate advice (requires affirmative misrepresentations) regarding OTC drugs that harms the patient. In Whiting v. Rite Aid Pharmacy,[12] the decedent's estate sued the pharmacist for a recommendation that the patient could safely take phenylpropanolamine and pseudoephedrine. The plaintiff contended that she informed the pharmacist of the decedent's prostate problems. The pharmacist denied the conversation occurred. The plaintiff asserted that the use of the drug exacerbated the patient's prostate condition, resulting in several surgeries, and ultimately, his death several years later. The pharmacy contended that **learned intermediary doctrine** protects pharmacists from such liability and the pharmacists' duty of care does not require giving adequate advice about OTC drugs. The court ruled the learned intermediary doctrine only applies to prescription drugs. Additionally, the court was clear in stating:

> 'Pharmacists in Utah clearly have duties regarding nonprescription drugs. If a pharmacist answers a customer's question and offers advice about nonprescription drugs, the pharmacist must advise and act in a non-negligent manner consistent with a reasonably prudent pharmacist's response to a customer's question about the safety of a nonprescription drug.'

Case Study 11–2

The health system pharmacist receives a prescription order for metformin 500 mg twice daily for a 55-year-old male patient who has severe renal impairment. The pharmacist dispenses the drug without checking the patient's renal function in the computer. The pharmacy department medication use manual policy for metformin requires the pharmacist to check and document the patient's creatinine clearance prior to dispensing metformin.

- *If the patient is harmed, did the pharmacist fall below the standard of care? Could the pharmacist be judged negligent?*

In Baker v. Arbor Drugs, Inc., the court ruled that by advertising its drug interaction software, the defendant pharmacy voluntarily assumed a duty to use its computer technology with due care. The pharmacy technician had overridden the drug interaction between tranylcypromine (Parnate®) and clemastine fumarate/phenylpropanolamine hydrochloride (Tavist-D®) that the system detected from the patient's medication profile. The patient committed suicide after suffering a stroke from the combination.[13] In another case, the pharmacist chose to override the computer alert regarding an interaction between tramadol and methadone, resulting in the patient's death. A 6-million-dollar verdict was returned against the pharmacy for failure to warn.[14]

❷ *There are a number of ways in which* **tort liability** *can relate to the provision of DI: incomplete information, inappropriate quality information, outdated information, inappropriate analysis or dissemination of information.*

INCOMPLETE DRUG INFORMATION

Is the pharmacist liable when the DI provided is incomplete? Should the pharmacist provide all the medication information via a DI sheet or patient package insert (PPI)? There have been several cases against pharmacists for failure to dispense mandatory PPIs for certain drugs that later caused harm. In Parkas v. Saary, the court addressed the issue of whether the pharmacist's failure to dispense the FDA-mandated PPI for progesterone was the proximate cause of a congenital eye defect that occurred.[15] Because congenital defects, but not eye deformities, were specified in the PPI, failure to provide the PPI could not be proven to be the proximate cause. Therefore, judgment was in favor of the pharmacy. In Frye v. Medicare-Glaser Corporation, the pharmacist counseled the patient regarding drowsiness with butalbital/aspirin/caffeine (Fiorinal®), but failed to provide a warning not to consume alcohol. The patient died presumably as a result of combining the drug with beer. Here, the DI provided was incomplete. The trial court did not find the pharmacist had a duty to warn.[16] The Omnibus Budget Reconciliation Act of 1990 contains mandatory patient counseling provisions. Although this case was decided before OBRA '90, the court's decision would probably not have changed as a result.

In a number of cases where the plaintiffs asserted that the pharmacist breached a duty to warn as required under OBRA '90, the courts have held that OBRA does not create an independent or private cause of action.[17–19] However, although only state Medicaid programs can violate OBRA '90, the state pharmacy laws promulgated under the OBRA '90 mandate may create a duty with regard to prospective drug utilization review (DUR) requirements.[17]

Other cases have found that pharmacists have a responsibility for patient counseling and drug therapy monitoring.[20] In Sanderson v. Eckerd Corporation, where the pharmacy advertised that its computer system would detect drug interactions or warn patients about adverse drug reactions, pharmacists were held liable when they failed to detect and warn the patient of a potential adverse reaction.[21] In Horner v. Spalitto, the court imposed a duty on a pharmacist to alert the prescriber when the dose prescribed is outside the therapeutic range.[22] In Happel v. Wal-Mart Stores, the pharmacy's computer system was overridden, and the pharmacist failed to warn a patient allergic to aspirin and ibuprofen of the potential for cross-allergenicity with ketorolac.[23] The court found a duty to warn when a contraindicated drug is prescribed. In Morgan v. Wal-Mart Stores, where the plaintiffs alleged that the pharmacist's failure to properly warn of the known dangers of desipramine was the proximate cause of the patient's death, the court held pharmacists have a duty beyond accurately filling a prescription "based on known contraindications, which would alert a reasonably prudent pharmacist to a potential problem."[24] However, the court did not find for the plaintiff opining that pharmacists do not have knowledge that desipramine may cause hypereosinophilic syndrome. Liability could also attach where there is a Risk Evaluation and Mitigation Strategy (REMS) requirement where either a pharmacist is required to provide a Medication Guide or where patient consent is required or for failure to adhere to some other component of the REMS program, such as patient or provider enrollment. In a recent case involving tardive dyskinesia from metoclopramide, the patient did receive a Medication Guide from the pharmacist. However, the pharmacy was sued for not providing verbal drug information about the risks. The learned intermediary doctrine resulted in a finding of no liability.[25] In two other recent cases, plaintiffs' claims of failure to provide a Medication Guide were not successful under learned intermediary and preemption defenses.[26,27]

Clearly, these cases demonstrate an expansion of pharmacist's duties from the nondiscretionary standard of technical accuracy to a discretionary standard that requires pharmacists to perform professional functions—that is, from a technical model to a pharmacist-supervised patient care model. Knowledge of, or access to, DI is becoming an important factor that courts consider in determination of the pharmacist's duty to warn.

In a case of first impression, a court decided whether a hospital pharmacist contacting a physician regarding a colchicine dosage had a duty of care to the physician to provide complete DI.[28] While the pharmacist advised regarding a correct oral dosage, he did not advise of the correct dose in a renally impaired patient. The plaintiff alleged that the hospital pharmacy's voluntary undertaking to provide DI, and the pharmacist's voluntary intervening between the patient and physician created a duty on the part of the pharmacist to the physician. This is different from other duty to warn cases where the plaintiff alleges the pharmacist has a duty to warn the patient. In this case, the plaintiff alleged the hospital's pharmacy voluntarily undertook to be a DI resource and the hospital pharmacist voluntarily intervened between the patient and physician, thereby creating a duty to the physician. The court, however, rejected the argument that a voluntary undertaking of a duty to a physician was created based on a pharmacist's interaction with the patient's physician. The court further held that the learned intermediary doctrine forecloses any duty of care on the part of the pharmacist to the patient, based on the pharmacist's statements to the physician. Significantly, the court commented that even if such a duty were placed on the pharmacist, the duty was not breached inasmuch as the pharmacist correctly followed the hospital's intervention policy.

In another recent case involving the pharmacist's duty to warn the prescriber, the patient received long-term intravenous gentamicin and vancomycin for osteomyelitis. The home infusion pharmacist suggested to the physician that the patient's serum creatinine be monitored. However, the pharmacist did not insist when the physician failed to do so and did not refuse to dispense the antibiotics. The patient developed vestibulopathy and there was a judgment against the pharmacist.[29]

While pharmacists are in a position to provide DI, providing the patient with all information may have a detrimental effect. In fact, it is the FDA's position that the information contained in professional labeling can be safely used only under the supervision of the licensed prescriber. It has, therefore, been the practice not to provide the patient with the professional labeling unless the patient specifically requests it. With regard to the duty to disclose to the patient low percentage risks, court rulings are inconsistent. One court allowed **strict liability** against a pharmacy. In Heredia v. Johnson, the pharmacist dispensed an otic solution without warning of the risk of tympanic membrane rupture and the need to discontinue the drug if certain symptoms appeared. The plaintiff claimed that because of the lack of warning he suffered from severe and permanent injury, including brain damage.[30] However, in Marchione v. State, a prison inmate alleged lack of informed consent based on failure of the prison physician to inform him about adverse effects of prazosin (Minipress®), which caused permanent impotence. The physician argued his duty was only to warn of severe or frequent adverse effects. The Marchione court concluded the physician need not disclose a laundry list of 31 remote adverse effects. The adverse effect had a reported incidence of only two or three cases out of several million prescriptions and was, therefore, rare. The plaintiff also did not have any unique risk factors that would increase the likelihood of the reaction occurring.[31] The courts seem to look at risk factors unique to the patient in deciding whether the health professional is required to indicate the likelihood of occurrence of the risks.

Hall and Honey[32] divided the risks associated with a particular drug into two groups: inherent or noninherent. Inherent risks are unavoidable, unique to the drug, and usually identified in the package insert (PI), but do not include probable or common adverse effects. However well a drug is researched, manufactured, and prescribed, it still may have the ability to produce certain adverse effects. Examples of inherent drug risks are stroke from oral contraceptives or teeth discoloration from tetracyclines. Noninherent risks are created by the particular drug in combination with some extrinsic factor about which the pharmacist should reasonably know, and include maximum safe dosages, interactions, patient characteristics influencing pharmacokinetics, and probable or common adverse effects. An example of noninherent risks would be nephrotoxicity from aminoglycosides in patients with renal impairment. The responsibility of the pharmacist to provide DI about noninherent risks is expanding.

What liability does the pharmacist incur for DI outside of the PI? Physicians may prescribe drugs as they see fit, without adhering to the specific therapeutic indications or dosing guidelines within the labeling. The FDA regulates the manufacture and promotion of drugs, not the practice of medicine. However, it has been held that a physician's deviation from the PI was **prima facie** (i.e., not requiring further support to establish validity, on its face value) evidence of negligence if the patient's injury resulted from the failure to adhere to the recommendations.[33] However, the states appear to be split on whether recommendations in a PI are prima facie evidence of the standard of care. It would be prudent for clinicians to consult the PI when responding to DI inquiries and include such information in the response, especially if the response contradicts what is in the PI.

A disciplinary action by a state pharmacy board highlights the importance of checking the PI or literature concerning the proposed use of a product. In re Michael A. Gabert,[34] a pharmacist received a prescription for 5% silver nitrate for bladder instillation. The pharmacist contacted a DI center and was told there was no literature supporting the proposed use. The pharmacist then requested evidence from the prescriber for such use and was referred to a published Mayo Clinic newsletter. The pharmacist did not seek or obtain a copy of the publication for the pharmacy records. Significant patient harm resulted when the solution was instilled into the patient's bladder. The Mayo Clinic newsletter pertained to silver argyrol, not silver nitrate.

INAPPROPRIATE QUALITY DRUG INFORMATION

It has long been recognized by law that false information provided to another could result in harm to the recipient if the recipient acted relying on the false information. Although **negligent misrepresentation** has not been applied to DI, there is no guarantee that it will not in the future.[35] The relevant law is the Restatement (Second) of Torts, §311, Negligent Misrepresentation Involving Risk of Physical Harm, which states:

> One who negligently gives false information to another is subject to liability for physical harm caused by action taken by the other in reasonable reliance upon such information[...] Such negligence may consist of failure to exercise reasonable care in ascertaining accuracy of the information, or in the manner in which it is communicated.[36]

Thus, the DI itself may be faulty for one or more reasons: it may be dated; it may simply be wrong; it may be incomplete and, therefore, misleading; or none may have been provided because of an incomplete search or incompetent searcher. Information negligence may occur because of: (1) **parameter negligence** (failure to consult the correct source) or (2) **omission negligence** (consulting the correct source, but failure to locate the correct answer[s]). A 1994 study evaluated the accuracy of a drug identification response by 56 DI centers. Approximately 30% correctly identified the investigational drug product; 67% could not make the identification; most importantly, 3.6% (two DI centers) made an incorrect identification. The study found inconsistencies in responses of DI centers.[37] Another study evaluated the quality of DI responses provided by 116 DI centers to multiple queries. The correct response rates varied from 5% for a question pertaining to erythromycin for diabetic gastroparesis to 90% for a drug interaction question pertaining to didanosine-dapsone. For each of three patient-specific questions, the percentages of centers eliciting vital patient data were 5%, 27%, and 86%. The findings suggest that many DI centers continue to fail to elicit patient-specific information necessary for informed responses and focus instead on procedural and technical matters.[38]

Quality issues also exist in references. As an example, despite the peer-review process, the structure of bilirubin was found to be incorrect in an article and the three leading biochemistry textbooks in the United States.[39]

DI of inappropriate quality is not limited to the print media. Several studies have evaluated the use of mobile device apps, such as Epocrates®, Medscape, Lexicomp®, Skyscape®, and MIMS for providing DI.[40] A recent quality assessment study of the top 100 apps in medical categories revealed deficiencies in appropriateness, reliability, usability, and privacy. For DI apps, most did not allow for product identification and did not provide supporting references for the DI. Apps with a drug interaction checker had only a ~67% overall quality rating, which the authors of the studies conclude may be providing unreliable DI to clinicians. Additionally, differences in functionality were found when using different platforms, such as Apple or Android versions.[41] Another quality study of 270 drug summaries in five online compendia found a median of 782 errors with the greatest number occurring with dosage and administration, patient education, and warnings and precautions. A majority were classified as incomplete, followed by inaccurate and omitted.[42]

Mobile device apps do not undergo any quality assessment and DI apps are no exception. FDA only regulates medical apps that are defined as medical devices where functionality could pose a risk to patient safety if they do not function as intended (e.g., smart phone app to evaluate electrocardiogram data).[43] The FDA has explicitly stated that it will exercise enforcement discretion for all other **mobile apps** including DI apps.

Inappropriate quality information may be the result of ghostwriting or publication marketing. Ghostwriting occurs when a pharmaceutical company develops the concept for an article to counteract criticism of a drug or embellish its benefits, hires a professional writing company to draft the article, retains a health professional to sign off as the author, and finds a publisher to unwittingly publish the work. In a recent product liability case, the court ordered the pharmaceutical company to disclose its documents pertaining to its ghostwriting practices.[44] In some instances, posters and meeting abstracts may actually be generated by pharmaceutical industry or incomplete and lacking in peer review. For example, the reader has no way of knowing whether the abstract results are reflective of the entire study population or merely a small subset.

Can pharmacists providing DI be held responsible for retrieving information that is itself inaccurate? What responsibility does the information producer incur for errors in information sources? An unskilled searcher or one with insufficient searching knowledge may not find correct or complete information, which can lead to the wrong answer. The fault can lie anywhere in the information dissemination chain, publication, collection, storage, retrieval, dissemination, or utilization. Errors are often encountered in DI databases.[45] DI pharmacists are constantly finding errors and reporting the errors to the vendor or publisher. For example, when completing a class review of potential probiotic agents for the drug formulary, it was noted that only capsules were listed for one product, although the product was available as a liquid and granules. Although very few cases have been brought before courts concerning the liability of print or online information sources, there is some case law to guide under the theory of strict liability.

Strict liability applies where a defective product proximately causes physical harm. Where the service rendered is deemed to be a professional service, the courts exhibit a reluctance to impose strict liability. With exceptions, persons physically injured because of their reliance on defective and unreasonably dangerous information have only negligence as a cause of action, and only against the author, not the publisher[46]; only if the publisher is negligent or offers intentionally misleading information, could it be held liable. This was tested in Jones v. J.B. Lippincott Co., where a nursing student was injured after consulting and relying on a nursing textbook that recommended hydrogen peroxide enemas for the treatment of constipation. The courts rejected the plaintiff's claim that strict liability should be applied to the publisher.[47] Similarly, in a German case, a misprint in a medical textbook resulted in the injection of 25% rather than 2.5% sodium chloride solution, injuring a patient. Again, the court rejected strict liability for the publisher on the basis that any medically educated person should have noticed the misprint.[48] In Roman v. City of New York, the plaintiff sued for an alleged misstatement in a booklet distributed by a Planned Parenthood organization that resulted in a "wrongful conception." The court found that "a publisher cannot assume liability for all misstatements, said or unsaid, to a potentially unlimited public for a potentially unlimited period."[49] In Winter v. G.R. Putnam's Sons, two people required liver transplants after collecting and eating poisonous wild mushrooms. They relied on an Encyclopedia of Wild Mushrooms in choosing to eat the mushrooms that caused this severe harm.[50] The court refused to hold the publisher liable and found a publisher has no duty to investigate the accuracy of information it publishes.

In Delmuth Development Corp. v. Merck & Co., the plaintiff claimed lost sales because of publication of erroneous information in the Merck Index. The court considered the duty of a publisher to a reader to publish accurate information in a compendium.[51] The court noted a publisher's right to publish without fear of liability is guaranteed by the First Amendment and societal interest. It further held that even if it had a duty to publish with care, the plaintiff could not claim suffered damages because of reliance on this information.

In 2015, an Austrian DI company, Diagnosia Enterprise, was sued by the global pharmaceutical company Sanofi for the way its product and its side effect profile were classified in a drug decision support software app. Sanofi sought an injunction at the time which was denied and Diagnosia refused to change the information regarding the drug. The case has apparently settled.[52] The case does have implications for other DI companies.

What liability is incurred by an author or publisher for publication of product comparisons? Recently, a pharmacy journal publisher and author were sued for defamation by a device manufacturer where the publication compared and opined on the performance of devices for compounding sterile products.[53] The court granted the defendants' motion to dismiss, stating lack of actual malice (a necessary element of defamation). In this ruling, the court protected the First Amendment rights of scientists to report product comparisons and the rights of publishers regarding the peer-review process and publication of such comparisons.[54]

In Libertelli v. Hoffman La Roche, Inc. & Medical Economics Co., the plaintiff became addicted to diazepam (Valium®) and sued the publisher of the Physician's Desk Reference (PDR).[55] The claim was based on the absence of warnings in the PDR regarding the addictive nature of the drug. The court dismissed the case against the publisher. Under a long line of cases, a publisher is not liable for matters of public interest if it has no knowledge of its falsity. Although some effort should be made to verify search results, the pharmacist cannot be held responsible for knowing and verifying the contents of all sources, whether in print or online. However, checking a second reference to verify information is prudent.

In a recent case, the patient developed Stevens-Johnson syndrome from lamotrigine and sued the prescriber, pharmacy chain, publisher, and software company for providing an abbreviated monograph sheet.[56] The software company had switched from a five-page monograph (with no sections for "Before Using This Medication," "Overdose," and "Additional Information") to a full eight-page monograph. To save printing costs, the pharmacy chain requested software customization so that it could continue to use the truncated monograph. The plaintiff claimed that she would not have taken the medication had she seen the redacted information. The publisher won on the basis of California law that it owed no duty to the plaintiff as it is neither a drug manufacturer nor a seller. The software company maintained that the DI monographs were protected by the First Amendment and it could not be held liable for omitting information. The court disagreed and this case is one of the first to hold a software vendor liable where it did not sell the plaintiff anything, did not write the monograph, and gave the pharmacy access to an abbreviated monograph meeting specifications set by the pharmacy itself. Evidence was, however, presented showing that the software company had requested and received a release of liability and an indemnity agreement from the pharmacy chain. Duty was found under the Good Samaritan liability, which holds that a person who undertakes to render services necessary to protect another is subject to liability resulting from failure to exercise reasonable care.[57]

Strict liability would appear applicable to software that is licensed without significant modification as a standard packaged system, as has been found with defective medical computer programs.[58] Clinicians providing DI should be aware of computer-related lawsuits that have arisen involving defects (or bugs) in software that caused erroneous results. These cases result in greater damage awards based on **consequential damages** (i.e., special as opposed to actual) suffered. An example of consequential damages would be damage to a firm's reputation. Perhaps the most widely cited software-related accidents involve malfunctioning computerized radiation machines where overdosages have caused patient deaths.[59] Radiation overdosages from faulty software continue to occur today; grim reminders of the problems faced by reliance on software.[60] In one particularly relevant case, the court held that the National Weather Service was liable for the deaths of four fishermen off Cape Cod, Massachusetts. The Weather Service had forecasted calm weather because of faulty software. Although the verdict was overturned on technical grounds, the U.S. District Court let stand the precedent holding an entity liable for information it provides.[61]

In another case, Jeppesen, an information provider, was held liable for an airplane crash caused by faulty data from the Federal Aviation Administration on flight patterns. A pilot used one of the faulty charts and crashed into a mountain, killing the crew and destroying the plane. The company paid $12 million in damages.[62] The court held the information provider strictly liable because the charts were considered a product. In Jeppesen, the mass production and mass marketing of the charts rendered them a product. Similarly, in Greenmoss Builders v. Dun & Bradstreet, the issue involved the erroneous listing of Greenmoss Builders as a company in bankruptcy in Dun & Bradstreet Business Information Report database. A jury awarded $350,000, including $300,000 in punitive damages. The case was appealed all the way to the Supreme Court, where Dun & Bradstreet lost the case.[63]

In Daniel v. Dow Jones & Co., Inc., where a subscriber brought action against a provider of a computerized database alleging that he relied on a false news report in making investments, the court found that the subscriber did not have a special relationship with the database provider necessary to impose liability for negligent misstatements. First Amendment guarantees of freedom of the press also protected the provider from liability.[64]

As mentioned previously, DI provided may be inaccurate because it is dated, incomplete, or wrong. For example, inappropriate quality information may occur because references are updated differently. Even electronic references are updated differently—some monthly, others weekly. Most DI services require documentation of an answer in at least two different sources. The double-check procedure is common practice when preparing chemotherapy and avoiding drug administration errors. In many of the cases described above, liability could have been prevented by checking the information in more than one reference or source. Thus, checking a DI response in several references is the standard of practice.

INAPPROPRIATE ANALYSIS/DISSEMINATION OF DRUG INFORMATION

Is liability for providing DI a rhetorical supposition or a real possibility? The responsibility of pharmacists providing DI goes beyond that of mere information intermediary, the person between the information producer and the user. Published studies for DI centers have reported that 41% to 83% of requested information is patient specific or judgmental in nature.[65] In addition to liability for the negligent information retrieval and dissemination, the pharmacist's role involves information interpretation, evaluation, and giving advice. This role falls into a consultative model and differs greatly from that of librarians. Librarians are not equipped to give advice. The pharmacist's role as evaluator and interpreter of the information creates a duty sufficient to sustain liability.

The paucity of case law in the area does not negate liability. The issue deserves consideration because of the potential for harm caused by DI provided by pharmacists. There have only been three cases, two cases involving poison information centers, one of which also was a DI center and a third involving the omission to provide DI while on rounds with the medical team. In Reben v. Ely, the plaintiffs filed suit against the DI center for injuries sustained by inadvertent administration of cocaine solution instead of acetaminophen to a 10-year-old patient. The local pharmacy had colored the 10% cocaine solution red and labeled it red solution to thwart abuse. When the nurse realized the mistake, she contacted the Arizona Poison and DI Center. The DI pharmacist described the symptomatology of cocaine overdose, but did not go far enough in recommending that the patient seek emergency care. The patient developed seizures and cardiopulmonary arrest with brain damage that required lifetime nursing care. At the trial, the expert witness testified that the DI center operated below the standard of care. The issue was not erroneous information, but whether the center went far enough in its responsibility in handling the call. The plaintiff was awarded $6.5 million; the DI center was held liable for $3.6 million.[66]

In another case, a lawsuit named a poison information center that was called for assistance when a student died after swallowing a toxic substance during a laboratory experiment. The poison center was named in the $2.5 million suit because it refused to release proof of its claim that the person who called had given the wrong name for the solution that the student drank.[67]

In a more recent case, the court denied the motion to dismiss a case where the pharmacist rounding with a medical team "should have known that the patient was receiving the wrong drug for his condition" and failed to make a recommendation.[68] How this case is decided may expand liability for incomplete DI where the pharmacist has proximity to the patient (e.g., rounds).

From a liability standpoint, there are disadvantages to the formal combination of poison control and DI centers. For example, poison inquiries usually require immediate answers in critical situations without written documentation and sometimes without supporting references.[69,70] The outcomes of poisonings (e.g., overdoses, suicide attempts) are more likely to result in patient morbidity and mortality and require medical backup for acute treatment decisions. Some states (e.g., Arkansas, Oregon, Washington, Arizona, New Jersey) have statutory provisions for joint poison control and DI centers. In several of these states, such as Arkansas, immunity from personal liability in judgment (in contrast to carelessness or inadvertence) would not be actionable as malpractice unless a lack of due care can be shown. However, not all DI centers are protected from liability. Additionally, there have been other lawsuits involving poison control centers, but these have mostly involved medical toxicologists serving as poison control center consultants, not DI pharmacists.[71]

Defenses to Negligence and Malpractice Protection

Even if the plaintiff can establish all the necessary elements of negligence, legal defenses can avoid or reduce liability. Some defenses might include a statute of limitations, comparative or contributory negligence, informed consent, or governmental immunity. It is important to keep in mind that there may be differences in both types of defenses to negligence and insurance coverage for individuals and employers. Further information on defenses will be described in the following sections.

DEFENSES FOR INDIVIDUALS

Assumption of the risk via informed consent and comparative or contributory negligence are defenses to negligence. Under informed consent, the defendant could assert that the patient knowingly assumed the risk for a new or experimental therapy or regimen. However, the risk the patient assumes does not include negligence on the part of the physician or pharmacist. There is no assumption of the risk for negligent behavior.

Comparative negligence is the allocation of responsibility for damages incurred between the plaintiff and defendant, based on the relative negligence of the two. **Concurrent negligence** is the wrongful acts or omissions of two or more persons acting independently, but causing the same injury. Under comparative or concurrent negligence, the pharmacist may also be held liable, either alone or together with the information requestor (e.g., physician and nurse), for inaccurate information or information that does not ensure maximal protection for the patient.

In the landmark case Harbeson v. Parke Davis, a federal court ruled that the doctrine of informed consent required a physician to furnish a patient contemplating pregnancy with information concerning the teratogenicity of the phenytoin she was taking. The physician had a duty to provide information reasonably available in the medical literature, but failed to do so. Even though the physician was not aware of the potential effects of phenytoin, studies were reported in the medical literature.[72] This case represents the only case in which a lack of a literature search resulted in liability.

Cases of **vicarious liability** are not new to medical malpractice. Vicarious liability is the attribution of liability upon one person for the actions of another. Through the doctrine of vicarious liability, a pharmacist could become associated with professional liability actions as part of a case against a hospital or a physician. Physicians have been found negligent for the negligence of nurses, therapists, and others working under their supervision. Significantly, no cases were found where physicians were found negligent from the negligence of pharmacists working under them. If a physician requests DI, he or she would also be held liable if a patient suffers because the search was deficient or the information incorrect. For example, in the Harbeson case, if the physician had requested the pharmacist to search for information about the teratogenicity of phenytoin and no references were found because of a faulty search, the pharmacist would share in the negligence together with the physician. The institution would probably also be named as a party in such legal action.

Delegation of authority does not mean abdication of responsibility. Under vicarious liability, a pharmacist who has not been personally negligent could be held responsible for the negligence of others. Supervision and adequate training of subordinates (e.g., interns, pharmacy technicians, other employees) are essential. Incompetence and substandard training of these individuals can lead to liability. An example might include a breach of confidentiality (e.g., revealing someone has a loathsome disease) by an employee.

From a legal standpoint, does charging a fee increase liability for the DI provider? Fee-based providers would appear to be at greater malpractice risk, especially if the relationship is a contractual one. If any of the contractual expectations are not met, the client has a contractual cause of action against the DI center. The courts will look to the terms of the agreement and the reasonable expectations of the parties. However, where bodily injury results, tort law may impose liability even where the defective information is given gratuitously and the DI provider derives no benefit from giving it.

A decision to comment on a physician's therapeutic recommendations, even if factually correct and in the patient's best interest, may result in a legal liability. Prescribers have brought defamation claims against pharmacies where the pharmacist made statements about the patient's physician who wrote the prescription. When the pharmacist wrote the words "pill mill" on the back of the prescription (libel), the defamation case was dismissed as only the defamed person can bring such a lawsuit.[73] In LeFrock v. Walgreen Co., the court held, however, that the pharmacist did not commit slander (oral defamation) against the physician as the necessary element of malice was missing.[74] In addition, the pharmacist's comments during the consultation were privileged. However, in another case, the judge denied the chain pharmacy's allegation that the pharmacist's comments about the patient's physician were protected by a privilege.[75] Pharmacists have a legal and professional responsibility to detect and resolve problems with drug therapy and screen prescriptions for controlled substances. Meeting that responsibility may involve strong language when consulting with patients. Without removing the fear of civil liability as to anything said during patient counseling, pharmacists can be placed in an untenable position. At least a qualified privilege should apply where the alleged defamatory statements bear some connection to the ordinary course and scope of the pharmacist's practice.

DEFENSES FOR EMPLOYERS

Is the provider the hospital, university, or pharmacy where the DI is provided, or the practitioner providing the DI? The employer-employee relationship is a significant factor under either common law **respondeat superior** doctrine or, alternatively, a theory of negligent hire or supervision. Respondeat superior refers to the proposition that the employer is responsible for the negligent acts of its agents or employees. The injured party may also sue the employer for its negligence in hiring or supervising the employee. Under a negligent hire theory, it must be shown that the employee was unfit for the position and that a reasonable, pre-employment interview or postemployment supervision would have discovered this fact.[76]

Although the person who provides the information is liable for the harm caused by it, the employer may also be held liable in the absence of sovereign or charitable immunity. For pharmacists providing DI employed by the government (e.g., Veteran's Affairs [VA] or Public Health Service [PHS]), there are statutes providing governmental immunity, also called sovereign immunity, from **civil liability**. Such immunity, however, will not protect an intentionally or grossly negligent person.

Even if the lawsuit is nonmeritorious, DI providers affiliated with hospitals or universities represent a deep pocket for contribution to the settlement. With exceptions, suing the practitioner alone would fail to provide a windfall settlement for plaintiffs. The board of directors/trustees of the hospital or university where the DI is provided would be jointly liable. Joint and several liability refers to the sharing of liabilities among a group of people collectively and also individually. If the defendants are jointly and severally liable, it means that the injured party may sue some or all of the defendants together, or each one separately, and may collect equal amounts or unequal amounts from each. In states where joint and several liability applies, the pharmacist provides additional assurance that there will be sufficient assets to recover. The DI provider will be held responsible for the standard of care in the response to DI inquiries and may be found negligent.

PROTECTING AGAINST MALPRACTICE

Methods to protect against lawsuits include contracts covering financial arrangements, adequate documentation, disclaimers, and insurance.[77] For example, a disclaimer can be placed on results of online searches stating that the data being provided are from a source believed to be reliable and factually correct.[78] The best way to avoid omission negligence is to learn from experience, anticipate mistakes that may appear in electronic sources, and keep abreast of changes in DI sources. Even if the delivery of false information is the result of inaccurate information itself, the pharmacist would likely be named as a defendant if the database producer were sued.

Adequate documentation may spell the difference between refuting or not refuting an unfounded claim of malpractice. Such documentation includes responses to inquiries, as well as a record of steps taken in a search. Designing and following procedures to document the research process can help avoid negligence. In Fidelity Leasing Corp. v. Dun & Bradstreet, Inc., the court looked at the operation procedures and adherence to them in the particular instance to determine liability for providing false information.[74]

The key to provision of quality DI is the availability of current, objective information. Procedures should be in place to ensure that data is continually reviewed and updated. Quality assurance (QA) standards for the timeliness, thoroughness, and accuracy of information could also insulate against liability.

Problem areas common to DI regardless of practice site include outdated files and incomplete documentation of responses to requests. With regard to inquiries about adverse reactions, details of the adverse event should be taken and reported to the FDA Adverse Event Reporting System (FAERS). Cases may be clinically urgent and the physician or nurse may have a patient waiting. Response via email, even with alerts attached, is not prudent in such situations as there is no guarantee that the caller is at their desk to receive such emails. All statements made should be traceable to the literature. Additionally, information should be confirmed with other references to ensure consistency between various resources. DI centers should address at least some of the items in Table 11-1.

Insistence on a good educational background for entry-level positions including PGY1 and, ideally PGY2 residencies in DI, followed by the continuing education of DI professionals, certification in online training courses, and good interpersonal communication skills, may also protect against malpractice. Several studies have shown that physicians who were sued frequently had poor interpersonal skills, i.e., patients did not like them.[79] It is also important to keep abreast of changes in sources of DI via regular advanced training, conferences, and reading. All courses in DI should teach situations in ethical conflict that will assist in the decision making and value judgments encountered in the provision of DI.

Under the tort law doctrine of respondeat superior, both the practitioner providing DI and the employer are jointly and severally liable for the damages. This enables the

TABLE 11–1.   QUALITY ASSURANCE AS A LIABILITY-REDUCING FACTOR

- Identify scope of activities and personnel requirements.
- Develop and follow policies and procedures or formal call triaging protocols.
- Keep standard operating procedure manual available for consultation.
- Avoid violations of statutes and regulations.
- Unapproved uses or doses should be well documented and if a use or dose differs from the labeling, the requestor must be so notified.
- Do not recommend a use or dose of a drug based solely on foreign literature or animal studies or questionable resources or references that are not peer reviewed.
- Never extrapolate pediatric or geriatric dosages from usual adult dosages.
- Maintain knowledge of the current literature, new drug applications and supplemental approvals, labeling changes, and new warnings.
- Do not present inadequate data or ignore contrary data.
- Avoid overly enthusiastic or exaggerated efficacy and safety claims.
- Do not attempt to diagnose or treat acute poisoning—direct such inquiries to a poison control center or an emergency room.
- Know the circumstances of the case and appropriate background information (e.g., knowledge of causality assessment scales [e.g., Naranjo Algorithm—see Chapter 19], laboratory findings, concurrent drugs necessary for adverse drug reaction inquiries.
- Exert special care for drug identification questions in view of the growth of counterfeit drugs.
- Responses of new employees, students, residents should be checked—document, document, document. Maintain reasonable response time; if necessary, prioritize requests.
- Obtain peer concurrence or outside professional consultation, if necessary.
- Develop a quality assurance (QA) mechanism to ensure that service is maintained at a high level of quality (e.g., periodic audits or surveys).
- Maintain up-to-date files and reference texts (e.g., paper files should be randomly checked to be sure that they contain articles at least as recent as 2 years old).
- For Internet-specific data-check currency, authorship, publisher, length of time site has existed, site reviews, links to/from other sites, biases/objectiveness, intended audience, quality of the writing, references provided (information without references should receive little weight in clinical decision-making), who maintains the site (owner/sponsor or whether the site has an expert advisory board), affiliations (commercial, organization "org", governmental "gov"), and seal of approval from organizations that review health care sites. (See Chapter 3 for further information regarding evaluating Internet websites.)

plaintiff to have access to the practitioner's personal assets where the employer's assets are not sufficient to cover an adverse judgment. Professional liability insurance provides protection to cover exactly this kind of liability. Consideration should be given to obtaining professional indemnity insurance for the DI practitioner.

Most policies now provide coverage on either an occurrence or claims-made basis. Occurrence means any incident that occurs during the policy period, no matter when the claim is filed, within the applicable statute of limitations. Claims-made policies cover only claims that are filed while the policy is active. To cover claims that are filed after a claims-made policy is terminated, the DI practitioner can purchase tail coverage from the insurer. Tail coverage insures for an incident that occurred while the insurance was in effect but was not filed by the time the insurer-policyholder relationship terminated. It is important to be aware of the limitations and exclusions in these policies, such as some policies no longer covering intravenous compounding. Many do not require the carrier to obtain the consent of the insured before settling a claim. In these policies, the right to protect one's reputation may conflict with the economic interest of the insurer to dispose of the claim as inexpensively as possible. Therefore, it is imperative that individuals obtain insurance coverage policies separate from those of their employers. Most common exclusions are coverage for dishonest, fraudulent, criminal, or malicious acts; property damage; and personal injury coverage. In these cases, the practitioner faces such liability alone, and in certain situations can be ruined financially.

Finally, limiting language in subscriber contracts (i.e., **exculpatory clauses**) may serve to restrict monetary awards in certain circumstances. Such clauses could be included in either contracts for subscribers or signed on acceptance of responses to inquiries. A provision could be included that specifically disclaims any responsibility to a third party who might rely on the information. Written information (e.g., a bulletin) should carry a disclaimer specifying that the DI provided is issued on the understanding that it is the best available from the resources available to the service at a particular time.

An attorney could draft a standard agreement providing that the application of the research by the recipient would not be subject to any implied warranty of fitness for that purpose. However, certain jurisdictions have held that contracts that purport to exculpate a party from negligence will be subjected to strict judicial scrutiny. Courts in certain jurisdictions have declared contracts that attempt to exempt a party's willful or grossly negligent conduct to be void. Further, no exculpatory clause will protect a pharmacist who is grossly or intentionally negligent.

Labeling and Advertising

The FDA defines labeling as written, oral, or electronic information used to supplement or explain a product regardless of whether the information accompanies the product. As such, even literature, textbooks, reprints of articles, scientific seminars may constitute labeling. Labeling requires full disclosure. Advertisements, on the other hand, require a fair balance, meaning there must be a discussion of both benefits and risks, so as not to be misleading, and substantial evidence from clinical trials must be included for comparative claims.[80] The FDA has issued a number of guidance documents pertaining to advertising with regard to Internet/social media platforms (e.g., messages on Twitter [i.e., tweets], individual product pages on social networking sites such as Facebook, blogs, microblogs, online communities, YouTube™, live podcasts, and online web banners).[80–83]

❸ *There are at least three key areas of labeling and advertising liability: the learned intermediary doctrine, which is a defense to failure to warn actions; the doctrine of overpromotion, under which adequate warning is alleged to have been diluted by communications failing to adequately convey the full impact of the warning; and promotion of off-label use or FDA unapproved indications.*

Direct-to-Consumer (DTC) Drug Information

In 1997, the FDA relaxed the standards for Direct-to-Consumer Advertising (DTCA).[84] DTCA involves magazine, television, website, cell phone, and text advertisements, suggesting the use of various prescription drugs for medical conditions the viewer might experience and also suggesting the viewer ask their physician if the medication would be appropriate for them.

Today, prescription drug advertising is a multibillion-dollar industry. Prescription drug advertising is governed by the Food, Drug, and Cosmetic Act (FDCA) and 21 U.S.C. §331, which prohibits the misbranding of a prescription drug.[85] The primary regulation aimed at pharmaceutical product advertising is found at 21 C.F.R. § 202.1 that pertains to all "advertisements in published journals, magazines, other periodicals, newspapers, and other advertisements broadcast through media such as radio, television, and telephone communication systems." These implementing regulations specify that prescription drug advertisements cannot omit material facts, and must present a fair balance between effectiveness and risk information. Further, for print advertisements, the regulations specify that every risk addressed in the product's approved labeling must also be disclosed in the advertisements. The regulations further require that the advertisement contain a summary of "all necessary information related to adverse effects and contraindications" or "provide convenient access to the product's FDA-approved labeling and the risk information it contains." DTCA of off-label uses of prescription drugs is prohibited.[86]

There is evidence that DTCA is becoming more aggressive.[87] The FDA has cited unsubstantiated safety claims and minimization of risk, including "websites that omit or bury important safety information," as areas of particular concern.[88] In some cases, the advertising does not focus on a product but rather on patient education. One company has developed a campaign to bring mental health educational forums to college campuses featuring free screenings for depression. In another case, a 24-hour television network directed to a captive audience (i.e., hospitalized patients) was launched. As federal regulations require patient education, this programming may be used by hospitals for patient education. Other manufacturers offer monetary rewards or gifts (e.g., free exercise video) to patients who visit their physician regarding the product or offer a rebate or sweepstakes opportunity if the patient completes a questionnaire. Manufacturers are also sending out video press releases about drugs that are often aired as news stories. Many advertisements provide an 800 number to encourage consumers to seek additional information about the products; others offer free USB drives or DVDs, brochures, and information packets discussing the product.[89] There also exist DI search tools and apps for use directly by consumers (e.g., PDR.net, http://www.pdr.net).[90]

Another popular DTCA vehicle is blog posts. For example, YouTube™ videos about products from patients are being posted on pharmaceutical company websites without review. Often these patient testimonials go well beyond what a company is permitted to advertise about the product. In general, patient testimonials minimize product risks and adverse events and are unbalanced. In August 2015, the FDA issued a guidance pertaining to risk information in DTCA via print.[91] In January and June of 2014, the FDA issued draft guidances on interactive promotional media such as firm-sponsored microblogs (e.g., Twitter), social networking sites (e.g., Facebook), and firm blogs.[82,83] In March 2012, the FDA issued a draft guidance on DTCA via television, but has not issued a final guidance. Nor has the FDA issued formal guidelines regarding online DTCA.

While DTCA bypasses the advice of the physician, only a few cases have created an exception to the learned intermediary doctrine on the ground that foundational tenets of the doctrine are no longer applicable in the context of DTCA. In Perez v. Wyeth Laboratories Inc.,[92] the New Jersey Supreme Court created an exception for Norplant®, an implantable contraceptive that provided contraception for up to 5 years, but was removable. The plaintiffs alleged personal injury and failure to warn of the contraceptive's adverse effects, including removal complications, which resulted in pain and scarring. The plaintiffs asserted that based on the mass advertising campaign to women that the pharmaceutical manufacturer had a duty to warn patients directly. According to the majority in Perez, the learned intermediary doctrine has four theoretical premises: (1) a reluctance to undermine the physician-patient relationship, (2) an absence for the need for the patient's informed consent, (3) the inability of drug manufacturers to communicate with patients, and (4) the complexity of the subject matter. The court asserted that each of these bases, except the fourth, is obviated in DTCA of prescription drugs. According to Perez, when direct advertising influences a patient to request a particular drug, and the physician does not adequately consult with the patient, "neither the physician nor the manufacturer should be entirely relieved of their respective duties to warn."[93]

Despite the ruling in Perez, two decades later, plaintiffs have not been able to convince many jurisdictions to recognize the DTCA exception to the Learned Intermediary Rule. Only a few courts other than Perez have allowed a DTCA exception for prescription drugs. Therefore, the duty to warn runs to the prescriber, not the patient.

Increasingly, the courts are holding that the pharmacist has a duty to warn patients and intervene on their behalf. In 1991, Pharmacists Mutual reported no claims involving drug utilization review. In 1999, drug review claims accounted for 9% of all pharmacist liability claims. A 2002 study by the same firm found that drug review claims were continuing in a straight-line increase.[94] In 2010, drug review claims at 7.9% represented the largest category of intellectual errors (as opposed to mechanical or dispensing errors). Counseling claims account for 1.6% of all claims.[95] In 2017, drug review claims rose to 8.3%, but counseling claims remained at 1.6% of all claims.[96]

In any event, pharmacists must remain vigilant to ensure that DTCA does not promote false expectations. Clearly, DTCA achieves its goals of encouraging consumerism, whereby patients go to seek prescription information from health professionals. DTCA increasingly leads patients to seek information that will confirm or refute the manufacturer's claims that differentiate a product from its competitors. When confronted with the influences of such advertising, pharmacists are on the front lines educating patients regarding these products, including the cost-effectiveness of prescription drug options. Pharmacists have a responsibility to provide objective information, to educate the patient, and to serve as a DI resource.[97] Refer to Chapter 25 for additional information.

DOCTRINE OF DRUG OVERPROMOTION

The doctrine of overpromotion is based on liability where an adequate warning is alleged to have been diluted by communications that do not adequately convey the full impact of the warning and are so overpromoting of a drug that members of the medical profession prescribe when it was not warranted. In other instances, overpromotion involves promoting a drug to a group for an off-label use. Recent examples include promoting an opioid indicated for cancer pain to nononcologists; promoting a birth control pill to treat premenstrual syndrome and/or acne; promoting an antipsychotic approved for bipolar disorder and schizophrenia for anxiety, obsessive compulsive disorder, dementia, and autism.

On August 9, 2003, Prescription Access Litigation Project filed the first class action lawsuit against a pharmaceutical company in connection with DTCA. The class action was brought for allegedly deceptive advertising and overpricing of Claritin®.[98] Plaintiffs alleged that the company's DTCA overstated the limited efficacy of its product and that the company deliberately left out any information about the drug's efficacy.

In yet other cases, the overpromotion failed to warn of the potential for serious adverse effects. While product liability laws vary by jurisdiction, counts of fraud/intentional misrepresentation, negligent misrepresentation, and breach of warranty are often found in the lawsuit pleadings. Another DTCA lawsuit involves Paxil®, one of the top selling drugs in the world.[99] Plaintiffs allege the drug causes withdrawal symptoms, such as severe nausea and other psychological problems, and that the company failed to tell plaintiffs, their physicians, or the public of this adverse effect.[94] If the adverse reaction is not listed in the labeling, the health care provider is exonerated, leaving the pharmaceutical company liable. Cases have involved tendon rupture from fluoroquinolone antibiotics, amputation from inadvertent promethazine intravenous extravasation,[100] and neuropathy and polyneuropathy from 3-hydroxy-3-methylglutaryl-Coenzyme A (HMG CoA) reductase inhibitors.[101]

Off-Label Use and Informed Consent

Off-label use involves use for indications not specifically approved by the FDA. It is an accepted principle that once the FDA approves a drug for marketing, a physician's discretionary use of that product is not restricted to the uses indicated on FDA-regulated labeling. This is particularly important in the areas of oncology, psychiatry (e.g., selective serotonin reuptake inhibitors [SSRIs]), and acquired immunodeficiency syndrome (AIDS), where a significant portion of drug use is off-label. While patients and medical innovation, in general, benefit from having their physicians informed about off-label uses, off-label use information from manufacturers has been restricted. In fact, manufacturer promotion of off-label use constitutes misbranding under the Food, Drug, and Cosmetic Act (FDCA).[102]

Under the 1997 Food, and Drug Administration Modernization Act (FDAMA), specifically Section 401, the FDA attempted to strengthen regulation of information pertaining to off-label uses.[103] One requirement under FDAMA was FDA review of material to be disseminated to ensure that it does not pose a significant risk to public health and is not false and misleading.[104] However, the authority of the FDA under the FDAMA to regulate the promotion of off-label uses was successfully challenged and Section 401 ceased to be effective on September 30, 2006.[105] In favoring the commercial free speech doctrine, the court ruled that the FDA had to permit drug company-sponsored advertisements for off-label use, as long as they were directed at physicians and not consumers.[106] In 2009, the FDA released a guideline allowing for distribution of reprints about off-label uses from peer-reviewed publications.[107] In February 2014, the FDA issued a new draft guidance regarding off-label use, updating the 2009 guidance. Major provisions of both guidelines, which refer to what is considered "Good Reprint Practices" and clarifying FDA's position on manufacturer dissemination of scientific journal articles, scientific or medical reference texts, and Clinical Practice Guidelines are found in Table 11-2.[108] The FDA agrees that off-label uses by unbiased researchers in bona fide published literature should be discussed.

In June 2018, the FDA issued a pair of guidelines that pertain to off-label use.[109,110] The first guidance, "Medical product communications that are consistent with FDA-required labeling—questions and answers" uses the term **CFL promotional communication** to refer to off-label advertising that is Consistent with FDA-required Labeling. A three-pronged factor analysis is applied to such communication to determine whether such advertising constitutes CFL promotional communication.[109] See Table 11-3. The second guidance "Drug and device manufacturer communication with payors, formulary committees, and similar entities—questions and answers" uses the term **Health Care Economic**

TABLE 11–2. MAJOR PROVISIONS OF THE 2009 AND 2014 FDA GUIDANCES FOR INDUSTRY—GOOD REPRINT PRACTICES FOR THE DISTRIBUTION OF MEDICAL JOURNAL ARTICLES AND MEDICAL OR SCIENTIFIC REFERENCE PUBLICATIONS, REFERENCE TEXTS, AND CLINICAL PRACTICE GUIDELINES ON UNAPPROVED NEW USES OF APPROVED DRUGS[108]

Journal Articles
- Article(s) should:
  - Be published by an organization with an editorial board.
  - Be peer-reviewed.
  - Be an unabridged reprint, copy of an article, or reference publication.
  - Be accompanied by the approved labeling and, when such information exists, a comprehensive bibliography of well-controlled clinical studies.
  - Be disseminated with a representative publication which reaches contrary or different conclusions.
  - Contain information that describes/addresses well-controlled clinical investigations.
- Article(s) should not:
  - Be a special supplement or funded by a manufacturer of the product that is the subject of the article.
  - Be primarily distributed by a manufacturer but should be generally available via other distribution channels.
  - Be written, edited, excerpted, or published specifically at the request of a manufacturer or edited or influenced by someone having a significant financial relationship with the manufacturer.
  - Be false or misleading or discuss a clinical trial that the FDA has indicated is not adequate and well-controlled.
  - Pose a significant risk to public health, if relied upon.
  - Be marked, highlighted, summarized, or characterized by the manufacturer.
- Not consistent with Good Reprint Practices are:
  - Letters to the editor.
  - Abstracts of a publication.
  - Reports of Phase I trials in healthy subjects.
  - Reference publications with little or no substantive discussion of relevant investigation or data.
- Articles should be distributed separately from information that is promotional:
  - They may not distribute in exhibit halls or during promotional speakers' programs.
  - Articles should not be attached to specific product information.
- Articles should be accompanied by a prominently displayed and affixed statement disclosing:
  - That the uses are off-label.
  - The manufacturer's interest in the subject drug of the article.
  - Any person known to the manufacturer as having a financial interest and the nature of that interest.
  - All significant risks/safety concerns known to the manufacturer.
  - Any author who has received financial compensation from the manufacturer and the nature and amount of same.

continued

TABLE 11–2. MAJOR PROVISIONS OF THE 2009 AND 2014 FDA GUIDANCES FOR INDUSTRY—GOOD REPRINT PRACTICES FOR THE DISTRIBUTION OF MEDICAL JOURNAL ARTICLES AND MEDICAL OR SCIENTIFIC REFERENCE PUBLICATIONS, REFERENCE TEXTS, AND CLINICAL PRACTICE GUIDELINES ON UNAPPROVED NEW USES OF APPROVED DRUGS[108] *(CONTINUED)*

Scientific or Medical Texts and Clinical Practice Guidelines[a]
- Should:
  - Be based on a systematic review of existing evidence.
  - Be published by an independent publisher.
  - Be the most current version.
  - Be authored, edited, and/or contributed to by experts.
  - Be peer reviewed by experts.
  - Be sold through the usual and customary independent distribution channels.
  - Be delivered separately from promotional material.
  - Contain a prominently displayed affixed statement identifying both the distributing manufacturer and that some of the uses are off-label.
  - Be disseminated with the approved product labeling.
- Should Not:
  - Be false or misleading.
  - Contain information that makes the product dangerous to health when used in the manner suggested.
  - Be primarily distributed by a manufacturer.
  - Be edited or significantly influenced by a manufacturer or any individuals having a financial relationship.
  - Be written or published at the request of a manufacturer.
  - Be abridged or excepted in any manner.
  - Be attached to any product information other than approved labeling.

[a]There are additional requirements for dissemination of chapters.

Information (HCEI). The guidance provides the FDA's thinking on communication to payors about unapproved drugs, devices, and off-label uses of approved products.[110] Examples of HCEI include an evidence dossier, a reprint from a peer-reviewed journal, a software package comprising a model with a user manual, a budget-impact model, a slide presentation, or a payor brochure. Moreover, medical science liaisons are permitted to provide off-label information in response to unsolicited medical inquiries. The types of nonpromotional information that can be provided include general education, report of a clinical trial, follow-up to a question originally posed to a sales representative, and advice for formularies. Insurers and government plaintiffs have increasingly attempted to claim a "formulary influence" theory of liability, alleging that manufacturers engaged in off-label promotion or kickbacks that caused states to wrongfully include a medication on their Medicaid formularies or gave medications preferred tier status. In one such case, however, United States ex rel. v. Solvay S.A., the product information sent to the P&T Committees was requested and the court held that any temporal relationship between sales representative visits to P&T Committee members was too tenuous.[111]

TABLE 11–3. THREE-FACTOR TEST FOR CONSISTENT WITH FDA-REQUIRED LABELING (CFL) COMMUNICATIONS[109]

Factor 1

If the answer to any of the following questions is yes, the product communication is not consistent with FDA-required labeling.

- **Indication**: Does the communication relate to a different indication than the one reflected in the FDA-required labeling?
- **Patient Population**: Is the patient population represented or suggested outside the approved patient population in the FDA-required labeling?
- **Limitations and Directions for Handling/Use**: Do the representations/suggestions in the communication conflict with the use limitations or directions for handling, preparing, and/or using the product reflected in the FDA-required labeling?
- **Dosing or Use Regimen/Administration**: Do the representations/suggestions conflict with recommended dosage or use regimen, route of administration, or strength(s)?

Factor 2

If the answer to the following question is yes, the product communication is not consistent with the FDA-required labeling.

Do the representations/suggestions about use of the product in the product communication increase the potential for harm to health relative to the information reflected in the FDA-required labeling?

Factor 3

If the answer to the following question is no, the product communication is not consistent with the FDA-required labeling.

Do the directions for use in the FDA-required labeling enable the product to be safely and effectively used under the condition represented/suggested in the product communication?

Problematic are responses to inquiries that are not really unsolicited or formulary advice that borders on preapproval promotion (known as new product seeding).[112] Additionally, pharmaceutical companies may freely distribute, to health professionals, copies of articles from peer-reviewed professional journals or reference textbooks containing discussions of off-label product usage. However, sales representatives are not permitted to use this information to promote the company's products. In December 2011, the FDA issued a draft guidance for industry entitled "Responding to Unsolicited Requests for Off-Label Information About Prescription Drugs and Medical Devices."[113] An entire section of this document is devoted to unsolicited requests for off-label information through emerging electronic media. The FDA is recommending that the public DI response to off-label information be limited to providing the firm's contact information and should not include any off-label information. This will ensure that the communication occurs solely between the firm and the individual who made the request and circumvents both broad distribution and issues regarding the enduring nature of online responses.

Researchers continually conduct studies to determine new uses for already marketed drugs and effective combinations of drugs for new indications with the results being published in the literature. Additionally, with up to 40% of all prescriptions being for off-label use, off-label use comprises a large component of providing DI, especially for queries that involve pediatrics.[114] These queries are often from physicians seeking evidence to support a particular off-label use. Problems arise when the off-label use is not really off-label, but rather, crosses the line and is experimental (in which case an Investigational New Drug Application and/or Institutional Review Board [IRB] approval for study is required).[125] Refer to Chapter 23 for more detailed information.

Unfortunately, once an off-label use becomes rampant, the market drives it and there remains little incentive for the pharmaceutical company to provide more data or conduct further research regarding that off-label use. This disincentive arises not only because of the expense involved in conducting clinical trials but also because trial results could actually have an adverse effect on sales by showing lack of efficacy or safety. For example, it was a study of rofecoxib (Vioxx®) for an off-label use that first uncovered the cardiovascular risks that eventually led to market withdrawal.[115]

Medicare Parts B and D are required to cover off-label uses of drugs in cancer treatment when the use is supported by a citation in at least one of the following references: American Hospital Formulary Service-Drug Information (AHFS-DI), Lexicomp® by Wolters Kluwer, The National Comprehensive Cancer Network's Drugs and Biologics Compendium (NCCN), IBM Micromedex® DRUGDEX® or Clinical Pharmacology by Elsevier/Gold Standard, or the use is supported by clinical research in peer-reviewed articles published in respected medical journals.[116] Medicaid utilized only AHFS Drug Information® and IBM Micromedex® DRUGDEX®.[117] When providing DI, it should be realized that not all compendia include revision dates for the monographs. Moreover, a recent study revealed that updated policies were not followed, certain off-label indications were excluded without rationale, and for common off-label cancer treatments, outdated literature and incomplete or inconsistent evidence was found in the compendia.[118] Under the Medicare Improvements For Patients and Providers Act of 2008 (MIPPA), the criteria for medically accepted off-label uses are now the same for both Medicare Part B and Part D.[119]

For noncancer Part B and Part D drugs, the off-label coverage is limited to uses in IBM Micromedex® DRUGDEX®, Lexicomp® by Wolters Kluwer, Clinical Pharmacology, or AHFS Drug Information, but only if the FDA has approved the drug for some other use. There is a divergence between Part B and Part D for the use of peer-reviewed literature to support off-label use of noncancer drugs. Peer-reviewed literature (excluding abstracts, meeting abstracts, and in-house publications) can be used to support Part B but not Part D. There is much litigation in this area and the question as to whether CMS reliance on proprietary compendia, not accessible to the public for Part D off-label approval raises serious due process issues.

Following these guidelines for DI queries pertaining to an off-label use would appear to be a prudent practice. Similarly, in providing responses to DI requests pertaining to off-label uses (including usages of off-label dosages), it is prudent to provide complete information, so that a decision may be made whether the information is enough to warrant a particular off-label use. For example, letters to the editor or abstracts would not be complete information. When there is another drug on the market with an approved-label use for the same indication that the off-label product is being considered, the response to the DI request should mention that labeled alternative.[120] Moreover, it is also important to be cognizant of the implications of disseminating off-label information in the context of patient safety and liability. Responding to consumer requests for information about off-label uses is not advised, simply because, unlike health professionals, most often they are not in a position to evaluate the literature and extrapolate to a particular situation.

Off-label use of pharmaceuticals has resulted in liability. For example, litigation involving gabapentin (Neurontin®), an antiepileptic drug linked to suicide and prescribed for numerous off-label uses, was one of the earlier off-label cases and resulted in a $21 million settlement. Another example is bevacizumab (Avastin®), an oncology drug, used off-label to treat macular degeneration, which caused blindness in some patients. Also, the U.S. Court of Appeals has ruled that off-label promotion may be treated as racketeering in civil litigation.[121] The 2018 ruling is based on a 2013 decision and is significant, in that it is the first time a third-party payor recovered for "damages" incurred by prescriptions of off-label promotional activities of a pharmaceutical company.

While there is no question that patients should be advised if a proposed treatment is truly investigational or experimental, off-label use is not necessarily experimental or investigational; thus, informed consent is not necessary whenever an off-label use is proposed.[122] Federal informed consent regulations governing investigational drugs do not apply to off-label use.[123] State-informed consent laws vary but usually require discussion of the nature, risks, benefits, and alternative modes of treatment. For example, the New York statute states:

> Lack of informed consent means the failure of the person providing the professional treatment or diagnosis to disclose to the patient such alternatives thereto and the reasonably foreseeable risks and benefits involved as a reasonable medical…practitioner under similar circumstances would have disclosed, in a manner permitting the patient to make a knowledgeable evaluation.[124]

Actions for informed consent are, therefore, limited to the nondisclosure of medical information. However, failure to disclose FDA status does not raise a **material issue of fact** as to informed consent. That is, it would not result in a **summary judgment** in a lawsuit.

Liability Concerns for Internet/Social Media Information

❹ *DI is currently being obtained from a number of Internet/social media and mobile apps, and there is a possibility of DI liability for information obtained from these sources.* Google Scholar, Wikipedia, RxWiki, PubDrug, and web citations, in general, are increasingly being accessed for handling DI queries. It has been reported that half of U.S. physicians use Wikipedia for medical information.[125] The percentage of those who use Wikipedia for DI is unknown. Recently, Internet/social media DI sources have appeared as references in publications.[126] More than 25% of the Internet's content involves health care and medical information.[127] The browser of Internet information resources can now expect to find full prescribing information for most heavily marketed drugs. The situation is complicated by links to investigational products or investigational uses and vice versa. The question is whether this is promotion of off-label uses.[128] Refer to Chapter 25 for further information on this topic.

Liability concerns arise in the area of whether a manufacturer's website content is considered labeling or advertising. It appears to be necessary to distinguish between Internet promotion directed to health professionals and consumers. DTCA on the Internet is considered labeling, rather than advertising and, as such, the FDA has principal authority to regulate it.[129]

On February 2004, the FDA issued new industry guidelines, entitled "Help-Seeking and Other Disease Awareness Communications by or on Behalf of Drug and Device Firms and Brief Summary: Disclosing Risk Information in Consumer-Directed Print Advertisements." While these guidelines are intended to improve the brief summaries of adverse effects that must be included in DTCA, they do not address Internet advertisements.

QUALITY OF INTERNET DRUG INFORMATION

Not all websites are reputable and currently there is no way to distinguish which sites providing DI are authoritative and which are not. Problems have arisen such as **hyperlink** obsolescence, defunct websites, broken links, altered content, and an inability to determine currency.[113] Moreover, it is common for websites to change or move.

Entries in Wikipedia, an encyclopedia project, recently ranked as one of the top ten sites visited, can be the subject of erroneous entries, fraud, conflict of interest, or even criminal mischief.[130] For example, pharmaceutical companies may edit or delete their product information as the site is user edited. Thus, sites such as Wikipedia are not authoritative and can only be supplementary to, rather than the sole source of DI.[131] In a recent study of the accuracy and completeness of DI in Wikipedia versus IBM Micromedex®

using package inserts as a standard comparator, Wikipedia was found to lack the accuracy and completeness of the clinical reference, IBM Micromedex®. Lower completeness, and importantly, accuracy scores for Wikipedia compared with IBM Micromedex® (mean composite scores 18.55 vs. 38.4, respectively; $p < 0.01$), led to the conclusion that Wikipedia is inappropriate for clinical decision-making.[132]

Google Scholar includes both published and unpublished (hence not peer-reviewed) information and, unlike PubMed®, it may not contain the latest literature. However, as the number of Internet-only journals not indexed in PubMed® increases, there will be increased reliance on Google Scholar as an easy-to-use source for locating primary literature. In fact, in a recent comparison with PubMed®, no significant differences were found regarding the number of primary literature articles, although PubMed® did retrieve more specific articles.[133]

What about liability for DI obtained from the Internet and electronic journals or apps (such as Epocrates®)? Is there a possibility of pharmacist liability occurring via cyberspace? As mentioned above, the Internet contains a growing hodgepodge of sources with little organization and uneven credibility. In fact, material on the Internet may contain innocent mistakes and/or deliberate fraud, as well as outdated material. Several situations may result in search results that are not comprehensive. Examples include faulty search strategies and failing to search for historical information. Many databases including PubMed® do not contain material prior to the 1940s. Searchers may not even be aware that pre-Internet or old nonelectronic material exists. Old MEDLINE® articles from 1949 through 1965 may not be updated with MeSH terms and may not contain searchable abstracts.[134] For e-books (i.e., online textbooks) with their own built-in search engine (e.g., Merck Manual), there is a possibility of patient harm occurring when the computer malfunctions. Currently, there are no laws pertaining to, and no means for, ensuring the accuracy of DI posed on the Internet. It is possible for information on the Internet to be false, misleading, corrupted by an outside source, or otherwise harmful to the reader to apply it to their specific situation. There is a potential for misinformation to be disseminated, while the reader unknowingly assumes the DI to be accurate and true via the Internet and related technologies.

The Health Summit Working Group, which consists of professional societies including ASHP, and the Health on the Net Foundation (HON) are currently working to improve the quality of DI on the Internet. HON has developed a code (HONcode) for quality and reliability which, if displayed, increases the likelihood that the information is reliable. A seal of approval may also be given from other organizations that approve health care sites such as Internet Healthcare Coalition, Verified Internet Pharmacy Practice Sites (VIPPS®), and Medical Matrix. Unfortunately, these instruments may be difficult to use and their actual validity is unclear. Additionally, a seal of approval should in no way replace critical clinical judgment of the content. Also, the application of the National Information

Infrastructure to consumer health information is one of the priorities of the federal government. Examples of website QA criteria are included in Table 11-1 and are found in Chapter 18.

Another venue where the quality of DI may be suspect is social media and/or email communication. Both the American Medical Association and the American Medical Informatics Association have issued guidelines for physicians using email to communicate with patients.[135] These guidelines encourage physicians to be cautious when using email because of the possibility of liability due to misunderstanding and privacy concerns.[136] Perhaps in the near future, health insurers will cover calls made to online pharmacists providing DI, much the same way as Medicare now covers teleconferencing.

The Internet is at the forefront of practice, where pharmacists will consult with each other, thereby learning from one another and benefiting their DI clients and patients.[137] Web applications facilitate interactive information sharing, such as **Wikis**, blogs, hosted-services, and networking sites. Specific examples include Vizient (formerly, the University Health System Consortium), WebMD, and Google Scholar. In the fast-paced practice of DI, Internet information may provide a quick starting point for an answer to a query. However, other non-web-based references should also be consulted. DI professionals should never rely solely on a search retrieved from Google Scholar to respond to a DI query. Additionally, when using Web citations, it is recommended to include the date accessed to provide readers with some indication of how current the information is (refer to Appendix 13-3).

TELEMEDICINE AND CYBERMEDICINE

Legal issues are emerging from e-health technologies, such as telemedicine and cybermedicine programs. **Telemedicine** is defined as the use of telecommunications and interactive video technology to provide health care services to patients who are at a distance. **Cybermedicine** is a broader concept that includes the marketing, relationship creation, advice, prescribing, and selling pharmaceuticals and devices in cyberspace. Therefore, telepharmacy is a subset of telemedicine and the terms are used interchangeably here. As telemedicine and cybermedicine expand, questions regarding liability for pharmacists providing DI on the Internet will need to be addressed. For example, health professionals, such as pharmacists, are licensed by states. Which state law applies when the pharmacist is located in New York, the patient is in Florida, and the website is maintained by a company in California? Who is liable for technical problems that make it impossible for the information to be received in a timely manner or for breaches of confidentiality caused by those who would invade private files? Already some sites offer fee-based live physician offices and nurse-triage services (e.g., Optum®

NurseLine) for self-diagnosis and health screening. Additionally, some DI providers provide information over the Internet.

Although the courts have yet to test liability for medical malpractice involving the practice of pharmacy or medicine on the Internet, such a case is bound to surface soon. The most important determination of whether there is such malpractice is whether or not a health care provider-patient relationship has been created by the consultation in the absence of physical contact. Hard copy printouts of Internet discussions would be discoverable before trial and could be uncovered in the defendant's computer files by a plaintiff's attorney. It is likely that where a physician consults with a pharmacist for DI via telemedicine, the pharmacist will not be deemed to have established a pharmacist-patient relationship. Telephone consultations between physicians are most analogous and have not been held to create a physician-patient relationship.[138] Similarly, as previously mentioned, no pharmacist-physician relationship has been found based on a provision of DI to the physician.[28] This is largely because of the public policy interest of promoting consultations, professional association, and education, as well as the assumed limited information conveyed to the consulting physician. However, in view of advancing technology where the patient's entire medical history and test results are available on the computer, this situation may change, especially where a consultation fee is involved. Also, where a pharmacist posts a website and is paid to provide DI, the courts will surely find such cybermedical consultation to create a pharmacist-patient relationship.

Although there have been several lawsuits for false information on online bulletin boards (e.g., Usenet News, CompuServe®), the basis of these lawsuits has been defamation, not malpractice.[139,140] The offering of general medical advice and judgments online (e.g., chat rooms) does not appear to be creating a formal physician-patient relationship. Nor does it appear that the giving of generic advice will generate liability for either the provider or the publisher. If, however, the information is fraudulent or quackery, then courts do have authority under both state and federal computer statutes to stop the activity. Similarly, Internet (or telephone) medical call centers, or triage services used by some health care plans can expect to be held liable when misdiagnosis occurs. On the other hand, liability is lessened where Internet discussions resemble an academic conference between health care providers, rather than a formal consultancy. Similarly, the issuance of a disclaimer in writing with the original subscription and with each message written may help insulate from any liability.

Some websites now carry disclaimers to protect the authors from liability. The limitation of the remedies available should be displayed prominently. A cap equal to the price of the service sold may be included. The following is an example:

Please read this agreement entirely and carefully before assessing this website. By accessing the site, you agree to be bound by the terms and conditions below. If you do not wish to be bound by these terms and conditions, you may not access or use this site. Our maximum liability to you under all circumstances will be equal to the purchase price you paid for any goods, services, or information.

This statement is then followed by disclaimers pertaining to accuracy, currency, copyright, no medical advice, no warranties, a disclaimer of endorsement, disclaimer regarding liability for third-party content, and a general disclaimer of liability including negligence with a statement that the user assumes all responsibility and risk for use.[141] It may also be desirable to include a provision that any dispute will be brought in the city of the site owner's principal place of business.

SOCIAL MEDIA

There is a growing use of social media that allows health professionals to share information with their colleagues and, more often recently, their patients. Social media allows for large groups of individuals to share information, expand contact, and serve as a means for professional news and a tool for discussion of pharmacy-related issues. Examples include Facebook®, LinkedIn®, Amazon.com®, Twitter®, YouTube, Pinterest®, blogs, and forums. In fact, most state pharmacy organizations have a Twitter® presence. A number of legal issues for DI pharmacists who use social media warrant consideration—ranging from patient privacy under HIPAA and state privacy torts, creation of a pharmacist-patient relationship to anti-kickback issues. Privacy controls vary by site and change frequently, but patient information must never be disclosed on such sites. Breaches can occur easily such as inquiring about how a patient's diabetes is on Facebook® or discussing celebrities getting medications in pharmacies. Posting of comments and breaches of patient confidentiality, especially by students, are common.[142] Even text-messaging with patients can present legal issues that health professionals may not have considered. In addition to the text messaged **protected health information (PHI)** not being accorded the necessary privacy and security protection, the health professional must always be certain that any information they send and receive must be added to the patient's medical and/or pharmacy profile and retained for the required period of time. While many health care professionals simply delete texts they have read, they may be violating the law. From a liability standpoint, not having a copy of texts a clinician has sent to or received from a patient who is suing him or her for malpractice is a precarious position and may amount to spoliation of evidence. Best practice is to retain posts and texts to and from patients and colleagues. There has been a recent increase in lawsuits brought under invasion of privacy. For discovery purposes, opposing counsel may review any public social network of a witness or party to discover social media posts.

While there are no legal rules on this, friending patients is not a good idea. ASHP has developed a statement on use of social media by pharmacy professionals.[143] However, there is still no clear picture of issues such as the duty to warn in social media.[144] While TJC originally opined against physicians or other health care providers texting orders to hospitals and other health care settings, it has since stated, "Licensed independent practitioners....may text orders as long as a secure text messaging platform is used and the required components of an order are included."[145]

Questions have also been raised whether providing DI over social media is tantamount to unlicensed practice in a state where the pharmacist is not licensed. Moreover, harmful patient-specific advice may lead to malpractice. Some pharmacists have placed a disclaimer on their blog to indicate "Reading this blog should not be construed to mean that you and I have a pharmacist-patient relationship." Besides privacy and negligence issues other liability may follow for defamation, copyright infringement, discrimination, or harassment.

Some pharmaceutical manufacturers have developed patient blogs and other social media websites especially for patients with chronic illnesses such as diabetes. In some cases, testimonials by what appear to be patients are actually being made by people paid or allied with the pharmaceutical company. While the effect of social media on patient care is currently unclear, the FDA is currently drafting guidelines to cover drug companies' social media presence.

Fraud and Abuse

Another consideration pertains to fraud and abuse laws, such as the anti-kickback laws.[146] The Anti-Kickback Statute prohibits physicians participating in the Medicaid and Medicare programs from submitting any false remuneration, including any kickback, bribe, or rebate to induce referrals of patients.[147] Certain aspects of e-health promotional and marketing tools, such as per-click payment arrangements, are particularly susceptible to violation of the Anti-Kickback statute. The violation occurs because the health care provider is receiving remuneration based on the referral rate provided by the fee charged per click. Likewise, promotional banners on a health care organization or pharmacist's website that link to a pharmacy or other type of patient care items are most likely in violation because the referring provider is receiving a benefit (i.e., per click arrangements involve the payment of a fee based on the clicking on a particular link on a website) in exchange for referrals.[148] Similarly, the provision of free email services, online publications, computer equipment, or other types of computer ventures are in violation of the Anti-Kickback statute when these companies sell items or services reimbursable under Medicaid or Medicare programs.

Another area of uncertainty pertains to the handling of links between web pages. A link is any component of a web page that connects to another web page. The issue of whether pharmaceutical manufacturers will be liable for material posted on sites they have not sponsored, but have merely linked to their own, is yet to be decided in the courts.

At least according to cases over the past few years, mere hyperlinking does not constitute copyright or trademark infringement.[149] Copyright law does not require that permission be obtained for linking, but if there is copyrighted graphic material, people will be reproducing and displaying copyrighted material they do not own. The copyright owner's permission needs to be obtained to use the graphic image, unless fair use is utilized (fair use is discussed further under the section for copyright law). Where the information being linked to is violating the copyright law, it is also possible that a website owner who links to a site containing infringing material may be liable for contributory copyright infringement. Contributory copyright infringement is established when a defendant, with knowledge of another's infringing activity, causes or materially contributes to the infringing conduct.

Moreover, whether deep linking (i.e., bypassing the homepage and linking to an internal page of the linked site) is copyright infringement is currently unclear.[150] However, if a web page specifically states, ask permission before linking, it is possible that linking to the site without the owner's permission may be trespass or breach of contract where there are terms of use to which were agreed.[151]

Additionally, certain businesses, who do not want their valuable content associated with or connected to certain sites, have brought legal action under theories of trademark, defamation, disparagement, unfair competition, false advertising, invasion of privacy, and other laws. In Playboy Enterprises, Inc. v. Universal Tel-A-Talk, Inc., an X-rated website linked to the Playboy website.[152] Playboy sued and proved that users of the site may be confused as to whether Playboy sponsored or endorsed the adult site. Playboy also proved that its trademark bunny logo would be blurred or tarnished by the association with the adult site. Also, in Coca-Cola Co. v. Purdy, the Court entered judgment for several well-known trademark owners on their infringement claims where an antiabortionist used a host of domain names incorporating their famous marks.[153] The antiabortionist linked the domain names (e.g., mycoca-cola.com) with a website associated with abortionismurder.com. According to the decision, the "quick and effortless nature of 'surfing' the Internet makes it unlikely that consumers can avoid confusion through the exercise of due care."[154]

The practice of using framing to incorporate third-party content into a website is also an area of unsettled law. The framing site can surround the framed pages with its own advertising, logos, or promotions. Framing may trigger a dispute under copyright and trademark law theories because a framed site arguably alters the appearance of the content and creates the impression that its owner endorses or voluntarily chooses to associate with the framer.[155] However, liability for framing has not been fully or clearly resolved by the courts.[156]

Advances in technology may render this dilemma moot. Technology now exists to keep undesired links or frames off a website. In any event, it is advisable not to link to or frame another website without the express (i.e., explicit, written) permission of that site. However, if a website owner is concerned about liability for links or frames, a prominently placed disclaimer may be added. Additionally, if a webmaster wants to obtain permission before someone links to their site, a request permission notice needs to be posted and require users to agree to the terms by clicking "I agree" on the homepage.

The Internet raises a variety of legal issues, most of which are unresolved but evolving. Future goals should be for pharmaceutical manufacturers to promote their products to consumers more responsibly, for the FDA to regulate DTCA more effectively, and for the medical and pharmacy communities to educate the public about prescription drugs more constructively.

Intellectual Property Rights

COPYRIGHT

The current copyright law is codified at 17 U.S.C.A. § 101 et seq. A copyright is a property right in an original work of authorship that is fixed in tangible form.[157] It is a statutory requirement that literary, dramatic, and musical works, for example, must have been recorded or produced in some physical object (or fixed) before copyright can subsist. A copyright holder in a work is granted certain exclusive rights to control use of the work created. A work of authorship must be original in order to qualify for copyright protection. This requirement has two facets. First, the author must have engaged in some intellectual endeavor of his or her own, and not just have copied from a preexisting source. Second, the work must exhibit a minimal amount of creativity. Copyright protection covers both published and unpublished works. Also, the fact that the previously published work is out of print does not affect its copyright. Works of authorship under copyright and items not entitled to copyright are found in Table 11-4.

❺ *Pharmacists providing DI must have a working knowledge of copyright law both to avoid liability and to protect their own literary works.* Under the 1976 Copyright Act, an author is protected as soon as a work is recorded in some concrete way. The process of registering for a copyright involves depositing material with the Copyright Office to be reviewed by an examiner, followed by publication with a copyright notice, usually the symbol ©. Under the Copyright Term Extension Act (CTEA) of 1998, such work is protected until 70 years after the death of the author or for 95 years for corporate copyright holders.

TABLE 11–4. COPYRIGHT PROTECTION

Works of authorship entitled to copyright protection include the following:

- Literary works
- Musical works, including any accompanying words
- Dramatic works, including any accompanying music
- Pantomimes and choreographic works
- Pictorial, graphic, and sculptural works
- Motion pictures and other audiovisual works
- Sound recordings
- Architectural works

Not entitled to copyright protection:

- Ideas, concepts, principles, or discovery
- Procedures, processes, systems, methods of operation
- Mere compilations of facts

In effect, the CTEA retroactively extended copyright terms by 20 years.[158] The constitutionality of CTFA has been challenged and upheld by the Supreme Court. The author or copyright owner has the exclusive right to make copies of the work, control derivative works or adaptations, and sue for damages and injunctive relief (an injunction is a judicial remedy issued in order to prohibit a party from doing or continuing to do a certain activity) against infringers. Public domain works may be copied and distributed without copyright permission. Works of the U.S. government (e.g., General Accounting Office [GAO] reports, Congressional Record, FDA releases) are considered part of the public domain.

Ownership of copyright usually rests with the author at the time when the work is created. The exception is a work made for hire (i.e., "a work prepared by an employee within the scope of the employment relationship, or a work specially ordered or commissioned for use as a contribution to a collective work, as part of a motion picture or other audiovisual work, as a translation, as a supplementary work, as a compilation, as an instructional text, as a test, as an answer material for a test, or as an atlas, if the parties expressly agree in a written instrument signed by them that the work shall be a work made for hire" [Copyright Law of the U.S., 17 U.S.C. Sec 106]).[159] Another exception is the first-sale doctrine, which, in effect, permits interlibrary loan of materials. Under the first-sale doctrine, a person who legitimately owns a copy of a work is one who purchased the work or otherwise acquired ownership of the work with the permission of the copyright owner, and has full authority to "sell or otherwise dispose of the possession of that copy."[160]

Since the Berne Convention in 1989, the copyright formalities of registration and notice have lost almost all their legal significance. Registration, although not mandatory, affords the copyright claimant certain advantages. For example, it prevents an infringer from pleading innocent infringement. Similarly, the only substantive legal effect of copyright registration is that attorney fees and statutory damages are only recoverable for post registration infringements. That is, U.S. authors must register before bringing suit. However, for works prior to 1989 and the Berne Convention, copyright can be lost if notice was omitted and that omission was not cured within 5 years of publication by registration and affixation of notice to the remaining copies.

Under the fair use provision of the 1976 Copyright Act, if a use is fair, permission of the copyright owner need not be received, nor royalties paid. Fair use is determined by a four-pronged test: (1) nature and character of use, (2) nature of the work, (3) the proportional amount copied, and, most importantly, (4) the effect on the market for the copied work.[161]

The first factor in the fair use analysis is the nature and character of the use. Uses for research, teaching, scholarship, and news reporting are more likely to be considered fair than strictly commercial uses. In addition, there is a narrow special exemption for educators. The mere fact that the use is educational and not for profit does not insulate the use from a finding of infringement.

The second factor in the fair use analysis is the nature of the work. This factor centers on whether a copyrighted work is creative or informational, and whether it is published or unpublished. The scope of fair use is greater when the copyrighted work is informational, because it is generally recognized that there is a greater need to disseminate factual material than works of fiction or fantasy.[162] An unpublished work is given greater copyright protection than a published work and is, therefore, less likely to be subjected to a valid assertion of fair use.[163] In Harper & Row Publishers, Inc. v. Nation Enterprises, Nation obtained an unauthorized manuscript of former President Ford's memoirs before they were published in a book form under a contract with Harper & Row. The fact that President Ford's memoirs had not yet been published by the time Nation published them was a deciding factor.[164] That is, in looking at the nature of the work, an unpublished work seems to be entitled to greater protection than a published work.

The third factor is the amount copied. There does not appear to be a minimal amount or threshold quantity (e.g., five sentences) standard where fair use will be presumed. Many copyrighted works are accessed through a campus license that overrides copyright. Libraries vigorously negotiate licenses for such materials. Although the statute itself does not set the maximum standards for educational fair use, Classroom Guidelines have been agreed upon by educational, author, and publisher organizations.[165] Multiple copies for classroom use, but not to exceed in any event more than one copy per pupil in a course, are permissible, provided each copy bears a copyright notice and meets the test of (1) brevity, (2) spontaneity, and (3) cumulative effect. For example, to meet the test of brevity the Classroom Guidelines prohibit multiple copying of complete articles longer than 2500 words. They prohibit copying excerpts longer than 1000 words or 10% of the work, whichever is shorter. For motion media, up to 10% or 3 minutes, whichever is less, in the aggregate of a copyrighted motion media work may be reproduced or otherwise incorporated as part of an educational multimedia project. To meet the test of spontaneity, the copying must be at the instance and inspiration of the individual teacher, where the teacher's decision to use the work in class does not allow for a timely reply to request for permission. To meet the cumulative effect requirement, the copying must be for only one course in the school, and except for current news periodicals, newspapers, and current news sections of periodicals, only one article or two excerpts therefrom may be copied from the same author, or three excerpts from the same collective work or periodical volume. Additionally, the copying must be for only one class term; and no more than nine instances of such multiple copying for one course during one class term. In other words, the copied material may only be used for one semester and permission for longer use must be obtained. Further, students may not be charged for the copy beyond the actual cost of photocopying.

Case Study 11–3

You are publishing a guide regarding "do not crush" drugs for which you will receive compensation. You are merely listing all drugs that should not be crushed. However, the material for this publication is derived from a number of published references, all of which are copyright protected. You adopt an entire table from one of the articles without permission. You also take several direct sentences without providing any source reference. One of the references you are using is out of print.

- *Which of these acts would constitute a violation of the copyright law? What steps should have been taken to avoid copyright violation?*

In Association of American Publishers v. New York University, the issue was the production and distribution of custom-made anthologies sold to students. Although the classroom guidelines allow students to make single copies for personal use, the court found infringement when anthologies were sold for profit.[166] The action was settled with the adoption of certain procedures by New York University.

The fourth factor in a fair use analysis is the impact the infringing work will have on the market or potential market of the copyrighted work. The Supreme Court has decided that all four factors of the fair use test should be given equal weight.[167] Under the Copyright Act of 1976, these four fair use factors provide a broad and flexible defense against copyright infringement.

Fair use is an equitable defense to copyright infringement, determined by the courts on a case-by-case basis. Unfortunately, in court decisions on educational photocopying to date, the ruling in almost every case has been against fair use. Copying by nonprofit medical libraries has been held to be a fair use where the photocopying of medical journals by federal nonprofit institutions was made solely for the purpose of medical research. In Williams & Wilkins Co. v. United States, the library was copying a single copy for each request and the court found that "medical science would be seriously hurt if such library photocopying were stopped."[168] In Williams & Wilkins, the copying of medical journals was by two governmental libraries, i.e., the National Institutes of Health (NIH) and the National Library of Medicine (NLM), a repository of much of the world's medical literature.[169] The public benefits of fair use apparently held considerably more weight than any commercial considerations presented before the courts. However, where the photocopying of medical journals by scientists occurred in a large for-profit company, the court decided the making of unauthorized copies of copyrighted articles published in scientific journals for use by research scientists was not fair use. The court determined that the publishers had created through the Copyright Clearance Center, Inc., a viable market for institutional users to obtain licenses to allow photocopying of individual articles. However, in Princeton University Press v. Michigan Document Services, Inc., the court held that a copy shop selling coursepacks, which are compilations of various copyrighted and uncopyrighted materials such as journal articles, sample test questions, course notes, and book excerpts, infringed the copyrights of several publishers.[170] In deciding this was not a fair use, the court noted that the copying was substantial and commercial. Similarly, in Basic Books v. Kinko's Graphic Corp., the court held that a copy shop's reproduction and sale of coursepacks to students was not a fair use of the copyrighted material.[171]

Course management systems and digital course packs, which post copyrighted articles, book excerpts, and research data, are used today by 90% of U.S. colleges and universities. Simply because the material is online does not mean it is free from copyright protection. Unless fair use or some other exemption applies, permission is required before posting.[172] When fair use does not apply, the institution must obtain permission from the rightsholder, who may charge a fee for such permission based on the amount of content and the number of people, usually students, who will view the content. Additionally, reporting of the same material for use in a subsequent semester requires a new permission. Moreover, it violates the intent and spirit of copyright law to use course management systems as a substitute for the purchase of books, subscriptions, or other materials when substantial portions of the material are required for educational purposes. When scanning in paper materials (such as textbooks) to create electronic copies, be sure that legally obtained copies of the work are used, either purchased or owned by the institution. All posted materials in a course management system should contain both the copyright notice from, and complete citation to, the original material, as well as a caution against further electronic distribution.[154] Instant permission may be obtained at http://www.copyright.com through the Copyright Clearance Center for use in course management systems, coursepacks, e-reserves, classroom handouts, and other formats.

The court has also ruled that there is only a limited copyright protection available to a compilation of works written by another author. In Silverstein v. Penguin Putnam, the plaintiff had compiled a collection of 122 unpublished Dorothy Parker poems.[173] He presented the compilation to Penguin, which rejected it and subsequently inserted the poems into a new edition of Parker's work published by Penguin. The court held that Silverstein would not be entitled to injunctive relief as he did not hold the copyrights on the poems. Thus, his efforts to gather the poems were not protectable in copyright. Additionally, the court looked at Silverstein's arrangement of the poems and found that Penguin did not copy his arrangement.

In 2008, in Warner Bros. Entm't Inc. v. RDR Books, a lexicon of terms from the Harry Potter series of books, initially posted on a free Internet website and then scheduled for publication, was held as copyright infringement.[174] The legal issues involved were whether there is a distinction in the law between digital and printed copyright and what is a third party's right to create a new reference book designed to help others better understand the original work (i.e., a study guide). The court held that the print version of the lexicon was not a derivative work, especially in view of the number of places where copying was deemed excessive. However, the court explicitly stated that authors do not have the right to stop the publication of reference guides and companion works.

Copyright infringement requires a showing of copying, which can be proven circumstantially by demonstrating that the defendant had access to the copyrighted work and that the defendant's work is substantially similar to that work. Copyright infringement for purposes of commercial advantage or private financial gain is punishable under 18 U.S.C. §2319. Although the act allows for damages of as much as $100,000 per infringement, innocent infringers (e.g., educators and universities) may be entitled to a remission of statutory damages. They are only liable for actual damages, such as profits earned by the infringer or profits denied to the copyright holder. This provision lowers the incentive for the publishing industry to sue. Recently, publishers have resorted to unsavory tactics in their attempts to control educational copying, such as sending letters threatening to sue copy shops for infringement unless they agree to pay royalties.

Newsletter copying is strictly prohibited and violators risk not only the statutory damages ($100,000), but can be subject to criminal penalties. These newsletters require a fee to be paid to the Copyright Clearance Center even for internal or personal copying and offer rewards to those who report violations. Washington Business Information, Inc. has won major payments in infringement actions against pharmaceutical manufacturers for photocopying its Food and Drug Letter.

Section 201(c) of the Copyright Act has produced electronic copyright issues for freelance articles and photography in electronic databases. Specifically, a series of cases involves whether or not permission is required from authors to place their articles on commercial databases or in the electronic public domain (e.g., MEDLINE®). In New York Times v. Tasini, the U.S. Supreme Court ruled that publishers cannot republish printed works electronically without obtaining permission from authors.[175] Tasini should not have much impact on new work as most publisher agreements now address electronic publication rights. Problematic, however, are older works published without a written agreement. The publishers argued unsuccessfully that the use of the articles in a database was no different from issuing a microfilm or microfiche copy of a newspaper. However, permissibility of electronic republication of an entire issue of a newspaper, magazine, newsletter without further payment to authors, remains unresolved.[176] Rather than attempt to contact freelancers and offer compensation for articles, some database producers have already begun to purge their databases of freelance contributions.

Photocopies fall within the territory of the Copyright Act. When sending copies of original articles, a statement to the effect that the copies are only for personal or private use must be made. The most effective way for any DI facility to protect itself against copy infringement lawsuits is to copy the page with the copyright notice and stamp the first page of the copies with a statement that the enclosed document is protected by copyright, thus putting the burden of responsibility on the recipient of the one copy. Such a notice might state, "This material is subject to the United States Copyright Law (17 U.S. Code): unauthorized copying may be prohibited by law."

The Computer Software Act of 1980 amended the Copyright Act to extend protection to computer software. However, copyright laws do not provide sufficient protection for information transmitted over the Internet and other information networks. Although copyright protection applies when copyrighted material is converted into a digital form, the havoc that cyberspace can wreak on copyright owner's rights cannot be overestimated. A debate is currently raging over whether existing copyright law can successfully adapt to the Internet.

Google settled two class action lawsuits regarding application of copyright protection to the indexing of scanned documents.[177,178] The lawsuits involve the Google Library Project, where in 2004, the company announced that it has entered into agreement with several libraries to digitalize books and other documents from those libraries' collections. The books and documents were also to be indexed for search purposes. Thus, the legal question of whether indexing for search purposes is fair use. Google was sued by publishers and authors when attempting to create an unprecedented extensive digitalized library of books. The authors and publishers claimed the scanning and indexing was not fair use but commercial in nature.[179] The case was settled and not decided by a court. However, the court denied the final settlement approval. Consequently, Google has now amassed a database of about 25 million books which no one is allowed to view.[180] Meanwhile, the

TABLE 11–5. MAJOR PROVISIONS OF THE TEACH ACT

- Expanded range of allowed works (e.g., nondramatic literary works; nondramatic musical works; audiovisual works).
- Expanded receiving locations. Educational institutions may now reach students through distance education at any location.
- Storage of transmitted content. Allows retention of the content and student access for a brief period of time especially with regard to digital transmission systems.
- Allows for digitalizing of analog works but only if the work is not already available in digital form.
- Educational institutions must now institute policies regarding copyright although the details of content of those policies are not provided.
- Transmission of content must be made solely to students officially enrolled in a course for which the transmission is made. Technological restrictions on access are required.

National Digital Public Library, and beginning in 2017, the National Digital Exchange, provides access to over 300,000 openly licensed titles.[181]

On October 3, 2002, Congress enacted the Technology, Education, and Copyright Harmonization (TEACH) Act, fully revising §110(2) of the U.S. Copyright Act governing the lawful uses of existing copyright materials in distance education. The TEACH Act defines the conditions and circumstances on which educators may clip pieces of text, images, sound, and other works and include them in distance education. Table 11-5 outlines the key provisions of the TEACH Act. If a particular use does not fit these conditions, one may still consider whether the use is a fair use.[182]

Access to works on the Internet or those publicly available does not automatically mean that these can be reproduced and reused without permission or royalty payment and, furthermore, some copyrighted works may have been posted on the Internet without authorization of the copyright holder. Publicly available is not to be confused with the legal concept of public domain, which comprises all works that are either no longer protected by copyright or never were. With the ease of retrieval of material electronically, copyright holders are likely to uncover those who are violating their copyright. Publishers who did not previously press for royalty payments of small segments of works can now trace the borrowing of snippets of text and create systems of payment and collection. Research downloading, with deletion of material after use, appears to be a fair use of the material. However, downloading to create a personal database and avoid payment of connect fees and higher user fees is illegal unless covered under special agreements between the database owner and subscriber. Also, linking to a work is always an option. Copyright law does not preclude anyone from linking to a copyright work on a website. However, it is important to remember that if the link contains copyrighted graphic material, it cannot be used without permission of the copyright holder. Recently, in Goldman v. Breitbart News Network, a case brought for copyright infringement for embedding a tweet that contained the plaintiff's copyrighted photo, the court did not find a triable copyright liability issue with regard to "embedding."[183] Further, although the Berne Convention is the principal copyright treaty, there is no such thing as an International copyright. The treaty obligates signatory countries to extend the protection of their copyright law to foreigners whose works are infringed within their borders.[184]

Current copyright law denies protection to compilations of facts unless such facts are arranged or organized with some minimal element of originality. Even then, it is the creative aspect of such arrangements or organization that may be protected and not the underlying facts themselves. Legislation has been repeatedly introduced, advocated primarily by large database companies, aimed at codifying into law a new unique form of intellectual property protection for databases. The situation is different in Europe where the European Union (EU) 1996 Database Directive grants copyright protection for the selection and arrangement of information in a European database, and calls downloading and hyperlinking unfair extraction of information.

Related to copyright infringement are plagiarism and fictitious reporting. Plagiarism is a legal offense or crime. The owner of a copyright (i.e., author) could sue the plagiarist in federal court for violation of the copyright. Fictitious reporting may simply constitute poor journalism or it may rise to the level of fraud or libel. Plagiarism involves not citing material while factitious reporting involves citing things that do not exist.

The definition of plagiarism is subjective and vague. History, facts, and ideas are not copyrighted, although they may be plagiarized. The addition of original material by the plagiarist in no way excuses the act of plagiarism. In fact, trivial changes in copied text, in an attempt to avoid copyright infringement, is specifically prohibited by the copyright law. Additionally, there is no fixed number or percentage of words that can be used without exposure to charges of plagiarism.[185] Verbatim quotes are permitted, provided they fall within the fair use protection. Software and web-based technologies (e.g., Turnitin®) now exist that can scan millions of documents almost instantly to compare what has been written before to what is being written today. Further information on plagiarism is contained in Chapter 13.

Privacy

HEALTH INSURANCE PORTABILITY AND ACCOUNTABILITY ACT OF 1996

Information security concerns are at the forefront of legal issues involved in electronic communications, specifically, questions of authenticity of medical or pharmacy records and confidentiality or privacy of the contents of medical and personal information of patients. Today, an individual's health information is often used for payment, QA, research, peer review, accreditation, and a multitude of other purposes. Further, communicating with patients using mobile devices such as iPhones, iPads, or Android phones is an increasing trend among health care providers.

Congress enacted the Health Insurance Portability and Accountability Act of 1996 (HIPAA).[186] While security and privacy under HIPAA are inextricably linked, there are distinctions. HIPAA Privacy Rule protects the privacy of individually identified health information. HIPAA Security Rule sets standards for the security of electronic protected health information (ePHI). The security rule standards define the administrative, physical, and technical safeguards (e.g., encryption) to protect the confidentiality, integrity, and availability of ePHI.

HIPAA's security standards are intended to protect the security of the environment in which health care information is maintained and transmitted. The privacy rule, by contrast, sets standards for how PHI should be controlled by setting forth what uses and disclosures are authorized or required and what rights patients have with respect to their health information. The privacy rule applies to information in any form, whereas the security rule only applies to ePHI.

Increased use of personal mobile devices such as tablets and smartphones by health care providers and professionals to access and exchange ePHI triggers the HIPAA security rule. In addition to the security risks inherent in the way these devices store data and/or lack of encryption software features, mobile devices are particularly vulnerable to loss and theft. The Office of the National Coordinator for Health Information Technology has outlined best practice steps organizations should take to manage mobile devices used by health care professionals.[187]

For pharmacies, the security standards are applicable only to ePHI, not paper, facsimile, nor telephone transmissions. HIPAA's privacy standards govern the use and disclosure of protected health information. Many aspects of HIPAA fall outside the scope of this chapter. In any event, reasonable steps should always be taken to ensure that fax, text, or email transmissions are sent to and received by the intended recipient. Examples of such steps for faxes include: confirming with the intended recipient that the receiving fax machine is located in a secure area or the intended recipient is waiting by the fax machine; preprogramming and testing fax numbers for frequent recipients of DI faxes to avoid errors associated with misdialing; double-checking the recipient's fax number prior to transmission; using a fax cover sheet with an erroneous transmission statement and advising to notify the sender immediately and arrange for return or destruction of the fax; promptly checking all fax confirmation sheets to determine that faxed material was received at the intended fax number.

Individual PHI is information, including demographic data, that relates to the following: the individual's past, present, or future physical or mental health or condition; the provision of health care to the individual, or the past, present, or future payment for the provision of health care to the individual, and that identifies the individual or for which there is a reasonable basis to believe it can be used to identify the individual.[188] Individually identifiable health information includes many common identifiers such as name, address, birth date, and social security number.

However, there are no restrictions on the use or disclosure of de-identified health information.[189] De-identified health information neither identifies nor provides a reasonable basis to identify an individual. There are two methods for de-identifying protected health information: the statistical method and the safe-harbor method via removal of certain identifiers.[190] De-identified data sets, which separate individuals' identities from their protected health information, are becoming increasingly available through the Centers for Medicare and Medicaid Services and the NIH.[191] This data is proving useful for outcomes and medical error research not associated with the original data collection protocol.

Under HIPAA, a covered entity may engage in research activities in four ways: (1) by using or disclosing only de-identified information, (2) by obtaining a waiver or an authorization from the individual to use and disclose the information for research purposes, (3) by obtaining a waiver of an authorization from an IRB, or (4) by representing that the use or disclosure is solely of the protected health information of a deceased individual. Clinical investigators are most likely to choose option 3.[192]

HIPAA specifically permits covered entities such as health care professionals or hospitals to report adverse events and other information relate to the quality, effectiveness, and safety of FDA-regulated products to both the manufacturers and directly to FDA. Under this exception, a pharmacist need not obtain an authorization from a patient before notifying a pharmaceutical company and the FDA that the patient had an adverse reaction to a drug manufactured by the drug company.[193] ❻ *It is important to keep in mind that the HIPAA Privacy Rule is not intended to disrupt or discourage adverse event reporting or DI in any way.*

In responding to DI questions, it is of utmost importance to obtain specific patient identification information including, but not limited to, patient name, age, height, weight, or medical record number. Nothing in HIPAA would diminish or affect that responsibility. In the DI arena, HIPAA allows disclosure of patient information for treatment, payment, and health care operations. Examples of health care operations include quality management, QA, outcomes evaluation, development of clinical guidelines, peer review, and credentialing. While not specifically mentioned, DI would appear to fall under both treatment and health care operations. In most instances, HIPAA should not affect DI requests from health care providers as patient identity is usually not required or is provided via medical record number only. However, when patient identifying information is communicated, protection of information within the DI center (or pharmacy) is an important HIPAA requirement. Policies and procedures governing use and disclosure of confidential information should be in place. These policies should include guidance on training and strategies for mitigating risks during all stages of the DI request processing (receipt, triage, and response). For example, procedures should be in place to verify the identity of the requestor of information. Patient information security safeguards should be in place, for example, requiring personal identifiers to be removed as soon as feasible, physical controls, software controls, and formal oversight.[194]

Case Study 11–4

A drug information question involves a patient who has a socially stigmatic disease. In responding to the question, the pharmacist needs to share the patient's PHI with the laboratory and pharmacokinetic services. However, in sharing this information the pharmacist discusses it as well as the diagnosis in an area where it was easily overheard by others not entitled to know. Additionally, the patient's personal information is faxed by the pharmacist to a fax machine in an unsecured area where many people have access to the fax machine.

- *Does HIPAA prohibit any of the pharmacist's actions?*
- *What safeguards should be taken when discussing the patient and his/her information?*
- *What reasonable steps are necessary to ensure that fax transmissions are sent and recorded by the intended recipient?*

There are several other situations in pharmacy practice where HIPAA compliance issues may be triggered. For example, in clinical case reports, whether for publication or teaching purposes, the patient should only be referred to via his or her initials, age or sex (e.g., RM, a 35-year-old female). When writing a case report or article for publication, always remove any patient identifiers. In some cases, patient consent may be required to publish the report.

HIPAA permits a pharmacist to counsel individuals other than the patient (e.g., a friend, family member, or neighbor picking up the patient's prescription) even though some of the patient's PHI may be revealed in such a situation. However, the regulation is clear that such disclosures must be limited and should only be made when the provider believes it is in the patient's best interest. For example, there can be no doubt that disclosing that the medication picked up is for treatment of HIV infection would not be necessary. Under HIPAA, personal representatives, defined as individuals legally authorized, under state or other applicable law, to make health care decisions on behalf of a patient, are to be treated in the same way as a patient. However, in some cases the personal representative's authority is limited to a specific matter, such as treatment for a life-threatening illness. In these cases, the personal representative may only access protected health information directly related to that illness. Additionally, many states have enacted laws that protect persons with illnesses that are seen as particularly stigmatizing, such as HIV, mental illness, and drug addiction. The Public Health Service Act and implementing regulations govern the confidentiality of substance abuse records maintained by federally assisted drug and alcohol abuse programs.[195]

Similarly, parents are considered the personal representative of a minor child and can access the minor's health records. Exceptions exist when the minor consents to health care and consent of the parent is not required under state or other law, or when the minor obtains health care at the direction of a court, or when the minor is emancipated. Other exceptions exist if a provider believes that a patient or minor is subject to abuse, neglect, or domestic violence by their personal representative.[196] Many states specifically authorize minors to consent to conceptive services, testing and treatment for HIV and other sexually transmitted diseases, prenatal care and delivery services, treatment for alcohol and drug abuse, and outpatient mental health care.

HIPAA also requires that pharmacies make a good faith effort to obtain a patient's acknowledgment that they have received a copy of the Notice of Privacy Practices. The notice describes how the pharmacy uses and discloses protected health information to carry out treatment, payment, or health care operations and the patient's rights. The notice is to be distributed to patients on or before the first treatment encounter. Where the prescription is being picked up by someone other than the patient, the pharmacy must attempt to deliver the notice to the patient. Examples of a good faith effort include providing the notice in the prescription bag or mailing the notice to the patient together with some type of return receipt means. However, the pharmacy is not in violation if the return receipt is not returned. The pharmacy need only document its efforts.[197]

Under HIPAA, pharmacists will be held accountable for handling confidential information properly. Civil and criminal penalties for violating patient confidentiality exist. A patient cannot use a HIPAA violation as a basis of a private lawsuit as there is no "right of private action." However, if the HIPAA violation amounts to negligence or malpractice then such cases may be brought under state laws. Plaintiffs use evidence of a HIPAA violation as proof of a breach of duty in negligence or state law invasion of privacy cases. Increasingly, HIPAA is being used as the basis of negligence claims.

In a recent interesting pharmacist employment case, pursuant to a discovery request, a pharmacy received a subpoena in a defamation case to provide records of patients who might have witnessed the defamatory statements made by the employer against the pharmacist. The employer refused to provide such records since they contain PHI. The court ruled that a covered entity may disclose PHI in any judicial proceeding in response to an order of a court or a discovery request that is not the subject of a court order if the covered entity receives satisfactory assurance from the requesting party that it has made reasonable efforts to obtain a qualified protective order that meets HIPAA requirements.[198]

HIPAA rules allow a covered entity to disclose PHI in response to a subpoena, discovery request, or other lawful process that is not accompanied by a court order, provided that the covered entity receives a written statement and accompanying documentation from the party seeking the information that reasonable efforts have been made either (1) to ensure that the individual(s) who are the subject of the information have been notified of the request, or (2) to secure a qualified protective order for the information.

COMMUNICATION PRIVACY

The Telephone Consumer Protection Act (TCPA) sets rules prohibiting unsolicited commercial faxes and text messages. A Federal Communication Commission (FCC) regulation implementing the act requires businesses and nonprofit groups to get signed written permission from clients or members before faxing unsolicited materials containing advertisements. Litigation under the TCPA is increasing, particularly in the area of junk fax class actions and insurance coverage for TCPA damages. There have also been a number of recent cases against pharmacies for sending robotexts to patients regarding pharmacy services or automated refill reminders without patients' consent.[199,200] The statute provides statutory damages of ~$16,000 for each violation, which are paid to the consumer.

Privacy is also an issue on the Internet (e.g., e-health sites) where the dominant privacy issue arises from the growing practice of data collection. Some websites are interactive; that is, they may require the patient to complete a survey or will send visitors a prescription refill reminder. These sites then link to privacy policies that address any concerns prospective patients may have about filling out an online survey. Disclosure of an online privacy policy together with an opt-out feature can provide assurances about the protection of consumer privacy and personal information. The policy should also address passive disclosure of information, e.g., from cookies (a feature which allows web servers to recognize a specific user or computer to access the website) or web server logs. Unfortunately, e-health sites were not included under HIPAA. Some of these e-health Internet sites violate their own privacy policies and transfer patient-identifiable information to third parties.[201]

Email use in health care has developed without encryption and HIPAA does not directly address email in any of its standards. However, because email may involve protected health information in electronic form, both HIPAA's privacy and security rules apply. The security of unencrypted email is low. Passwords, firewalls, and other conventional network security should exist to secure electronic DI communications.[202]

There has also been litigation in this area. In re Pharmatrak Inc. v. Privacy Litigation, the plaintiffs alleged that numerous pharmaceutical companies secretly intercepted and accessed their personal information through the use of computer cookies and other devices,[203] in violation of state and federal laws such as the Electronic Communications Privacy Act.[204]

Industry Support for Educational Activities

Many pharmacists attend conferences, sometimes funded by pharmaceutical companies to further their professional education. Dialogue between health professionals and the pharmaceutical industry is an opportunity to pass along scientific and educational information, and product risks and benefits. Such dialogue encourages and supports medical research, while providing the health professional with an opportunity to address questions, discuss issues, and offer expertise.

GUIDELINES AND GUIDANCE

❼ *The FDA, the American Council for Continuing Medical Education (ACCME) and the Pharmaceutical Research and Manufacturers of America (PhRMA)[205] have established educational policies, guidelines, or guidances which allow communication between industry and the continuing medical education (CME) providers* with the proviso that the final decisions and control rest with the accredited provider. The Office of Inspector General (OIG) issued a Guidance that prohibits the pharmaceutical industry from direct communication with CME providers and calls for an intermediary organization to develop CME programs.[206] The following factors are provided in the OIG Guidance: Does the arrangement skew clinical decision-making? Is the information complete, accurate, and non-misleading? Does the arrangement have the potential to be a disguised discount or result in inappropriate over- or underutilization? Does the arrangement raise patient safety, quality, or care concerns? Importantly, for pharmacists providing DI as industry clinical education consultants or medical liaisons, the Accreditation Council for Pharmacy Education (ACPE) no longer accredits pharmaceutical and biomedical manufacturers.[207] However, not all states actually require all of a pharmacist's continuing education activities to be accredited by the ACPE.[208]

The PhRMA Code on Interactions with Healthcare Professionals, which became effective in July 2002, and updated in January 2009 and again in September 2019 is the most specific and stringent and deals with various interactions between industry and health care professionals, such as informational presentations, professional meetings, consultant activities, scholarships and educational funds, and educational and practice-related items.[209] Scholarships for pharmacists, students, and residents to attend selected educational conferences may be provided. Salient features of the latest PhRMA Code are found in Table 11-6 and at: https://www.phrma.org/-/media/Project/PhRMA/PhRMA-Org/PhRMA-Org/PDF/A-C/Code-of-Interaction_FINAL21.pdf.

The FDA Guidance seeks to draw a distinction between educational activities that the FDA considers nonpromotional and those it considers promotional. The distinction is important, especially with regard to off-label uses, which can be an important component of educational activities. The FDA's Factors to Determine Independence of the Educational Activity are found in Table 11-7.[210]

Some health care institutions have established their own best practices approach to developing ethical guidelines for pharmaceutical industry support. The practice involves a process similar to weighing the risks and benefits of a particular medication or therapeutic intervention, whereby each proposal for support can be viewed as having potential value, which may or may not outweigh any potential drawbacks inherent in the involvement of funding from a for-profit company. Often a committee assesses proposals based on the apparent balance between these factors and a set of guidelines developed by the institution.[211]

In general, most policies and procedures prohibit acceptance of commercial support of educational activities if such acceptance would appear to (1) create an atmosphere limiting academic freedom and the free exchange of ideas and information, (2) introduce bias or otherwise threaten objectivity, (3) create a conflict of interest, or (4) be in conflict with the mission and profit status of the health care organization.[212]

RELATIONSHIP TO THE ANTI-KICKBACK STATUTE

Particular arrangements between pharmacists and the pharmaceutical industry pose potential risks under the Anti-Kickback Statute. The Anti-Kickback Statute makes it a criminal offense to knowingly and willfully offer, pay, solicit, or receive any remuneration (in cash or in kind) to induce (or in exchange for) the purchasing, ordering, or recommending of any good or service reimbursable by any federal health care program.[213] Funding that is conditioned, in whole or in part, on the purchase of product implicates the statute, even if the educational or research purpose is legitimate. Several cases hold that intent is improper if one purpose, not the sole or even primary purpose, is to induce the purchase or recommendation of a company's goods or services.[214,215] When a grant is provided to a customer or potential customer, it may violate the Anti-Kickback Statute if one purpose is to induce the customer to buy the company's product. Educational grants, for example, were at the heart of the $161 million Caremark, LLC settlement[216] and research grants were at the heart of the $450,000 Hoffman-La Roche, Inc. settlement.[217] Furthermore, to the extent the manufacturer has any influence over the substance of an educational program or the presenter, there is a risk that the educational program may be used for inappropriate marketing purposes.

In the area of DI, specific practices that may be problematic under the Anti-Kickback Statute include gifts, use of pharmacists who are customers as consultants or members of

TABLE 11–6.   PHRMA CODE ON INTERACTIONS WITH HEALTH CARE PROFESSIONALS

- Formulary Committees/Clinical Practice Guidelines (CPG)
  - Such individuals may serve as speakers or consultants to pharmaceutical companies, but all such relationships must be disclosed to the committees they sit on.
  - Upon disclosure, such individuals must follow the procedures for that Formulary/CPG Committee which may include recusing themselves from decisions relating to the medicine for which they have provided speaking or consulting services.
- Gifts
  - Generally prohibited.
  - Exceptions—$100 or less that benefits patients or educate health care professionals; e.g., medical textbooks or anatomical models permitted, but not a DVD or CD player or stethoscopes that are primarily used for treating patients.
  - Pens, pads, etc., no longer permitted.
  - Product samples allowed.
- Meals
  - Modest meals (as judged by local standards) accompanying informational presentations.
  - Are provided in a manner conducive to informational communication.
  - Can only be offered occasionally.
  - Can only be **directly** provided in-office or inhospital settings (no restaurants or resorts; "take out" or "dine & dash" meals are not appropriate).
  - Cannot include spouses or other guests.
- Entertainment
  - Prohibited (regardless of value).
  - Prohibited for consultants as well.
  - May sponsor meals or reception at conferences
- Spouses.
  - Never appropriate for lodging, travel, meals, entertainment.
- Consultants
  - Must be bona fide via written contract, appropriate venue (e.g., resorts are not appropriate venues), and selection criteria related to purpose of service.
  - Compensation must be reasonable and based on fair market value.
  - Reimbursement for travel, lodging, and meals must be reasonable.
  - Special disclosure requirements for health care professionals that set up formularies or develop clinical practice guidelines—disclosure requirements extend 2 years beyond the terms of any speaker or consultant arrangements.
  - Legitimate need identified in advance of entering into agreement required (token consulting or advisory arrangements are not permitted).
  - Number of consultants cannot be greater than number reasonably needed to achieve purpose.
- Financial Sponsorship of Educational Conferences
  - Support should be provided to CPE sponsor, not individual speaker/author.
  - Sponsor should control selection of content, faculty, educational materials, and venue.
  - Faculty, but not attendees or spouses, may be paid/reimbursed for time, travel, and lodging.
  - Exception—companies may pay for travel/lodging for students to attend educational conferences; educational institutions must select individual students.

continued

TABLE 11–6. PHRMA CODE ON INTERACTIONS WITH HEALTH CARE PROFESSIONALS (*CONTINUED*)

- Speaker Programs and Speaker Training Meetings.
  - Ensure neither an inducement nor reward for prescribing a particular product.
  - Should be modest by local standards
  - Should occur in a venue and manner conducive to informational communication (again, no resorts)
  - Should provide scientific or educational value
  - Can recommend to continuing education providers topics of interest that manufacturer would sponsor
  - Companies must develop policies addressing speakers (e.g., must be separate from CME activities)
  - Speakers should recuse themselves from decisions about the medications for which they have provided speaking/consulting services

TABLE 11–7. FACTORS USED BY THE FDA TO DETERMINE INDEPENDENCE OF AN EDUCATIONAL ACTIVITY

- Control of content and selection of faculty: Is there scripting or other actions designed to influence the content by the supporting company?
- Disclosures: Does it include company funding the program, relationship between provider(s) and presenters to the supporting company, and off-label discussion?
- The focus of the program: Does the title accurately represent the presentation? Is there fair-balanced educational discussion?
- Relationship between provider and supporting company: Is there a legal, business, or other relationship between the parties?
- Provider involved in sales or marketing: Are provider employees also doing marketing or promotional programs?
- Provider's demonstrated failure to meet standards: Does the provider have a history of biased programs?
- Multiple presentations: Do they serve public health interests?
- Audience selection: Is the audience generated by sales or marketing departments to influence marketing goals?
- Opportunities for discussion: Is there an opportunity for meaningful discussion?
- Dissemination: Is the supporting company distributing additional information after the activity; unless requested by participant and then through an independent provider?
- Ancillary promotional activities: Are promotional activities taking place in the educational meeting room?
- Complaints: Are provider(s), faculty, or others complaining about the supporting company?

speaker's bureaus, and questionable research grants. Problems under the Anti-Kickback Statute could arise where the DI pharmacist participates in any of these activities and also advises on formulary choices or is a member of a formulary committee or subcommittee or is involved with purchasing decisions. If a product or service is recommended and the recommender stands to make financial gain from it, and that service is paid for in part or in whole by the federal government, that person may be violating the Anti-Kickback Statute. Similarly, no gifts should be accepted if there are strings attached.

Educational activities or speakers can be funded by the pharmaceutical industry, whereas promotional marketing activities that purport to be of an educational purpose but serve no direct patient benefit are prohibited. Hiring DI pharmacists under the guise of a consultant or advisor, or focus group participant or advisory board member, or even as a speaker at a meeting, could be considered payments for referrals. Similarly, compensating DI pharmacists as consultants, when all they do is attend conferences primarily in a passive capacity, is suspect. Other suspect activities include compensation for speaking, researching, listening to marketing pitches, or providing preceptor, shadowing, or ghostwriting services. However, where the pharmacist is compensated for actual, reasonable, and necessary services, the activities may be considered legitimate.

The Anti-Kickback Statute prohibits involvement with research contracts that come through a pharmaceutical company's marketing department, research not reviewed by the manufacturer's scientific or medical department, research that is unnecessarily duplicative or not needed for any purpose other than the generation of business, and postmarketing research used as a pretense for product promotion.[218] Manufacturers should use firewalls (i.e., ethical barriers prohibiting exchange of confidential information between different departments of an organization) for marketing and grant-funding activities to demonstrate that grants are bona fide and not improperly influenced by marketing considerations. The Anti-Kickback Statute requires that grants be given in exchange for fair market value research consideration. This is often difficult to accomplish, since the precise costs and schedules of research activities are not knowable in advance and sometimes not conducive to being reduced to written agreements.

Conclusion

By now, the reader has undoubtedly discovered that the liability aspects of DI include more than just negligence. Liability for off-label uses, consumer advertising, copyright infringement, liability issues unique to the Internet, privacy concerns, and industry support for educational activities are all connected to DI practice. The DI practitioner and pharmacists in general must at least have a working awareness of these areas. DI services provide a foundation for the provision of pharmacist supervised patient care. To date, pharmacists providing DI have only speculated about and not actually faced malpractice lawsuits. Hopefully, this chapter has shed some light on how courts would react to malpractice suits against pharmacists for negligent provision of DI. However, legal precedents cannot be relied upon to predict the future. There is no way to predict how a court will rule in a particular case. What can be done to avoid malpractice and other causes of action? First, always strive for excellence. Second, have good relations with requestors and make sure they are aware of alterations or modifications in information systems and sources. Third, make no outrageous claims about the accuracy and thoroughness of the information provided. Finally, pharmacists should carry their own malpractice insurance policy.

The future of pharmacists as DI providers clearly lies in their ability to provide consultative DI services. While in the past, most of the reported appellate decisions against pharmacists have involved routine dispensing errors, not mistakes in DI or other expanded practice areas, in the future this situation may change. Pharmacists should not be preoccupied with the risk of incurring liability, but should take the necessary steps to limit exposure and develop an appreciation of modern legal philosophy. Definitive guidelines need not emerge only through court decisions. It remains most important that DI be recognized as a liability-reducing factor for the institution and personnel who provide health care to patients.

Self-Assessment Questions

1. All of the following would result in holding the pharmacist providing drug information to a higher standard **EXCEPT**:
   a. The drug information query pertains to nuclear pharmacy and the pharmacist completed a residency in this specialty and is a Board Certified Nuclear Pharmacist (BCNP).
   b. The pharmacist knows the patient is pregnant and ibuprofen is prescribed.
   c. The pharmacist passed the pharmacy licensure exam with a perfect score.
   d. The pharmacist runs a drug information center.
   e. The pharmacist is aware that the patient is on oral contraceptives and aprepitant is prescribed.

2. Under which of the following scenarios is court likely to decide a pharmacist had a "duty to warn" a patient?
   a. The patient is prescribed a sulfa-based antibiotic. A sulfa allergy is found in the computer system. The pharmacist overrides the computer system's flag and dispenses the drug. The patient develops Stevens-Johnson syndrome and dies.
   b. A manufacturer of metoclopramide fails to update its labeling to include tardive dyskinesia. A pharmacist dispenses the drug and does not provide a patient warning regarding tardive dyskinesia, which the patient then develops.
   c. The pharmacist dispenses trazodone and fails to warn the patient about priapism from the drug. The package insert does not mention this adverse effect and the patient develops priapism.
   d. The patient denies having a penicillin allergy. Amoxicillin is dispensed and the patient develops an anaphylactic reaction.
   e. The patient undergoes surgery at a hospital and receives aprepitant postoperatively prior to discharge. No one counsels the patient regarding the drug

interaction with oral contraceptives and the need to use a second form of birth control for 28 days. The patient becomes pregnant.

3. Which of the following drug information scenarios may result in vicarious liability?
   a. The pharmacist undertakes to warn the patient about the adverse effects from ciprofloxacin, but fails to warn of tendonitis.
   b. The pharmacist is too busy to counsel the patient on the warning against sunbathing while on doxycycline. She instructs the pharmacy technician to counsel the patient instead. The technician instructs the patient not to take a bath while taking the drug. The patient goes to the beach and harm results.
   c. The pharmacist receives a drug information query from a prescriber asking what the common adverse effects of metformin are. The pharmacist provides the correct response; the prescriber counsels the patient incorrectly.
   d. b and c
   e. a and c

4. All of the following are Health Care Economic Information (HCEI) **EXCEPT**:
   a. A slide deck showing the economic consequences of absent work days as a result of signs and symptoms associated with a disease for which the drug is indicated.
   b. Studies regarding the treatment impact of the drug on length of hospital stay.
   c. A payor brochure based on drug utilization data from a health plan database.
   d. An evidence dossier assessing patient compliance/adherence with a drug for its approved indication.
   e. A reprint that states that the drug in question "Allows health care providers to optimize pain relief."

5. Which of the following statements is/are **FALSE**:
   a. The drug information consultation between the pharmacist and patient has been determined by courts to be privileged.
   b. Since the drug information provided is oral and not written, no liability can attach.
   c. A malpractice case is brought against the pharmacist who failed to warn the patient about driving while taking the medication. The pharmacist is not protected via his professional liability insurance policy if the lawsuits brought after the policy expired, even if the event occurred while the policy was effective.
   d. b and c are false.
   e. a, b, and c are false.

6. A violation of the anti-kickback statute would occur when:
   a. The pharmacist contacts the patient's physician to recommend the patient be switched to a particular drug within a therapeutic class. For each patient, the pharmacist is able to obtain a switch, he/she receives a fee from the pharmaceutical company.
   b. A hospital pharmacist is preparing the monograph for P&T and making the recommendation whether the hospital should add the medication to formulary or not. The pharmacist's spouse is employed by the pharmaceutical company that manufactures the medication.
   c. Compensation is provided to a drug information pharmacist by a pharmaceutical editor to ghost write a review article about their new product. The pharmaceutical company makes the final decision regarding the article content.
   d. b and c
   e. a, b, and c

7. Which of the following is correct with regard to off-label use of medication?
   a. An investigational new drug application (IND) is needed before a medication may be prescribed for an off-label use.
   b. Patient-informed consent is necessary before a pharmacist should recommend an off-label use to a prescriber.
   c. Off-label use of a medication is common in certain patient groups such as pediatric patients.
   d. Off-label refers to the fact that the use is not listed in any drug information reference.
   e. None of the above.

8. Problems using the Internet for responding to drug information queries include:
   a. Information may contain innocent or deliberate mistakes.
   b. There are no laws for assuring the accuracy of information on the Internet.
   c. May include unpublished (not peer reviewed) information.
   d. The information may be outdated or not evidence-based.
   e. All of the above.

9. DM is a new pharmacist at XYZ Hospital. During his first week, he identifies a great case report for publication. He takes a photo of a mole on the patient's face and talks about his patient case in the elevator. He leaves his computer with patient information open unattended while he grabs lunch. At lunch, he sees Dr. Jones so they sit alone together and discuss the mutual patient. When DM presents his case, he invites Dr. Jones to the presentation. The first slide reveals the patient's medical record number. When he publishes the case report, he

includes a patient identifier. How many separate violations of HIPAA has pharmacist DM committed?
a. Three
b. Four
c. Five
d. Six
e. Eight

10. Which of the following would constitute fair use under the copyright law?
   a. Obtaining a copyright to prohibit use of a list of medications that cause seizures.
   b. Scanning and distributing to all drug information colleagues an entire chapter from Drug Information: A Guide for Pharmacists.
   c. You, Professor Lee, photocopy an excerpt from an article which is about 3% of the work. You will only be using the excerpt for one lecture of a course for one semester only.
   d. You, Professor Lee, photocopy without permission multiple copies of a 6000-word article every semester for classroom use in both your therapeutics and communication classes.
   e. Your colleague has written an article which is currently unpublished. He requests that you critique it and you borrow several paragraphs verbatim in your new book.

11. Which of the following would **NOT** constitute a product communication that is Consistent with FDA-Required Labeling (CFL)?
   a. A firm's communication describes a rate of occurrence of headache observed in clinical practice and this rate is slightly higher than that in the FDA-required labeling.
   b. A product communication provides information from a head-to-head study indicating that a manufacturer's drug approved to treat hypertension in adults has superior efficacy to another drug that is approved for the same indication.
   c. FDA-required labeling for a product identifies nausea as a potential adverse reaction and further indicates that the product can be taken with or without food. A firm's product communication provides information about how taking the product with food might reduce nausea.
   d. A product is approved for cardiovascular disease. A firm's communication provides information about using the product to treat diabetes.
   e. Information on long-term safety of a product approved for chronic use in FDA-required labeling is based on a 24-week study. A firm provides postmarketing information for its product regarding safety over 18 months.

12. Which of the following statements is **INACCURATE** under HIPAA?
    a. Permits pharmacists to report adverse events to manufacturers and directly to the FDA without patient authorization.
    b. HIPAA allows disclosure of patient information in the handling of drug information queries but requires protection of information within the drug information center.
    c. Permits communication which discloses PHI between a pharmacist and other health care professionals with regard to a specific patient's therapy.
    d. HIPAA privacy standards do not apply to email or social media communication.
    e. All the above statements are allowed under HIPAA.

13. Which of the following actions would constitute a HIPAA violation?
    a. You publish a case report and identify the patient by his initials.
    b. You fax a response to a drug information query containing PHI to an incorrect fax number.
    c. You are conducting research using de-identified health information. You lose the flash drive containing this information.
    d. A patient you are following develops a serious, unexpected adverse drug reaction. You report the reaction to the FDA.
    e. a and b are HIPAA violations.

14. Which of the following is in accordance with the 2019 PhRMA Code on Interactions with Health Care Professionals?
    a. A weekly meal of lobster and steak is offered in connection with informational presentations by field sales representatives at ABC hospital pharmacy.
    b. Inexpensive opera tickets are provided periodically to Directors of Pharmacy who are on the pharmaceutical company's speaker's bureau.
    c. Continuing medical education (CME) grants are awarded by a pharmaceutical company's marketing department.
    d. Honoraria is provided to nonconsultant health care professional attendees at pharmaceutical company-sponsored meetings.
    e. Pharmaceutical company support is provided for third-party educational conferences.

15. In which of the following scenarios would education be considered promotional activities?
    a. A portion of the presentation content is directed or scripted by the pharmaceutical company.
    b. Promotional activities are taking place in the educational meeting room.
    c. Disclosures do not mention that the pharmaceutical company has funded the program.

d. Educational session evaluations report that the session was biased toward a particular product.

e. All of the above.

REFERENCES

1. Ghaibi S, Iperna H, Gabay M. ASHP guidelines of the pharmacist's role in providing drug information. Am J Health-Syst Pharm. 2015;72:573-7.
2. Southwick AF. The law of hospital and health care administration. 2nd ed. Ann Arbor: Health Administration Press; 1988.
3. Nathan JP, Gim S. Responding to drug information requests. Am J Health-Syst Pharm. 2009;66:706, 710-1.
4. Joint Commission of Pharmacy Practitioners. The Pharmacist's Patient Care Process. 2014 May 29.
5. Baker K. OBRA '90 mandate and its impact on pharmacist's standard of care. Drake Law R. 1996;44:503, 508.
6. Burns K, Spies A. A pharmacist's duty to warn: trying to make sense of all the legal inconsistencies. Rx Ipsa Loquitur. 2008;35:1-2.
7. Kelly WN, Krause EC, Krowinski WJ, Small TR, Drane JF. National survey of ethical issues presented to drug information centers. Am J Hosp Pharm. 1990;47:2245-50.
8. Doppelparker Case, OLG Karllsrule GRUR 1979 P267.
9. Perkins E. Johns Hopkins' tragedy: could librarians have prevented a death? [Internet]. [Cited 2017 Mar 18]. Available from: http://newsbreaks.infotoday.com/NewsBreaks/Johns-Hopkins-Tragedy-Could-Librarians-Have-Prevented-a-Death-17534.asp
10. 805 S.W.2d, 380 (Tenn. Ct. App. 1991).
11. 453 N.Y.S.2d 121 (1987).
12. Whiting v Rite Aid Pharmacy, 2014 U.S. Dist. Lexis 87354 (D. Utah, Jun 24, 2014).
13. 544 N.W.2d 727, 731 (Mich. Ct. App. 1991).
14. Fink JL. Ignore computer alerts at your peril? Pharm Times. 2013 Jan:56.
15. 191 A.D.2d 178, 594 N.Y.S.2d 195 (1993).
16. 579 N.E.2d 1255 (Ill. App. 1991) reversed by 605 N.E.2d 557 (Ill. 1992).
17. Brushwood DB. Pharmacist malpractice liability: no loopholes in OBRA-90's proDUR requirement. Pharmacy Today. 2019;25(19):38.
18. Deed v. Walgreens, 2004 WL 2943271 (Conn. Super. Ct.).
19. K-Mart v. Chamblin, 612 S.E.2d 25 (Ga. Ct. App. 2005).
20. Brushwood DB, Belgado BS. Judicial policy and expanded duties for pharmacists. Am J Health-Syst Pharm. 2002;59:455-7.
21. 780 So.2d 930 (Fla. App. 2001).
22. 1 S.W.3d 519 (Mo. App. 1999).
23. 737 N.E.2d 650 (Ill. App. 2000).
24. 30 S.W.3d 455 (Tex. App. 2000).
25. Urbaniak v. American Drug Stores, LLC, (Il. App. 2019) 180248.

26. Tutwiler v. Sandoz, Inc, 726 F. Appx. 753719024 (11th Cir. 2018).

27. McDaniel v. Upsher-Smith Labs, Inc., 893 F. 3d 941 (6th Cir. 2018).

28. Larrimore v. Springhill Memorial Hospital. LEXIS 38:008 WL 54 2000 (Ala. 2008). CV-02-3205, 1051748.

29. HPSO Cases. Pharmacists and medical malpractice: case Study with risk management strategies [cited 2019 Sep 15]. Available from: http://www.hpso.com/landing/pharmacist-legal-case-study-v2-index?refID=BP1BWi

30. 827 F. Supp. 1522 (D. Nev. 1993).

31. 598 N.Y.S.2d 592 (App. Div. 1993).

32. Hall M, Honey W. The evolving legal responsibility of the pharmacist. J Pharm Market Manage. 1994;8:27-41.

33. Brushwood DB. The pharmacist's drug information responsibility after McKee v. American Home Products. Food Drug L J. 1993;48:377-410.

34. In re Michael A. Gabert, No. 92 PHM 21 (Wis. Pharmacy Examining Bd., Dec. 14, 1993).

35. Rees W, Rohde NF, Bolan R. Legal issues for an integrated information center. J Am Soc Info Sci. 1991;42:132-6.

36. Restatement (Second) of Torts, Section 311, 1982.

37. Beaird S, Coley R, Blunt JR. Assessing the accuracy of drug information responses from drug information centers. Ann Pharmacother. 1994;28:707-11.

38. Calis KA, Anderson DW, Auth DA, Mays DA, Turcasso NM, Meyer CC, Young LR. Quality of pharmacotherapy consultations provided by drug information centers in the United States. Pharmacotherapy. 2000;20:830-6.

39. McDonagh AF, Lightner DA. Attention to stereochemistry. Chem & Engin News. 2003 Feb. 3, p. 2.

40. Aungst TD. Medical applications for pharmacists using mobile devices. Ann Pharmacother. 2013;47:1088-95.

41. Loy JS, Ali EE, Yap KY. Quality assessment of medical apps that target medication-related problems. J Manage Care Spec Pharm. 2016;22(10):1124-40.

42. Talwar SR, Crudele NT, Dankiewicz EH, Crudele NT, Haddox JD. Implementing a process to review product-specific misinformation in online drug information compendia. Ther Innov Reg Sci. 2015;49:262-8.

43. U.S. Food and Drug Administration. Mobile medical applications: guidance for industry and Food and Drug Administration staff. 2015 Feb.

44. In re Prempro Products, 03-CV-015070-WRW, U.S. Dist Ct., E.D. Arkansas (Jul 17, 2009).

45. Clauson KA. Pharmacists: are your drug information databases accurate? U.S. Pharmacist. 2008 Sep:54-63.

46. Gray JA. Strict liability for the dissemination of dangerous information? Law Lib J. 1990;82:497-517.

47. 694 F. Supp. 1216 (D. Md. 1988).

48. Bundesqe Richtsaf. Neue Juristische Wochenschrift (1970), 1973.

49. 110 Misc.2d 799, 442 N.Y.S.2d 945 (N.Y. Sup. 1981).

50. 938 F.2d 1033 (9th Cir. 1991).

51. 432 F. Supp. 990 (E.D.N.Y. 1977).

52. Sanofi Sues Decision Aid Maker for "Injurious Falsehood." Pharmafile. Available from: http://www.pharmafile.com/news/198126/sanofi-sues-decision-aid-maker-injurious-falsehood

53. Containment Technologies v. ASHP, 2009 US Dist LEXIS 25421 (Mar 26, 2009), 2009 US Dist LEXIS 76270 (Aug 26, 2009).

54. Talley CR. Affirming science and peer-review publishing. Am J Health-Syst Pharm. 2009;66:896.

55. Prod. Liab. Rep (CCH), Section 8968 (S.D.N.Y., Feb 20, 1981).

56. Hardin v. PDX, Inc., No. A137035, 2014 WL 2768863 (Cal. Ct. App., Jun 19, 2014).

57. Restatement (Second) of Torts Sec. 324A.

58. Brannigan VM, Dayhoff RE. Liability for personal injuries caused by defective medical computer programs. Am J L Med. 1981;122:132-3.

59. Joyce EJ. Software bugs: a matter of life and liability. Datamation. 1987 May 15:88-92.

60. Gage D, McCormick J. Case 108-we did nothing wrong. Panama's Cancer Institute. Baseline. 2004;28:32-47.

61. Cuzamanes PT. Automation of medical records: the electronic superhighway and its ramifications for health care providers. J Pharm Law. 1997;6:19.

62. Brocklesby v. Jeppesen, 767 F.2d 1288 (9th Cir. 1985), cert. denied, 474 U.S. 1101 (1986).

63. 472 U.S. 749 (1985).

64. 137 Misc.2d 94, 520 N.Y.S.2d 334 (N.Y. Civ. Ct. 1987).

65. Amerson AB. Drug information centers: an overview. Drug Info J. 1986;20:173-8.

66. 705 P.2d 1360 (Ariz. Ct. App. 1985).

67. Rumore MM, Rosenberg JM, Costa JG. The pharmacist and the law: legal aspects of providing drug information. Wellcome Trends Hosp Pharm. 1989 Dec;6-8.

68. Gallegos v. Wood, 2016 U.S. Dist. LEXIS 48150 (D. N.M., Mar 31, 2016).

69. Gough AR, Healey KM, Rupp SR. Poison control centers, from aspirin to PCBs and the scarlet runner beam: a study of legal anomaly and social necessity. Santa Clara L R. 1983;23:791-809.

70. Brushwood DB, Simonsmeier LM. Drug information for patients: duties of the manufacturer, pharmacist, physician, and hospital. J Leg Med. 1986;7:279-341.

71. Curtis JA, Greenberg MI. Legal liability of medical toxicologists serving as poison control center consultants: a review of relevant legal statutes and survey of the experience of medical toxicologists. J Med Toxicol. 2009;5(3):144-8.

72. 656 P.2d 483 (Wash. 1983).

73. Collins v. Walgreen Co., 2013 U.S. Dist LEXIS 81422 (E.D. Cal., Jun 10, 2013).

74. LeFrock v. Walgreen Co., 77 F. Supp.3d 1199 (M.D. Fla. 2015).

75. Goulmamine v. CVS Pharmacy, Inc., 3:15-cv-00370-REP (U.S. Dist. VA, Oct 9, 2015).

76. Gray JA. The health sciences librarian's exposure to malpractice liability because of negligent provision of information. Bull Med Libr Assoc. 1989;77:33-7.

77. Mintz AP. Information practice and malpractice. Libr J. 1985:38-43.

78. Fidelity Leasing Corp. v. Dun & Bradstreet, Inc., 494 F. Supp. 786 (E.D. Pa. 1980).

79. Baker KR. Do people sue people who counsel? Drug Topics. 2007 Dec 3:4.

80. Food and Drug Administration [Internet]. Center for Drug Evaluation and Research, Office of Medical Policy, Division of Drug Marketing, Advertising and Communications, Comparative Advertising, Fair Balance, and the Patient-Consumer; c2003 [cited 2019 Sep 15]. Available from: http://www.fda.gov/downloads/AboutFDA/CentersOffices/OfficeofMedicalProductsandTobacco/CDER/UCM213627.pdf

81. Food and Drug Administration. Guidance for industry: internet/social media platforms with character space limitations—presenting risk and benefit information for prescription drugs and medical devices. 2014 Jun.

82. Food and Drug Administration. Guidance for industry: fulfilling regulatory requirements for postmarketing submissions of interactive promotional media for prescription human and animal drugs and biologics. 2014 Jan.

83. Food and Drug Administration. Guidance for industry: internet/social media platforms—correcting independent third-party misinformation about prescription drug and medical devices. 2014 Jun.

84. Food and Drug Administration. Guidance for industry: consumer-directed broadcast advertisements. 1997 Aug 8.

85. 21 U.S.C. § 352(n).

86. 21 C.F.R. § 202.1(e).

87. Wilkes MS, Bell RA, Kravitz RL. Direct-to-consumer prescription drug advertising: trends, impact, and implications. Health Aff. 2000:19:110-28.

88. Anon. FDA officials describe agency actions on problematic drug promotion activity. BNA Pharm Law Industry Report. 2003 Sep 19;1(35):1006.

89. Schwartz TM. Consumer-directed prescription drug advertising and the learned intermediary rule. Food Drug L J. 1991;46:829-37.

90. PDRnet. PDR Network [cited 2019 Sep 15]. Available from:https://www.pdr.net/

91. Food and Drug Administration. Guidance for industry: brief summary and adequate directions for use—disclosing risk information in consumer-directed print advertisements and promotional labeling for prescription drugs. 2015 Aug.

92. 161 N.J. 1, 734 A.2d 1245 (N.J. 1999).

93. Ferrelli JJ. Perez creates exception to learned intermediary doctrine. New Jersey Law J. 1999 Sep 20.

94. Gebhart F. Here comes the judge. Drug Topics. 2005:26-32.

95. Pharmacist's Mutual [Internet]. [Cited 2019 Sep 15]. Available from: https://apps.phmic.com/RMNLFlipbook/06_2011/index.html

96. Pharmacist's Mutual [Internet]. [Cited 2019 Sep 9]. Available from: apps.phmic.com/rmn/flipbook/04_2016/drilling-down-on-drug-errors.html

97. Rumore MM. Direct-to-consumer advertising of prescription drugs: emerging legal and regulatory issues. Hosp Pharm. 2004;39:1058-68.

98. New Jersey Citizen Action v. Schering-Plough Corporation. 367 N.J. Super. 8, 842 A.2d 174 (App. Div. 2004). Available from: http://www.prescriptionaccess.org/lawsuitssettlements/past_lawsuits?id=0011

99. Anderson v. SmithKline Beecham Corp., W.D. Wash. No. CV 03-2886-L (Sep 22, 2003).

100. Wyeth v. Levine 129 S. Ct. 1187, 1200 (2009).

101. Patsy BM, Furburg CD, Ray WA, Weiss NS. Potential for conflict of interest in the evaluation of suspected adverse drug reactions: cerivastin and risk for rhabdomyolysis. JAMA. 2004;292:2585-90.

102. FDC Act § 312.7.

103. 21 U.S.C. §§ 360.999, 403 (1998).

104. 21 C.F.R. § 99.101(a)(3)-(4).

105. Ward SM. WLF and the two-click rule: The First Amendment inequity of the Food and Drug Administration's regulation of off-label drug use information on the Internet. Food Drug L J. 2001;56:41-56.

106. Kennedy D. The old file-drawer problem. Science. 2004;305:451.

107. Dept. HHS, Food and Drug Administration, Office of the Commissioner. Guidance for industry. Good reprint practices for the distribution of medical journal articles and medical-scientific reference publications on unapproved new uses of approved drugs and approved or cleared medical devices. 2009 Jan.

108. Dept. HHS, Food and Drug Administration, Office of the Commissioner. Guidance for industry. Distributing scientific and medical publications on unapproved new use-recommended practices. 2014 Feb.

109. Dept. HHS, Food and Drug Administration, Center for Drug Evaluation and Research, Center for Biologics Evaluation and Research, Center for Veterinary Medicine, Center for Devices and Radiological Health. Guidance for industry. Medical product communications that are consistent with FDA-required labeling—questions and answers. 2018 Jun.

110. Dept. HHS, Food and Drug Administration, Center for Drug Evaluation and Research, Center for Biologics Evaluation and Research, Center for Veterinary Medicine, Center for Devices and Radiological Health. Guidance for industry. Drug and device manufacturer communications with payors, formulary committees, and similar entities—questions and answers. 2018 Jun.

111. United States ex rel. King v. Solvay S.A., No. 06-2662, 2016 U.S. Dist. LEXIS 14804 (Feb 8, 2016 S.D. Tex.).

112. The Medical Science Liaison: Examining the Role. CME Briefing, 2002 Jul-Sep:3-5.

113. Dept. HHS, Food and Drug Administration, Center for Drug Evaluation and Research, Center for Biologics Evaluation and Research, Center for Veterinary Medicine, Center for Devices and Radiological Health. Guidance for industry. Responding to unsolicited requests for off-label information about prescription drugs and medical devices. 2011 Dec.

114. American Academy of Pediatrics. Policy Statement 2002;110-1, 2002 July 18:1-3.

115. Fugh-Berman A, Melnick D. Off-label promotion, on-target sales. PLoS Med 2008;5(10) [cited 2019 Sep 15]. Available from:http://www.medscape.com/viewarticle/704698

116. Understanding the approval process for new cancer treatments [Internet]. Bethesda (MD): National Cancer Institute; c2004 [cited 2019 Sep 15]. Available from: http://www.cancer.gov/clinicaltrials/learningabout/approval-process-for-cancer-drugs/page1

117. Brown L. Gain a solid understanding of compendia and its impact on patient access. Formulary. 2012;47:252-6.

118. Abernethy A, Raman G, Balk EM, Hammond JM, Orlando LA, Wheeler JL, Lau J, McCrory DC. Systematic review: reliability of compendia methods for off-label oncology indications. Ann Intern Med. 2009;150:336-43.

119. P.L. No. 110-275. Medicare Improvements for Patients and Providers Act of 2008. 2008 Jul 15.

120. Vivian JC. Off-label use of prescription drugs. US Pharm. 2003;28:508.

121. Kaiser Foundation Health Plan et al. v. Pfizer Inc., et al. 11-1904 and 11-2096 (1st Cir. 2013).

122. Beck JM, Azari ED. FDA, off-label use, and informed consent: debunking myths and misconceptions. Food Drug L J. 1998;53:71-103.

123. 21 C.F.R. pt. 50.

124. N.Y. Pub. Health L. § 2805-d(1) (McKinney 1993).

125. Institute of Medicinal Science Institute for Healthcare. Engaging patients through social media. IMS Institute Report. Parsippany (NJ): IMS Institute for Healthcare Informatics; 2014. p. 17-25.

126. Edmunds MW, Scudder L. Using web citations in professional writing. J Prof Nursing. 2008;24:347-51.

127. Wood JM, Dorfman HL. Dot.com medicine: labeling in an Internet age. Food Drug L J. 2001;56;143-78.

128. Moberg MA, Wood JW, Dorfman HI. Surfing the Net in shallow waters: product liability concerns and advertising on the Internet. Food Drug L J. 1998;53:213-24.

129. 21 U.S.C. §§ 351-354 (1994).

130. Deugan L, Powe N, Blakey B, Makary M. Wiki-surgery? Internal validity of Wikipedia as a medical and surgical reference. J Am Coll Surg. 2007;205 (Suppl):576-7.

131. Clauson KA, Poten HH, Boulos MK, Dzeno Wagis JH. Scope, completeness, and accuracy of drug information in Wikipedia. Ann Pharmacother. 2008;42:1814-21.

132. Reilly W, Jackson W, Berger V, Candelaria D. Accuracy and completeness of drug information in Wikipedia medication monographs. J Am Pharm Assoc. 2017;57(1):193-7.

133. Freeman MK, Lauderdale SA, Kendrach MG, Woolley TW. Google Scholar versus PUBMED in locating primary literature to answer drug-related questions. Ann Pharmacother. 2009;43:478-84.

134. Adams SR. Information quality—liability and corrections. Online. 2003 Sep/Oct:16-22.

135. Kane B. Guidelines for the clinical use of electronic mail with patients. White paper. JAMA. 1998;5:104-11.

136. Gulick PG. E-health and the future of medicine: the economic, legal, regulatory, cultural, and organizational obstacles. Alb L J Sci Tech. 2002;12:351-60.

137. Engstrom P. Can you afford not to travel the Internet? Med Econ. 1996;73:173-80.

138. Lopez, et al. v. Aziz, 852 S.W.2d 303, 304 (Tex. App. 1993).

139. Cubby v. CompuServe, 776 F. Supp. 135,140 (1990).

140. Stratton Oakmont Inc. and Daniel Porush v. Prodigy Services Co. & Others (NY Sup. Ct. 1995).

141. Terms of Use Agreement. HealthActCHQ™ Inc. [cited 2019 Sep 15]. Available from: http://www.healthact.com/terms.php

142. Muhlen MV, Ohno-Machado L. Reviewing social media use by clinicians. J Am Med Inform Assoc. 2012;19:777-81.

143. American Society of Health System Pharmacists. ASHP statement on use of social media by pharmacy professionals. Am J Health-Syst Pharm. 2010;74:145-8.

144. Clauson KA, Seamon MJ, Fox BI. Pharmacist's duty to warn in the age of social media. Am J Health-Syst Pharm. 2010;67:1290-3.

145. Update: texting orders. Joint Commission Perspectives. 2016;36(5):15.

146. Kalb PE, Bass IS. Government investigations in the pharmaceutical industry: off-label promotion, fraud and abuse, and false claims. Food Drug L J. 1998;53:63-70.

147. 42 U.S.C. § 1320a-7b(b)(1) (1994).

148. Huntington S. Presentation to the American Bar Association Health Law Section, Emerging professional liability exposures for physicians on the Web, 2001 Jun 8.

149. Warnecke M. Tested IP litigation storm of '04: Fair use principles prove their pluck. Patent, Trademark, Copyright J. 2005;69:369.

150. Ticketmaster Corp. v. Tickets.Com, Inc., 2003 U.S. Dist. LEXIS 6483 (C.D. Cal. 2003).

151. eBay, Inc. v. Bidder's Edge, Inc., 100 F. Supp. 2d 1058 (N.D. Cal. 2000).

152. 1998 U.S. Dist. LEXIS 17282 (E.D. Pa. 1998).

153. D Minn., No. 02-1782 ADM/JGL, 2005 Jan 28.

154. Warnecke M. Effortless nature of Web surfing makes it unlikely consumers can avoid confusion. Patent, Trademark, Copyright J. 2005;69:363-4.

155. Millstein JS, Neuberger JD, Weingart JP. Doing business on the Internet. New York: Law Journal Press, 2004, § 3.02[17][a][iii].

156. Futuredontics, Inc. v. Applied Anagramics, Inc., 1998 U.S. App. LEXIS 17012 (9th Cir. 1998).

157. 17 U.S.C. § 102.

158. Eldred v. Ashcroft, 239 F. 3d 373 (D.C. Cir. 2001).

159. 17 U.S.C. § 106.

160. 17 U.S.C. § 109(a).

161. 35 U.S.C. § 107.

162. College Entrance Examination Boear v. Pataki, 889 F. Supp. 554, 568 (N.D.N.Y. 1995).

163. Epstein E, Zulieve AJ. The Fair Use doctrine: commercial misappropriation and market diversion. Isaacson Raymond [Internet]. [Cited 2019 Sep 15]. Available from: http://www.isaacsonraymond.com/Articles/tabid/123/articleType/ArticleView/articleId/9/The-Fair-Use-Doctrine-Commercial-Misappropriation-And-Market-Diversion.aspx

164. 471 U.S. 539 (1985).

165. Guidelines for classroom copying in not-for-profit educational institutions. H.R. Rep. No. 1476, 94th Cong., 1st Sess. § 68-70 (1976).

166. Latman A, Gorman R, Ginsberg JC. Copyright for the nineties. 3rd ed. Charlottesville (VA): Michie;1989:655-6.

167. Campbell v. Acuff-Rose Music, 510 U.S. 569, 578 (1994).

168. 420 U.S. 376 (1975).

169. Perlman R. Williams & Wilkins Co. v. United States; photocopying, copyright, and the judicial process, 1975 Sup. Ct. Rev. 1976;355.

170. 74 F. 3d 1512 (6th Cir. 1996).

171. 758 F. Supp. 1552 (S.D.N.Y. 1991).

172. Copyright Clearance Center. Using course management systems. Guidelines and best practices for copyright compliance [cited 2019 Sep 15]. Available from: http://www.copyright.com/content/cc3/en/toolbar/education/resources/reprints_and_reports.html

173. 2004 WL 1008314 (2d Cir., May 7, 2004).

174. No. 07 Civ. 09667 (S.D.N.Y., Sep 8, 2008).

175. New York Times Co, Inc., et al. vs. Tasini et al. FindLaw® for Legal Professionals [Internet]. Thomson Reuters; c2013 [cited 2019 Sep 15]. Available from:http://caselaw.lp.findlaw.com/scripts/getcase.pl?court=US&vol=000&invol=00-201

176. Greenberg v. National Geographic, 201 U.S. App. LEXIS 4270 (11th Cir. 2001).

177. The Authors Guild, Inc. et al. v. Google Inc, Case No.05 CV 8136 (S.D.N.Y.).

178. Google Book Search Copyright Class Action Settlement [cited 2019 Sep 15]. Available from: www.googlebooksettlement.com

179. Persky AS. Paper or plastic? Google's plan to digitalize materials pits book lovers v. book innovators. Washington Lawyer. 2009 Jun:35-40.

180. Somers J. Torching of the Modern Day Library of Alexandria. The Atlantic. 2017 Apr 20.

181. The National Digital Exchange [cited 2019 Dec 6]. Available from: https://exchange.dp.la/.

182. Crews KD. New copyright law for distance education: The meaning and importance of the TEACH Act [Internet]. American Libraries Association; c2004 [cited 2019 Sep 15]. Available from: http://www.ala.org/Template.cfm?Section=distanceed

183. Goldman v. Breitbart News Network, CV-0-3144, (S.D.N.Y. 2017).

184. Smedinghoff TJ, editor. Online law. New York: Addison Wesley Press; 1996. 139 p.

185. Pack R. Honest writers. Washington Lawyer. 2004:21-26.

186. Health Insurance Portability and Accountability Act of 1996, Pub. L. No. 104-191, 110 Stat. 1936 (1996) (codified as amended in scattered sections of 18, 26, 29 and 42 U.S.C.A.); 42 U.S.C.A. § 1320d to 42 U.S.C.A. § 1320d-8.

187. Barrett C. Healthcare providers may violate HIPAA by using mobile device to communicate with patients. ABA Health eSource. 2011;8(2):1-5.

188. 45 C.F.R. § 160.103.

189. 45 C.F.R. §§ 164.502(d)(2), 164.514(a) and (b).

190. Daniels JG. Health care privacy and HIPAA. In: Cronin KP, Weikers RN, editors. Data security and privacy law. West Group; 2002.

191. Clause SL, Triller DM, Bornhorst CP, Hamilton RA, Cosler LE. Conforming to HIPAA regulations and compilation of research data. Am J Health-Syst Pharm. 2004;61:1025-31.

192. 45 C.F.R. § 164.512(i)(1)(i).

193. 45 C.F.R. § 164.512(b)(1)(iii).

194. Car J, Sheikh A. Email consultation in health care: 2. Acceptability and safe application. BMJ. 2004;329:439-42.

195. 42 U.S.C.A. § 290dd-2.

196. Bishop S. Interactions with individuals other than the patient, Part 2: Caregivers, personnel representatives, and minors. Pharm Today. 2003;4.

197. Bishop S. Interactions with individuals other than the patient, Part 1: Notice of Privacy Practices and medication counseling. Pharm Today. 2003;4.

198. Hughes v. WalMart Stores, East, LP, No. 2:CV-225, M.D. Ala. 2018 U.S. Dist LEXIS 176369 (Oct 15, 2018).

199. Thompson v. CVS Pharmacy, Inc, 6:204cvo2081 (M.D. Fla., Dec 19, 2014).

200. Kolinek v. Walgreen Co., 2014 WL 3056813 (N.D. Ill., Jul 7, 2014).

201. California Healthcare Foundation [Internet]. Oakland (CA): California Health Care Foundation; 2017. Achieving the right balance: Privacy and security policies to support electronic health information exchange. 2012 Jun [cited 2019 Sep 15]; [about 2 screens]. Available from: http://www.chcf.org/publications/2012/06/achieving-right-balance

202. Baker DB. Provider-patient e-mail: with benefits come risks. J Am Health Info Mgmt Assoc. 2003;74:22-9.

203. D. Mass, No. 00-11672-JLT (Nov 6, 2003).

204. 18 U.S.C. § 2510 et seq.

205. Pharmaceutical Research and Manufacturers of America Code on Interactions with Healthcare Professionals. 2002 Jul [updated 2009 Jan; updated 2019 Sep; cited 2019 Dec 6]. Available from: https://www.phrma.org/-/media/Project/PhRMA/PhRMA-Org/PhRMA-Org/PDF/A-C/Code-of-Interaction_FINAL21.pdf

206. Health and Human Services, OIG Compliance Program for Pharmaceutical Industry; 2003 Apr.

207. Accreditation Council for Pharmacy Education [Internet]. Accreditation Standards and Criteria; c2005 Jan [cited 2019 Sep 15]. Available from: http://www.acpeaccredit.org/ceproviders/standards.asp.

208. 2018 National Association of Boards of Pharmacy (NABP) Survey of Pharmacy Law. Mount Prospect (IL): NABP; 2018.

209. Cutting the strings on gifts and other questionable marketing practices: PhRMA takes a stand. CME Briefing. 2002;1-6.

210. FDA guidance for industry-supported scientific and educational activities, 1997.

211. Steiner JL, Norko M, Devine S, Grottole E, Vinoski J, Griffith EE. Best practices: developing ethical guidelines for pharmaceutical company support in an academic health center. Psychiatr Serv. 2003;54:1079-89.

212. Rosner F. Pharmaceutical industry support for continuing medical education programs: a review of current ethical guidelines. Mt. Sinai J Med. 1995;62:427-30.

213. 42 U.S.C. § 1320a-7b(b).
214. U.S. v. Greber, 760 F.2d 68 (3d Cir. 1985).
215. U.S. v. LaHue, 261 F.3d 993 (10th Cir. 2001).
216. In re Caremark Int'l, Inc. Derivative Litig., 698 A. 2d 959 (1996).
217. Drug firm settles kickback charges. The Palm Beach Post, 1994 Sep 6:4B.
218. Astrue MJ, Szabo DS. Pharmaceutical marketing and the anti-kickback statutes. Food Drug Cosmet Med Device Law Dig. 1993;10(2):57-60.

SUGGESTED READINGS

1. Reilly T, Jackson W, Berge V, Candelario D. Accuracy and completeness of drug information in Wikipedia medication monographs. J Am Pharm Assoc. 2017;57(1):193-7.
2. Chew SW, Khoo CS. Comparison of drug information on consumer review sites versus authoritative health information websites. J Assoc Info Sci Tech. 2016;67(2):333-49.
3. Gershman J. 6 Tips for managing a drug information center. Pharmacy Times. 2018 Feb 8.
4. Anderson R. The difference between copyright infringement and plagiarism and why it matters. J Periop Nursing. 2016;29(4):50-1.
5. Dept. HHS, Food and Drug Administration, Center for Drug Evaluation and Research, Center for Biologics Evaluation and Research, Center for Veterinary Medicine, Center for Devices and Radiological Health. Guidance for industry. Responding to unsolicited requests for off-label information about prescription drugs and medical devices. 2011 Dec.
6. Tyrawski J, DeAndrea DC. Pharmaceutical companies and their drugs on social media: a content analysis of drug information on popular social media sites. J Med Internet Res. 2015;17(6):e130. Published online 2015 Jun 1; doi:10.2196/jmir.4357.
7. American Society of Health System Pharmacists. ASHP statement on use of social media by pharmacy professionals. Am J Health-Syst Pharm. 2010;74:145-8.

12

Chapter Twelve

Ethical Aspects of Drug Information Practice

Elyse A. MacDonald

Learning Objectives

After completing this chapter, the reader will be able to:

- Explain characteristics that differentiate an ethical deliberation from other types of decision-making.
- Interpret and make use of ethics rules, principles, and theories to analyze identified ethical dilemmas.
- Identify and analyze examples of ethical dilemmas that may arise for health professionals when providing drug information, in various practice settings and for various types of clients and circumstances.
- Identify micro, meso, and macro levels of ethical decision-making that may occur during the provision of pharmacy practice.
- Use the described process of ethical analysis in order to propose and justify a specific decision or course of action in an ethical dilemma case.
- Describe resources and structures that can prepare, guide, and support clinicians faced with ethical dilemmas during the course of providing drug information.

Key Concepts

❶ Ethical deliberations may be differentiated by three characteristics: they are ultimate (fundamental); the issue is universal; and the welfare of all affected parties is considered.

❷ Ethical judgments may occur at micro, meso, or macro levels of health care decision-making.

❸ Professional ethics is different from the law.

❹ The primary focus will be on the health care professional's identification, interpretation, specification, and balancing of pertinent ethical rules and principles.

❺ The application of a proposed process of ethical analysis is demonstrated for identifying, analyzing, and resolving ethical dilemmas that may arise during the health care professionals' provision of drug information.

❻ The first process step requires identification and evaluation of pertinent background information to ensure that the facts of the specific case are understood, and to assess whether a true ethical dilemma exists.

❼ Sometimes, the professional will find it necessary and valuable to more consciously deliberate on how various ethical theories suggest that the relevant rules and principles should be prioritized or balanced.

❽ Health care professionals need training, resources, and support to prepare them to effectively address those ethical dilemmas they confront.

Introduction

♦ WHAT IS ETHICS AND WHAT IS NOT

The Ethics Course Content Committee of the American Association of Colleges of Pharmacy (AACP) described **ethics** as "the philosophical inquiry of the moral dimensions of human conduct."[1] They mentioned that Aristotle taught ethics as "an eminently practical discipline..." dealing "with concrete judgments in situations in which action must be taken despite uncertainty."[1] These authors indicated that the term "ethical" is often used synonymously with the term "moral" to describe an action or decision as good or right. They further stated that ethics is not the study of moral development, and it is not the law.

Veatch stated that "an ethical, or moral, issue involves judgments between right and wrong human conduct or praiseworthy and blameworthy human character."[2] This author indicated that an ❶ *ethical deliberation may be differentiated from other endeavors by three characteristics: (1) it is ultimate or fundamental, there is no higher standard against which to measure the rightness of the decision or action; (2) the issue is universal; the parties involved in the dilemma do not consider it simply a difference of opinion or taste—each party believes there is a right or wrong answer—even if they disagree about what the answer is; and (3) the deliberation takes into account the welfare of all involved or affected by the judgment at hand.* Those who provide drug information (DI) typically rely on an intuitive sense of these characteristics. They have the feeling that the situation being confronted is a big deal, and somehow anticipate that they should not address personal preference in the matter at hand.

DIFFERENT LEVELS OF ETHICS

Evolving literature has described that ❷ *ethical judgments may occur at micro, meso, or macro levels of health care decision-making.*[3-14] A traditionally recognized **micro** level of health care–related decision-making involves decisions made at the individual, professional, or the patient level of health care. A less commonly discussed **meso** level of decision-making (with some literature using the term "organizational" for similar purpose) is variably described as occurring at the institutional/organizational level or at community/regional levels. **Macro**-level decision-making often sets policy for the health system, as a standard established for an entire profession, or through government as law/regulation for the society as a whole.

Health care providers may be involved in ethical decision-making at each of these levels related to the provision of or access to drug information. Primarily, micro-level ethical decision-making scenarios will be presented in this chapter. However, certain scenarios involving meso- and macro-level ethical decision-making will also be addressed. For example, a physician, nurse, and pharmacist may all be participating on a **pharmacy and therapeutics committee** that is developing an organizational policy regarding the use of pharmaceutical samples within hospital clinics, or in a large independent clinic practice. The policy also addresses the use of in-house professionals versus industry detailers to provide information about new drug products. Each of these professionals may have competing priorities and concerns that add ethical dimensions to their decision-making on this proposed policy.[10] This example constitutes a meso level of ethical decision-making for these professionals. A clinician participating on a national task force charged with developing policy related to **medication therapy management** services (with inherent drug information access) as part of a health care reform model will have macro-level ethical decisions to make relative to balancing patient needs, professional identity, and societal economic constraints.[9]

DIFFERENCE BETWEEN ETHICS AND LAW

❸ *Professional ethics is different than the law.* The law might be defined as rules of conduct imposed by society on its members. By contrast, professional ethics has been defined as "rules of conduct or standards by which a particular group in society regulates its actions and sets standards for its members."[15] Both constitute macro-level policy making, across society or across an entire profession. Law involves written rules set by the whole society (or its representatives) that address responsibilities of that society's members. Professional ethics focuses on explicit or implicit rules and standards set by a professional subgroup of society, and addresses the responsibilities of only those who are members of that subgroup. Certain ethical standards of a given profession may be institutionalized as law by society as a whole. However, professional ethical standards (e.g., do no harm or preserve life) are often impossible to fully regulate by law. Meeting an ethical standard also goes beyond legal requirements; indeed, our ethical beliefs may on occasion command our civil disobedience (e.g., a prison pharmacist who refuses to dispense drugs to be used in legal executions). On the other hand, as will be discussed further below, law also represents one aspect of the culture within which ethical decisions are made. In considering the cultural perspectives of a given dilemma, relevant legal requirements must be identified and considered when one seeks to make an ethical decision.

ETHICAL DILEMMAS WHEN PROVIDING DRUG INFORMATION

This chapter will present case scenarios representing ethical dilemmas. These scenarios will be used to demonstrate a specific method for analyzing ethical dilemmas confronted by health care professionals providing drug information. The discussion will address ethical dilemmas encountered by generalist and specialist patient care providers providing drug information, as well as examples drawn from the experiences of drug information specialists. All health care professionals provide drug information and must address the ethical dilemmas that arise in the course of providing this service. Many of these scenarios represent examples of micro-level ethical dilemmas that primarily involve an interaction between a drug information provider and the direct recipient of the information. Other scenarios where health care professionals may be providing or determining access to drug information occur at meso (organizational) or macro (societal) levels of ethical decision-making. While perhaps less immediately obvious as an ethical dilemma to some individuals involved, these may constitute dilemmas that have even further reaching impacts for both individual professionals and impacted groups. These larger dilemmas may often seem beyond the scope of individual decision-making, but indeed ultimately are primarily addressed through the contributed actions or decisions of individuals, typically as they interact in some group process. Of course, all ethical dilemmas, by definition, have some implications beyond the welfare of the most immediate individuals involved. The list of example dilemmas provided in Table 12-1 includes scenarios from each of these levels. These dilemmas might arise in a wide variety of settings and circumstances where health care is practiced or health care policy is set. It is important to identify the level of ethical decision-making that each example seems to represent, and consider what ethical issues might exist for each scenario.

TABLE 12–1. EXAMPLES OF ETHICAL SITUATIONS IN HEALTH CARE

- The hospital practitioner is asked to provide information that might be used to speed the end of life of a terminal patient.
- The community pharmacist or physician is requested by a patient to critique another health care provider's drug therapy recommendation.
- The drug information pharmacist is confronted by an administrator pressuring for a certain formulary recommendation that is more focused on cost-containment than evidence-based.
- The home health care practitioner is asked to positively present questionably substantiated information on the efficacy of a given therapy, in order to support insurance reimbursement for a truly needy patient.
- Practitioners working in industry are asked to prepare a consumer product education and promotion piece according to directions that do not adhere to Food and Drug Administration (FDA) or World Health Organization (WHO) guidelines for balanced presentation of both the benefits and the risks associated with the drug product being advertised.
- The health care professional practicing in any patient care setting, who experiences another episode (in a repetitious pattern) where his or her patients would benefit from additional drug information, but who finds workload demands to be an impossible barrier to providing more than the minimum, legally required information.
- An oncology pharmacist receives orders for a chemotherapy regimen that is also being used in a clinical trial, but the oncologist does not want to enroll the patient in the trial.
- The hospital pharmacist is asked to compound a medication for which there is little to no safety and efficacy data, based on the pharmacist's review of existing literature.
- The hospital only has enough of an oncology medication to treat one patient, but there are three patients who need treatment. The drug information pharmacist is asked to review literature to help decide which patient receives the medication.

In the eighth (2019) edition of Principles of Biomedical Ethics,[16] Beauchamp and Childress addressed the following aspects of the moral life: moral norms, moral character, and moral status. The responsibilities (based on principles and rules) and rights of the health care provider and other involved parties will be addressed in this chapter as considerations that must be dealt with in the course of responding to a specific dilemma. Beauchamp and Childress have covered this content since the fifth edition of their textbook. While acknowledging their importance, this chapter will not address the roles of character, moral virtue, or emotions in ethical decision-making by health care professionals. One might say that they constitute the provider's inherent moral perspective that will direct and support his or her decision-making. The remainder of this chapter is intended to prepare and assist the pharmacist and other health care professionals providing drug information to analyze and address dilemmas, such as those listed above. ❹ *The primary focus will be on the health care professional's identification, interpretation, specification, and balancing of pertinent ethical rules and principles* as he or she seeks to determine and justify what he or she considers the right decision or the best course of action.

Basics of Ethics Analysis

This section briefly presents relevant terminology and definitions used in the field of ethics, as well as an overview of a specific process of analysis that may be used in assessing ethical dilemmas. In the section following this one, specific case scenario demonstrations of this process for analysis will be presented.

● DEFINITIONS USED IN THE FIELD OF ETHICS

Beauchamp and Childress[17] defined ethics as "a generic term for several ways of examining the moral life." These authors described a process of deliberation and justification that is necessary when confronting a moral dilemma. They stated, "When we deliberate ... we are considering which judgment is morally justified ...." They indicated that, "Particular judgments are justified by moral rules, which in turn are justified by principles, which ultimately are defended by an ethical theory." These authors presented a hierarchical diagram that depicts this approach to analysis (Figure 12-1). This figure continues to represent key aspects of ethical deliberation, although Beauchamp and Childress have evolved a more complex conceptual approach in later editions of their text. A later article by Beauchamp further addresses the need to consider these principles and rules within the specific context of the case at hand, in order to fully realize their action-guiding potential.[18]

The authors referred to these hierarchical levels of analysis (particularly rules and principles) as action-guides, which are used to justify a particular judgment. They describe a rule of ethics as specific to context and relatively restricted in scope; for instance, the moral rule about confidentiality that specifically addresses a patient's right to consent prior to release of privileged information.[17] Principles are more broad and fundamental in scope; for example, the principle of respect for **autonomy**, which is the patient's right to decide on personal issues. They describe ethical theories as "integrated bodies of principles and rules ... that may include mediating rules that govern cases of conflicts." The

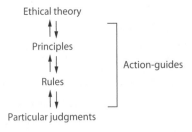

Figure 12–1. Hierarchical levels of ethical analysis.

prominent rules and principles guiding ethical decision-making by health care professionals can generally be placed within one of two broad ethical theories: **consequentialist** theory or **deontological** (derived from the Greek word "deon," meaning duty) theory.[17] Multiple versions exist of each of these broad categories.

Consequentialist theories describe actions or decisions as morally right or wrong based on their consequences, rather than on any intrinsic features they may have. The two cardinal principles of consequentialist theory are **beneficence** (do that which promotes a good outcome) and **nonmaleficence** (do that which minimizes bad outcomes). Consequentialist theories focus on this one feature of an act, its consequences. For example, an informed consent ethical rule can be of value within consequentialist theory because consent generally results in improved compliance and outcomes—good consequences. However, if informed consent was likely to result in a bad outcome, it would not be justifiable within consequentialist theory. A mediating rule utilized by many advocates of consequentialist theory is to hold nonmaleficence as more important, or more foundational, than beneficence.

Duty-driven (deontological) theories look more to intrinsic qualities of an act or decision to assert its moral rightness or wrongness. Deontological theory considers other inherent features of an act, besides consequences, as also relevant and often of greater importance. For example, in various forms of deontological theory, the act is considered inherently wrong if it is dishonest or breaks confidentiality, or if it does not respect individual autonomy. Conflicts between different rules are mediated by appealing to more foundational, underlying principles such as adherence to justice or to respect for persons.

Conscious recognition of the pertinent action-guides, and understanding mediating rules that operate within the health professional's preferred ethical theory or theories, can help providers honestly and equitably analyze the ethical dilemma, and better comply with the imperative characteristics of ethical deliberation (see the beginning of this chapter).

OVERVIEW OF A SUGGESTED PROCESS OF ANALYSIS TO BE USED WHEN AN ETHICAL DILEMMA ARISES

In the article "Hospital pharmacy: what is ethical?," Veatch[2] indicated that often people reach a particular ethical decision without a great deal of conscious deliberation, through moral intuition, and without subsequent challenge from any external party. However, on occasion, when pondering a certain ethical judgment, they are called on (internally or externally) to analyze and justify the basis for their conviction. He suggested that when this occurs, it is first important to understand the facts of the specific case. He then described progression through three additional process stages of reflection (on ethical rules, principles, and theories) by which we may identify, analyze, and present reasons for our judgment. In the same report, the author also emphasized the importance in one's reflection to consider the points of view of all parties impacted. As stated earlier in this chapter, this is one of the key characteristics distinguishing an ethical deliberation. A survey of the book Cross-Cultural Perspectives in Medical Ethics, 2nd ed.,[19] demonstrates that there are many commonalities, but also important differences across the ethical perspectives of different cultures. These cultural perspectives must be considered if all parties' points of view are to be considered.

In this section ❺ *the application of a proposed process of ethical analysis is demonstrated for identifying, analyzing, and resolving ethical dilemmas that may arise during health professionals' provision of drug information.* These steps of analysis are derived from the writings of Veatch, Beauchamp, and Childress, as well as other authors.[2,17,19–21] The process may be summarized as follows:

I. Identification of relevant background information
   A. Factual details of the issue at hand
   B. Consideration of who is affected by the ethical issue
   C. Learn and respectfully address the cultural perspectives (including applicable legal requirements) for those affected by the dilemma
II. Identification and justification of the relevant moral rules and principles (action-guides) pertinent to the case
III. Deliberation, through the use of moral intuition and application of ethical theory, on how to rank/balance the rules and principles pertinent to the case in order to resolve the ethical dilemma

Step I. Identification of Relevant Background Information

❻ *The first process step requires identification and evaluation of pertinent background information to ensure that the facts of the specific case are understood and to assess whether a true ethical dilemma exists.* This first step deserves careful consideration and research. Once the facts of a case are known, the moral concerns may be resolved. This step has been divided into three parts: (1) data gathering, (2) consideration of the welfare of all affected parties, and (3) respect for the cultural perspectives of these parties.

Health care professionals already use data gathering when they apply a systematic approach to answering any drug information question (see Chapter 2). When addressing a potential ethical dilemma, the providers must learn about the factual details of the issue, who is directly involved, and whether there is conflict in factual understanding among the involved parties in the issue. For example, does the parent who calls to ask about the medication recently prescribed for her teenager already know that the teenager is taking a birth control pill prescribed by a gynecologist (rather than a dermatologist for acne) and simply wants to know the name of the product?

If the matter still seems to involve an ethical dimension once data gathering clarifies the facts, the next step is to consider the rights and responsibilities of all affected parties. As previously mentioned, this has been described as an essential component of any ethical deliberation.[2] The health care provider, the direct client (patient or parent in the case just described), other indirect but individual clients (e.g., any existing or unborn children, parent paying for service provided to the child patient or the patient's spouse), other health professionals (e.g., the patient's physician), other societal groups (e.g., other patients who might be harmed by an incompetent practitioner), and any higher power recognized by the health professional have rights and/or responsibilities that should be considered.

Finally, during first consideration of any potential ethical issue, the provider should take into account the cultures of the affected parties.[20] In his reviews of the foundations of modern medical ethics theories, Veatch[19,21] described how the unique perspectives of Western, Chinese, Hindu, Jewish, Catholic, Protestant, and other cultural groups have affected the formulation of their dominant medical ethics traditions. Other cultural classifications might include socioeconomic status, political affiliation, age category, and racial or ethnic group.

In a very interesting case study, Carrese and associates[22] discussed the ethical obligations of medical professionals in caring for those of a different ethnic culture. In this case, a young Laotian mother used a traditional Mien folk cure to treat her infant. The treatment involved placing several small burns on the child's abdomen to treat *gusia mun toe*, an apparently transient, but very distressing, colic-like ailment. The cure resulted in several small scars, but no other obvious ill effects. The mother indicated that the cure worked. The physician recognized the value in supporting the positive impacts of the woman's attachment to her cultural support group. However, the physician was confronted with the dilemma of how to respond to this mother's revelation of a culturally promoted treatment measure that was not scientifically supported and could be dangerous. Sometimes, culturally based actions may conflict with the professional's goal to avoid harm and promote benefit. However, failing to consider a cultural perspective may also have harmful effects or disrupt the trust between patient and health care professional. An extended discussion of how differing cultural perspectives affect ethical decision-making is beyond the scope of this chapter. However, the health care professional should strive to be aware of and respect the cultural perspectives of the affected parties when contemplating an ethical dilemma. The interested reader is encouraged to refer to the resources cited here and above for further discussion of cultural factors in ethical analysis.[19,21]

One final issue should be addressed relative to cultural considerations. The legal requirements of the society within which an ethical dilemma occurs are part of the culture and must be identified. A specific ethical decision will not always exactly conform to the existing legal requirements of society. The ultimate nature of ethical deliberations may result in decisions that are more demanding than the legal requirements and, unfortunately, may even occasionally involve perceived or true conflict with specific legal requirements. This may involve, for instance, a decision not to divulge confidential communications between a professional and client, which may or may not be acceptable within the law. In another case, the health professional may decide not to provide information related to abortion or capital punishment, even though these activities are acceptable within the law. Obviously, legal requirements cannot be ignored or dismissed lightly when making a specific ethical decision.

Step II: Use of Rules and Principles (Action-Guides) to Assist in Analysis of an Ethical Dilemma

If the dilemma persists, once the available background information has been identified and considered, proceed with the process of full ethical deliberation. Veatch[2] suggests that the involved party/parties can proceed as far as necessary through successive stages of general moral reflection assessing at the level of moral rules and then at the level of ethical principles, within their accepted ethical theory. These might be described as the action-guides referred to by Beauchamp and Childress.[17] This second process step of analysis will look at moral rules that may apply to the specific case and more general pertinent ethical principles. Definitions are provided at the end of this section for a number of ethical rules and principles that are considered particularly relevant to decision-making by practitioners.

Specific action-guides may be considered a rule within one ethical theory and a principle within another. For example, **veracity** (truth telling) as mentioned above may be considered by some ethicists to be a specific moral rule and by others to be a general principle, depending on which ethical theory is followed. For the practitioner immediately involved in analyzing a specific ethical dilemma, defining the relevant action-guides as rules or principles is important only to the extent that this helps in assessing which are more fundamental to the issue at hand. Therefore, in this chapter, both rules and principles will be included within the same process step of ethical analysis.

Examples of moral rules within biomedical ethics include a confidentiality rule dictating that patient-entrusted information should not be disclosed or an informed consent rule that addresses the individual's right to information before agreeing to a specific medical procedure. Unfortunately, there is no definitive list universally defining all moral rules and, sometimes, multiple pertinent rules can be in conflict. Furthermore, there are acceptable exceptions to most moral rules. For instance, disregarding the informed consent rule might be justifiable in an acute situation to protect the life of the client, suffering may be necessary in order to achieve cure of serious disease, and many consider killing justified under certain circumstances. Therefore, there may not be a specific rule that resolves a particular ethical dilemma.

When such a circumstance arises, the practitioner may begin a more general level of analysis by looking at the ethical principles that apply to the case. Sometimes, the involved parties can reach an acceptable resolution to an ethical dilemma once they recognize the broader relevant ethical principles. In a given dilemma, the professional may decide that the primary principle is to respect the autonomy of the client and that requires providing complete information enabling the client to make an informed decision. In another dilemma, if do no harm is considered the most fundamental ethical principle, decisions or acts that deny this principle would be considered unethical. It becomes immediately obvious, however, that relevant ethical principles such as these may also come into conflict. This problem can be demonstrated by the following example: The professional may believe that full disclosure will result in nonadherence by the patient, with significant risk of resultant harm. The practitioner therefore confronts two conflicting principles: respecting client autonomy by providing full disclosure versus the duty to do no harm.

Step III: Ethical Theory as a Means to Clarify or Resolve Ethical Dilemmas

This third step of ethical analysis reveals how relevant moral rules and principles interact within the preferred ethical theory to address the given dilemma. When confronted with conflicting ethical rules or principles, the practitioner may simply resolve the dilemma through his or her moral intuition of the right thing to do; even if unconsciously, this reflects the individual's at least temporary affiliation to some theory of what constitutes good versus bad or right versus wrong. ❼ *Sometimes, the professional will find it necessary and valuable to more consciously deliberate on how various ethical theories suggest that the relevant rules and principles should be prioritized or balanced.* According to Veatch,[2] this process step can lead to more rational and honest decision-making or action-taking. He suggests that these ultimate deliberations at the level of ethical theory will be affected by our most basic religious and/or philosophical commitments. It is important that the practitioner recognizes and acknowledges the impact on decision-making of his or her own personal ethical perspective. Those dilemmas that cannot be fully resolved can at least be viewed with greater clarity.

Veatch[21] states that, "The components of a complete theory will answer such questions as what rules apply to specific ethical cases, what ethical principles stand behind the rules, how seriously the rules should be taken, and what constitutes the fundamental meaning and justification of the ethical principles." In this reference and another text, the author reviews the foundations of consequentialist, deontological, and other ethics theories particularly relevant to health professionals, including: the Hippocratic tradition; Judeo-Christian and other religious-based traditions; the philosophies of the modern secular West; and medical ethics theories outside the Anglo-American West, including Socialist, Islamic, Hindu, African, Chinese, and Japanese traditions.[19,21] Frequently, versions of the broad consequentialist and deontological theories are expressed in various ways across these traditions. Keep in mind the core of the various **Hippocratic Oaths**, since this has been the central ethical tradition of Western medicine: "Those who have stood in that (Hippocratic) tradition are committed to producing good for their patient and to protecting that patient from harm."[21] In Hippocratic tradition, there is also a special emphasis placed on the responsibility of the health care professional to the specific patient versus obligations to other less directly affected parties or to society in general. A contract theory of medical ethics has also been proposed, which describes an implicit (unwritten) contract between health professionals and patients.[21] This modern theory is of special relevance to the pharmacist providing drug information as a service within an implicit pharmaceutical care contract.[21,23] First of all, this theory represents a shift in thinking for those pharmacists who might have considered their primary obligation to be to the prescriber rather than to the patient. Furthermore, this contract between patient and professional suggests an obligation for more substantive communication with patients and a higher level of caregiving than some pharmacists have previously felt obligated to offer. The reader is referred to foundational writings by Veatch, as well as those of Beauchamp and Childress, for a more in-depth discussion of various medical ethics theories.[17,19,21]

AN ANNOTATED LISTING OF RULES AND PRINCIPLES (ACTION-GUIDES) APPLIED IN MEDICAL ETHICS INQUIRY

The following rules and principles (action-guides) of ethical conduct will be described and subsequently used in the analysis of case scenarios provided in the next section. Their description will necessarily be brief. The reader is referred to other sources to read more about these rules and principles.[17,21]

1. *Nonmaleficence*—A basic principle of consequentialist theory; encompasses the duty to do no harm. This tenet has a long history as part of the Hippocratic tradition, where it has often been described in terms of the health care provider's duty to the individual patient. The principle is also cited as justification for actions benefiting all. Sometimes, application of the principle requires addressing conflicts between the needs of one and all.[16]

2. *Beneficence*—Another basic principle of consequentialist theory that expresses the duty to promote good. Again, conflict can arise between what constitutes good for one individual versus the larger societal group. Good or bad consequences are also of importance within deontological theories, but are evaluated along with other principles that may be considered of equal or greater importance.[16]

3. *Respecting the patient-professional relationship*—A moral rule, often referring to respect for the physician-patient relationship, but also applicable to other

professional-patient relationships, as well. This rule has been mentioned in published reports of ethical dilemmas arising during the provision of drug information.[24-26] As expressed in Hippocratic traditions, this rule indicates that the physician's primary duty is to the patient and tends to give the physician, rather than the patient, control in the relationship, which may be judged paternalistic by some. This rule is particularly noted in duty-driven (deontological) ethical theories that consider the professional's duty to the patient, but also supports consequentialist theory to the extent that good outcomes are enhanced.

4. *Respect for autonomy*—A principle described particularly within deontological theory. This principle is founded on a belief in the right of the individual to self-rule. It speaks to the individual's right to decide on issues that primarily affect self.

5. *Consent*—A moral rule related to the principle of autonomy which states that the client has a right to be informed and to freely choose a course of action; for example, informed consent to receive a therapy or procedure.

6. *Confidentiality*—A moral rule, also related to the principle of autonomy, which specifically addresses the individual client's right to give or refuse consent relative to release of privileged information.

7. *Privacy*—Another rule within the principle of autxonomy, more generally relating to the right of the individual to control his or her own affairs without interference from or knowledge of outside parties. This rule has been addressed in deliberations on the rights of individuals with AIDS versus those of their potential sexual contacts.

8. *Respect for persons*—A principle expressing duty to the welfare of the individual, particularly described within religion-based deontological theories. This principle may also be expressed within dignity of life or sanctity of human life principles. It has common elements with the respect for autonomy principle, but addresses more directly a belief in the inherent value of human life, independent of characteristics or abilities of the specific human being.

9. *Veracity*—This term addresses the obligation to truth telling or honesty. Veracity is considered an ethical principle within deontological theory. However, it is considered a useful rule within consequentialist theory, to the extent that it promotes good.

10. *Fidelity*—Another principle of moral duty in deontological theory that addresses the responsibility to be trustworthy and keep promises. This principle also relates to a duty of reciprocity—consideration of the other's point of view. Recent descriptions of care by health care professionals focus on the relationship with the patient and the need to develop an ethical **covenant** between the parties in

the relationship.[23,27] This covenant details the characteristics of a relationship requiring fidelity and reciprocity, in which each party takes on certain responsibilities and gives up certain rights in order to achieve specific good outcomes (consequentialist theory). Success of this contract depends in good measure on consideration by each party of the other's point of view.

11. *Justice*—This concept has been presented within various principles that relate to fairness and tendering what is due, resource allocation and providing that to which the individual is entitled. A number of more fundamental justice theories have also been developed to connect and justify these various principles.[17] Moral decision-making at the meso and macro level will frequently cite justice as a main justification for particular decisions. A more thorough discussion on justice-related principles and theories is beyond the scope of this chapter. However, several texts that address this topic can provide much assistance to those health professionals preparing for roles at these levels of ethical decision-making, or to those who teach such professionals.[28,29]

These are certainly not the only relevant rules or principles, nor are they necessarily universally accepted definitions. However, these action-guides seem particularly pertinent to medical ethics inquiry. Furthermore, several of these rules and principles have been specifically discussed in published reports that describe ethical dilemmas encountered by drug information specialists.[24,25] Such dilemmas have also been described in situations where practitioners are providing drug information directly to patients, either from a formal drug information center or during the process of providing patient care.

DEMONSTRATION OF CASE ANALYSIS

The following examples demonstrate ethical dilemmas that might arise for professionals providing drug information. These cases will be used to demonstrate the aforementioned process of analysis for the practitioner(s) addressing an ethical dilemma.

Case Example 12–1 (Micro-Level Case)

Mrs. Burns, a new patient at the medical center, calls the Drug Information Center (DIC), which the medical center advertises as a resource for both patients and professionals. The patient said to Dr. Pike, a drug information pharmacist, she is concerned about whether she should take the amoxicillin plus clavulanate just prescribed for her by Dr. Stills, her family practitioner (who practices at the center where the DIC is located).

■ ANALYSIS

Step #1 Identification of relevant background information.

A. Factual details of the issue at hand: The drug information practitioner learns the following information through discussion with the patient:
   1. Mrs. Burns is approximately 8 weeks pregnant; she wonders if this medication is safe for the baby.
   2. She says she is being treated for acute bacterial rhinosinusitis.
   3. She mentions that she has only recently begun seeing Dr. Stills, as her family just moved into town about 3 months ago.
   4. Mrs. Burns indicates that Dr. Stills knows she is pregnant. He is managing her pregnancy.
   5. She states that she asked him about the safety of the drug, but he rather impatiently brushed off her questions by asking "don't you trust me?"
   6. Dr. Pike may decide that it is necessary to consult professional resources to evaluate whether the therapy appears to be appropriate. She should not hesitate to ask the patient for some reasonable time period in which to investigate the pertinent information before providing an answer.
   7. Dr. Pike will need to consider whether any identified risks are likely to be known to the physician.
   8. Dr. Pike may decide that further facts must be obtained through direct discussion with Dr. Stills.

B. Identification of who is affected by any ethical issue considered to be present: As the drug information provider reflects on this patient's inquiry, it is helpful to consider who might be impacted by her response:
   1. Herself, relative to her own desire to do right; any relationship between her and her patient, any relationship between her and the physician.
   2. Mrs. Burns relative to the consequences of any harm to her infant or of inadequate treatment of the infection, and relative to her future relationships with both the physician and the drug information provider.
   3. Mrs. Burns' infant, relative to the consequences of any harmful or beneficial effects of the drug, or of inadequate treatment of the mother's infection.
   4. Dr. Stills, relative to the consequences of prescribing a potentially inappropriate therapy during the woman's pregnancy, and relative to the effects of any drug information provided on the patient-physician relationship.
   5. Mrs. Burns' family, significant others, and society in general, relative to the impacts of either delivery or abortion of a child with harm from the therapy, or from inadequate treatment of the woman's infection.

C. Consideration for the cultural perspectives of those affected by the dilemma.

Dr. Pike will consciously or unconsciously act within her own cultural and religious framework, and her understanding of her legal obligations. Awareness of her own perspective, as well as consideration of the cultural perspectives of others who may be affected, is important if she is to pursue a truly ethical course of action. To repeat Veatch's words differentiating ethical deliberations, "The deliberation takes into account the welfare of all involved or affected."[2] Each involved party's welfare is affected by his or her cultural perspective. Cultural, religious, and legal perspectives that the clinician must be aware of in this case might include:

1. Perspectives regarding parental responsibility to the unborn infant versus self.
2. Perspectives and legal requirements relative to both the DI provider and physician's obligations to the patient and to her infant.
3. Perspectives about the role and authority of the physician and of the DI provider.

D. Consideration of the level of decision-making involved in responding to any ethical dilemma recognized by the DI practitioners.

Within the context of this DI professional's job description, or the charge of the particular case, it should be fairly obvious whether micro-, meso-, or macro-level decision-making activities are involved. However, a clinician may be involved in micro-level decision-making activities related to individual patients, but also have obligations to the pharmacy and therapeutics committee within the health organization (meso level), or perhaps even beyond as a policy committee member for his or her national professional organization (macro level). By definition, all ethical dilemmas tend to have implications beyond the context of just two individuals (note from the first page of this chapter that ethical deliberations consider the welfare of all involved or affected by the judgment at hand), but meso- and macro-level decision-making will always affect various population groups, as well as the individuals within those groups.

Step #2 Identification and justification of the relevant moral rules and principles (action-guides) pertinent to the case at hand.

If the background facts of Mrs. Burns' inquiry do not dismiss the DI provider's ethical concerns, Dr. Pike will find it helpful to consider the various rules and principles discussed above in order to clarify the dimensions of her concern. It is most useful to first identify all potentially pertinent action-guides, and seek an understanding of how fundamentally each applies to the situation.

Ethical action-guides that seem pertinent to this inquiry include the following:

1. *Informed consent*—A moral rule supporting Mrs. Burns' right to be informed and freely choose whether to take the amoxicillin plus clavulanate in relation to other available options.

2. *Respect for the patient-professional relationship*—This rule addresses the obligation of Dr. Pike to support the professional relationship between Mrs. Burns and Dr. Stills. It also requires Dr. Pike to respect her own professional relationship with the patient. Increasingly, professionals within all health care professional groups are interpreting this ethical rule to define their obligation to the patient as primary. Such an interpretation represents a departure for many health care providers from a historical orientation of their primary obligation being to the physician.

3. *Veracity*—Addresses the responsibility of Dr. Pike to tell the truth to Mrs. Burns. This may be considered a basic principle of obligation within deontological theory, or a useful rule within consequentialist theory (to the extent that it promotes good).

4. *Nonmaleficence*—A basic principle of consequentialist theory that would base a decision to divulge information on minimizing the potential for harm.

5. *Beneficence*—This consequentialist principle would base the decision regarding what information to divulge on the potential to promote good. Beneficence and nonmaleficence can be considered together in judging the ethical response to the dilemma faced by Dr. Pike.

Dr. Pike must consider the potential benefits of the prescribed therapy for Mrs. Burns, and address the potential harm resulting from exposure of her infant to amoxicillin plus clavulanate. Consideration of other available alternatives for therapy is also pertinent. Frequently such consideration takes place, at least initially, in the face of inadequate and conflicting information. Dr. Pike will also need to decide what constitutes harm and good for Mrs. Burns versus all others who may be affected.

6. *Fidelity/reciprocity*—A principle of obligation to an ethical covenant between Dr. Pike and Mrs. Burns (within deontological theory), which may suggest a requirement for full disclosure of information. However, to the extent that this covenant asks that each party take on certain responsibilities and give up certain rights in order to achieve specific good outcomes full disclosure of potentially harmful information may not be required. If Dr. Pike were concerned that Mrs. Burns may decide to forgo any treatment, there could be the potential of negative consequences for both Mrs. Burns and her infant.

7. *Justice*—This principle is considered of intrinsic value within certain deontological theories, and addresses the right of Mrs. Burns (and other affected parties) to be given what is due—entitlement to information may be considered justice in this case. Certainly, the time and expertise of Dr. Pike might be legitimately considered due to her patient.

8. *Autonomy*—This principle is directly applicable to the dilemma of Dr. Pike, as was the related rule of informed consent, based on a belief in Mrs. Burns' right to decide on issues that primarily affect her. The principle of autonomy has support within both deontological (as an intrinsic good) and consequentialist (if it is likely

to promote good consequences) theories. However, competing interests (e.g., Mrs. Burns and her infant), and the individual's capability to be truly autonomous (e.g., the infant in this case), are factors that often complicate the application of this principle in medical ethics.

The reader may believe that other ethical rules or principles are pertinent to this case. If so, they should also be considered as the analysis proceeds.

Step #3 How should these rules and principles be ranked or balanced against each other in order to resolve the ethical dilemma?

This step may sometimes be accomplished rather easily through the use of moral intuition. At other times, careful consideration of ethical theory can suggest the more fundamental action-guides to be applied. In some cases, it may be necessary to balance similarly weighted principles against each other, identifying when the weight of one versus another might be considered greater.

The rules and principles that Dr. Pike considers pertinent to her dilemma over how to respond to the inquiry by Mrs. Burns could be ranked as shown in Figure 12-2.

■ SUMMARY

In the case of Dr. Pike and Mrs. Burns, autonomy, justice, and nonmaleficence may be considered the primary principles that must be balanced against each other. Autonomy and justice are both valued principles within various deontological theories. Nonmaleficence and beneficence are the cornerstone principles of consequentialist theory. The principle of justice also seems to be inherent in the contract theory of medical ethics described by Veatch.[2] The other relevant rules and principles above support these primary principles and inform how they apply to specific ethical dilemmas. The Code of Ethics for Pharmacists (see Appendix 12-1) approved in 1994 provides further support for these fundamental principles and clearly indicates that the primary obligation of Dr. Pike is to Mrs. Burns rather than to Dr. Stills.[15,16] It may be surmised that all of the fundamental principles seem to support honestly discussing the benefits and risks of the therapy with the patient. However, if there

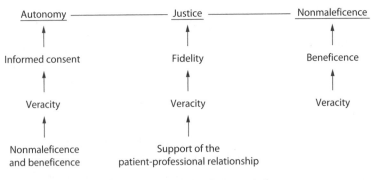

Figure 12–2. Possible hierarchy of "action-guides" in case.

were no good alternative therapies for Mrs. Burns' infection, and Dr. Pike was concerned that probable nonadherence constituted a greater risk to her and/or her baby, the decision would become more difficult. Once Dr. Pike has considered the facts of the case, who will be affected by her action, the cultural perspectives and legal requirements for the affected parties, and the relevant action-guides, she should have more clarity on what constitutes the ethical action. Finally, the personal beliefs and values of Dr. Pike relative to these principles of patient autonomy, promotion of justice, and the importance of potential consequences will all affect her ultimate ethical decision. It must be emphasized that she will make some response, even if only by avoiding the patient's question.

It is not likely that all will agree on the provided ranking or balancing of the pertinent rules and principles in this case, nor will there be universal agreement about what constitutes the right resolution to the ethical dilemma presented. It is necessary to remember that an ethical issue has been defined as one where most agree that there is a right answer, but cannot always agree on what that answer is.

Case Example 12–2 (Meso-Level Case)

Drs. Watt, Joseph, and Stockton are a physician, a nurse practitioner, and a pharmacist, respectively. These individuals are members of a project team who work for a multinational pharmaceutical company along with advertising, communications, and legal and technical production staff. The team has just been brought together and charged to prepare a new advertisement piece for a new cholesterol-lowering drug product. The promotional piece will be targeted toward consumers in the United States and also India; therefore, two different versions will be created. One version will meet the USFDA guidance on drug promotion rules by including a description of safety issues. The other version will omit the safety information because it will be used in India where guideline adherence is not monitored as closely (for additional information on drug promotion, see Chapter 25).

ANALYSIS

Step #1 Identification of relevant background information.
A. Factual details of the issue at hand.

During project group discussion, and based on their research, the health care professional members of the work group clarify their understanding of current USFDA guidance on drug promotion,[30,31] and WHO criteria for ethical medicinal drug promotion that are available to the world community.[32] They confirm that the FDA educates the pharmaceutical industry and health care professionals about what constitutes misleading prescription drug promotion, and takes action in response to complaints about instances of nonadherence with promotion guidelines in the United States.[33] The health care professionals of the project group also review two published reports analyzing compliance with WHO guidelines in India.[34,35] It appears from this research and an earlier study from India[36] that there has been an ongoing history of wide noncompliance with the WHO guidelines among companies marketing drugs in India.

B. Identification of who is affected by any ethical issue considered to be present: As these drug information developers work on creating the advertisement, it is again helpful to consider who might be impacted by the included and excluded information.

Certainly, the patient will be affected by the information included and excluded in the drug advertisement. There are advocates for and opponents against direct-to-consumer advertising (DTCA).[37] Advocates of DTCA suggest increased patient knowledge aids in patient ownership of their own health care and helps them make better choices. Opponents of DTCA argue the information in the advertisements may be misleading. Additionally, opponents suggest the prescriber-patient relationship may be negatively impacted.[37]

The medical professionals prescribing the promoted drugs may also be impacted in their ability to make evidence-based decisions on appropriate use of the drug. Their credibility may also be questioned if their prescribing practices are found to be deficient, especially if patients are demanding to be prescribed this new medication based on the placement of information in the advertisement. Furthermore, the prescriber's patients may be impacted to the extent that lack of full knowledge of the potential benefits and harms of the drug may negatively affect the outcomes of the therapy. A survey with 160 responses from physicians detailed the prescribing habits of those physicians who met with pharmaceutical sales representatives (PSRs).[38] The authors concluded that there is an association with a change in prescribing habits when a physician meets with PSRs.[38] This information suggests the potential for society, in general, to be negatively impacted by drug promotional materials that encourage prescribing of higher cost drugs, and the potential for lost productivity from workers who do not gain optimal disease state management.

C. Consideration of the cultural perspectives of all those affected by the dilemma.

The professional and cultural perspectives of both the project team professionals and the prescribers/patients must be considered, as well as the overall cultural norms of populations in the two countries.

The health care professionals confronting this potential ethical dilemma will need to address the cultural and professional standards and codes that they have subscribed to as licensed members of their professions. Indeed, it might be argued that these standards, in addition to their clinical experience, are reasons for their presence on this work group. These norms may be different in India versus the United States with respect to prescriber use and dependence on promotional materials as a main source of information about new drugs available for prescribing. The typically wide gap in social and educational status between the medical practitioner in India and his/her patients may also result in a greater tendency to follow the physician's directions without question. By comparison, in the United States, attitudes are often quite different, and there is also greater access for the patient to secondary sources of information. These factors may all lead to somewhat greater risk of negative impacts felt by prescribers and patients in a country where provided promotional materials are incomplete and even misleading, but may be the only written drug information available.

D. Consideration of the level of decision-making involved in responding to any ethical dilemma recognized by the DI practitioners.

These authors designated the case above as one involving a meso level of ethical decision-making by the concerned practitioners, because the activities involve workers within one specific drug manufacturing company. When considering the wide reach of actions taken by this group across the greater organizational system of the multinational company, and the multiple countries where the system operates, some might also appropriately judge this to involve a macro level of decision-making.

Step #2 Identification and justification of the relevant moral rules and principles (action-guides) pertinent to the case at hand.

Some might claim that the charge of this work group is wholly about advertising and marketing of a product, and as such claims no particular ethical demand on the producers of the advertising piece. Such an interpretation would require an assessment of the company's and the professionals' obligations to the WHO Guidelines, as well as other governmental and professional guidelines on drug information. There appears to be fairly clear ethical issues for these health care professionals, as they consider their roles in determining content of the planned promotional material. A brief listing of a few ethical rules and principles is provided below that should probably be considered by them as they consider their ethical responsibilities in preparation of the advertisement.

1. *Veracity*—Does this basic principle of obligation within deontological theory constitute a duty for these professionals, impelling them to advocate for complete and truthful information to be provided, in keeping with WHO guidelines? Within consequentialist theory, veracity also holds value as an ethical rule to the extent that it promotes better prescribing by the medical professionals using the promotional materials.
2. *Nonmaleficence*—A basic principle of consequentialist theory that would base a decision to divulge more complete and accurate information on minimizing the potential for harm. This principle appears to have relevance for the project group professionals to consider.

3. *Justice*—This principle within certain deontological theories addresses whether it is just to provide a higher level of educational content only subject to enforced regulation and guidelines, without regard to possible innate rights of access to such information by health care providers and patients in a country with less stringent safety protections. Basic fairness would seem to be relevant when the more informative and complete materials are being prepared and could perhaps be made available without a great deal of additional cost or effort.

4. *Respect for autonomy*—The principle described in deontological theory suggests the patient has a right to self-rule and a right to be involved in his or her own health care decisions. How could the patient make an informed decision regarding the new medication if the information is incomplete?

The reader is encouraged to consider other ethical rules and principles that may apply to this case, as well as think about what seems to be a general tendency by some to dismiss the professional and ethical obligations of licensed health care professionals producing such materials for advertising purposes.

Step #3 How should these rules and principles be ranked or balanced against each other in order to resolve the ethical dilemma?

The reader will need to consider these rules and principles, as well as any others considered pertinent, in order to reach his or her own conclusions about the professionals' ethical responsibilities to the ultimate beneficiaries (or victims) of these information services. How does one think he or she would view his or her role and responsibilities if he or she were a health care professional providing drug information in circumstances such as these?

■ SUMMARY

The reader is encouraged to apply this process of analysis to two additional case scenarios. Imagine a set of circumstances that might provide the background context behind each case, and carry out an ethical analysis in light of this context. The reader might perhaps then vary some important aspect of the background context to determine whether this affects the analysis of the ethical dimensions of the case. As each case is considered, also assess at what level of health care (micro, meso, or macro) does the ethical decision-making seem to apply.

Case Study 12–1 (Micro Level)

A study evaluating a new medication for hypercholesterolemia includes a whole-genome sequencing component. The consent document includes a separate section for study subjects to consent to the genomic testing, but the consent document did not address what to do if there is an incidental genomic finding (IGF). During the study, there is an IGF of *BRCA* gene (indicates a substantially increased risk of developing breast cancer) in a female subject who consented to the whole-genome sequencing. Does the study team have an ethical responsibility to inform the subject of this finding?

1. Assess whether this drug information request constitutes a potential ethical dilemma, based on the three characteristics that differentiate such a situation.
2. What background information might you want to obtain to clarify this information request? (Imagine a background with details that might establish this as an ethical dilemma for you.)
3. If you can imagine this scenario to constitute an ethical dilemma for the study team, identify whether you consider it a situation requiring decision-making at a micro, meso, or macro level.
4. Consider what moral rules and principles are likely to apply to this issue.
5. Assuming that some of these relevant action-guides conflict with others, describe further deliberations by which the clinician might prioritize or balance these conflicts in order to reach a decision on how to respond to the information request.
6. What organizational strategies might best prepare the study team to most effectively respond to ethical dilemmas such as this one?

Refer to the article "Management and return of incidental genomic findings in clinical trials" by C Ayuso and associates for further information regarding IGF during clinical trials.[57]

Case Study 12–2 (Micro Level)

A nurse on one of the medical-surgical units of your hospital calls you, the on-call pain pharmacist, with a question. She has a patient who she believes is being undertreated for pain. The patient is a young female who was admitted the previous evening after a car accident. She is a frequent patient in the ER, known to have a drug problem, including a variety of street products. She does not believe that the patient is in withdrawal, but does think she is getting inadequate pain medications for the severe bruises, scrapes, and a broken arm. However, the admitting physician is quite adamant that he will not enable the patient's drug habit, and maintains that perhaps living with some pain will encourage the patient to mend her ways. The nurse asks you to intervene with the physician to convince him that additional pain therapy is indicated, medically and ethically, for this patient.

1. Assess whether this drug information request constitutes a potential ethical dilemma, based on the three characteristics that differentiate such a situation.
2. What background information might you want to obtain to clarify this information request? (Imagine a background with details that might establish this as an ethical dilemma for you.)
3. If you can imagine this scenario to constitute an ethical dilemma for the pain management nurse, identify whether you consider it a situation requiring decision-making at a micro, meso, or macro level.
4. Consider what moral rules and principles are likely to apply to this issue.
5. Assuming that some of these relevant action-guides conflict with others, describe further deliberations by which the clinician might prioritize or balance these conflicts in order to reach a decision on how to respond to the information request.
6. What organizational strategies might best prepare this nurse specialist to most effectively respond to ethical dilemmas such as this one?

Refer to the article "Ethical dilemmas: controversies in pain management" by Janet Brown to read the analysis of a similar case.[58]

Case Study 12–3 (Meso Level)

Dr. Blake, who is a drug information pharmacist, is asked by a hospital administrator to review and encouraged to recommend a medication for formulary. This medication is not as effective, is less expensive, and has a more adverse events compared with a medication in its same class already on the formulary. Dr. Blake discovers a conflict of interest as the spouse of the hospital administrator works for the pharmaceutical company of this new medication being considered for formulary.

● ■ ANALYSIS

1. Assess whether this drug information request constitutes a potential ethical dilemma, based on the three characteristics that differentiate such a situation.
2. What background information might you want to obtain to clarify this information request? (Imagine a background context with details that might establish this as an ethical dilemma for you.)

3. If you can envision this scenario to constitute an ethical dilemma for this health care professional, identify whether you consider it a situation requiring decision-making at a micro, meso, or macro level.
4. Consider what moral rules and principles are likely to apply to this issue.
5. Assuming that some of these relevant action-guides conflict with others, describe further deliberations by which the clinician might prioritize or balance these conflicts in order to reach a decision on how to respond to the information request.
6. What organizational strategies might best prepare this pharmacist to most effectively respond to ethical dilemmas such as this one?

Case Study 12–4 (Macro Level)

A physician in the urology department of the hospital is prescribing a parenteral agent called nudrugumab for patients with a certain urological condition. There are limited data supporting the use of the agent for the urologic condition, and the product is compounded. It is unknown if the patients know this is an unlabeled use for this unapproved medication. The physician approached his state representative regarding how to change the state law. The use of this new agent is escalated to the Chief of Pharmacy and Chief Medical Officer who will meet to discuss the situation.

● ■ ANALYSIS

1. Assess whether this drug information request constitutes a potential ethical dilemma, based on the three characteristics that differentiate such a situation.
2. What background information might you want to obtain to clarify this information request? (Imagine a background context with details that might establish this as an ethical dilemma for you.)
3. If you can envision this scenario to constitute an ethical dilemma for this health care professional, identify whether you consider it a situation requiring decision-making at a micro, meso, or macro level.
4. Consider what moral rules and principles are likely to apply to this issue.
5. Assuming that some of these relevant action-guides conflict with others, describe further deliberations by which the clinician might prioritize or balance these conflicts in order to reach a decision on how to respond to the information request.

6. What organizational strategies might best prepare this pharmacist to most effectively respond to ethical dilemmas such as this one?

Resources for Use by Professionals Seeking to Learn More about Medical Ethics, as Applied to Issues Involving Provision of Drug Information

❽ *Health care professionals need training, resources, and support to prepare them to effectively address the ethical dilemmas they confront.* The first goal in learning more about medical ethics should be to learn to recognize opportunities for ethical deliberation when they are confronted. Situations will arise where ethical judgments will be made that have moral consequences—with or without the conscious understanding of the parties involved. It is just as important that professionals are prepared to deal with these situations, as it is for them to learn how to address efficacy and safety concerns relative to drug therapies. This section of the chapter offers a survey of medical ethics resources that can assist practitioners who personally desire to learn how to better recognize ethical situations and how to respond to them, or who will be teaching others in formal settings or informally in the workplace.

Formal coursework, inservices, or continuing education opportunities can teach skills that will aid professionals in handling ethical dilemmas related to work responsibilities involving provision of drug information. Thornton and associates[20] discussed what should be taught in basic ethics education that takes place within and outside the academic environment. Their review of important elements to be included in ethics education is worthwhile reading for anyone who may desire to participate in these teaching activities. They also refer the reader to other useful resources on the topic. In Davis's manual on patient-practitioner interactions, the author presents an easy to understand description of the stages of moral development, comparing two commonly identified models proposed by Piaget and by Kohlberg.[39] This information is valuable to assist in gaining insight into one's personal moral development, as well as that of others. This workbook, published by a physical therapist for the purpose of assisting in the professional socialization process, also offers a description of moral values associated with development as a professional. The author goes on to present a framework for resolving ethical dilemmas that has similar elements to those presented in this chapter; she also provides exercises that could be readily adapted for use in various health care professionals' education or even for professional inservices.

Haddad and associates[1] provided a comprehensive guideline on pharmacy ethics course content; this is also valuable reading for those wishing to address ethics topics in continuing education of health care professionals. This guideline describes examples of educational methods including case presentation and debate; scenario building, with identification and discussion of potential ethical issues; and role-playing activities. The authors indicate that such educational methods should involve group participation to conduct the analysis of sample cases for the ethical issue being discussed. Writing techniques, such as a 5-minute write exercise prior to discussion, can serve to focus the participant's ideas and facilitate the resultant discussion.[40] The guideline also provides an extensive bibliography of resource materials. Two other texts, one edited by Haddad[41] and the third edition of Case Studies in Pharmacy Ethics by Veatch and Haddad,[42] provide further discussion of teaching methods and many case examples of ethical dilemmas confronted by pharmacists.

Pirl[15] described the use of role-playing assignments for pharmacy students. This article also listed case scenarios that could be used in continuing education programs for any practitioners who are exploring ways to resolve ethical dilemmas arising in their provision of drug information. Smith and associates[43] wrote a book on pharmacy ethics that also provides background discussion and case examples that relate to many target areas of health care practice, including providing responses to drug information inquiries. This resource can be very useful for various practitioners who need to address ethical issues in their particular area of practice. Case discussion activities should always respect the privacy of individual practitioners and patients who have been involved in any specific case with ethical dimensions.

Students and practitioners also require education about their ethical obligations when receiving and passing on manufacturer's drug information at micro, meso, or macro levels of practice. Monaghan and associates[44] addressed this issue in their report, "Student understanding of the relationship between the health professions and the pharmaceutical industry." This cross-sectional survey of pharmacy, nursing, and medical students identified deficiencies in student knowledge and attitudes about ethical aspects of professional interactions with drug companies. Over reliance on potentially biased or incomplete promotional materials provided by industry representatives may lead professionals to make less than optimal therapeutic decisions or recommendations for their patients. It may also lead professional consultants or institutional leaders to recommend institution-wide (meso-level) therapeutic policies such as formulary approvals that do not reflect the best available evidence. Physicians were 13 times more likely to request that drugs manufactured by specific companies be added to the formulary if they had met with industry representatives from that company. The FDA provides information and tools for health care professional education on what to expect in compliant product promotion literature, and guidance on reporting "Bad Ad" materials.[31,33]

As they prepare drug information, health care professionals must also be vigilant about the potential for ethical lapses such as scientific misconduct to impact the evidence available to them from the drug therapy literature. Samp and associates[45] identified 73 drug study articles published in the general biomedical literature between 2000 and 2011 that were classified as representing scientific misconduct. Steen also identified about 800 articles indexed on PubMed that were retracted for fraud or error between 2000 and 2010.[46] Research misconduct (fabrication or falsification of data) was generally intentional with a greater number of authors and where the first author was an author in another retracted paper. While learning of such publication-related ethical lapses would not inherently constitute an ethical dilemma for the drug information provider, deciding whether and how to correct faulty drug information developed from such materials might indeed constitute such a dilemma.

Information technology is an integral part of the provision of drug information by health care professionals. Sometimes technology is used as a tool to access literature and other information sources used by the professional responding to an inquiry. In other cases, the professional may use the Internet to offer drug information to various target audiences, both professional and the lay public. Anderson and Goodman authored a book Ethics and Information Technology: A Case-based Approach to a Health Care System in Transition.[47] This book addresses many ethical issues of pertinence to health care professionals, related both to web-based services and drug information. Case studies on topics such as provision or use of inaccurate information, conflicts of interest, issues of confidentiality and data sharing, and ethical standards that have been set for health websites are presented.

Poirier and Laux[48] have discussed redesign of a drug information resources course to meet the needs of nontraditional Doctor of Pharmacy students. This report describes addition of a course section where ethical issues associated with drug information questions received at the author's practice site were used to demonstrate how to deal with such situations. The authors used self-study, computer-assisted instruction, and recitations to teach the course. Published descriptions of ethical dilemmas arising during the provision of drug information may be used to build case discussions. These scenarios are helpful for educators of both traditional and nontraditional students, as well as for inservices aimed at practicing health care professionals.[24–26]

Structures That Support Ethical Decision-Making

Berger describes the need for an ethical covenant between the pharmacist and the patient who is being provided pharmaceutical care.[23] This term suggests an implicit contract between client and health care provider that broadly describes the relationship involved whenever a pharmacist provides drug information. Within this contract, the service recipient has a right to receive competently provided information as well as respectful treatment. He or she also has the obligation to provide background information needed by the pharmacist. Likewise, the pharmacist has the right to adequate background information (and respectful treatment as well), and the obligation to give competent, trustworthy, and caring service. Recognition of this implicit contract can occasionally suggest corrective action to resolve or avoid perceived ethical dilemmas. Such recognition is especially helpful when there has been a failure to adequately communicate, or there has been a lack of mutual respect in the interaction. Pharmacists also have a revised Code of Ethics for Pharmacists available to them since 1994, which may serve as a general guide to those obligations implicit to the patient-pharmacist relationship.[49,50] The text of this Code is provided in Appendix 12-1. While specific documents will not be reviewed here, there are Codes and Ethical Standards set forth by associations for nurses and physicians that describe the rules of relationship with clients who are requesting drug information among other services.

It is also important to establish organizational structures that guide and support the practitioner providing drug information (in any setting), when he or she is faced with an ethical dilemma. Some formal structures, such as ethics committees[51,52] and other policy setting bodies (e.g., pharmacy and therapeutics committees), are generally available in larger hospitals. Formal attention to education and anticipatory planning activities on how to address ethical conflict situations is also needed within smaller hospitals and care centers, the chain pharmacy setting, or in small independent or nonprofit health care organizations (e.g., independent community pharmacies, rural hospitals). A report on a survey of medicine information pharmacists, conducted in the United Kingdom, assessed perceptions of possible ethical scenarios involving lay callers, and asked about respondents' training to address such situations.[53] The authors described considerable variation in how specific scenarios were addressed, and a minority of the respondents had received training in this area. It is also imperative that pharmacists and other health care professionals participate in policy setting that may affect how they are expected to practice.

Both the organization and the individual practitioner have an obligation to plan in advance how they will handle situations where ethical conflict might arise, particularly relative to compliance with any policy affecting the employee's patient care obligations.

An article, "Promising, professional obligations, and the refusal to provide service," by Alexander maintained that the professional "may not override the obligations derived from a prior act of promising to abide by the values, norms, and procedures that define their professional roles as instantiated within a specific practice," suggesting that the professional should leave the organization if they cannot conform to the expectations of their role within that practice.[54] In practice, pharmacists and other practitioners may have to deal with a specific ethical dilemma very rapidly and alone in order to decide or act in a timely manner. Case law may vary among the different states, and policies and procedures will vary by company. It is important for health care professionals to understand their obligations under law versus their own personal beliefs. Policies and procedures to inform and support the clinician in overall client interactions, and in ethical analysis and decision-making, can better prepare the practitioner to address the real-life dilemmas he or she will encounter. Practitioners should be involved early (whatever their side in the issue) to make their voices heard during initial policy development (a meso-level activity within the organization, or perhaps a macro-level one if contributing to policy development for the whole profession or in law). They must also keep themselves informed about existing organizational policies in order to protect themselves and their patients. In the opinion of these authors, after the fact controversy over unfamiliar policies does not serve the needs of practitioners, patients, or organizations.

Organizations can assist professionals by sponsoring the creation of explicit policies addressing certain issues that have demonstrated a history of ethical controversy. For example, in the American Society of Health System Pharmacists (ASHP) "ASHP guidelines on the pharmacist's role in providing drug information" it is explicitly stated that "Consideration should be given to the ethical and legal aspects of responding to medication information requests."[55] In relation to the emergency contraception case mentioned above, a written policy might state that clinicians may refer questions (to another practice colleague or perhaps at a minimum back to the prescriber), where provision of an answer would violate their personal ethics. This could at least partially resolve a potential dilemma for the practitioner who has been asked to provide information that involves ethical conflict. A policy that states practitioners are not required to answer questions from a client who refuses to provide required background information could guide response in the dilemma of dealing with an unidentified client who wants to know how long amphetamine can be detected in the urine. Another policy might address adequate staffing requirements to ensure the community pharmacist has adequate time to perform counseling services. Of course, the legal and ethical rights of clients have to be recognized during development of such policies. These authors believe that all health care professionals, including pharmacists, should demand the right to a major role in organizational policy development that affects their practice, preferably with input from client/patient representatives. To be useful, organizational policies must be developed with attention to avoiding what constitutes infringement on the domain of personal ethics (such as a personal prohibition against euthanasia).

Finally, institutions engaged in the professional education of health care practitioners must provide foundational education in the area of ethics. Organizations employing these practitioners should continue this education through the use of various continuing education programs that foster increasing skills in application of ethical principles to practical decision-making.[56]

Conclusion

Many health care professionals will be called on to provide drug information. On occasion, they will encounter ethical dilemmas regarding what information, if any, should be provided. It is important that the practitioner approach such moments prepared to, often quickly, identify the pertinent facts, analyze relevant points of the situation, and rank or balance the pertinent ethical rules and principles that are involved. The individual professional must recognize his or her rights and responsibilities relative to the client, to other involved individuals and populations, to society as a whole, and to any higher power to whom the practitioner feels accountable. Organizations can assist employee professionals by formal identification and orientation on certain implicit and explicit policies. Furthermore, opportunities for deliberate study and rehearsal of important analytic steps are important to help practitioners be prepared to address ethical dilemmas that arise when providing drug information.

Self-Assessment Questions

1. Characteristics that differentiate an ethical deliberation from other decision-making endeavors include which of the following? (Choose all that apply.)
   a. The issue is universal with any parties involved agreeing that there is a right or wrong answer.
   b. The issue has been addressed in law with penalties identified for failure to comply with the legal directive.
   c. The welfare of all parties affected by the judgment at hand is considered.
   d. The issue is fundamental with no higher standard against which to measure the rightness of the decision.

2. A retail pharmacist receives two prescriptions for two different patients for an oral oncology agent. The agent is on national shortage, and the pharmacist only has enough to fill one of the prescriptions. More product is not expected for a few months, and other pharmacies in the area are unable to procure the medication. What level of ethical decision-making comes into play while the pharmacist decides who receives the oncology medication?
   a. Micro level
   b. Meso level
   c. Macro level
   d. No ethical dilemma exists

3. Assuming you decide that the case in Question #2 involves an ethical dilemma for the pharmacist, which of the following ethical rules or principles do you think would potentially apply to the situation? (Choose all that apply.)
   a. Consent
   b. Fidelity
   c. Respect for persons
   d. Veracity

4. A new policy is presented to the Pharmacy & Therapeutics (P&T) Committee regarding the administration of the influenza immunization by certified pharmacy technicians in the outpatient pharmacy. A physician and nurse who are members of the P&T committee strongly disapprove of this new policy. They believe the law does not permit pharmacy technicians to administer this vaccine. What level of ethical decision-making is described in this situation?
   a. Micro level
   b. Meso level
   c. Macro level
   d. None of the above

5. A practitioner is asked by administration to present an in-service for department colleagues on a recently approved drug product that may have applicability for use in the department's target population. The clinician is expected to present a set of materials provided by the administrator. What would be a first step in determining whether this is an ethical dilemma for the presenter?
   a. Considering who might be affected by the dilemma
   b. Considering the cultural perspectives of those attending the presentation
   c. Determining what ethical rules seem to be at play in this situation
   d. Seeking the factual details relative to the content provided by the administrator

6. Based on question #5, assume the practitioner does ultimately feel that he is confronting an ethical dilemma in being asked to present drug information with which he disagrees. Which of the following organization policies might be useful to support this professional in addressing his dilemma? (Choose all choices that apply.)
   a. A policy that requires supervisor approval of all educational content presented by staff professionals
   b. A policy that supports staff professional's freedom to independently develop educational content of drug information provided in group settings, subject to review by designated expert reviewers
   c. A policy establishing a mediation process for resolving conflict between staff professionals and administrative supervisors
   d. A policy mandating education for administrative and professional staff on shared governance and professional rights and responsibilities

7. Which of the following statements are true when describing ethics?
   a. Philosophical inquiry on the moral dimensions of human conduct.
   b. The terms "ethical" and "moral" have substantially different meaning.
   c. Ethics involves the study of moral development.
   d. Ethics involves concrete judgments on the legal aspects of situations.

8. Ethical issues might arise around which of the following kinds of issues in relationship to the provision of drug information?
   a. Decisions by the health professional on whether to provide drug information.
   b. Decisions on policies related to access to drug information.
   c. Both answers in a and b may involve ethical issues.
   d. Neither answer in a or b is likely to involve ethical issues.

9. Identification of relevant background information when analyzing an ethical dilemma includes which of the following statements? (Choose all that apply.)
   a. Determine the applicable moral rules in the case.
   b. Determine the factual details of the issue at hand.
   c. Consider who is affected by the ethical issue.
   d. Identify the cultural perspectives of the dilemma.

10. The purposes for identifying relevant background in analyzing a potential ethical dilemma include which of the following? (Choose all that apply.)
    a. Knowledge of available background information sometimes alleviates any moral concerns about the issue.
    b. Background information typically clarifies what parties might be affected by decisions made or actions taken.
    c. Background information generally leads to resolution of a recognized ethical dilemma without further analysis.
    d. Background information normally facilitates the drug information provider in addressing the dilemma in a culturally sensitive manner.

11. A spouse comes into the outpatient pharmacy and asks the pharmacy intern if his wife is taking an oral contraception pill. Which of the following moral rules or principles apply to this situation? (Choose all that apply.)
    a. Privacy
    b. Beneficence
    c. Confidentiality
    d. Justice

12. A pediatric pharmacist is conducting a medication reconciliation for a 15-year-old patient. The patient mentions she takes three herbal products and oral contraceptive pills (OCPs). The patient does not want her mother to know about the

OCPs. What additional information is needed before considering any ethical concerns the pharmacist may have about this situation?

a. The reason why the patient does not want the pharmacist to speak with the mother

b. Potential drug-drug interactions between the herbal products and OCPs

c. Possible side effects of the herbal products

d. Indications for the herbal products

13. Considering question 12, which of the following ethical principles or rules do you think would be most pertinent to this case?

a. Nonmaleficence

b. Consent

c. Privacy

d. Beneficence

14. A medical oncology physician is the primary investigator for an investigator-initiated trial evaluating a combination of chemotherapy agents (new agent plus standard of care) for pancreatic cancer. Oncology guidelines were updated to include a different combination of chemotherapy agents (different agent plus standard of care). The investigator wants to enroll the patient in the trial instead of starting therapy per the updated guidelines. Which of the following action-guides is likely to be prioritized in this ethical dilemma?

a. Respecting the patient-professional relationship

b. Nonmaleficence

c. Confidentiality

d. Consent

15. You are a clinic pharmacist working collaboratively with a physician in a pain clinic. A patient reports having uncontrolled chronic pain secondary to a car accident 3 years ago. The patient reports she tried medical marijuana while on vacation, and her pain was significantly less. The patient currently takes less than 45 mg morphine milligram equivalents, and she would like some additional pain control. The physician is able to write a letter of recommendation for medical marijuana per state law; however, the health system does not support providers writing these letters. What level of ethical decision-making would this scenario constitute if there is an ethical dilemma?

a. Micro level

b. Meso level

c. Macro level

d. None because there is no ethical dilemma

REFERENCES

1. Haddad AM, Kaatz B, McCart G, McCarthy RL, Pink LA, Richardson J. Report of the ethics course content committee: curricular guidelines for pharmacy education. Am J Pharm Educ. 1993;57(Winter Suppl):34S-43S.

2. Veatch RM. Hospital pharmacy: what is ethical? (Primer). Am J Hosp Pharm. 1989;46:109-15.

3. Wilson R, Rowan MS, Henderson J. Core and comprehensive health care services: 1. Introduction to the Canadian Medical Association's decision-making framework. Can Med Assoc. 1995;152(7):1063-6.

4. Smith L, Morrissy J. Ethical dilemmas for general practitioners under the UK new contract. J Med Ethics. 1994;20:175-80.

5. Dierchx de Casterle B, Meulenbergs T, van de Vijver L, Tanghe A, Castmans C. Ethics meetings in support of good nursing care: some practice-based thoughts. Nurs Ethics. 2002;9(6):612-22.

6. Kirby J, Simpson C. An innovative, inclusive process for meso-level health policy development. HEC Forum. 2007;19(2):161-76.

7. Martin D, Singer P. A strategy to improve priority setting in health care institutions. Health Care Anal. 2003;11(1):59-68.

8. Goold SD. Trust and the ethics of health care institutions. Hastings Cent Rep. 2001;6:26-33.

9. Nunes R. Evidence-based medicine: a new tool for resource allocation? Med Health Care Phil. 2003;6:297-301.

10. Coyle SL, for the Ethics and Human Rights Committee, American College of Physicians-American Society of Internal Medicine. Physician-industry relations. Part 1: Individual physicians. Ann Intern Med. 2002;136:396-402.

11. Kenny N, Joffres C. An ethical analysis of international health priority-setting. Health Care Anal. 2007;16:145-60.

12. Ruger JP. Ethics in American Health 1: ethical approaches to health policy. Am J Pub Health. 2008;98(10):1751-6.

13. Ruger JP. Ethics in American Health 2: an ethical framework for health system reform. Am J Pub Health. 2008;98(10):1756-63.

14. Khushf G. The case for managed care: reappraising medical and socio-political ideals. J Med Phil. 1999;24(5):415-33.

15. Pirl MA. An ethics laboratory as an educational tool in a pharmacy law and ethics course. J Pharm Teach. 1990;1(3):51-68.

16. Beauchamp TLC, Childress JF. Principles of biomedical ethics. 8th ed. New York: Oxford University Press; 2019.

17. Beauchamp TLC, Childress JF. Principles of biomedical ethics. 4th ed. New York: Oxford University Press; 1994.

18. Beauchamp TL. Principles or rules? In: Kopelman L, editor. Building bioethics. Great Britain: Kluwer Academic Publishers; 1999. p. 15-24.

19. Veatch RM. Cross-cultural perspectives in medical ethics. 2nd ed. Sudbury (MA): Jones and Bartlett Publishers; 2000.

20. Thornton BC, Callahan D, Nelson JL. Bioethics education: expanding the circle of participants. Hastings Cent Rep. 1993;23(1):25-29.

21. Veatch RM. A theory of medical ethics. New York: Basic Books Publishers; 1981.

22. Carrese J, Brown K, Jameton A. Culture, healing, and professional obligations. Hastings Cent Rep. 1993;15:7.

23. Berger BA. Building an effective therapeutic alliance: competence, trustworthiness, and caring. Am J Hosp Pharm. 1993;50:2399-2403.

24. Arnold RM, Nissen JC, Campbell NA. Ethical issues in a drug information center. Drug Intell Clin Pharm. 1987;21:1008-11.

25. Kelly WN, Krause EC, Krowsinski WJ, Small TR, Drane JF. National survey of ethical issues presented to drug information centers. Am J Hosp Pharm. 1990;47:2245-50.

26. Schools RM, Brushwood DB. The pharmacist's role in patient care. Hastings Cent Rep. 1991;12:7.

27. Haddad AM. Reflections on the pharmacist-patient covenant. Am J Pharm Educ. 2018;82(7):6806.

28. Powers M, Faden R. Social justice. The moral foundations of public health and health policy. New York: Oxford University Press; 2006.

29. Bayer R, Gostin LO, Jennings B, Steinbock B, editors. Public health ethics. Theory, policy and practice. New York: Oxford University Press; 2007.

30. U.S. Food and Drug Administration. Guidance for industry presenting risk information in prescription drug and medical device promotion: DRAFT GUIDANCE: Food and Drug Administration; 2009 [cited 2013 Oct 18]. Available from: http://www.complianceonline.com/articlefiles/FDA_Guidance_Presenting_Risk_Information_Labels_Drugs_Devices.pdf

31. ComplianceOnline.com. Risk information in prescription drug & medical device ads, promotional labeling—what the FDA expects. ComplianceOnline; 2011 Nov [cited 2016 Sep 15]. Available from: http://www.complianceonline.com/ecommerce/control/article Detail?contentId=12737&catId=10002

32. World Health Organization. Ethical criteria for medicinal drug promotion. Geneva: World Health Organization; 1988 [cited 2016 Sep 15]. Available from: http://apps.who.int/medicinedocs/documents/whozip08e/whozip08e.pdf

33. U.S. Food and Drug Administration. Truthful prescription drug advertising and promotion. Food and Drug Administration; 2018 Jun [cited 2020 Mar]. Available from: https://www.fda.gov/drugs/office-prescription-drug-promotion/truthful-prescription-drug-advertising-and-promotion

34. Khakhkhar T, Mehta M, Shah R, Sharma D. Evaluation of drug promotional literatures using WHO guidelines [Internet]. J Pharm Negative Results. 2013; 4:33-8. Available from: http://www.pnrjournal.com/article.asp?issn=0976-9234;year=2013;volume=4;issue=1;spage=33;epage=38;aulast=Khakhkhar

35. Dhanaraj E, Nigam A, Bagani S, Singh H, Tiwari P. Supported and unsupported claims in medicinal drug advertisements in Indian medical journals. Indian J Med Ethics. 2011;8(3):170-4.

36. Lal A. Information contents of drug advertisements: an Indian experience. Ann Pharmacother. 1998;32:1234.

37. Womack CA. Ethical and epistemic issues in direct-to-consumer drug advertising: where is patient agency? Med Health Care Philos. 2013;13:275-80.

38. Lieb K, Scheurich A. Contact between doctors and the pharmaceutical industry, their perceptions, and the effects on prescribing habits. PLoS One. 2014;9(10):e110130.

39. Davis CM. Patient practitioner interaction: an experiential manual for developing the art of health care. Thorofare (NJ): Slack; 1989.

40. Coach R. 5-minutes to monitor progress. Teaching Prof. 1991;5(9):1-2.

41. Haddad AM, editor. Teaching and learning strategies in pharmacy ethics. 2nd ed. Binghamton (NY): Pharmaceutical Products Press; 1997.

42. Veatch RM, Haddad AM. Case studies in pharmacy ethics. 3rd ed. New York: Oxford University Press; 2017.

43. Smith M, Strauss S, Baldwin HJ, Alberts KT. Pharmacy ethics. New York: Pharmaceutical Products Press; 1991.

44. Monaghan M, Galt KA, Turner P, Houghton B, Rich E, Markert R, Bergman-Evans B. Student understanding of the relationship between the health professions and the pharmaceutical industry [Internet]. Teach Learn Med. 2009;15(1):14-20. Available from: http://www.tandfonline.com/doi/pdf/10.1207/S15328015TLM1501_04?needAccess=true

45. Samp JC, Schumock GT, Pickard AS. Retracted publications in the drug literature. Pharmacotherapy. 2012;32(7):586-95.

46. Steen RG. Retractions in the scientific literature: do authors deliberately commit research fraud? J Med Ethics. 2011;37:113-7.

47. Anderson JG, Goodman KW. Ethics and information technology: a case-based approach to a health care system in transition. New York: Springer-Verlag; 2002.

48. Poirier TL, Laux R. Redesign of a drug information resources course: responding to the needs of nontraditional PharmD students. Am J Pharm Educ. 1997;61:306-9.

49. Vottero LD. Code of ethics for pharmacists. Am J Health Syst Pharm. 1995;52:2096-2131.

50. American Pharmacists Association. Code of ethics 1994 [updated 1994 Oct 27; 2010 Mar 26]. Available from: http://www.pharmacist.com/code-ethics

51. Mappes TA, Zembaty JS, editors. Biomedical ethics. 3rd ed. New York: McGraw-Hill; 1991.

52. Mappes TA, Degrazia D, editors. Biomedical ethics. 5th ed. Boston (MA): McGraw-Hill; 2001.

53. Wills S, Brown D, Astubry S. A survey of ethical issues surrounding supply of information to members of the public by hospital pharmacy medicines information centres. Pharm World Sci. 2002;24(2):55-60.

54. Alexander JK. Promising, professional obligations, and the refusal to provide service. HEC Forum. 2005;17(3):178-95.

55. Ghaibi S, Ipema H, Gabay M. ASHP guidelines on the pharmacist's role in providing drug information. Am J Health Syst Pharm. 2015;72:573-7.

56. Gettman DA, Benson B, Nguyen V, Luu SN, editors. Use of motivational techniques by drug information center personnel to respond to calls involving perceived ethical dilemmas [Abstract]. ASHP Midyear Clinical Meeting; 2000.

57. Ayuso C, Millan JM, Dal-Re R. Management and return of incidental genomic findings in clinical trials. Pharmacogenomics J. 2015;15:1-5.

58. Brown J. Ethical dilemmas: controversies in pain management. Adv Nurse Pract. 1997:69-72.

SUGGESTED READINGS

1. Wills S, Brown D, Astbury S. A survey of ethical issues surrounding supply of information to members of the public by hospital pharmacy medicines information centres. Pharm World Sci (The Netherlands). 2002;24(Feb):55-60.

2. Kelly WN, Krause EC, Krowsinski WJ, Small TR, Drane JF. National survey of ethical issues presented to drug information centers. Am J Hosp Pharm. 1990;47:2245-50.

3. Beauchamp TLC, Childress JF. Principles of biomedical ethics. 6th ed. New York: Oxford University Press; 2012.

4. Veatch RM, Haddad A. Case studies in biomedical ethics. 2nd ed. New York: Oxford University Press; 2015.

5. Ethical criteria for medicinal drug promotion [Internet]. Geneva: World Health Organization; 1988 [cited 2013 Oct 18]. Available from: http://apps.who.int/medicinedocs/documents/whozip08e/whozip08e.pdf

13

Chapter Thirteen

Professional Communication of Drug Information

Patrick M. Malone • Meghan J. Malone

Learning Objectives

● *After completing this chapter, the reader will be able to:*

- State reasons both for and against writing professionally.
- Describe the various steps of professional writing.
- Identify the order for authors in a professional paper.
- Describe the importance of knowing the audience.
- Describe various writing styles and their differences.
- Explain where to find a publication's requirements for submission.
- Describe what an article proposal consists of and why it is used.
- Explain the need for continued practice to develop good writing skills.
- List the components of both a research and review paper.
- Explain the general guidelines for writing.
- Explain the absolute importance of revision.
- Explain the steps in creating a website or newsletter.
- Describe how to prepare audiovisual materials for a poster or platform presentation and place those items on a website.
- Describe techniques for creating an abstract for an article.
- Describe how to correctly cite reference materials.

Key Concepts

❶ Essentially any time a professional takes pen, stylus, word processor, or any other writing implement in hand to fulfill professional duties, it is considered professional writing.

❷ When writing, it is best to keep things as simple and direct as possible.

❸ With the probable exception of policy and procedure documents, the two most important paragraphs in any document are the first and last.

❹ If the information is taken from a specific source, even if it is reworded, the original author should be given credit via citation.

❺ In many cases, revision of a document will be necessary.

❻ Instead of concentrating on the technology, it is best to concentrate on the message.

❼ Professional writing is a skill necessary for every health care professional.

Introduction

A common thought when considering the topic of **professional writing** is "That doesn't apply to me, I'm not writing for a journal," but professional writing is certainly not limited to journal articles or books. It includes writing evaluations of medications for consideration on a hospital formulary, writing policies and procedures for the preparation of an intravenous admixture, reporting the results of the latest sales to the home office, writing for a professional website, responding to a drug information question via email, preparing a written performance evaluation, writing in a chart, writing a paper for a class, preparing slides or posters for a presentation, writing a letter of recommendation,[1] and many other things. ❶ *Essentially any time a professional takes pen, stylus, word processor, or any other writing implement in hand to fulfill professional duties, it is considered professional writing.* When writing, although the format changes, the general principles remain the same. So, whether the objective is to write the ultimate book on the practice of medicine or to prepare a label for a prescription vial, a health care professional must know how to write professionally.

Although some may say the purpose of writing is to keep a job or to pass a course, there are, generally, four larger purposes for the existence of written material: to inform, instruct, persuade, or entertain. The first three items are those usually considered in professional writing, although including the fourth, whenever possible and appropriate, will help keep people interested in what they are reading.

There are also some advantages to professional writing, besides those mentioned above. For example, writing is often used to evaluate an employee for promotion in many jobs. In academia, there is always the concept of publish or perish. Pharmacy technicians are also encouraged to write as a means of advancement.[2] Additionally, writing gives the authors the opportunity to share their knowledge or ideas,[3] obtain gratification or satisfaction,[4] and improve their knowledge. It may even lead to some fame or notoriety in a field.

Unfortunately, there are disadvantages to professional writing. The major problem is that any significant amount of writing often involves a great deal of time and a lot of potentially frustrating work, because few people are natural writers. The author must practice becoming proficient at writing, which will involve false starts, numerous drafts, roadblocks, and other problems.[5] If that is not enough, writing exposes a person to criticism and possible rejection. Although at one time authors were paid to publish articles, today it is not unheard of that authors may have to pay to have their article published.[6,7]

At best, the direct financial rewards are likely to be few in professional writing. Indirectly, writing may lead to pay increases and promotions. However, because writing is a professional necessity, it is unavoidable. It can be made easier by following the correct procedures, which will be covered in this chapter.

Steps in Writing

As each step in professional writing is covered in this section, the emphasis will be on writing items likely to be encountered in a professional practice setting, although additional steps that are necessary when writing for publication will be mentioned.

PREPARING TO WRITE

The first step in writing is to know the purpose—why something needs to be written in the first place. It is necessary at this time to have a good idea of the expected endpoint, which is important, no matter what is being done. For example, someone learning to mow grass with a lawn mower may be concentrating on the ground near the mower and end up wandering all over the lawn, thinking he or she is going straight. However, by concentrating on going to a specific point on the far end of the lawn, rather than looking just in front of the mower, the row will probably be mowed fairly straight. Similarly, throughout the whole writing process it is necessary to keep in mind the endpoint to keep from wandering all over the place. If the item being written is for publication, rather than just something required for work, it will also be necessary to pick the topic and, perhaps, submit an **article proposal** (see Figure 13-1). Although the writing is considered to be more important than the idea, it is still essential to have a good idea or topic that is of interest to prospective readers before starting[8]; it can even cover an old topic, as long as the topic is covered in greater depth, in a new way, or is addressed to a different group. In other

Although not all professionals write articles for journals or books, those who do need to occasionally complete another step in addition to those outlined in the main text of this chapter. One difference is the potential need to write an article proposal to the publisher. This simply is a letter asking the publisher whether there would be any interest in publishing something on a specific topic written by the person who is inquiring. As might be expected, this step is generally not necessary if writing a description of original research, but would be important when writing a review article or even a descriptive article. The letter should contain certain information, which will be described below, and be addressed to an appropriate editor. If possible, it is also a good idea to talk to an editor before submitting your proposal. For example, the proposal for the first edition of this book originated after a discussion with the editor at a publisher's booth in the American Society of Health-System Pharmacists Midyear Clinical Meeting Exhibitor's Area.

In the written proposal, the prospective author should first briefly explain the basic idea that is to be covered in the article or book, including a working title. Similarly, a description of the approach the author wishes to take in covering the subject should be described. Although this description should be kept brief, it must provide enough information for the publisher to determine whether the topic and approach are even appropriate for their publication. In the case of a book, it is important to include a table of contents that is descriptive enough to be useful to reviewers who will be advising the publisher on the need for such a book. Related to that need, it is also necessary to describe why the proposed article or book will be important to the publisher's customers (sometimes referred to as a needs assessment). This is the sales pitch. It is necessary to briefly show that there is nothing similar, or as good, currently available in the literature for the intended audience.

Although the above is the meat of the proposal, there are several other items that should be included. These include the time necessary to complete the article or book (be realistic), the approximate length of the work, and a statement of the authors' qualifications, including any previous publications.

There are several good reasons for submitting a proposal. The first is simply to avoid work if the editor decides that there is no need for such a publication (although an author should not hesitate to send the proposal to another publisher, if it still seems that the topic is important). Second, and perhaps most important, it allows the editor(s) to make suggestions. By following those suggestions, an author is more likely to be successful in getting work published. Finally, if the idea is accepted, the acceptance letter will provide motivation.

Figure 13–1. Article proposal to publishers.

words, it should contribute something to the literature and not merely be confirmatory.[9] It should also be pointed out that in the case of clinical trial results, it can be important to publish articles showing that something did not work, although in the past such topics have often been avoided.[10]

- It is also necessary to decide whether there needs to be a **coauthor**. This may be easy to resolve, depending on who is working on the project. However, even if no one else has been involved, it may be a good idea to look for a coauthor. An inexperienced writer (e.g., a student or someone early in his or her career) would benefit from working with an experienced author.[11] Additionally, working with someone will give a different perspective (especially if working with practitioners from many disciplines) and, hopefully, lessen the work for each person. Finally, it is sometimes a necessity to include coauthors for political reasons (as in "Would you prefer to share the credit or work nights and holidays for the rest of your life?"). Although this last reason should not exist, it does. Coauthors who are not direct contributors to the written work may be considered honorary authors and are relatively common,[12] although this is considered to be inappropriate.[13] A variety of other problems with authorship credit are also seen.[14-16] The best outcome is that everyone must do part of the writing[17] and that authors be listed in the order of their contributions to the project. This does not always happen.[18,19] In some cases (e.g., non-English-speaking authors), pharmaceutical manufacturers may want ghostwriters to write an article for the researchers, but even they agree that original authors must prepare the first draft of editorials or opinion pieces.[20] The ghostwriters should also be appropriately acknowledged.[10] Although arguments may be made,[21-27] there is no valid reason for someone to be listed as an author in excess of his or her contribution to the writing and submission of the work for publication.[28-31] The only exception would be if the publisher has other specific rules. For example, some journals may want to list contributors with an explanation of what they contributed (e.g., writing, origination of study idea, data collection). Generally, ALL the following must be met for an individual to be given credit as an author[31,32]:

- Conception and design of the study, or analysis and interpretation of the data in the study.
- Writing or revising the article.
- Final approval of the version that is published.
- Agreement to be accountable for all aspects of the work, which includes ensuring questions related to accuracy or integrity are investigated and resolved. In addition, an author must be able to identify which sections of an article are the responsibility of each named author.

Things that do not qualify a person to be listed as an author include[30-32]:

- Acquisition of funding
- General supervision of the research group
- Writing assistance, editing, and proofreading

Individuals that do not meet the first qualifications should be listed in the acknowledgments section. It is necessary to obtain the permission of an individual before that person is acknowledged. Also, the **primary author** should be able to explain the order in which the authors are listed. Additionally, journals may require one or more authors to be guarantors, who will be taking responsibility for the work as a whole, including legally.[31]

It should also be mentioned that there can be too many authors and acknowledgments.[33] Some scientific papers list a tremendous number of authors for a particular paper, and the number of authors has grown over the years.[34] It is obvious that 20 authors could not have written a three-page paper. Some of this may be a result of job requirements that include publishing a certain number of articles, leading to demands by individuals to get their name listed on any article they can. Again, authors should contribute to the written work in some significant way, as defined above. In some cases it may be necessary to just name the group performing the research, with a few of the most responsible individuals specifically named, and list others as acknowledgments, sometimes by group, institution, or type of contribution.[29,33,35] Others may be listed as clinical investigators, participating investigators, scientific advisors, data collectors, or other appropriate titles.[31] In relationship to authorship, remember the people taking credit are also taking responsibility—they need to make sure that the work is clear and not subject to misinterpretation (i.e., do not write something that is designed to mislead the reader into believing something that has not been proven).[36]

Before the first word is written, it is necessary to know the audience, which involves knowing the type of person who will be reading the final document and where it will be published. Keep in mind that the word *published* was chosen for a specific reason. Whether the final product appears in the New England Journal of Medicine, the IV Room Policy and Procedure Book, or even the label on a prescription vial, it is published. It is necessary to aim the work at the audience. At a broad level, written work should not be submitted for possible publication in a journal that does not cover the topic; it is no more appropriate to submit an article on preparation of cardioplegic solutions to the Journal of Urology than it is to type a monthly fiscal report on prescription labels. An author needs to be sure to review a journal and its Instructions for Authors before attempting to write an article for submission to that journal.[37]

More specifically, it is necessary to aim both the writing style and depth of information toward the audience. If something is written for physicians, it is not likely to be understood by laypeople. Conversely, items written for laypeople may not satisfy the needs of physicians. It is certainly appropriate to have a secondary audience in mind. For example, a report written for physicians may be of interest to pharmacists and nurses. However, make sure the secondary audience is not served at the expense of the primary audience.

Regarding writing style, there are three types of writing styles commonly used by health care professionals: **pure technical style**, **middle technical style**, and **popular technical style** (see Table 13-1).[38]

Pure technical style is used by business or technical professionals when they are writing for other professionals in the same or similar fields. For example, an article published in American Journal of Health-Systems Pharmacy, American Journal of Nursing, or Journal of the American Medical Association would normally be written in this style.

TABLE 13–1. TYPES OF TECHNICAL WRITING

- Pure technical style—used by professionals addressing other professionals in the same field
- Middle technical style—used by professionals addressing professionals in other fields
- Popular technical style—used by professionals addressing laypeople

There are several characteristics of this style. First, the authors can use technical jargon because they can expect the readers will understand it. Second, it is written in formal English. Third, it is written in the third person; words such as I, we, us, and you are eliminated. Finally, there is a general lack of slang or contractions. The great majority of writing done by health care professionals will be in this style, because it is usually other health care professionals who will be reading their work.

Middle technical style is very closely related to pure technical style. This style is used by authors when they are writing for readers with a variety of technical backgrounds, with everyone having some unifying factor. For example, a report regarding a hospital's medication error reports might be presented to the hospital's pharmacy and therapeutics (P&T) committee. That committee is made up of physicians, nurses, hospital administrators, pharmacists, and other professionals. Although each has a background that makes their membership on the committee appropriate, not all of them would understand what Lactated Ringer's solution is, as would most physicians, nurses, and hospital pharmacists. Therefore, it is necessary to better explain, or sometimes avoid, some technical areas or specific abbreviations. Otherwise, this writing style is very similar in most respects to pure technical style.

Finally, popular technical style is used in anything meant for the general public. Common language is used throughout. For example, a patient information sheet would need to be written in this style. A widely available example would be the articles on medical subjects that have appeared in Consumer Reports® over the years. Information that is written in this style will use less complicated words and be less formal in its presentation.

It should be pointed out that usual technical writing differs greatly from what most people learn in high school English class or college composition courses. Although there is often a tendency to protest the formality of professional writing styles at first, the reality of the situation is that those styles must be followed for a piece of written material to be accepted.

The next step is to know the requirements of the publisher. Whether the work is for the department's policy and procedure manual or a journal, chances are that there is a format that needs to be followed. In the case of a journal, directions on the format to follow will typically be published on the journal's website. Also, specific guidelines are followed by a number of professional journals, both for general format and statistical reporting. Many journals have approved those guidelines and expect that all work submitted for publication will follow them. Many journals follow a format called the Recommendations for the Conduct, Reporting, Editing, and Publication of Scholarly Work in Medical Journals[31] (previously, the Uniform Requirements for Manuscripts Submitted to Biomedical Journals) published by the International Committee of Medical Journal Editors (ICMJE)[32]. This standardization makes it easier on the prospective author; one style can be learned and followed, regardless of the journal. Other publications that can be helpful are Scientific Style and Format: The CSE Manual for Authors, Editors, and Publishers prepared by the Council of Science Editors; The American Medical Association Manual of Style; The Modern Language Association (MLA) Style Manual; and the Publication Manual of the American Psychiatric Association.

In the case of reports, policy and procedure manuals, and similar documents, it is best to see what has been done in the past. If this is the first time an item is being prepared, it is advisable to try to see what has been done in other places and prepare something similar that meets the perceived needs. If writing something for work, do not be afraid to try to improve the format to make it more usable. However, be aware that it may be necessary to get any changes in format approved by the appropriate individual(s) or committee(s). Whenever possible, follow the Recommendations for the Conduct, Reporting, Editing, and Publication of Scholarly Work in Medical Journals[31] format used by the medical journals, because it is the standard for biomedical writing.

GENERAL RULES OF WRITING

Once the preparation is completed, it is time to start writing. Unfortunately, there is no easy way to learn how to write professionally; it just requires a lot of practice. However, a number of rules can be followed (see Table 13-2). This section covers some of the general rules, with information on how to prepare specific items (e.g., introduction, body, conclusion, references, **abstracts**) being covered later.

- **Rule 1**: Organize the information before starting to write, including preparing an outline.[5] In the past, this was an onerous task that few performed. However, with modern word processing software, the outline becomes part of the finished product, so it does not amount to any significant extra work. Minimally, the different sections should be listed to create some order to the layout of the work (remember, keep in mind the endpoint). Overall, the goal is to prepare a document that is clear, concise, complete, and correct. The two latter items depend, to a large part, on preparation. The former items, however, can be helped by following some simple rules.
- **Rule 2**: Do enough research before getting started. Research in this regard means obtaining whatever information—whether records, articles, performance evaluations, financial reports, or anything else—necessary to prepare the item. Although

TABLE 13–2. CHECKLIST IN PREPARATION OF WRITTEN MATERIALS

- Do research first
- Put oneself in the reader's position
- Use proper grammar and spelling
- Make the document look professional
- Follow the appropriate format and style
- Keep things simple and direct
- Keep the document as short as possible
- Avoid abbreviations and acronyms
- Avoid the first person (e.g., I, we, us)
- Use active sentences
- Avoid slash construction (e.g., he/she, him/her, and/or)
- Avoid contractions (e.g., don't, can't)
- Cite other references wherever appropriate (and get permission to do so where appropriate)
- Write things in whatever order is easiest, but make sure the entire document is well organized
- Give credit where it is due
- Get any necessary copyright permissions
- Get everything down on paper before revising
- Edit, Edit, Edit!

it is likely that additional research will be necessary to fill in the fine points at some point in the process, most information should be gathered ahead of time. It is impossible to be organized if there is nothing collected, and a document that is not organized will generally not be worth much.

Rule 3: The author should put him or herself in the reader's position. What does that reader want and how does he or she want it presented?

Rule 4: Use proper spelling and grammar. This is easier than in the past because word processing programs check both; however, it is still necessary to double check because the computer is likely to overlook things. For example, a properly spelled, but incorrect, word will be missed (e.g., two instead of to, trail instead of trial, ration instead of ratio). Unfortunately for some writers, appearances count greatly. The writer may know more about a subject than anyone else, but if poor grammar and spelling permeate the document, it is unlikely that anyone will read or believe the information presented.[39] It will be dismissed as probably wrong, based on grammar and spelling alone. In a case where the finished product will be published in a language other than the writer's native language, the writer should have the work read and edited by someone for whom the language is their first language.

Rule 5: The writing should try to be entertaining. Professional writing tends to be a bit dry; thus, an attempt should be made to make it as enjoyable and easy to read as possible while staying cautious with humor and within limits of professionalism and good taste. It should also be unpretentious, direct, and accurate.[40]

- **Rule 6**: The document should look presentable; otherwise, it is not professional. The sad truth is that people will assume that if an author was sloppy with the appearance of the document, he or she was probably sloppy with the information. That may not be so, but that assumption will ruin a good, but sloppy, document.

- **Rule 7**: ❷ *When writing it is best to keep things as simple and direct as possible.*[41–44] This has been referred to as the KISS (Keep It Simple, Stupid) principle. There is a temptation to use big words that sound impressive, but doing so is more likely to confuse than impress. Emails should be written at the third-grade reading level in order to get people to respond.[45] Related to that, keep documents as short as possible.[46] If a document is long, subheadings should be used. This can be part of the outline step, mentioned earlier. Also, consider whether tables, figures, or graphs would make the document simpler and easier to understand. Tables can be particularly useful in documents containing a great deal of data.

- **Rule 8**: Avoid using abbreviations or acronyms. If it is necessary to do so, state the full form of the word or term the first time that it is mentioned in the document, followed by the abbreviation in parentheses (e.g., acquired immunodeficiency syndrome [AIDS]). The only exceptions to this rule are units of measurement (e.g., mL, mg). Express units of measurement using the metric system. Clinical chemistry and hematologic measurements should be in terms of the International System of Units (SI), although alternative units may be requested in some cases.

- **Rule 9**: Use an appropriate "voice" in writing. Completely avoid writing in the first person and avoid the second person whenever possible. Search via the word processor to find all occurrences of *I, me, we, us,* and *you.* If those words are found, try to rewrite the sentence to avoid them. Also, it is preferable to avoid using the passive voice throughout[47]; again, a grammar checker can help. Avoid both contractions and slash construction (e.g., *and/or, he/she* [use *he or she*], *this/that*). Finally avoid sexism. This means to avoid using words like only *he* or *she* (both genders should be included in a statement, except where inappropriate). For example, using *he* in a case report of a patient with testicular cancer is quite appropriate. Also, in the past it was usually considered inappropriate to use *their* instead of *his or her* to get around the problem, although a recent publication says that this is now considered to be appropriate.[48]

- **Rule 10**: Be sure to give credit where it is due. This does not mean just making sure the listed authors wrote part of the document. It includes using citations that can be included as endnotes, or possibly footnotes, for all information obtained from one or a limited number of sources. If there is extensive quoting, permission to do so should be obtained by writing to the person or organization holding the copyright on the material. Endnotes are something most people dreaded in the past. They waited until the end, because the articles should be cited in the order they appear in the document. By that time, it was difficult to go back and do it. Now, it is much easier with word processors; it is possible to insert the citations as the document is prepared and let the software worry about making sure they are in the correct order. There are even add-on programs for word processors that give additional functions in managing the references, although it is necessary to be careful in using them, since the document may not be fully accessible if it is then emailed to someone who does not possess a copy of that add-on. In cases like that, it would be best to use the built-in endnote feature of programs like Microsoft® Word.

Related to the endnotes, everything that is stated should be supported by objective evidence. When writing a paper based on scientific literature, that evidence must be shown in the citation endnotes. To reemphasize, any unreferenced statement of fact is for all practical purposes worthless. However, it is necessary to make sure information is extracted from the original article and expressed properly (remember to avoid plagiarism, which will be discussed in more detail later in the chapter). Some writers will improperly twist facts, whether inadvertently or not, to support their assertions.[49]

Rule 11: Work through the document in whatever order seems easiest.[5] In preparing a drug evaluation for a pharmacy and therapeutics committee, 50 articles might be used. At first, the collection of articles may look like an impossible task, but after sorting the articles into groups (whether electronically or physically) that correspond to the sections, start with the smallest group or the easiest information. By the time the document is finished, the writer may be surprised to find out that it was much easier than they expected.

Rule 12: Edit the document thoroughly. At first, a writer should simply try to make sure that all of the information is down on paper.[5] Once that occurs, go back and revise, and perhaps reorganize the document. Waiting a few days before revising the document can be very beneficial. After some time away from the project, errors practically jump off the page. It is also a good idea to have someone else who has not been involved with the writing read the document. Something that seems quite clear to the author may not actually be clear at all. Also, the author may be mentally inserting words or sentences that were inadvertently omitted. Having someone edit the document can be humbling, but helpful. Be sure to provide the product in a format that will make things easier for the person reviewing the document. A typed, double-spaced manuscript will make it easy to read and provide room for comments. Even better, electronic versions of a document can be reviewed directly on a computer using "comment" or "track changes" features. The reviewer can put in comments or suggested wording changes electronically and then return the document. The writer can then go through the document making changes or simply accepting proposed changes with the click of a button. Often, the use of the electronic reviewing mechanism will be quicker, easier, and provide much clearer suggestions.

The three most important things in real estate may be location, location, location, but the three most important things in writing are edit, edit, edit. This can be particularly important when multiple authors have contributed different sections since it will be necessary to make sure that the various contributions fit well together, including the style of writing.[50] It may be best for either the first author or most senior author to edit for consistency. Also, remember editing includes paring out unnecessary words, sentences, and larger sections. It is not sufficient to settle for good enough—do your best. Look at it this way: the boss or editor is only going to do so much editing before giving up. The trick is to make sure that the document is well prepared and does not need that much editing.

SPECIFIC DOCUMENT SECTIONS

A typical document consists of three main parts—the introduction, body, and conclusion. In the case of a clinical study, it is recommended to follow the IMRAD structure that divides a paper into Introduction, Methods, Results, and Discussion,[31] which is the standard for such papers.[51] In the case of instructional design and assessment, the IDEAS (Introduction, Design, Evaluation, Assessment, and Summary) format has been recommended.[52] Other parts, such as references, tables, figures, and abstracts may also be necessary. These will be discussed in later sections and in the appendices of this chapter. It should also be noted that a number of the points in Chapters 4, 5, and 6 are applicable to writing of journal articles. There are various other important guidelines for writing articles, which include the following:

- International Committee of Medical Journal Editors (http://www.icmje.org) —the standards available at http://www.icmje.org/icmje-recommendations.pdf are used by hundreds of health-related journals; articles submitted to those journals must follow the directions provided.
- Consolidated Standards of Reporting Trials (CONSORT) statement (http://www. consort-statement.org) —contains a checklist for contents of a clinical trial to report when publishing and flow diagram illustrating recruitment, randomization, and analysis of subjects enrolled in a trial.[53-63] Extensions to this statement are also available for such things as cluster trials, noninferiority and equivalence trials, N-of-1 trials, herbals, etc. (http://www.consort-statement.org/extensions).

- Preferred Reporting Items for Systemic Reviews and Meta-Analysis (PRISMA)[64,65] (http://www.prisma-statement.org/)
- The Strengthening the Reporting of Observational Studies in Epidemiology (STROBE) Statement—guidelines for reporting observational studies along with extensions (https://www.strobe-statement.org/index.php?id=strobe-home)
- CARE Case Report Guidelines—extensions available for this (https://www.care-statement.org/)
- AGREE Reporting Checklist for practice guidelines (https://www.agreetrust.org/resource-centre/agree-reporting-checklist/)
- Revised Standards for Quality Improvement Reporting Excellence—SQUIRE 2.0—for reporting quality improvement studies (http://squire-statement.org/index.cfm?fuseaction=Page.ViewPage&PageID=471)
- Consolidated Health Economic Evaluation Reporting Standards (CHEERS) Statement—for economic reporting (https://www.ispor.org/heor-resources/good-practices/article/consolidated-health-economic-evaluation-reporting-standards-(cheers)—explanation-and-elaboration)
- Conference on Guideline Standardization (COGS) standards (http://gem.med.yale.edu/cogs/)
- Good Publication Practice Guidelines (GPP3) for pharmaceutical companies (http://www.ismpp.org/gpp3)[66]
- AMA Manual of Style (https://www.amamanualofstyle.com/)
- A compilation of over 400 standards for reporting medical studies may be found at http://www.equator-network.org/

An example question layout that includes an introduction, body, and conclusion section is shown in Appendix 13-1.

Introduction

3 *With the probable exception of policy and procedure documents, the two most important paragraphs in any document are the first and last.* It is vital to start out strong, to encourage the reader to continue reading. Otherwise, the work will end up in that collection of articles that everyone intends to read someday, but seldom does. The first paragraph should also inform the reader of what they can expect in the rest of the document; it should be like a road map that shows what is to be accomplished in the document. The introduction should have a clear objective for the existence of the document. Many people neglect the need to state a clear objective, which leaves the reader to flounder and wonder whether there really is a purpose to the document. In a research article, the introduction will also contain the hypothesis being investigated. In a policy and procedure document, it may simply be a description of what the remainder of the document will cover. The introduction should also contain background information about the topic that provides a good information base for the reader. In the case of a research article, it should also show where there is a gap in the literature that the study is intending to address.[9] The amount of background information has to be a balance—enough to show the reader that the writer has done an appropriate amount of research, but yet not so exhaustive as to bore or overwhelm the reader with unnecessary details.[67] Overall, the introduction should be short but contain properly referenced background material and show the reader where the document is headed.

The introduction should generally not be a conclusion; some writers are so anxious to jump to the end that they put the conclusion first. Admittedly, the BLOT (bottom line on top) concept has its purpose in some documents (e.g., policy and procedures, formulary monographs), but that should be a conscious decision. If the introduction amounts to a conclusion, many people will read no further, making the remainder of the document a waste of time and effort.

Body

The body of the document contains all the details. In a research article, the body may be divided into the methods, results, and, possibly, discussion sections, although the latter section may be incorporated into the conclusion. Details of what should be included in a research study are covered in Chapter 4. A requirement for data sharing is also important to consider.[68] In other documents, the body will probably be divided into whatever sections are appropriate or logical. A number of rules can be followed in preparing the body of a document.

The first rule is that, while it is important to be concise, all necessary information must be presented. Again, keep an eye on the desired endpoint, and do not stray from the subject unless it is absolutely necessary. Including unnecessary information, even if it is interesting, will tend to confuse or obscure the important points. Also, be sure to provide a balanced coverage of the material and avoid unsupported bias.[10] In the case of a research article, the methodology section should be complete enough that the reader would be able to duplicate the study.[9]

It is important to cover the information in a logical order, so that it flows easily from one point to another. A common mistake, when learning to write professionally, is to skip back and forth between subjects. For example, someone might insert a point about dosing in the middle of indications, when dosing is discussed at another point in the document.

Material that can identify patients should be left out of any work, unless it is absolutely necessary to include. If that is not possible, informed consent must be obtained[31] and pertinent legal procedures must be followed (see Chapter 11 (legal chapter is now Chapter 11)). The authors should also disclose any approval of a study by institutional review boards (IRB) and their following of other rules related to protection of study subjects (both human and animal).[31]

Writers should also put the information in their own words. Perhaps out of lack of confidence, a number of professionals are tempted to simply quote other authors word for word. However, by presenting the information in their own words, writers demonstrate that they understand the topic. ❹ *Remember, though, that if the information is taken from a specific source, even if it is reworded, the original author should be given credit via citation.*

It is necessary to expand on the topic discussed in the previous paragraph because there seems to be much confusion about it and there are many cases where the rules against copyright infringement and plagiarism are broken. Plagiarism can be considered the copying of another's words or ideas, without properly giving credit. Copyright violations consist of copying another's work, even with appropriate quotations and citation, without permission. They are similar; however, it is possible to commit either plagiarism or copyright violations without committing the other. Self-plagiarism, where an author copies material that he or she previously had published in one journal to use in a publication in another journal, is a concern and can lead to copyright violations.[69] It appears that plagiarism is becoming more frequent and many people do not understand that it is wrong to copy work without proper attribution, even something from a source written by many anonymous people (e.g., Wikipedia, Yahoo! Answers, and Answers.com).[70,71]

Sometimes those infractions are rather blatant, such as the cases documented in the news about students downloading papers from the Internet and presenting them as their own or simply retyping a previously published article (an attempt to prevent this can be seen on the Internet at http://www.plagiarism.com, http://www.plagiarism.org, or http://www.turnitin.com). Interestingly, although there might be suspicions that this is more prevalent with online classes, a study found that it was more likely to occur with traditional campus students.[74] Another website, http://www.ithenticate.com/ is a resource to check if published material is plagiarized. Other times, the infringement is quite accidental. For example, it was once brought to the attention of the famous science fiction writer, Isaac Asimov, that a short story he wrote was similar to an article that had been published 10 years previously.[75] Dr. Asimov went back and found the article and read it, realizing that he had read it when it first came out and had forgotten about it. When he wrote his story 10 years later, he did not realize that portions of it could be considered plagiarism. Although he had no intention of infringing upon the other author's work, Dr. Asimov made sure that the story was never reprinted and even wrote an article discussing the problem. Even Shakespeare has been shown to have been influenced by another author and may have crossed the line into plagiarism.[76] This shows how easy it is to inadvertently cross the line into copyright infringement or plagiarism, and there are many examples that would fall in between the extremes given above.[77] Therefore, it is necessary for the author to be on guard and to try to prevent the problem in the first place. Also, be aware that journals will retract articles with plagiarism. In one bizarre case, an Indian journal retracted an article that turned out to be plagiarized—the article retracted was a guideline on avoiding plagiarism.[78]

A few general rules can act as a guide to prevent plagiarism.

- Use quotations and seek permission: When copying wording directly from another's work, it should be in quotations (or otherwise shown to be a quote) and a citation should be used to give credit to the original author(s). Also, if a significant amount of a work published in the last 100 years is quoted, it is probably necessary to get permission from the copyright holder, which may require paying a fee.[79] Exactly what is a significant amount is debatable; however, it would be best to err on the side of asking for permission if a quotation is more than a few sentences. Reproducing an entire chart, table, figure, and so on should normally require asking for permission. A letter to the copyright holder will prevent problems; publishers often have forms to request permission. Some special cases need to be mentioned. First, U.S. government documents are not copyrighted, so only quotation marks and citations are necessary. Second, if it is impossible to locate a copyright holder (e.g., the publisher went out of business without transferring copyrights), the writer should at least be able to document a thorough effort to obtain permission. Finally, there are special legal requirements for use of copyrighted materials in online education, covered in the Technology, Education and Copyright Harmonization (TEACH) Act. Further information on this can be found in Chapter 11.
- Avoid extensive quotations: If a writer cannot put something in his or her own words, does that person truly understand the material? In any writing, there really is very little reason to provide quotations. The author should try to put things in his or her own words whenever possible.
- Use original publications: Paraphrased information should have the original publication(s) cited, if it comes from one or a limited number of sources. If the material came from a review article, cite that article, not the original study that was not consulted. It is worth mentioning that in the case of unusual information, reading and citing the original study is preferable to just using a review article, because the review may be inaccurate.
- Be sure to follow publishers' rules or licenses, which may be stricter and may not allow any reproduction of material. An author must obtain permission from publisher, even if it is that author's original work, for use in a different publication to avoid copyright violations.[69]
- Always cite everything: It is necessary to always cite others work, even on slides[80] and even if it is the author's own previously published work to avoid self-plagiarism.[69]

- To help decide if something needs citation, a flowchart tool is available at https://thevisualcommunicationguy.com/2014/09/16/did-i-plagiarize-the-types-and-severity-of-plagiarism-violations/.

In preparing certain documents (e.g., written answers to questions), there may be very little information available as only one or two research articles may have been written on the topic. If so, it will often be desirable to summarize the articles in detail, including most of the information presented in an abstract (see Appendix 13-2). In general, the information presented will summarize how many and what type of patients (i.e., inclusion and exclusion criteria), the drug or procedure being investigated, the results (e.g., efficacy, adverse effects), and the conclusions of authors of referenced articles. It is also important to point out any noticeable flaws in the paper. An example would be:

> Smith and Jones performed a double-blind, randomized comparison of the effects of drug X and drug Y in patients with Tsutsugamushi disease. Patients were required to be between 18 and 70 years old, and could not have any concurrent infection or disorder that would affect the immune response to the disease (e.g., neutropenia, AIDS). Twenty patients received 10 mg of drug X, three times a day for 15 days. Eighteen patients received 250 mg of drug Y, twice a day for 10 days. The two groups were comparable, except that the patients receiving drug X were an average of 5 years younger ($p < 0.05$). Drug X was shown to produce a cure, both in terms of symptoms and cultures in 85% of patients, whereas drug Y only produced a cure in 55.5% of patients. The difference was statistically significant ($p < 0.01$). No significant adverse effects were seen in either group. Although it appears that drug X was the better agent, it should be noted that drug Y was given in its minimally effective dose, and may have performed better in a somewhat higher or longer regimen.

A list of material to be covered in a review of an article similar to that above is found in Table 13-3.

It should go without saying, but it is necessary to state that information in any written document or presentation needs to be correct and not invented. This has become more common and has been written about in regard to politicians[81]; however, it can also be pertinent to professional communications. There have been situations documented where researchers have falsified information about research. In some cases, this has led to controversy about responsibility,[82] retractions of an article,[83] loss of a job,[84] a ruined career,[85] and even suicide.[86] It just needs to be stated that information presented needs to be correct, as far as the author can verify, and stated as clearly as possible to avoid deception. That may lead to undesirable results, but it is best to be truthful in the long run for the sake of everyone. If it is a minor case of inadvertent human error, any necessary correction should be published as soon as possible and, if serious, a retraction should be published, as would be the case if scientific misconduct is present.[31] Related to this, there

TABLE 13–3. ITEMS TO INCLUDE IN WRITTEN REVIEW OF A JOURNAL ARTICLE

Items to Include	Examples
Main author of article and a reference number	Johnson *et al.*[2] Smith and associates[24]
Type of article	Clinical study, case report, case series, review, meeting abstract
Research design (if appropriate)	Blinding, randomization, experience report, descriptive report
Objective or purpose of the report	Population, disease or condition, intervention, comparison (if appropriate), outcome (primary and secondary)
Description of groups studied	Size of groups, age, sex, disease state(s), other pertinent demographic characteristics, inclusion and exclusion criteria
Any important confounding factors	Smoking, age, general health
Description of treatment being studied	Drug, dose, administration route, dosing interval, treatment duration
What was measured as an indicator of effect/outcome variables	Measurements appropriately matched with outcomes
Results	Efficacy, adverse effects, safety, adherence, drop-outs (reasons)
Author conclusions	
Strengths and weaknesses of the study	See Chapters 4 and 5 (note: these comments can be located in conjunction with any of the above items)

is a case where multiple journal articles were retracted because the author managed to arrange for numerous false reviewers for the journal, including the author reviewing his own paper.[87] This should also never be done.

Conclusion

A conclusion should be placed at the end of the body of the document, except for certain documents (e.g., policy and procedures). This conclusion should follow logically from the information presented and should serve to summarize that information. No new information should be presented in the conclusion. Remember, the conclusion should also correspond with the objective stated in the introduction.[88] It is worth noting that in clinical consultations, a common mistake is to write the conclusion in a general manner, rather than addressing the specific patient in question, which is what the reader wants to hear about. The author must remember to address the specific patient's situation.

Many writers are tempted to avoid formulating a conclusion. Various reasons include not feeling qualified to make a conclusion for the reader, not wanting to restate what has already been stated, laziness, not knowing how to write one, and so on. This is improper.

The readers need something to bring their thoughts together at the end, and the author is in the perfect position to provide this closure. However, the author should also be careful to avoid extrapolating beyond the information available.

Other Items

If written works include endnotes, the references should be found following the conclusion (see Appendix 13-3 for more information on how to prepare a **bibliography**). Use of bibliographic software, such as EndNote (Clarivate Analytics—http://www.endnote.com), or Zotero (Roy Rosenzweig Center for History and New Media—http://www.zotero.org/) can be helpful in this process.[20] Other items may also be necessary, depending on the document, such as tables, graphs, figures, disclaimers, conflicts of interest, source(s) of support, author information, statement of authorship, copyright transferal, and so forth.[31] They will not be dealt with here, other than to say that those items should supplement or clarify (not distort or misrepresent), and not simply duplicate material in the text portion of a piece of written work, although there may be overlap as an author explains data or expands on the material presented.

SUBMISSION OF THE DOCUMENT

Once the document is completed, proofread, and edited, it is ready to be submitted, whether this is to a supervisor or a journal. In the latter case, you may need to include a cover letter that serves as an introduction to the document. In the former case, it will be possible to be less formal. Also, it should be noted that when submitting an item to a journal it may be necessary to include transfer of copyright forms, conflict of interest disclosures (including financial and personal)[17,31,89–91] or other items, which will be found in the instructions for authors for that journal (usually found on the publication's website). The conflict of interest may be reported by the publisher in the final publication, but this is variable.[92] In addition, be sure to precisely follow the journal's Instructions for Authors to improve chances for acceptance.[93] Unless given a special circumstance, articles should not be submitted to more than one journal at the same time (note: prior publication of an abstract does not mean that submission of a full article is duplication, and publication in a second language is often considered acceptable).[10,17,94] If duplicate submission is determined to be necessary, the rules outlined in the Recommendations for the Conduct, Reporting, Editing, and Publication of Scholarly Work in Medical Journals must be followed.[31] Also, the article should not be broken down into many small articles and submitted over time, unless submission as a whole would result in a publication that would be too long or complex, or would significantly delay the publication of important findings.[95]

PEER REVIEW

If the document is to be published in a peer-reviewed publication (most biomedical journals, but not magazines), it will undergo a peer-review process as the name implies. The peer-review process is that by which **referees**, also referred to as reviewers and content experts, review, comment, and provide insights regarding the merit of the document for potential publication in the journal. On a local level, reviewers are the people that a writer may ask to look at a report before the boss gets it. Whatever arena, whether local or international, a person should also be willing to be a reviewer at that level. To be a reviewer for a journal (which produces **refereed publications**), a person usually can simply write a letter stating interests, qualifications, and experience to the editor of the journal, and ask to be considered for the journal's reviewer list. If the person has adequate credentials, the journal will usually be happy to have that person as a reviewer.

Anyone who is a reviewer should be up front about such things as lack of expertise, conflict of interest,[31,91] or inability to complete a review within a reasonable time, and should be willing to step aside as a reviewer of a particular paper if those are problems.[96] Also, a reviewer should treat anything submitted to him or her as a confidential document. Characteristics needed by a peer reviewer include: knowledge of the topic area and its literature, timeliness, detailed analytic ability, provision of clear recommendations, ability to point out both good and bad aspects, and good language skills.[97]

It should be pointed out that people who act as reviewers for papers should follow the procedures discussed in Chapters 4 and 5. Specific directions will also be received from the editor and may involve preparing comments for both the editor (to discuss matters, such as ethics, with the editor alone) and for the author(s) (this latter document is also used by the editor). It may be required that the latter be signed or unsigned. Also, as with any quality assurance procedure, the reviewer should treat it as an opportunity to provide constructive, as opposed to destructive, criticism.[98] Finally, for those who are reviewers for journals, it is recommended to get new people involved in the process, such as residents or new practitioners, so that they can learn how to be a reviewer.[99]

Further information on how to do a peer review may be found in Chapter 10.

It is beyond the scope of this chapter, but if further information is needed on being an editor of a biomedical journal, the reader should consult the website of the World Association of Medical Editors (http://www.wame.org).

REVISION

❺ *In many cases, revision of the document will be necessary.* This may be due to a difference in opinion or different perception of need. Although an author should never change a document to say something he or she believes is wrong, minor revisions are often necessary to improve clarity or make the document more appropriate in some other manner. The comments given with the request for revision are likely to be helpful,[100] and they should be taken seriously. Even if it is felt that the person who read and commented on the paper is wrong, all concerns should be addressed. If a comment is truly wrong, it may still indicate that the work was not clear in a particular area and needs some other appropriate revision to clarify the material. Changes should be made, based on the comments and completed within the time limits given.[101]

Sometimes, however, a document may be rejected entirely. This can be for any of the following reasons[38]:

- The document is not up to standards (i.e., too much work to correct or edit). It should be noted that the peer-review process should not be treated as a service of a journal to take a rough draft and make it into a finished document. A well-written paper should be submitted initially.[102]
- The idea or research the document is based on is too weak.
- The idea is inappropriate for that forum of publication.
- A similar article has been recently prepared (and possibly published) by someone else in that forum.
- The article does not fill an important gap in the body of literature.

The first two bullet points are considered the most common reasons for rejection.[9] In the case of the first item, major revisions would be necessary before resubmitting to the boss or a journal. The second reason may also prompt major revisions, or even cause an author to stop working on the document. An article submitted to a journal but rejected for the third and fourth reasons is not necessarily bad. It may be possible to submit it to another appropriate journal after only minor changes. In the case of the final reason, it may be possible to change the focus or expand the coverage of the article to make it useful.

GALLEY PROOFS

A term well known to authors who have published articles or books is **galley** (or page) **proofs**. This is a final copy of the document, as it will appear when published. It is the responsibility of the author(s) to carefully check to make sure there have been no mistakes made in typesetting. Although it may seem like a lot of work, everything must be checked, including the references, which frequently contain errors.[103–108] This step is necessary to prevent problems later. Although documents ready for distribution at work are generally not referred to as galley proofs, it is still necessary to carefully check those items.

Case Study 13–1

Your supervisor comes to you and lets you know that you are assigned to write a policy and procedure for a new product that is to be carried in the institution; however, the product requires specific safety precautions when used by patients. This is to be approved and available when the product is first stocked.

- *What are your first steps?*
- *You have progressed to the point where you have the material gathered to prepare your policy and procedure. What should be done at this stage?*
- *Once the document is written, what needs to be done next?*

Specific Documents

NEWSLETTERS AND WEBSITES

Newsletters, whether printed or electronic, can be a part of any pharmacy practice, but have probably been encountered most frequently in hospitals as a method for communicating pharmacy and therapeutics committee actions and other drug-related topics to the medical, pharmacy, nursing, and other health care provider staffs. Newsletters have also been seen from community pharmacies[109,110] (addressed to patients and/or physicians), nursing homes, drug companies, pharmacy organizations, and government or regulatory bodies. Wherever newsletters are found, their reason for existence is likely to be one or more of the following reasons: to communicate information to a target group, advertisement, or compliance with legal and accreditation standards. Nowadays, the electronic versions of newsletters can provide direct links to further information and even such benefits as videos.

In many cases, newsletters are now replaced by a website. Such sites can serve the same purposes, but can also have some specific advantages and disadvantages. For example, websites take very little effort for distribution, because all they take is a computer with access to the Internet, which also makes minor updates very easy. Also, the material can take a greater variety of forms, including audio and video. The website can be used to sell products. Within institutions, the material can be kept available for health care providers to review for an indefinite time period, thereby preventing problems when somebody wants another copy of an old article or when nurses are trying to make sure they have all the publications for an accreditation visit. In regard to disadvantages, it should be noted that consulting a website does take more effort, because it does not just fall into people's hands when they open their mailboxes. Also, there are still some people who do not use the Internet and would, therefore, not be able to consult the site. Finally, it will be necessary to have a plan to regularly review the web pages to determine if they require updates or even elimination.

Whatever the reason for the existence of a newsletter or website, the same set of steps generally applies to their preparation.[111-115] These steps will be covered individually in the remainder of this section.

Define the Audience

Who will, or at least should, be reading the newsletter or accessing the website? It may be physicians, pharmacists, nurses, other health care professionals, the lay public, other groups, or some combination of these. The target group(s) will influence decisions made in the other steps.

Define the Goals

The goal can be any of the reasons mentioned previously, but generally includes informing and educating the reader, and also to report news (including changes in policies and procedures, laws, etc.). With websites, it can also be to directly sell products or gather information.

Identify Constraints

No matter what kind of newsletter or website is produced, there are always going to be constraints that will limit what it can contain and how good it will be.

> **Constraint 1**: Time. It seems like every year people are busier and have less time to do things that they want or need to do. This includes preparing a newsletter or keeping up a website (must be done continuously), which can take a significant amount of time if it is done right. It will be necessary to have time to write, type, edit, typeset, and perform other functions in publishing the newsletter—and all those things have to be done in time to get the finished result to the printer, so that it can be ready for distribution on time. With a website, it is necessary to write the material, figure out the layout or organization, and prepare it on the computer. It is generally best, when beginning publication of a newsletter, to have it come out at longer intervals. If the newsletter is well received it is found that there is enough time, and there is enough material, publication frequency can be increased. Overall, it is better to find it necessary to speed up publication frequency, rather than spread it out (people might get the idea the newsletter ceased publication).

Constraint 2: Personnel. People who can, or will, be involved with publishing the newsletter or website, particularly the editor-in-chief and webmaster, are in short supply. This is a case where the phrase, "many hands make light work" may be applicable. If a group of dependable people are willing to work together to make sure the articles get written, the job may be easier. Generally, there are two extremely hard parts to publishing a newsletter or website, neither of which is the actual writing. One of them is coming up with topic ideas; the other is to make it look good. If others are at least willing to help here, it can be a great aid to the editor of the newsletter. If possible, people from all groups served by the newsletter should be asked for topics, if not entire articles. Residents and students can also contribute articles. If a health care professional oversees the newsletter or website, some other possible places for help include an institution's public relations department, if available, and clerical help (to do the typing, formatting, copying, distribution, etc.). Keep an eye on the time necessary for health care professional (e.g., pharmacy, nursing) staff to produce the newsletter or website, because this is likely to be the costliest item.

Constraint 3: Money. As has been said, "There is no such thing as a free lunch." This also applies to newsletters and websites. There is always some cost involved. Although personnel costs are likely to be the largest expense, the computer equipment, and printing or duplication charges (for printed newsletters) can be significant. If the printing is to be done by an outside agency it is best to check on such items as the effect of order size (number of copies) and type of paper (e.g., plain vs. glossy, 8½ in × 11 in vs. 11 in × 17 in vs. A4, colors), stapling or binding on the cost. It is preferable to get bids from at least three printers, if not done by the author's company. Another item to consider is method of delivery (e.g., personal vs. first-class mail vs. second-class mail). All these items do add up and, depending on the budget, it may be necessary to sell advertising space to cover the costs.

Constraint 4: Resources. It is necessary to look at what equipment or resources are available. If possible, the use of a high-end word processing program or desktop publishing program with a laser or inkjet printer will allow production of a high-quality, professional newsletter quicker and at a lower cost. This equipment may be all that is necessary for a website, if the computer has some type of Internet connection.

Newsletter/Website Design

While it might be easy to believe substance is more important than appearance, it eventually becomes noticeable that many people do not bother looking at the substance if the appearance is poor or unprofessional. Therefore, one of the most important things is to make the publication look appealing.[116,117] People tend to throw away newsletters that look sloppy or unprofessional, and do not bother with websites that are not exciting, easy to use, and neat. Even if the publication looks good it may[118-120] or may not[121,122] have any impact on health care professionals; but without looking professional it is highly unlikely to even have a chance.

A few general rules can help make a newsletter or website more appealing. These will be covered in the remainder of this section. However, for a more in-depth look at this subject, the reader is directed to references specializing in the subject.[123,124] A particularly detailed document is available on the Internet at https://guidelines.usability.gov.

- **Rule 1**: Keep the publication consistent. This means not only from month to month, but also from page to page. This does not mean that improvements cannot be made from time to time. Nor does it mean that each page must look exactly like the previous one. Instead, it means that it should have its own style that is recognizable by the reader, and that the various pages must fit with one another. The easiest way to do this, with either a newsletter or website, is to create a template, style sheet, or theme (these terms overlap somewhat). Many pieces of software make this possible for either type of publication. A template is a file that contains material that appears the same from issue to issue—the term is often associated with a newsletter, although there may also be template files for websites. Examples of this can be a newsletter or website's masthead (main heading), the listing of editors, footers at the bottom of each page, number of columns, and so on. A theme should be similar to a template, but may be used more frequently when discussing a website. Style sheets define how specific paragraphs or other parts of the newsletter or websites will look (they would often be incorporated into the template or theme). For example, a style might be called "Heading 1," and by using this style for each article's title, the look remains the same from page to page, and issue to issue. This style can include such items as what the font looks like (e.g., typeface, font size, bold, italic, underlined, superscript, subscript), and what the paragraph looks like (e.g., left justified, right justified, centered, line spacing, space before or after), in addition to other items (e.g., whether the section is to be located in a particular part of the page, borders). A style manual should be established or at least a commercially available style manual, such as the American Medical Association Manual of Style, should be used. Whatever the editor(s) establish should be reasonably simple and elegant (i.e., do not get carried away—a couple of different fonts on a page are fine, but 10 fonts look terrible).

- **Rule 2**: Use appropriate software and equipment. A high-end word processor or desktop publishing program and a laser printer can be used.[125,126] This can allow a pharmacy to turn out a product that looks typeset at a fraction of the cost. As mentioned, there are a variety of low (or no) cost website software tools. Some are specific, whereas others are incorporated into word processors, web browsers, or other software.

- **Rule 3**: Make the newsletter or website look good. For example, use white space properly. Do not just crowd in as much material as possible on the page. The reader will have a hard time following if it is too crowded and may just give up. Layout really is a difficult problem and requires at least a little artistic ability to do well. If lack of artistic ability is a problem, it is probably a good idea to look over other newsletters or websites from various sources to try to come up with ideas concerning what looks good. Minimally, most newsletters should at least be set up in two columns to allow easier reading. Other, more artistic, items to consider are asymmetrical layout (not having the two sides of each page look the same from a distance, perhaps using a narrow column for graphics or titles along one edge), different column widths, teasers (statements taken from the text that may pique the curiosity of the reader enough to read the article), surrounding boxes and columns with rules, and artwork or graphics.[127] The programs used to prepare either newsletters or websites can also have samples that can be used to prepare a professional looking end product.

Next on the list for newsletters or websites is to design a masthead. As mentioned, the masthead is essentially the part of the first page of the newsletter that gives the name of the publication, volume, issue, date, and so on. This may be at the top of the page or down one side of the first page. On a webpage, it would be material on the home page. It is a good idea to consider having this done professionally because it is a one-time expense and can be a major factor in the appearance of the newsletter. Sometimes it is good to have a multicolored masthead that is preprinted on blank stock paper, in the case of printed newsletters. The newsletter text can then just be photocopied onto the paper and look much more professional. Material to be put into the masthead, or at least be included somewhere in the newsletter includes the newsletter or website name (be descriptive, but do not get cute—remember this is a professional publication), name and address of the department or organization, names of editor and editorial staff (give credit or blame where it is due), and frequency of publication. The name of the publication, along with some way of identifying the issue and page, should be placed on every page of the newsletter, so that the source of information can be identified if the page is photocopied or torn out.

Much of the material in a masthead should also be contained on the home page, if not every page, of a website. Again, getting professional design help, at least at first, may be of value. Also, following the guidelines of the Health on the Net Foundation Code of Conduct (http://www.hon.ch/HONcode/Conduct.html) in designing the web page is appropriate.

In general, software themes available will help create a professional looking site if professional help is not available. However, some specific items that need to be considered for a website include the following[128,129]:

- Provide information that is good, credible, timely, and original. Share everything possible.
- Custom tailor information to consider user preferences.
- Break up tables for readability.
- Related to the previous item, optimize the other aspects of the page to improve download times.
- Make the page easy to read—good contrast between the text and background including the colors (remember that some people are color blind and may not be able to distinguish some colors, rendering some things unreadable), not too busy.
- Use self-generating content—make the site interactive.
- Web pages should be well organized—both the pages by themselves and how the pages are interconnected on the site.
- Consider selling things, if appropriate.
- Make sure everything works, from all likely browsers.

In designing the newsletter or website, effort should also be placed in deciding on a name. A local or institutional newsletter will often have a name related to the organization and the purpose of the newsletter. A website may be similarly named, but there is an opportunity to go farther. In this case, the Uniform Resource Locator (URL) should be considered. This is the address of the website on the intranet and/or the Internet. An institution may already have a registered URL, and the department web page may simply be under that name (e.g., https://www.yourorganizationname.org/pharmacy). However, independent community pharmacies, ambulatory clinics, physician offices, etc., can also register an unused name on the Internet and have that address (e.g., https://www.johns-pharmacy.com). There is now a .pharmacy domain available, rather than just using .com.

It has been alluded to, but it is necessary to make a very specific decision on how the newsletter is to be printed, if it will be printed. While typesetting still produces the best looking newsletter, it is quite easy to get a good looking final product using a good photocopy machine. Also, even if the department produces the original copy on its computer, the file can be taken to a service bureau that can essentially produce a typeset copy. It is necessary to determine the paper to be used (glossy paper is not going to be used if you are photocopying). Most newsletters are 8½ × 11. in size, but that does not mean the paper is that size. It is better to use 11 in. × 17 in. paper for multipage newsletters and just fold the sheets. That looks much better than simply stapling the corner. Also, it is possible to provide an electronic storage file to some professional printers for them to print good looking final copies.

Newsletter/Web Page Content

Before getting into items that a newsletter or website should or can contain, it is necessary to discuss some general rules that deal with any article.[130]

First, it is a good idea to have a number of short articles, rather than one long article.[117,131] People will take a look at a short article and mentally decide if they have the time to read it, whereas a long article may be dismissed immediately ("If I'm going to read something that long, it will be out of New England Journal of Medicine!") or put aside to read when they have time. As a matter of fact, some recommend that newsletters should not exceed two pages (one sheet, front and back)[130] and one hospital cut their newsletter to one page (for P&T News) and replaced the remaining articles with a page to fit into a Drug Therapy Pocket Guide that consisted of useful tables (e.g., sodium content and neutralizing capacity of different antacids).[132] Use catchy titles to draw the reader into reading the article right then.

Use proper writing techniques, as described earlier in this chapter. Be clear, concise, and complete—do not waste the reader's valuable time. Also, be unbiased—support the article with facts. Be positive—talk about 90% adherence, rather than 10% nonadherence.

Finally, be sure the newsletter or website is properly edited. Have multiple people read and edit the newsletter or web pages before publication. Having more people read it makes it more likely that simple mistakes will be noticed and corrected. In particular, the editors should check for spelling, grammar, and readability. Also, it is a good idea to have people from each target group as editors, particularly physicians.[133]

The actual content of a newsletter or website is one of the two most difficult areas for the editor (the other being that the newsletter should look good). Coming up with new ideas on a regular basis can be rather difficult. A list of possible areas to cover is included in Table 13-4. If possible, material that was prepared for a different audience can be recycled for the newsletter or website readers. For example, material from the pharmacy and therapeutics committee meeting might be turned into a short review of a drug. Whenever possible, the material presented should be topics not available to the audience from another source, or material that is prepared in a format that will be of greater value to the readers than that same topic area as presented by other publications. Whatever the topics used, it is a good idea to survey the readers on a regular basis to make sure their needs are being met.

If a website provides a link to an outside website that is not under control of the same group, it is recommended that a disclaimer be published along with it stating that the original website does not endorse or take responsibility for the contents of that external site.[31]

TABLE 13–4. WEBSITE OR NEWSLETTER TOPICS[111,112,117,130]

- Adherence
- Advances in therapeutics
- Adverse drug reactions
- Calendar of events
- Clinical guidelines
- Clinical pearls
- Compliance
- Drug abuse
- Drug shortages
- Drugs withdrawn from market
- Effects of external events on jobs
- Food and Drug Administration (FDA) warnings
- Job-related information
- New information sources
- New legal or regulatory requirements
- New services
- News from other departments
- Organization's stand on issues
- Patient safety
- Personnel policies
- Pharmacoeconomics
- Pharmacogenomics
- Pharmacy and therapeutics committee actions and news
- Productivity improvement
- Professional announcements
- Review of drugs or drug classes
- Quality assurance
- Quality improvement

Newsletter Distribution

All the above work will be for nothing if the readers do not get the newsletter. A good distribution system must be developed. Sometimes it can be as simple as sticking the newsletters in individual mailboxes, setting out piles of newsletters, or using intraorganizational mail systems. If it is necessary to use the post office, it would be a good idea to check on the possibility of second class or bulk mail, which can save money. More often, newsletter publications are distributed by email[134] or other computerized methods.[135] It may also be useful to distribute information with **QR (Quick Response) codes** that will make it easier to download information via a smartphone or tablet. Whatever method used, it is important to make sure the readers get the newsletter. Also, make sure they get the newsletters on a regular cycle so that they know when to anticipate the arrival of the publication.

Case Study 13–2

Your supervisor lets you know that you are in charge of a new website.

- *What are the first steps to do?*

PRESENTATIONS

A health care professional may have the opportunity to give a formal presentation at some point in a career. This could be simply where the health care professional works or at a national meeting. Although fear of public speaking is an extremely common occurrence, a speaker who prepares should do well. The problem may simply be fear of the unknown and having some simple directions may be of immense help. Overall, the main concern should be to know the topic. If someone knows enough to be asked to talk, chances are that person will know quite a bit about a topic, or will be able to learn enough about the topic. Alternately, the potential presenter may volunteer to give a presentation on an interesting topic or one in which the person has done a lot of work (e.g., a new method of practice or a new practice area). After that, most of the concern will deal with looking good. This includes a variety of items, many of which involve professional writing, and will be dealt with in the remainder of this section.

In cases where a person is asking to speak, a proposal will need to be submitted. This describes the proposed topic, which should be of interest to the target audience. The directions given by the organization preparing the meeting will need to be followed. Beyond that, the skills described earlier in this chapter and appendices will need to be used.

Next, it may be necessary to write an abstract that the organization providing the presentation forum will use to inform potential attendees about the presentation. Each organization may have a format to be followed in creating the abstract. Regarding the content of the abstract, the writer might use the information presented in Appendix 13-2. Ideally, an abstract should be prepared after the presentation is done to best reflect what was said. However, abstracts may be requested more than six months before the presentation, so in this case it will serve more as a planning document. It may be best to create a brief outline of the presentation (at least the topics to be covered) and then write the abstract.

It may also be necessary to prepare learning objectives to describe what the attendee will be able to do as a result of participating in the program. The objectives should state that behavior in objective, measurable terms. For example, an objective may state that the attendee can explain, list, or identify something. It will not say that the attendee knows, understands, or learns, because those are not measurable. The objectives should relate directly to the program and should be adequately broken down to cover the different areas of the presentation. Refer to the beginning of any of the chapters of this book for examples of objectives. Also, refer to Bloom's Taxonomy of Educational Objectives and Appropriate Verbs for more details.[136] This information could also be used for objectives written for other documents.[137]

Occasionally, the presenter may be requested to provide self-assessment questions. Often these will be multiple choice or true/false, to simplify assessment. Those questions should be clearly stated and measure that the attendee has met the objectives. Efforts should be made to make the questions clear. Also, they should avoid the use of NOT or EXCEPT because these terms can lead to confusion. Writing good questions can be extremely difficult, so testing the questions out on others before the presentation may help improve the quality.

The speaker may also have to prepare a brief biography to be used in the introduction. This includes a few items about the speaker's background, such as title and current position. Also, some information that gives the audience an idea of why the speaker is qualified to make a presentation is useful.

Presentations can usually be broken down into platform or poster presentations. The former is a more formal, oral presentation that typically requires some sort of audiovisual component and is often presented in a room set up for an audience. The latter requires the presenter to place a summary of the material to be presented on a poster (or series of small posters) that will be displayed on a bulletin board–type display (usually provided by the organization) that will be 3–4 feet high and 6–8 feet wide. In that situation, the attendees can walk through a group of such presentations, stopping to look at any that appeal to them and ask the presenter questions. Also, a QR code on the poster may allow the attendee to download further information or the poster itself using a smartphone or tablet.

Many of the rules described in the main part of this chapter relate to preparing the presentation materials, including slides, posters, and other audiovisual materials. However, a few other rules need to be mentioned.

- The presenter should learn the circumstances under which the presentation is to be given. That includes whether it is a platform or poster presentation.
- The presenter should learn what equipment will be provided (e.g., computer projector, microphone, size of board for poster presentation).
- If the presenter needs other items, they should be made clear to the organization. For example, it is common for presenters to want to use computer projection equipment, which may present certain technical requirements for both the equipment and support people. Also, the presenter may need such things as power outlet strips, extension cords, wireless microphones (many good speakers prefer

to move about on the stage or in the audience and are frustrated by a podium microphone that requires them to stand in one place behind a podium), Internet connection, connections from a computer to the room sound system, Bluetooth®, Wi-Fi, USB connection, DVD player, cables, remote device to advance slides, audience response systems, and other items. The presenter's own needs and desires should be taken into account, in addition to those of the audience. It is necessary to be very specific, since the people organizing the meeting may not understand the requirements. For example, a speaker requesting an Internet connection may arrive to find a connection that is too slow for streaming video or one that has security restrictions preventing access to necessary Internet sites.

- If the speaker is doing a poster presentation, it is necessary to remember to bring pushpins to mount the poster on the provided display board.
- The audience should be considered. One common complaint when a speaker flies in for a presentation is that they may not know anything about local circumstances, including simple social skills that are expected (e.g., foreign countries). It is best if the speaker tries to find out more about the audience and the situation, adjusting the presentation to take those items into account.[138]
- If necessary, the setup of the room should be specified (e.g., theater style, discussion tables, screen placement).

All the above should be double checked at the location of the presentation after arrival, but in plenty of time to correct any problems. Speakers may also want to take advantage of a Speaker Ready Room that many organizations offer to review slides, etc. As a side note, checking in with those arranging the presentation is necessary so that they will not be worried about your arrival and they will be able to clear up any last-minute items.

The speaker then needs to develop the presentation, doing appropriate research and preparation, using skills described earlier in this chapter and in the following sections. The presentation should also be rehearsed adequately. The next steps will discuss preparation of audiovisual materials, which can enhance the audience's ability to understand and retain the material.[139,140]

Platform Presentations

When giving platform presentations, it is usually necessary to prepare audiovisual materials and, possibly, handouts. Most office software suites (e.g., Microsoft Office, Google Docs, Apple iWork) have very powerful tools to create slides and other materials. These also have professionally designed templates that provide good layouts for materials, including color and background choices. The programs may also guide the user to follow general rules, such as avoiding a busy slide that will be unreadable from the back of a large room.[141] Also, the programs can be used to do everything from creating simple slides to multimedia extravaganzas—the former being learned in a few minutes, with the more advanced features available for those who need or desire them. Be aware, however, that it is necessary to use only those features that truly add to the presentation and to avoid having fancy effects in slides just for the sake of the effects.[141] **❻** *Instead of concentrating on the technology, it is best to concentrate on the message.*[142] This will also have the advantage of having fewer things that might go wrong in a presentation.

When starting to prepare audiovisuals, it is necessary to determine what type of equipment, software, and situation will be found at the location where the presentation will be given. The most desirable type of audiovisual is the use of a computer with a projector and appropriate software to give the presentation. It is also possible to project slides from a smartphone or tablet (e.g., Android or iOS) that is properly equipped,[143] although the presentation may not be able to use some advanced features, such as the embedding of multimedia items.[144] When information or software is available on the Internet, it can be demonstrated. Also, in cases where a discussion ensues, it is possible for the presenter to use a word processor, presentation program, or other software to record items on the screen for users to read during or after the session. It is even possible to not only record the information on the screen during the presentation, but to also make it immediately available on the Internet at the end of the program, including audio and video. Some disadvantages include the cost of the equipment for the organizing group, the need for greater technical skills by both the presenter and organizing group, the potential for technological problems (e.g., a computer that refuses to boot, corrupted data, an Internet connection that does not work), and it may be necessary for the presenter to bring a notebook computer with appropriate software and data. Fortunately, the technical support people for professional meetings are familiar with the equipment and the equipment itself is often dependable.

When preparing the slides themselves, the presenter will have to prepare an outline to guide what is to be presented and determine the information to be presented in each slide. Some general rules can be mentioned.145

1. Start with an introduction that explains and gives an overview of what will be learned.[146]
2. Limit each slide to a topic. Sometimes this will be an **overview**, but specifics should be limited to a discrete topic. One or two minutes of presentation material per slide is appropriate. If it is necessary to refer to a previous slide, just make a duplicate that is inserted at the appropriate location.
3. Be sure to reach a conclusion that summarizes the information, rather than just having an abrupt end.[146]
4. Keep things simple. The program may be able to do many things (e.g., 20 fonts in 16 million colors), but they may not be desirable. Typically use one font

(perhaps with bold or underline in a few specific places for emphasis) and limited graphics.

5. Limit the amount of information presented on each slide.[141] A rule of thumb is no more than about five bulleted points per slide and no more than about five words per bulleted point. Any more than that quickly becomes confusing or unreadable. The font should be at least 16 point on PowerPoint, except perhaps for the citation for a table or graph. Generally, if someone in the back of the room has to squint or it takes more than 10 seconds to read a slide, there is too much information on it.[147] It has been theorized that a portion of the blame for the loss of the space shuttle, Columbia, was due to the information necessary for National Aeronautics and Space Administration (NASA) engineers being hidden in small print on an extremely busy slide.[148] While the consequences for most presentations are not nearly as large, it is still important that slides enhance the provision of the appropriate information, rather than obscure it. In general, by using the templates available in PowerPoint, it is likely that the slides will be readable.

6. Use a sans-serif font, such as Arial.

7. Consider using a theme in the program that will provide colors that go together well and contrast enough to be legible. Colors and color combinations must be carefully considered because they may have emotional overtones or, in cases of color-blind attendees, may not even be distinguishable.[149]

8. Consider graphics. They can make the slide more pleasing to the eye, but they also need to be as simple as possible. If cartoons are included to entertain the audience, make sure they are related to the talk and, preferably, help to make a point. Usually, it is good to avoid such things as cartoons and clip art, which may be distracting. Also, pictures of landscapes or the presenter's institution may be desired by the presenter, but serve only to distract from the presentation and should be avoided. In general, the best way is to include graphics (e.g., graphs) that add to the presentation. Remember that if copyrighted material will be used, it is necessary to get permission to reproduce the material.

9. Consider embedding sound or video in the presentation, if it adds to the presentation. That sounds difficult, but may be done with a few clicks of the mouse. It will be necessary in this case to make sure the computer for the presentation is connected to the room's sound system so that attendees can hear the audio.

10. Embed links to appropriate websites in the presentation. This can be particularly useful if an electronic version of the handout is provided to attendees.

11. Save the presentation several ways. Even if it is on the computer hard drive, it may become corrupted or the computer can break. Perhaps also bring it on a USB drive so that someone else's computer can be borrowed if necessary. Also, in case the computer to be used in the presentation does not have presentation

software, it might be necessary to use the feature in many presentation software packages that creates a run-time presentation that does not require the actual software. In some cases, putting the slides on a web server in presentation format may work, although accessing the slides and web pages over the Internet can be a risky proposition. Also, as mentioned previously, the presentation might be given using a smart phone or tablet device.

Other items to consider include the following:

- Make sure to carry the presentation materials personally and do not check them as luggage, since they may be lost. Also, be careful not to damage the materials being carried.
- Make the presentation interactive—ask the audience questions and take input, or have the audience work on some project during the presentation. This is now a requirement of continuing education programs and will help the audience retain the information being presented.
- In all but a very small room, be sure to use the microphone. Speakers may not want to be bothered or may feel it is a sign of weakness to use a microphone, but they need to remember that the microphone is there to help the audience, not the speaker, and should be used so that everyone in the back of the room can hear over the ventilation system, etc.
- Keep to the slides, if at all possible, but do not read the slides—use the slides as speaking points for the oral presentation information and to organize your thoughts.[141] However, a speaker who simply reads the slides to the audience will likely be perceived as both unknowledgeable about the subject and boring.
- Do not read a prepared script, unless it is the norm in a particular environment. Actors and politicians can read such scripts and sound natural, but most speakers cannot do so. Instead use the slides (preferable) or a simple outline. The presentation software will allow easy preparation of handouts and speakers notes that can be used.
- Consider the delivery of the material, including pitch, power, pace, poise, and confidence.[150]
- Be prepared for technological disaster.[142] Even when using something as simple as a projector, the bulb can burn out. When using more equipment and more complex equipment, the potential for equipment failure rapidly increases. Whenever possible, have backup equipment, but also have a backup plan so that the presentation can proceed without any equipment. Just making sure to have a printed copy of the slides can save a presentation.
- Dress professionally.
- Make eye contact with the audience and be cheerful.

- Avoid distracting the audience with unnecessary words (e.g., um, like) or unnecessary body movements (e.g., rocking, tapping, rubbing hands), but be sure to move around if possible and do not hide behind the podium.

It may be desirable, or even a requirement, to prepare a handout for the audience, in which case, the presenter can consider the following styles[151]:

- *Outline*—a reference document that gives the audience a guide to where the speaker is going in text form. This can often be prepared by importing the slide content from the presentation software to a word processor. Some presentation programs will also prepare the document itself.
- *Full-text handout*—this is essentially a transcription of the speech. While helpful as a reference document, it is probably of more use to politicians when they wish to avoid being misquoted. This is seldom seen in the health care field because the presenter will not be able to make last minute changes and the audience will likely read ahead and become bored. Interestingly, a comment heard when such documents are presented is that the speaker did not know the material, because all the person did was read the handout, even though the speaker was the one who wrote it!
- *Slide reproduction*—this is becoming more popular and easier; presentation programs allow easy slide handout preparation. This does give the attendee all the information, including graphics, but will likely require more paper.
- *Partial text handout*—this can be something of a combination of the above, where only a portion of the presentation is on the handout.

In any of the above, it is good to consider the following[151]:

- Consider whether it is necessary to provide references or supplemental readings.
- Make sure the handout follows the order of the presentation. If it does not, the attendee may become confused and annoyed.
- Make it look good, using skills mentioned elsewhere in this chapter. Allow plenty of room for the attendee to take notes.

The speaker may also use the handout as a set of speaker notes, but care should generally be taken to avoid just reading the handout to the audience, except in the case of full-text handouts, for the reasons previously mentioned.

The skills necessary to give the presentation itself are beyond the scope of this chapter that deals with the preparation and distribution of written material. New presenters may wish to read a book or pamphlet on how to give effective talks. Also, Toastmasters International (https://www.toastmasters.org) is a group that will help individuals develop their speaking skills. Many organizations have a chapter of this organization. These aids will provide guidance on such skills as what level of sophistication to use in speaking, how to stand (e.g., do not hide behind the podium, make eye contact), what language to use, how to use humor and other techniques to entertain the audience, how to address questions (including so-called sniper questions that tend to disrupt speakers due to the level of difficulty and how they are thrown into the middle of the presentation),[152] how to avoid distractions by having everyone turn off phones,[153] and so forth. Also, some of the references used in preparation of this chapter provide many additional suggestions.[139,151]

Poster Presentations

Preparing a poster requires the presenter to first determine what is to be included. Typically, the information will be similar to that found in an abstract, but with an expansion of the various sections. There are likely to be tables, bulleted points, and figures. Overall, the information to be presented must be brief, so that it can be read within a couple of minutes by an individual passing by the display. Therefore, large amounts of text are undesirable. A poster presentation will not likely contain nearly as much information as a formal journal article, but will contain many of the same sections. It will serve as a place for discussion to begin between the presenter and interested individuals.

Preparing posters was at one time a very difficult prospect. This has changed with the availability of presentation and high-end word processing or publishing software on computers. A large, one-piece poster that is typically about 3 × 6 feet may be made using this software. Although the final poster must be printed by a graphics firm (e.g., printer, architectural drawing firm), the cost can be reasonable to produce a very attractive poster. This may also be done over the Internet. The initial preparatory work can also be done by various firms, but it is less expensive to do this yourself. The software necessary would be either desktop publishing software (e.g., Adobe® PageMaker, Microsoft Publisher, and Microsoft PowerPoint) or a high-end word processor (e.g., Microsoft Word). Lay out the page in these programs so that it is in landscape format (i.e., sideways from the normal typed page). The top of the page will have a centered title in large print, with the author names, institution, city, and so on centered in a smaller font below the title. Often, it is desirable to place graphics to one or both sides of that information, such as the symbol(s) for the authors' institution(s). Under that, the page may be divided up into three or so columns and the information laid out in a logical order, including tables and figures, which generally read from top to bottom and left to right. It may be desirable, once finished, to print out the final copy. One can produce a copy that fits on typical 8½ in. × 11 in. paper that can be reproduced and distributed to interested individuals at the meeting. It may also be on larger paper (e.g., 11 in. × 17 in.), if there is a suitable high-quality printer available.

Some general suggestions for posters include[154]:

- Limit the number of full sentences.
- Use appropriate white space.

- Use 24-point font or larger.
- Use a serif font (e.g., Times New Roman).
- Use graphics resolution of at least 150 dpi.
- Include a QR code that allows downloading of a copy of the poster or further information.

Whatever method is used, the final product will need to be transported to the meeting (poster tubes are available for little or no cost from many graphics firms). It is preferable to carry such posters on airplanes, rather than to check them, because they may be crushed in the baggage areas or lost. High-resolution cloth posters are becoming popular alternatives to paper posters due to their damage resistance. It is also possible to have the printer send the poster directly to the location of the presentation, although this would preclude the possibility of checking it ahead of time. The presenter should also remember to bring push pins to mount the presentation at the meeting and business cards to give to anyone requesting them. The presenter should show up early enough for the presentation to mount the poster to the bulletin board before meeting attendees are allowed in the area and will be expected to remain with the presentation to answer questions during the assigned time. Although many people may be the authors of a presentation, it is not uncommon that only one or two attend the meeting and give the presentation.

Web Posting

After a presentation, consider making the material available on the Internet. Some organizations make at least some presentation materials available that way. Copyright restrictions may prevent individuals from posting the material, but technology makes it easy when it is allowable. Text documents or graphic images, such as posters, are easily placed on a website. Even full-slide presentations can be placed on a website, using streaming audiovisual. A variety of software can be used to prepare such streaming presentations that can include slides and an audiovisual recording of the presenter. This can even be done concurrently with the presentation (live streaming), with a recording being made for later viewing. The equipment needs are relatively minor (i.e., computer, presentation software, microphone, inexpensive computer video capture device). For the actual Internet streaming, the appropriate streaming software, running on a file server, is necessary. For those who do not have the appropriate streaming software, just placing the slides themselves, as a downloadable file or in presentation format, can be an easy process using the original software used to prepare the slides. Even the simplest website can then be used to give access to the material.

Case Study 13–3

You are preparing a platform presentation for a national professional meeting for the first time.

- *What are some things that should be considered in slide preparation?*

Conclusion

❼ *Professional writing is a skill necessary for every health care professional.* It simply consists of following the accepted rules for writing that have been established by the profession to prepare a written item that is clear, concise, complete, correct, and in the appropriate format.

Self-Assessment Questions

1. Which of the following items are a type of professional writing?
   a. An article published in a professional journal
   b. A budget report
   c. A patient information sheet
   d. A performance evaluation of a new employee
   e. All of the above

2. All of the following are necessary for credit as an author EXCEPT?
   a. Writing or revising article
   b. Acquisition of funding
   c. Final approval of the version published
   d. Accountability for all aspects of the work
   e. All of the above

3. When writing a document that is intended for an audience of pharmacists, physicians, and nurses, which style of writing should be employed?
   a. Pure technical style
   b. Middle technical style
   c. Popular technical style

4. Which guideline tends to be used the most in writing for medical and pharmacy journals?
   a. American Medical Association Manual of Style
   b. MLA Handbook for Writers of Research Papers
   c. Publication Manual of the American Psychiatric Association (APA)
   d. Scientific Style and Format: The CBE Manual for Authors, Editors, and Publishers
   e. Recommendations for the Conduct, Reporting, Editing, and Publication of Scholarly Work in Medical Journals

5. It is necessary to only define unusual abbreviations in a document, since nearly every reader will understand common abbreviations, such as the use of AIDS for Acquired Immunodeficiency Syndrome.
   a. True
   b. False

6. When writing a document, it is not necessary to provide a citation to a personal communication (e.g., email, letter), since that is not a refereed publication.
   a. True
   b. False

7. In most cases, when writing up an answer to a question for another health care practitioner, the first paragraph of the paper should contain the summary of the information contained in the body to make things simpler and faster to read.
   a. True
   b. False

8. Copyright violations and plagiarism are not the same. It is possible to commit one while avoiding the other.
   a. True
   b. False

9. The CONSORT statement provides what?
   a. A Code of Conduct for websites
   b. A web hosting site for medically related websites
   c. Standards for reporting clinical trials
   d. a and b
   e. None of the above

10. Which of the following is an appropriate objective for a presentation? The attendee will:
    a. List the steps for preparation of the intravenous form of drug X
    b. Know the steps for preparation of the intravenous form of drug X
    c. Learn the steps for preparation of the intravenous form of drug X
    d. Understand the steps for preparation of the intravenous form of drug X
    e. None of the above are appropriate.

11. When preparing slides for presentations, it is best to provide as many details on each slide as possible, even if the font must be smaller than normal.
    a. True
    b. False

12. You are going to provide a 1-hour CE presentation. How many slides should you likely be preparing?
    a. 10
    b. 50
    c. 100
    d. 150

13. Which of the following is true when giving a presentation?
    a. It is best to avoid the use of a microphone, if possible, since most people do not know how to use it for the best effect and it is just another technology that may fail. Most of the time the speaker can just raise his or her voice so that everyone can hear.
    b. Microphones are placed in a room for the convenience of the audience, not the presenter. If there is a microphone present, the speaker should always use it.
    c. Ask the audience whether you should use the microphone.
    d. Run a test prior to the presentation and ask an assistant to see if you sound loud enough.

14. Presentation handouts should:
    a. Follow the order of the presentation.
    b. Provide the full text of the speech.
    c. Supplement, but not replace the presentation.
    d. a and c.
    e. All of the above.

15. Conclusions should be left relatively vague in order to allow the reader to draw their own conclusions from the body of a document.
    a. True
    b. False

REFERENCES

1. Kelley KW, Liles AM. Writing letters of recommendation: where should you start? Am J Health-Syst Pharm. 2012;69:563-5.
2. Thordsen DJ. Preparing an article for publication. J Pharm Technol. 1986;Nov/Dec: 268-75.
3. Generali JA. Why publish? Hosp Pharm. 2008;43(11):868.
4. Moghadam RG. Scientific writing: a career for pharmacists. Am J Health-Syst Pharm. 2003 Sep 15;60:1899-1900.
5. Armbruster DL. Starting the writing process. J Pediatr Pharmacol Ther. 2003;8(3): 210-1.
6. Fye WB. Medical authorship: traditions, trends, and tribulations. Ann Intern Med. 1990;113:317-25.
7. Gannon F. Ethical profits from publishing. EMBO Rep. 2004;5(1):1.
8. Nahata MC. Publishing by pharmacists. DICP Ann Pharmacother. 1989;23:809-10.
9. Persky AM, Romanelli F. Insights, pearls, and guidance on successfully producing and publishing educational research. Am J Pharm Educ. 2016;80(5):Article 75.
10. Wager E, Field EA, Grossman L. Good publication practice for pharmaceutical companies. Curr Med Res Opin. 2003;19(3):149-154.
11. Morris CT, Hatton RC, Kimberlin CL. Factors associated with the publication of scholarly articles by pharmacists. Am J Health-Syst Pharm. 2011;68:1640-5.
12. Dotson B, Slaughter RL. Prevalence of articles with honorary and ghost authors in three pharmacy journals. Am J Health-Syst Pharm. 2011;68:1730-4.
13. Sadler TR. Publishing in academia: woes of authorship, figures, and peer review. Drug Inf J. 2011;45:145-50.
14. Wilcox LJ. Authorship. The coin of the realm, the source of complaints. JAMA. 1998;280:216-17.
15. Hoen WP, Walvoort HC, Overbeke AJ. What are the factors determining authorship and the order of the authors' names? A study among authors of the Nederlands. Tijdschrift voor Geneeskunde (Dutch J Med). 1998;280:217-8.
16. Zoog HB, Chang T. Interpretation and implementation of good publication practice. Drug Inf J. 2011;45:137-44.
17. Committee on Publication Ethics (COPE). Guidelines on good publication practice. Cope Report. 2002:48-52.
18. Shapiro DW, Wenger NS, Shapiro MF. The contributions of authors to multiauthored biomedical research papers. JAMA. 1994;271:438-42.
19. Flanagin A, Carey LA, Fontanarosa PB, Phillips SG, Pace BP, Lundberg GD, Rennie D. Prevalence of articles with honorary authors and ghost authors in peer-reviewed medical journals. JAMA. 1998;280:222-4.
20. Wager E. Raising the quality of publications: now we have GPP! Qual Assur J. 2003;7:166-70.
21. Peterson AM, Lowenthal W, Veatch RM. Authorship on a manuscript intended for publication. Am J Hosp Pharm. 1993;50:2082-5.

22. Carbone PP. On authorship and acknowledgments. NEJM. 1992;326:1084.

23. Hart RG. On authorship and acknowledgments. NEJM. 1992;326;1084.

24. Pinching AJ. On authorship and acknowledgments. NEJM. 1992;326:1084-5.

25. Canter D. On authorship and acknowledgments. NEJM. 1992;326:1085.

26. Rennie D, Yank V, Emanuel L. When authorship fails: a proposal to make contributors accountable. JAMA. 1997;278:579-85.

27. Fathalla MF, VanLook PF. On authorship and acknowledgments. NEJM. 1992;326:1085.

28. The International Committee of Medical Journal Editors. Statement from the International Committee of Medical Journal Editors. JAMA. 1991;265:2697-8.

29. Hasegawa GR. Spurious authorship. Am J Hosp Pharm. 1993;50:2063.

30. Rennie D, Flanagin A. Authorship! Authorship! Guests, ghosts, grafters, and the two-sided coin. JAMA. 1994;271:469-71.

31. International Committee of Medical Journal Editors. Recommendations for the conduct, reporting, editing, and publication of scholarly work in medical journals [Internet]. International Committee of Medical Journal Editors; 2018 Dec [cited 2019 Feb 11]. Available from: http://icmje.org/icmje-recommendations.pdf

32. International Committee of Medical Journal Editors. Uniform requirements for manuscripts submitted to biomedical journals: writing and editing for biomedical publication [Internet]. Philadelphia: International Committee of Medical Journal Editors. 2009 Nov [cited 2010 Nov 16]. Available from: http://www.icmje.org/index.html

33. Kassirer JP, Angell M. On authorship and acknowledgments. NEJM. 1991;325:1510-2.

34. Drenth JPH. Multiple authorship: the contribution of senior authors. JAMA. 1998;280:219-21.

35. Kassirer JP, Angell M. On authorship and acknowledgments. NEJM. 1992;326:1085.

36. Foote MA. Medical writing: looking back, moving forward. Drug Inf J. 2011; 45:121-3.

37. Foote MA. How to write a better manuscript. Drug Inf J. 2009;43:111-4.

38. McConnell CR. From idea to print: writing and publishing a journal article. Health Care Supervisor. 1984;2:78-94.

39. Burnakis TG. Advice on submitting papers. Am J Hosp Pharm. 1993;50:2523.

40. Higa GM. Scientific publications and scientific style. W V Med J. 1995;91:198-9.

41. Crichton M. Medical obfuscation: structure and function. NEJM. 1975;293:1257-9.

42. Jones DE. Last word. Omni. 1980;2(12):130.

43. Hamilton CW. How to write effective business letters: scribing information for pharmacists. Hosp Pharm. 1993;28:1095-1100.

44. Albert T. The fear of writing—it's not as hard as pharmacists seem to think. Pharmaceut J. 2003 Jan 11;270:55-6.

45. Tsukayama H. How to write emails if you want people to actually respond [Internet]. Wash Post. 2016 Feb 16 [cited 2016 Jun 22]. Available from: http://washington-post.com/news/the-switch/wp/2016/02/16/want-to-get-more-responses-for-your-emails-write-like-a-third-grader/.

46. Baker SJ. Getting published. Aust J Hosp Pharm. 1994;24(5):410-5.

47. Hamilton CW. How to write and publish scientific papers: scribing information for pharmacists. Am J Hosp Pharm. 1992;49:2477-84.

48. Guo J. Sorry, grammar nerds. The singular "they" has been declared Word of the Year [Internet]. Wash Post. 2016 Jan 8 [cited 2016 Jun 22]. Available from: http://www.washingtonpost.com/news/wonk/wp/2016/01/08/donald-trump-may-win-this-years-word-of-the-year/.

49. Ingelfinger FJ. Seduction by citation. NEJM. 1976;295:1075-6.

50. Roederer M, Marciniak MW, O'Connor SK, Eckel SF. An integrated approach to research and manuscript development. Am J Health-Syst Pharm. 2013 Jul 15;70:1211-8.

51. Sollaci LB, Pereira MG. The introduction, methods, results and discussion (IMRAD) structure: a fifty-year survey. J Med Libr Assoc. 2004;92(3):364-7.

52. Poirier T, Crouch M, MacKinnon G, Mehvar R, Monk-Tutor M. Updated guidelines for manuscripts describing instructional design and assessment: the IDEAS format. Am J Pharm Educ. 2009;73(3):Article 55.

53. Schulz F, Altman DG, Moher D. CONSORT 2010 statement: updated guidelines for reporting parallel group randomized trials. Ann Intern Med. 2010;152(11):1-7.

54. Moher D, Hopewell S, Schulz KF, Montori V, Gøtzsche PC, Devereaux PJ, Elbourne D; Egger M, Altman DG; CONSORT Group. CONSORT 2010 explanation and elaboration: updated guidelines for reporting parallel group randomized trials. BMJ. 2010;340:c869. doi:10.1136/bmj.c869.

55. Campbell MK, Elbourne DR, Altman DG, for the CONSORT Group. CONSORT statement: extension to cluster randomized trials. BMJ. 2004;328:702-8.

56. Piaggio G, Elbourne DR, Altman DG, Pocock SJ, Evans SJ; CONSORT Group. Reporting of noninferiority and equivalence randomized trials. An extension of the CONSORT Statement. JAMA. 2006;295:1152-60.

57. Gagnier JJ, Boon H, Rochon P, Moher D, Barnes J, Bombardier C; CONSORT Group. Reporting randomized, controlled trials of herbal interventions: an elaborated CONSORT Statement. Ann Intern Med. 2006;144:364-7.

58. Boutron I, Moher D, Altman DG, Schulz KF, Ravaud P; CONSORT Group. Methods and processes of the CONSORT Group: example of an extension for trials assessing nonpharmacologic treatments. Ann Intern Med. 2008;148:W-60-W-66.

59. Ioannidis JP, Evans SJ, Gøtzsche PC, O'Neill RT, Altman DG, Schulz K, Moher D; CONSORT Group. Better reporting of harms in randomized trials: an extension of the CONSORT Statement. Ann Intern Med. 2004;141:781-8.

60. Hopewell S, Clarke M, Moher D, Wager E, Middleton P, Altman DG, Schulz KF; CONSORT Group. CONSORT for reporting randomized controlled trials and conference abstracts: explanation and elaboration. PLoS Med. 2008;5(1):e20. doi:10.1371/journal.pmed.0050020.

61. von Elm E, Altman DG, Egger M, Pocock SJ, Gøtzsche PC, Vandenbroucke JP; STROBE Initiative. The Strengthening the Reporting of Observational Studies in Epidemiology (STROBE) statement: guidelines for reporting observational studies. Ann Intern Med. 2007;147:573-7.

62. Vandenbroucke JP, von Elm E, Altman DG, Gøtzsche PC, Mulrow CD, Pocock SJ, Poole C, Schlesselman JJ, Egger M; STROBE initiative. Strengthening the Reporting of Observational Studies in Epidemiology (STROBE): explanation and elaboration. Ann Intern Med. 2007;147:W-163-W-194.

63. Zwarenstein M, Treweek S, Gagnier JJ, Altman DG, Tunis S, Haynes B, Oxman AD, Moher D; CONSORT group. Improving the reporting of pragmatic trials: an extension of the CONSORT Statement. BMJ. 2008;227:a2390. doi:10.1136/bmj.a2390.

64. Moher D, Cook DJ, Eastwood S, Olkin I, Rennie D, Stroup DF. Improving the quality of reports of meta-analyses of randomised controlled trials: the QUOROM statement. Lancet. 1999;354:1896-900.

65. Moher D, Liberati A, Tetzlaff J, Altman DG. The PRISMA Group (2009) preferred reporting items for systematic reviews and meta-analyses. The PRISMA Statement. PLoS Med. 2009;6(7):e1000097. doi:10.1371/journal.pmed.1000097.

66. Graf C, Battisti WP, Bridges D, Bruce-Winkler V, Conaty JM, Ellison JM, Field EA, Gurr JA, Marx ME, Patel M, Sanes-Miller C, Yarker YE; International Society for Medical Publication Professionals. Good publication practice for communicating company sponsored medical research: the GPP2 guidelines. BMJ. 2009;339:b4330. doi:10:10.1136/bmj.b4330.

67. Talley CR. Perspective in journal publishing. Am J Hosp Pharm. 1993;50:451.

68. Tiachman DB, Sahni P, Pinborg A, Peiperl L, Laine C, James A, Hong S-T, Halleamlak A, Gollogly L, Godlee F, Frizelle FA, Florenzano F, Drazen JM, Bauchner H, Baethge C. Data sharing statements for clinical trials. A requirement of the International Committee of Medical Journal Editors. JAMA. 2017 Jun 27;317(24):2491-2.

69. LaRochelle JM, King AR. Avoiding plagiarism. Hosp Pharm. 2011;46(12):917-9.

70. Gabriel T. Plagiarism lines blur for students in digital age. New York Times. 2010 Aug 1 [cited 2010 Aug 2]; [4 p.]. Available from: http://www.nytimes.com/2010/08/02/education/02cheat.html?_r=1&scp=1&sq=plagiarism%20lines%20blur&st=cse

71. Turnitin.com [Internet]. Oakland (CA): iParadigms, LLC; c1998-2012. Plagiarism and the web: a comparison of internet sources for secondary and higher education students; 2011 [cited 2012 Jun 13]; [about 10 p.]. Available from: http://pages.turnitin.com/rs/iparadigms/images/Turnitin_WhitePaper_SourcesSECvsHE.pdf

72. Mapes D. Steal this story? Beware Net's plagiarism "cops" [Internet]. MSNBC. 2009 Sep 10 [cited 2019 Jul 25]; [3 p.]. Available from: http://www.nbcnews.com/id/32657885/ns/technology_and_science-tech_and_gadgets/t/steal-story-beware-nets-plagiarism-cops/#.XToFHOhKiWk

73. Ware J. Cheat wave. Yahoo! Internet Life. 1999;5(5):102-3.

74. Stuber-McEwen D, Wiseley P, Hoggatt S. Point, click, and cheat: frequency and type of academic dishonesty in the virtual classroom. Online J Dist Learning Admin. 2009 Fall [cited 2009 Sep 17]; XII(III); [10 p.]. Available from: http://www.westga.edu/~distance/ojdla/fall123/stuber123.html

75. Asimov I. Gold: The final science fiction collection. New York: HarperPrism; 1995.

76. Blanding M. Plagiarism software unveils a new source for 11 of Shakespeare's plays. NYTimes. 2018 Feb 7 [cited 2019 Jan 29]. Available from: https://www.nytimes.com/2018/02/07/books/plagiarism-software-unveils-a-new-source-for-11-of-shakespeares-plays.html

77. Willful infringement. [Cited 2004 Aug 9]. Available from: http://www.willfulinfringement.com/.

78. Development of a guideline to approach plagiarism in Indian scenario: retraction. Indian J Dermatol. 2015 Mar-Apr;60(2):210.

79. Ardito SC, Eiblum P, Daulong R. Conflicted copy rights. Online. 1999 May/June;23(3): 91-5.

80. Crawford M. Are you committing plagiarism? Top five overlooked citations to add to your course materials [Internet]. Message to: Patrick M. Malone. 2010 Sep 29. [4 p.].

81. Milbank D. Hope Hicks told the truth about lying for Trump. Now she's gone. Wash Post. 2018 Feb 28 [cited 2019 Jan 29]. Available from: https://www.washingtonpost.com/opinions/hope-hicks-says-she-lies-for-trump-thats-encouraging/2018/02/28/09e61982-1cc3-11e8-9de1-147dd2df3829_story.html?utm_term=.28a0fc53c5c0

82. Barbash F. Scientist falsified data for cancer research once described as "holy grail", feds say. Wash Post. 2015 Nov 9 [cited 2019 Jan 29]. Available from: https://www.washingtonpost.com/news/morning-mix/wp/2015/11/09/scientist-falsified-data-for-cancer-research-once-described-as-holy-grail-feds-say/?utm_term=.e423b3825222

83. Doshi P. No correction, no retraction, no apology, no comment: paroxetine trial reanalysis raises questions about institutional responsibility. BMJ. 2015;351:h4629. doi:10.1136/bmj.h4629.

84. Abbott A. Japanese scientist resigns as "STAP" stem-cell method fails. Nature. 2014 Dec 19 [cited 2019 Jan 29]:doi:10.1038/nature.2014.16631. Available from: https://www.nature.com/news/japanese-scientist-resigns-as-stap-stem-cell-method-fails-1.16631

85. McCoy T. How Japan's most promising young stem-cell scientist duped the scientific journal Nature—and destroyed her career. Wash Post. 2014 Jul 3 [cited 2019 Jan 29]. Available from: https://www.washingtonpost.com/news/morning-mix/wp/2014/07/03/how-japans-most-promising-young-stem-cell-scientist-duped-the-scientific-journal-nature-and-destroyed-her-career/?utm_term=.cc585eaaea27

86. McCoy T. Famed Japanese stem-cell scientist dies in apparent suicide amid retraction scandal. Wash Post. 2014 Aug 5 [cited 2019 Jan 29]. Available from: https://www.washingtonpost.com/news/morning-mix/wp/2014/08/05/famed-japanese-stem-cell-scientist-dies-in-apparent-suicide-amid-retraction-scandal/?utm_term=.112dffe77bb0

87. Barbash F. Scholarly journal retracts 60 articles, smashes "peer review ring". Wash Post. 2014 Jul 10. Available from: https://www.washingtonpost.com/news/morning-mix/wp/2014/07/10/scholarly-journal-retracts-60-articles-smashes-peer-review-ring/?utm_term=.976aa7ab89da

88. Gousse G. Advice on submitting papers: I. Am J Hosp Pharm. 1993;50:2523.

89. World Association of Medical Editors. Policies for Medical Journal Editors, prepared by the WAME Ethics and Policy Committee [Internet]. Chicago: World Association of Medical Editors; 2016 [cited 2019 Jul 25]. Available from: http://www.wame.org/policies

90. International Committee of Medical Journal Editors. Conflict of interest. Am J Hosp Pharm. 1993;50:2398.

91. Davidoff F, DeAngelis CD, Drazen JM, Hoey J, Højgaard L, Horton R, Kotzin S, Nylenna M, Overbeke AJ, Sox HC, Van Der Weyden MB, Wilkes MS; International Committee of Medical Journal Editors. Sponsorship, authorship, and accountability. Lancet. 2001 Sep 15;358:854-6.

92. Krimsky S, Rothenberg LS. Financial interest and its disclosure in scientific publications. JAMA. 1998;280:225-6.

93. Laniado M. How to present research data consistently in a scientific paper. Eur Radiol. 1996;6:S16-8.

94. DeAngelis CD. Duplicate publication, multiple problems. JAMA. 2004;292:1745-6.

95. Stead WW. The responsibilities of authorship. J Am Med Inform Assoc. 1997;4:394-5.

96. Hasegawa GR. How to review a manuscript intended for publication. Am J Hosp Pharm. 1994;51:839-40.

97. Janke KK, Bzowyckyj AS, Traynor AP. Editors' perspectives on enhancing manuscript quality and editorial decisions through peer review and reviewer development. Am J Pharm Educ. 2017;81(4):Article 73.

98. Hoppe S, Chandler MJJ. Constructive versus destructive criticism. Am J Health-Syst Pharm. 1995;52:103.

99. Baker DE. Peer review: personal continuous quality improvement. Hosp Pharm. 2004;39:8.

100. Garfunkel JM, Lawson EE, Hamrick HJ, Ulshen MH. Effect of acceptance or rejection on the author's evaluation of peer review of medical manuscripts. JAMA. 1990;263:1376–8.

101. Baker WL, DiDomenico RJ, Haines ST. Improving peer review: what authors can do. Am J Health-Syst Pharm. 2017;74:e517-20.

102. Hasegawa GR. An editor's perspective on peer review. Am J Health-Syst Pharm. 2017;74:e530-4.

103. Evans JT, Nadjari HI, Burchell SA. Quotation and reference accuracy in surgical journals. JAMA. 1990;263:1353-4.

104. Roland CG. Thoughts about medical writing. XXXVII. Verify your references. Anesth Analg. 1976;55:717-8.

105. Biebuyck JF. Concerning the ethics and accuracy of scientific citations. J Anesthesiol. 1992;77:1-2.

106. McLellan MF, Case LD, Barnett MC. Trust, but verify. The accuracy of references in four anesthesia journals. Anesthesiology. 1992;77:185-8.

107. de Lacy G, Record C, Wade J. How accurate are quotations and references in medical journals. Br Med J. 1985;291:884-6.

108. Doms CA. A survey of reference accuracy in five national dental journals. J Dent Res. 1989;68:442-4.

109. Seltzer SM. Desktop publishing in a drug store? Am Druggist. 1987:196:64, 66.

110. Srnka QM, Scoggin JA. 10 ways to distribute newsletters to build sales volume. Pharm Times. 1984;50;71-2, 74.

111. Making the media. The pharmacy newsletter. Hosp Pharm Connection. 1986;2(3):11-2.

112. Kaldy J. Effectively creating a pharmacy newsletter. Consult Pharm. 1992;7(6):700, 697-8.

113. Goldwater SH, Haydon-Greatting S. How to publish a pharmacy newsletter. Am J Hosp Pharm. 1991;48:2121, 2125.

114. Almquist AF, Wolfgang AP, Perri M. Pharmacy newsletters—the journalistic approach. Hosp Pharm. 1988;23:974-5.

115. Schultz WL, Dendiak ST. Pharmacy newsletters: a needed service. Hosp Pharm. 1975;10(4):146-7.

116. Plumridge RJ, Berbatis CG. Drug bulletins: effectiveness in modifying prescribing and methods of improving impact. DICP Ann Pharmacother. 1989;23:330-4.

117. Appearance and content attract newsletter audience. Drug Utilization Review. 1988;4(4):45-8.

118. Lyon RA, Norvell MJ. Effect of a P&T Committee newsletter on anti-infective prescribing habits. Hosp Formul. 1985;20:742-4.

119. Fendler KJ, Gumbhir AK, Sall K. The impact of drug bulletins on physician prescribing habits in a health maintenance organization. Drug Intell Clin Pharm. 1984;18:627-31.

120. May JR, Andrusko KT, DiPiro JT. Impact and cost justification of a surgery drug newsletter. Am J Hosp Pharm. 1984;41:1837-9.

121. Ross MB, Volger BW, Bradley JK. Use of "dispense-as-written" on prescriptions for targeted drugs: influence of a newsletter. Am J Hosp Pharm. 1990;47:2519-20.

122. Denig P, Haaijer-Ruskamp FM, Zijsling DH. Impact of a drug bulletin on the knowledge, perception of drug utility, and prescribing behavior of physicians. DICP Ann Pharmacother. 1990;24:87-93.

123. Parker RC. Looking good in print. 4th ed. Scotsdale (AZ): The Coriolis Group, LLC; 1998.

124. Baird RN, McDonald D, Pittman RK, Turnbull AT. The Graphics of Communication: Methods, Media and Technology. 6th ed. New York: Hartcourt Brace Jovanovich College Publishers; 1993.

125. Don't let cost prohibit publication of pharmacy-related newsletter. Drug Utilization Review. 1988;4(4):48-9.

126. Utt JK, Lewis KT. Using desktop publishing to enhance pharmacy publications. Am J Hosp Pharm. 1988;45:1863-4.

127. Pfeiffer KS. Award-winning newsletter design. Windows Mag. 1994;5(8):208-18.

128. What makes a great web site? [Cited 1999 May 13]; [1 screen]. Available from: http://webreference.com/greatsite.html

129. Tweney D. Don't be a slow poke: keep your site up to speed or lose visitors. InfoWorld. 1999;22;21(12):64.

130. Tullio CJ. Selecting material for your newsletter. Hosp Pharm Times. 1992;Oct: 12HPT-16HPT.

131. Journalism pro offers editing tips for effective pharmacy newsletters. Drug Utilization Review. 1988;4(4):49-50.

132. Mitchell JF, Cook RL. Pharmacy newsletters: time for a new approach. Hosp Formul. 1985;20:360-5.

133. Ritchie DJ, Manchester RF, Rich MW, Rockwell MM, Stein PM. Acceptance of a pharmacy-based, physician-edited hospital pharmacy and therapeutics committee newsletter. Ann Pharmacother. 1992;26:886-9.

134. Craghead RM. Electronic mail pharmacy newsletters. Hosp Pharm. 1989;24:490.

135. Mok MP, Castile JA, Kowaloff HB, Janousek JR. Drugman—a computerized supplement to a hospital's drug information newsletter. Am J Hosp Pharm. 1985;42:1565-7.

136. Bloom BS, editor. Taxonomy of educational objectives, Handbook 1: cognitive domain. New York: David McKay; 1956.

137. Medina MS. Using the three e's (emphasis, expectations, and evaluation) to structure writing objectives for pharmacy practice experiences. Am J Health-Syst Pharm. 2010 Apr 1;67:516-21.

138. Speaking abroad. How to prepare when you're presenting over there. Presentations. 1999;13(6):A1-15.

139. Spinler SA. How to prepare and deliver pharmacy presentations. Am J Hosp Pharm. 1991;48:1730-8.

140. Simons T. Multimedia or bust? Presentations. 2000;14(2):40-50.

141. Buchholz S, Ullman J. 12 commandments for PowerPoint. Teaching Prof. 2004;18(6):4.

142. Zielinski D. Technostressed? Don't let your gadgets and gizmos get you down. Presentations. 2004 Feb:28-35.

143. Malone PM. Slides, files and keeping up. Adv Pharm. 2004;2(2):175-80.

144. Goldstein M. PDA presenting has come a long way, but still has drawbacks. Presentations. 2003 Nov:22.

145. Lewis B. Presenting smarter: keep the joint running. Minneapolis (MN): IS Survivor; 2018 Jul 2:3.

146. Medina MS, Avant ND. Delivering an effective presentation. Am J Health-Syst Pharm. 2015;72:1091-4.

147. Endicott J. For the prepared presenter, fonts of inspiration abound. Presentations. 1999;13(4):22-3.

148. Bullet points may be dangerous, but don't blame PowerPoint. Presentations. 2003 Nov:6.

149. The psychology of presentation visuals. Presentations. 1998;12(5):45-51.

150. DeCoske MA, White SJ. Public speaking revisited: delivery, structure and style. Am J Health-Syst Pharm. 2010 Aug 1;67:1225-7.

151. Engle JP, Firman SC. Perfecting pharmacist presentation skills. Am Pharm. 1994;NS34(7):60-4.

152. Simons T. For podium emergencies. Presentations. 2003 Nov:24-29.

153. Hill J. The attention deficit. Presentations. 2003 Oct:27-32.

154. McClendon KS, Sover KR. Tips for a successful poster presentation. Am J Health-Syst Pharm. 2014;71:449-51.

Chapter Fourteen

Media Relations

Erin R. Fox • Linda S. Tyler

Learning Objectives

After completing this chapter, the reader will be able to:

- Discuss the importance of working effectively with the media.
- Plan methods to interact with the media effectively.
- Develop ways to address potential barriers to working with the media.

Key Concepts

❶ Health care practitioners have an important story to tell, if you do not tell your own story, someone else will tell the story for you. And they may not get it right!

❷ Work with the organization or institution's resources before accepting any media requests.

❸ Develop a plan and key messages before talking with the media.

❹ Be cognizant of deadlines and follow-up requests.

❺ Stories can help your patients, organization, community, and profession, and shape public policy.

Introduction

A key competency for health care practitioners is to advocate for our patients, organizations, community, and our profession. In fact, it is considered a professional obligation for pharmacists.[1] It is important to take a stand on key health care issues that affect patients (e.g., drug shortages, drug pricing). Yet for most health care practitioners, the thought of talking to someone from the media is frightening, if not paralyzing. What many do not recognize is that we advocate for our patients and community frequently, but may not think of this advocacy as a strategy to further our aims. They may not think they have anything to say. In the case of pharmacists, they are the most accessible clinicians providing health care in communities and are painfully aware of the issues that affect patients, the health care teams, and communities. ❶ *Health care practitioners have an important story to tell, if you do not tell your own story, someone else will tell the story for you. And they may not get it right!*

Working with the Media

PLANNING

If asked to speak with the media, do not miss an opportunity to do so if the topic is right and you have support and approval from your supervisor and media relations department.[2] If not familiar with the topic, seize the opportunity to facilitate getting the right person in your organization to work with the media. Likewise, there may be an opportunity to ask for coverage of a specific topic (push a story). Most organizations have resources available to help with media requests. ❷ *Work with the organization or institution's resources before accepting any media requests.* At a minimum, it's important to obtain permission first, and to be clear if you are speaking on behalf of yourself and your expertise, or if you are speaking on behalf of the organization. In most cases, you will not be speaking on behalf of your organization. Get to know the media relations and government affairs professionals within your organization. Let them know you are willing to help work with media inquiries. Likewise, let them know what the current issues are for you. Meet regularly to keep each other informed. Inquire if they have media training opportunities. If not, ask them for hints in working with the media. See if they will help practice and role-play a media opportunity.

Case Study 14–1

You receive a call from your public relations department from the local television station about a recall of blood pressure medications. They ask if you can be ready to be on camera in 90 minutes.

- *What should you think about before accepting this request?*

BEFORE THE INTERVIEW

Two important details are essential before agreeing to work with a reporter. First, understand the story they are covering, and second, know their deadline.[3] A reporter may simply be doing some background on a future story, or they may have a story mostly complete and are just looking for one more quick comment.[4] Either way, it's worth doing some research to see if the reporter has covered the issue before and what their stance might be. The next step is to know the story. ❸ *Develop a plan and key messages before talking with the media.* Think about your key messages and try to distill the ideas into three key points. Draft your key messages and practice them—this is the best chance you have at not having your words taken out of context. Establish the time and length of the interview and ask for questions ahead of time, if possible. Your organizational resources may be able to help you with some of these activities and support you through the process.

Case Study 14-2

An investigative reporter from STAT news emails you about a new Food and Drug Administration (FDA) black box warning for increased risk of death being added to a gout medicine. He is working on a story to run in the next few weeks on how black box warnings are mainly ignored by most providers and wonders if you can comment.

* *What should you think about before accepting this request?*

DURING THE INTERVIEW

Be sure you communicate why the audience should care about your key message and keep the message short and memorable. A mix of facts plus a story about how those facts are impacting your patients or practice works well. For example, you could mention a specific recall and why it occurred as well as what actions the FDA is taking. Next, provide some context for how that recall is affecting your patients such as having to switch prescriptions or provide a notification.

An interview is not a conversation. The reporter will ask questions. You need to develop skill in using these questions as a vehicle to communicate your message. Keep your message simple. Stay on track with your key points during the interview. You may be repeating these key messages several times during the interview. Treat each time as if it is the first time you are using them. This may be a story you have discussed many times—but this is the first time the reporter you are working with has heard it. Use this as an opportunity to educate the reporter. Remember, few in the media have advanced science degrees or in-depth knowledge of the subject matter. Most are generalists and cover a number of different "beats." Be cautious, but honest, when talking with reporters. You are always on the record unless you say so, so make sure to use key points and beware of slipping into slang as you may see yourself quoted in a way that you did not intend.

Before starting, take a deep breath, relax, and smile. Communicate clearly, consistently and accurately. Minimize the filler words such as the "uhs," "ums," "duhs," and "okays" as examples. Adapt to both the audience and the medium. Often, how something is said matters as much, or more, than what is said. Be positive throughout the interview. Relax, breathe, speak slowly, and pause occasionally. Answer back the question in a complete sentence. This gives the chance to both confirm the question and organize your response. Do not let your guard down and fall victim to casual conversation. It is a standard interviewers' ploy to get you comfortable and get you to talk candidly. If you stick to the talking points, you will avoid this trap.

Be sure to listen to the question the reporter is asking. Clarify the question if not understood. Often times we may want to jump in and start answering the question before the reporter has finished the question and, in doing so, we answer a different question than what the reporter was asking. Reporters, in clarifying their stories, often present things in ways that may seem like a "trap," leading you to phrase things in ways that can easily be taken out of context or answer questions that were not really asked. Here are some hints on potential problem areas.

- The hypothetical. Do not respond to hypothetical questions. These start out as: "So what would happen if ..." Respond by stating that you cannot comment on the hypothetical question, but you can discuss XXX and then emphasize your key points.
- Commenting on what others say. Often times the reporter will comment on what others are saying about the topic. You should respond that while you do not know what others are saying or you cannot comment on what others are saying, you can tell the reporter XXX and then discuss your key points.
- Paraphrasing. A reporter may paraphrase what you said to confirm what you said. If it is not accurate, take the opportunity to say, "No that is not what I am saying. What I am saying is XXX (emphasize your key points)."
- Unclear questions. Reporters may ask a question unclearly. It is okay to respond with your understanding of what the question is by stating, "I think your question is XXX." This gives you the opportunity to make sure you are responding to the question the reporter is really asking.

When necessary, say "I do not know" or "I'll have to check on that." Know your counterarguments and be prepared to back up what you say. Reporters may ask you for suggestions for other people to speak with, so be ready with a recommendation if you feel comfortable. Also, be willing to provide follow-up information or additional background to help the story. Do not repeat negative questions or statements. Do not lose your cool during an interview—the reporter has the ultimate control on how your message comes out.

At the end of the interview, the reporter may ask you if you have anything to add. This is a great opportunity to reiterate your key messages. Have an answer to the question: "What else should I know about this?"

You will not generally get the opportunity to review the interview that will be published, though you may be contacted by fact checkers. You will appear inexperienced if you ask to review it before it goes to press or is aired. It will discourage news outlets from using the piece.

TIPS FOR SPECIFIC SITUATIONS

Be flexible. You have to make time for interviews. ❹ *Be cognizant of deadlines and follow-up requests.* Working with radio, television, and "print" media outlets require different strategies. Below are some tips for working with each of these.

Television is in general the most time consuming with a very short timeline. With local television, you may receive a request to be on camera within 1–2 hours. National television may have longer deadlines, especially for investigative stories, but you still may be asked to be ready for the camera within a short timeline. How you look and your professional image matters. Bright colors and pastels look best on TV; avoid wearing white or all black. Avoid wearing clothes with patterns, such as herringbone as they create a "shimmer" effect on TV cameras. Follow the camera crew instructions. Do not try to look at the camera. Maintain eye contact with whosoever is asking the questions. Sometimes you will be working with a reporter in person, but not always. Have good posture and do not fidget. If you have the opportunity to select the setting, choose a chair without wheels so you will not be tempted to roll back and forth on camera. If you are not on live TV, it is absolutely okay to ask to start over. Do not let the mistake fluster you or affect the overall interview. Everyone makes mistakes. Most TV reports are looking for simple "sound bites." This is not a time to go into detailed explanations. By the time the story is edited, you will probably only be on camera 15–30 seconds. However, if you are on live TV, you will not have this option. TV stations do not run corrections. If you feel you were misrepresented, consider it a lesson learned with that particular reporter. Each reporter has a different acumen for reporting science-based stories.

Radio is also typically a short turnaround—in fact, sometimes you may be asked to "go live" within seconds of answering the phone. Live radio while scarier is often better, in that your comments cannot be edited (or cut short or possibly taken out of context). Use a landline for the interview as it will provide a higher, more reliable sound quality than cell phones. In some cases, you may be asked to record a voice memo on your smart phone during the interview in addition to the landline call, or you may be asked to download an app for your smart phone. Your interview may not air for days or weeks. You may also be asked to visit a local radio station, which increases the time commitment. As with television, if you are not live it is okay to ask to start over. Stick to your talking points and have them in front of you if possible. Use verbal illustrations. You will have to create a picture with your words. Modulate your voice—smile and exude lots of energy!

For print, newspapers, or online outlets, the reporter will usually be calling you and you will discuss the story over the phone. The timelines for print media vary widely. A reporter may be working on developing a story and may have several weeks of time. In other cases, the reporter may be trying to file a story that same day and will ask for a quick turnaround. Talking on the phone allows you the option to keep your message points in front of you. You will want to stick to these points and reiterate them at every opportunity. Newspapers will seldom run corrections—follow up quickly if an error has been made or you have been misquoted or taken out of context.

What if the media is not calling you—but you have a great story to tell? You have the opportunity to highlight issues that are important to you and your organization, and most importantly your patients. You can work with your public relations department to "pitch" a story to the media. Another way to pitch a story is to use social media. Twitter works well for this purpose as you can tag a specific reporter who may be interested, or you may be contacted by a reporter who wants to learn more about the topic. Think about: "Who decides the news?" As much as we would like to influence the news, few of us have that opportunity. News is what is new or newsworthy to the reporters, producers, or editors of a media outlet. It is often something that is unreported, interesting, simple, or what sells. It is necessary to adapt our message considering these realities.

Case Study 14–3

Your organization is short on prefilled syringes of 50% Dextrose. The reason is because the main manufacturer is having quality problems at the factory. You are frustrated that this emergency medication is unavailable, but do not see any news stories about it. You believe that this problem should not remain invisible and want to pitch a story to the media.

- *What should you think about before talking to your public relations department?*

AFTER THE INTERVIEW

Whenever you work with a reporter, you will want to use it as an opportunity to build trust for future stories. Offer to be a resource in the future. You are looking to establish long-term relationships and contacts with the media. If you promised to provide additional details, do so as quickly as possible. Make yourself available to clarify any points as the writer is working on the story. If you are active on social media, "follow" the reporter on Twitter. Post the story to your social media sites and tag the reporter. For example, you could tweet something like "Thanks to @reporter for covering this important story on _____." Make sure you include the link. This also works well for LinkedIn.

Summary

Working with the media can be time consuming and may put you outside of your comfort zone. However, be open to working with the media. You may think that you could never make a difference. The old adage, "never say never," applies. Regardless of where you are in your career, you have the opportunity to make a difference. Working with the media is an opportunity to highlight important issues. ❺ *Stories can help your patients, organization, community, and profession, and shape public policy.*

Self-Assessment Questions

1. Who is in the best position to advocate for patients concerning medication-use issues?
   a. Nurses
   b. Pharmacists
   c. Physicians
   d. Representatives from pharmaceutical companies

2. For which of the following professions is it considered a professional obligation to advocate for medication-related issues?
   a. Hospital administrators
   b. Nurse practitioners
   c. Pharmacists
   d. Physicians

3. If you are called to speak with the media, but it is not a topic you are familiar with, which of the following would be the best course of action?
   a. Ask the student on rotation with you to research the topic and speak with the reporter.
   b. Facilitate finding a media contact that would be better suited to speak on the topic.
   c. Speak on the topic anyway, since you still know more on the topic than most.
   d. Tell the reporter that you cannot help them.

4. Who within your organization would be the best resource within your organization to support you in efforts to talk with the media?
   a. Chief medical officer
   b. Purchasing department
   c. Public relations department
   d. Security department

5. Before accepting an opportunity to work with a reporter, what things are the most important for you to understand?
   a. Determine if the reporter will be talking with you or wanting to video tape you as well.
   b. Know if the reporter has worked on similar stories or not.
   c. Know the reporter's background and how long they have worked as a reporter.
   d. Understand the story they are covering and the deadline.

6. In preparing for the story, what will be the most useful for you to have?
   a. Conduct a literature search on the topic.
   b. Develop three key messages concerning the topic.
   c. Have available primary literature on the topic.
   d. Prepare a thorough literature review on the topic.

7. Which of the following is the most useful technique to help talking points connect with audience?
   a. Describe what another pharmacist thinks about the topic.
   b. Discuss the primary literature on the topic.
   c. Quote expert researchers concerning the topic.
   d. Tell a story about your patients and how they are impacted.

8. Which of the following best describes the nature of reporter deadlines?
   a. Reporters are often under a lot of pressure to meet their deadlines so have little flexibility in working with you.
   b. Usually the date is flexible and the reporter is willing to work around your schedule within a few days.

   c. Reporters will ask you when you are available and develop their story within your requirements.

   d. If you are not available, reporters can usually wait and find another time.

9. When preparing to be on TV, what outfit would be the best choice to wear?
   a. A new suit jacket in a hound's-tooth print
   b. A light tan suit jacket
   c. An all-black suit with black shirt
   d. A white shirt

10. The best way to build trust with a reporter after an interview so they're more likely to contact you again in the future is to:
   a. Send them an email pointing out better scientific phrasing.
   b. Tell your friends about the story.
   c. Tweet their story linking the reporter's handle to the story.
   d. Do nothing; you did them a favor by being in their story.

REFERENCES

1. Little J, Ortega M, Powell M, Hamm M. ASHP statement on advocacy as a professional obligation. Am J Health-Syst Pharm. 2019;76(4):251-3.
2. Peters HP, Brossard D, Cheveigne S, Dunwoody S, Kallfass M, Miller S, Tsuchida S. Science communication: interactions with the mass media. Science. 2008;321(5886):204-5.
3. Larsson A, Appel S, Sundberg CJ, Rosenqvist M. Medicine and the media: medical experts' problems and solutions while working with journalists. PLoS One. 2019;14(9):e0220897.
4. Waddell C, Lomas J, Lavis JN, Abelson J, Shepherd CA, Bird-Gayson T. Joining the conversation: newspaper journalists' views on working with researchers. Healthcare Policy. 2005;1(1):123-39.

Chapter Fifteen

Pharmacy and Therapeutics Committee

Patrick M. Malone • Mark A. Malesker • Indrani Kar •
Danial E. Baker • Sunil Kumar Jagadesh

Learning Objectives

● *After completing this chapter, the reader will be able to:*

- Describe the pharmacy and therapeutics (P&T) committee.
- Define the functions of the P&T committee.
- Describe attributes and structure of a P&T committee likely to promote its ability to function successfully.
- Describe where and how the P&T committee fits into the organizational structure of a health care institution or other groups.
- Describe how the pharmacy department participates in P&T committee activities.
- Describe and explain the concepts of drug formularies and drug formulary systems, and how pharmacy participates in their establishment and maintenance.
- Describe how P&T committee activities contribute to the quality improvement of medication use.
- Describe how to develop policies and procedures for the process of medication use.

Key Concepts

❶ A **pharmacy and therapeutics (P&T) committee,** or its equivalent, oversees all aspects of medication use within an institution, health plan, or health care system.

❷ While P&T committees have traditionally been associated with institutional pharmacy, other organizations (e.g., pharmacy benefit managers, outpatient infusion centers, specialty pharmacies) and governmental agencies (e.g., Indian Health Service, Veterans

Affairs, and Department of Defense) are using P&T-type committees in an attempt to improve drug therapy while lowering costs.

❸ More than one formulary may be necessary for an institution or health system.

❹ Although it is common for pharmacists to downplay or misunderstand the importance of P&T committee support in comparison to other clinical activities, such support is vital for pharmacy to impact patient care.

❺ A P&T committee may find it necessary to create ad hoc committees to address various issues, depending on their complexity and size.

❻ Typically, P&T committee functions include determining what drugs are available on **formulary**, who can prescribe specific drugs, policies, and procedures regarding drug use (including pharmacy policies and procedures, clinical protocols, standard order sets, and clinical guidelines), what to do about counterfeit drugs or drug shortages, performance improvement, as well as quality assurance activities (e.g., drug utilization review/drug usage evaluation/medication-use evaluation, as well as compliance surveillance), adverse drug reactions/medication errors, dealing with product shortages, and education in drug use.

❼ A variety of topics regarding the quality of medication use, inclusive of applicable medication metrics, are normally part of the activities of a P&T committee.

Introduction

When considering how a clinician can have an impact on a patient's drug therapy, it is common to consider the individual practitioner caring for a specific patient or, perhaps, a small group of patients. Certainly, the clinician can have a deep impact this way, but he or she does have the disadvantage of dealing with a very limited number of patients. In order to efficiently impact a population of patients, a different approach is necessary. Fortunately, there is the opportunity to participate in the activities of ❶ *a P&T committee or its equivalent, which generally oversees all aspects of medication use in an institution, health plan, or health care system.* The definition of medications is generally very broad in this case, and includes prescription medications, nonprescription medications, vaccines, diagnostic agents (including contrast media), radioactive agents (diagnostic or therapeutic), nutraceuticals, enteral nutrition, parenteral nutrition, and anesthetics. Prescribers and pharmacists have collaborated to implement cost-effective prescribing practices and assess clinical outcomes through educational initiatives, administrative programs to restrict ordering practices, use of formularies and prescribing guidelines, and financial incentives.[1-3]

Before proceeding, it must be stated that while this chapter deals with the P&T committee, which is usually the group responsible for overseeing all aspects of drug therapy in an organization, there is sometimes a similar body referred to as the formulary committee. This latter group deals strictly with determining which drugs are carried within an institution or organization (perhaps with some involvement with drug-related policies, such as tablet splitting, quantity per co-pay, and prior authorization), whereas the P&T committee has numerous other tasks, covering all aspects of drug therapy (e.g., adverse drug reaction [ADR]/medication error monitoring, quality assurance, policy and procedure approval), although the exact group of functions may vary from place to place.[4] Depending on the institution or overarching health system with multiple institutions, some institutions use a formulary committee, since other bodies may perform the additional P&T committee tasks described later in this chapter, while other health care groups may use both committees. For example, the formulary committee may function as a subcommittee reporting to the P&T committee. All structures described above apply to single institutions up to large health systems. A single institution with a formulary and/or P&T committee may address issues for the individual institution as a whole, whereas a health system representing a group of institutions addresses issues specific to the health system. In a health system structure, a system P&T committee makes formulary decisions for the system. Individual institutions making up the health system may also employ local P&T committees to address local issues, such as restricting medications further and assessing medication safety reports. It is important to note that local P&T committees generally do not supersede system P&T committee decisions, similar to state and federal law, although in some cases the system body may cede oversight of a specific group of medications to the local body. That is because the one institution may be the only one with the specialty area that would need them and, therefore, they have the expertise to best determine which agents should be approved for formulary inclusion. In this chapter, anything discussed regarding medication availability within an institution or health system applies to both bodies, whereas all other items are for the P&T committee only.

Case Study 15-1

You are the P&T secretary and manage the nonformulary review process for medications that haven't been evaluated by the formulary process. You receive a request from one of your pharmacists at an off-site infusion center if they can order a drug, luspatercept.

- *What is reviewed first?*
- *What steps are followed?*
- *What is important for future discussion?*

❷ *While P&T committees have traditionally been associated with institutional pharmacy, other organizations (e.g., pharmacy benefit managers, outpatient infusion centers, specialty pharmacies) and governmental agencies (e.g., Indian Health Service, Veterans Affairs, and Department of Defense) are using P&T-type committees in an attempt to improve drug therapy while lowering costs.* Some places where such committees are seen include **managed care organizations (MCOs)**,[5] insurance companies, pharmacy benefit management (PBM) companies, unions, employers,[6] state Medicaid boards, state departments of public institutions,[7] Medicare,[8] long-term care facilities,[9] ambulatory clinics,[10] and even community pharmacies.[11] Much of this chapter will use examples from institutional practice and managed care, simply because much of the published literature deals with those areas of practice, and it is the most likely setting in which prescribers and pharmacists will be directly involved in P&T committee activities. However, the concepts covered are applicable to any P&T or equivalent committee and comply with recommendations of the American Medical Association (AMA),[12,13] the American Society of Health-System Pharmacists (ASHP),[14] The Joint Commission [TJC, formerly the Joint Commission on Accreditation of Healthcare Organizations (JCAHO)],[15] and the Academy of Managed Care Pharmacy (AMCP).[16,17]

The role of the P&T committee has continuously expanded over the years and now encompasses a great number of functions and activities that cover all aspects of overseeing drug therapy. As some of these are of sufficient size and importance, they are covered separately in other chapters (e.g., drug monographs, quality assurance). In addition, there are a number of areas (e.g., investigational drugs) in which P&T committees play a secondary role, and these too are covered in other chapters. This chapter will serve to provide a base to tie together discussion of all of these areas and a number of smaller functions or activities that will be covered as a portion of this chapter. The information is appropriate both for those just learning about the concepts and also for those individuals who are involved with P&T committee activities.

Organizational Background

ORIGIN OF THE P&T COMMITTEE

The concept of a P&T committee represents a unique niche within the structure of a hospital or hospital system. The current role of a hospital in western countries[18] began about 200 years ago, at a time when very few efficacious medications were available, although drug formularies had been developed during the Revolutionary War to list the drugs available.[19] It has also been noted that a **drug formulary** was developed for all municipal hospitals in New York City at Bellevue Hospital in 1868.[20] Drug formularies were required for participation in the Medicare program in 1965.[21] The original hospital was a place to receive basic health care when a person had no extended family to provide the basic needs of good health. After infection control became a recognized concept and anesthesia for surgery evolved around 1900, the value of the modern hospital progressively became a recognized need for all segments of society. The origins for standards of how a hospital functioned subsequently developed during the first half of the twentieth century. This began with the early efforts of the American College of Surgeons in the United States to develop the first accreditation standards for hospitals. Later, the Joint Commission on Accreditation of Hospitals (JCAH), now known as TJC, evolved to centralize the basic requirements for the functional character of a U.S. hospital. The concept of the P&T committee originated and evolved to help hospitals meet various standards regarding drug therapy. The first P&T committee was formed at Bellevue Hospital in New York City in the mid-1930s.[19,22] While it dealt with true compounding formulas, it was originally founded to ensure quality and efficacy of those products, which is still a significant function of P&T committees.

In keeping with the social origins of the hospital, the legally sanctioned or licensed privilege of being a professional health care provider evolved.[18] Both the physician and pharmacist were considered unique for the needs of society. Minimum standards evolved, including the accreditation of their training as a basis for being licensed. Originally, physicians and pharmacists functioned primarily as independent professionals. The nature of a physician's independence was legally defined to further support their obligations to a patient. Many states in the United States legally prohibited a physician from being employed by a corporation. Eventually, these laws were all repealed, but they had the effect of creating the basis for a medical staff as being a separate legal entity within a hospital. The medical staff reflected the legally evolving traditions of a physician, and indirectly the pharmacist, as being independent professionals committed only to the care of a patient without unnecessary outside influences. This evolution has had a major impact on the organizational structure of hospitals.

ORGANIZATIONAL STRUCTURE OF P&T COMMITTEE

A typical hospital organization is shown in Figure 15-1. The board of directors divides the functions of its organization into two entities. First, the administration of the hospital operates as a typical business with a chief executive officer, chief operating officer, and so forth. Second, the board of directors authorizes that a medical staff be formed that reports separately to the board of directors. While the medical staff as a whole is ultimately in charge of all clinical aspects of care in the hospital, in most institutions this is unworkable without an administrative structure of some kind. Therefore, the medical staff may elect officers and either elect or appoint somebody to oversee all aspects of patient care. In this

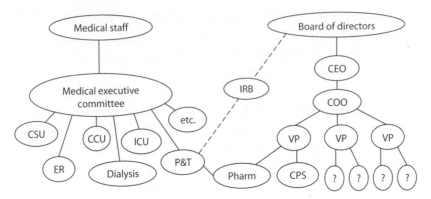

Figure 15–1. Hospital organization. CCU, Coronary Care Unit Committee; CEO, Chief Executive Officer; COO, Chief Operating Officer; CPS, Central Processing & Supply; CSU, Cardiac Surgery Unit Committee; ER, Emergency Room Committee; ICU, Intensive Care Unit Committee; IRB, Institutional Review Board; Pharm, Pharmacy Department; P&T, Pharmacy & Therapeutics Committee; VP, Vice President; ?, Other Hospital Departments.

example, the term **medical executive committee** is used for that body, although the name and exact function may vary. The medical staff functions to certify the credentials of its members, establish their scope of practice where appropriate, monitor the quality of health care provided by its members, and maintain the means to collaborate with the administration of the hospital.

In modern medicine, there are so many clinical areas to consider that it is unrealistic for one committee to adequately oversee all aspects of patient care, except in very small institutions. For this reason, various subcommittees of the medical executive committee are usually necessary, as can be seen in Figure 15-1. As a means to coordinate the needs of the medical staff and the operation of the hospital pharmacy, the modern P&T committee developed. From the traditions established by TJC and ASHP, the P&T committee developed as a function of the medical staff's responsibilities. This committee or related committees may have other names, such as the drug and therapeutics committee in other countries,[23,24] but the functions are the same. While the P&T committee has been referred to in TJC accreditation standards in the past, it is no longer specifically required and may be replaced by some other committee(s) or body(ies),[15,25,26] although the P&T committee concept is supported by many national and professional organizations.[27] A formulary is an absolute requirement of TJC, and which committee manages it depends on how the organization functions.[15] Given the continuing growth in the number, complexity, and expense of medications, both the importance and number of functions of the P&T committee have continued to increase. Example policy and procedures to set up a P&T committee are described in Appendix 15-1, but the following will serve as a general description of P&T committees and their actions. Regardless of the way P&T committee functions are organized, they should be laid out in detail in the medical staff bylaws of an institution.

● Health System P&T vs. Local P&T

In some cases, the P&T committee may represent multiple hospitals and medical centers that comprise a health system, rather than just representing a specific institution. While the philosophy of operating one P&T committee within this corporate structure seems reasonable, this is not often implemented without obstacles that will require careful coordination to overcome,[28] and decentralization of these efforts is one option depending on the structure.[29] Different patient populations, medication needs, cross-hospital physician participation, meeting time, length and location of meetings, and differing clinical cultures within a specific institution are examples of barriers that may be present for one committee to represent multiple hospitals with no local-level committee. The use of differing electronic medical record systems between hospitals may complicate matters. In all likelihood, a method to distribute materials, have discussions, and vote may need to be set up electronically in order to allow virtual meetings over the Internet between widely scattered facilities.[30] The P&T model may need to be revised to work with these challenges.[28,31-36] A hybrid model where the system-wide P&T provides oversight, structure, and manages a system formulary, but local-level P&T committees refine the implementation of the formulary and focus on medication safety and quality at the local level, may offer a more practical path than the elimination of local-level P&T committees entirely. In very rare cases, health systems may give individual hospitals the opportunity to determine whether they will use the system P&T committee or establish their own, although this was more likely to be seen in the past.[37] Alignment of a health system's individual hospitals within a system P&T structure and formulary has been a source of significant cost savings for multihospital health systems.[28,38]

● P&T Committee Membership

Although it is easy to assume from its name that the P&T committee is organizationally a part of the pharmacy department, such is not the case, as was mentioned above. Instead, it is usually a medical staff entity and, perhaps, only one or two pharmacists may actually be members of the committee (possibly *ex officio* members without voting privileges). Commonly, the pharmacy director or clinical coordinator, serving as the committee's secretary (e.g., taking minutes, collating, and arranging the agenda), may be the sole official pharmacy representative. Other pharmacists may also attend to act as consultants to the committee, often having great impact on the committee's decisions, even if they cannot officially vote. In many institutions, it is usually the pharmacist that prepares the evaluation of a medication for formulary consideration, possibly in collaboration with physicians.[39] Fortunately, in larger institutions, it appears that more pharmacists are now becoming full members of P&T committees.[40] As institutions expand the number of pharmacists supporting the formulary structure, this allows appropriate focus and value to be placed on literature evaluation and providing expertise in literature evaluation. This allows for focus on better support for appropriate medication use, guideline/policy development, therapeutic interchanges, and management of nonformulary medications that lead to an improved formulary and cost savings opportunities.[41,42]

Typically, the voting members of an institutional P&T committee are limited to members of the medical staff, although there may be a few voting or nonvoting members from other groups, including pharmacy, nursing, etc. Membership is mostly composed of physicians (preferably a wide variety of physicians from various areas of practice or multiple chief medication officers from multiple hospitals), but usually includes at least one pharmacist and often members from other areas of the hospital (e.g., nursing, administration, radiology, respiratory therapy, dietary, quality assurance, medical records, laboratory, and risk management).[43] If there is a specialty pharmacy in the system, that group may also be represented in addition to the standard pharmacy. Other individuals that might be considered for membership or service as consultants include a pharmacoeconomics specialist, a medical ethicist, and an ambulatory or community pharmacist.[44]

Encouraging a smaller number of physician members to participate more fully may help to address a wide variety of issues, and calling in physicians to consult with the committee on an as needed basis may enhance the committee's efficiency.[45] When possible the committee's membership should be made up of individuals who are committed to rational drug therapy, evidence-based principles, and the institution or health system's patients at-large.[46] As an example, the U.S. Department of Defense has procedures for appointment of members, including nonphysician members, of the P&T committee.[47] The procedures are available on the Internet https://www.health.mil/About-MHS/OASDHA/Defense-Health-Agency/Operations/Pharmacy-Division/DoD-Pharmacy-and-Therapeutics-Committee-2021).

Efforts should be made to ensure that the physician chosen to be chair of the committee is an advocate of the pharmacy department and institution or health system. It is possible for the medical executive committee of the medical staff to pass a resolution to approve a policy broadening the voting members of the P&T committee (e.g., director of pharmacy, hospital vice president) or delegating the functions of the P&T committee to the hospital. In this latter arrangement, the medical staff would reserve the right to terminate the policy if the P&T committee fails to support the needs of the medical staff. If the P&T committee is a hospital committee, rather than medical staff committee, a pharmacist or nurse might more easily obtain voting privileges, given appropriate physician quorum requirements in the authorizing policy.

The P&T committee of MCOs and government bodies often have similar membership to that in institutional committees; however, there may be a requirement for at least some of the members to be independent practitioners and retail pharmacists (i.e., having no financial ties to the organization or group that sponsors the P&T committee).[43,48,49] In accordance with the 2003 Medication Modernization Act (MMA), the use of formularies is an essential component to the PBM.[43]

Reporting Structure of P&T Committee

Once the general organizational setting of the P&T committee has been determined, the operating policy of the P&T committee requires careful attention to two key issues. The first key issue is obvious—to whom does the P&T committee report and to what degree can the decisions of the P&T committee be overturned by another segment of the organization. It is important to point out that, in general, the P&T committee may act only as an advisory body to the medical executive committee. Decisions of the P&T committee may not be considered final (and therefore not be implemented) until they are reviewed and approved by the medical executive committee. In this situation, a report is forwarded from the P&T committee after each meeting to the medical executive committee. In addition, an annual report of the P&T committee may be prepared for both internal review and review by the medical executive committee. This annual report is time consuming in preparation, but is a very important means of tracking P&T activities and action over time. Utilizing project management software at an institution may improve how P&T activities are tracked over time and lead to a more efficient annual report.

The second issue is that the P&T committee will likely be successful based on the leadership qualities of its members, secretary, and the chairperson. The roles of the chairperson and secretary include developing the respect and involvement of all members of the committee and providing leadership surrounding formulary decisions.

❻ *More than one formulary may be necessary for an institution or health system* (e.g., Medicare Part D or specialty hospitals may be a factor). As **biosimilars** become more prevalent or a unique service line requires special focus, a **drug formulary** may be necessary for these medications. For example, a specialty medication formulary would provide focus to a complex medication process from prescription to dispensing. Alternatively, a P&T committee may choose to focus on a smaller number of comprehensive formularies (e.g., adult and pediatrics, or academic medical center and community). The P&T committee further manages the drug formulary by providing usage guidelines, policies or procedures (e.g., intravenous to oral conversion, renal dosing programs, therapeutic substitutions, biosimilar interchange programs, antibiotic stewardship), or restrictions to guide medication use (e.g., prior authorization, limiting access to specific medical specialties or outpatient-only). These items of formulary management may be automated within the hospital's electronic medical record and drug information resource, such as Lexicomp® or Micromedex®. By incorporating medication-use guidance directly into the information source at the point of prescribing and the electronic medical record, prescribers are made aware of the P&T committee's expectations for medication use. This passive display of information may be incorporated into a protocol or order set, which guides a practitioner to the appropriate medication use actively. In summary, the P&T committee provides leadership to formulary management, with the guidance of the chair.

A P&T committee must also maintain oversight of insurance payor impact on the hospital formulary.[50] This is particularly important with P&T committee's continued focus on cost savings initiatives like biosimilars, or when the health system includes both hospitalized and ambulatory patients. A particular biologic reference product may have several biosimilars available on the market. Each one may be supported in a different fashion by multiple payors and have different reimbursement models than the reference product. Each organization will need to develop a strategic approach to manage these various facets to remain nimble in the changing biosimilar market and maintain appropriate medication use.[51-54]

PHARMACY BENEFIT MANAGEMENT (PBM) P&T COMMITTEE ORIGIN

Evolution of PBM

The origin of the PBM organizations dates back to the late 1960s. Their primary focus was on claims administration for insurance companies. Later, it became a challenge for the insurance companies to efficiently manage the increase in drug coverage in the private sector, when the prescription volume was high and the cost per claim was low.[55] The plastic drug benefit card began in the 1970s and changed the way many prescriptions were bought and paid for by the insurance company and employee. From then on, any employee with an ID card, using a pharmacy network, only had a small copayment.[55] In addition, administrative costs for the third-party payer, whether it is the insurance company, health plan, or employer, were reduced, with the PBM creating pharmacy networks and mail service benefits. Pharmacy networks are a group of pharmacies that are under contract with the insurance company, health plan, and/or their contracted PBM partner to promote prescription services at a negotiated discounted fee.[56] Mail service is a program offered by the PBM, whereby pharmaceutical agents, both prescription and nonprescription, are offered through the mail.[56]

In the late 1980s, the introduction of real-time electronic claims processing began. Not only was there two-way communication between the pharmacy and the PBM for claim processing, but also for clinical information. In the 1990s, the PBM companies moved toward a greater emphasis on patient health by offering a variety of new services in addition to the claims processing. Since 2000, there has been an emphasis on consumer behavior modification, enhanced patient interventions, physician connectivity, clinical consulting, disease management, and retrospective drug utilization review (DUR; see Chapter 18 for further information), to name a few.[55]

Drug Formularies in PBM

One of the key functions of a PBM is to design, implement, and administer outpatient drug benefit programs for employers, MCOs, and other third-party payers. PBM companies manage prescription drug benefits separate from other health care services (i.e., physician and hospital services).[56] Determining which medications are most cost-effective, without compromising patient care, is one of the key elements for controlling the cost of a prescription drug benefit.[6,57,58] PBM companies accomplish this by developing drug formularies.[6] Formularies define what medications are covered (i.e., paid for) and provide the main component of the pharmacy benefit. Specific PBM drug payment and management activities occur within this formulary structure, such as therapeutic interchange and disease management programs. Eighty to one hundred percent of PBM-covered lives receive some type of formulary management service.[6,56] The use of drug formularies is unlikely to go away, but instead become more regulated by governmental oversight (e.g., Centers for Medicare and Medicaid Services (CMS) evaluation of Medicare Part D plans).[59]

P&T Committee in PBM

Development and maintenance of drug formularies for third-party payers is an ongoing process. The formulary must be continuously updated to keep pace with new drugs, therapies, medication shortages, prices, recent clinical research, changes in medical practice, evidence-based treatment guidelines, updated Food and Drug Administration (FDA) information,[60] and even civil rights issues.[61] PBM companies use a panel of experts called the P&T committee to develop and manage their drug formularies. P&T committees may be even more important to PBM companies under the Accountable Care Act (ACA).[62] Many times individuals with special clinical expertise are consulted when considering medications within a specific therapeutic class.[60] Meetings are usually held on at least a quarterly basis, and not only are drug formulary recommendations made, but this group also provides input into other clinical areas, such as development of disease management programs, tablet-splitting programs, quantity per co-pay, and prior authorization.[6,55,56,59,60]

Many PBM companies establish their own P&T committee to evaluate the efficacy, safety, uniqueness, cost of therapeutic equivalent drugs, and other appropriate criteria. In addition, PBM companies work with the health plan, employer, or insurance company P&T committee to develop drug formularies using the same evaluation process. This can result in drug formularies that can vary considerably in coverage.[63] In any case, if the P&T committee determines that one drug provides a clear medical benefit over the other therapeutically equivalent drugs in that same therapeutic category, the drug is usually added to the formulary.[6] However, if there are drugs in the same therapeutic category that have very similar efficacy and safety profiles and no unique properties that would make it a better drug, then the net cost becomes a deciding factor as to which drug should be added to the formulary.[6] There has been some discussion as to whether drug costs are weighted too heavily, while drug efficacy and other clinical information is weighted too lightly, when it comes to drug formulary decisions.[55,56,64] The committee leadership needs to recognize the potential for conflicts of interest between efficacy and economic interests of the PBM and to establish collaboration as the basis for resolving conflicts that arise. However, some P&T committees make their formulary status recommendations solely based on drug's safety and effectiveness and a separate group (e.g., business decisions team) makes the final decision based on economic considerations.

Me-too drugs are drugs that are structurally very similar to an already known drug that has only minor differences. Many drugs come in two versions: an L-isomer (left) and an R-isomer (right). An example of a me-too drug is esomeprazole (Nexium®), the L-isomer of omeprazole (Prilosec®, the R- and L-isomers). Both drugs are used to treat gastroesophageal reflux disease (GERD). When a comparative analysis was conducted looking at drugs approved for marketing between January 2007 and July 2008, those that had a different chemical entity and a separate mechanism of action accounted for 69%; however, they offered no clinical improvement over those already on the market. Forty-four percent offered some type of new convenience, but only 13% offered greater efficacy.[65] For this reason, PBM companies may include only one of the products as the preferred drug.

In the case of a health plan, employer, or insurance companies with their own P&T committee, the drug formulary recommendations made by the PBM P&T committee are reviewed by the organization's P&T committee. This committee will then determine if the PBM's recommendations are accepted or rejected.

Pharmacy Support of the P&T Committee

ROLE OF PHARMACISTS IN P&T COMMITTEE

❹ *Although it is not uncommon for pharmacists to downplay or misunderstand the importance of P&T committee support in comparison to other clinical activities, such support is vital for pharmacy to impact patient care.* It is easy to lose sight that the P&T committee's role is to provide adequate care for large patient populations, while the individual practitioners provide care for individual patients. P&T committee support and participation can have far-reaching effects on the overall quality of drug therapy in an institution and health system, and must be given a great deal of attention, since the benefits of its function serve to build collaboration, transparency, and trust among the institutional divisions of authority for drug therapy within health care. While such attention is time consuming,[66] it can be of value to the pharmacy. This is an opportunity to present recommendations to a decision-making body, and P&T committees often accept pharmacists' recommendations[67,68]; therefore, pharmacy departments can have a great and far-reaching impact on drug therapy through this mechanism. The pharmacist has the opportunity to be informed and develop important relationships with other health care professionals while serving as a liaison for the interprofessional committee that is focused on patient outcomes.[69]

● Steering Committee for Formulary Management

Some pharmacists who participate in P&T committee activities serve their function by providing information requested by physicians and considering drugs for formulary approval only following physician requests. This can rapidly deteriorate into crisis management, where the pharmacy department reacts to problems and fights each fire as it occurs. A proactive approach for a pharmacy department is more efficient and effective[70,71] and seeks to address issues (e.g., changes in drugs carried on the formulary, new policies and procedures, standard class reviews and guideline reviews, quality assurance activities) before they become immediate needs. TJC accreditation requirements include annual evaluation of all drugs and/or drug classes.[15] Through prospective actions with the P&T committee, it is possible for the pharmacy to obtain physician support for their clinical activities and be better prepared for medication management overall.

In the specific instance of P&T committee support, one or more pharmacists must be identified to conduct the necessary planning. This may consist of a pharmacy-based steering committee and might include administrators, purchasing agents, clinicians, informatics specialists, and drug information specialists. These individuals must develop and regularly evaluate data sources to anticipate prescribers' needs[72] (see Table 15-1)

TABLE 15–1. AREAS WHERE PHARMACISTS SHOULD BE SUPPORTING A PHARMACY AND THERAPEUTICS COMMITTEE

- Planning future agendas (including medications, policies and procedures, quality assurance, and other subjects to be addressed)
- Gathering data to create drug monographs and other necessary documents
- Evaluating medications for formulary adoption, deletion, and/or restrictions
- Preparing and conducting quality assurance programs (including drug usage evaluation and monitoring of adverse effects and medication errors)
- Preparing policies and procedures
- Communicating information from the P&T committee to other areas of the institution
- Creating electronic and/or hardcopy versions of the formulary
- Preparing education for individuals involved in medication use
- Collaborating with interdisciplinary groups to manage content, including safety issues
- Sharing best practices, near misses, or other safety information across a health system
- Continuously tracking new FDA drug approvals, new dosage forms, medication shortages
- Developing strategy for new types of medications (e.g., biosimilars)
- Project management for medication use and process improvement
- Budget projection

TABLE 15–2. FDA CLASSIFICATION BY CHEMICAL TYPE

Type	Definition
1	New molecular entity not marketed in the United States
2	New salt, ester, or other noncovalent derivative of another drug marketed in the United States
3	New formulation or dosage form of an active ingredient marketed in the United States
4	New combination of drugs already marketed in the United States
5	New manufacturer of a drug product already marketed by another company in the United States
6	New indication for a product already marketed in the United States (note: this category is no longer used)
7	Drug that is already legally marketed without an approved NDA • First application since 1962 for a drug marketed prior to 1938 • First application for DESI (Drug Efficacy Study Implementation)-related products that were first marketed between 1938 and 1962 without an NDA • First application for DESI-related products first marketed after 1962 without NDAs. In this case, the indications may be the same or different from the legally marketed product
8	Over-the-counter (OTC) switch
9	New indication submitted as separate NDA, which is consolidated with original NDA after approval
10	New indication submitted as a separate NDA, but not consolidated with original NDA

Source: Drugs@FDA frequently asked questions [Internet]. Washington: Food and Drug Administration; [updated 2015 Mar 27; cited 2016 Jul 18]. Available from: http://www.fda.gov/Drugs/InformationOnDrugs/ucm075234.htm#chemtype_reviewclass

and specific methods, using lean methodology, have been developed to standardize the method by which such a group can work.[73] For example, it is necessary to assess what drugs have been recently approved by the FDA to identify drugs for possible formulary inclusion. FDA approval often occurs about 3 months or longer before commercial availability and is published on the FDA website (http://www.accessdata.fda.gov/scripts/cder/drugsatfda/index.cfm). Therefore, there is time for the drug to be considered for formulary addition before the first physician request or the first orders arrive from the nursing units, which necessitates a review under TJC standards.[15] In a case where it is not possible to consider a drug before it is commercially available, it has been suggested by some that drugs rated P (priority) by the FDA be made available to prescribers until the drug can be fully considered (the FDA classification codes are listed in Tables 15-2 and 15-3, with the priority vs. standard explanation provided in Table 15-3).[74] This latter procedure may be effective, but considering the drug before commercial availability is preferable, since, if the ultimate P&T committee decision is to leave the drug off the drug formulary it may cause problems for patient and conflicts with various prescribers. An advantage of a proactive review process makes it easier to implement the formulary decision, especially if a prior authorization or interchange program is going to be implemented, and to make sure that the correct information is in the electronic ordering (i.e., electronic

TABLE 15–3. FDA CLASSIFICATIONS BY THERAPEUTIC POTENTIAL

Type	Definition
P	Priority handling by FDA—before 1992 this had two categories:
	A—Major therapeutic gain
	B—Moderate therapeutic gain
S	Standard handling by FDA—before 1992 this was referred to as class C, which indicated the product offered only a minor or no therapeutic gain
O	Orphan Drug

Source: Drugs@FDA frequently asked questions [Internet]. Washington: Food and Drug Administration; [updated 2015 Mar 27; cited 2016 Jul 18]. Available from: http://www.fda.gov/Drugs/InformationOnDrugs/ucm075234.htm#chemtype_reviewclass

health record) and delivery (i.e., infusion pumps, if required) systems. While proactive review is helpful, P&T committees may choose to review a medication for formulary addition only after receiving an official request. This enhances physician engagement in the P&T process, but also requires an efficient nonformulary support process for medications not yet available on the drug formulary.

It has been suggested that an objective way to determine which medications should get priority review (i.e., review as quickly as possible by the P&T committee), standard review (i.e., review later, as there is time to evaluate), or no review by the committee is useful. These decisions could be made using a weighted spreadsheet that evaluates each product based on the amount of quality evidence regarding the medication, the population affected, the severity of the disease to be treated, the potential therapeutic benefit, adverse reactions, cost impact, patient preference, and current availability of alternatives on the formulary.[75] Something like that may be helpful, if it becomes difficult to determine priorities; however, the subjective characteristics of the categories evaluated may make some people doubt the final rating of products or be time efficient.

Some P&T committees may alternatively require physician requests for medications to be reviewed for addition to the drug formulary, which is a more reactive process to market changes and available treatments, but it allows the P&T committee to remain focused on the immediate needs of the institution. A fine line between managing the immediate needs and future needs should be developed by the P&T committee. Some P&T committees review medications only after having been available on the market for 6 months or a year. In addition, class reviews, which will be discussed later in the chapter and in Chapter 16, assist with the proactive review of potential formulary opportunities in medication-use guidance, cost savings, and potential additions/deletions from formulary. The P&T committee's process for reviewing medications should be determined by the committee and written into the policy and procedure governing the committee.

Tracking Medication Usage

It is also important to track utilization and appropriate use of drugs. For example, the use of nonformulary drugs or off-label use of approved drugs should be tracked within the institution (a nonformulary drug is a product that has not been approved for use within an institution and off-label usage is prescribing for a use other than the use approved by the P&T committee or the FDA[76]).[77,78] If patterns of increased use are noted, a reason for that use should be identified. If the use is inappropriate, the physician(s), which may be in one specific group, should be contacted and given information about alternative formulary agents. In some cases, new information may be available showing a new advantage or use for a drug, which can lead to its reconsideration for formulary adoption. Related to this is the necessity to regularly consider the material being promoted by the drug company representatives. It is worth mentioning that some hospitals will restrict pharmaceutical representative's access to the institution or restrict the drugs that may be promoted by those representatives to only items approved for use in the hospital, in order to proactively manage this situation and facilitate compliance with the formulary. (See Chapter 25 for further information.)

There may also be new indications or other information that will increase demand for nonformulary items or off-label utilization. It is important to remember that formularies cannot be static, but require continued attention and reevaluation. If there are sufficient changes noted in the use(s) of a particular class of drugs, it is useful to review the class as a whole to decide which drug(s) are to be retained on the formulary. TJC requires annual review of all medications,[10-15] which assists in reviewing new available information (e.g., labeling changes or warnings from postmarketing surveillance) that may necessitate changes in formulary items in a particular class, including additions, deletions, and therapeutic interchange opportunities. Other items, such as trends in reported ADRs in the institution or published data for new products with little information in the literature on first approval, may also be useful in determining products for P&T committee consideration or reconsideration.[79] Although there must be a mechanism by which prescribers can request that drugs be added to the formulary, all of the above methods and others can help the pharmacy anticipate physician needs, allowing time for information gathering, evaluation of products, and P&T committee consideration before the need becomes too urgent to permit proper consideration.

To guide the clinician into considering the logic of requesting the addition of items to the drug formulary, a specific request form may be useful. Items that a physician may be required to fill out or attach to the form are listed in Table 15-4.[80] An example form is provided in Appendix 15-2.

Planning P&T Committee Meetings

The P&T committee should be kept advised by the above-mentioned pharmacy-based steering committee of future plans, so that it can be aware that a rational planning process is

TABLE 15–4. ITEMS THAT MAY BE ON A REQUEST FOR FORMULARY CONSIDERATION FORM

- Date and time of request
- Name of product (e.g., generic, brand, chemical)
- Source of product (e.g., manufacturer, distributor)
- Specific information about drug product (e.g., class of drug, mechanism, adverse effects, clinical studies)
- Anticipated use of drug (e.g., what type of patient, how often)
- Comparable drugs already on the formulary
- Why the product is needed
- What drugs could be removed from the formulary (medication category review)
- What restrictions, policies, cautions, guidelines, etc., are necessary
- How the drug fits into any clinical guidelines
  - Evidence of unforeseen benefits, even if guidelines do not mention the medication
- Action requested (e.g., addition, deletion, restriction)
- Conflict of interest disclosure

governing its agenda. Also, it is a good idea for one or more representatives of this steering committee to meet with the pharmacy director, chair of the P&T committee, and, potentially, a representative of the hospital administration on a regular basis to assist with planning and ensure their concerns are addressed. This meeting could be held shortly before the P&T committee actually meets to present preliminary formulary evaluations, medication-use evaluation (MUE) material, and policy and procedure documents for an initial review, allowing modifications addressing physician and administration concerns to be made before formal committee review and action. During this meeting, plans for future months can be made or adjusted as the circumstances dictate. It is also valuable to visit with the key thought leaders in the institution, especially the specialist that might be involved with prescribing the drug, to understand their thoughts and concerns prior to the committee meeting. It may also decrease potential conflict once decisions are made. For example, if changes to the cephalosporins carried on the drug formulary or their permitted uses (e.g., restrictions to particular uses or prescribing groups) are considered, the infectious disease specialists should be contacted to provide input. (Note: This does not necessarily mean that recommendations are changed to account for physician preferences, but that their preferences and concerns are specifically addressed in the evaluation.)

Regarding quality assurance activities, the pharmacy department should obtain data to guide the selection of upcoming quality assurance programs. This will be covered in greater detail in Chapter 18.

Reimbursement

Methods of reimbursement for formulary medications may be incredibly complex, with specific rules dependent on the medication or third-party payer.[64,125] Therefore, pharmacists may have to devote a great deal of effort into investigating it for specific new medications that may be considered for use. A P&T committee may employ restrictions to an approved prior authorization for certain medications where reimbursement is imperative.[53] Especially as formulary management expands to encompass more than inpatient medication use, such as outpatient and health plan formularies, reimbursement will continue to be a crucial component of analysis.[81] One resource is the CMS' Medicare Part B Drug Average Sales Price (ASP) data (https://www.cms.gov/Medicare/Medicare-Fee-for-Service-Part-B-Drugs/McrPartBDrugAvgSalesPrice. This information is freely available and helps clarify how Medicare will cover and reimburse medications. This document is updated four times a year. A P&T committee may evaluate a medication that has not been added to the Medicare ASP data file. In the event that an institution still needs to determine reimbursement, methods for estimation should be developed. One option is taking 106% of the Wholesale Acquisition Cost, when no ASP price is available.[82] Incorporation of economic information (e.g., cost savings, reimbursement) into a formulary evaluation improves the robustness of the evaluation.[83]

Guiding Medication-Use Policies and Procedures

The pharmacy should also investigate which medications need specific policies and procedures developed to guide their use and monitoring. This may be done when the drug is first being evaluated for formulary addition or later if problems (e.g., increased ADR reports, medication errors, and overuse) are noted. For example, concerns about a new anticoagulation therapy leading to increased morbidity and mortality through improper use might prompt the P&T committee to approve specific protocols for the use of the agent. They may be even more pertinent when a regulatory body focuses on a specific class of medications, such as TJC's National Patient Safety Goal surrounding anticoagulation. Policy and procedure documents are covered later in the chapter. Information on preparing policies and procedures can be found in Chapter 21.

Finally, it is extremely important for the P&T committee to make sure that all prescribers are informed about the actions taken, although the major stakeholders will likely be aware of potential changes early in the process. Often the pharmacy is heavily involved in providing this information to prescribers. While a great deal of effort is placed on communication within the committee itself, it is also necessary to keep the entire medical staff informed. This may be accomplished through medical department meeting presentations, emails, websites, newsletters (refer to Chapter 13), online formulary, or other mechanisms.

AD HOC COMMITTEES

⑤ *A P&T committee may find it necessary to create ad hoc committees to address various issues, depending on their complexity and size.* Some of the common committees are discussed below. Institutions may or may not use these committees (sometimes referred to as subcommittees) and their exact use varies from place to place, depending on their needs or desires.[4]

Adverse Reactions

A comprehensive ADR monitoring and reporting program is an essential component of the P&T committee (see Chapter 19 for further information about ADRs and how they are handled). A subcommittee may be helpful to review the entire ADR data for trends and any necessary actions that need to be taken. The P&T committee will usually report the ADR data on a monthly or quarterly basis. Following approval of this report, the P&T committee is responsible for the dissemination of information to the medical staff and other health professionals in the institution. This includes recommending processes to cut the rate of preventable ADRs. This subcommittee may be combined with the medication errors subcommittee.[15,84]

Anticoagulation

The anticoagulation subcommittee is responsible for policies and procedures to maintain compliance with TJC Goal 3E, now called TJC National Patient Safety Goal 03.05.01.[15,85] This goal is to reduce the likelihood of patient harm associated with anticoagulation therapy. The subcommittee can also participate in improvement processes to maintain standards with quality organizations, such as the National Quality Forum (NQF) and the Surgical Care Improvement Project (SCIP). Standard orders and policies to follow evidence-based guidelines of the American College of Chest Physicians (ACCP) are also developed by this subcommittee. Pharmacists have an important role on this committee. Most hospitals have pharmacists dedicated to anticoagulation monitoring and education.

Antimicrobial/Infectious Disease

Antibiotics are an important category of formulary medications.[86] Frequent category review and revision is necessary and complex.[87] Cunha has defined five factors to consider when reviewing antimicrobial agents for formulary inclusion: microbiologic activity,[88] pharmacokinetic and pharmacodynamic profiles,[89] resistance patterns,[90,91] adverse effects,[92] and cost to the institution.[93] The P&T committee or a subcommittee of the P&T may be responsible for developing appropriate antibiotic selection and use in both inpatient and outpatient settings.[94,95] Some institutions may rely on input from the infection control committee regarding antimicrobial formulary management and appropriate utilization. Multidisciplinary antimicrobial use committees or antibiotic stewardship programs have limited inappropriate prescribing of antimicrobials and increased the medical staff's knowledge on appropriate antibiotic use.[93,96,97]

The main purpose of the antimicrobial/infectious disease subcommittee is to promote antimicrobial stewardship to ensure cost-effective therapy and improve patient outcomes, along with reducing the development of resistance to the antimicrobials. Antimicrobial stewardship promotes and optimizes antimicrobial therapy consistent with the hospital's/ health system's **antibiograms**. Guideline development and education is provided to the medical staff as well as to other health care professionals. The subcommittee is also involved in the enforcement of formulary agent use, substitution policies, therapeutic interchange, and restrictions for antibiotics. In addition, review and feedback on prescribing patterns is provided to the medical staff regarding antimicrobial therapy.[98–100] Use of P&T formulary and policy decisions has been shown to be successful in controlling antimicrobial use in hospitals.[101,102] TJC and CMS now requires Antimicrobial Stewardship in institutions and ambulatory care settings, which will allow this subcommittee to serve as a backbone for decisions and implementation of this type of program.[103]

Medication Safety

A medication safety committee (sometimes called safety committee, medication error prevention, safe medication administration committee, or medication misadventure subcommittee) should be multidisciplinary in nature. This subcommittee reviews medication misadventures and medication errors that occur within the institution or health care system. They may also review adverse drug reactions (instead of an adverse reaction committee), drug-drug interactions, drug dispensing processes, medication errors (see Chapter 20 for more information), look-alike/sound-alike medications, high-alert medications, acceptable medical abbreviations, and communication errors. It may also be appropriate for them to review protocols to improve medication safety, such as the settings for intravenous (IV) fluid pumps.

A safety report will commonly be presented to the P&T committee on a monthly, quarterly, or semiannual basis. Following approval of this report, the P&T committee is responsible for the dissemination of information to the medical staff and other health professionals in the institution. This includes recommending processes to cut the rate of preventable medication safety issues. In some places, a medication error reduction plan (MERP) is prepared to identify process improvements that have been made and those that are planned. When evaluating drug cost strategies, patient safety should always be a priority.[104] TJC Accreditation Process Guide for Hospitals addresses the potential for adverse drug events.[15,105] Also, as explained in the next chapter, patient safety will be evaluated whenever a product is considered for formulary addition. Review of relevant policies and implementation of national safety recommendations, such as yearly best practices published by the Institute for Safe Medicine Practices (ISMP), are important functions of this subcommittee to additionally assess safety of products on formulary.[106]

Medical Devices

The FDA definition of a medical device is[107]:

- "an instrument, apparatus, implement, machine, contrivance, implant, *in vitro* reagent, or other similar or related article, including a component part or accessory which is: recognized in the official National Formulary, or the United States Pharmacopoeia, or any supplement to them,
- intended for use in the diagnosis of disease or other conditions, or in the cure, mitigation, treatment, or prevention of disease, in man or other animals, or
- intended to affect the structure or any function of the body of man or other animals, and which does not achieve its primary intended purposes through chemical action within or on the body of man or other animals and which is not dependent upon being metabolized for the achievement of any of its primary intended purposes."

The P&T committee or a subcommittee may be responsible for the approval of some medical devices within an institution. This subcommittee is often multidisciplinary and is given the opportunity to review medical devices before purchases are made or contracts are signed. The committee is also responsible for reviewing the safety information associated with these devices, because adverse medical device events are an important patient safety issue. Devices that contain medications, such as topical hemostats that contain thrombin, may also be reviewed by the committee or by the transfusion service committee described below. When an institution does not have a separate committee under P&T for medical devices, some institutions may split consideration of this topic between the supply chain and P&T. Interdisciplinary collaboration on medication products that are not strictly medications is imperative and can easily be overlooked.

Nutrition

As nutrition of the hospitalized patient evolved and became more complex, the role of the pharmacist on a nutrition support team became more justified. Their role started out improving the ordering process for parenteral nutrition and communicating these changes to the pharmacy staff for proper preparation. Today, pharmacists on the nutritional team assist in the clinical management of parenteral nutrition patients, parenteral nutrition research, and continual involvement with improving the safety of parenteral nutrition use.[108] TJC, in their National Patient Safety Goals (NPSG), once addressed the safe use of parenteral nutrition feeding solutions,[109] but even though that has been removed, one of the responsibilities of the P&T committee is to oversee and approve the components of the parenteral nutrition solutions, usually in cooperation with dietitians.

Oncology Committee

Care of oncology patients is complex and requires smooth transitions between inpatient and outpatient settings. In addition, the ever-changing oncology protocols and increasing number of new agents, which are often very toxic and expensive, makes this an area where the P&T committee will find having a subcommittee is important. This subcommittee is charged with reviewing the use of oncology agents, appropriate restrictions for use, and need by location. An interdisciplinary group of oncologists, oncology pharmacists, oncology nurses, and electronic medical record colleagues are key to seamlessly developing and implementing formulary decisions related to oncology products and related supported care.

Pediatrics

Consideration of medications for pediatric patients is different from adult use. There is often a lack of published information and doses of medications may require compounding, in addition to other differences. Therefore, if pediatric patients are a portion of the patients in an institution that deals with patients of all ages, it may be necessary to have a subcommittee to specifically consider pediatric therapeutics, since usual committee members may lack the necessary expertise.

Quality Assurance of Medication Use

A subcommittee of the P&T committee may be placed in charge of planning and overseeing the plan for quality assurance regarding drug therapy. Details about this activity are found in Chapter 18. This committee may develop criteria for a drug-use evaluation, collect the data, interpret the data, and develop necessary recommendations regarding the appropriate use of medication.

Specialty Pharmacy

Specialty pharmacies deal with medications requiring special handling, storage, and distribution requirements, along with medications to treat complex conditions that may be chronic and rare. They work to make sure medications are used appropriately and, therefore, avoid unnecessary costs. While this may be accomplished through normal mechanisms, some institutions may have a specific specialty pharmacy that is separate. In a case like that, they may also include a subcommittee of the P&T committee to consider the special circumstances and needs addressed by that specialty pharmacy.

Transfusion Service Committee

Hospitals often have a transfusion service committee charged with reviewing the use of blood and blood derivative products. Many of these products overlap with medications and may also be classified as medications. Therefore, it is necessary for this type of committee to work with or, possibly, be combined with the P&T committee in order to oversee the proper use of such products.[110]

Frequently, departments or service lines (e.g., oncology, cardiology, psychiatry/mental health, critical care, radiology, neonatology/pediatrics, neurology, surgery, women's health) are asked for input regarding the formulary management within their specialty area of practice. Depending on the volume of activity, there may be an ad hoc committee formed for any of those groups.

P&T Committee Meeting

Before beginning the description of a typical P&T committee meeting, it is important to note that a smoothly functioning P&T committee has certain needs. The committee will need the support of its parent organization. A room for the meetings should be carefully selected (see Appendix 15-3). The agenda for the meeting should be prepared in advance by the committee's secretary and sent to the members. Most often, as mentioned previously, an informal meeting of the supporting pharmacists and others is required between P&T committee meetings to plan the activities necessary to support the agenda. The chair of the committee may also attend such planning meetings to ensure that priority issues are addressed before the meeting.

Formulary reviews represent a special concern when sending out an agenda, since they may trigger the outside influences of dedicated pharmaceutical marketing efforts if companies learn from committee members that their products or their competitor's products are being evaluated. Efforts must be made to make sure the committee is not distracted by outside influences, such as the pharmaceutical industry and advertisements. Some institutions do not disclose the membership of their P&T or formulary committee to decrease the risk of these types of influences. An important consideration in the selection of the committee's members should be their ability to be independent thinkers and their understanding of the confidentially of the materials used in the decision-making process. Timing of the committee members' access to the support materials is important. If not distributed prior to the meeting, they won't have adequate time to review and make an informed decision. If materials are distributed too far in advance, there is a risk of unanticipated distribution or disclosure of information. The same problem exists for the minutes of the committee meetings. Committee meeting minutes may not adequately describe the full basis of a decision and may be misinterpreted. As a result, the minutes might be open to inappropriate projection regarding the basis for the P&T committee decision process. Some institutions simply make the minutes a pure recording of the decisions, eliminating any information about the discussion to avoid this problem. Though minutes pose the above challenges, some institutions use more detailed minutes to provide full transparency of their formulary decision-making process, along with providing additional information about any necessary details regarding discussion of issues. A sample set of minutes is provided in Appendix 15-4, and a stepwise process to writing minutes is available.[111]

Along with sending an agenda to members, a reminder phone call, email, text, and/or fax may be useful to facilitate attendance. Each P&T committee meeting requires extensive preparation by the pharmacists involved in its affairs. Specifically, management of the formulary requires extensive background research and the preparation of written reports for any addition or deletion. Similarly, quality-related functions require time-consuming review of patient records. It has been noted that literature review is the most highly valued work in a P&T committee. This helps to avoid bias and the halo effect, where members might have bias when not all information is presented or the expert is acting on emotion or anecdote, rather than on any additional knowledge.[42,112] Finally, the P&T committee functions are peripherally related to other affairs of the parent organization, for example, the standard order set preparation by other segments of a hospital. This requires special attention in order to prevent the use of nonformulary products. These items will be discussed in greater detail in the next section. Finally, the chair or secretary should be skilled at guiding an efficient meeting (see Appendix 15-5). In respect of the time commitment for members, meetings should always start and end at the scheduled times.

P&T Committee Functions

⑤ *Typically, P&T committee functions include determining what drugs are available on formulary, who can prescribe specific drugs, policies, and procedures regarding drug use (including pharmacy policies and procedures, clinical protocols, standard order sets, and clinical guidelines—see Chapter 8 for the latter), what to do about counterfeit drugs or drug shortages (see Chapter 17), performance improvement as well as quality assurance activities (e.g., drug utilization review/drug usage evaluation/medication usage evaluation, as well as compliance surveillance—see Chapter 18), adverse drug reactions/medication errors (see Chapters 19 and 20), and education in drug use.*[15,113,114] Many of those functions are related to quality assurance activities, because they are designed to improve the quality of drug therapy. Because the functions may improve drug therapy quality, they may actually provide some legal protection for an institution, as long as the reason for decisions is not strictly based on financial considerations.[115] P&T committee functions can also include investigational drug studies; however, that is often delegated to the **institutional review board (IRB)** that oversees all investigational activities in the hospital (see Chapter 23). In addition, some P&T committee functions may be delegated to subcommittees (e.g., quality assurance, antibiotic, and medication errors subcommittees)[116]; however, this can be cumbersome and is often avoided, except in larger institutions. P&T committees should recognize principles of epidemiology and pharmacoeconomics in the decision making whenever possible.[117-121] A standardized safety assessment tool has been developed to evaluate potential formulary agents as well.[122]

According to TJC, the medical staff, pharmacy, nursing, administration, and others are to cooperate with each other in carrying out the previously mentioned functions.[15] Although the medical staff normally takes overseeing drug therapy very seriously and expects to approve all activities of the P&T committee, it is common for the pharmacy department to complete much of the preparation work for the committee. Although pharmacists are generally charged with the preparation work, institutions may employ a specific pharmacist to manage the P&T committee functions or pay pharmacists to do this work as part of their salary. Physicians usually do not obtain any direct monetary compensation for this committee's work, although such compensation may be considered by an institution to encourage more physician participation. Physician participation in committees may be a result of medical staff bylaws to maintain credentials.

FORMULARY MANAGEMENT

Drug Formulary

Wherever a **drug formulary system** is in place, the drug formulary usually is published in electronic format (e.g., website, intranet, or other software, particularly software used to order medications for patients). It should be readily available to all individuals who interact with medication use as part of their daily functions. In its simplest form, the drug formulary contains a list of drugs, which can also potentially include natural products, alternative products, blood derivatives, radiologic products (both diagnostic and therapeutic), and other diagnostic items that are available under that formulary system and reflect the clinical judgment of the medical staff.[123,124] It may also contain medication-associated products or devices (e.g., spacer tubes for inhalers). While traditionally this would be a list of products that will be routinely stocked in the pharmacy, this has evolved to include a compilation of medications that are approved for routine use in the institution or system.[125] In that case, there may be some products that are considered formulary, but are not routinely stocked because they are rarely used and can be obtained with adequate speed. Conversely, a few products may be considered nonformulary because they should only be used if the formulary product is not appropriate, but they may be stocked in small supplies due to the urgency of need when they are used.

The formulary list will normally be arranged alphabetically and/or by therapeutic class (e.g., American Hospital Formulary Service [AHFS] classification), and usually contains information on the dosage forms, strengths, names (e.g., generic, trade, chemical), and ingredients of combination products. Many drug formulary publications contain a great deal of more material related to the drugs, including a summary of indications, side effects, dosing, use restrictions, costs, and other information.[126] This may be done through interlinks with commercially available information products. Formularies may also be referred to as preferred medication lists or **preferred drug product** lists.[19]

Definition of Formulary System

A related term, the formulary system, can be thought of as a method for developing the list, and sometimes even as a philosophy.[127] In theory, a well-designed drug formulary can guide clinicians to prescribe the safest and most effective agents for treating a particular medical problem, at the most reasonable cost.[128-134] Some people in the past have argued that the formulary system itself does not work because it is not properly implemented and recommended replacing it with counterdetailing by pharmacists or, more likely now, computers at the time a prescription order is written (see Chapter 25 for further information).[135] However, this has not been established as a substitute and it is likely that a combination will result in the best patient care at the least cost. An article indicating that formularies may ultimately result in higher patient costs was written by Horn and associates.[136] While this may be one of the best articles on the topic and the author has defended criticism of the article,[137] there are nevertheless various deficiencies in the study that make it uncertain whether it was truly the drug formulary or other factors that lead to increased costs.[138-141] Horn and associates[142] also published a similar study conducted in the ambulatory environment, which appears to have similar results and deficiencies. In the case of national drug formularies, there has been a positive effect on prescribing habits shown in Canada.[143] A study of formulary use in the western Pacific region found that they are commonly used in the hospital setting, but questioned their effectiveness, since in that area the products on the formulary are often not connected to treatment guidelines or the best evidence for treating disease.[144] Further research is needed before a definite conclusion may be reached on the effectiveness of formulary management.[145] For now, a well-constructed formulary is still believed to improve patient care while decreasing costs and remains a requirement of accreditation organizations. It serves as a focus for building comprehensive drug therapy options.

Decision-Making in the Formulary System

The goal of the formulary system is to provide a decision-making process leading to the selection of medications necessary for the treatment of any disease states likely to be seen in that institution.[129] In some cases, decisions for formulary addition can be made for entire groups of institutions, for example, the U.S. Veteran's Affairs has combined the formularies of all of its component parts.[146] These formulary medications should be the most efficacious, safe, and cost-effective agents with the fewest side effects or drug interactions.[15] Other factors should also be taken into consideration, such as the variety of dosage forms available for the medication, estimated use, convenience, dosing schedule, compliance, abuse potential, physician demand, ease of preparation, storage requirements, and risks.[147] Economic factors should not be the sole basis for this evidence-based process.[129] Typically, only two or, perhaps, three drugs from any drug class are added to the formulary. Some would argue that only one agent is necessary from any class; however, some patients will not respond and/or tolerate certain agents, so at least one secondary agent is usually desirable. Therapeutic redundancy must be minimized, however, by excluding superfluous or inferior preparations. This should improve the quality of prescribing and also lead to improved cost-effectiveness, both by eliminating less cost-effective agents that do not improve patient care and by assisting patients to become well faster. To analyze potentially conflicting literature and strength of recommendation, a grading system has been developed for review of potential formulary additions.[148]

Whether an institution has a strict formulary with a minimum number of items or a less-restricted formulary that excludes items that are significantly inferior is sometimes a matter of philosophy. The former will cut down the pharmacy department's inventory and often save money through avoidance of highly priced products, but may only be practical in closed **health maintenance organizations (HMOs)** where the same formulary is used in both the inpatient and ambulatory environments. In cases where prescribers are free to prescribe any products they prefer in the ambulatory environment, they have been shown to have difficulty in remembering what products are contained on the formularies of third-party payers.[149] Therefore, the increased time necessary for pharmacists to contact prescribers for order changes may lead to the disruption of patient care and increased costs. As a result, a less restricted formulary may be more practical and incorporation of payor coverage review into formulary evaluation is needed. As an example, a patient is admitted to the hospital on a nonformulary medication. While there would be other satisfactory medications in the same therapeutic category on the formulary, some think it may be best to simply allow use of the nonformulary product, rather than adding another complicating factor to the patient's hospital treatment by attempting to change therapy. Pharmacist and physician time would also be saved. A more contemporary approach is available to facilities with computerized physician order entry (CPOE). The challenge of prescribers remembering which medication within a class is available is reduced, and order sets can guide clinicians to formulary products. Medication orders can be programmed to list the patient's home medication if a substitution was made and a double check can be performed upon discharge medication reconciliation. Less storage space, smaller medication inventories, and significant cost savings may be achieved under this model that approaches a strict or closed formulary.

Even in cases where an institution has a strict and enforced closed drug formulary, it should be noted that there are occasions when it is necessary to prescribe a drug that is not on the drug formulary. This might be due to a patient with a rare illness, a patient who does not respond or has intolerable side effects to the formulary drugs, a patient stabilized on a nonformulary medication where it would be difficult or dangerous to change, a conflict between the institutional formulary and the patient's insurance company formulary,[150] or some other valid reason. A mechanism must be in place to promptly obtain the particular drug when it is shown to be necessary (the National Committee for Quality Assurance [NCQA] requires such a mechanism for HMOs,[151] as does TJC for hospitals,[15] but it must try to prevent prescribers from ordering nonformulary drugs "because I said so!"). Some institutions require specific request forms to be filled out (see example in Appendix 15-2), sometimes with approval from the physician's department head, or at least require a consultation between a pharmacist and the physician before the drug is obtained. Also, patients may be charged more for the nonformulary medications. In some HMOs and insurance company plans, the prescribers or pharmacies may be financially penalized for use or overuse of nonformulary medications.[152] Whatever mechanism is used, it is important to make requesting nonformulary medications transparent, but difficult to obtain unnecessary medications; otherwise the benefits of the formulary system may be negated.[77] Also, it is necessary to track nonformulary drugs use and frequency, which may lead to a worthwhile addition to the drug formulary.[153]

Misconceptions about the Formulary System

Some prescribers feel that a drug formulary serves only to keep costs down, at the expense of good patient care.[154] These prescribers must be reassured that there is evidence to support that a good formulary does keep expenses down[155] without negatively affecting care,[156] although in some cases the costs are merely transferred to other hospital expenses.[157,158] One study demonstrated that a well-controlled formulary or therapeutic substitution (substituting a different medication that is effective for the disease being treated for the one ordered by the physician) results in 10.7% lower drug costs per patient day, and both a well-controlled formulary and therapeutic substitution together could cause 13.4% lower drug costs per day.[159]

Some prescribers do not support formularies, because they consider them to be a limitation to their authority.[154] It is necessary to keep in mind that when prescribers become a part of a medical staff or sign up to participate in some managed care group, they are given privileges not rights. The privileges generally do include limitations on what medications they can prescribe, and when and how they can prescribe them. If a drug formulary system is run well there is little reason to feel there are inadequate drugs available; however, it does take some effort for the physician to learn to use the drugs available rather than the drugs they normally prescribe. An effort must be made to collaborate with prescribers to reassure them that every effort is being made to ensure the best drugs are available for the patients. Additionally, all changes to the drug formulary must be quickly and effectively communicated to the prescribers to avoid confusion. A lack of such communication can negate some of the benefits of the formulary and lead to poor physician/pharmacist relations.[157] Also, it is important for prescribers to be aware that it is the medical staff that affirms P&T decisions, in order to avoid pharmacy being perceived as the sole participant in decisions for the institution and as a barrier to physician requests.[160]

Prescribers entering prescription orders into the computer can immediately be informed of formulary drug choices and guided in their therapeutic decisions. However, pharmacists may have to tactfully contact the prescriber about nonformulary drugs in order to make a formulary system work.

Similarly, pharmacies filling prescriptions for an HMO must be kept informed of the formulary status of drugs. One suggestion is to have a help desk to answer pharmacist questions and to provide information.[161]

Contents of the Drug Formulary

Oftentimes, drug formularies will contain other information, such as ancillary information about the P&T committee and pharmacy department, policy and procedure information (e.g., how to obtain nonformulary drugs, how to request a drug be placed on the formulary), laboratory test information, dietary supplement charts, pharmacokinetic information, approved abbreviations, sodium content, nomograms, dosage equivalency charts, apothecary/metric equivalents, drug-food interactions, skin test directions, cost data, antibiograms, antimicrobial therapy charts, and any other brief clinical information tables felt to be necessary. Use of linking in websites or specific computer programs can make such information much more readily available and usable, since users can navigate back and forth between these tables and the drug list. MCOs may need to include the procedure they use to limit choice of drugs by prescribers, pharmacists, and patients.[16,162]

In institutional pharmacies, a hardcopy book once was normally published once a year. Often it was published in a pocket-size format that could be carried in lab coats by prescribers, pharmacists, and nurses. There may also have been a larger loose-leaf binder published that could be updated regularly throughout the year. Such a book is no longer justified.[163] It is now common for this information to be available electronically. The electronic form can be made more widely available and can be kept continually up to date by making changes, as necessary, in one central location. Also, the electronic formulary coupled with physician order entry may lead to the most efficient and effective way to encourage or enforce the use of formulary items,[164–166] although there is some evidence that electronic messages may be ignored by physicians.[167] Also, other information can be included to improve drug therapy. For example, this may include a requirement for a consultation by a specialist or pharmacokinetic monitoring. For outpatient drug formularies this may include quantity level limits and requirements for **prior authorizations**.

Preferably, the pharmacy can use the information on their computer system to create a formulary that is constantly up-to-date. The information can be accessed as part of the prescription order software and/or it may be interfaced with web software.[168] The latter makes it possible to embed other information easily, but may take further work by the pharmacist. In any case, this information should be available to the physician and other health care professionals wherever necessary—even by wireless connection or on a mobile device. As a side note, many institutions do not want information about their formularies readily available to individuals not directly associated with the institution (e.g., pharmaceutical manufacturers, pharmaceutical representatives, product vendors), but this should not be a problem using Virtual Private Network (VPN) software and firewalls to secure the data—allowing access to only qualified individuals. Increasingly, prescribers access this information using smart phones or tablets.

PBM companies, in conjunction with an organization, may publish a **patient pocket formulary** or informational website in addition to the formulary for prescribers and provided online for pharmacies. These patient pocket formularies or websites may contain the top therapeutic categories and other information as well. Within these categories are the key drugs in that specific therapeutic class as well as the designated preferred products and the associated patient cost index. Patients may have access to the PBM formulary list via the plan's website. Patients are encouraged to take the pocket formularies on their physician visits as a means of ensuring formulary compliance when discussing therapeutic options. Prescribers may also have the capability of prescribing online, whereby the physician enters the prescription in an electronic device and instant messaging occurs alerting the physician to potential drug interactions or formulary status of the prescription, allowing the physician to change the prescription immediately and eliminating the need for a pharmacist to call the prescriber.[56,169]

In addition to pocket formularies, one method whereby the pharmacist educates the physician about formulary drugs is academic detailing. Through mailings, phone conversations, and personal visits, the pharmacist discusses with the physician his or her prescribing patterns and, using evidence-based medical literature, supports the rational for preferred formulary product selection and clinically appropriate, cost-effective prescribing without compromising quality (see Chapter 25 for more information).[56]

It is recommended to use a combination of methods to make sure prescribers are informed about formulary information, including electronic resources, academic detailing, educational programs, and any other available methods.[170]

Evaluating Drugs for Formulary Inclusion

The establishment and maintenance of a drug formulary requires that drugs or drug classes be objectively assessed based on scientific information (e.g., efficacy, adverse effects, cost, contribution to some critical treatment pathway,[171] ease of preparation/use, and other appropriate items), not anecdotal physician experience.[112,127,172] Also, it must be noted that the safety of medications is an important consideration and that decisions must not be made purely based on cost.[173] When costs are considered, it needs to be an evaluation of all costs to the institution, not just the cost of the medication itself, and may include such diverse things as laboratory monitoring costs, length of therapy, nursing care demands, and rehospitalization rates.[174] Medication selection and procurement were specifically added to TJC accreditation process under medication management in the 2009 standards.[175] There is an emphasis in the literature that P&T committee activities should be a result of evidence-based decisions.[129,176] Regarding the formulary process, TJC standard MM.02.01.01 calls for written criteria for addition or deletion of medications.[15] Any health care practitioner who is involved with ordering, dispensing, administering, and monitoring medications needs to be involved with the development of the criteria.[15,175] A process must also be in place to monitor patient responses to a new medication. All formulary medications and all categories of the AHFS therapeutic classification are to be reviewed in some fashion at least annually based on safety and efficacy information in order to comply with TJC standards and to maintain the most effective and safe formulary.

Evaluation Criteria

According to TJC, the criteria used for approving addition of a drug to a formulary minimally should include the following[15]:

- Indications for use
- Effectiveness
- Drug interactions
- Potential for errors and abuse[177]
- Adverse drug events
- Sentinel event advisories
- Population(s) served (e.g., pediatric, geriatric)
- Other risks
- Cost

A procedure for preparing the written evaluation of drug products is found in the next chapter; however, this section will go further into how the P&T committee should use that information and other items to do the actual evaluation.

When a P&T committee considers a drug for formulary adoption, it is quite common for the discussion to include statements such as "In my clinical experience...," which often leads the discussion into rather subjective areas. Though clinical experience adds an important component to a discussion, this should not be the sole basis for a formulary review. Additionally, physicians commonly request drugs after they have met with the pharmaceutical company representative or received compensation from the drug company (e.g., speaking fees and travel funds to a meeting).[167,178] CMS provides a transparent tool for searching financial relationships of physicians with manufacturers (https://www.cms.gov/openpayments). In addition, medications may be requested and added to a formulary simply because they are new, even when they clearly are not superior and cost more.[179] Valid formulary decisions should always be based on objective evidence, particularly clinical studies,[180] rather than a few cases of clinical experience by a physician or a representative.[129] Efforts must be made to guide discussions to scientific information for an effective and comprehensive review.[128]

In some cases, this is rather difficult because many new drugs have limited published information, when they are first commercially available. The information that is available is generally placebo-controlled studies that are funded by the manufacturer, although this is clearly not possible with some agents, such as those for oncology. In situations such as this, the decision on formulary addition may need to be postponed until adequate information is available. It may be recommended that consideration of any new product be delayed until it has been on the market for at least 1 year, unless it is a treatment that is significantly different from those already available.[181] In at least one case, it has been bluntly stated that a P&T committee should show leadership by restricting the availability of a drug product if there is no convincing evidence that the product offers meaningful benefits over other available products.[182] Sometimes the decision cannot wait, as is the case with many managed care companies, who need to review a drug before a patient picks up the drug from the pharmacy, so that appropriate coverage determination can be made.[15,175]

The P&T committee's decision-making process needs to be structured in a manner that is objective and data driven, and takes into account the lack of data.[129] A committee may make a decision and then place the product on a 6-month follow-up for an additional review, after which time additional prescribing and patient use data or clinical trial data may be available.

While there is a temptation to think that anything new is better, which is an attitude that is certainly advocated by pharmaceutical company representatives with new products to sell, it cannot be assumed and must be proven. In some cases, experts have determined that the new products pose no significant advantages to the patients to justify the costs.[183–185] Often, manufacturers try to get products approved and on the market that may be in a different strength or dosage form, a single isomer of a product, a new indication for a product, or even an extended-release version of a product (sometimes several different extended-release versions).[186] All of the products potentially need to be given consideration by a P&T committee. However, with a lack of published trials and, in many cases, objective and reliable data, the P&T committee faces the challenge of creating a sound drug formulary that represents the needs of an organization or patient population in an objective manner that encompasses current clinical practice, established guidelines of patient care, and a thorough risk-benefit analysis of the drug product.[27] Some places have even tried computerized methods to make more objective decisions[187,188]; however, there does not seem to be any data demonstrating the superiority of such a method. Similarly, there are processes called System of Objectified Judgment Analysis (SOJA), which uses a computer program to score different aspects of drugs in the same class to determine the best product,[189,190] and multiattribute utility technology.[191]

To summarize, TJC Accreditation Process Guide for Hospitals addresses the elements of performance for selecting and procuring medications.[15] Elements of this performance that provide additional information to that already covered are the following:

1. Members of the medical staff, licensed independent practitioners, pharmacists, and staff involved in the ordering, dispensing, administering, and/or monitoring the effects of medications develop written criteria for determining which medications are available for dispensing or administering to patients.
2. The hospital develops and approves criteria for selecting medications, which, at a minimum, include the following:
   • Indications for use
   • Effectiveness
   • Drug interactions
   • Potential for errors and abuse
   • Adverse drug events
   • Sentinel event advisories
   • Populations(s) served (pediatrics, geriatrics)
3. Before using a medication new to the hospital, the hospital determines a method to monitor the response of the patient.
4. The hospital maintains a formulary, including medication strength and dosage.
5. The hospital makes its formulary readily available to those involved in medication management.
6. The hospital standardizes and limits the number of drug concentrations available to meet patient care needs.
7. The hospital has a process to select, approve, and procure medications that are not on its formulary.
8. The hospital implements the process to select, approve, and procure medications that are not on its formulary.
9. Medications designated as available for dispensing or administration are reviewed at least annually based on emerging safety and efficacy information.
10. The hospital has a process to communicate medication shortages and outages to licensed independent practitioners and staff who participate in medication management (see TJC Standard MM.02.02.01).

Conflict of Interest

Also, it is necessary to determine whether individuals (or their spouses or domestic partners, if applicable) involved in the discussion and decision about a drug's formulary status have a **conflict of interest** and avoid that biasing factor. This could include receiving some direct or indirect compensation from having a drug available, e.g., stock in a company, honoraria for speaking, consulting fees, and gifts or grants from a company.[114,181,192-194] Nationally, this is considered to be a significant problem.[195] The P&T committee has the responsibility to identify and address conflict of interest issues in the decision-making process.[129] A conflict of interest policy, requiring regular disclosure of any possible conflicts, should be established and declared in writing annually.[27,196,197] An example form to gather information about conflicts of interest is found in Appendix 15-6. Also, the ProPublica website (https://projects.propublica.org/docdollars/) and CMS website (https://www.cms.gov/openpayments/) disclose payments to prescribers from some pharmaceutical companies. In certain cases, regular voting P&T committee members may have to abstain from the vote, if they disclose a possible conflict of interest, or the committee may vote to determine whether the conflict is considered to be significant enough to prevent voting by the individual in question. There is concern at a federal, state, and institutional level regarding potential conflict of interest. In 2009, some drug manufacturers made public their financial relationship with health care providers.[198] There is also concern that P&T committees of the PBM companies may be financially influenced by drug manufacturers.[199] Unlike the traditional health insurers, the U.S. Department of Defense solicits input from various providers and beneficiaries. In addition, they provide beneficiaries and their representatives an opportunity to comment on the committee recommendations prior to final approval. However, this has not deterred their placement in a category where they will provide the lowest reimbursement for the product.[200]

Other Aspects of Formulary Evaluation

Several other areas need to be considered, which will be explained below.

Patent Expiration

Patent expiration is a common question that should be considered for all products or drug classes undergoing formulary review, since the introduction of generic products after that date may lead to decreasing prices. Patent expiration information can be found at https://www.accessdata.fda.gov/scripts/cder/ob/index.cfm.

Orphan Drug Status

Similarly, whether a medication is granted orphan drug status is an issue. In just the first half of 2019, 35 novel drugs that were approved were for orphan diseases, which allows pharmaceutical companies to have high profits.[201] This too can greatly affect the cost of medications for an institution, including for older products that might have previously been marketed for a much lower cost.[202]

High-Alert or Hazardous Medications

TJC Medication Management Standards are focused on medication safety (see TJC Standard MM.04.01.01). High-alert medications are those where there is a high likelihood of errors and/or sentinel events, potential for abuse, or other adverse events. A listing of high-alert medications is available from ISMP (www.ismp.org/tools/highalert-medications.pdf). Hazardous medications by definition of exposure to animals or humans have the potential to cause cancer, developmental or reproductive toxicity, or organ damage. Lists of hazardous medications are available from the National Institute for Occupational Safety and Health (NIOSH) (https://www.cdc.gov/niosh/docs/2016-161/pdfs/2016-161.pdf). Institutions must define how they will determine which formulary medications are hazardous, especially if they are not on the NIOSH list. An institution can choose to consider all medications hazardous or use an assessment of risk evaluation that develops handling criteria in a standard manner. The NIOSH list includes three categories of hazardous, chemotherapy, nonchemotherapy, and reproductive risk and includes handling precautions for them. This process is dictated by United States Pharmacopeia/National Formulary (USP/NF) under chapter <800>. The definition of a medication goes beyond prescription products and the FDA classification as drugs. The following are also considered medications: herbal/alternative therapies, vitamins, nutraceuticals, nonprescription products, vaccines, diagnostic and contrast agents, radioactive agents, respiratory treatments, parenteral nutrition, blood derivatives, intravenous (IV) solutions, anesthetic gases, sample medications, and anything else deemed by the FDA to be a drug.[175] The pharmacist is required to review the appropriateness of all medication orders, prospectively before a medication is dispensed.[15,175,203]

Complementary and Alternative Medicine

While it is desirable to evaluate herbal or other alternative medicine products,[204–206] some institutions may instead handle them as nonformulary requests or investigational drugs.[207] Although alternative and herbal medications may seem somewhat unusual for the P&T committee to address, they can still be treated much the same way as any drug product, perhaps with additional evaluation of the purity and composition of the products (Natural Medicines Medical Literature section of Chapter 5 for additional details regarding how to evaluate these products).[208] Some pharmacies also have other policies and procedures,[209] perhaps some that are highly restrictive,[210] including requiring pharmacists to verify labeled product ingredients.[211]

Potential Medication Errors

The possibility of a new drug product leading to medication errors should also be considered in the evaluation of products. For example, difficulty in dosing or administration (including programming IV infusion pumps), boxed warnings, look-alike and sound-alike names, the need for extra monitoring, unusual storage requirements, and other issues such as Risk Evaluation and Mitigation Strategy (REMS) requirements may be considered.[212]

Patient Affordability

In addition to considering the cost of drug products in the institution, it is necessary to consider the cost to the patient, once he or she returns home. If a product is so expensive that an uninsured or underinsured patient cannot afford it in the ambulatory environment, it may not be appropriate to place the patient on that drug in the hospital. However, in some cases, pharmaceutical companies may offer assistance to this type of patient.

"Right to Try" Laws

A newer concept that needs to be considered is "Right to Try" legislation being adopted by some states that allow patients to try experimental medications without approval of the FDA.[213] This may be more of an issue for the IRB in an institution, but the P&T committee may be involved.

Open versus Closed Formularies

When setting up a drug formulary, there are several things to consider. First is whether it will be an open or **closed formulary**.[214] The **open** (or voluntary) **formulary** is defined as including any drug on the market that is available, and some would argue that the term "open formulary" is really an oxymoron.[128] One exception to this definition is that the NCQA states that an open formulary for an MCO can be a list of recommended drugs, as long as there are no requirements concerning its use.[215] A closed (or restricted) formulary means that only a limited number of agents are available.[123] This is certainly preferable, because such agents should be chosen by objective evidence in the scientific literature. The evidence should support the superiority of the agents over other similar drugs, and can result in cost savings.[216] Closed formularies have become much more common in HMOs.[217,218] In some instances of closed formularies, patients may have access to non-formulary or nonpreferred drug products by paying a substantially higher copayment, by paying the difference between the formulary and nonformulary products in addition to the copayment, or by paying for the nonformulary drug in its entirety unless there is a prior authorization to allow this drug.[55]

Issues may arise with a closed or restricted formulary, in that it may be too restrictive for those patients who cannot afford the drug, even though the drug is still available on a closed formulary. A growing health policy concern is the ability to successfully appeal for coverage of a nonformulary product. Newer breakthrough medications and biotechnology products are making their way onto the market. Although clinically valuable, they are very expensive. In addition, PBM companies have managed or preferred formularies. In a managed or preferred formulary, interventions may be used to encourage prescribers to use the preferred products. Some of these interventions for prescribers include academic detailing, prior authorizations, and coverage rules. For pharmacies this may mean a higher dispensing fee for formulary compliance. For the patient this may mean higher copayments if the formulary or preferred product is not used.

Unlike hospitals, PBM companies along with their clients (i.e., health plans) place their formulary and nonformulary medications into tiers with an associated copayment with each tier. This tier copayment structure came about in response to the rising cost of prescription drugs. The first tier is generally reserved for generic drug products. This tier usually has the lowest copayment (e.g., $15.00). The second tier is usually reserved for those name brand drugs that are formulary (e.g., $40.00). This tier has a higher copayment than the first tier due to the added cost of the brand name drug. The third tier is reserved for those drug products that are nonformulary brand names. This copayment is significantly higher than the other two tiers (e.g., $80). However, some third tier copayments may be calculated as a proportion of the drug cost, even as much as one-third as a form of coinsurance, or require paying for the drug in its entirety. The reason for the copayment structure is to encourage the patient to use the most clinically appropriate, cost-effective drug without compromising quality care.[55] Decisions as to the tier placement of a drug product may be dependent on comparative effectiveness research.[219]

The **closed formulary** can also be broken down into what is referred to as **positive or negative formularies**. This is the method by which the formulary is developed. A positive formulary effectively starts with a blank sheet of paper and specifically adds agents. While this is probably the best method to limit the number of drugs available, it is often not very popular when first implementing the formulary because every agent must be considered. That means the physicians must even make specific decisions on whether they should add such things as acetaminophen and amoxicillin to the formulary. Therefore, in hospitals just establishing a formulary, it is often more popular and easier to use a negative formulary system. This essentially starts with the current hospital drug stock, with each drug class being evaluated to eliminate agents that are not necessary.[220] The first steps in this process may be as simple as eliminating multiple salts/esters of the same drug. Then classes of drugs with multiple similar products could be addressed (e.g., analgesics, antacids, laxatives, vitamins, and topical steroids). While in some ways this process is easier, it is also likely to result in a much bigger formulary, since the decision will be made as to what drugs are definitely not needed, rather than which drugs the institution definitely needs. However, the specific institution's situation will need to be assessed before the method of determining the formulary items can be decided on. Overall, the goal is to provide an optimal array of agents; it is easy to end up with too many duplicative agents; however, having a greater number of agents to choose from can lead to better patient care in some areas.[221,222]

While a drug formulary system provides medication-use guidance, a drug formulary does not require a hospital to stock the product. A formulary medication may not always be available in the pharmacy for a variety of reasons. The P&T committee should work closely with pharmacy management to maintain an expectation of medication stock, if stock specifically affects the safety and need of patients. For example, an antidote for snake bites on formulary should be available at the hospital, if snake bites are common in the community the hospital serves, however, if such bites are seen, but not common, it may be appropriate to classify the product as formulary, but only have it available at one of several hospitals, with mechanisms set up to obtain the antivenom common stock quickly when necessary.

Regardless of which formulary type a P&T committee maintains, managing the use of medications on formulary is accomplished in a number of ways. Particularly, restrictions based on criteria, such as service type, patient type, or medication criteria, provide the means by which a P&T committee guides practitioners to appropriate medication use. Such restrictions can result in more appropriate use of various medications and substantial cost savings.[223] The types of restrictions allowed by a P&T committee should be developed by the voting membership. In addition to restrictions in one or more formularies, a P&T committee may choose to maintain an emergency review process for nonformulary medications for documentation of nonformulary use. This process is required by TJC, so that appropriate patient care can be provided, despite the time constraints of the P&T process.[15]

Therapeutic Interchange

Definition of Therapeutic Interchange

The AMA[12,214] defines therapeutic interchange as "authorized exchange of therapeutic alternatives in accordance with previously established and approved written guidelines or protocols within a formulary system." An example would be the use of cefazolin in specific doses whenever any other first-generation injectable cephalosporin is ordered.

Note that therapeutic interchange is different from biosimilar substitution in which the FDA has determined that specific biologic products are similar except for minor differences in clinically inactive components, with no meaningful differences between the biologics in safety, purity, and potency.[224,225] Biosimilar substitution may allow something very similar to therapeutic interchange, even in community pharmacies, depending on state and federal laws that are being updated to allow for it.[226,227] A P&T committee can assess biosimilars as a candidate for therapeutic substitution and approve the protocol within the formulary system, regardless of state law. It is important to note that the evaluation of a biosimilar should follow the normal process of evaluating a product for formulary. There are unique items to consider during this review, such as indications for use, immunogenicity, transitions of care, and nomenclature (e.g., biosimilars are given a four-letter suffix to distinguish the products from the originator product and other biosimilars of the same biologic).[228]

Benefits of Therapeutic Interchange

Therapeutic interchange is used in nearly 90% of U.S. hospitals[229] to take advantage of cost savings,[230–232] improved patient outcomes, decreased adverse effects, decreased inventory, fewer medication errors,[233] or other benefits. Therapeutic interchange has been shown to decrease costs without adversely affecting patient outcomes.[71,234] There is even reason to believe that when therapeutic interchange is properly performed, and not entirely based on financial considerations, it may produce lower legal liability on an institution,[115] although there are no published legal cases regarding therapeutic interchange to demonstrate either increased or decreased legal liability.[235] Interdisciplinary teams should develop protocols and comprehensive therapeutic assessments in collaboration to result in an effective and supported therapeutic interchange.

Several medication classes may be the target of therapeutic interchange, and an aggressive intravenous to oral conversion may be part of this process.[236] The most common classes of drugs for therapeutic interchange are, in order: H_2 antagonists, proton pump inhibitors, antacids, potassium supplements, cephalosporins, and hydroxymethylglutaryl-coenzyme A reductase inhibitors.[237] Some drug classes, such as low-molecular-weight heparins, which at first glance may appear to be possible places for therapeutic interchange, may be found to be unacceptable after a closer inspection.[237]

Therapeutic interchange is considered acceptable to the AMA, unlike therapeutic substitution, which they define as the "act of dispensing a therapeutic alternative for the drug product prescribed without prior authorization of the prescriber" (note: prior authorization may be a blanket authorization, not a specific authorization for each case[238]).[239] Therapeutic interchange has also been found to be acceptable by other organizations, including the American College of Clinical Pharmacy (ACCP), American College of Physicians (ACP),[240] ASHP, American Pharmacists Association (APhA), American Association of Colleges of Pharmacy (AACP), AMCP,[241] and the American Society of Consultant Pharmacists (ASCP).[242,243] The ACCP spells out the concept of therapeutic interchange in great detail and suggests that it not only be conducted under the auspices of a P&T-type committee, but also that it specifically include a drug usage evaluation (DUE—see Chapter 18), a set method for informing the physicians and other staff that interchange is taking place (should be well planned and thorough[244]), and a mechanism under which the therapeutic interchange policies may be overridden in specific cases.

Decisions for Therapeutic Interchange

Evaluations for therapeutic interchange should also consider medical, legal, and financial evaluations.[237] Other practical aspects, such as communication forms, policies and procedures, medical staff bylaw changes, and other items, may need to be addressed by the institution.[245] Electronic means to provide authorization for a therapeutic interchange is an option[246] that is likely to have become common. Outside of an institution (e.g., ambulatory environment), therapeutic interchange may not be as easy to implement due to practical procedure methods and because patients are not as closely monitored; however, it may still be possible.[247,248] In the ambulatory situation, the AMA states that therapeutic interchange recommendations must be approved by the majority of physicians affected and must otherwise follow similar standards to that described for inpatient settings.[214]

The consideration of certain therapeutic agents for interchange may result in strong differences of opinion among medical staff members regarding their appropriate use. The process for evaluating any product should be followed, along with efforts being made by committee members to actively approach appropriate influential individuals to manage expectations and assess individual thoughts on an interchange prior to formulary discussion. Through anticipatory, structured negotiation, it is more likely that rational and balanced decisions will be made. Also, it is necessary to take into consideration whether a short-term interchange of products, while the patient is in a hospital, may cause confusion or other difficulties when the patient returns to the outpatient environment and may be restarted on the original agent.[249] Working with the physicians to resolve this issue is a necessity for the long-term care of patients.

Generic substitution can also be considered by the P&T committee, but many pharmacies consider generic substitution to be one of their responsibilities and do not take such decisions to a P&T committee for approval. An exception may be drugs with narrow therapeutic indexes (e.g., anticonvulsants, immunosuppressants for transplant patients), where a P&T committee may determine a list of products where generic substitution is not allowed,[250] although the FDA insists that such precautions are unnecessary.[251] In relation to generic substitution, it must be mentioned that pharmacies must determine quality suppliers. The ASHP has guidelines for this function.[252] Also, states may have a variety of laws governing generic substitution. They may also publish so-called positive and negative formularies, which differ in definition from those terms used elsewhere in this chapter, in that they are lists of drugs that may or may not be substituted for one another, respectively.[235]

In some instances, prescribers may prefer that no generic substitution or therapeutic substitution occur on a written order or prescription by indicating "Dispense as Written" (DAW) on that document. This can occur in the inpatient setting as well as the outpatient setting. Depending on the state, dispense as written is synonymous with the following: no substitution, do not substitute, medically necessary, brand necessary/medically necessary, no drug product selection, brand medically necessary, substitution prohibited without permission of physician or patient, or no substitution/brand necessary.

In most states, the law provides that pharmacists can use a generic version of any medication on a prescription or medication order if the physician has not precluded that action by indicating DAW. In the outpatient setting, in general, if a patient wants a generic medication, they should be sure that their pharmacist knows of their desire.

In some benefit plans, if the physician requests a brand name medication when a generic equivalent is available, the patient member may be responsible to pay the difference in cost in addition to the generic copayment. In some instances, members may not be required to pay this cost difference, if their physician documents that the brand name medication is necessary.

Case Study 15–2

As a pharmacist practicing in a large health system at an outpatient dialysis clinic at the main hospital, a request is presented by the patient's insurance to use a biosimilar (epoetin alfa-epbx [Retacrit]) instead of epoetin alfa (Epogen). The nonformulary review process approved use of the biosimilar in this patient.

- *What is important for a formulary process to consider when evaluating the biosimilar for formulary addition?*
- *What strategies might the P&T committee employ with biosimilars?*
- *What implementation strategies might be needed for successful biosimilar adoption?*

Nonformulary Usage

Many institutions track the drug use patterns of prescribers, as was mentioned previously in describing the tracking of nonformulary drug products.[253] Annually, a listing of nonformulary products and expenses should be made available to the P&T committee. It is helpful if the pharmacy director can report the total cost of nonformulary items as a percent of the total budget, particularly since the cost can exceed the cost of carrying the nonformulary product on the formulary.[254] Also, it is important to include whether nonformulary drug usage has led to medication errors, since there was at least one report that such nonformulary use resulted in a 28% error rate.[253] Ideally, a report of the number involved and costs of nonformulary orders will be made available to each prescriber. This process is helpful in improving the appropriate use of medications and has also been linked to the prescriber credentialing process.[255] The process can also be used to reevaluate whether nonformulary items should be made available on the drug formulary.

Unlabeled Uses

While some third-party payers may attempt to limit the use of drugs to only FDA-approved indications, this may unnecessarily restrict use of products for indications that may have significant literature support. This should not be supported.[256] However, as will be discussed in more detail in the next chapter, it is sometimes necessary for institutions to specifically restrict drugs to specific uses, if there is a high probability they may be used inappropriately. Such restrictions may be totally unrelated to approved labeling, since product use may be permitted for unlabeled indications if there is adequate literature support and, conversely, may not be permitted at least without special approval within the institution, for FDA indications when there may be more appropriate drugs available. An institution may use monitoring of off-label use of medications to determine if they should be allowed or otherwise addressed.[257]

New Product Introductions

When new drug products are added to the formulary, it is best to prepare prescribers, nurses, and others.[167] Initially, it is necessary to inform affected individuals that the drug will be available as of a specific date. That could be immediately or at some time in the near future. There are various reasons for a delay. For example, a drug may have been approved by both the FDA and the P&T committee, but the company may not have yet made it commercially available because they have not yet produced a sufficient supply, they are not yet ready to start their marketing efforts, or the Drug Enforcement Agency (DEA) needs to make its final ruling. In some cases, it is necessary for specific equipment to be obtained and installed. Such was the case a number of years ago, when Fluosol®-DA was made available for a limited period of time. This parenteral product required very specialized preparation method involving a warm water bath and percolating a mixture of gases through an intravenous bag under sterile conditions. Few, if any, pharmacies had the necessary equipment at the time of introduction, and it would have taken some time to get the equipment, set it up, and train pharmacists and technicians in its use, requiring a delay in making the product available in an institution.

In addition to equipment acquisition time, hospitals using electronic medical records, smart pump technology, patient education tools, and formulary management software to electronically list formulary changes may need time for those items to be updated. This includes building automated formulary restrictions into an electronic medical record, thereby providing prescribers the information at the point of prescription. Each of these areas may have their own processes to update each system. Another important reason for the delay includes the time it takes to inform all individuals who will be involved in prescribing, preparing, and administering the drug of drug availability and education in proper use. These education efforts may be provided through websites, portals, email, newsletters, memos, educational programs, or other methods. The method chosen should generally be a standard method used within the institution and should be appropriate for the specific medication product introduction. In cases where a product is particularly complicated, dangerous, or prone to misuse, several methods of instruction, perhaps along with prescribing restrictions, should probably be employed. Further information about websites and newsletters is found in Chapter 13.

POLICIES AND PROCEDURES

Occasionally, policies and procedures must be developed to support the rational use of medications. While the pharmacy department may decide they need to have their own policies and procedures for internal functions, that is not the focus of this discussion.[258] Instead, policies and procedures for the use of medications in an institution, clinic, and so forth will be discussed, since that is often provided through a P&T committee.

TJC recognizes the potential for medication errors and promotes written policy to minimize errors (see TJC Standard MM.04.01.01). TJC has specifically stated that they expect policies and procedures for the following types of orders[15]:

- As needed (prn) medications
- Standing orders
- Automatic stop
- Titrating
- Taper
- Range
- Compounded or admixed drugs
- Medication-related devices
- Investigational medications
- Herbal products
- Medications at discharge or transfer[76]

Definitions of Policies and Procedures

To begin this discussion, the definitions for policies and procedures should be considered.[259] A policy is a broad general statement that describes the goals and purposes of the document. The procedures are specific actions to be taken. In some ways, policies and procedures may resemble a cookbook-type approach, in that a set of steps to be accomplished are described in order. Taken together, these policies and procedures may be a logical, step-by-step explanation of why and where a product may be used, how to use it, and who is to follow the policy (i.e., there may be different portions of the document addressed to pharmacists, technicians, nurses, prescribers, and others),[260] along with a brief introductory statement describing why the process is necessary.

• Before developing a specific policy and procedure, the first step should be deciding whether it is necessary at all. This can be looked at as a risk-benefit decision. For example, is there sufficient risk that a particular medication will be used incorrectly (e.g., prepared wrong, administered wrong, used for an inappropriate indication) to make it worthwhile to develop a policy and procedure? Generally, the answer will be no, but in a certain number of cases, policies and procedures may be necessary. Examples of where a policy and procedure may be necessary include thrombolytic agents (where the drug can cause serious or fatal effects if used improperly), antibiotics (where it is found that expensive, broad-spectrum antibiotics are being used where amoxicillin should suffice), injectable drugs (where specific individuals who will administer the medication and the process, including programming infusion devices, will be defined),[261] and even for drugs where reimbursement may be a problem. All policies and procedures may be surveyed by CMS and TJC. As such, P&T committees may choose to develop guidelines, which at times are incorrectly called policies and procedures, as opposed to policies and procedures to guide appropriate medication use. The challenges of education and availability of these guidelines apply. Another method to identify needed policies is addressing required documents from accreditation agencies, like Joint Commission and the Board of Pharmacy in the state. This helps to create an efficient list of policies that meet the needs of the organization and serve as a core baseline during an accreditation visit.

Developing Policies and Procedures

• Once a decision is reached to develop the policy and procedure or guideline, a logical and orderly course should be followed. A proactive, rather than reactive, approach should be employed, when determining if a policy is needed. The policy should be reviewed by the normal drug formulary process, where a mechanism is set up to help determine policy need, evaluate content, and approve the policy. In many cases, a policy and procedure for use of drugs likely to be misused may be developed in conjunction with its consideration for addition to the drug formulary.

• As in any process, it is first necessary to decide who will be coordinating the effort and the likely endpoint. That person, or designee, will then need to investigate various sources for background material necessary to develop the policy and procedure. This might include completing a literature search, talking to experts in the field, collaborating with other institutions who have already developed policies on the same topic, reviewing published professional material (e.g., https://www.ashp.org/Pharmacy-Practice/Policy-Positions-and-Guidelines) or clinical guidelines (e.g., https://guidelines.ecri.org/), and checking the institution's requirements for developing policies and procedures. If the policy and procedure is for a hospital group, other institutions in the group must also be involved. In particular, it is necessary for the person developing the policy and procedure to have good communications with those who will be affected to avoid confusion and enhance likelihood of policy and procedure utilization. Where the policy and procedure fits in relation to other institutional policies and procedures will also have to be evaluated. Finally, a document should be written, reviewed, and revised, using many of the skills outlined in Chapters 13 and 21.

As part of the process of preparing the policy, it is important to be clear how the policy will be applied, and if there may be exceptions. For example, institutions have policies for the automatic stop of specific medications (e.g., stopping an antibiotic after 7 days). The policy should only be applied in cases where it will improve drug therapy. There also needs to be a mechanism to make sure that such an automatic stop, which may be programmed into the computer system, does not cause harm to particular patients[262] (e.g., patients with osteomyelitis receiving antibiotics for an extended period of time).

Implementation of Policies and Procedures

Once the policy and procedure is finished, it will need to be approved by the same process that drug formulary changes go through (i.e., P&T committee, medical executive committee). Some facilities or organizations also have policy approval bodies that have other reporting structures. It is important to understand the appropriate process for policy approval. The approval and/or effective date for the policy and procedure should be recorded on the document itself to ensure it is not confused with earlier or later documents. A plan for implementing the policy and procedure and educating those involved should also be developed. Forms may need to be prepared and distributed. The policy and procedure should be made available to all people affected by the policy (preferably on the computer network or intranet), and educational programs will need to be planned and given.

Once the policy and procedure is implemented, perhaps in conjunction with the first appearance of a particular agent on the drug formulary, the policy and procedure should be evaluated to determine if it is being properly followed and having the desired effect as a part of a quality assurance plan. A method to enforce compliance with the policies and procedures is required, and it is necessary for legal reasons to demonstrate that this enforcement method is used.[260] Also, the policy and procedure will need to be reviewed, revised (if necessary), and reapproved on a regular basis (preferably once a year). As part of that process, the actual need for the policy and procedure should be reconsidered. The policy and procedure should be eliminated if no longer needed. One way to determine whether the policy and procedures are consulted is if they are on a web server, where the number of times the specific page is opened is recorded. Superseded copies (i.e., previous versions) of the policies and procedures should be kept on file for background and for legal purposes, but should not be available as live documents for use.

It is also necessary to have policies and procedures for the operation of the P&T committee itself (see Appendix 15-1 for policies and procedures for setting up a P&T committee). Some examples of other policies and procedures that may need to be developed include how new drugs are requested for addition to the formulary, how nonformulary drugs can be used, what procedure is used to evaluate new drugs,[175] the composition of the committee, and other committee functions (e.g., conflict of interest). These have been discussed elsewhere in the chapter and will not be dealt with further at this point.

Each organization should proactively create and maintain policies that meet regulatory requirements (e.g., documentation required for TJC) and describe the formulary management process at the organization for transparency.

For more information on writing policies and procedures, please refer to Chapter 21.

CLINICAL GUIDELINES

P&T committees may be involved with the development, alteration (to fit local circumstances), and/or approval of evidence-based clinical guidelines. The reader is directed to Chapter 8 to obtain further information.

STANDARD ORDER SET DEVELOPMENT

Many prescribers, both in their offices and in institutions (e.g., hospital and nursing home), make use of something called standard orders. This usually consists of a form, preprinted hardcopy, or electronic checklist, which lists orders that are often written for specific patients under certain circumstances. This can include medications, laboratory tests, x-rays, other diagnostic tests, diet restrictions, preoperative preparation, restrictions, and many other things. For example, there may be a specific set of orders for all patients a prescriber admits to the hospital in general or for a specific diagnosis, or a set of orders for a patient who is scheduled to undergo a specific procedure, such as an operation or colonoscopy. Standard order sets are commonly used for some medications, such as total parenteral nutrition solutions and oncology agents, where the order can be complex and confusing, perhaps resulting in dangerous medication errors. Standard order sets may also be used to limit doses and concentrations of intravenous solutions to correspond to policies and procedures. The prescribers using the standard order sets can simply indicate which of the items they wish their patients to receive and provide various necessary details, such as dose or duration. The use of standard order sets can be a very good practice, since they act like checklists used by pilots or astronauts— saving time and ensuring that important items are not inadvertently missed or misused.

This can be particularly important in the use of drugs that can be dangerous or ineffective if not properly used, such as chemotherapeutic regimens in oncology patients. However, the disadvantage is that the standard order sets do take time to establish and maintain, and may not keep up with actual practice standards depending on review/ update process, therefore, contributing to the perpetuation of outdated or inappropriate practices.

While many P&T committees do not address standard order sets directly, leaving them to the individuals or groups that use them or collaborating with other groups specifically designed to look at order sets, it is something that still needs to be considered for several reasons. First, P&T committees are responsible for overseeing all things related to medication use in an institution. Second, the standard order sets include medications, which should only be medications on formulary. If medications are included in standard order sets and are medications that have been removed from formulary, P&T committees should integrate into those discussions to prevent errors. The same thought process is applied to adding medications to standard order sets that are not yet added to formulary. These situations require the P&T committee to make a special effort to communicate with those individuals or groups with standard order sets. This communication should begin prior to medication-related recommendations. The formulary and order set processes are likely separate, which may delay the frequency of changes based on meeting times of the affected groups, the time it takes to have new standard order set sheets either printed or put on the computer system, and the necessity to adequately train personnel in the use of the updated order sets. In all likelihood, it may take several months after a decision by the P&T committee before the changes can be put into effect. Practitioners should be made well aware of the expected timeline for completion, when such a time difference exists in formulary approval and actual implementation of operations for a formulary change that affects a standard order set. Finally, P&T committees may find that products on standard order sets may be used in ways that are not supported by the medical literature and/or hospital policy, which means that they need to make sure the prescribers or groups that use those orders make necessary changes.

Optimally, individuals or groups using standard orders should be required to review and reapprove their use on a regular basis (probably at least once a year). These standard order sets usually go through an institutional standard order sets committee. In any case, TJC requires a specific policy and procedure for how institutions handle standard order sets.[175] Any changes should be reported to the affected groups (e.g., nursing units, pharmacy, and information technology) and to the P&T committee in cases where the standard order sets include drugs. All standard order sets should include their revision date, to make sure that old copies are not inadvertently used. Old copies of the orders must be maintained for medicolegal purposes, with the length of time for keeping such records to be determined by the institution's legal counsel.

CREDENTIALING AND PRIVILEGES

Health care institutions are required by various groups to verify that prescribers and other health care professionals have the credentials to practice.[263] This can include degrees, licenses, training, and experience. Based on the credentials, professionals may be given credentialing and privileges to practice within that institution and perform certain activities.[264] Please note that this term is privilege, not right. For example, while all physicians may have the same license, only those trained in surgery may be allowed to do more than very minor surgical procedures (e.g., suturing lacerations and removing minor skin growths). There may be even more specific rules, such as those preventing a thoracic surgeon from performing neurosurgery. These privileges can also extend to drugs. For example, it may be decided within the P&T committee that only oncologists have privileges to prescribe most antineoplastic agents. This type of policy and procedure is the basis for some restrictions that may be placed when a drug is considered for formulary addition. In addition to restrictions placed within an institution, restrictions may be enforced from outside the institution.

It also must be mentioned that policies and procedures may be in place within an institution to permit pharmacists to perform certain operations, whether that is the preparation of particular agents or performing specific clinical functions (e.g., intravenous to oral conversion, renal dosing, vancomycin dosing, lab monitoring, TPN ordering, and anticoagulant dosing).[263] Institutions may have a method by which pharmacists are credentialed to perform such services. Further credentialing of pharmacists may be necessary in the future as pharmacist interdependent prescribing becomes more common.[265]

QUALITY IMPROVEMENT WITHIN THE P&T COMMITTEE—INTERNAL AUDIT

❼ *A variety of topics regarding the quality of medication use, inclusive of applicable medication metrics, are normally part of the activities of a P&T committee*, especially timely communication issues. Many of these activities are covered in Chapter 18; however, the items described in the following sections may be considered to be specific to the P&T committee.

Medication Quality Assurance

In addition to determining which medications are available and providing direction in their use, it is required that the quality of use is regularly measured in whatever areas are felt to be necessary, including MUE, DUE, and other similar activities. The P&T committee will likely be involved in this, although coordination of such efforts, including preparing an annual plan of quality assurance activities, may be through other groups, such as a quality assurance committee. The initial plan may be developed by pharmacists, but multidisciplinary feedback is essential before the focused areas of evaluation are finalized. Ideally, all practice areas of the medical staff are given opportunity for input into these focused evaluations. The project list should be continually reviewed and allow for special urgent projects when necessary. If a project is not completed during the year, it may be reconsidered for the next year. DUE criteria selected for continuous improvements should meet TJC accreditation requirements. DUE activities may be used to identify ADRs, contain cost, and expand clinical pharmacy activities.[266] Even if the P&T committee does not direct quality assurance efforts, they must be kept informed of the information gathered and the medication-related quality improvement efforts that are being instituted. This way the P&T committee can be supportive of such efforts directly (e.g., making changes to the drug formulary or policies and procedures to improve medication use) or less directly (e.g., providing statements supporting such activities). Quality assurance is a large topic and further information is available in Chapter 18.

Adverse Drug Reactions

The P&T committee has a responsibility to review adverse reaction data in an institution to identify trends. One tool they can employ is to monitor the use of medications, sometimes referred to as tracer drugs, to treat the symptoms and side effects of other medications.[267] For example, the monitoring of epinephrine, flumazenil, phytonadione, or protamine to try to detect allergic responses, benzodiazepine overdoses, warfarin overdoses, or heparin overdoses, respectively. The topic of ADRs is covered more in Chapter 19.

Medication Error Incidents

Data collected regarding medication errors, even near misses, may be reported to the P&T committee and, probably, for investigational drugs, to the IRB. A systematic method to collect data about medication errors must be set up within an institution, perhaps using internal incident report forms employed by the institution to track all unusual occurrences regarding patients. All incidents are reviewed by severity (e.g., none, minimal, moderate, major, death) and by process (e.g., prescribing, transcription, dispensing, administration, other). A multidisciplinary review of all incidents should take place and trends in the specific quality indicators should be shared with the entire professional staff. High-alert medications (e.g., narcotics, patient-controlled analgesia, insulin, anticoagulants, electrolytes, neuromuscular blockers, thrombolytics, and chemotherapy) should be benchmarked and followed to identify trends to improve the medication management system and ultimately enhance patient safety.

Another monitoring consideration is related to errors with medical devices and may also be monitored by these committees. A study completed in a 520-bed tertiary teaching institution demonstrated that more intensive surveillance methods yielded higher rates of medical device problems as compared to voluntary reporting.[268]

The topic of medication errors is covered in more detail in Chapter 20.

Illegible Handwriting, Transcription, and Abbreviations

It is important to work with the medical staff and all other health professionals regarding illegible handwriting and transcription errors in places where computerized electronic order entry is not utilized, although this has rapidly disappeared. A task force assigned by the P&T committee may be given the charge of evaluating and trending illegible handwriting, followed by developing process improvement measures. A report can be made to the P&T on an ongoing or quarterly basis. An education process must be in place for those individuals who consistently demonstrate poor handwriting. Hands-on reminders have been helpful or, in some extreme cases, handwriting school is recommended. In addition, institutions have adapted TJC unapproved abbreviation list.[15] Unacceptable abbreviations may have an intended meaning but often are potentially misinterpreted and can lead to serious complications. In many institutions, the nurse or pharmacist must clarify the order with the prescriber, when an unapproved abbreviation is written. In some cases, the only effective prevention of this problem has been when the medical staff has determined through the P&T committee that orders containing unapproved abbreviations are completely invalid and must be rewritten by the physician without the inappropriate abbreviation.[269] The addition to the formulary of look-alike, sound-alike medications is discouraged.[270–273] In most cases now, institutions have implemented computerized physician order entry (CPOE), which eliminates the problem of illegible handwriting and decimal point errors, thus reducing medication errors,[274] although implementation costs are considerable, and some institutions may have felt that it was not worth the effort and expense.[275] Also, CPOE may lead to other errors that may turn up in the monitoring for medication errors. In addition, health care practitioners may still be commonly using unacceptable abbreviations in fields where they can input free text.

Timeliness

The time for medication orders to be filled and sent to the floor may be tracked by the P&T committee. One area of importance is the response time sequence for a stat (immediate) order. The time should be evaluated from the time the order was written, to when the order was filled, to when the patient receives the medication. There are many obstacles in the order process and getting the medication to the patient. Each institution should have a standard expectation of the turnaround time for stat orders and a policy that will assure that the medication is dispensed and administered promptly. Benchmarking should be done to make sure the policy is followed.

Although not quite as imperative, the timeliness of ordinary order fulfillment must also be evaluated for appropriateness, although this is likely to be a pharmacy department quality assurance function.

Counterfeit Drug Products

Counterfeit drugs can be considered to be those that do not contain the ingredients claimed on the labeling, perhaps having no active ingredients, incorrect dose, or even other drugs.[276] Counterfeit drugs appear to be an increasing problem, although the actual incidence is unknown.[277] The ASHP partners with the FDA in a program to keep pharmacists informed about entrance of counterfeit drug products into the nation's drug supply. The ASHP planned to provide rapid alerts to hospital pharmacy departments about counterfeit drug incidents.[278] Also, there are methods being developed or implemented that will help to ensure the pedigree of products, particularly those imported from foreign countries, to help avoid counterfeit products. This may include the use of radio frequency identification (RFID) tags to help track products.[279] Regulations are being phased in through 2023 and it is unlikely that it will be known how successful they are until some later date.

The FDA website may be consulted at https://www.fda.gov/safety/medwatch-fda-safety-information-and-adverse-event-reporting-program and the SafeMedication website is found at http://www.safemedication.com/safemed/MedicationTipsTools/WhatYouShouldKnow/RecognizingCounterfeits.aspx for updated lists of counterfeit products. Because of the potential problems associated with counterfeit drug products, the P&T committee must be kept informed of any situations that affect the institution, as should the medical staff as a whole.[277] This topic also may be handled with medication errors, since it leads to such errors. With the approval of the Drug Supply Chain Security Act (DSCSA), several requirements are now in place to prevent counterfeit product from reaching a hospital. A number of companies have developed software to collect the required medication tracking data for auditing purpose by the FDA or other organizations attempting to reduce medication counterfeiting. Hospitals need to evaluate their suppliers to ensure compliance with DSCSA standards and to implement procedures to restrict access for staff to place orders through less reputable, or gray market, vendors. Staff education on how to detect potentially counterfeit medication products is another risk mitigation strategy that can be coordinated with the P&T committee as drug procurement can involve other departments like radiology, supply chain, and physician offices. Additional information on this topic may be found in Chapter 17.

Drug Shortages

Product shortages should be continuously monitored by the pharmacy department in an organized fashion; this is a TJC requirement.[114,175,280] Information on this can be found at http://www.fda.gov/Drugs/DrugSafety/DrugShortages/default.htm or http://www.ashp.org/shortages. It is possible to get a free notification of these shortages. In the past, there has been a trend toward more frequent medication shortages.[281] However, more recent data in the previously mentioned websites suggests a decrease in shortages. In some cases, evaluation of information may show that acceptable alternative products or treatments may be interchanged for products affected by a shortage. The appropriate health care professionals (e.g., prescribers, drug information service, pharmacy director, and buyer) need to be immediately notified of product shortages that may have an effect on therapeutic outcomes, along with plans or recommendations on how to address the situation.[282] In some instances, the chief of the medical staff and even the ethics committee may be consulted when policies need to be put into place to ration drug supplies. The shortage of intravenous immunoglobulin (IVIG) intermittently over the years has necessitated a complete medical staff and pharmacy department agreement for appropriate patient selection for treatment.[283] This shortage required product rationing with the available supply. Unfortunately, few therapeutic alternatives are available for an IVIG shortage. Methods of alerting medical staff of shortages include personal communication, the use of posters or message boards in key areas of the hospital (e.g., medical staff lounge, dictation area, parking garage, and high traffic areas), email, smartphone notification, computer/tablet notification during physician order entry, and the use of newsletters or faxes. This becomes more complex in a large health system, which may experience shortages in different fashions at separate hospitals in the system. A guideline is available from the ASHP to aid in determining how to handle a variety of types of shortages.[280]

In today's health care environment, it is essential to keep medication shortages as a standard agenda item for each P&T meeting. Products with limited availability and products that are not available need to be evaluated constantly. Formulary alternatives for these product shortages then need to be communicated to the medical staff. Further information on this topic may be found in Chapter 17.

Safety Alert

A variety of other safety-related items are also important to P&T committees, including recalls, black box warnings, FDA safety communications, REMS (see Chapter 24),[173] and product shortages, which will be covered in the following subsections and in Chapter 17. The items covered in this section can also be considered related to ADRs and medication errors, since some portions fit under those categories. Also, this information is included in drug evaluation monographs (see Chapter 16).

Recalls

TJC Accreditation Process Guide for Hospitals requires that a policy and procedure be in place, and be implemented when necessary, to retrieve recalled or discontinued medications. This policy must involve notification of prescribers and patients.[15] The pharmacy department constantly reviews medication products recalled by the manufacturer or the FDA due to a safety issue.[280] This information is provided to the pharmacy by the wholesaler and the manufacturer. If a product lot number involved in the recall is found in the pharmacy inventory, that product should be removed from the inventory immediately and recalled from other areas of the institution that may stock it.[175] In the outpatient environment, a recall from consumers may be necessary. A report of medications that have been pulled from the pharmacy inventory should be made available to pharmacy operations and the P&T committee, and the committee may need to decide whether or not to identify patients who may have been affected by the safety issue. Further actions would be based on these findings. The P&T committee chair should be contacted when a patient has significant consequences in relation to a product recall. When a product recall requires the removal of a product treating a disease with limited alternative treatments from the pharmacy inventory, therapeutic alternatives must be made known to the prescribers.[10]

The safety of medications is under constant evaluation, and the safety of new agents cannot be known until the product has been on the market for a period of time.[284] Some newly reported serious adverse effects result in black box warnings being inserted in the product labeling or REMS requirements, which may necessitate action up to the withdrawal of the medication from the market, as was done with propoxyphene.[285] The reason for the black box name is that the warning is set off from the rest of the information in the package insert by a thick black box that is drawn around it. It is the responsibility of the P&T committee to review safety data for every medication on the formulary. Many P&T committees have a standing agenda item to review all new black box warnings or newly released FDA safety alerts for medications (obtainable from http://www.fda.gov/Safety/MedWatch/default.htm). The P&T committee needs to review the safety data and make any formulary, policy and procedure, and/or other changes as required. The black box safety data of formulary products need to be disseminated to the medical staff, including any special restrictions or actions taken on a specific product.[15]

Case Study 15–3

The health system is interested in updating the formulary status for cytomegalovirus immune globulin (Cytogam). The P&T committee decides to restrict the medication to infectious disease (ID) and requires that ID be consulted before any doses are provided to the patient.

- *How will this restriction be implemented?*
- *What needs to be documented for P&T?*
- *How is information shared?*

Communication within an Organization

INSTITUTIONAL REVIEW BOARD

While P&T committees are generally responsible for overseeing all aspects of medication use in a hospital, they often turn the major responsibility for overseeing investigational drug use over to an IRB. The IRB should provide a regular overview of its actions to the P&T committee for review, but oftentimes this is all that is done. Further information about IRBs can be found in Chapter 23.

COST, BUDGET, AND FORECASTING

How does the P&T committee actively balance its quality promoting activities as well as the economic requirements of its parent organization? For an individual hospital, this is probably an easier task as long as the economic pressures on the hospital's margin are manageable. As previously mentioned, a closed formulary can result in lowered costs within an institution.[216] However, the P&T committee decisions will be more difficult for the PBM function of a health insurance company or HMO. In the latter situation, the pressures of cost containment, the contents of an insurance plan's Certificate of Benefits, and the applicable payer regulations represent formidable obstacles for building broad support for the decisions of a PBM's P&T committee. In comparison to institutional formularies, PBM companies have instituted tier-based formularies that encourage the use of more cost-effective agents to control prescription costs and improve therapy.[286,287] In spite of the economic influences on the P&T committee functions of a PBM, there is no end to opportunities for quality improvement by a PBM since there is no other organization that has the ability to access outpatient medication use to the same extent. Regardless of the organizational setting, the requirements for quality as a basis for decisions should be the chief focus of a P&T committee. Obviously, this is a potentially moving target because of the need to achieve a balance between the ethical standards involved in health care. The vested interests of the parent organization, patient's needs and expectations, the professional activities of physicians, pharmacists, and nurses, the pharmaceutical companies, and the requirements of society may be very difficult to reconcile.

National drug expenditure projection data, and the factors likely to influence drug costs for a particular year, can be reviewed by the P&T committee on a yearly basis. Also, it is necessary to keep hospital administrators informed of drug costs and the measures in place to contain costs.[288] An opportunity to inform frontline prescribers of increased drug costs exists in integration with the electronic medical record. In CPOE, a medication order not only can list medication-use guidance (e.g., restriction, guideline, order set) to coach appropriate use, but also include cost information. An institution includes dollar signs next to high-cost medications in the CPOE system in order to inform prescribers of high-cost items.[289,290] An understanding of current trends is also essential for formulary management.[291–293] With knowledge of cost trends, available resources and reports from group purchasing organizations, and historical purchase data from the hospital, pharmacy leaders must attempt to request a rational drug budget and justify the request.

LIAISON WITH OTHER ELEMENTS OF THE ORGANIZATION

Within any organization, it is often found that the root of problems is communications or, perhaps more often, a lack thereof. Unfortunately, the solution is not simply an increase in communication efforts in general. Instead, the need is for increasing appropriate communication, along with decreasing inappropriate communication. Some specific things have to be kept in mind.

All individuals involved in drug therapy should receive concise and effective communication about medication-related matters.[194,294] Often, this may simply be a list of new drugs available to practitioners, along with any policies and procedures. Newsletters and educational presentations may also be valuable, depending on the circumstances. Electronic methods of communication are increasingly important, but the use of in-person counter detailing may be necessary (see Chapter 25).[170]

In addition to making sure that information is provided to those needing it, be sure the amount of material is not overwhelming, otherwise it will be ignored. A news program on television a number of years ago described a situation that the military found regarding its pilots in Vietnam. They had a tape from the cockpit of an aircraft that had been shot down. Those listening to the tape could clearly hear the warning alarm letting the pilot know that a radar missile was locked on his aircraft and posing an imminent danger; however, it was also clear that the pilot did not even realize that warning was happening because of everything else going on. He mentally tuned out the warning and was shot down as a result. It became clear to those training pilots that it was necessary to limit the amount of information to whatever is most important, so that those items were noticed. This is also important in communicating P&T committee materials.

In addition, it is important to keep certain materials confidential for various reasons. In the case of quality assurance materials, keeping materials suitably confidential may protect that data from legal discovery in court (see Chapter 11 and consult attorneys for specifics). Also, some P&T committees keep the agenda and handouts confidential by not sending them to committee members in advance and by collecting the materials at the end of the meeting in order to destroy them. By doing so, they can often avoid pressure put on the committee by pharmaceutical company representatives, who may be trying to have their products included on the formulary, while having their competitor's products excluded. The disadvantage, of course, is that committee members are not able to prepare for a meeting in advance. In relationship to this, it is often a good idea to make sure the pharmaceutical company representatives do not know the members of the committee and who is preparing the evaluation of a particular product, since that can lead to the evaluator being pressured to sway his or her opinion about a particular product. Many hospitals even fully ban pharmaceutical representatives from the hospital to avoid issues.

Finally, an annual report of the P&T committee may be prepared for both internal review and review by the medical executive committee. This annual report is time consuming in preparation but is a very important means of tracking P&T activities and actions over time.

Overall, it is necessary for the chairperson and secretary of the P&T committee to work in cooperation with other appropriate individuals and groups to make sure that essential information is provided wherever needed, while minimizing the amount of extraneous material.

SYNCHRONIZATION OF DATABASES

Although it is more common to think of communication in regard to people, another important area of communications to be addressed is that between electronic databases. The pharmacy computer system may have to communicate with a whole hospital system or other computer systems. It is important to make sure all of these electronic systems are also synchronized, preferably automatically, although the interfaces required to facilitate synchronization may be cost or time prohibitive.[295] In addition, they may introduce medication errors if they are not done properly.

Case Study 15-4

The hospital formulary's preferred intravenous proton pump inhibitor is pantoprazole. As the clinical pharmacy manager, a notice from the ASHP daily bulletin notes there is a current shortage.

- *What steps do you take to investigate?*
- *You learn stock is relatively low and no new stock is expected for several weeks. What is your next step?*
- *How is this recommendation reviewed?*

Conclusion

The pharmacy department can have a major impact on the quality of drug therapy in an institution through participation in P&T committee functions and activities described in this chapter, many of which are related to the management of information or are commonly performed by drug information practitioners. While there are many appropriate ways that may be used in addition to those outlined above, those described can be successfully used to improve drug therapy. Pharmacists trained in literature evaluation provide unbiased support for a P&T committee and formulary process that oversees medication use (addition/restriction/deletion of medications, guidelines, class reviews, policies, medication-use evaluations, etc.). The process implements these decisions into all relevant areas of an organization (e.g., smart pumps, electronic medication record, online portal) to maintain an objective, interprofessional, and patient-focused formulary. A P&T committee and formulary process must strategically manage cost savings, medication use, and medication safety for an organization.

Study Questions

1. What is the P&T committee, what are its functions, and how does the committee relate to a pharmacy department?
2. How should a pharmacy/pharmacist be involved in supporting a P&T committee?
3. Define drug formulary and formulary system. How do those items relate to one another?
4. Define open versus closed formularies, including the specific types of closed formularies.
5. What methods can a P&T committee employ to manage and disseminate information about appropriate medication use?
6. Define a restriction and provide an example.
7. How does a P&T committee improve the quality of medication use in a hospital?
8. Define policy. Define procedure.
9. What are the steps in preparing a policy and procedure?
10. Name and briefly explain four policies and procedures that may be implemented by a P&T committee.
11. How does an institutional P&T committee differ from one in a PBM?

12. Who must a P&T committee communicate with? What should they communicate and how should they communicate?
13. What is considered a conflict of interest?
14. What other areas of a hospital need to be updated after a medication has been added to formulary?

Self-Assessment Questions

1. The P&T committees are utilized in the following organizations:
   a. Hospitals
   b. Health systems
   c. Veterans Affairs
   d. Outpatient infusion centers
   e. Pharmacy Benefits Management companies
   f. All of the above

2. The focus of a P&T committee includes:
   a. Implementing cost-effective prescribing practices
   b. Usage of guidelines
   c. Completion of medication-use evaluations
   d. Collaboration to oversee medication use at an institution
   e. All of the above

3. The Pharmacy and Therapeutics Committee (P&T) can be defined as:
   a. A committee that oversees all aspects of medication therapy in an institution, including development of a formulary, related policies, order sets, guidelines, and quality assurance
   b. A committee that oversees medication and nonmedication procedures of the institution
   c. A committee that oversees only the medications that are carried in a hospital
   d. A committee that oversees only the quality of medication utilization
   e. A committee that oversees only medication errors

4. The P&T committee may act only as:
   a. An advisory body to the medical executive committee
   b. An advisory body to the administration
   c. An advisory body to the board of trustees
   d. An advisory body to the pharmacy

5. The functions of a P&T committee include:
   a. Determining what medications are available
   b. Providing medication-use guidance at point of dispensing
   c. Quality assurance activities
   d. Policies and procedures regarding drug use
   e. All of the above

6. A system P&T committee does the following:
   a. Manages a system formulary for multiple hospitals
   b. Negates the need for a local P&T committee at individual hospitals
   c. Conducts business in person
   d. Coordinates root cause analysis

7. The P&T committee is commonly:
   a. A delegated committee on behalf of a medication executive committee
   b. Led by a well-respected chair
   c. Well-versed in new issues facing medication use, for example, payor impact on ambulatory medications
   d. All of the above

8. The pharmacist serves several functions on a P&T committee, including:
   a. Gathering drug information for a medication review
   b. Completing a medication-use evaluation
   c. Determining which medication should be reviewed
   d. All of the above

9. Preparation by the pharmacist for a P&T committee meeting includes:
   a. Creation of an agenda and content without a prior meeting with the chair of impacted specialty
   b. Presentation of medication-use evaluation results for one hospital in a system-for-system action
   c. Transparent communication of all actions to committee members and medical executives
   d. A solely reactive approach to medication evaluation

10. A P&T's quality improvement functions include:
    a. Drug use review
    b. Compliance surveillance
    c. Medication error analysis
    d. Education
    e. All of the above

11. One of the core elements of a pharmacist's role in P&T is:
    a. Attending patient care rounds
    b. Giving medication education lectures
    c. Communicating all P&T decisions with medical staff including making a formulary available to staff (preferably in an electronic format)

12. The P&T process includes:
    a. Written criteria for addition and deletion of medications
    b. Process for development of criteria
    c. Process to monitor patient responses to medications
    d. An annual review of the formulary
    e. All of the above

13. A medication-use evaluation requires:
    a. An initial plan
    b. Development of criteria
    c. Evaluation of patient charts or available data
    d. Development of process improvement plan
    e. All of the above

14. A drug formulary and a formulary system relate to each other in that:
    a. A drug formulary is a list of available medications under the formulary system which is the method for developing the drug list that reflects the clinical judgment of the medical staff.
    b. A drug formulary comes before a formulary system.
    c. The formulary system provides for a drug formulary that serves only to keep costs down at the expense of patient care.
    d. Where there is a drug formulary system in place there is never a drug formulary published.

15. Pharmacy/pharmacists support the P&T committee by:
    a. Having the P&T committee part of the pharmacy department
    b. Serving as chairperson
    c. Being involved in the rational planning process for each meeting agenda
    d. Only addressing medications to be stocked in the pharmacy

Acknowledgment

Paul Nelson, MD for his assistance on previous editions of this book.

REFERENCES

1. Shulkin DJ. Enhancing the role of physicians in the cost-effective use of pharmaceuticals. Hosp Formul. 1994;29:262-73.
2. Nair KV, Ascione FJ. Evaluation of P&T committee performance: an exploratory study. Hosp Formul. 2001;3:136-46.
3. Zellmer WA. Dr. Avorn's wake-up call to pharmacy. Am J Health-Syst Pharm. 2004;61:2010.
4. Nair KV, Coombs JH, Ascione FJ. Assessing the structure, activities, and functioning of P&T committees: a multisite case study. P&T. 2000;25(10):516-28.
5. Redman RL, Mays DA. Data analysis: drug information services in the managed care setting. Drug Benefit Trends. 1997;9:28-40.
6. Sroka CJ. CRS report for Congress: pharmacy benefit managers. Washington, DC: Library of Congress; 2000 Nov 29.
7. Gourley DR, Halbert MR, Hartmann KM, Malone PM. Development and implementation of a P&T committee for state institutions. Hosp Formul. 1981;16(2):143-4, 149-51, 154-5.
8. McCutcheon T. Medicare prescription drug benefit model guidelines. Washington, DC: United States Pharmacopeial Convention; 2004.
9. Stefanacci RG. The expanding role of P&T committees in long-term care. P&T. 2003;28:720-3.
10. Feldman L. Pharmacists' role in the pharmacy and therapeutics committee. Pharm Times. 2004 Feb:26.
11. Jenkins A. Formulary development by community pharmacists. Pharmaceutical J. 1996;256:861-3.
12. AMA Board of Trustees. Drug formularies and therapeutic interchange H-125.991 [Internet]. Chicago (IL): American Medical Association; 2010 [cited 2020 Jan 27]. 1 p. Available from: https://policysearch.ama-assn.org/policyfinder/detail/Drug%20Formularies%20 and%20Therapeutic%20Interchange%20H-125.991?uri=%2FAMADoc%2FHOD.xml-0-227. xml
13. H-125.991 drug formularies and therapeutic interchange [Internet]. Chicago (IL): American Medical Association; 2000 [cited 2004 Mar 9]. 2 p. Available from: https:// policysearch.ama-assn.org/policyfinder/detail/Drug%20Formularies%20and%20 Therapeutic%20Interchange%20H-125.991?uri=%2FAMADoc%2FHOD.xml-0-227.xml
14. Formulary management (medication-use policy development) [Internet]. Bethesda: American Society of Health-System Pharmacists; 2004 [cited 2019 Nov 12]. 1 p. Available from: https://www.ashp.org/-/media/assets/policy-guidelines/docs/policy-positions/ policy-positions-formulary-management.ashx?la=en&hash=DC8648C51DA367C6BDFFB 29C8C61643DA6DFA35E%20%20%20?

15. TJC—The Joint Commission comprehensive accreditation and certification manual [Internet]. Accreditation requirements for hospitals [Internet]. Oakbrook Terrace (IL): The Joint Commission; 2013 Jan 1 [cited 2012 Dec 14]. Available from: https://e-dition. jcrinc.com/MainContent.aspx

16. Format for formulary submissions. Version 4.0. Alexandria (VA): Academy of Managed Care Pharmacy; 2016.

17. The AMCP format for formulary submissions. Version 4.1. Select provisions for public comment. Alexandria (VA): Academy of Managed Care Pharmacy; 2019.

18. Raffel MW, Barsukiewicz CK. The US health system: origins and functions. Albany (NY): Delmar; 2002.

19. Balu S, O'Connor P, Vogenberg FR. Contemporary issues affecting P&T committees. Part 1: The evolution. P&T. 2004;29:709-11.

20. Worthen DB. The amazing Charles Rice and Bellevue Hospital [Internet]. Pharm Pract News. 2010;37(06):[2 p.]. Available from: https://www.google.com/ search?rlz=1C1GCEA_enUS850US851&q=Worthen+DB.+The+amazing+Charles+Rice+a nd+Bellevue+Hospital+2010+pharmacypractice&tbm=isch&source=univ&sa=X&ved=2a hUKEwiCr_GO47DlAhXsJzQIHYjSA1UQsAR6BAgREAE&biw=1920&bih=977#imgrc=V m3jfD5SyQZDRM

21. Condition of participation: pharmaceutical services. Fed Regist. 1986;51:22042.

22. Millano C. Bellevue Hospital: the birthplace of formulary medicine? Pharm Pract News. 2004;31:14.

23. Plumridge RJ, Stoelwinder JU, Rucker TD. Drug and therapeutics committees: the relationships among structure, function, and effectiveness. Hosp Pharm. 1993;28:492-3, 496-8, 508.

24. World Health Organization, Management Sciences for Health. Drug and therapeutics committees—a practical guide. Geneva (Switzerland): World Health Organization; 2003.

25. Doherty EC. The JCAHO agenda for change: what changes in pharmacy and P&T activities do you need to prepare for in 1994. Hosp Formul. 1994;29:54-68.

26. The Joint Commission on Accreditation of Health care Organizations. 1995 Comprehensive Accreditation Manual for Hospitals. Oakbrook Terrace (IL): Joint Commission on Accreditation of Healthcare Organizations; 1994.

27. Academy of Managed Care Pharmacy. Principles of a sound drug formulary system. 2000 [cited 2004 Mar 18]. Available from: https://www.ashp.org/-/media/assets/policy-guidelines/docs/endorsed-documents/endorsed-documents-principles-sound-drug-formulary-system.ashx

28. Leonard MC, Thyagarajan R, Wilson AJ, Sekeres MA. Strategies for success in creating an effective multihospital health-system pharmacy and therapeutics committee. Am J Health-Syst Pharm. 2018;75(7):451-5.

29. Eavy GR, Swinkey NJ, Rehan A. Decentralizing the P&T committee: rationale and successes. Formulary. 2000;35:752-69.

30. Al-Jedai AH, Algain RA, Alghamidi SA, Al-Jazairi AS, Amin R, Bin Hussain IZ. A P&T committee's transition to a complete electronic meeting system—a multisite institution experience. P&T. 2017;42(10):641-6, 651.

31. Mubarak-Shaban H, Billups SJ. The pharmacy and therapeutics committee within a hospital corporation: challenges and solution. P&T. 1998;23(6):309-10, 332.

32. Herbert WJ, Mahaney LM. Consolidating P&T committees in an integrated health care system. Formulary. 1996;31:497-504.

33. Cano SB. Formularies in integrated health systems: Fallon health care system. Am J Health-Syst Pharm. 1996;53:270-3.

34. Rizos AL, Levy E, Furnier J, Crowley K. Formularies in integrated health systems: Sharp HealthCare. Am J Health-Syst Pharm. 1996;53:274-8.

35. Barkley GL, Krol G, Anandan JV, Isopi M. An integrated health care system's attempt to create a unified formulary. Formulary. 1997;32:60-74.

36. Jarry PD, Fish L. Insights on outpatient formulary management in a vertically integrated health care system. Formulary. 1997;32:500-14.

37. CHI Health Pharmacy and therapeutics committee [Internet]. CHI Health. 2016 July [cited 2016 Aug 10]; [5 p.]. Available from: https://chihealth-all.policystate.com/policy/253510/

38. Glowczewski JE, Osborne SM. Aligning health system formularies for cost savings. Pharm Purchas Prod. 2015;12(11):4-8.

39. Anagnostis E, Wordell C, Guharoy R, Beckett R, Price V. A national survey on hospital formulary management processes. J Pharm Pract. 2011;24(4):409-16.

40. Mannebach MA, Ascione FJ, Gaither CA, Bagozzi RP, Cohen IA, Ryan ML. Activities, functions, and structure of pharmacy and therapeutics committees in large teaching hospitals. Am J Health-Syst Pharm. 1999;56:622-8.

41. Helmons PJ, Kosternik JGW, Daniels C. Formulary compliance and pharmacy labor costs associated with systematic formulary management strategy. Am J Health-Syst Pharm. 2014;71:407-15.

42. Rodriguez R, Kelly BJ, Moody M. Evaluating the training, responsibilities, and practices of P&T committee members and nonmember contributors. J Manag Care Spec Pharm. 2017;23:868-74.

43. Balu S, O'Connor P, Vogenberg FR. Contemporary issues affecting P&T committees. Part 2: Beyond managed care. P&T. 2004;29:780-3.

44. Solow BK. P&T committees today: ensuring they bring value to your organization. Am J Pharm Benefits. 2009;1(4):189-90.

45. Teagarden JR. How many members should be on a P&T committee. P&T Society. 2003 Fall.

46. Miller WA. Making the pharmacy and therapeutics committee more effective. Curr Concepts Hosp Pharm Manage. 1986;Summer:10-15.

47. Bono RC. Charter Department of Defense pharmacy and therapeutics committee [Internet]. Washington; 2015 Dec 18 [cited 2019 May 20]; [5 p.]. Available from: https://health.mil/Reference-Center/Policies/2015/12/18/DoD-Pharmaceutical-and-Therapeutics-Committee-Charter

48. Barlas S. Role of P&T committees in Medicare: how much authority, accountability? P&T. 2004;29:678.

49. Cross M. Increased pressures change P&T Committee makeup. Managed Care. 2001:10(12):18-30.

50. Heindel GA, McIntyre CM. Contemporary challenges and novel strategies for health-system formulary management. Am J Health-Syst. Pharm. 2018;75(8):556-60.

51. Smeeding J, Malone D, Rachandani M, Stolshek B, Green L, Schneider P. Biosimilars: considerations for payers. P&T. 2019;44(2):54-63.

52. Ventola CL. Evaluation of biosimilars for formulary inclusion: factors for consideration by P&T committees. P&T. 2015;40(10):680-9.

53. Trovato A, Choudhary K, Fox ER. Development and implementation of a strategy to ensure outpatient access to medications started in the inpatient setting. Am J Health-Syst Pharm. 2019;76(6):334-5.

54. Leber MB. Considerations for adding biosimilars to formulary. Pharm Purch Prod. 2017;14(12):24.

55. The ABCs of PBMs. A discussion featuring Peter D. Fox, Ph.D., Terry S. Latanich, Chris O'Flinn, J.D. LLM, and Phonzie Brown. Washington, DC: The George Washington University. National Health Policy Forum. Issue Brief No. 749; 1999 Oct 27.

56. Lipton HL, Kreling DH, Collins T, Hertz KC. Pharmacy benefit management companies: dimensions of performance. Annu Rev Public Health. 1999;20:361-401.

57. Cross M. Do P&T committees have enough power? Manage Care. 2007;16(4):28-30.

58. Reinke T. PBMs just say no to some drugs—but not to others. Manage Care. 2015;24(4):24-6.

59. Teagarden JR. Perspectives on prescription drug benefit formularies. Hosp Pharm. 2004;39:1102-25.

60. PricewaterhouseCoopers. The value of pharmacy benefit management and the national cost impact of proposed PBM legislation. Pharmaceutical Care Management Association; 2004 Jul.

61. Barlas S. Formulary policies a battleground in HHS proposal on nondiscrimination. Are tiering and cost sharing civil rights issues? P&T. 2016;41(3):173-5,193.

62. Barlas S. HHS proposes formulary changes for marketplace health plans. P&T committees would take on a more visible role. P&T. 2015;40(2):119-22.

63. Regnier SA. How does drug coverage vary by insurance type? Analysis of drug formularies in the United States. Am J Manage Care. 2014;20(4):322-31.

64. Vogenberg FR, Marcoux R, Rumore MM. Systemic market and organizational changes: impact on P&T committees. P&T. 2017;42(1):28-32.

65. Carroll J. Plans look askance at me-too medications. Manage Care. 2008;17(1):37-42.

66. Butler CD, Manchester R. The P&T committee: descriptive survey of activities and time requirements. Hosp Formul. 1986;21:89-98.

67. Chi J. When R.Ph.s talk P&T committees listen. Hosp Pharm Rep. 1994;8(5):1, 7-8.

68. Gannon K. More power to you. Pharmacists flex their muscles and exert greater influence on P&T committees. Hosp Pharm Rep. 1998;12(2):18-20.

69. 5 best practices for P&T committee members [Internet]. University of Wisconsin-Madison. [Cited 2019 Jul 3]. Available from: https://ce.pharmacy.wisc.edu/blog/5-best-practices-for-pt-committee-members/

70. Chase P, Bell J, Smith P, Fallik A. Redesign of the P&T committee around continuous quality improvement principles. P&T. 1995;20(10):25-26, 29-30, 32, 34, 37-8, 40.

71. Croft CL, Crane VS. Redesign of P&T committee functions and processes: a model. Formulary. 1998;33:1105-22.

72. Crane VS, Gonzalez ER, Hull BL. How to develop a proactive formulary system. Hosp Formul. 1994;29:700-10.

73. Karel LI, Delisle DR, Anagnostis EA, Wordell CJ. Implementation of a formulary management process. Am J Health-Syst Pharm. 2017;74(16):1245-52.

74. Poirier TI, Vorbach M, Bache T. Linking a policy on nonformulary drugs to the FDA's therapeutic–potential classification system. Am J Hosp Pharm. 1994;51:2277-8.

75. Abu Esba LC, Almodaimegh H, Alhammad A, Ferwana M, Yousef C, Ismail S. P&T committee drug prioritizations criteria: a tool developed by a Saudi health care system. P&T. 2018;43(5):293-300.

76. Rich DS. Pharmacies' noncompliance with 2009 Joint Commission hospital accreditation requirements. Am J Health-Syst Pharm. 2009;66:e27-30.

77. Green JA, Chawla AK, Fong PA. Evaluating a restrictive formulary system by assessing nonformulary-drug requests. Am J Hosp Pharm. 1985;42:1537-41.

78. Hailemeskel B, Kelvas M. Nonformulary drug requests as a guide in formulary system management. Am J Health-Syst Pharm. 1999;56:818, 820.

79. Adding drugs to the formulary: your work is never done. Hosp Pharm. 1999;34(7):828.

80. Shea BF, Churchill WW, Powell SH, Cooley TW, Maguire JH. P&T committee overview: Brigham and Women's Hospital. Pharm Pract Manag Q. 1998;17(4):76-83.

81. Stefanacci RG. Dealing with new formulary types: health system outpatient formularies. J Clin Pathways. 2018;4:34-5.

82. Chen M. Medicare biosimilar reimbursement: Hopes for cost savings, a dream deferred [Internet]. Managed Care. 2018 Apr 18 [cited 2019 Nov 27]. Available from: https://www.managedcaremag.com/pharmdcorner/medicare-biosimilar-reimbursement-hopes-cost-savings-dream-deferred

83. Picone MF, Hayes GL, Wisniewski CS. Use of economic predictions to make formulary decisions. Am J Health-Syst Pharm. 2019; 76(suppl 1):S15-20.

84. McCain J. P&T Committees in position to reduce medication errors. Manage Care. 2004;13(6):39-42.

85. National Patient Safety Goal for anticoagulant therapy. R3 Report. 2018 Dec 7 [cited 2019 Sep 26]; [1-4 p.]. Available from: https://www.jointcommission.org/assets/1/18/R3_19_Anticoagulant_therapy_FINAL2.PDF

86. Cunha BA. Principles of antibiotic formulary selection for P&T committees. P&T. 2003;28(6):396.

87. Empey KM, Rapp RP, Evans ME. The effect of an antimicrobial formulary change on hospital resistance patterns. Pharmacotherapy. 2002;22(1):81-7.

88. Cunha BA. Principles of antibiotic formulary selection for P&T committees. Part 1: Antimicrobial activity. P&T. 2003;28(6):397-9.

89. Cunha BA. Principles of antibiotic formulary selection for P&T committees. Part 2: Pharmacokinetics and pharmacodynamics. P&T. 2003;28(7):468-70.

90. Cunha BA. Principles of antibiotic formulary selection for P&T committees. Part 3: Antibiotic resistance. P&T. 2003;28(8):524-7.

91. Polk RE. Antimicrobial formularies: can they minimize antimicrobial resistance? Am J Health-Syst Pharm. 2003;60(Suppl 1):S16-S19.

92. Cunha BA. Principles of antibiotic formulary selection for P&T committees. Part 4: Antimicrobial side effects. P&T. 2003;28(9):594-6.

93. Cunha BA. Principles of antibiotic formulary selection for P&T committees. Part 5: The cost of antimicrobial therapy. P&T. 2003;28:662-5.

94. Motz JC. Influence of the P&T committee on antibiotic selection in a staff model HMO. P&T. 1998;23(8):411-8.

95. DiLiegro N, Groves AJ, Caspi A. Cost savings from an antimicrobial-monitoring program. P&T. 1998;23(8):419-24.

96. Carlson JA. Antimicrobial formulary management: meeting the challenge in a health maintenance organization. Pharmacotherapy. 1991;11(1 pt 2):32S-35S.

97. Quintiliani R, Quercia RA. How to create a therapeutics committee that is scientifically and economically sound. Formulary. 2003;38:594-602.

98. Owen RC, Shorr AF, Deschambeault AL. Antimicrobial stewardship: shepherding precious resources. Am J Health-Syst Pharm. 2009;66(suppl4):S15-22.

99. Lesprit P, Brun-Buisson C. Hospital antibiotic stewardship. Curr Opin Infect Dis. 2008;21:344-9.

100. Drew RH. Antimicrobial stewardship programs: how to start and steer a successful program. J Manag Care Pharm. 2009;15(2)(Suppl):S18-S23.

101. Chen AWJ, Khumra S, Eaton V, Kong DCM. Snapshot of antimicrobial stewardship in Australian hospitals. J Pharm Pract Res. 2010;40(1):19-25.

102. Deuster S, Roten I, Muehlebach S. Implementation of treatment guidelines to support judicious use of antibiotic therapy. J Clin Pharm Ther. 2010;35:71-8.

103. Approved: new antimicrobial stewardship standard [Internet]. The Joint Commission. 2016 [cited 2017 Sep 18]. Available from: https://www.jointcommission.org/assets/1/6/New_Antimicrobial_Stewardship_Standard.pdf

104. Culley CM, Carroll BA, Skledar SJ. Formulary decisions for pre-1938 medications. Am Health-Syst Pharm. 2008;65(15): 1368-83.

105. Medication errors and adverse drug events [Internet]. Rockville (MD): PSNet; 2019 Jan [cited 2019 Sep 26]; [6 p.]. Available from: https://psnet.ahrq.gov/primer/medication-errors-and-adverse-drug-events

106. Targeted medication safety best practices for hospitals [Internet]. Institute for Safe Medication Practices. c2018 [cited 2020 Jan 27]. Available from: https://www.ismp.org/sites/default/files/attachments/2019-01/TMSBP-for-Hospitalsv2.pdf

107. Medical device overview [Internet]. Silver Springs (MD): Food and Drug Administration. 2018 Sep 14 [cited 2020 Jan 28]; [7 p.]. Available from: https://www.fda.gov/industry/regulated-products/medical-device-overview#What%20is%20a%20medical%20device

108. Mirtallo JM. Advancement of nutrition support clinical pharmacy. Ann Pharmacother. 2007;41:869-872.

109. The Joint Commission. 2010 Provision of Care, Treatment and Services. The Joint Commission Web. [Cited 2010 Oct 21]. Available from: http://www.jointcommission.org

110. Fagan NL, Malone PM, Baltaro RJ, Malesker MA. Applying the principles of formulary management to blood banking. Transfusion. 2013;53:2094-7.

111. Anagnostis E. Writing meeting minutes for a pharmacy and therapeutics committee and its subcommittees. Am J Health-Syst Pharm. 2015;72:95-9.

112. Austin JP, Halvorson SAC. Reducing the expert halo effect on pharmacy and therapeutics committees. JAMA. 2019;321(5):453-4.

113. ASHP statement on the pharmacy and therapeutics committee. Am J Hosp Pharm. 1992;49:2008-9.

114. Ventola CL. An interview series with members of the ASHP Expert Panel on Formulary Management. Part 1: Linda S. Tyler, Pharm.D. P&T. 2009;34(11):623-31.

115. Brushwood DB. Legal issues surrounding therapeutic interchange in institutional settings: an update. Formulary. 2001;36:796-804.

116. Mutnick AH, Ross MB. Formulary management at a tertiary care teaching hospital. Pharm Pract Manag Q. 1997;17(1):63-87.

117. Dore DD, Larrat EP, Vogenberg FR. Principles of epidemiology for clinical and formulary management professionals. P&T. 2006;31(4):218-26.

118. Suh D, Okpara I, Agnese WB, Toscani M. Application of pharmacoeconomics to formulary decision making in managed care organizations. Am J Managed Care. 2002;8(2):161-9.

119. Odedina FT, Sullivan J, Nash R, Clemmons CD. Use of pharmacoeconomic data in making hospital formulary decisions. Am J Health-Syst Pharm. 2002;59:1441-4.

120. Getting the most out of formularies involves a bit of economic training. Manage Care. 2015;24(4):9-10.

121. Studdert AL, Gong CL, Srinavas S, Chin AL, Deresinski S. Application of pharmacoeconomics to formulary management in a health system setting. Am J Health-Syst Pharm. 2019;76(6):381-6.

122. Pick AM, Massoomi F, Neff WJ, Danekas PL, Stoysich AM. A safety assessment tool for formulary candidates. Am J Health-Syst Pharm. 2006;63:1269-72

123. Barr B. Open and closed. Pharmaceutical Representative [Internet]. 2007 May 1 [cited 2008 Jul 14]; [4 p.]. Available from: http://www.pharmexec.com/open-and-closed

124. ASHP statement on the formulary system. Am J Hosp Pharm. 1983;35:326-8.

125. Heindel GA, McIntyre CM. Contemporary challenges and novel strategies for health-system formulary management. Am J Health-Syst Pharm. 2018;75(8):556-60.

126. ASHP technical assistance bulletin on drug formularies. Am J Hosp Pharm. 1991; 48:791-3.

127. ASHP guidelines on formulary system management. Am J Hosp Pharm. 1992;49:648-52.

128. Rucker TD, Schiff G. Drug formularies: myths-in-formation. Med Care. 1990;28:928-42.

129. Tyler LS, Cole SW, May JR, Millares M, Valentino MA, Vermeulen LC Jr, Wilson AL. ASHP guidelines on the pharmacy and therapeutics committee and the formulary system. Am J Health-Syst Pharm. 2008;65:1272-83.

130. Grissinger M. The truth about hospital formularies. Part I. P&T. 2008;33(8):441.

131. Lehmann DF, Guharoy R, Page N, Hirschman K, Ploutz-Snyder R, Medicis J. Formulary management as a tool to improve medication use and gain physician support. Am J Health-Syst Pharm. 2007;64:464-6.

132. ASHP statement on the pharmacy and therapeutics committee and the formulary system. Am J Health-Syst Pharm. 2008;65:2384-6.

133. Rubino M, Hofman JM, Koseserer LJ, Swendryznski RG. ASHP guidelines on medication cost management strategies for hospitals and health systems. Am J Health-Syst Pharm. 2008;65:1368-84.

134. Keedy CA, Schnibben AP, Crosby JF Jr, McGlasson ACL, Misher A. Am J Health-Syst Pharm. 2018;75(23):1854,1856.

135. Chi J. Hospital consultant foresees dim future for drug formularies. Drug Topics. 1999 April 19:67.

136. Horn SD, Sharkey PD, Tracy DM, Horn C, James B, Goodwin F. Intended and unintended consequences of HMO cost-containment strategies: results from the managed care outcomes project. Am J Manag Care. 1996;2:253-64.

137. Horn SD. Unintended consequences of drug formularies. Am J Health-Syst Pharm. 1996;53:2204-6.

138. Goldberg RB. Managing the pharmacy benefit: the formulary system. J Manag Care Pharm. 1997;3(5):565-73.

139. Formulary effectiveness: many questions, but few clear answers. Consult Pharm. 1996;11(7):635.

140. Curtiss FR. Drug formularies provide a path to best care. Am J Health-Syst Pharm. 1996;53:2201-3.

141. Formularies and generics drive up health resource use, study suggests. Am J Health-Syst Pharm. 1996;53:971-5.

142. Horn SD, Sharkey PD, Phillips-Harris C. Formulary limitations and the elderly: results from the managed care outcomes project. Am J Manag Care. 1998;4:1105-13.

143. Marra F, Patrick DM, White R, Ng H, Bowie WR, Hutchinson JM. Effect of formulary policy decisions on antimicrobial drug utilization in British Columbia. J Antimicrob Chemother. 2005;55:95-101.

144. Penm J, Chaar B, Dechun J, Moles R. Formulary systems in the Western Pacific Region: exploring two Basel Statements. Am J Health-Syst Pharm. 2013;70:967-79.

145. Hepler CD. Where is the evidence for formulary effectiveness. Am J Health-Syst Pharm. 1997;54:95.

146. VHA formulary management process. Washington: Department of Veterans Affairs; 2009.

147. Kelly WN, Rucker TD. Considerations in deciding which drugs should be in a formulary. J Pharm Pract. 1994;VII(2):51-7.

148. Corman SL, Skledar SJ, Culley CM. Evaluation of conflicting literature and application to formulary decisions. Am J Health-Sys Pharm. 2007;64:182-5.

149. Shih Y-C T, Sleath BL. Health care provider knowledge of drug formulary status in ambulatory care settings. Am J Health-Syst Pharm. 2004;61:2657-63.

150. Muirhead G. When formularies collide: hospitals vs. health plans. Hosp Pharm Rep. 1994;8(10):1, 8.

151. 1999 accreditation standards address public concerns, says NCQA. Am J Health-Syst Pharm. 1998;55:2221, 2225.

152. Bruzek RJ, Dullinger D. Drug formulary: the cornerstone of a managed pharmacy program. J Pharm Pract. 1992;V(2):75-81.

153. North GLT. Handling nonformulary requests for returning or transfer patients. Am J Hosp Pharm. 1994;51:2360, 2364.

154. Davis FA. Formularies: a dangerous concept for patients. Priv Pract. 1991 Sep:11-17.

155. Palmer MA, Hartman SK, Gervais S. Introducing a formulary system in long-term care facilities: initial experience. Consult Pharm. 1994;9:307-14.

156. Shulkin DJ. Enhancing the role of physicians in the cost-effective use of pharmaceuticals. Hosp Formul. 1994;29:262-73.

157. Pearce MJ, Begg EJ. A review of limited lists and formularies. Are they cost-effective? Pharmacoeconomics. 1992;1:191-202.

158. Sloan FA, Gordon GS, Cocks DL. Hospital drug formularies and use of hospital services. Med Care. 1993;31:851-67.

159. Hazlet TK, Hu T-W. Association between formulary strategies and hospital drug expenditures. Am J Hosp Pharm. 1992;49:2207-10.

160. Pickette S, Hanish L. Dealing with demands for nonformulary drugs. Am J Hosp Pharm. 1992;49:2920, 2923.

161. Corliss DA. Computer-assisted help desk for handling drug benefits. Am J Health-Syst Pharm. 1997;54:1941-42, 1945.

162. NCQA draft accreditation standards for 2000 address formularies. Am J Health-Syst Pharm. 1998;55:1266-7.

163. Le AG, Generali JA. From printed formularies to online formularies. Hosp Pharm. 2004;38:1003.

164. Navarro RP. Electronic formulary control. Med Interface. 1997;10(8):74-6.

165. Drug czars, electronic formulary systems increase formulary compliance. Formulary. 1997;32:171-2.

166. Ukens C. Hospital finds computer carrot can save drug dollars. Hosp Pharm Rep. 1994;8(6):20.

167. Computerized drug cost information fails to sway physician prescribing. Am J Health-Syst Pharm. 1999;56:1183-4.

168. Sears EL. Development and maintenance of an online formulary for a large health system. Am J Health-Syst Pharm. 2008;65:510,512.

169. E-prescribing applications help physicians with Vioxx recall. Pharm Pract News. 2004;31(11):67.

170. Patel B, Pichardo RV. Improve formulary adherence through effective provider engagement. Formulary. 2012;47:400-1.

171. McCaffrey S, Nightingale CH. How to develop critical paths and prepare for other formulary management changes. Hosp Formul. 1994;29:628-35.

172. Current formulary decision-making strategies and new factors influencing the process. Formulary. 1995;30:462-70.

173. Raber JH. The formulary process from a risk management perspective. Pharmacother. 2010;30(6 Pt 2):42S-47S.

174. Shulkin D. Reinventing the pharmacy and therapeutics committee. P&T. 2012 Nov;37(11):623-4, 649.

175. Rich DS. New JCAHO medication management standards for 2004. Am J Health-Syst Pharm. 2004;61:1349-58.

176. Neumann PJ. Evidence-based and value-based formulary guidelines. Health Aff (Millwood). 2004;23(1):124-34.

177. Murri NA, Somani S. Implementation of safety-focused pharmacy and therapeutics monographs: a new University Health System Consortium template designed to minimize medication misadventures. Hosp Pharm. 2004;39:654-60.

178. Chren M-M, Landefeld CS. Physicians' behavior and their interactions with drug companies. JAMA. 1994;271:684-9.

179. Bach PB, Saltz LB, Wittes RE. In cancer care, cost matters. New York Times. 2012 Oct 14:A25.

180. Haslé-Pham E, Arnould B, Späth H-M, Follet A, Duru G, Marquis P. Role of clinical, patient-reported outcome and medico-economic studies in the public hospital drug formulary decision-making process: results of a European survey. Health Policy. 2005;71:205-12.

181. Ventola CL. An interview series with members of the ASHP Expert Panel on Formulary Management. Part 3: Sabrina W. Cole, Pharm.D. P&T. 2010;35(1):24-8.

182. Shrank WH. Change we can believe in: requiring better evidence for formulary coverage. Am J Pharm Benefits. 2009;Fall:134-6.

183. Asmus MJ, Hendeles L. Levalbuterol nebulizer solution: is it worth five times the cost of albuterol? Pharmacother. 2000;20:123-9.

184. Desloratadine (Clarinex). Med Lett. 2002;44(W1126B):27-9.

185. Escitalopram (Lexapro) for depression. Med Lett. 2002;44(W1140A):83-4.

186. Most medications approved in the 1990s not new, but modified versions of older drugs, report states [Internet]. Menlo Park (CA): kaisernetwork.org; 2002 May 29 [cited 2004 Apr 22]. Available from: http://khn.org/morning-breakout/dr00011414/

187. Senthilkumaran K, Shatz SM, Kalies RF. Computer-based support system for formulary decisions. Am J Hosp Pharm. 1987;44:1362-6.

188. Computer tool lets P&T members assess Tx classes with their own weightings, product ratings. Formulary. 2000;35:603.

189. Janknegt R, Steenhoek A. The system of objectified judgement analysis (SOJA). A tool in rational drug selection for formulary inclusion. Drugs. 1997;53(4):550-62.

190. Janknegt R, van den Broek PJ, Kulberg BJ, Stobberingh E. Glycopeptides: drug selection by means of the SOJA method. Eur Hosp Pharm. 1997;3(4):127-35.

191. Zachry WM III, Skrepnek GH. Applying multiattribute utility technology to the formulary evaluation process. Formulary. 2002;37:199-206.

192. Berghelli JA. Conflict of interest policy approved. P&T. 1995;20:497.

193. Alpert JS. Doctors and the drug industry: how can we handle potential conflicts of interest? Am J Med. 2005;118:88-100.

194. Ventola CL. An interview series with members of the ASHP Expert Panel on Formulary Management. Part 2: J. Russell May, Pharm.D. P&T. 2009;34(12):671-7.

195. Campbell EG. Doctors and drug companies—scrutinizing influential relationships. NEJM. 2007;357(18):1796-7.

196. Palmer MA. Developing a conflict-of-interest policy for the pharmacy and therapeutics committee. Am J Hosp Pharm. 1987;44:2012-4.

197. Fredrick DS, Maddock JR, Graman PS. Hashing out a policy on conflicts of interest for a P&T committee. Am J Health-Syst Pharm. 1995;52:2791-2.

198. Campbell EG. A national survey of physician-industry relationships. NEJM. 2007;356:1742-50.

199. Barlas S. Inspector General cautions PBMs on formulary decision making. P&T. 2003;28(6):367.

200. Trice S, Devine J, Mistry H, Moore E, Linton A. Formulary management in the Department of Defense. J Managed Care Pharmacy. 2009;15(2):133-46.

201. Total number of orphan drug approvals in the month requiring exclusivity determinations. [Internet]. U.S. FDA; 2019 Jun 30 [cited 2019 Nov 12]. Available from: https://www.accessdata.fda.gov/scripts/fdatrack/view/track.cfm?program=osmp&id=OSMP-OOPD-Number-orphan-drug-approvals-in-the-month

202. Johnson CY. High prices make once-neglected 'orphan' drugs a booming business. [Internet]. Wash Post. 2016 Aug 4 [cited 2016 Aug 10]. Available from: https://www.washingtonpost.com/business/economy/high-prices-make-once-neglected-orphan-drugs-a-booming-business/2016/08/04/539d0968-1e10-11e6-9c81-4be1c14fb8c8_story.html

203. JCAHO unveils medication-management standards. Am J Health-Syst Pharm. 2003;60:1400-1.

204. Cardinale V. Alternative medicine: the law, the marketplace, the formulary. Hosp Pharm Rep. 1999;13(7):15.

205. Is alternative medicine poised for hospital formularies. Drug Util Rev. 1999;15(5):65-8.

206. Brubaker ML. Setting up the herbal formulary system for an alternative medicine clinic. Am J Health-Syst Pharm. 1998;55:435-6.

207. Beal FC. Herbals and homeopathic remedies as formulary items. Am J Health-Syst Pharm. 1998;55:1266-7.

208. Johnson ST, Wordell CJ. Homeopathic and herbal medicine: considerations for formulary evaluation. Formulary. 1997;32:1166-73.

209. Malesker MA, Meyer RT, Kuhlenengel LJ, Galt MA, Nelson PJ. Development of an alternative medication use policy [abstract]. ASHP Midyear Clinical Meeting. 1998; 33(Dec):P-406R.

210. Walker PC. Evolution of a policy disallowing the use of alternative therapies in a health system. Am J Health-Syst Pharm. 2000;57:1984-90.

211. Ansani NT, Ciliberto NC, Freedy T. Hospital policies regarding herbal medicines. Am J Health-Syst Pharm. 2003;60:367-70.

212. Pick AM, Massoomi F, Neff WJ, Danekas PI, Stoysich AM. A safety assessment tool for formulary candidates. Am J Health-Syst Pharm. 2006;63:1269-72.

213. Dennis B, Cha AE. "Right to Try" laws spur debate over dying patients' access to experimental drugs [Internet]. Wash Post. 2014 May 16 [cited 2016 Aug 10]. Available from: https://www.washingtonpost.com/national/health-science/right-to-try-laws-spur-debate-over-dying-patients-access-to-experimental-drugs/2014/05/16/820e08c8-dcfa-11e3-b745-87d39690c5c0_story.html

214. H-125.911 Drug formularies and therapeutic interchange [Internet]. Chicago (IL): American Medical Association; [cited 2004 Apr 23]. Available from: https://policysearch.ama-assn.org/policyfinder/detail/Drug%20Formularies%20and%20Therapeutic%20Interchange%20H-125.991?uri=%2FAMADoc%2FHOD.xml-0-227.xml

215. NCQA draft accreditation standards for 2000 address formularies. Am J Health-Syst Pharm. 1999;56:846.

216. Chiefari DM. Effect of a closed formulary on average prescription cost in a community health center. Drug Benefit Trends. 2001;13:44-5, 52.

217. Survey reveals continued HMO shift toward closed and partially closed formularies. Formulary. 1997;32:781-2.

218. Survey finds HMOs, PBMs still moving to restricted formularies, quickly advancing in informatics. Formulary. 1998;33:622, 625.

219. Doyle JJ. The effect of comparative effectiveness research on drug development innovation: a 360° value appraisal. Comp Effectiveness Res. 2011;1:27-34.

220. Abramowitz PW. Controlling financial variables—changing prescribing patterns. Am J Hosp Pharm. 1984;41:503-15.

221. Open formularies improve oncology outcomes in capitated care system. Formulary. 1996;31:878, 881.

222. TennCare formulary restrictions hurt patient care, survey says. Formulary. 1996;31(6):443.

223. Vincent WR III, Huiras P, Empfield J, Horbowicz KJ, Lewis K, McAneny D, Twitchell D. Controlling postoperative use of i.v. acetaminophen at an academic medical center. Am J Health-Syst Pharm. 2018;75(8):548-55.

224. Traynor K. Virginia passes nation's first biosimilar substitution law. Am J Health-Syst Pharm. 2013;70:834-6.

225. Labeling for biosimilar products. Guidance for industry. Washington (DC): U.S. Department of Health and Human Services, June 2018.

226. Blank C. Arizona passes pharmacy biosimilar law [Internet]. Drug Topics. 2016 Jun 2 [cited 2016 Aug 10]. Available from: https://www.drugtopics.com/associations/arizona-passes-pharmacy-biosimilar-law

227. Gabay M. Biosimilar substitution laws. Hosp Pharm. 2017;52(8):544-5.

228. Ventola CL. Evaluation of biosimilars for formulary inclusion: factors for consideration by P&T committees. P&T. 2015;40:680-9.

229. Schachtner JM, Guharoy R, Medicis JJ, Newman N, Speizer R. Prevalence and cost savings of therapeutic interchange among U.S. hospitals. Am J Health-Syst Pharm. 2002;59:529-33.

230. Bowman GK, Moleski R, Mangi RJ. Measuring the impact of a formulary decision: conversion to one quinolone agent. Formulary. 1996;31:906-14.

231. Chase SL, Peterson AM, Wordell CJ. Therapeutic-interchange program for oral histamine H_2-receptor antagonists. Am J Health-Syst Pharm. 1998;55:1382-6.

232. Therapeutic substitution could lower prescription drug spending. Avoidable brand-name costs reached $73 billion in three years, study finds [Internet]. Managed Care. 2016 May 10 [cited 2016 Aug 10]. Available from: http://www.managedcaremag.com/news/therapeutic-substitution-could-lower-prescription-drug-spending

233. Stoysich A, Massoomi F. Automatic interchange of the ACE inhibitors: decision-making process and initial results. Formulary. 2002;37:41-4.

234. Frighetto L, Nickoloff D, Jewesson P. Antibiotic therapeutic interchange program: six years of experience. Hosp Formul. 1995;30:92-105.

235. Vivian JC. Legal aspects of therapeutic interchange [Internet]. U.S. Pharm. 2004 Aug 15 [cited 2004 Oct 22]; [6 screens]. Available from: http://www.uspharmacist.com/index.asp?show=article&page=8_1129.htm

236. Janifer AN, Chatelain F, Goldwater SH, Mikovich G. Reengineering hospital pharmacy through therapeutic equivalency interchange while maintaining clinical outcomes. P&T. 1998;23(2):78-82, 85-8, 90-2.

237. Merli GJ, Vanscoy GJ, Rihn TL, Groce JB III, McCormick W. Applying scientific criteria to therapeutic interchange: a balanced analysis of low-molecular-weight heparins. J Thromb Thrombolysis. 2001;11(3):247-59.

238. Reich P. Therapeutic drug interchange. Med Interf. 1996;9(5):14.

239. H-125.995 Therapeutic and pharmaceutical alternatives by pharmacists [Internet]. Chicago (IL): American Medical Association [cited 2019 Nov 12]. Available from: https://policysearch.ama-assn.org/policyfinder/detail/Drug%20Formularies%20and%20Therapeutic%20Interchange%20H-125.995?uri=%2FAMADoc%2FHOD.xml-0-227.xml

240. American College of Physicians. Therapeutic substitution and formulary systems. Ann Intern Med. 1990;113:160-3.

241. Therapeutic interchange [Internet]. Alexandria (VA): Academy of Managed Care Pharmacy; 2012 June [cited 2019 Nov 12]. Available from: https://www.amcp.org/

policy-advocacy/policy-advocacy-focus-areas/where-we-stand-position-statements/therapeutic-interchange-0

242. American College of Clinical Pharmacy. Guidelines for therapeutic interchange. Pharmacother. 1993;13(2):252-6.

243. Massoomi F. Formulary management: antibiotics and therapeutic interchange. Pharm Pract Manag Q. 1996;16(3):11-8.

244. Heiner CR. Communicating about therapeutic interchange. Am J Health-Syst Pharm. 1996;53:2568-70.

245. Rosen A, Kay BG, Halecky D. Implementing a therapeutic interchange program in an institutional setting. P&T. 1995;20:711-7.

246. Kielty M. Improving the prior-authorization process to the satisfaction of customers. Am J Health-Syst Pharm. 1999;56:1499-1501.

247. Carroll NV. Formularies and therapeutic interchange: the health care setting makes a difference. Am J Health-Syst Pharm. 1999;56:467-72.

248. Nelson KM. Improving ambulatory care through therapeutic interchange. Am J Health-Syst Pharm. 1999;56:1307.

249. D'Amore M, Masters P, Maroun C. Impact of an automatic therapeutic interchange program on discharge medication selection. Hosp Pharm. 2003;38:942-6.

250. Banahan BF III, Bonnarens JK, Bentley JP. Generic substitution of NTI drugs: issues for Formulary Committee consideration. Formulary. 1998;33:1082-96.

251. FDA comments on activities in states concerning narrow-therapeutic-index drugs. Am J Health-Syst Pharm. 1998;55:686-7.

252. ASHP guidelines for selecting pharmaceutical manufacturers and suppliers. Am J Hosp Pharm. 1991;48:523-4.

253. Pummer TL, Shalaby KM, Erush SC. Ordering off the menu: assessing compliance with a nonformulary medication policy. Ann Pharmacother. 2009 July/Aug;43:1251-7.

254. Sweet BV, Stevenson JG. Pharmacy costs associated with nonformulary drug requests. Am J Health-Syst Pharm. 2001;58:1746-52.

255. Tse CST, Roecker W, Benitez M, Musabji M. How to tie a drug therapy improvement program to physician credentialing. Hosp Formul. 1994;29:646-56.

256. ASHP statement on the use of medications for unlabeled uses. Am J Hosp Pharm. 1992;49:2006-8.

257. Skledar SJ, Corman SL, Smitherman T. Addressing innovative off-label medication use at an academic medical center. Am J Health-Syst Pharm. 2015;72:469-77.

258. Steinberg SK. The development of a hospital pharmacy policy and procedure manual. Can J Hosp Pharm. 1980;XXXIII(6):194-5, 211.

259. Ginnow WK, King CM Jr. Revision and reorganization of a hospital pharmacy and procedure manual. Am J Hosp Pharm. 1978;35:698-704.

260. Van Dusen V, Pray WS. Issues in implementation and enforcement of hospital pharmacy policies and procedures. Hosp Pharm. 2001;36(4):398-403.

261. Piecoro JJ Jr. Development of an institutional I.V. drug delivery policy. Am J Hosp Pharm. 1987;44:2557-9.

262. Grissinger M. Eliminating problem-prone, automatic stop-order policies. P&T. 2004;29:344.

263. Galt KA. Credentialing and privileging for pharmacists. Am J Health-Syst Pharm. 2004;61:661-70.

264. Galt KA. Privileging, quality improvement and accountability. Am J Health-Syst Pharm. 2004;61:659.

265. Abramowitz PW, Shane R, Daigle LA, Noonan KA, Letendre DE. Pharmacist interdependent prescribing: a new model for optimizing patient outcomes. Am J Health-Syst Pharm. 2012;69:1976-81.

266. Sass CM. Drug usage evaluation. J Pharm Pract. 1994;7(2):74-8.

267. Orsini MJ, Funk Orsini PA, Thorn DB, Gallina JN. An ADR surveillance program: increasing quality, number of incidence reports. Formulary. 1995;30:454-61.

268. Samore MH, Evans RS, Lassen A, Gould P, Lloyd J, Gardner RM, Abouzelof R, Taylor C, Woodbury DA,Willy M, Bright RA. Surveillance of medical device-related hazards and adverse events in hospitalized patients. JAMA. 2004;291:325-34.

269. Traynor K. Enforcement outdoes education at eliminating unsafe abbreviations. Am J Health-Syst Pharm. 2004;61:1314, 1317, 1322.

270. Baker De. Sound-alike and look-alike drug errors. Hosp Pharm. 2002;37:225.

271. Vaida AJ, Peterson J. Common sound-alike, look-alike products. Pharm Times. 2002;68:22-3.

272. Starr CH. When drug names spell trouble. Drug Topics. 2000;144:49-50, 53-4, 57-8.

273. Cohen M. Medication error update. Consult Pharm. 1997;12:1328-9.

274. Soulliard D, Hong M, Saubermann L. Development of a pharmacy-managed medication dictionary in a newly implemented computerized prescriber order-entry system. Am J Health-Syst Pharm. 2004;61:617-22.

275. First Consulting Group. Computerized physician order entry: costs, benefits and challenges. A case study approach. Long Beach: First Consulting Group; 2003.

276. Combating counterfeit drugs. A report of the Food and Drug administration [Internet]. Washington (DC): U.S. Department of Health and Human Services; 2004 Feb [cited 2019 Nov 12]. Available from: https://www.fda.gov/media/77086/download

277. Generali JA. Counterfeit drugs: a growing concern. Hosp Pharm. 2003;38:724.

278. Young D. FDA urges adoption of anticounterfeit technologies by 2007 [Internet]. Bethesda (MD): American Society of Health-System Pharmacists; 2004 Feb 19 [cited 2004 Mar 8]. Available from:https://www.ashp.org/news/2004/02/19/fda_urges_adoption_of_anticounterfeit_technologies_by_2007

279. Redwanski J, Seamon MJ. Impact of counterfeit drugs on the formulary decision-making process. Formulary. 2004;39:577-9, 583.

280. Fox ER, McLaughlin MM. ASHP guidelines on managing drug product shortages. Am J Health-Syst Pharm. 2018;75(21):1742-50.

281. Fox ER, Tyler LS. Managing drug shortages: seven years' experience at one health system. Am J Health-Syst Pharm. 2003;60:245-53.

282. Leady MA, Adams AL, Stumpf JL, Sweet BV. Drug shortages: an approach to managing the latest crisis. Hosp Pharm. 2003;38:748-52.

283. Schrand LM, Troester TS, Ballas ZK, Mutnick AH, Ross MB. Preparing for drug shortages: one teaching hospital's approach to the IVIG shortage. Formulary. 2001;36:52-9.

284. Lasser KE, Allen PD, Woolhandler SJ, Himmelstein DU, Wolfe SM, Bor DH. Timing of new black box warnings and withdrawals for prescription medications. JAMA. 2002;287:2215-20.

285. Gandey A. Propoxyphene withdrawn from US market [Internet]. Medscape. 2010 Nov 19 [cited 2010 Nov 19]; [2 p.]. Available from: http://www.medscape.com/viewarticle/732887_print

286. Huskamp HA, Deverka PA, Epstein AM, Epstein RS, McGuigan KA, Frank RG. The effect of incentive-based formularies on prescription-drug utilization and spending. NEJM. 2003;349:2224-32.

287. Thomas CP. Incentive-based formularies. NEJM. 2003;349:2186-8.

288. Crane VS, Hull BL, Hatwig CA, Teresi M, Croft CL. Presenting drug cost information to a board of directors: a case example. Formulary. 2001;36:857-64.

289. Helmons PJ, Coates CR, Kosterink JGW, Daniels CE. Decision support at the point of prescribing to increase formulary adherence. Am J Health-Syst Pharm. 2015;72:408-13.

290. Rattles by drug price increases, hospitals seek ways to stand guard [Internet]. Washington Post. [Cited 2016 Jun 29]. Available from: https://www.washingtonpost.com/national/health-science/rattled-by-drug-price-increases-hospitals-seek-ways-to-stay-on-guard/2016/03/13/1c593dea-c8f3-11e5-88ff-e2d1b4289c2f_story.html

291. Hoffman JM, Shah ND, Vermeulen LC, Hunkler RJ, Hontz KM. Projecting future drug expenditures-2004. Am J Health-Syst Pharm. 2004;61:145-58.

292. Shah ND, Vermeulen LC, Santell JP, Hunkler RJ, Hontz K. Projecting future drug expenditures—2002. Am J Health-Syst Pharm. 2002;59:131-42.

293. Shah ND, Hoffman JM, Vermeulen LC, Hunkler RJ, Hontz K. Projecting future drug expenditures—2003. Am J Health-Syst Pharm. 2003;60:137-49.

294. Mora MW. How P&T committees can be effective change agents: part 1. Am J Pharm Benefits. 2010;2(2):99-100.

295. Brookins L, Burnette R, De la Torre C, Dumitru D, McManus RB, Urbanski CJ, Vrabel RB, Wolfschlag RP, Tribble DA. Formulary and database synchronization. Am J Health-Syst Pharm. 2011;68(3):204,206.

16

Chapter Sixteen

Drug Evaluation Monographs

Patrick M. Malone • Mark A. Malesker • Indrani Kar •
Danial E. Baker • Sunil Kumar Jagadesh

Learning Objectives

After completing this chapter, the reader will be able to:

- Describe and perform an evaluation of a drug product for a drug formulary.
- List the sections included in a drug evaluation monograph.
- Describe the overall highlights included in a monograph summary.
- Describe the recommendations and restrictions that are made in a monograph.
- Describe the purpose and format of a drug class review.
- Describe and perform an evaluation of a therapeutic interchange.

Key Concepts

❶ The establishment and maintenance of a drug formulary requires that drugs or drug classes be objectively assessed based on scientific information (e.g., efficacy, safety, uniqueness, cost), not anecdotal prescriber experience.

❷ The drug evaluation monograph provides a structured method to review the major features of a drug product.

❸ A definite recommendation should be made based on need, therapeutics, side effects, cost, and other items specific to the particular agent (e.g., evidence-based treatment guidelines, dosage forms, convenience, dosage interval, inclusion on the formulary of third-party payers, hospital antibiotic resistance patterns, potential for causing medication errors), usually in that order.

④ The recommendation must be supported by objective evidence.

⑤ The most logical decision to benefit the patient and the institution should be recommended to the pharmacy and therapeutics (P&T) committee.

⑥ Cost is heavily emphasized in formulary decisions and must be properly accounted for, given the complexities of drug acquisition pricing, payor coverage, cost to the hospital, and reimbursement.

⑦ Preparation of a drug evaluation monograph requires a great amount of time and effort, using many of the skills discussed throughout this text to obtain, evaluate, collate, and provide information. However, the value of having all of the issues evaluated and discussed can be invaluable in providing quality care.

Introduction

❶ *The establishment and maintenance of a* **drug formulary** *requires that drugs or drug classes be objectively assessed based on scientific information (e.g., efficacy, safety,[1] uniqueness, cost), not anecdotal prescriber experience.* A rational evaluation of all aspects of a drug in relation to similar agents provides the most effective and evidence-based method in deciding which drug is appropriate for formulary addition. In particular, it is necessary to consider need, level of evidence for the drug's efficacy, effectiveness, safety, risk, and cost (overall, including monitoring costs, discounts, rebates, economic impact on other medical costs, and so forth)—often in that order, although a committee may mostly be concerned about efficacy/indications, evidence of need, operational issues, cost, and safety.[2] Some other issues that are evaluated include dosage forms, packaging, requirements of accrediting or quality assurance bodies, evidence-based treatment guidelines, prescriber preferences, regulatory issues (including risk evaluation and mitigation strategies [REMS]), distribution pathways, patient/nursing convenience, advertising, possible discrimination issues,[3] consumer expectations,[4] and patent expiration dates for similar drugs or treatments. Additional issues are continually added to the depth of a drug review, including assessment of risk to meet new regulatory requirements from the USP <800> (i.e., hazardous drug handling), considerations for **biosimilars**, and standardized financial reimbursement assessments. There is increasing emphasis on evaluating clinical outcomes from high-quality trials, continuous quality assurance information, real-world comparative efficacies,[5] pharmacogenomics, and quality of life.[6]

Purpose of Drug Evaluation Monographs

When completing an evaluation, special consideration should be given to how a drug, if added to formulary, will safely be implemented at the institution. All drug evaluations will have many similar components, but the emphasis and impact of those components may be different for each type of institution (e.g., hospital, managed care organization, outpatient surgery center, long-term care facility, pharmacy benefit manager, specialty pharmacy program). A hospital or outpatient surgery center may need to consider such questions of policies and procedures for administration and special considerations that need to be added to the electronic medical record (e.g., restrictions placed on use, administration instructions). In addition, their economic evaluation within a hospital may cover short time frames, while an outpatient formulary will need to consider short- and long-term cost considerations along with drug, patient, and disease factors that may influence patient adherence. Example questions should be considered that may need to be addressed in the drug evaluation monograph (e.g., Does the medication need an order set? Will the medication be stocked? Does the medication need to be added to tools like a smart pump?). An example of a new medication that posed challenges to incorporation into electronic order sets and the smart pump library was angiotensin II (GIAPREZA) which is dosed as ng/kg/minute. In this case it was necessary to delay use after formulary approval to complete nursing education and program the pumps to include ng dosing capabilities. What warnings, reports, restrictions, etc., must be put into affected computer systems? Does the institution require a medication-use guideline for this medication? Is a REMS program required? In the event the institution is not reimbursed for services provided, should the medication be added to formulary from an ethical standpoint? What restrictions should be considered and why? Even the potential effect that a drug addition to formulary may have on the public image of the institution (e.g., abortion-related products, gene therapies, and gender change therapies) may impact the pharmacy and therapeutics (P&T) committee's decision. This is particularly relevant to medications with a high cost and for an orphan disease state. For example, onasemnogene abeparvovec-xioi (Zolgensma) is a medication for spinal muscular atrophy (SMA). It is marketed as a curative dose for patients with SMA and costs more than $2.1 million per dose. An in-depth **drug evaluation monograph** can be prepared to assist in this process as described below. ❷ *The drug evaluation monograph provides a structured method to review the major features of a drug product.* Once a monograph is prepared, it can easily be used as a structured overview of a drug product. That allows for easy comparison or contrast to other products that may be used for the same indication or that are in the same product class. The monograph format can also be used to evaluate a biosimilar product, where the new biologic product is very similar to a reference product, other than possible minor differences in clinically inactive components.[7] In the case of a biosimilar, the product would most likely be compared to the reference product and there would be additional consideration of the interchange of the products within the institution. Other important considerations for a biosimilar monograph include assessment of the literature used for Food and Drug Administration (FDA) approval, acceptability of extrapolation of data to other approved FDA indications, allowance of substitution under state law, insurance coverage in the region of the institution, reimbursement compared to the reference product, and method of incorporation into the electronic medical record.[8,9]

When a P&T committee reviews an entire class of drugs, a drug class review is prepared instead of a single drug evaluation monograph. **Drug class reviews** are often lengthier than a single-product drug evaluation monograph; however, they can use a similar structure and format. Hospitals, health systems, and managed care organizations are required by accreditation standards to review their formulary annually. One method to accomplish this is reviewing the formulary through annual drug class reviews. How often an entire class of drugs is reviewed within the required frame is determined by the institution and may be based upon any new agents, utilization of agents within the category, and primarily cost.[10] This review process gives an organization the opportunity to reevaluate the formulary status of products in light of new publications or trials, new products that have entered the market, safety warnings from the FDA, or the potential to delete particular products from the class. Samples of drug class reviews prepared by the U.S. Department of Veterans Administration are available on the Internet at http://www.pbm.va.gov/clinicalguidance/drugclassreviews.asp. Similar to drug class reviews, developing a therapeutic interchange, addition of restrictions, or removal from formulary recommendation can follow the same structure and format as a drug monograph. This structure allows for appropriate efficacy, safety, and cost review to be completed. Presentation of all formulary reviews to the P&T committee is essential. These types of reviews, as outlined above, include (a) addition to formulary, (b) removal from formulary, (c) therapeutic interchange, and (d) drug class review considerations. Contemporary strategies with these types of reviews include addition of guidelines, criteria for high-cost medications, reimbursement, **white bagging** potential (i.e., receiving a medication from the pharmacy [usually specialty pharmacy] and taking it to the physician's office for administration), and monitoring.[11] A standardized, defined process within the workflow of formulary management within an organization is important and must be continually managed.[12]

Sources of Drug Monographs

Commercially prepared monographs can be obtained from various sources (e.g., Wolters Kluwer [https://www.wolterskluwercdi.com/facts-comparisons-online/formulary/] has monographs available from Facts & Comparisons® eAnswers and Lexicomp Online) and can be used as is or with modifications to suit the needs of the institution. If this latter method is used, be aware that the quality of the commercial monographs may vary, even from the same publisher, and they may need extensive updating. Often, writing a new drug evaluation monograph may be easier than improving a commercial monograph. Whether or not the monograph is commercially available or prepared by a member from within the organization, the material should reflect the local conditions, current prescribing practices, and nature of the organization. As such, this material may be classified as confidential and not for dissemination by the organization, and is owned by the P&T committee as a means of executing its functions per policy and procedure. In order to prevent unwarranted dissemination of institution- and committee-owned materials, especially to drug company representatives, some institutions distribute this material for review during a P&T committee meeting, and then require the materials to be returned at the end of the meeting, rather than providing materials ahead of time. This would have the disadvantage in that it would be difficult to fully review the prepared material, so other strategies are sometimes employed. Some institutions number each monograph with a unique numbering system to assist in tracking the return of P&T committee documents, although this may be seen more in state Medicaid situations. In other cases, the material may be only available through a secure intranet system.

Contents of the Drug Monograph

Although there are recommendations concerning monograph contents,[4,13] information that may be valuable and specific to an institution, and necessary for an objective review of the product, is commonly missing.[14] An outline of a sample monograph is found in Appendix 16-1. Each of the sections of this monograph will be discussed below. An example of some of the information found in the various parts of a monograph is provided in Appendix 16-2. This sample monograph meets or exceeds the recommendations of the American Society of Health-System Pharmacists (ASHP),[13] and should serve as a good example for most circumstances. Additional guidance from ASHP is available at https://formularytoolkit.org/. Guidelines published by the Academy of Managed Care Pharmacy (AMCP)[4,15] and The Joint Commission (TJC)[10] are also noted and discussed for situational applicability. The AMCP format is the recommended standard for manufacturers to submit data to managed care organizations. It is designed to restrict the marketing-related emphasis and maximize evidence-based information and full disclosure impact of the company in providing information. While it has applicability as to how an institution may evaluate a drug, it also has restrictions as to the amount of information that it can cover, which may make it undesirable in some cases. It is always worthwhile for an organization to review these types of documents to assure their information is comprehensive and is not missing critical information that may not have been discovered in their review process. It may be worthwhile for institutions or other organizations to request this information from the drug company, preferably, well in advance of the time it is needed. Note, in some cases this request may require signing a nondisclosure agreement, since it may contain proprietary information.[4] However, these types of documents are not generally distributed to the members of the P&T committee, but are used by the developers of the organization's drug monographs.

The precise monograph should be tailored to the needs of the institution, organization, and patient population. Several sections not recommended by ASHP have been added to the monograph described in this chapter to increase the utility of the monograph for other sites of practice, including ambulatory clinics, pediatric institutions, long-term care facilities, standalone psychiatric hospitals, rehabilitation centers, managed care or pharmacy benefit managers, or even Medicare or Medicaid formularies. Also, in some cases, the information has been divided into multiple sections or subsections to increase clarity. The format recommended in this chapter can also be used to evaluate whole classes of drugs. In most cases, a specific drug is compared with others in the same class. The only difference in a class review is that one drug is not receiving the greatest attention; all drugs are being compared with equal attention. Comparative charts and tables are often more prevalent in drug class reviews, as they can serve as a concise method to compare features of the products in a particular drug class. This format can also be used to evaluate biosimilars, therapeutic interchanges, and any potential removals from formulary. Monograph expectations on length and depth vary greatly between institutions. Regardless of these factors, the monograph is a tool to effectively and efficiently review information in a manner that assists the P&T committee in evaluating the evidence for a recommendation.

Specific formats, differing somewhat from the one presented here, may be required by organizations or governments. For example, Australia (http://www.tga.gov.au/industry/pm-argpm.htm),[16] Ontario, Canada (http://www.health.gov.on.ca/en/pro/programs/drugs/dsguide/docs/dse_guide.pdf),[17] and the United Kingdom (https://www.nice.org.uk/process/pmg19/chapter/1-acknowledgements)[18] have specific, published guidelines that need to be followed for a drug product to be considered for their formularies. The process recommended in this chapter appears to be common in both Canada and the United States, and has been recommended in Australia.[19] Where appropriate, features of these formats have been incorporated into the description presented in this chapter. While the format described in this chapter does provide much of the information in those government standards, with the exception of details about product manufacturing and specific pricing for the particular country, the order and amount of information is often different, and the reader is referred to those standards for details.

♀ Importance of the Drug Monograph

The drug monograph is a powerful tool for the pharmacy organization to guide the rational development of a drug formulary. Although the pharmacy department may have few, if any, votes in the ultimate adoption of a formulary agent, the monograph, which is prepared by the pharmacist, provides background and evidence used by the P&T committee and guides the evaluation process. It is likely to be a major factor in the final decision. While monograph preparation can be very time consuming, it is extremely important to support rational medication therapy and should be given proper attention to provide a fair and balanced evaluation of the drug or drug class. The structured evaluation process of a drug monograph, in many cases, is the only time a full, fair, and balanced review of a drug that may be presented to a practitioner. Pharmacists have a unique role in the preparation of a monograph, in that they view the drug product from a whole and macroeconomic view—all aspects of the drug product are objectively reviewed in a monograph, whereas oftentimes when a prescriber is presented information about a new drug product, they may be basing their use or nonuse of the product on a single study, package insert data, pharmaceutical representative information, or some other microeconomic view of a drug product that may or may not represent the full utility of the drug product.[20,21]

In addition to FDA-regulated drug products, health care professionals need to be aware of complementary and alternative medicine use, along with the responsibilities and implications that it has for pharmacy services. These products can only be marketed as dietary substances, since the FDA does not regulate herbal products, so manufacturers and distributors cannot make specific health claims. However, they may be commonly used, such as melatonin being used in intensive care units to prevent delirium. Although there may be minimal scientific evidence regarding efficacy and safety of these products, pharmacists must provide information relating to all therapeutic agents that patients are receiving, preparing a drug monograph for the P&T committee, much the same as for any FDA-approved product. This can also follow the format described in this chapter.[22]

Even more complications may result if there is a request to consider medical marijuana for a hospital formulary. To begin with, some states may allow medical marijuana to be used medicinally or recreationally, even though it is considered to be a Schedule I controlled substance federally and, therefore, not truly legal in the United States. Medical marijuana may be available from a dispensary, but would not be available from a pharmacy. In addition, there are claims made for the product that are not widely supported by high-quality medical studies. While it may be difficult to do a full rational review of such a product, it should be treated professionally and be fully considered. However, a P&T committee may determine that it will not be evaluated and will be considered a nonformulary item, due to the legal issues surrounding it. It may be useful for the P&T committee to consider such issues in advance of receiving requests for such products and work collaboratively with the institution's legal department to follow appropriate policies surrounding medical marijuana at the hospital. With changing regulations regarding hemp (e.g., hemp < 0.3% tetrahydrocannabinol is now federally legal and may be legal in some states), it is crucial for organizations to also consider the efficacy, safety, and policy needs of these products prior to patients requesting to use them in their institution. Additionally, FDA-approved medications derived from marijuana or hemp (e.g., cannabidiol [Epidiolex]) that have an appropriate DEA schedule allowing use, may be evaluated using a monograph like any other medication review. It is important to distinguish FDA-approved drugs in this area versus medical marijuana or hemp, which is unregulated by the FDA like a medication.

The following sections describe the parts of the drug monograph, as shown in the appendices. Please note that skills in information retrieval (see Chapter 3), drug literature evaluation (see Chapters 4 and 5), professional writing (see Chapter 13) and areas covered in various other chapters must be employed when preparing a drug evaluation monograph.

Summary Page

The first page of the monograph is essentially a summary of the most important information concerning the drug, and includes a specific recommendation of the action to be taken on the product. The summary itself is a brief overview of the important aspects of the drug product. Some P&T committees only review this first sheet; however, the remainder of the document should be prepared in order to completely evaluate a drug product and to provide a record of all that was taken into consideration. The summary and recommendation could be placed at the end of the monograph, but it is probably best to keep it on the front to make it easier to refer to during the P&T committee meeting. The summary may also be used during the P&T committee meeting, while the full monograph may support subcommittee discussions.

FORMAT OF SUMMARY PAGE

The format of the summary page usually begins with general institutional information. Following the name header, specific introductory information about the product is included. The generic name, trade name, and manufacturer are self-explanatory, but the classification may require some explanation. This is meant to give the readers a quick way of classifying the agent.

Determining Drug Classification

The summary page includes the drug's prescription or controlled substance status, **American Hospital Formulary Service (AHFS) classification**, the United States Pharmacopeia–Drug Classification (USP-DC), and FDA classification. It may also contain other classification schemes used by particular organizations, such as the Veterans Affairs. Managed care organizations may use more detailed drug product identification schemes, such as those established by First Databank, Inc. (http://www.fdbhealth.com).

The AHFS classification can be found in the AHFS Drug Information reference book, published by ASHP or available online (http://www.ahfsdruginformation.com/) for subscribers. This classification can help the reader determine where a new agent falls in therapy. Often, new drugs will be evaluated for possible formulary addition before they are actually placed in AHFS Drug Information. Classification for many new agents is available at http://ahfs.ashp.org/drug-assignments.aspx before the listing is added to AHFS Drug Information. If the AHFS classification cannot be identified, it will be necessary to consult the therapeutic classification table in the front of the AHFS Drug Information reference book to decide where the product fits. The classification of similar products listed in AHFS Drug Information can also be checked before deciding where to categorize the new product. One AHFS category often overlooked is blood products. The FDA classifies blood and blood derivatives as medications. Even if these products are stored in the blood bank at some organizations, TJC recognizes formulary oversight responsibility by the pharmacy department.[23]

The USP-DC can be found at https://www.usp.org/health-quality-safety/usp-drug-classification-system.

The FDA classification is given to nonbiologic products during the review process and is finalized when the new drug application (NDA) is approved. This classification gives some idea of the importance of the product. The classification consists of Chemical Type classification (see Table 16-1) and Therapeutic Rating classification (see Table 16-2). An FDA classification of 1P (or 1A prior to 1992) would indicate a drug that was given a priority review status by the FDA. This means that the product offered a therapeutic advance over existing products in the market, may be for a new disease state, or may represent a new drug class. The FDA generally reviews these products in an expedited manner, often not requiring as many clinical trials or a lower number of patients enrolled in the trials before the drug is approved to be on the market. In contrast, a classification of 2S (or 3C prior to 1992) is likely a me-too product, meaning that it is an additional product in a class of medications that is already on the market and is similar in many ways to the other products already marketed. These products are generally reviewed by the FDA in a standard review manner and do not receive an expedited review process.

Knowing and understanding the FDA classification status of a product can assist a reviewer in preparing the drug evaluation monograph in several ways. First, if the reviewer

TABLE 16-1. FDA CLASSIFICATION BY CHEMICAL TYPE

Type	Definition
1	New molecular entity (NME) not marketed in the United States
2	New salt, ester, or other noncovalent derivative of another drug marketed in the United States
3	New formulation or dosage form of an active ingredient marketed in the United States
4	New combination of drugs already marketed in the United States
5	New manufacturer of a drug product already marketed by another company in the United States
6	New indication for a product already marketed in the United States (note: this category is no longer used)
7	• Drug that is already legally marketed without an approved NDA • First application since 1962 for a drug marketed prior to 1938 • First application for DESI (Drug Efficacy Study Implementation)-related products that were first marketed between 1938 and 1962 without an NDA • First application for DESI-related products first marketed after 1962 without NDAs. In this case, the indications may be the same or different from the legally marketed product
8	Over-the-counter (OTC) switch
9	New indication submitted as separate NDA, which is consolidated with original NDA after approval
10	New indication submitted as a separate NDA, but not consolidated with original NDA

Drugs@FDA frequently asked questions [Internet]. Washington: Food and Drug Administration [updated 2015 Mar 27; cited 2016 Jul 18]. Available from: http://www.fda.gov/Drugs/InformationOnDrugs/ucm075234.htm#chemtype_reviewclass.

TABLE 16-2. FDA CLASSIFICATIONS BY THERAPEUTIC POTENTIAL

Type	Definition
P	Priority handling by the FDA—before 1992 this had two categories: A—Major therapeutic gain B—Moderate therapeutic gain
S	Standard handling by the FDA—before 1992 this was referred to as class C, which indicated the product offered only a minor or no therapeutic gain
0	Orphan drug

Drugs@FDA frequently asked questions [Internet]. Washington: Food and Drug Administration [updated 2015 Mar 27; cited 2016 Jul 18]. Available from: http://www.fda.gov/Drugs/InformationOnDrugs/ucm075234.htm#chemtype_reviewclass.

knows that the product being reviewed has an FDA classification status of 1P, the reviewer will often have to compare the product to a drug outside of the class of the product being reviewed. For example, if a new class of antibiotics was developed and called ketolides, the reviewer will not have any other drugs in the class with which the product can be compared, and therefore he or she may need to search for studies or review articles of products that fall in other classes of antibiotics, such as the macrolides. Oftentimes in cases in which cancer chemotherapy medications are approved for a treatment that was previously treated by nondrug therapy, a surgical procedure or radiation therapy may be the best comparator for the product. In the case of products that are given an FDA classification status of 2S, the reviewer generally will be able to prepare a head-to-head comparison of the product to another product that is in the same drug class. For example, if a new hydroxymethylglutaryl-Coenzyme A (HMG-CoA) reductase inhibitor was approved by the FDA, the reviewer would normally want to compare the product with other HMG-CoA reductase inhibitors. Sometimes, when 1S or standard review products enter the market, if there are already a number of similar products available in the market, the manufacturer will conduct trials with the product compared with others in the same class. This product is generally then referred to as the comparator or gold standard product. The reviewer will want to discuss the comparator product and any other similar agents in the class. This can assist the decision makers in the P&T committee in reviewing the new product, if they are already familiar with other products in the class.

Comparative Analysis

A particular institution may request additional or specific information that may be relevant to include in the introductory information. Additional product introductory information may include the product's patent exclusivity date and/or the product's patent expiration date. This information can generally be located on the FDA's website at http://www.accessdata.fda.gov/scripts/cder/drugsatfda/index.cfm. It is also common to provide a list of similar agents.

The summary itself is a brief overview of the important aspects of the drug product. If there are similar products or different drugs used for the same indication, it is important to state how the drug being reviewed compares to those products. If a comparison between the agent in question and some other treatment is possible, that comparison must make up the bulk of the section, just as the comparison must be a prominent feature in every other section of the document. The summary will include information on the efficacy, safety (e.g., adverse effects and drug interactions),[24] uniqueness, cost, treatment need in the institution, inpatient versus outpatient needs, potential for inappropriate use,[25] and other factors, such as the likelihood patients would be more compliant with one agent or another[26,27] or how the therapy fits into published clinical guidelines. When possible, it is also good to include the consideration of patient preferences,[28] which may be related to any aspect of the medication. Information should be limited in this section to those items where a drug has a definite advantage/disadvantage or, if products are similar, where there would be concerns about the possibility of a clinically significant difference. Items that are not clinically significant and not likely to be of concern should be left out of the summary to avoid distractions, except, perhaps, for a general statement saying there are no significant differences in certain areas. In cases where the new drug under evaluation is indicated for a disease that has normally received nondrug treatment (e.g., surgery, radiation, physical therapy), the drug should be compared to that standard treatment. It is worth pointing out that the summary should be just that—a summary of the material presented in the body of the document. Similar to the conclusion of a journal article, this is not the place to put new material or, for that matter, to provide citations; both of those items belong in the body.

FORMULARY RECOMMENDATION

❸ *Finally, a definite recommendation should be made based on need, therapeutics (including outcome data and the use of evidence-based clinical guidelines), adverse effects, cost (full pharmacoeconomic analysis, if possible), and other items specific to the particular agent (e.g., evidence-based treatment guidelines, dosage forms, convenience, dosage interval, inclusion on the formulary of third-party payers, hospital antibiotic resistance patterns, potential for causing medication errors),*[29] *usually in that order.*[30,31] Recommendations should be specific to the circumstances in the institution, hospital system, third-party payer plan, and/or other organization in which it is being considered. In hospitals, it may be useful to list the indications for use that the drug the P&T committee is approving. This should be a specific list, although it is acceptable to give a blanket authorization to FDA-approved indications in general. The list may include off-label indication reviews as well as the dosage forms being approved for formulary addition.[32] Note that the requirement that drugs be approved for specific indications may be practical only in hospitals where computerized prescriber order entry is available and the prescriber has to state the indication when ordering. It may not be efficient to maintain an indication list for all recommendations and approvals, unless required for appropriate use of the medication.

Tiered Formulary Decisions by Third-Party Payer Health Plans

The decision related to potential formulary inclusion is generally considered separately from the health plan's drug management strategies, such as co-pays and tiered coverage. The group making the decision may also use the drug evaluation monograph along with the P&T committee's decision, the plan's policies and procedures, and financial evaluation (including rebates) to decide which tier is assigned to the drug. When making formulary recommendations, as it pertains to third-party payers (e.g., insurance companies), consideration should also be given to the placement of the formulary agent into a multitiered copayment system, where the copayment varies according to the cost of the drug and/or formulary status. The patient member is required to pay these varying amounts of copayment out-of-pocket at the time when the prescription is filled. In general, if the drug is a generic, the placement is at the first tier that has the lowest copayment. If the drug is a brand name drug preferred by the health plan, it is usually placed in the second tier with a higher copayment. All other brand name, nonpreferred drugs are usually placed in the third tier with the highest copayment. Drugs in the third tier, the nonpreferred agents, usually have therapeutic alternatives in either the first or second tier. Patient members are encouraged to talk to their prescribers or pharmacists about switching to the more cost-effective, therapeutic alternative drugs in the lower tiers.[33,34]

Tier designation or formulary status may change, based on the discretion of the health plan and/or pharmacy benefits manager (PBM), in the absence of significant new clinical evidence.[35] Quality-of-life information and patient preferences should be considered, if possible. Recommendations for third-party payers may also include a step-therapy approach, quantity limits on the prescription, prior authorization, and coverage rule criteria in order for the drug to be covered. Third-party payers may require some drugs to have a prior authorization before being dispensed. In the community pharmacy setting, prior authorization (also known as prior approval) is usually required for those drugs that are of high cost and/or are likely to be used inappropriately. Examples include various biologics for treating rheumatoid arthritis, compounded medications, newer long-acting opioids, newer drug formulations, newer atypical antipsychotics, and growth hormones. Prior authorization requires that predetermined criteria must be met by the member before the drug can be covered by the third-party payer. As an example, the member may be required to try an established, less expensive drug therapy first. If this drug therapy proves to be ineffective or if the patient is unable to tolerate the therapy, then the third-party payer may cover a newer, more expensive therapeutically equivalent drug.[36] Prior authorization continues to be important in hospital settings providing outpatient infusion and specialty care to patients. Incorporating the prior authorization process into the monograph review is crucial for managing nuances related to coverage and addition of these types of medications to formulary.[37]

In some cases, an institution may have a subformulary that is available for only a specific group of patients (e.g., Medicaid, pediatric).[38] Recommendations to conduct drug-use evaluation on the drug (see Chapter 18), clinical guidelines to be followed (see Chapter 8), and how prescribers are to be educated about the new drug and other items may also be necessary. Education may range from a simple newsletter, email, web page, or memorandum to a specific educational program and certification required before a prescribing.[39]

Some people strongly object to placing specific recommendations in the document, because the recommendation in a monograph may differ from the final recommendation approved by the P&T committee. Others do not feel it is appropriate for them to make these recommendations before committee review; however, the person preparing the monograph is in the best situation to advance a logical recommendation. Also, without a recommendation, the discussion does not have a foundation to begin with. In addition, the lack of a specific recommendation allows emotion, conjecture, and anecdotes to overcome evidence and science. From the pharmacists' perspective, the expectation that a prepared monograph includes a formulary recommendation can vary with the culture of the specific organization. This opportunity is welcomed because provision of a specific recommendation is one of the best opportunities for pharmacists to have a deep and wide-ranging impact on patient care, and should not be neglected.

Input and Support from Nonmember Expertise

❹ *The recommendation must be supported by objective evidence* (presented in the summary). Subjective factors that are likely to be significant from the point of view of all involved parties (i.e., physicians, pharmacists, nurses, and patients) should also be considered. Dieticians and respiratory therapists may not be regular members of the P&T committee; however, they may be called upon for input regarding nutritional supplements or respiratory medications. Decision analysis can be used to show the best drug at the least cost (effectively, this is pharmacoeconomic analysis—see Chapter 7 for details).[36,40-43] Other factors may also be considered and given weight to indicate importance (e.g., multiattribute utility theory).[44] These methods may be commonly seen in managed care.[45] They look at the possible decisions and their likely outcome, allowing a decision to be made that is likely to lead to the most desirable outcome. Meta-analysis may also find a place in the decision-making process[46]; however, appropriate evaluation of a meta-analysis is important if being utilized. Tentative recommendations should be discussed with appropriate physicians and any clinical pharmacists specializing in that area of therapy before the recommendation is finalized. For example, if a cardiac medication is being evaluated, one or more cardiologists should be consulted to identify their concerns and desires. That does not mean the recommendation should necessarily be changed to what a prescriber wants. If the objective evidence supports the original recommendation, that is the one that should be made; however, it is necessary to demonstrate that the prescribers' concerns were addressed. In a health system, considerations should be given to concerns that affect the entire system, when creating a recommendation. This may include reviewing the recommendation with specialists in the appropriate areas from all hospitals in the system that may have a need for the agent(s). This can be challenging, so the need to leverage physician, pharmacy, and nursing leadership to build consensus is essential. A pharmacist trained in literature evaluation is well positioned to support this work, which incorporates an unbiased review and pharmacoeconomic analysis[47] that includes appropriate discussions with relevant colleagues to develop the most robust and needed recommendation for the organization.[48,49]

It is important to minimize opportunities for a pharmaceutical representative to influence any decision, so that clinical evidence is the basis of a recommendation. Overall, the items most likely to be added to the formulary include those that are effective, unique, that serve the specific population, that are most cost-effective and, unfortunately, those with the biggest marketing drive by the marketer. Multiple ingredient products or products that are the extended-release or other variations on the patent of a product are least likely to be added in the institutional setting.[50]

Types of Formulary Recommendation

The recommendation should be a logical conclusion supported by the objective evidence and the needs of the health care system, including health care staff needs, distribution concerns, drug administration, and drug availability. Whenever possible, at least for recommendations prepared for an institutional pharmacy, it is best to follow or adapt the ASHP guidelines for recommendations, which would place the drug into one or a combination of the following groups[13]:

- Added for uncontrolled use by the entire medical staff.
- Added for monitored use—No restrictions placed on use, but the drug will be monitored via a quality assurance study (e.g., drug usage evaluation, medication usage evaluation) to determine appropriateness of use. This is a tie-in to the institution's quality assurance/drug usage evaluation process.[51] Note: this category does not mean that the patient is monitored, since that is necessary for every drug. It means that the quality and appropriateness of how the drug is used is monitored.
- Added with restrictions—The drug is added to the drug formulary, but there are restrictions on who may prescribe it and/or how it may be used (e.g., specific indications, certain physicians or physician groups, certain policies to be followed, specific locations for use, certain medication-use guidelines). Example: neuromuscular blocking agents being restricted to anesthesiologists or specific anti-infective medications being restricted to infectious disease physicians.
- Conditional—Available for use by the entire medical staff for a finite period of time. This may be particularly important during a heightened market, where shortages are common; however, it should be used carefully, since it may be very difficult to eliminate a product once it has been available at all. For example, use of peramivir (Rapivab) during influenza season during oseltamivir shortage.
- Not added/deleted from formulary—Nonformulary medications are not routinely stocked and, when ordered, the prescriber needs to provide justification for use and recognize procurement may take 24 hours or longer.
- Nonstocked, nonformulary—Medications that are not added to formulary and are deemed nonstocked are not used regardless of the justification for use. This is a category that should be used sparingly, unless the medication is unsafe for patients.
- Therapeutic interchange with a preferred agent for the institution's formulary.

Note, there may be different recommendations presented for specific strengths, forms, sizes, and so forth of a drug being reviewed. However, being that specific may not result in any real benefit and may only make things more complicated to manage, with little improvement in drug therapy or decrease in costs.[52]

• Most drugs should be added for uncontrolled use or, at the other extreme, not be added, simply because the other categories cause greater work for the pharmacy or other departments. As a side point, if a recommendation to not add the drug to the formulary is approved, it is often good to require a time period before the drug can be considered again (typically 6 months) to prevent political pushback and subsequent approval of a less-than-desirable drug, due to a request for review every month.

• Being added for uncontrolled use does not mean that the medication is always stocked in the institution; some rarely used products may officially be formulary, but not normally stocked, as long as they can be obtained promptly when needed. For example, snake antivenom may be officially on the formulary in all hospitals in a city where snake bites are seldom seen, but only stocked by one particular institution, which then provides it to other hospitals immediately, when needed. Also, in the case where a product may be nonformulary, it may still occasionally be stocked by an institution when it would be necessary to obtain it immediately in an emergency situation. The reasoning is that there may be a formulary medication normally used, but a rare patient may not be able to use it due to history of therapeutic failure or intolerance, so a nonformulary medication would be stocked in very small quantities to serve the immediate needs in that rare case until an adequate supply can be obtained for that patient. In this situation, it is important to monitor nonformulary use and use the drug evaluation process to add needed medications to formulary. Increased use of a rare nonformulary medication may indicate that it needs to be added to formulary, so that appropriate operational items are in place for safe use in the future.

Monitored use is occasionally needed if there is concern that a drug might be used in some inappropriate manner or has a great risk for adverse events. A limited drug usage evaluation would be conducted until it is evident that the drug is being appropriately used or not causing adverse events. One example where monitored use might be considered is an expensive biotechnology product that only has one labeled indication, but multiple investigational uses, where it could be inappropriately prescribed without an investigational protocol. Also, a toxic product might be monitored to see if adverse effects are appropriately addressed by the prescriber. When electronic drug usage evaluation is available, monitoring may be used to a greater extent, but is seldom justified in systems requiring the pharmacist to manually collect data. Instead, frequent drug usage evaluations will necessitate the importance of data availability as opposed to a manual collection process. Newer products, such as interfaced clinical surveillance software systems, can gather data without a manual chart review. A true chart review's importance should not be minimized; instead, because it takes substantial time to complete, a manual chart review should be used to evaluate medication use when the data cannot be obtained any other way.

Conditional addition to the formulary is a less common type of recommendation of last resort, simply because it is much easier to keep a drug off the formulary rather than try to delete an inappropriate drug that is already being used. This type of approval might be used when it is very difficult to clearly determine whether an agent will benefit the institution, if available data are limited at the time of the P&T meeting, or if there is a shortage situation where a normally nonformulary medication needs to become the formulary agent of choice, while the current formulary agent of choice is on shortage. If conditional approval is given, it is necessary to specify when the P&T committee will reconsider whether the drug should be retained on the formulary.

Recommendations to Add with Restrictions

The recommendation to add with restrictions deserves more explanation. Occasionally, there are drugs that should be added to a drug formulary, but are dangerous[53] or prone to misuse or overuse. This could include agents such as antineoplastics, thrombolytics, and fourth- or fifth-generation cephalosporins.[54] In such cases, it may be desirable to limit the use of the drugs in some manner.[55] For example, the antineoplastics might be limited to prescriptions from oncologists or a defined group that might include a few physicians who are not oncologists (e.g., rheumatologists using methotrexate), and may be required to have written or electronic orders (i.e., verbal orders not being accepted) to eliminate errors and for dose verification. Specific antibiotics might be limited to either infectious disease physicians or to specific, culture-proven diagnoses (this could be done in conjunction with the TJC requirement to approve drugs for specific indications[10]). Often antibiotics may be restricted to a specific length of therapy, after which a new order must be provided or the original order will automatically be discontinued. Accreditation requirements now have institutions maintain an antimicrobial stewardship program, where restrictions and monitoring of antimicrobials is imperative. Other restrictions could include specific floors/areas of the institution or that the physician must receive counterdetailing by the pharmacist before the drug is dispensed (see Chapter 25).[56]

One method of restriction involves formularies for managed care organizations, where they may employ any number of restrictions. There may be a cap or limitation on the price, quantity, or on how many times a patient may receive a drug (e.g., one-time use for nicotine patches to quit smoking) or on how much a patient may receive at one time (e.g., 3-month supply). A medication may be subject to prior authorization or precertification before the drug can be made available to a patient. There may be step therapy or medications, which have to be tried and failed before a specific agent may be available for coverage for a patient. Additionally, practitioners (e.g., prescribers, pharmacists) may receive financial or other incentives to cut back on the use of specific products.[57] Whenever possible, these types of restrictions should be based on objective data, such as the FDA-recommended maximum dose limitations or prescribing contraindication that can be obtained from medication-use evaluation.

Some prescribers will object to restrictions, but remember that the prescribers are given privileges to prescribe specific drugs and not rights, which allows the use of restrictions. Usually, this is not an issue, because good prescribers realize there is a reason for the restrictions. The real problem, however, is the desire to use this category much too often in an attempt to ensure proper use of all drugs. While restrictions can be effective in changing usage of specific formulary agents,[58] every time a restricted drug is prescribed, more time and effort by the pharmacy, managed care organization, and, perhaps, the prescriber is required to ensure compliance with restrictions. At the very least, a policy and procedure or guideline, and probably appropriate forms or, more likely, computer restriction methods, will need to be developed or adapted and be presented as part of the drug recommendation to the P&T committee. Additionally, overuse of restrictions with lack of coordination in a health system leads to confusion in the types of restrictions an organization uses. Aligning formulary restrictions across an entire health system assists with clarity to both prescribers and pharmacists.[59] A cost-benefit analysis may also need to be conducted to ensure that the restriction is valid, meaning that it does assist in curbing inappropriate prescribing or use of an agent or that the restriction does not cost more than any potential overuse of the product. A drug-use evaluation may also be performed to assess the usefulness of the restriction. If the results of the drug usage evaluation suggest an acceptable level of appropriate use, the P&T committee may need to reconsider the restriction placed on the product or the restriction could be costing the institution more to administer and monitor than it is saving or avoiding. Therefore, unless the computer system can eliminate much of the effort or support staff in meeting the restriction, there needs to be great restraint used when deciding to recommend that a drug be added to the drug formulary with restrictions.

Oftentimes, adding a drug to formulary with monitored use may be a viable alternative to restrictions. A twist to the restrictions or monitoring types of approval is the use of critical or clinical pathways (clinical guidelines) within an institution or health system.[60,61] In this case, a drug may be approved for use in a particular manner for the treatment of a particular disease. These critical pathways may be established for several target populations or target diseases, where additional guidance of patient treatments can result in significant improvement in patient care and/or significant decreases in costs. Because a great deal of time is necessary to develop and manage these critical pathways, they will most likely only be seen in a few areas of any institution at any given time. The recommendation should state if the drug is to be used as part of some clinical guidelines or disease state management (DSM) program.[62] The reader is referred to Chapter 8 on clinical guidelines for further information. In managed care organizations, critical pathways may be incorporated into the use parameters of a drug, through prior authorization or precertification criteria. These are specific criteria that must be met, based on clinical guidelines, current medical practices, and product prescribing information before a product is deemed medically necessary for use.

Considerations for Formulary Deletion

While the decision to add or delete a drug from the formulary is seldom black or white, a general guideline may be helpful. If the drug is less expensive or the same price as others and is more efficacious or safer—addition to the formulary is appropriate. If the drug is more expensive without added benefit, such as increased safety or effectiveness—do not add to the formulary (or deletion from the formulary is appropriate). For example, new tetracycline derivatives omadacycline (Nuzyra®), eravacycline (Xerava™), or the aminoglycoside plazomicin (Zemdri™), are often not added to drug formularies due to lack of distinguishing features, monitoring, or safety. The problem comes when the drug is more expensive and also has more benefits. For example, sugammadex (Bridion) may be added to the formulary to be used as an alternative to neostigmine, which may have limited availability on the market. In that case, the careful analysis of the literature and weighing of the institution's needs must be carried out. This is the gray area that has no right answer, but the most appropriate decision must be found. This latter decision may also involve conditional or monitored use. For medications administered primarily in an outpatient setting, reimbursement for the medication, the cost to the patient, patient insurance payor coverage of the medication, and any current or potential bundled-pricing contracts also must be factored into the decision.

Whenever a recommendation is made to add a new agent, consideration should be given to the possibility of removing agents that will no longer be necessary or, in the case of a PBM, moving the agent to a different classification for reimbursement. This whole process can be used as a way of removing extraneous agents on the formulary; however, removal of agents can be difficult if the products are frequently prescribed. (Note: It is often worthwhile to annually review a list of products that have seen little or no use in the previous year in an attempt to remove these products from the formulary.[63]) Whether removing agents individually or through a review of an entire therapeutic class, there needs to be adequate information presented to the P&T committee to show that the product is no longer necessary.

The reasons for removal may include superior agent(s) on the formulary, safety, low or no use, and/or high cost.[64] A timetable for deleting these agents from the formulary must then be developed, and the prescribers must be informed when the agent will no longer be available. The TJC medication management standards require health care organizations to review medications that are available for dispensing or administration on at least an annual basis for safety and efficacy information.[10] Many managed care organizations, health systems, and individual hospitals accomplish this via the use of the drug class review or analysis of inventory/purchasing reports on a scheduled basis. The drug classes may be placed on a schedule for review in which all classes are reviewed over the course of the year. Another option is reviewing the purchased medications over the past year at a hospital and reviewing the most purchased versus least purchased to help make surrogate decisions about potential formulary recommendations. Another process is using clinical surveillance systems that provide usage information and cost information in real time. No matter what system an institution/organization chooses to use to delete or review agents, the use should be monitored, and follow-up is necessary to ensure the formulary deletions proceed smoothly.[65] Communication of these deletions can generally appear in newsletters, emails, websites, and the institutional intranet. If a product is used by only one particular prescriber, personal contact may be best to communicate the change as well as to provide information to the prescriber of alternative products.

Consideration for Therapeutic Interchange

Finally, therapeutic interchanges must be considered (see Chapter 15).[66,67] If this concept is acceptable to the institution, and legal in the state, it may be appropriate that the new drug be used to substitute for a less desirable agent, or vice versa. In that case, a separate policy and procedure or guideline for handling that interchange needs to be prepared and considered at the same time. Please refer to Chapter 15 for further information on this subject. Also, there may be other policies and procedures or clinical guidelines that may need approval as part of the recommendation, including the requirement for availability and use of concomitant drug therapy (e.g., perhaps a requirement that antiemetic therapy needs to be given prophylactically prior to the administration of a new cancer chemotherapy agent). It is worth noting that a therapeutic interchange is perhaps the least expensive method to deal with orders for nonformulary drug products and it provides clear guidance to providers and pharmacists on the preferred product on formulary.[68]

All of the material on recommendations presented above may be confusing. ❺ However, to state it simply, *the most logical decision to benefit the patient and the institution should be recommended to the P&T committee.*

Body of the Monograph

CONSIDERATIONS FOR MONOGRAPH PREPARATION

Many parts of the body of the monograph are self-explanatory from their names and will not be discussed in detail. Some specific points, however, do need to be made about the body. First, the body may not always be reviewed by the P&T committee and, even if presented, it may be covered only briefly. The body needs to be written as a means to compile the information for reference and further information and should be part of a robust conversation at least at the subcommittee level of the P&T process, or possibly for the whole committee in the case of institutions with no P&T subcommittees. Importantly, it serves as a way of bringing all of the information together in a logical order for preparation of the summary. Some P&T committees will want to review the data presented in the body of the monograph, but all need to know that the clinical data were reviewed adequately. Other times, an abbreviated monograph may be presented to the P&T committee, and the full monograph is presented to the chair.

Second, efforts must be made to ensure that the drug in question has been adequately compared with other therapies (whether drug, surgical, radiation, or something else), if applicable. The person preparing a monograph must go through each section and ask "Have comparisons been made between this drug and the appropriate alternative therapy?" If not, there should either be a good reason for the lack of comparison or some explanation must be put in the section. Sometimes, there will be no published comparison with other drugs or therapies. For example, when conivaptan (Vaprisol) was first marketed, there were only comparisons to placebo available, but physicians wanted to know how the drug compared to hypertonic saline in hyponatremia. In that case, that limited information may have been used because sometimes there is no alternative. Indirect methods of comparison may also be necessary (e.g., comparing hypertonic saline to placebo, and then comparing conivaptan to hypertonic saline by way of the placebo comparison). Sometimes, no comparison at all is available. For example, when onasemnogene abeparvovec-xioi (Zolgensma®) was added to the market, it had no comparison product in true comparative trials. Instead, a phase I study led to FDA approval. Other analyses were done afterward comparing to nusinersen (Spinraza®) and cost-effectiveness. If at all possible, studies directly comparing the drug being evaluated to the standard of therapy should be used. Also, if there are outcome studies data, those can be important to put in the evaluation, including such hard to quantify items as quality of life.[69] When direct comparisons are not available, any literature evaluating the drug and other comparators (e.g., quality of life, cost-effectiveness) add to the review. Third, every item should be addressed, even if only to state that information was not available or that it is not applicable (e.g., absorption of intravenous [IV] drugs). This follows the rule that "if it was not written down, it was not done," or in this case was not reviewed. This is imperative for documentation of full analysis of a medication, especially if questions arise after formulary addition.

Finally, the source of the information should be mentioned—any important statement of fact must be referenced, or must be suspected of being inaccurate. The package insert (now often available from http://www.accessdata.fda.gov/scripts/cder/drugsatfda/index.cfm or https://dailymed.nlm.nih.gov/dailymed/ for newly approved products) will serve as a basis for some of the information, particularly to define what is the

FDA-approved information, but other references must be used to fill in the gaps and to back up that information. Other information can be obtained from the manufacturer, as stated in the Format for Formulary Submissions, Version 4.1 by the AMCP[4] (an example letter requesting such information is available as a part of that document), but the person preparing the monograph should also personally complete an adequate literature search to identify clinical trials related to the medication for review.

SECTIONS OF DRUG MONOGRAPH

Pharmacologic Data

- The Pharmacologic Data section is often one of the shortest sections. A simple one-paragraph explanation of the proposed mechanism of action and how it differs from the comparator agent(s) usually will suffice for the drug in question. More information may be needed if the agent is being compared to a drug with an entirely different mechanism of action (e.g., comparing a new drug in a previously unknown class of antineoplastics to whichever antineoplastic is currently being used in the treatment of a particular tumor). If the agent under consideration is an antibiotic, the spectrum of activity should be discussed, which will be much longer.

Therapeutic Indications

- The therapeutic indications section normally requires the most work. This section may be broken into three main subsections. The first is a brief coverage of the indications that the drug has been used to treat. It is necessary to clearly indicate which uses are FDA approved, non-FDA approved but reasonably supported and likely to be seen, and those that are early in investigation. Non-FDA-approved indications or possible uses may be difficult to find for new drugs; however, a literature search may be conducted to determine if any abstracts or case reports have been published for uses that were not approved by
- the FDA. It is important to list these non-FDA-approved uses as they may be helpful in determining possible restrictions to place on the drug in the recommendations section of the monograph, and it will be necessary to consider which, if any, of those uses will be approved for orders in an institutional pharmacy or health system.[70]

An example would be a new agent that is approved for a single indication. If it is a relatively new alternative to another agent, many prescribers may want to use it for investigational uses in patients in which the other agent is indicated, but not tolerated. Doses may be different in those indications. The P&T committee should review available data to determine if these investigational or off-label uses will be allowed if the new agent is on formulary. In general, investigational uses are to follow an institutional review board (IRB)-approved protocol (see Chapter 23) and may not be fully managed by a P&T committee under those circumstances; however, physicians commonly do prescribe medications for well-known, but unapproved uses. In some cases, the nonapproved use may become the most common use. For example, gabapentin was only FDA-labeled for use as an anticonvulsant for many years, until later it became regularly used neuropathic pain. Also, non-FDA-approved uses are vital when evaluating medications in a pediatric institution or various other subpopulations. Often, if non-FDA-approved uses are found to have therapeutic benefit, they will be studied further and manufacturers will submit a request to the FDA to add indications for the product. In addition, it may be very difficult to monitor off-label uses. Therefore, the consideration of other uses is important when considering possible future use of the product. They can have an impact on use of an agent for an institution. If no off-label uses are noted when the reviewer is researching the product, it is appropriate to note that fact in the evaluation.[71]

The second subsection will explain how the product and any comparison products fit into any published clinical guidelines (see Chapter 8). This should include methods for treatment of the condition, both pharmacologic and nonpharmacologic treatment approaches. An excellent source of these guidelines is the ECRI Guidelines Trust (https://guidelines.ecri.org/), which replaced the National Guidelines Clearinghouse as a source for evidence-based clinical guidelines. The use of clinical guidelines is important for a P&T committee's consideration. The inclusion of clinical guidelines allows the reader to see the product's anticipated place in therapy. If the product will be a new first-line agent, an agent should often be available for second- or third-line therapy after other agents have failed. The product's place in therapy for a particular disease or indication can play an important role in budgetary decisions when determining the usage potential of a particular product. A pharmacy department may want to increase their budget in anticipation of a new drug that will see a lot of usage for a particular condition. For example, if a new vaccine was developed to help reduce or prevent Alzheimer's disease, a nursing home or long-term care pharmacy provider may want to increase their medication budget to allow for a larger supply of the product to be on hand. However, if a product is for an indication that occurs in less than 1% of a specific gender of a particular ethnic group, the recommendation for the product may be to not add it to the formulary. Many hospitals have stringent budget requirements. Increasing the drug budget may not be possible, which places more emphasis on appropriate use and robust medication evaluation.

The third subsection will be abstracts of clinical studies supporting the various uses (see Chapter 13 for further information on how to prepare an abstract of a study). In the rare case where a product only has one indication, data from several studies on that indication should be reviewed in the monograph. If there are multiple indications, at least one well-conducted study for each FDA-approved or the most used indication is usually reviewed. More can be added, but may be redundant and provide no added benefit. If there are several similar studies, one may be covered in depth with a statement at the end of the paragraph that the use is supported by other studies, providing citations. In the case of a medication with several high-quality studies with differing results, it may be necessary to cover each of those studies. If one well-conducted study for an indication cannot be found, several lower-strength studies may be needed to provide sufficient information. Whenever possible, clinical comparison studies should be used. When reviewing newly approved drugs, it is not unusual to find that no comparison studies have been published. In that case, a simple efficacy study should be used. In some cases, it may be necessary to use a meta-analysis or case report, simply because the disease state is rare, and a typical clinical study cannot be performed. Conceivably, a meta-analysis could be performed on several small, but high-quality studies, by the author of the drug evaluation monograph, if there is adequate information in the published study. However, this would take time and expertise that may not be readily available. Overall, the quality of the information needs to be evaluated, using the skills described in Chapters 4 and 5.

In cases where no human trials are available, unless there are extenuating circumstances, the drug should generally not be added to a drug formulary until sufficient published information is available. An example of extenuating circumstances would be when a new drug is available for a previously untreatable illness. In that case, the philosophy of anything-is-better-than-nothing may apply and may require an ethics discussion within the organization to justify the addition to formulary. Also, products are sometimes approved on a fast track through the FDA because they treat a very serious, but relatively untreatable disease (e.g., certain cancers, Alzheimer's disease). These drugs may be approved based on a surrogate endpoint (i.e., not the ultimate desirable endpoint, such as length of life in cancer patients, but something that is more easily measured) or with an agreement that further studies be conducted. In cases like this, it may be desirable for the P&T committee to wait until further studies are conducted, unless circumstances dictate otherwise. Information about requirements for individual agents may be found on the FDA website at http://www.accessdata.fda.gov/scripts/cder/pmc/index.cfm.[72] Orphan drugs are approved with little clinical data for small populations of patients with rare diseases (200,000 or fewer Americans) with a list of the diseases found at https://www.fda.gov/industry/designating-orphan-product-drugs-and-biological-products/orphan-drug-designation-disease-considerations. Those drugs approved as orphan drugs may be found at https://www.accessdata.fda.gov/scripts/opdlisting/oopd/index.cfm.

The information should be presented in a manner that is similar to the description of abstracts given in the appendices to Chapter 13, making sure all information is covered. When reviewing the clinical study, the person writing the drug evaluation monograph should point out strengths and weaknesses of the studies, along with applicability of the information to the patients that are covered by the drug formulary. This evaluation may be vital in arriving at the final recommendation. In some cases, the quality, quantity, and consistency of the literature are formally graded and given a score, in a way similar to the described evaluation of articles in Chapter 8 on evidence-based clinical guidelines, which is then used in the final evaluation of the product.[73]

A new item to consider in this section is pharmacogenomics, which should be discussed when available. Pharmacogenomics has been defined as the individualization of drug therapy based on individual's genetic information.[74,75] Numerous articles have been cited showing the benefits of pharmacogenomics in potentially improving therapy and reducing adverse drug reactions.[76–78] If the genetic makeup of patients is a factor in how the medication is to be used,[79,80] such clinical study information should be presented in this section. In addition, where appropriate, pharmacogenomic information should be presented in other appropriate sections, such as pharmacokinetics, adverse effects, summary, and so forth. Pharmacogenomics is rapidly becoming a standard of practice for many disease states and drugs. The FDA's website contains a table that includes genes and affected drug products.[81] The National Institutes of Health (NIH) and the FDA have announced a joint venture regarding the scientific and regulatory structure needed to support advancements in personalized medicine. Other sources of information include the International Society for Pharmacoeconomics and Outcomes Research (ISPOR) (http://www.ispor.org) and The Pharmacogenomics Knowledgebase (http://www.pharmgkb.org/). There are no specific methods for incorporation of pharmacogenomic information in a drug evaluation monograph. Since the information can be limited to various areas of the evaluation, it can be placed in the therapeutic information or other sections, wherever it fits best. Quite often, if any information is available, it will be under all three subsections of the therapeutic information section and perhaps other places.[82]

In cases of pediatric drug use, studies may focus on adult literature and the data for pediatric literature may be available in abstracts or poster presentations only. The situation may be the same in other areas where there may not be a great deal of information on the use of the product under review. For these cases, a summary of evidence table, such as the one in Table 16-3, may be beneficial to include in the product review, which should cover material whether it is positive or negative. This provides a concise overview of all the available literature, as well as a rating system for the weight of evidence that is available for a particular indication in the pediatric population. It also contains a comparative summary, in a tabular formation, of the literature and evidence available in the adult population. In cases in which published clinical trials are not available, the summary of evidence table serves to provide the P&T committee with an overview of the data available (Table 16-4).

Another new type of publication that may be of interest in this section is comparative effectiveness research, which helps in analyzing competing treatments for specific illnesses[5] and may be available in the FDA-approval packages for as many as half of all

TABLE 16–3. SUMMARY OF EVIDENCE TABLE

	Summary of Evidence	
	Place Drug Name here	
Literature Type	Comments	Weight of Evidence[a]
Pediatric Evidence		
Efficacy		
Controlled trials		
Published reports		
Abstract		
Uncontrolled trials		
Published reports		
Abstract		
Experience reports		
Published reports		
Abstracts		
Local specialist experience		
Safety		
Published		
Abstract		
Local specialists' experience		
PK/Dosing		
Published		
Abstract		
Adult Evidence		
Efficacy		
Evaluative reviews		
Controlled trials		
Other		
Summary comments:		

[a]Levels of evidence: Good; Fair; Poor; None.
DB = double-blind; F/U = follow-up studies; PC = placebo controlled; Ra = randomized.

new drug products that are approved.[83] This is different from efficacy trials, in that it often consists of a great number of patients who are typical of the patients receiving the medications in normal practice (i.e., they are considered to be real-world patients and may have other confounding disease states, etc.). Often this information is developed from cohort studies, systematic reviews, observational studies, or meta-analyses, using large numbers of patients. Insurance company data may be used for obtaining information to conduct these trials, and it is worth noting that these studies are much less likely to be commercially funded than normal efficacy trials.[84] While these studies are

TABLE 16–4. EXAMPLE SUMMARY OF EVIDENCE TABLE

	Summary of Evidence	
	Zonisamide (Zonegran®)	
Literature Type	Comments	Weight Of Evidence[a]
Pediatric Evidence		
Efficacy		
Controlled trials		
Published reports	Two trials; total $n = 333$ subjects; generalized and partial; intellectual disability and/or refractory	Good documentation of efficacy
Abstract		
Uncontrolled trials		
Published reports	One review/study and two study reports on use for infantile spasms; total $n = \sim 109$	Good documentation for efficacy; poor for safety
Abstract	(Much of the pediatric literature is from Japan, with limited availability in English language)	Poor documentation
	14 prospective, open-label Japanese trials involving 1237 subjects were reviewed in an Epilepsia abstract	Response ($\downarrow$ by $> 50\%$):
		Generalized: 47%, 152/325
	Direct study review available for some trials	Partial: 63%, 578/912
Experience reports		
Published reports	Two reports; total $n = 4$ infants with infantile spasms	Good documentation for these cases
Abstracts	Eight abstracts; total $n = 135$; most were pediatric	Poor documentation of varied experience from multiple independent groups
Local specialist experience	Not indicated (NI)	
Safety		
Published	Ten case/case series reports published, with extensive description of adverse events	Good documentation of ADR experience reports
Abstract	Two U.S. summaries of Japanese safety experience; first—four data sources, $n = 2574$; second—14 studies, $n = 1237$. Likely overlap between two reports	Poor documentation; rather extensive experience
Local specialists' experience	NI	

continued

TABLE 16–4. EXAMPLE SUMMARY OF EVIDENCE TABLE *(CONTINUED)*

Summary of Evidence		
Zonisamide (Zonegran®)		
Literature Type	**Comments**	**Weight Of Evidence**[a]
PK/Dosing		
Published	Two reports; total $n = 194$; children and adults	Good documentation; limited data
Abstract	~ Six reports; children and/or adults; drug interaction re effects on PKs	Poor documentation of limited data
Adult Evidence		
Efficacy		
Evaluative reviews	Cochrane Review of adjunctive use for refractory partial epilepsy in three Ra studies; total $n = 499$; 12-week duration An assessment of Japanese experience was compared against clinical guidelines for AED use (established by the International League Against Epilepsy); $n = 1008$ (ped $n = 403$)	Reviewer conclusions: Effective as adjunctive treatment for refractory partial seizures Authors concluded that zonisamide was effective against both partial and refractory generalized seizures
Controlled trials	Deferred review; FDA approved for adjunctive therapy of partial seizures in adults	Good documentation, based on FDA approval
Other		
Summary comments:	Extensive, independent pediatric reports of efficacy in a variety of seizure types, both published and abstracts; demonstrated benefit in refractory seizure types, including infantile spasms; substantial published experience literature on a variety of adverse events, generally documenting reversibility with dosage adjustment or discontinuation. Limitations in evaluation: multiple publications representing the same subjects	

[a]Levels of evidence: Good; Fair; Poor; None.
DB = double-blind; F/U = follow-up studies; PC = placebo controlled; Ra = randomized.

useful for practical data and to help discover rare adverse effects, they also do suffer from the weaknesses inherent in any cohort trial or meta-analysis (see Chapter 5 for further information). Although they may be available as part of FDA-approval packages, they are also relatively rare in the literature, even though it is believed that they can help obtain formulary addition for drug products[85] and are more commonly being used for formulary decisions made by national committees in countries such as Britain, Australia, and Canada.[86] They may also be used by third-party payers to determine the payment-tier placement of products.[87] Overall, it is anticipated that these trials will help to identify overuse, misuse, and underuse of various treatments,[88] and may be seen more commonly in the future.

In preparing the therapeutic use section, it may also be useful to review materials that were presented to any FDA Advisory Committees, which may be found at https://www.fda.gov/advisory-committees.

Other information may also be covered in the therapeutics section, including quality-of-life studies.

Pharmacokinetics

The Bioavailability/Pharmacokinetics section is similar to what would be found in most tertiary publications, but the information may be difficult to find for some new drugs. In some cases, a new dosage form may be considered in a drug evaluation. For example, when a drug is released in IV form, its use may be entirely different from the oral form, so the P&T committee might separately consider it. A change in route, however, does not necessarily mean that elimination is significantly different in the same patient population. Therefore, oral data may be more useful than no information. Whenever possible, a table comparing the drug in question to other products or formulations may be helpful.

Dosage, Administration, and Supply

The Dosage Form section is a good place to point out the limitations in dosage forms available for some drugs. For example, perhaps the drug in question is available only as an oral solid, but its comparator agent is available in oral solid, oral liquid, and injectable forms, which could be an advantage. This section can also be used to discuss unusual preparation directions or pointing out which product would be easier, quicker, and less expensive to prepare. Additionally, this section should state if the product has any limitations on access (i.e., the product is only available from a registry or available to select facilities), distribution, supply limitations, or possible anticipated shortages.[89] This section can also cover the handling of medications that have a high-risk for serious injury if misused or pose a risk to employees when handling the medication (see https://www.cdc.gov/niosh/review/peer/isi/hazdrug2018-pr.html). In addition, the dosage form section should also address special provisions for the procurement, storage, ordering, dispensing, and monitoring of these high-risk agents. Medication error problems in this area may be addressed by professional practice procedures describing product labeling and packaging, nomenclature, compounding and dispensing, education, administration, monitoring, and use. Specific recommendations are available regarding antineoplastic agents that address health care professionals, organizations, and patients.[90]

Known Adverse Effects/Toxicities

When presenting the information in the Known Adverse Effects/Toxicities section, serious and/or common adverse effects for both the specific drug and the drug class should be the focus. Whenever possible, incidence and severity should be included. An incidence comparison table listing the agent under consideration and other similar agents may be an efficient and informative method to show the material. If there are many rare, minor adverse effects, a statement to that effect can be listed at the end of the discussion. Conversely, other agents may have very little information available on adverse effects, simply because they are too new. In that case, it may be necessary to discuss adverse effects common to that class of agent, making it clear that they have not yet been seen with the new drug, but are possible. The new agent should be compared to other agents used for the same indication to determine whether there are any advantages. Keep in mind that these tables can be deceiving, because older agents may have 20 years of side effect reports, whereas, a number of adverse effects of the new agent may not yet be discovered.

Also, TJC requires patient safety information to be addressed in all monographs, including sentinel event advisories.[10] It has been recommended that a list of possible safety problems be compiled. This may include concerns in such areas as ordering, transcribing, order entry, storage, order verification, compounding, dispensing, administration, and monitoring.[91] It may be good to consider **Risk Evaluation and Mitigation Strategies (REMS)** information from the FDA in this section (e.g., tolvaptan [Jynarque®] concern with liver injury).[92] Some drugs may be added to the formulary simply because of improved patient safety, even though that comes at an increased cost.[1] Besides the package labeling, other sources of this information can be found at:

- Institute for Safe Medication Practices (ISMP): http://www.ismp.org
- MedWatch: http://www.fda.gov/medwatch
- United States Pharmacopeia: http://www.usp.org/

Once the list of possible safety concerns has been compiled, even a tally of the number of items can be helpful, but it also may be that specific items cause an overriding concern. In response, P&T committees have implemented safety-focused drug monographs, which include information regarding medication errors.[93]

The Patient Monitoring Guidelines and Patient Information sections listed are items not suggested by ASHP. These sections were originally added for use in the ambulatory care environment, although they can be quite informative in any practice area.

One new area would include pharmacoinformatics issues and IV pump library issues, which are having an increasing impact on the use of medications in institutions.[94] As mentioned previously, an example of challenges incorporating a new medication into the electronic medical record order set and smart pump library was angiotensin II (GIAPREZA) which is dosed as ng/kg/minute. It may be necessary to make a delay in use after approval as part of the recommendation to complete nursing education and getting the pumps reprogrammed to include an ng dose.

Contraindications

A list of the known contraindications must be provided.

Drug Interactions

A list of common and/or severe drug interactions must be provided. Usually this is done with a brief explanation of the interaction and, perhaps, what to do about it. It may be done referring to drug classes as a whole.

Patient Safety Information

There may be overlap of the information in this section with that in the previous several sections. However, it is important to make clear what is shown to be important by such groups as the Institute for Safe Medication Practices (ISMP), MedWatch, FDA Patient Safety News, United States Pharmacopeia Patient Safety Program, and National Institute for Occupational Safety and Health (NIOSH).

Patient Monitoring Guidelines

This section includes effectiveness, adverse effects, compliance, and other appropriate items.

Patient Information

This section is particularly important in the ambulatory environment. It briefly includes information usually found in a patient package insert.

Guideline/Order Set

This section includes guideline(s) or order set(s) needed and how operations will be affected if the drug is added to formulary. It will include any pharmacoinformatics issues and IV pump library issues.

Cost Comparison

The final section is the cost comparison, where the product being reviewed is compared in price to other similar products. Typically, three or four medications (possibly including both trade name and generic products) are compared, although sometimes it is necessary to compare a dozen or more products or dosage forms. Preferably, a pharmacoeconomic analysis should be prepared[95] (see Chapter 7) because the seemingly more expensive agent may turn out to be less expensive, as it decreases the length of hospitalization, degree of monitoring, or number of adverse events that would otherwise occur.[96–98] Such an analysis is considered to be important by the majority of institutions[99] and managed care organizations.[100] It may, however, take a considerable amount of time to prepare and sometimes the assumptions made in preparing the analysis will be challenged by attendees.[101] Sometimes, it may even be necessary to provide a spreadsheet to show what effect changes in assumptions may have on the economic analysis. In the case of drug evaluation monographs prepared in the method of the AMCP guidelines, the information in this section may provide detailed abstracts of pharmacoeconomic studies, in a manner similar to that seen for clinical studies in the Therapeutics section.[4] Overall, the items included in the analysis should make sense to those doing the evaluation.[102] It should be noted that the assumptions intrinsic in any pharmacoeconomic analysis are considered pseudoscience by some and are discouraged,[103,104] even though they may be the best information available on which to make important financial decisions.

Often, a full pharmacoeconomic review is not practical because of lack of time or expertise, although most large hospitals do report doing a formal economic analysis of some kind for each drug reviewed for possible formulary addition.[105] With particularly expensive products, a comprehensive pharmacoeconomic analysis becomes necessary.[106,107] Even when a full pharmacoeconomic analysis is not practical, any pertinent information that could be used in a full analysis should be included. This includes hospital medication cost, impact to length of stay or disease state, and reimbursement coverage. After all, sometimes the most expensive (per dose) drug product may actually be much less expensive in the long run, because of increased or faster efficacy, decreased incidence of adverse effects, or lower monitoring costs. It is relatively seldom that a simple comparison of cost per tablet/capsule between two products will correctly compare their financial impact on an institution.

In some cases, a simple price comparison can be prepared using the cost of the drugs and the frequency of administration. Health systems may be challenged with a medication cost analysis, since each hospital comprising the health system may purchase the medication at a different price. System-wide contracting agreements may mitigate this issue, but there will likely remain a gap for facilities that have **340b** program pricing and for those that do not. In these cases, the unique costs and current or estimated purchase volume must be evaluated to make sure that a rational decision is made. Such a price comparison must also consider that the patient may be getting medications both within an institution and after returning home, because institutional pharmacies may get considerable discounts. If at all possible, the patient costs based on locally common insurance companies/pharmacy benefit management companies and Medicare need to be considered, since that may affect home compliance with medications.[108–113] Therefore, both the institution's cost for the medication, likely **group purchasing organization (GPO)** pricing, and the average wholesale price (AWP) should be considered. Some medications are extremely inexpensive to the institution, making it tempting to include those agents on the formulary instead of similar therapeutic agents. However, if the AWP is excessively high, the patient may not be able to afford the product in the community, which could quickly lead to readmission into the hospital, when the patient's disease is no longer being treated. In those cases, it may not be an appropriate product to carry on the formulary, or the patient will need a prescription for the appropriate product on discharge. Also, the differences in package sizes and frequency of administration must be considered. In most cases, products can be compared on the cost of a typical day's therapy at a relatively normal dose; however, in some cases, a different approach may be necessary. For example, an antineoplastic agent may need to be compared with other agents based on a per-cycle or per-cost of therapeutic regimen basis. Another example that results in unusual cost comparisons is Nexplanon® (an implantable contraceptive agent). The cost of both the drug and the implantation procedure need to be compared to a 3-year supply of other contraceptive agents. In cases like this, over a period of years, it may be necessary to include calculations of inflation or other factors likely to change over the time period.[114]

Other costs should also be considered when possible, such as drug preparation costs, administration costs, laboratory tests, monitoring requirements, and changes of length of stay/therapy—after all, it is not a savings overall if costs are simply shifted from the pharmacy (i.e., drug price) to the laboratory (i.e., monitoring costs).[115] Increasingly, theranostics (also known as pharmacodiagnostics—which is defined as the analysis of a patient's genome in order to personalize medical treatment using pharmacogenomics) will be a substantial cost that needs to be included in the analysis.[116] Some pharmacies even include such items as the cost to order and hold the drug, and the cost of preparing the evaluation of the drug for the P&T committee.[117] Also, it may be necessary to take into account some items more difficult to assess, such as the probability and cost of therapeutic failure in comparison to other similar agents, impact of specific drug therapy on other health care costs (a drug may be cheaper, but require an increase in the cost of other nondrug therapy for the patient), and the cost of adverse drug effects.[118] Because these items may depend on the characteristics of the patients (e.g., age, socioeconomic status, education level), the costs used are going to be uncertain. In some cases, however, they will be important in the final formulary decisions. A drug that at first glance appears more expensive may be found to actually cost the institution less in the end.[96] Also, it is necessary to consider nondrug therapy (e.g., surgery, radiation therapy, physical therapy) in the comparison, when they are legitimate alternatives to drug therapy. Overall, the goal is to ensure that the comparison makes sense and takes into consideration all of the relevant economic factors. ❻ *Cost is heavily emphasized in formulary decisions and must be properly accounted for, given the complexities of drug acquisition pricing, payor coverage, cost to the hospital, and reimbursement.* Some drugs cost thousands of dollars per dose, and that can quickly deplete a pharmacy department's budget and significantly affect the economic status of an institution. Using a standard method to vet financial information helps an institution perform a due diligence review and include medication cost, reimbursement picture for outpatient care, bundled payments, and cost to the patient.

Overall

Of importance, a drug evaluation monograph follows a general pattern and sequence of content as outlined in this chapter. The depth, length, and expected template for use will differ between institutions, but should be appropriate, efficient, and approved for use at the institution. For example, some places prefer bullet points and tables to present information, while others expect a longer paragraph review. Refer to the institution for the guidance on a drug evaluation monograph.

Monographs should also include operational items for discussion and vetting. These include how a medication will appear in the electronic medical record, how order sets may be impacted, including a financial clearance process for outpatient care, impact of contracting, and education plans after approval. Incorporation and preparation of these items lend an additional lens to the normal drug monograph and give the P&T committee an opportunity to provide any suggestions for improvement of implementation once a drug is approved.

Distribution of Drug Formulary

One thing to take into consideration with a drug formulary is how it is to be made available to the members of a P&T committee. In the past, it would have naturally been by paper copy. However, particularly with distributed hospital systems, it may be necessary to have an electronic copy that may be made available.[119] This system may provide restrictions on when it is available and how it is available (e.g., it may not be printable) in order to prevent copies getting to drug company representatives. Such a system may also be sophisticated enough to assist in interchange of documents in more than one direction, online discussions and even secret ballots.

Conclusion

❼ *Preparation of a drug evaluation monograph requires a great amount of time and effort, using many of the skills discussed throughout this text to obtain, evaluate, collate, and provide information. However, the value of having all of the issues evaluated and discussed can be invaluable in providing quality care.*

Case Study 16–1

You are a recent graduate who just completed a PGY1 residency. You have accepted a position at a local hospital medical center as a clinical pharmacist. One of your first assignments is to prepare and present a medication monograph on a new oral direct thrombin inhibitor that was just approved by the FDA. You will have 10 minutes to present at the next pharmacy and therapeutics committee meeting that will be held next week. The only piece of information that you are given is the request to add this drug to formulary. All medications are reviewed for the outpatient pharmacy as well.

1. Having reviewed the request, what are the steps to add this drug to the formulary?
2. What are the essential elements of a medication monograph?
3. What sources of information do you need to develop a complete evidence-based medication monograph?

Case Study 16–2

Following the development of the drug evaluation monograph, you are then asked to prepare a concise high-level summary page of this medication monograph.

1. What are the elements of a high-level summary page?
2. You are planning to use this monograph for your inpatient as well as the outpatient pharmacies. What information should be included as it relates to the outpatient dispensing of this medication?
3. What are the different types of formulary status recommendations and how do they differ?

Case Study 16–3

After your success with the drug evaluation monograph and the high-level summary, you have now been asked to evaluate the cost of a new chemotherapy medication that has just received FDA approval. Your work will then be turned over to others for the creation of a full drug evaluation monograph. It is important to be aware that your hospital is part of a health system with a system-wide formulary so the following information will be important for your analysis of the cost of the new medication "Chemotherapy 1":

- GPO price: $10000 per 100 mg vial
- 340b price: $9000 per 100 mg vial
- Ten hospitals in the health system and two qualify for 340b pricing
- Anticipated annual use will be in 70 patients
- Average dose is 300 mg per patient × 28 doses
- Medicare reimbursement is $950 per 10 mg
- Your hospital markup for drug prices is two times cost
- Private insurance companies on average pay 53% of what they are charged for outpatient medications
- Medicare accounts for 50% of patient volume and the other 50% is private insurance
- 304b facilities account for 10% of health system oncology volume
- The health system charges all patients the GPO price for medications and passes on the 340b savings in other ways:
  1. What is the annual cost impact if this medication is added to formulary?
  2. How will the health system be reimbursed for this medication?
  3. What other considerations are important as the cost data is prepared for the monograph?

Case Study 16–4

As a pharmacist practicing in a large health system at an outpatient dialysis clinic at the main hospital, a request is presented by the patient's insurance to use a biosimilar epoetin alfa-epbx (Retacrit) instead of epoetin alfa (Epogen). The nonformulary review process approved use of the biosimilar in this patient.

1. What is important for a formulary process to consider when evaluating the biosimilar for formulary addition?
2. What is important to review for payor coverage?
3. What should the cost analysis include?

Case Study 16–5

The health system treats patients with SMA. A new medication, onasemnogene abeparvovec-xioi (Zolgensma), is now available. It is marketed as a curative dose for $2.1 million per dose.

1. What are important items to consider for the monograph?
2. How would a medication like this be implemented?
3. How should this medication be monitored?

Case Study 16–6

As the formulary pharmacist, you are supporting multiple drug evaluation monographs, class reviews, annual analysis, etc.

1. What tools are available to stay organized?
2. How are medication reviews prioritized?
3. What are some ways to remain efficient?

Self-Assessment Questions

1. Medications or medication classes considered for a medication formulary should be objectively assessed based on:
   a. Scientific information
   b. Anecdotal prescriber experience
   c. Manufacturer information
   d. Published review
   e. All of the above

2. The summary page of a medication monograph:
   a. Provides a summary of the most important information concerning the medication

b. Completely evaluates a medication product

c. Provides a record of all that was taken into consideration

d. Includes items that are not clinically significant

3. The body of the monograph does which of the following:

a. Brings all the information together in a logical order

b. Adequately compares the medication to other therapies

c. Only addresses certain items

d. Includes the source of the information

e. a and b

4. Hospitals and health systems review the medication formulary at least annually as required by The Joint Commission.

a. True

b. False

5. A medication monograph provides a tool for the pharmacy to:

a. Guide the rational development of a medication formulary

b. Provide a full, fair, and balanced review of a medication

c. View medications from a whole and macroeconomic view

d. All of the above

6. Pharmacogenomics is the study of:

a. Medication indications and nonapproved indications

b. Medication cost

c. Medication tier placement

d. Individualized drug therapy based on an individual's genetic makeup

7. When making formulary recommendations as it pertains to third-party payers, consideration should be given to the placement of the formulary agent into a multitiered copayment system where the copayment varies according to the cost of the drug and/or formulary status.

a. True

b. False

8. Future medication monographs may be expected to include clinical outcomes, continuous quality assurance information, pharmacogenomics, and quality-of-life issues.

a. True

b. False

9. A drug evaluation monograph cannot be used to evaluate a therapeutic interchange.

a. True

b. False

10. There is only one format, length, and style that a drug evaluation monograph should follow.
    a. True
    b. False

11. When evaluating the price of a medication for a monograph to be used for a health system, the following must be considered:
    a. Each hospital's individual price
    b. 340b status of the hospital
    c. If the medication will primarily be used inpatient or outpatient
    d. Common insurance company/Medicare prices in the area
    e. All of the above

12. All hospitals qualify for 340b medication pricing and it should be consistently used when evaluating medication costs.
    a. True
    b. False

13. A biosimilar medication and therapeutic interchange review does not require a standard analysis of cost information or insurance coverage.
    a. True
    b. False

14. Developing a monograph review in a PBM should include:
    a. QALY analysis
    b. Clinical evidence review
    c. Insurance tier/prior authorization
    d. All of the above

15. A robust recommendation results from:
    a. A pharmacist trained in literature evaluation incorporating unbiased review
    b. Pharmacoeconomic analysis
    c. Discussions with colleagues
    d. All of the above

Acknowledgment

The assistance of Linda K. Ohri, PharmD, MPH in preparation of this chapter in previous editions is acknowledged.

REFERENCES

1. Raber JH. The formulary process from a risk management perspective. Pharmacotherapy. 2010;30(6 Pt 2):42S-47S.

2. Schiff GD, Tripathi JB, Galanter W, Paek JL, Pontikes P, Fanikos J, Matta L, Lambert BL. Drug formulary decision-making: ethnographic study of 3 pharmacy and therapeutics committees. Am J Health-Syst Pharm. 2019 Apr 15;76(8):537-542.

3. Barlas S. Formulary policies a battleground in HHS proposal on nondiscrimination. Are tiering and cost sharing civil rights issues? P&T. 2016 Mar;41(3):173-5, 193.

4. Format for formulary submissions, version 4.1. Alexandria (VA): Academy of Managed Care Pharmacy; 2019.

5. Schumock GT, Pickard AS. Comparative effectiveness research: relevance and applications to pharmacy. Am J Health-Syst Pharm. 2009;66:1278-86.

6. Wade WE, Spruill WJ, Taylor AT, Longe RL, Hawkins DW. The expanding role of pharmacy and therapeutics committees. The 1990s and beyond. PharmacoEconomics. 1996;10(2):123-8.

7. Labeling for biosimilar products. Guidance for Industry. Silver Springs (MD): U.S. Department of Health and Human Services; 2018 Jul.

8. Smeeding J, Malone D, Rachandani M, Stolshek B, Green L, Schneider P. Biosimilars: considerations for payers. P&T. 2019;44(2):54-63.

9. Leber MB. Considerations for adding biosimilars to formulary. Pharm Purch Prod. 2017;14(12):24.

10. TJC—The Joint Commission comprehensive accreditation and certification manual. Accreditation requirements for hospitals [Internet]. Oakbrook Terrace (IL): The Joint Commission; 2013 Jan 1 [cited 2012 Dec 14]. Available from: https://e-dition.jcrinc.com/MainContent.aspx

11. Heindel GA, McIntyre CM. Contemporary challenges and novel strategies for health-system formulary management. Am J Health-Syst Pharm. 2018;75(8):556-60.

12. Karel LI, Delisle DR, Anagnostis EA, Wordell CJ. Implementation of a formulary management process. Am J Health-Syst Pharm. 2017;74(16):1245-52.

13. ASHP technical assistance bulletin on the evaluation of drugs for formularies. Am J Hosp Pharm. 1991;48:791–3.

14. Majercik PL, May JR, Longe RL, Johnson MH. Evaluation of pharmacy and therapeutics committee drug evaluation reports. Am J Hosp Pharm. 1985;42:1073-6.

15. Academy of Managed Care Pharmacy. Therapeutic interchange. 2003 Feb [cited 2010 Nov 5]; [2 p.]. Available from: http://www.amcp.org/WorkArea/DownloadAsset.aspx?id=18745

16. Australian regulatory guidelines for prescription medicines [Internet]. Woden, Australia: Australian Government, Department of Health and Ageing, Therapeutic Goods Administration; 2019 Feb 8 [cited 2019 Jun 19]. Available from: https://www.tga.gov.au/publication/australian-regulatory-guidelines-prescription-medicines-argpm

17. Ontario guidelines for drug submission and evaluation. Toronto: Ministry of Health and Long-Term Care; 2006.

18. Guide to the process of technology appraisal [Internet]. London: National Institute for Clinical Excellence; 2018 [cited 2019 Jun 19]. Available from: https://www.nice.org.uk/process/pmg19/chapter/1-acknowledgements

19. Duguid MJ. Evaluating new medicines for use in Australian hospitals: lessons from North America. J Pharm Pract Res. 2010;40(2):124-9.

20. Groves KE, Fanagan PS, MacKinnon NJ. Why physicians start or stop prescribing a drug: literature review and formulary implications. Formulary. 2002;37(4):186–8, 190-4.

21. Strite S, Stuart ME, Urban S. Process steps and suggestions for creating drug monographs and drug class reviews in an evidence-based formulary system. Formulary. 2008;43:135-6, 139-40,142,144-5.

22. Cohen KR, Cerone P, Ruggiero R. Complementary/alternative medicine use: responsibilities and implications for pharmacy services. P&T. 2002;27(9):440-6.

23. Fagan NL, Malone PM, Baltaro RJ, Malesker MA. Applying principles of formulary management to blood banking. Transfusion. 2013;53(9):2094-7.

24. Chan L-N. Consider potential for drug interactions during formulary review. Am J Health-Syst Pharm. 2000;57:391.

25. Schiff GD, Galanter WL, Duhig J, Koronkowski MJ, Lodolce AE, Pontikes P, Busker J, Touchette D, Walton S, Lambert BL. A prescription for improving drug formulary decision making. PLoS Med. 2012 May;9(5):e1001220.

26. Feldman JA, DeTullio PL. Medication noncompliance: an issue to consider in the drug selection process. Hosp Formul. 1994;29:204-11.

27. Sesin GP. Therapeutic decision-making: a model for formulary evaluation. Drug Intell Clin Pharm. 1986;20:581-3.

28. Abu Esba LC, Almodaimegh H, Alhammad A, Ferwana M, Yousef C, Ismail S. P&T committee drug prioritization criteria: a tool developed by a Saudi health care system. P&T. 2018 May;43(5):293-300.

29. Cohen MR. Adding drugs to the formulary: your work is never done. Hosp Pharm. 1999;34:828.

30. Hedblom EC. Pharmacoeconomic and outcomes data in the managed care formulary decision-making process. P&T. 1995;20:462-4, 468, 471–3.

31. Klink B. Formulary influences. Drug Top. 1998;142(20):72.

32. Rich DS. Pharmacies' noncompliance with 2009 Joint Commission hospital accreditation requirements. Am J Health-Syst Pharm. 2009;66:e27-e30.

33. Abourjaily P, Kross J, Gouveia WA. Initiatives to control drug costs associated with an independent physician association. Am J Health-Syst Pharm. 2003;60:269-72.

34. Gleason PP, Gunderson BW, Gericke KR. Are incentive-based formularies inversely associated with drug utilization in managed care? Ann Pharmacother. 2005;39:339-45.

35. Reissman D. Issues in drug benefit management. Drug Benefit Trends. 2004 Dec:598-9.

36. Sroka CJ. CRS report for Congress: pharmacy benefit managers. Washington (DC): Library of Congress; 2000.

37. Trovato A, Choudhary K, Fox ER. Development and implementation of a strategy to ensure outpatient access to medications started in the inpatient setting. Am J Health-Syst Pharm. 2019;76(6):334-5.

38. Tyler LS, Cole SW, May JR, Millares M, Valentino MA, Vermeulen LCJr, Cole SW. ASHP guidelines on the pharmacy and therapeutics committee and the formulary system. Am J Health-Syst Pharm. 2008;65:1272-83.

39. Dedrick S, Kessler JM. Formulary evaluation teams: Duke University Medical Center's approach to P&T committee reorganization. Formulary. 1999;34:47-51.

40. Kresel JJ, Hutchings HC, MacKay DN, Weinstein MC, Read JL, Taylor-Halvorsen K, Ashley H. Application of decision analysis to drug selection for formulary addition. Hosp Formul. 1987;22:658-76.

41. Szymusiak-Mutnick B, Mutnick AH. Application of decision analysis in antibiotic formulary choices. J Pharm Technol. 1994;10:23-26.

42. Basskin L. How to use decision analysis to solve pharmacoeconomic problems. Formulary. 1997;32:619-28.

43. Kessler JM. Decision analysis in the formulary process. Am J Health-Syst Pharm. 1997;54(Suppl 1):S5-S8.

44. Schumacher GE. Multiattribute evaluation in formulary decision-making as applied to calcium-channel blockers. Am J Hosp Pharm. 1991;48:301-8.

45. Barner JC, Thomas J III. Tools, information sources, and methods used in deciding on drug availability in HMOs. Am J Health-Syst Pharm. 1998;55:50-56.

46. Gibaldi M. Meta-analysis: a review of its place in therapeutic decision-making. Drugs. 1993;46:805–18.

47. Studdert AL, Gong CL, Srinavas S, Chin AL, Deresinski S. Application of pharmacoeconomics to formulary management in a health system setting. Am J Health-Syst Pharm. 2019;76(6):381-6.

48. Austin JP, Halvorson SAC. Reducing the expert halo effect on pharmacy and therapeutics committees. JAMA. 2019;321(5):453-4.

49. Rodriguez R, Kelly BJ, Moody M. Evaluating the training, responsibilities, and practices of P&T committee members and nonmember contributors. J Manag Care Spec Pharm. 2017;23:868-74.

50. Gannon K. Uniqueness of a drug key to formulary inclusion. Hosp Pharm Rep. 1996;10:27.

51. Chase P, Bell J, Smith P, Fallik A. Redesign of the P&T committee around continuous quality improvement principles. P&T. 1995;20(1):25-26, 29-30, 32, 34, 37-38, 40.

52. Ain KB, Pucino F, Csako G, Wesley RA, Drass JA, Clark C. Effects of restricting levothyroxine dosage strength availability. Pharmacotherapy. 1996;16(6):1103-10.

53. Limit potential dangers by restricting problem drugs on formulary. Drug Util Rev. 1997;13(4):49–51.

54. Anassi EO, Ericsson C, Lal L, McCants E, Stewart K, Moseley C. Using a pharmaceutical restriction program to control antibiotic use. Formulary. 1995;30:711-4.

55. Berndt EM. Drug expenditures. A medical center's experience with antibiotic cost-saving measures. Drug Benefit Trends. 1997;9:32-6.

56. McCloskey WW, Johnson PN, Jeffrey LP. Cephalosporin-use restrictions in teaching hospitals. Am J Hosp Pharm. 1984;41:2359-62.

57. Goldberg RB. Managing the pharmacy benefit: the formulary system. J Manag Care Pharm. 1997;3(5):565-73.

58. Hayman JN, Sbravati EC. Controlling cephalosporin and aminoglycoside costs through pharmacy and therapeutics committee restrictions. Am J Hosp Pharm. 1985;42:1343-7.

59. Solano S, Dow J, Audley T, Bangalore N. Aligning formulary restrictions across a health system and improving access to and clarity of medication restrictions. P&T. 2019 Jan/Feb;44(2):64-8.

60. McCaffrey S, Nightingale CH. The evolving health care marketplace. How to develop critical paths and prepare for other formulary management changes. Hosp Formul. 1994;29:628-35.

61. Dana WJ, McWhinney B. Managing high cost and biotech drugs: two institutions' perspectives. Hosp Formul. 1994;29:638-45.

62. Armstrong EP. Disease state management and its influence on health systems today. Drug Benefit Trends. 1996;8:18-20, 25, 29.

63. Persson EL, Miller KS, Nieman JA, Sgourakis AP, Akkerman SR. Formulary evaluation using a class review approach. Experience and results from an academic medical center. P&T. 2013 Apr;38(4):213-6.

64. Kelly WN, Rucker TD. Considerations in deciding which drugs should be in a formulary. J Pharm Pract. 1994 ;VII(2):51-7.

65. Lemay AP, Salzer LB, Visconti JA, Latiolais CJ. Strategies for deleting popular drugs from a hospital formulary. Am J Hosp Pharm. 1981;38:506-10.

66. Boesch D. Formularies and therapeutic substitution: gaining ground in long-term care. Consult Pharm. 1994;9:284–97.

67. Therapeutic interchange [Internet]. Alexandria (VA): Academy of Managed Care Pharmacy; 2012 Jun [cited 2017 Sep 22]; [2 p.]. Available from: http://www.amcp.org/WorkArea/DownloadAsset.aspx?id=18745

68. Helmons PJ, Kosterink JW, Daniels CE. Formulary compliance and pharmacy labor costs associated with systematic formulary management strategy. Am J Health-Syst Pharm. 2014 Mar 1;71:407-15.

69. Lewis BE, Fish L. Drug approvals. Formulary decisions in managed care: the role of quality of life. Drug Benefit Trends. 1997;9:41–7.

70. Skledar SJ, Corman SL, Smitherman T. Addressing innovative off-label medication use at an academic medical center. Am J Health-Syst Pharm. 2015;72:469-77.

71. ASHP statement on the use of medications for unlabeled uses. Am J Hosp Pharm. 1992;49:2006–8.

72. Marchand HC, Rose BJ, Fine AM, Kremzner ME. The U.S. Food and Drug Administration: drug information resources for formulary recommendations. J Manage Care Pharm. 2012 Nov/Dec;18(9):713-8.

73. Corman SL, Skledar SJ, Culley CM. Evaluation of conflicting literature and application to formulary decisions. Am J Health-Syst Pharm. 2007 Jan 15;64:182-5.

74. Feero WG, Guttmacher AE, Collins FS. Genomic medicine: an updated primer. N Engl J Med. 2010;363:301-4.

75. Hamburg MA, Collins FS. The path to personalized medicine. N Engl J Med. 2010;363:301-4.

76. Philips KA, Veensta DL, Oren E, Lee JK, Sadee W. Potential role of pharmacogenomics in reducing adverse drug reactions: a systemic review. JAMA. 2001;286:2270-9.

77. Meyer UA. Pharmacogenetics and adverse drug reactions. The Lancet. 2000;356(9242): 1667-71.

78. Empey PE. Genetic predisposition to adverse drug reaction in the intensive care unit. Crit Care Med. 2010;38(6):S106-S116.

79. Morrow TJ. Implications of pharmacogenomics in the current and future treatment of asthma. J Managed Care Pharm. 2007;13(6):497-505.

80. ASHP Statement on the pharmacist's role in clinical pharmacogenomics. Am J Health-Syst Pharm. 2015 Apr 1;72:579-81.

81. U.S. Food and Drug Administration. Table of valid genomic biomarkers in the context of approved drug labels. 2020 Feb 5 [cited 2020 Apr 13]. Available from: http://www.fda.gov/Drugs/ScienceResearch/ResearchAreas/Pharmacogenetics/ucm083378.htm

82. Poppe LB, Roederer MW. Global formulary review: how do we integrate pharmacogenomics information. Ann Pharmacother. 2011 Apr;45:532-8.

83. Goldberg NH, Schneeweiss S, Kowal MK, Gagne JJ. Availability of comparative efficacy data at the time of drug approval in the United States. JAMA. 2011 May 4;305(17):1786-9.

84. Hochman M, McCormick D. Characteristics of published comparative effectiveness studies of medications. JAMA. 2010 Mar 10;303(10):951-8.

85. Brixner DI, Watkins JB. Can CER be an effective tool for change in the development and assessment of new drugs and technologies. J Manage Care Pharm. 2012 Jun;18(5):S6-S11.

86. Clement FM, Harris A, Li JJ, Yong K, Lee KM, Manns BJ. Using effectiveness and cost-effectiveness to make drug coverage decisions. A comparison of Britain, Australia, and Canada. JAMA. 2009;302(13):1437-43.

87. Doyle JJ. The effect of comparative effectiveness research on drug development innovation: a 360° value appraisal. Comp Effectiveness Res. 2011;1:27-34.

88. Comparative effectiveness research: paving the way for evidence-based decision making. Managed Care. 2011 Aug;20(7 Suppl 4):2-7.

89. Leady MA, Adams AL, Stumpf JL, Sweet BV. Drug shortages: an approach to managing the latest crisis. Hosp Pharm. 2003;38:748-52.

90. Goldspiel B, Hoffman JM, Griffith NL, Goodin S, DeChristoforo R, Montello M, Chase JL, Bartel S, Patel JT. ASHP guidelines on preventing medication errors with chemotherapy and biotherapy. Am J Health-Syst Pharm. 2015;72:e6-e35.

91. Pick AM, Massoomi F, Neff WJ, Danekas PI, Stoysich AM. A safety assessment tool for formulary candidates. Am J Health-Syst Pharm. 2006;63:1269-72.

92. Milenkovich N. Ready or not, here come the REMS. Drug Top. 2009 Oct:65.

93. Murri NA, Somani S, University HealthSystem Consortium Pharmacy Council Medication Management/Quality Improvement Committee. Implementation of safety-focused pharmacy and therapeutics monographs: a new University HealthSystem Consortium template designed to minimize medication misadventures. Hosp Pharm. 2004;39(7): 653–60.

94. Karel LI, Delisle DR, Anagnostis EA, Wordell CJ. Implementation of a formulary management process. Am J Health-Syst Pharm. 2017 Aug 15;74(16):1245-52.

95. Sanchez LA. Pharmacoeconomics and formulary decision-making. PharmacoEconomics. 1996;9(Suppl 1):16–25.

96. Heiligenstein JH. Reformulating our formularies to reflect real-world outcomes. Drug Benefit Trends. 1996;8:35, 42.

97. Shulkin D. Reinventing the pharmacy and therapeutics committee. P&T. 2012 Nov;37(11):623-24, 649.

98. Studdert AL, Gong CL, Srinivas S, Chin AL, Deresinski S. Application of pharmacoeconomics to formulary management in a health system setting. Am J Health-Syst Pharm. 2019 Mar 15;76(6):381-6.

99. Odedina FI, Sullivan J, Nash R, Clemmons CD. Use of pharmacoeconomic data in making hospital formulary decisions. Am J Health-Syst Pharm. 2002;59:1441-4.

100. Suh D-C, Okpara JRN, Agnese WB, Toscani M. Application of pharmacoeconomics to formulary decision making in managed care organizations. Am J Manage Care. 2002;8(2):161-9.

101. McCain J. System helps P&T committees get pharmacoeconomic data they need [Internet]. Managed Care. 2001 Apr [cited 2007 Jul 17]; [14 p.]. Available from: http://www.managedcaremag.com/archives/0104/0104.amcp.html

102. Getting the most out of formularies involves a bit of economic training. Manage Care. 2015 Apr;24(4):9-10.

103. Langley PC. Supporting formulary decisions: the discovery of new facts or constructed evidence? [Internet]. Inov Pharm. 2016;7(2): Article 15. Available from: http://pubs.lib.umn.edu/innovations/vol7/iss2/15

104. Langley PC. Modeling imaginary worlds: Version 4 of the AMCP Format for Formulary Submissions [Internet]. Inov Pharm. 2016;7(2): Article 11. Available from: http://pubs.lib.umn.edu/innovations/vol7/iss2/11

105. Mannebach MA, Ascione FJ, Gaither CA, Bagozzi RP, Cohen IA, Ryan ML. Activities, functions, and structure of pharmacy and therapeutics committees in large teaching hospitals. Am J Health-Syst Pharm. 1999;56:622-8.

106. Shepard MD, Salzman RD. The formulary decision-making process in a health maintenance organisation setting. PharmacoEconomics. 1994;5:29-38.

107. Johnson JA, Bootman JL. Pharmacoeconomic analysis in formulary decisions: an international perspective. Am J Hosp Pharm. 1994;51:2593-8.

108. Heindel GA, McIntyre CM. Contemporary challenges and novel strategies for health-system formulary management. Am J Health-Syst Pharm. 2018;75(8):556-60.

109. Tseng C-W, Mangione CM, Brook RH, Keeler E, Dudley RA. Identifying widely covered drugs and drug coverage variation among Medicare Part D formularies. JAMA. 2007 Jun 20;297(23):2596-2602.

110. Barlas S. Medicare quietly forces changes to federal formulary requirements. P&T. 2018 Jul;43(7):400-2, 428.

111. Barlas S. Talk of a "default" drug formulary rattles the industry. P&T. 2018 Feb;43(2): 89-91, 110.

112. Vogenberg FR, Marcoux R, Rumore MM. Systemic market and organizational changes: impact on P&T committees. P&T. 2017 Jan;42(1):28-32.

113. Plotzker RM. Formulary snafus [Internet]. Medscape. 2018 Jun 5 [cited 2019 Jul 2]. Available from: https://www.medscape.com/viewarticle/897468_print

114. Basskin L. Discounting in pharmacoeconomic analyses: when and how to do it. Formulary. 1996;31:1217-27.

115. Macklin R. Understanding formularies. Drug Store News Pharmacist. 1995;5:82–88.

116. Vogenberg FR, Barash CI, Pursel M. Personalized medicine. Part 1: Evolution and development into theranostics. P&T. 2010 Oct;35(1):560-2, 565-7.

117. Myers CE, Pierpaoli P, Smith MA. Measurement of formulary inclusion costs. Hosp Formul. 1981;16:951-3, 957-8, 967-8, 970-1, 975-6.

118. Crane VS, Gonzalez ER, Hull BL. How to develop a proactive formulary system. Hosp Formul. 1994;29:700-10.

119. Al-Jedai AH, Algain RA, Alghamidi SA, Al-Jazairi AS, Amin R, Bin Hussain IZ. A P&T committee's transition to a complete electronic meeting system—a multisite institutional experience. P&T. 2017;42(10):641-6, 651.

120. Drugs@FDA frequently asked questions [Internet]. Washington (DC): Food and Drug Administration [updated 2015 Mar 27; cited 2016 Jul 18]. Available from: http://www.fda.gov/Drugs/InformationOnDrugs/ucm075234.htm#chemtype_reviewclass.

17

Chapter Seventeen

Drug Shortages and Counterfeit Drugs

Erin R. Fox

Learning Objectives

After completing this chapter, the reader will be able to:

- Describe the reasons why drug shortages occur.
- Describe actions taken to ameliorate the drug shortage problem.
- Formulate management strategies for drug shortage situations.
- Analyze drug shortage situations for potential medication-safety implications.
- List methods for identifying and reporting potential counterfeit drugs.

Key Concepts

1. Drug shortages are a significant public health problem, affecting patients, clinicians, and all aspects of the medication supply chain.

2. The leading cause of drug shortages is manufacturing problems, mostly related to quality or not following the Food and Drug Administration's (FDA's) Current Good Manufacturing Practices (CGMPs).

3. The FDA works to prevent shortages by expediting reviews of new manufacturing sites, processes, or new products.

4. Every health care setting should have a plan that addresses how drug shortages are managed.

5. Managing drug shortages requires complex problem-solving skills. Health care professionals must assess how a shortage will impact patient care, medication safety, and workflow in order to develop the best management plan.

❻ Drug shortages increase the risk of medication errors and can result in delayed patient care or adverse patient outcomes.

❼ Most counterfeit medications found in the United States are purchased over the Internet, or from unlicensed or foreign suppliers.

Introduction

❶ Drug shortages are a significant public health problem, affecting patients, clinicians, and all aspects of the medication supply chain. Defining a drug shortage is not easy as the definition can differ depending on perspective. At the most basic level, a shortage exists if a medication is not available for a patient. However, there can be many reasons besides a shortage that a medication may not be available. Short-term situations where a medication is not ordered or delivered on time are common. Most health care organizations use just-in-time inventory systems to prevent the cost burden of excess inventory, but this system can result in short-term shortages. Likewise, weather delays can prevent deliveries from wholesalers, also resulting in short-term shortages. This chapter will address longer-term drug shortages that impact the entire supply chain on a national scale.

Drug Shortages

DEFINITION OF A DRUG SHORTAGE

There are two key sources of information regarding drug shortages. The FDA (https://www.fda.gov/drugs/drug-safety-and-availability/drug-shortages) and the American Society of Health-System Pharmacists (ASHP) (https://www.ashp.org/Drug-Shortages/Current-Shortages) both provide information about drug shortages on frequently updated websites.[1] The University of Utah Drug Information Service (UUDIS) provides drug shortage content for ASHP. These data are recognized by the Government Accountability Office (GAO) as the most comprehensive source of drug shortage information.[2] Both sources differ with regard to their definition of a drug shortage. The FDA defines a shortage as "a situation in which the total supply of all clinically interchangeable versions of an FDA-regulated drug is inadequate to meet the current or projected demand at the patient level."[3] The UUDIS and ASHP define a shortage as "a supply issue that affects how the pharmacy prepares or dispenses a drug product or influences patient care when prescribers must use an alternative agent."[3] The differences in definitions mean that ASHP reports higher drug shortage totals than the FDA. National tracking of drug shortages began in 2001. Figure 17-1 shows the historical trends of the number of new drug shortages on an annual basis. Figure 17-2 shows the number of active and ongoing shortages by quarter. These figures are updated quarterly by UUDIS and hosted on the ASHP Drug Shortage Resource Center (https://www.ashp.org/drug-shortages). The trend in mid-2019 is a decrease in the number of total new drug shortages occurring each year and an increase in the number of ongoing active drug shortages.

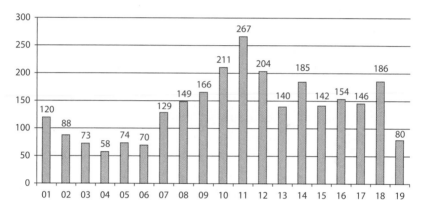

Figure 17–1. Number of new national drug shortages starting in each calendar year, January 2001 to June 30, 2019. Data are from the University of Utah Drug Information Service.

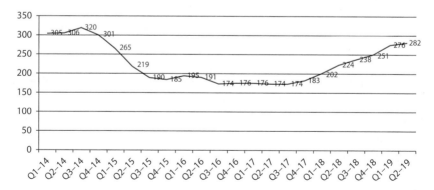

Figure 17–2. Number of active drug shortages by quarter through June 30, 2019. Q1-14 indicates January through March 2014; Q2-14, April through June 2014; Q3-14, July through September 2014; Q4-14, October through December 2014. Data are from the University of Utah Drug Information Service.

Case Study 17–1

During rounds, one of the team members mentioned that they read on a listserv that amphotericin B was in short supply. The team is concerned because results from the patient's blood sample show an infection that is only susceptible to amphotericin B. You volunteer to find out if the medication is available.

- *What sources are available to determine if a product is in short supply?*

CAUSES OF DRUG SHORTAGES

Drug manufacturers do not have to provide specific reasons for shortages, even to the FDA.[4] The FDA may know the reasons but cannot always provide detailed public information as the manufacturer may consider the information to be proprietary. Shortages can result from natural disasters that affect areas with concentrated manufacturing, such as the fluids shortages that resulted from Hurricane Maria affecting plants in Puerto Rico. Follow-on shortages can also occur when a shortage of one product creates a shortage of an alternative. In general, these are fairly uncommon reasons for shortages. The most frequent reason for a drug shortage is some type of quality problem. The 2019 report from the interagency Drug Shortage Task Force led by FDA identified three root causes for drug shortages: economics (lack of incentives to manufacture low-profit drugs), quality (lack of incentives or rewards for companies to invest in quality systems), and logistic and regulatory challenges to market recovery.[4] ❷ *According to the FDA, the leading cause of drug shortages is manufacturing problems, mostly related to quality or not following the FDA's Current Good Manufacturing Practices (CGMPs).*[4] Injectable products are particularly susceptible to quality problems and therefore may cause drug shortages due to the increased difficulty in manufacturing and higher likelihood of being sole-source products. Between 2013 and 2017, 62% of all drug shortages were caused by quality issues.[4] The specific reason for a shortage is almost never known. For example, a drug company may state that manufacturing problems are causing a shortage but the company does not reveal the root cause of the manufacturing problem.

Clinicians can follow a limited amount of quality data that the FDA provides regarding manufacturers, by reviewing FDA-issued **warning letters** and **483 inspection reports** (http://www.fda.gov/ICECI/EnforcementActions/WarningLetters/). Not all reports are posted by FDA; however, these data can provide some picture of a manufacturer's quality and may potentially be used to identify additional reasons for drug shortages. The reason for the limited information is that drug manufacturers consider many things propriety and therefore the reports redact this information. Examples of items that are considered to be proprietary include the list of products manufactured at a specific factory and the manufacturer of the product. U.S. labeling laws do not require that prescribing information (i.e., package insert) includes the name of the manufacturer or location of the factory. Despite these limitations, clinicians who are interested in the quality of drug manufacturing and drug shortages should sign up on the FDA's website to receive FDA's alerts regarding warning letters and 483 inspections (http://www.fda.gov/ICECI/EnforcementActions/WarningLetters/).

PREVENTING DRUG SHORTAGES

The FDA works diligently to prevent shortages from happening in the first place. A key aspect in their work is advanced notice that is required for successful prevention. ❸ *The key ways that the FDA prevents shortages is to expedite reviews of new manufacturing sites, processes, or new products.*[1] The FDA can also prevent shortages by using their regulatory discretion to allow a product with a minor problem to be distributed. Examples of this type of prevention strategy include allowing syringes with glass particles on the market. To prevent a shortage, the FDA allowed the product to be distributed with instructions to filter prior to administration and a **Dear Health Care Provider letter**. Once a shortage has started, it is more difficult for the FDA to ameliorate the situation, but they can allow companies to import products that meet FDA standards. Importing products is not always an available strategy as the FDA often cannot find another supplier with sufficient supplies to share with the United States. The FDA posts information about the availability of imported products on their drug shortage website, including any packaging or labeling differences. Examples of past imports include propofol, saline, sodium bicarbonate, and bleomycin.

A number of actions have occurred to attempt to improve the drug shortage problem. One of the key actions occurred on July 12, 2012 when the FDA Safety and Innovation Act was passed by Congress.[5] This legislation requires manufacturers to provide the FDA with advanced notice (6 months or as soon as possible) of any potential supply disruption. Ever since this law was passed, the FDA has been able to prevent more shortages, and the overall number of drug shortages has decreased. The International Society for Pharmaceutical Engineering (ISPE) has also been working on the drug shortage problem.[6] This organization focuses on helping manufacturers improve their overall quality systems.

MANAGING DRUG SHORTAGES

Despite advocacy by health care professionals and prevention strategies from the FDA, drug shortages impact health systems on a daily basis. ❹ *Every health care setting should*

TABLE 17–1. KEY ACTIVITIES DRUG SHORTAGE TEAM MEMBERS MUST ACCOMPLISH

- Gather data on amount of product on hand, typical usage, and monitor drug shortage information
- Contact wholesaler or manufacturers to ensure backorders are in place
- Purchase alternatives
- Make decisions such as changing the stocking location to a centralized location, or changing preparation or dispensing methods
- Evaluate medication-safety risks
- Make changes to technology
- Facilitate conservation and rationing decisions by contacting the Ethics Committee or Pharmacy and Therapeutics Committee
- Communicate shortage management plan to all stakeholders

have a plan that addresses how drug shortages are managed. Some accrediting bodies such as The Joint Commission require policies for managing drug shortages. The first step is to build a team of health care professionals to manage drug shortages.[3] The team should include people who can make decisions and quickly access information, such as purchase history or usage. Team members should understand the organization's process for change as well as how to expedite that process if needed. One person may be delegated to lead the team, but an effective drug shortage management team will include both decision-makers in the administration and informal leaders, such as clinical specialists or frontline staff. This group should also develop a list of stakeholders for specific clinical areas that can be called upon to weigh in on potential management strategies for specific situations. For example, identify key clinicians in specific clinical areas such as Anesthesia and Infectious Diseases that frequently suffer drug shortages. Communication is an essential component of the drug shortage management team. Make sure each member understands their role and shares information with the rest of the team in a timely manner. Table 17-1 identifies key actions required of drug shortage team members. Ensure each activity has a designated person to follow through on these actions.

Some organizations may choose to use compounding pharmacies to help manage drug shortages. In November 2013, Congress passed the Drug Quality and Security Act. One section updated the Federal Food, Drug and Cosmetic Act adding a new section 503B addressing a new type of compounder.[7] Compounding pharmacies fall into two categories: 503A and 503B. The 503A compounders must compound products based on a patient-specific prescription. The 503B compounders are also known as outsourcing facilities. Unlike the 503A compounders, 503B facilities must follow CGMPs and can only compound copies of commercial products if they are listed on the FDA Drug Shortage Website. The 503B outsourcing facilities must register with the FDA and are subject to inspections. Compounding is not always a solution for a drug shortage. There is often a significant delay in obtaining product from a 503B facility as the company has to wait for a product to be listed on the FDA shortage site, then manufacture the product.

TABLE 17–2. STEPWISE APPROACH TO DEVELOPING A DRUG SHORTAGE MANAGEMENT PLAN

Action	Resources for Information
Determine the amount of product on hand.	• Purchasing staff
• Estimate how long that product will last.	• ASHP and FDA shortage websites
• Estimate quantity and timing of next delivery.	
Determine the clinical impact of the shortage.	• Clinical knowledge
• How essential is the product? Is it life-saving or curative? Can treatment be postponed?	• Frontline staff
	• ASHP website for alternatives
• Are there clear alternatives?	• Professional Society websites for guidance on management
• Which clinicians or patients are most impacted?	
Determine any potential medication-safety risks posed by the drug shortage.	• Clinical knowledge
	• Medication Safety Officer
• If using an alternative, identify any differences in dosing, adverse effects, or drug interactions.	
• Is a different strength or formulation being used?	
• Are there potential look-alike or sound-alike differences?	
Determine whether any changes are needed to the overall workflow.	• Operations managers
• Should the shortage item be stored in a central location to ease tracking?	• Informatics
• Does the shortage affect any technology?	
• Is there beyond use dating for a compounded product replacing a commercial product?	
Determine how remaining products should be utilized.	• Ethics Committee
• Is conservation or rationing the best strategy?	• P&T Committee
	• Stakeholder clinicians

❺ *Managing drug shortages requires complex problem-solving skills. Health care professionals must assess how a shortage will impact patient care, medication safety, and workflow in order to develop the best management plan.* Table 17-2 outlines key steps to developing a drug shortage management plan. For example, is this a shortage of a product that has clear and effective alternatives, or is this a shortage that may delay treatments or cause patient harm? Analyze which patients and clinicians will be impacted the most by the shortage. Review potential medication-safety concerns that this shortage may pose.

Case Study 17–2

Your organization has discovered that a shortage of amphotericin B exists. The purchasing staff states that there is approximately a 20-day supply left at current usage rates. The next delivery date is unknown.

- *What are the next steps in managing this drug shortage? Which clinicians should you contact first?*

Once a plan is in place, it is essential to communicate effectively based on your audience.[3] Target communications when possible to avoid information overload. Share information in formal and informal ways. Use multiple methods to share the message such as rounds, team huddles, email, intranet blogs, or even paper or white boards. Make sure the communication provides details about the management strategy. If an alternative is recommended, make sure to include any differences in dosing, adverse effects, or drug interactions. If the product is going to be reserved for specific patients to conserve supplies, make sure to include criteria for use and a method for clinicians who would like an exception. The health system's Ethics Committee should be involved in decisions to ration drug products.[8] See Chapter 12 for additional information on ethical dilemmas in pharmacy practice.

IMPACT OF DRUG SHORTAGES

Drug shortages impact patient safety in two major ways. ❻ *Drug shortages increase the risk of medication errors and can result in delayed patient care or adverse patient outcomes.* Drug shortages pose high medication-safety risks because they can affect each step of the medication use process. Clinicians have attempted to identify the key safety risks of drug shortages through a Failure Modes and Effects Analysis. These data show that the highest risk points during a shortage are using a different concentration or using an alternative.[9] Medication errors and deaths have occurred when clinicians were unfamiliar with the dosing of an alternative agent.[10,11] Patient safety is also at risk when shortages cause treatment delays. For example, there may be missed opportunities to immunize, clinical trials may be delayed when the standard of care is not available, and delays in obtaining antimicrobials or chemotherapy agents may be life-threatening or affect the potential chance for a cure.[12-15]

Case Study 17–3

Your organization has suffered multiple shortages in the past week. You speak with the purchasing staff who provide you with and update on what products they have been able to obtain. They tell you about how they have purchased heparin vials since the premixed bags are not available. They have also purchased dopamine 200 mg/250 mL premixed bags because it was the only strength available and you are almost out of dopamine 800 mg/250 mL premixed bags.

- *What patient safety concerns do you have? What technology may be affected by these substitutes?*

Counterfeit Drugs

The World Health Organization (WHO) notes that **counterfeit drugs** affect every region of the world.[16] The WHO defines these products as "substandard, spurious, falsely labelled, falsified, and counterfeit" (SSFFC) products. The medications may not contain the right amount of **active pharmaceutical ingredient**, or may not contain the correct active ingredient at all. Products might contain fillers like chalk or even toxic chemicals. All types of medicines are falsified including expensive medications as well as generics. The most commonly reported counterfeit medications worldwide are antimicrobials. ❼ *Most counterfeit medications found in the United States are purchased over the Internet or from unlicensed or foreign suppliers.* In 2015, the FDA found a counterfeit version of Botox® that was sold by an unlicensed, foreign supplier. The FDA also found counterfeit Cialis® in 2015 that had been purchased by a single consumer from an Internet pharmacy (http://www.fda.gov/Drugs/ResourcesForYou/Consumers/BuyingUsingMedicineSafely/CounterfeitMedicine/). The FDA recommends patients or health care providers to purchase medications only from state-licensed pharmacies or Internet pharmacies with the Verified Internet Pharmacy Practice Sites Accreditation Program seal (https://nabp.pharmacy/programs/vipps/). The WHO provides recommendations to help identify counterfeit medications such as ensuring the package is in good condition, reviewing security seals, and checking that batch numbers and expiration dates match between the internal and external packages (http://www.who.int/medicines/regulation/ssffc/en/).[17] Health care providers can report potential counterfeit medications to FDA via **MedWatch** (http://www.fda.gov/Safety/MedWatch/). Ways of tracking medications within the medication supply lines to prevent the substitution of counterfeit products have been investigated, including the use of radio-frequency identification tags (RFID tags). In November 2013, Congress approved the Drug Supply Chain Security Act (DSCSA) with a goal of developing electronic methods to identify and trace prescription drugs as they are distributed through the United States.[17] Some elements are required as of 2015 such as providing a transaction statement for each product tracing from the manufacturer to dispenser. Additional standards will be phased in through 2023, including an overall system for product tracing. Notably, this regulation does not provide traceable information from where the product originated from (such as raw material source or manufacturing plant). The "trace" begins with the manufacturer selling the product and ends at the dispenser.

Conclusion

Drug shortages and counterfeit drugs pose significant public health risks. Clinicians can minimize the impact of drug shortages on their patients and practices by developing clear plans to manage the shortages. Health care providers can minimize the potential risks of counterfeit medications by purchasing medications from recommended sources and reviewing medication packaging for potential tampering or falsification.

Self-Assessment Questions

1. The trend in drug shortages for 2019 is one of:
   a. Decreasing new shortages and increasing active shortages
   b. Increasing new shortages but decreasing active shortages
   c. Slight increase in new shortages and decreasing active shortages
   d. Decreasing new shortages and a gradual decrease in active shortages

2. Most shortages have occurred due to:
   a. Raw material shortages
   b. Natural disasters
   c. Manufacturing or quality problems
   d. Corporate decisions

3. Package inserts must include which of the following items:
   a. Name of the company that manufactured the drug
   b. Location of the factory
   c. Country of origin for the active pharmaceutical ingredient (API)
   d. None of the above

4. The FDA can help prevent drug shortages by:
   a. Prioritizing approvals of new products
   b. Forcing companies to increase production
   c. Forcing companies to continue to produce a drug
   d. Decreasing drug prices

5. The FDA can help alleviate an ongoing drug shortage by:
   a. Requiring companies to manufacture additional product
   b. Fining companies that don't provide advanced notice of a shortage
   c. Allowing companies to import products that meet FDA criteria
   d. Overriding patents and approving new formulations

6. The Drug Supply Chain Security Act (DSCSA) intends to track prescription drugs from:
   a. The source of raw material to the patient
   b. The manufacturer selling the product to the dispenser
   c. The factory to the dispenser
   d. The source of raw material to the dispenser

7. A drug shortage policy has which of the following characteristics?
   a. Required by the Joint Commission
   b. Required by the FDA
   c. Required by wholesalers
   d. Required by group purchasing organizations

8. Members of a drug shortage team should do which of the following?
   a. Put a positive spin on communications by overestimating the supply on hand
   b. Consider making changes to the stocking locations
   c. Remove the product from formulary
   d. Rely on word of mouth to get the message out

9. Clinicians should exercise particular care at what point during a shortage?
   a. After the P&T Committee decides on an allocation strategy
   b. Selecting when to remove stock from the automated dispensing cabinets
   c. Selecting when to begin drawing up doses to conserve product
   d. At the beginning and end of a shortage

10. What information is necessary when assessing the potential impact of a drug shortage at an individual health system?
    a. Amount and location of inventory on hand
    b. Status of drug in short supply—unapproved or approved
    c. Whether or not FDA considers the drug medically necessary
    d. Whether the drug is available as a brand or generic product

11. The FDA's drug shortage information is different from that of the ASHP's because:
    a. The FDA provides detailed alternatives.
    b. ASHP does not include vaccines or biologics.

c. The FDA focuses on medically necessary drugs and information provided by the manufacturer.

d. The ASHP website is only updated monthly.

12. Important considerations in determining the potential clinical impact of a shortage include:
a. Whether an alternative is available
b. Identifying which patients will be most impacted
c. Determining if the product is life-saving or curative
d. All of the above

13. A Failure Modes and Effects Analysis identified which of the following items as the greatest medication-safety risks during a drug shortage?
a. Using different concentration or an alternative drug
b. Purchasing a more expensive product that is not on contract
c. Dispensing the product in a syringe instead of a vial
d. Changing the storage location of a product.

14. Clinicians should report suspected counterfeit drugs to:
a. FDA's MedWatch program
b. The Federal Bureau of Investigation
c. The Federal Trade Commission
d. The wholesaler

15. Patients who purchase medications on the Internet should look for the following to ensure that they do not receive counterfeit medications:
a. Consumer star ratings
b. Pharmacies with best customer service ratings
c. Pharmacies with the Verified Internet Pharmacy Practice Sites Accreditation Program Seal (VIPPS)
d. Pharmacies with locations listed in Canada

REFERENCES

1. Fox ER, Sweet BV, Jensen V. Drug shortages: a complex health care crisis. Mayo Clin Proc. 2014;89(3):361-73.
2. Drug shortages: public health threat continues, despite efforts to help ensure product availability [Internet]. United States Government Accountability Office. 2014 Feb [cited 2016 Nov 10]. Available from: https://www.gao.gov/products/gao-14-194
3. Fox ER, McLaughlin MM. ASHP guidelines on managing drug product shortages. Am J Health-Syst Pharm. 2018;75(21):1742-50.

4. Drug shortages: root causes and potential solutions [Internet]. U.S. Food and Drug Administration. 2019 Oct 29 [cited 2019 Dec 5]. Available from: https://www.fda.gov/media/131130/download

5. Food and Drug Administration Safety and Innovation Act (FDASIA). U.S. Food and Drug Administration [Internet]. 2012, 2015 Oct [cited 2016 Nov 10]. Available from: https://www.fda.gov/regulatory-information/selected-amendments-fdc-act/food-and-drug-administration-safety-and-innovation-act-fdasia

6. ISPE Drug Shortages Initiative: FAQs. International Society for Pharmaceutical Engineering (ISPE) [Internet]. 2015 [cited 2016 Sep 10]. Available from: https://ispe.org/initiatives/drug-shortages-faqs

7. Compounding Laws and Policies. U.S. Food and Drug Administration [Internet]. 2018 [cited 2019 Dec 4]. Available from: https://www.fda.gov/drugs/human-drug-compounding/compounding-laws-and-policies

8. Unguru Y, Fernandez CV, Bernhardt B, Berg S, Pyke-Grimm K, Woodman C, Joffe S. An ethical framework for allocating scarce life-saving chemotherapy and supportive care drugs for childhood cancer. J Natl Cancer Inst. 2016;108(6).

9. MacDonald EA, Fox ER, Tyler LS. Drug shortages: process for evaluating impact on patient safety. Hosp Pharm. 2011;46(12):943-51.

10. Institute for Safe Medication Practices. Drug shortages: national survey reveals high level of frustration, low level of safety. ISMP medication safety alert! Acute Care. 2010;15(15).

11. Institute for Safe Medication Practices. A shortage of everything except errors: harm associated with drug shortages. ISMP medication safety alert! Acute Care. 2012;17(8).

12. McBride A, Holle LM, Westendorf C, et al. National survey on the effect of oncology drug shortages on cancer care. Am J Health-Syst Pharm. 2013;70(7):609-17.

13. Goozner M. Drug shortages delay cancer clinical trials. J Natl Cancer Inst. 2012;104(12):891-2.

14. Griffith MM, Gross AE, Sutton SH, Bolon MK, Esterly JS, Patel JA, Postelnick MJ, Zembower TR, Scheetz MH. The impact of anti-infective drug shortages on hospitals in the United States: trends and causes. Clin Infect Dis. 2012;54(5):684-91.

15. Gogineni K, Shuman KL, Emanuel EJ. Survey of oncologists about shortages of cancer drugs. N Engl J Med. 2013;369(25):2463-4.

16. Substandard, spurious, falsely labelled, falsified and counterfeit (SSFFC) medical products [Internet]. World Health Organization. 2016 Jan [cited 2016 Sep 13]. Available from: http://www.who.int/mediacentre/factsheets/fs275/en/

17. Drug Supply Chain Security Act (DSCSA). U.S. Food and Drug Administration [Internet]. 2019 [cited 2019 Dec 4]. Available from: https://www.fda.gov/drugs/drug-supply-chain-integrity/drug-supply-chain-security-act-dscsa

SUGGESTED READINGS

1. American Society of Health-System Pharmacists Drug Shortage Resource Center. Available from: https://www.ashp.org/Drug-Shortages

2. Food and Drug Administration—Drug Shortages. Available from: http://www.fda.gov/Drugs/DrugSafety/DrugShortages/

3. American Society of Health-System Pharmacists Guidelines for Managing Drug Product Shortages. Available from: https://www.ashp.org/Drug-Shortages/Shortage-Resources

4. The World Health Organization Substandard, Spurious, Falsely labelled, Falsified and Counterfeit (SSFFC) Medical Products. Available from: http://www.who.int/medicines/regulation/ssffc/en/

5. National Association of Boards of Pharmacy's Verified Internet Pharmacy Practice Sites (VIPPS) Program. Available from: https://nabp.pharmacy/programs/vipps/

Chapter Eighteen

Quality Improvement and the Medication Use System

Jennifer K. Thomas • Rachel Digmann

Learning Objectives

After completing this chapter, the reader will be able to:

- Explain the changing environment for quality measurement and performance reporting in health care.
- Define quality and value in the context of health care services.
- Define quality measures and explain their development.
- Delineate the concepts of structure, process, and outcomes for quality assessment.
- Describe a systematic method for quality improvement.
- Define health equity and health disparities and how to improve health quality for all groups.
- Explain the role of performance indicators in quality improvement.
- Draft a performance indicator related to the medication use system.
- Discuss quality improvement techniques applied in drug information practice.

Key Concepts

❶ The term "value" has been assigned many definitions, but within health care, it usually reflects the ratio of quality and costs (value = quality/cost).

❷ Significant drivers for greater transparency in the quality and value of health care services include the federal government, employers that provide health care benefits, and accreditation organizations such as The Joint Commission (TJC).

❸ Quality improvement is prospective, continuous, team oriented, nonpunitive, systems oriented, customer focused, and data driven.

❹ A common methodology for quality improvement is known as FOCUS-PDCA (Find, Organize, Clarify, Understand, Select, Plan, Do, Check, Act).

❺ Donabedian's framework for quality assessment in health care includes the key elements of structure, process, and outcomes.

❻ Performance indicators are used to measure quality as part of the "Check" function of quality improvement. The indicators are an aspect of care and typically focus on the process or outcomes of a care system.

❼ Performance indicators can be subdivided into sentinel (occurrence of a serious event) or aggregate categories. Aggregate indicators are further divided into continuous or rate-based indicators.

❽ A commitment to health equity and the elimination of health disparities are necessary to achieve optimal health for all.

❾ Medication use evaluation is often part of an organization's overall performance improvement program that uses definitions of safe and effective use of medications to assess components of the medication use process.

❿ Performance, as demonstrated by data collected in the performance improvement process, not meeting the defined standard or threshold, or falling outside the control limits (for ongoing or follow-up assessments) indicates that intervention to improve performance is necessary.

Introduction

Value-driven health care is being touted as the future model for health care in the United States.[1,2] ❶ *The term "value" has been assigned many definitions, but within health care, it usually reflects the ratio of quality and costs (value = quality/cost).* Thus, value is optimized by enhancing quality while minimizing cost. Although it was traditionally assumed that higher quality would only be possible through higher expenditures, the medical community has learned that improving the quality of care may lead to long-term control of health care costs. Health care administrators have long been attentive to measuring expenditures on care and have developed cost-accounting systems that have allowed determination of costs of procedures, drugs, and various care models. However, the health care system has only recently developed explicit measures of quality. By measuring this missing piece of the value equation, it is now possible to achieve a more balanced perspective on health system performance.

The Changing Environment for Health Care Quality

The measurement of quality within health care settings has expanded rapidly during the previous two decades. ❷ *Significant drivers for greater transparency in the quality and value of health care services include the federal government, employers that provide health care benefits, and accreditation organizations such as The Joint Commission (TJC).* Accreditation standards for many providers have been amended to require providers to collect performance data. The federal government is the major driver of health care quality measurement and is accelerating change through implementation of the value-based model of care defined by the Affordable Care Act (ACA) and the Centers for Medicare & Medicaid Services (CMS) Quality Strategy 2016 which identified six priorities defined initially from the National Quality Strategy (NQS).[3,4] Specifically, goals are identified that tie payment to performance in the Medicare Fee-for-Service (FFS) program with an invitation to private payers to match or exceed these goals. To achieve the payment tied to quality outcomes, there are six focus priorities of the NQS: (1) make care safer by reducing harm in care delivery, (2) ensure care is patient/family centered, (3) promote effective communication and coordination of care, (4) promote effective prevention and treatment for the leading causes of mortality starting with cardiovascular disease, (5) work with communities to promote best practices for healthy life, and (6) making quality care more affordable. The national health care landscape, policies, and programs continue to evolve and the NQS' aims and focus continue through the CMS value-based programs. These value-based programs are extensive and defining each is beyond the scope of this chapter, but these programs cover virtually every sector of care in the U.S. health care arena. The value-based programs include: End-Stage Renal Disease Quality Incentive Program (ESRD QIP), Hospital Value-Based Purchasing (VBP) Program, Hospital Readmission Reduction Program (HRRP), Value Modifier (VM) Program also known as the Physician Value-Based Modifier (PVBM), Hospital-Acquired Conditions (HAC) Reduction Program, Skilled Nursing Facility Value-Based Program (SNF VBP), Home Health Value-Based Program (HHVBP), Alternative Payment Models (APMs), and Merit-Based Incentive Payment System (MIPS); the latter two fall under the Quality Payment Program (QPP) for physician practices.[5] All the federal quality measures and/or value-based programs include meaningful measures for improvement in the quality of medication use. To help achieve quality goals providers are incentivized by associated Medicare payment adjustment. A payment adjustment is determined by the final score associated with a unique clinician or clinician group identifier. The score is used to determine whether a positive, negative, or neutral adjustment will be applied to the covered professional services furnished within the performance year. For example, a provider may select the quality measure for patients with a diagnosis of hypertension whose blood pressure is adequately controlled, defined as <140/90 mmHg, during the measurement period. Providers will receive a positive payment adjustment to their Medicare payments for meeting the quality goals. Conversely, the provider may be penalized or receive a negative payment adjustment if the quality performance goals are not met. In each value-based purchasing program, the incentive programs' adjustments are specified by law, and some performance scores and payment adjustments are phased in over time, such as the QPP incentives. Using medication management as an example of a dimension of quality of care, the programs incorporate a medication measure included in the overall performance score. In the hospital, examples of payment adjustments for Medicare for inpatient services include the "communications about medications" in the Hospital VBP Program,[6] for the Skilled Nursing Facility Quality Reporting Program (SNF QRP) there is a "drug regimen review" measure,[7] for home health agencies the "improving oral medication use" measures,[8] and for QPP MIPS physician practices "medication reconciliation postdischarge" measures.[9] The MIPS program and the APM are defined in the Medicare Access and CHIP Reauthorization (MACRA) legislation (CHIP is the Children's Health Insurance Program).[10] The QPP, starting in 2017, initiates payment to eligible professionals (physicians, physician assistants, nurse practitioner, clinical nurse specialist, nurse anesthetist) through either MIPS, if they bill Medicare Part B above a specific threshold and have greater than a specified number of FFS patients, or via the APM if they are part of a group using an innovative payment model, such as accountable care organizations (ACO). ACOs are doctors, hospitals, and other health care providers that form groups to provide coordinated patient care with reimbursement tied to quality performance and the goal of reducing the cost of health care.

Case Study 18–1

Your hospital's Board and Executive Leadership have identified several performance measures for the 2022 performance year (CMS identifies and defines measures for the program 2 years beyond the measurement period, 2020) to improve the total performance score results and payment, in the Hospital VBP program performance period year into 2020. One of the measures identified for improvement is the "communication about medications" dimension of the Person and Community Engagement: Hospital Consumer Assessment of Healthcare Providers and Systems (HCAHPS) measure. On the most recent Hospital VBP report the "communications about medications" result was 63.4%. The floor result was 33.19% (the worst performing hospital's results), the achievement threshold was 63.83% (the 50th percentile of hospital's performance), and the benchmark was 74.75% (the mean of the top decile of all hospital's performance). The hospital's Quality and Safety Committee is charged with identifying process improvement to improve the hospital's rate to 70%.

CMS and other organizations display public reports about the quality of care across multiple care settings for each of the following: hospitals,[11] long-term care facilities,[12] health plans,[13,14] home health agencies,[15] dialysis facilities,[16] and physicians.[17,18] Additionally, many public and private purchasers (e.g., insurance companies) of health care services have begun to demand evidence of quality and value,[19,20] and consumers selecting plans in the recently established ACA Health Insurance Marketplace (also known as Health Insurance Exchange) may select their plan based on quality "star ratings." Each plan receives a star rating of 1–5 based on criteria of performance, such as customer service, customer complaints, cost, quality, and safety. The reporting of star ratings for the exchange plans began as a phased-in pilot in 2016 with two states, Virginia and Wisconsin, and expanding to five states with the addition of Michigan, Montana, and New Hampshire in 2019. From 2020 forward, all health insurance exchange plans are to use and report the star ratings.[21,22] Individual State exchanges, such as the Maryland Health Connection, also have star ratings.[23] While many care settings and providers are being directly measured with attribution of their quality of care, such as Hospital Compare, Physician Compare, Nursing Homes compare, and others, as previously listed in this chapter, which have comparison quality data available for viewing at those respective websites, there is no "Pharmacy Compare" website at this time. Pharmacies and pharmacists are currently only indirectly assessed because pharmacists and pharmacies are not covered as a provider under Medicare statute. However, measuring pharmacy/pharmacist performance with attribution of the quality of pharmacy-provided care is occurring as indicated below through pharmacy organizations and health insurance plans.

The Pharmacy Quality Alliance (PQA) was established in 2006 as a public-private partnership with CMS shortly after the implementation of the Medicare Part D Prescription Drug Benefit. PQA develops consensus-based measures for medication safety, adherence, and appropriate use. Most PQA measures are for evaluating health plan performance and quality improvement.[24] The initial testing of PQA performance measures took place in 2007,[25] and several demonstration projects have been conducted to show how community pharmacies can be included in performance measurement systems.[26] PQA began work in 2019 to develop a set of pharmacy performance measures that would be appropriate for pharmacy accountability, once assessed against standard measure criteria and endorsed by PQA membership.[27] Although CMS is not publicly reporting on the quality of individual pharmacies, it has included several PQA-developed health plan quality measures within the Medicare Part D Plan ratings.[28] The inclusion of the PQA quality measures, such as the adherence measure for diabetes classes of medications and the adherence of statin use, measured at the Part D Plan level, helps to assess the percent of patients taking their medications as prescribed. Emphasis by the Part D Plans to improve medication use adherence indirectly impacts and measures how pharmacists/pharmacies influence appropriate medication use. Higher adherence rates are better.[29] As the scrutiny of prescription drug plans increases, plans are beginning to require participation of their preferred network pharmacies in quality measurement programs, including medication adherence, **medication therapy management (MTM)**, and generic medication utilization. These plan sponsors are assessing pharmacy performance[30,31] and may report this data to the public. An enhanced MTM program, a 5-year pilot program beginning in January 1, 2017 and ongoing through December 2021, includes Medicare Part D prescription drug plans selected for participation by the **Centers for Medicare and Medicaid Innovation (CMMI)**. The program aim is to determine if incentives for Part D stand-alone prescription drug plans will promote MTM enhancements and reduce medical costs. Participating Plans achieving decreased medical expenses (among these decreased hospital admissions and emergency room visits) through the enhanced MTM services will obtain incentive payments.[32] The first performance year 2017 of the enhanced MTM demonstrated participants in the model spent approximately $325 million less than the anticipated spending benchmark across the 1.7 million beneficiaries enrolled in participating plans.[33] Thus, all sectors of health care are affected by the rapidly expanding trend of quality measurement and public reporting of performance data.

Case Study 18–2

You are the manager for pharmacies in the preferred pharmacy network for a Medicare Part D Plan participating in the enhanced MTM program pilot. You are responsible for your pharmacists completing comprehensive medication reviews and targeted medication reviews to achieve or exceed performance thresholds, so the Plan receives incentive payments. What specific process will you implement to identify Plan patients for enhanced MTM services? Upon which medication-related problems will you focus your efforts?

This chapter will focus on the measures of quality in the medication use system and the use of these measures in improving the quality of medication use. The term "performance" will be used interchangeably with quality within this chapter, although understanding that performance can also refer to the overall value of the health care system is important.

Purpose of Measuring Quality

Quality, like value, has been defined in different ways. Although the definitions for quality may vary, the purpose of measuring quality is to identify problems in a system (also known as opportunities for improvement) and to monitor improvements in quality as systems are modified.[34] Although quality improvement is the goal of collecting performance data, the mechanisms for using performance data in achieving quality improvement may vary. For example, the performance data may be used directly by a health care organization to identify opportunities for improvement and to gauge the impact of changes in its policies or procedures.

Performance data may also be used by external entities (e.g., a regulatory or accrediting body) to determine whether a health care organization should retain its accreditation or certification. The data may also be used to determine payments to providers (e.g., pay for performance), or the data may be used by employers, governments, or the public for determining which providers to use.

When comparative data on the performance of health care providers are released to payers and patients, it is presumed that the providers in a competitive environment will improve quality to maintain market share.

Quality Measures

The development and use of **quality measures** for assessing different aspects of health care as provided by practitioners in different care settings allow us to quantify performance compared with benchmarks. In order to measure performance that is comparable across the spectrum of performance, benchmarks are often established using historical data.[35,36]

Creation and development of quality measures is a continuous process. The federal government drives the measures development, primarily as the Congressional laws for Medicare programs require oversight of the taxpayer outlays and assessment of the performance of these programs. The five-star ratings programs are measures of the quality and safety performance of each program. The most recent Medicare laws, Medicare Part D as previously stated required medication measures for assessing the Part D Plans. Under the ACA the Health Insurance Exchanges are assessed by the star ratings program. As the government payment of health care services moves from quantity of services to quality of services, the new MACRA MIPS program assesses physicians and other providers of Medicare Part B services with a composite score that is a hybrid score to indicate both performance and reductions in cost. For each of the star ratings programs reviewed above, there is a continuous PDCA (plan–do–check–act is an iterative four-step management method used for continuous improvement of processes and products). PDCA measures development and assesses intended quality and safety outcomes, and, most recently, has also assessed cost reductions while maintaining quality and safety performance. Various stewards or measure developers undertake quality measure development. CMS and other payers of health care services issue requests for proposals (RFPs) from organizations who can provide services, via awarded contracts, as defined by law and/or when requirements arise for measure development teams to be formed. The intended entities or providers of the performance measures are generally required to use the measurement sets as conditions of participation (COP); for example, for hospitals to receive Medicare payments they must collect, measure, and report data (data via identified medical claims for a specific process of care) for the hospital performance measures set (e.g., fibrinolytic therapy post-MI or upload of collected data through Quality Net-CMS's Medicare quality reporting program).[37] Other performance measures created by accrediting organizations such as TJC are also required for use by hospitals or organizations accredited by TJC. CMS and TJC have worked together to align their respective measures into a harmonized measure sets, completely identical, such as for the core measures disease performance measurement for acute myocardial infarction and heart failure care. The alignment reduced the burden for providers (hospitals, other entities) of data collection and reporting for performance measurement.[38] Measure stewards, as described above, invite participating experts, representatives from areas of practice, organizations, and stakeholders, including patient and family advocacy groups to reach consensus in developing applicable measures. These contracts for measure development are won by a variety of companies or organizations including universities, quality improvement organizations, organizations with missions of quality, such as the National Committee for Quality Assurance (NCQA), the Agency for Healthcare Research and Quality (AHRQ), TJC, and PQA, to name a few. The final measures created under these contracts are submitted for consideration of endorsement to the National Quality Forum (NQF). The NQF, under contract of the U.S. Department of Health and Human Services, is responsible for creating, prioritizing, and maintaining a portfolio of quality and efficiency measures across care settings and providers. AHRQ also maintained a measures listing, the National Quality Measures Clearinghouse, but funding to support the AHRQ listing ended in July 2018.[39] Endorsement of the measures indicates the performance measures are likely to achieve the intended goal of efficient, safe, quality care. If the measures are endorsed by the NQF, the steward maintains and updates the measures, as necessary. The NQF currently categorizes measures into clinical conditions/topic areas, by care setting, and into one of the six NQS priorities: affordable care, effective communication and care coordination, health and wellbeing, patient safety, person and family-centered care, and prevention and treatment of cardiovascular disease (diseases as leading causes of mortality). An example of a cross-cutting medication safety and care coordination measure is the "medication reconciliation postdischarge" measure (measure steward: NCQA, NQF# 0097). The measure description: The percentage of discharges for patients 18 years of age and older for whom the discharge medication list was reconciled with the current medication list in the outpatient medical record by the prescribing practitioner, clinical pharmacist, or registered nurse. This measure is a process measure, identifying the medication reconciliation is performed and documented in the record. The reader is encouraged to view a searchable listing of measures through the Quality Positions System (QPS), an NQF website available under the measures, reports, and tools on the NQF website (http://www.qualityforum.org/QPS/).[40]

Another nationally recognized measure developer is NCQA. HEDIS is one of health care's most widely used performance improvement measure sets and is a trademark developed and maintained by NCQA. HEDIS stands for "Healthcare Effectiveness Data and Information Set." HEDIS is a tool used by many health plans, including Medicare, Medicaid, and commercial payers, in the United States to measure performance of managed care and services. NQF reports that an estimated 90% of health plans use HEDIS measures sets and approximately three-quarters of HEDIS measures are NQF endorsed. HEDIS users in the United States collect the HEDIS data and report the data to NCQA that aggregates, analyzes, and provides individual uses reports as well as aggregate summary results reports allowing easy comparison of different plans based on their performance. Health plans also use the HEDIS results to identify the crucial areas that need improvement in order to ensure quality. Consumers and employers use the HEDIS data to choose the best health plans that suit their specific needs.[41] The results of a HEDIS measure of adolescent immunizations demonstrate the impact of measurement and improvement over time. As an example, the results of a HEDIS measure of adolescent immunizations, specifically meningococcal (MCV) immunization, can be used to compare rates of age-appropriate vaccinations by health plan. For adolescent MCV immunization, results are reported by year and by plan. In 2018, commercial health maintenance organization (HMO) rate was 83.5 as compared to Medicaid HMO rate of 81.3. In 2017, commercial HMO rate was 81.1 as compared to Medicaid HMO rate of 79.6. Each year identifies an incremental improvement as compared to initial year of 2010 when commercial HMO rate was 55.2 and Medicaid HMO rate was 56.3.[42]

Quality Improvement

Practitioners are sometimes confused when faced with the myriad of quality-related acronyms being used today, such as CQI (continuous quality improvement), QI (quality improvement), QA (quality assurance), QAPI (quality assurance, performance improvement), TQM (total quality management), SPC (statistical process control), and PDCA (Plan, Do,

TABLE 18–1. **ATTRIBUTES OF CONTINUOUS QUALITY IMPROVEMENT**

Characteristic	Description
Prospective	Forward thinking; always looking for better ways to provide care.
Continuous	A standard element of practice rather than a onetime effort.
Team oriented	A collaborative effort of all employees and management; recognizes the unique and valuable knowledge of each team member.
Nonpunitive	Employees should be rewarded for identifying problems/mistakes and not be fearful of discussing operational problems.
Systems oriented	Focus of improvement efforts is on the process or system of care rather than the elimination of bad employees.
Customer focused	All team members are focused on fulfilling the needs of the customer (e.g., patient, physician, other team members).
Data driven	Evaluates performance based on objective data.

Check, Act). Things become even murkier when many different quality-related philosophies are added, along with blurry distinctions between quality improvement, quality assurance, and quality control.

Quality improvement can generally be characterized by certain attributes, which are listed in Table 18-1. Concisely stated, ❸ *quality improvement is prospective, continuous, team oriented, nonpunitive, systems oriented, customer focused, and data driven.* Although there are a variety of methods, the quality improvement process is typically implemented via the PDCA or PDSA cycle, also called the Deming Cycle (although Deming referred to it as the Shewhart Cycle).[43,44] This cyclical process involves four key elements: *Plan, Do, Check (or Study),* and *Act.*

To apply PDCA to a new health care service, *Plan* would entail designing a new approach for providing the service that leads to an improvement in quality. This approach would include guidelines or procedures for how care will be provided and plans for how the care process will be evaluated. The *Do* step in the cycle concerns the implementation of the new plan, while *Check* refers to an objective evaluation of the plan. Once the performance of the plan has been checked, the performance data can be *Acted* upon to standardize the new plan (if it led to improvement) or the existing plan can be further revised and the PDCA cycle can be repeated.

❹ *A common methodology for quality improvement is known as FOCUS-PDCA (Find, Organize, Clarify, Understand, Select, Plan, Do, Check, Act).* It is an extension of the PDCA cycle[45] (Figure 18-1). This approach was developed by the Hospital Corporation of America to facilitate quality improvement efforts in their hospitals. The first step of FOCUS-PDCA is to *Find* the process that will be targeted for improvement (e.g., the pharmacokinetic service referral process). The second step is to *Organize* a team to study the problem (e.g., pharmacists, physicians, nurses, unit clerks). Next, *Clarify* the team's

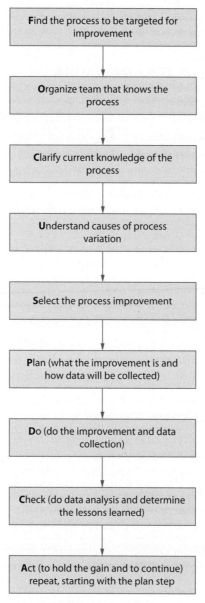

Figure 18–1. FOCUS-PDCA®.

understanding of the process (i.e., ensure that everyone has a common understanding of how the referral process is being carried out, perhaps using a flow diagram). Then, seek to *Understand* the root causes of variation in performance (i.e., identify problems such as a poorly designed workflow, inadequate training, or unclear roles and determine why they occur). Finally, *Select* the parts of the structure or process to change. Once the target for change has been selected, a new *Plan* can be formulated for how the process will change and then continue the PDCA cycle through the *Do, Check*, and *Act* steps.

MEASURING QUALITY IN THE MEDICATION USE SYSTEM

One of the most challenging elements of quality improvement is measuring the quality of care. Donabedian[46] suggested that the evaluation of medical care quality could be best accomplished by subdividing care into three parts. ❺ *Donabedian's framework for quality assessment in health care includes the key elements of structure, process, and outcome.* The Donabedian framework also can be used to evaluate the quality of the medication use system.[47]

Structure refers to the characteristics of providers, the tools and resources at their disposal, and the physical or organizational settings in which they work.[47] Examples include professional licensure or certification, computer systems for tracking patient information, patient counseling areas, and human resource policies. The elements of structure create the environment for care. These structural elements may be necessary to provide optimal care, but their presence does not ensure optimal care.

Process refers to the set of activities that occur between patient and provider, encompassing the services and products that are provided to patients and the way the services are provided. Experts often group the specific elements of care processes within two domains: *technical* or *interpersonal*. The technical domain of patient care may include gathering patient information, entering prescription information into computers, reviewing patient records, checking prescription labels, evaluating a patient's laboratory results, identifying and resolving potential drug-related problems, and answering patient questions. The interpersonal domain of patient care includes the ability of the practitioner to express empathy, listen attentively, and develop a caring relationship with the patient. The process of care is often the primary focus of quality improvement efforts as practitioners strive to do what is best for patients. Care processes can be directly evaluated by using the norms or standards that exist across the health care system (e.g., what is commonly accepted as good care) or indirectly evaluated by determining their impact on outcomes.

The term *outcomes* was originally defined by Donabedian as "a change in a patient's current and future health status that can be attributed to antecedent health care."[46] Lohr also characterized outcomes in terms of the consequences of medical care for patients (e.g., death, disability, disease, discomfort, and dissatisfaction).[48] In later years, the use of this term has broadened to encompass the economic, clinical, and humanistic consequences of health care processes (ECHO model).[49] In the ECHO model, outcomes may include:

- Economic consequences (e.g., costs of care)
- Clinical measures or endpoints (e.g., blood pressure, glycosylated hemoglobin [HgbA1c], pain, mortality—see Chapters 4 and 5)
- Humanistic issues (e.g., patient satisfaction, health-related quality of life)

Outcomes are sometimes classified as *intermediate* or *long-term*.[50] This terminology results from considering the link between process and numerous outcomes as a causal chain of events. Intermediate outcomes may occur between the health care process and long-term or ultimate outcomes. For example, providing patient counseling services regarding the appropriate use of blood glucose meters (the process) will lead to better adherence to the meter (an intermediate outcome), which leads to more appropriate adjustments of medications (another intermediate outcome) that lead to better glycemic control (another intermediate outcome) that could, in turn, lead to better health-related quality of life (the long-term outcome). Thus, when evaluating the linkage of the *process* with long-term *outcomes*, identifying potential intermediate outcomes along the causal path between the process and long-term outcomes may be useful.

Performance Indicators

Within the cycle for continuous quality improvement, quality is often monitored using **performance indicators**.[51,52] ❻ *Performance indicators are used to measure quality as part of the "Check" function of quality improvement. The indicators are an aspect of care and typically focus on the process or outcomes of a care system,* although they can also focus on structure. Typically, they measure specific processes or steps within a process that are known to be associated with an important outcome. For example, to evaluate the process of responding to a drug information request, one could identify a few key steps within the process that can be easily measured (e.g., in what percentage of cases was the desired timeline for a response documented, in what percentage of cases was the desired timeline met?).

Although one might think that outcomes are the ideal indicator of health care performance, they are often more difficult to measure than specific health care functions and may not always be directly, or independently, caused by the process of interest. Process indicators are useful for quality improvement when the:

- Outcome is difficult to measure.
- Outcome is far removed in time from the process (e.g., 10-year survival in cancer).
- Outcome is influenced by many factors other than the process.
- Process, by itself, is of interest (e.g., it is required to be measured for accreditation by TJC, as it reflects an issue of social justice, such as racial inequities in receiving specific elements of care).[53]

Therefore, if one wanted to improve the quality of care for patients with diabetes, it may be more useful to assess the appropriateness of adjustments in insulin doses than to measure the rate of hospitalizations during a 5-year period for patients in the diabetes care program. We can assess the process of care delivered or the difference in care by measuring the appropriateness of adjustments in insulin doses across many different population groupings such as age groups, race/ethnicity, or by socioeconomic category. This is not to suggest that evaluating outcomes is unwise. If outcomes can be directly linked to the process and can be evaluated in a timely, efficient, and reliable manner, they become powerful tools for quality improvement.

● ❼ *Performance indicators are typically categorized as either sentinel or aggregate measures.*[51,54,55] **Sentinel indicators** *reflect the occurrence of a unique, isolated, and serious event that requires further investigation (e.g., adverse drug-related event, death), whereas* **aggregate indicators** *provide a summary of the frequency, or timeliness, of a process by aggregating numerous cases. Aggregate indicators are further divided into continuous or rate-based indicators.* **Continuous indicators** provide a simple count, or time estimate, related to a process (e.g., average turnaround time on medication orders), whereas **rate-based indicators** usually measure the proportion of activities, or patients, that conform to a desired standard (e.g., the proportion of stat orders that are dispensed within 15 minutes). Thus, the rate-based indicators are generally expressed as a ratio. The denominator within the ratio should be the total number of patients within the target population, while the numerator should be the number of patients who received (or failed to receive) the desired test or who achieved a specified goal.[55] For example, if it is necessary to construct an indicator for medication errors, the numerator would be the number of medication errors within a defined time period and the denominator would be the total number of error opportunities (e.g., number of prescriptions filled) during the same time period. This facilitates the comparison of error rates over time even as prescription volume fluctuates.

Selecting and Defining an Indicator

● Characteristics for an ideal indicator have been proposed by several authors and organizations.[50–57] In general, it is necessary to seek indicators that are clearly defined, quantitative, reliable, clinically meaningful, and actionable. Kerr and associates[58] also suggest using indicators where the link between process and outcome is clearly established and the link between an indicator and a potential quality improvement response is evident. Thus, the indicator provides clinically meaningful and actionable information. Indicators should be selected based on their usefulness to quality improvement efforts. The indicator should help determine where potential problems are occurring within the process. For example, it may be useful to know that only 30% of patients reported that they were provided with adequate answers to their questions about medications. The method with which drug-related information is provided to patients can then be changed. However, knowing that only 30% of patients with diabetes had received a microalbumin test would not be as helpful if there is no control of when that test is ordered.

● Providing definitions for any variables that are not intuitive will also be necessary. **Medication error** means different things to different people; therefore, if it is necessary to construct an indicator for medication errors, the staff would need to be informed what constitutes an error (see Chapter 20). It is also necessary to identify inclusion or exclusion criteria. The patients to be included within an indicator must be determined. Even for disease-specific indicators, it is necessary to decide whether to combine data for all patients with the disease or to subdivide the analyses for different types of patients with that disease. For example, it may be possible to divide patients with diabetes into at least three subgroups: Type 1, Type 2, and gestational. Other questions include the following: are people of all ages included? Are only those who attended all diabetes education sessions or anyone who completed even a portion of the program included? The answers to these questions may depend on the indicator. The key is to compare apples to apples. If, for example, the standard for HgbA1c testing is different for patients with gestational diabetes compared with Type 1 or Type 2 diabetes, then a person would not want to combine HgbA1c data from all these patients into a single indicator.

To judge the quality of performance from the indicator data, having a frame of reference will be necessary. Thus, current performance data can be compared with previous performance (i.e., was there an improvement over time?) or with an external criterion or standard (i.e., benchmark); both comparisons can be useful. For example, it is possible to track the proportion of patients who reached the target HgbA1c during the previous 2 years (e.g., 45% of patients last year vs. 62% of patients this year). However, whether this year's result, 62% of patients reaching the target, is considered good, fair, or poor performance is less clear. To determine this, compare the success rate with that of other programs. If the latest data from surrounding health plans indicate that 60% of their enrollees with diabetes have achieved the same target for HgbA1c, the person could assert that performance is at least as good as the standard. Ideally, the goal will be to continually improve success rate, regardless of the minimal standard.

Sources for Indicator Data

Data for constructing indicators can come from numerous sources. The most common sources of performance data are (1) medical or prescription records, (2) administrative claims, (3) operations records, and (4) patient reports. Each of these sources has strengths and weaknesses. Medical records provide rich information about an individual patient; however, the aggregation of data from written documents can be very slow and labor intensive. As advances in health information technology lead to widespread adoption of electronic medical records, the use of medical records for performance review will become increasingly attractive.

Administrative claims are available in electronic format, so data across providers and across an entire patient population can be easily aggregated and analyzed. However, administrative claims lack in-depth information and may contain some inaccuracies in coding. Thus, indicators built solely on administrative claims are limited in their usefulness for problem solving.

Operations records refer to data that are collected as part of the process of care. For example, a hospital pharmacy may document the time that a medication order was received and the time that the medication was dispensed. If the pharmacy has a predetermined standard for the timeliness of medication-order turnaround, then a performance indicator could be developed to show the proportion of medications that were dispensed within the designated time frame.

Patient-reported data can also be valuable in assessing several subdomains of quality. Patient satisfaction measures are the most common way of collecting patient feedback on care. Satisfaction is an important outcome of care because patients who are dissatisfied with services are more likely to complain to external entities (e.g., regulatory agencies, employers) and are more likely to discontinue using services. Patients can also be asked questions about specific steps in the process of care to identify the source of quality deficits (e.g., were you asked if you had any questions about your medication?). The most commonly used tools for gathering patient feedback are within the Consumer Assessment of Healthcare Providers and Systems (CAHPS) family of surveys (http://www.ahrq.gov/cahps/index.html).[59] CAHPS contains surveys for health systems, physicians, and other facilities and clinicians. PQA has developed a CAHPS-like survey tool to gather patient feedback on ambulatory pharmacy services.[60]

The best method for collecting performance data is to use a hybrid approach wherein several different sources of data are used to examine the same care process. This allows for a more reliable and broad-based perspective on performance. This is important because different data sources have been found to provide different estimates of the quality of care.[61,62] For practical purposes the ability to collect and report data from an electronic system would be ideal for efficiency and accurate comparison from standard coding of data elements, that is when standard coding has been built into the electronic health records or pharmacy information systems. Obviously, standard coding is not universal across informatics systems at this time, but the benefits of interoperability for timely collection and reporting and comparing performance data across entities will be significant. The previously described MACRA MIPS[10] program for quality performance measurement of providers of Medicare Part B includes improving interoperability as one of its aims for sharing of information and coordination of care across the care continuum. The electronic health records vendors are incorporating standard coding of data elements to meet the interoperability and quality measurement aims.[10] Pharmacy informatics systems are beginning to include structured, standardized coding, "pharmacy value sets" through the efforts of the Pharmacy e-Health Information Technology (eHIT) Collaborative. Specifically, the inclusion of the Systematized Nomenclature for Medicine Clinical Terms (SNOMED CT)[63] is a standardized terminology of over 300,000 clinical codes. The Pharmacy eHIT Collaborative has created a subset of the SNOMED CT codes as a "pharmacy value set" for pharmacies, such as a list of codes for drug therapy problems and drug therapy recommendations. These code sets will allow capture of pharmaceutical care data for interoperability and measurement.[64]

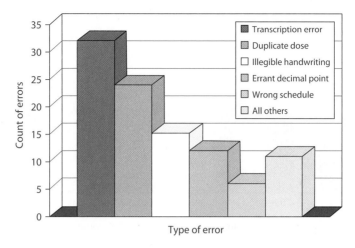

Figure 18–2. Pareto chart: Factors contributing to improper dose errors.

Interpreting Indicator Data

The collection of performance data is good, but data are most useful when transformed into interpretable and actionable information. Several tools can help transform data into easily interpreted information. These tools include Pareto charts, bar charts, scatter diagrams, regression analyses, run charts, and control charts. Detailed information on the use of these tools can be found elsewhere, including Appendix 18-1[65]; however, examples for a few of the tools are shown in Figures 18-2 through 18-6.

Pareto charts are vertical bar graphs with the data presented so that the bars are arranged from left to right on the horizontal axis in their order of decreasing frequency. This arrangement helps to identify which problems to address in what order. By addressing the data represented in the tallest bars (e.g., the most frequently occurring problems or contributing factors), efforts can be focused on areas where the most gain can be realized. Pareto charts are commonly used to identify issues to address, delineate potential causes of a problem, and to monitor improvements in processes. An example of a Pareto chart is shown in Figure 18-2. This example illustrates frequently occurring factors that contribute to improperly dosed medication errors. By looking at transcription errors as a contributing factor on which to focus quality improvement efforts, the quality improvement team will generally gain more than they would by tackling the smaller bars.

Bar charts and scatter diagrams are particularly useful for displaying data for sentinel events. If a pharmacy wanted to evaluate data on medication errors, a bar chart could show the distribution of errors by day of the week or by time of day (Figure 18-3). Displaying the rate (i.e., percent of doses dispensed in error) rather than a simple count of errors helps control for fluctuations in the workload across days of the week. This might help to pinpoint whether errors were more likely to occur during days or shifts. If so, the

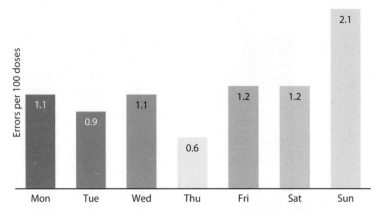

Figure 18–3. Bar chart showing percentage of doses dispensed in error.

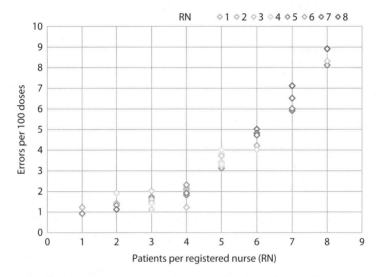

Figure 18–4. Scatter diagram to depict relationship of error rate and workload.

staff could then investigate why the errors were higher at times. The frequency of errors could also be depicted on a scatter diagram. A scatter diagram illustrates the relationship of two variables. For example, a nursing home might be interested in whether the frequency of errors is related to staffing levels. A scatter diagram could be constructed wherein the number of errors was shown on the vertical (y) axis and the staffing level on the horizontal (x) axis (Figure 18-4). The data points are plotted to show the number of errors at each level of staffing.

Run charts and control charts are useful for depicting trends in rate-based indicators. Both charts illustrate the trend in a variable over time; however, the control chart also

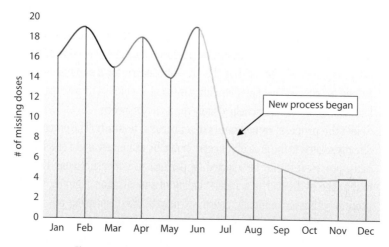

Figure 18–5. Run chart depicting rate of missing doses over time.

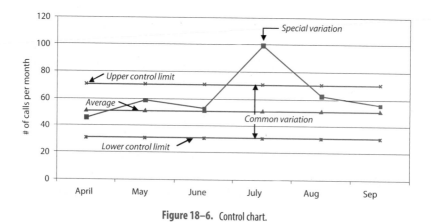

Figure 18–6. Control chart.

shows the extent of variation in the trend by placing control limits above and below the trend line (typically at two standard deviations from the mean). In most cases, a simple run chart will suffice for visualizing a trend. For example, if a health system wanted to examine the impact of changing the medication delivery process on the rate of missing doses of medications, the rate could be calculated for each month and trended over time (Figure 18-5).

Constructing Process Indicators

A stepwise approach to constructing a rate-based process indicator is outlined here.[66]

1. **Identify an area of concern.** The area of concern may be identified from internal reports of quality-related problems or from external mandates (e.g., requirements

for accreditation). Often, these concerns relate to areas in which errors have occurred with great frequency or in which the clinical consequences of suboptimal quality are substantial. For illustrative purposes, patient's understanding of a medication regimen will be used as the area of concern for a community pharmacy. Asking for suggestions for where improvement should occur from patients, front-line staff, or clinicians can help identify the area of concern.

2. **Select the process, or segments of a process, to study.** The process(es) most directly related to the area of concern should be examined, and a specific segment of the process(es) may be selected for performance measurement. For example, in the case of the patient's understanding of a medication regimen, the relevant process within a community pharmacy may be the dispensing process and the specific segment of the process for assessment may be patient counseling.

3. **Determine what can be measured to evaluate the process.** For patient counseling, it is possible to measure the frequency of patient counseling events, the accuracy of information provided to patients, or the patient's knowledge about the medication regimen. Those performing the assessment should then select the measures that are most likely to be reliable, are feasible to collect, and facilitate a valid assessment of the quality of the counseling segment of the dispensing process. In this example, the rate of patient counseling might first be selected for measurement because it should be easily and reliably collected and will provide a valid assessment of whether counseling was occurring (although it would not tell the effectiveness of counseling).

4. **Define the numerator for your indicator.** For an indicator, the numerator should reflect the number of times that a selected event occurred. For the patient counseling indicator, the numerator could be the number of patient counseling events within a specified time interval (e.g., 1 month). To accurately determine the number of counseling events, defining what is and what is not a counseling event is important. For example, must a counseling event involve oral communication between patient and pharmacist, or will the provision of a written pamphlet suffice? If oral communication is required, how much communication is necessary to be considered a counseling event? Do certain elements of drug information need to be conveyed for the event to be counted? Ensuring that all employees have a clear understanding of the definition of counseling is important to reduce inaccuracies in counting the events.

5. **Define the denominator for your indicator.** For an indicator, the denominator should represent the eligible population or the total number of opportunities in which the numerator could have occurred. For the counseling indicator, the denominator could simply be defined as the number of prescriptions dispensed in a time period (e.g., 1 month). However, it is necessary to refine this number to enhance the validity of our inferences about the quality of counseling. Should both

new and refill prescriptions be included in the denominator? If the patient declines the offer to counsel, should they be included in the denominator? If the patient receives five prescriptions at one time, will they be counted as one counseling opportunity or as five counseling opportunities? Having clear inclusion and exclusion criteria will be important to the interpretability of the indicator.

6. **Determine the method for data collection.** Numerous methods may exist for collecting data for a specific indicator. For the counseling indicator, the denominator could be derived from automated reports of new (and perhaps refill) prescriptions. If the pharmacy has a mechanism for tracking patients who were offered but declined counseling, then the prescriptions for those patients could be subtracted from the denominator. The numerator in the counseling indicator could be measured in several ways. A pharmacist could record on a notepad, or electronic record, whether he or she counseled the patient. Alternatively, the pharmacy could select a time period during which an external data collector would document the frequency of counseling. This could entail direct observation of the pharmacist–patient encounters or could entail the data collector asking the patients whether they had been offered counseling and had received counseling about their medications. In the latter approach, the patient could also be asked whether he or she understood the information that they were provided. A step further would be to assess the patient's understanding, although that would take more time and, therefore, may not be possible. Each of these methods has strengths and limitations.

7. **Select tools to display the indicator data.** After the data are collected, displaying the results in a manner that provides an efficient assessment of quality would be helpful. This can be accomplished by comparing the results with an external benchmark or by comparing the most recent results with previous results for the same provider. Currently, the only external benchmark that exists for the example may be a regulatory requirement for counseling. For example, the state of Michigan requires pharmacists to counsel 100% of patients who receive a new prescription unless the patient meets certain exemption criteria. However, a more useful comparator may be the prior performance of the pharmacy. Thus, plotting the counseling rate on a run chart each month may eventually provide the pharmacy with insight on whether the counseling rate is improving or declining. If the rate is declining, then further investigation could reveal the potential causes of the change in performance and actions taken to improve performance.

Quality Indicators and Measures Evaluation

A quality indicator or measure may be identified and defined internally by the health care provider, the facility, the system, or plan. However, more frequently, providers are assigned specific nationally recognized indicators or measures by which their performance will be determined. As previously mentioned, the NQF, the NCQA, and PQA are sources of developed endorsed quality measures. These endorsed measures are required by agencies, health insurers, and others to assess performance of providers, facilities, care settings, or plans. Several examples of medication-related measures with descriptions are provided in Table 18-2.

TABLE 18-2. EXAMPLE MEDICATION MEASURES AND EVALUATION

Measure Name	Measure Description	Setting[a]	Evaluation Domain[b]
High-risk medication (HRM)	Percent of plan members who received prescriptions for certain drugs, high-risk medications as included in the American Geriatrics Society Beers Criteria, with a high risk of serious side effects, when there may be safer drug choices	Medicare Part D star rating	Drug pricing patient safety
Medication adherence for diabetes medications	Percent of plan members with a prescription for diabetes medication who fill their prescription often enough to achieve proportion of days covered (PDC) of 80% or more	Medicare Part D star rating	Drug pricing patient safety
Medication adherence for hypertension renin angiotensin system antagonists (RASA)	Percent of plan members with a prescription for a renin angiotensin system blood pressure medication who fill their prescription often enough to achieve proportion of days covered (PDC) of 80% or more	Medicare Part D star rating	Drug pricing patient safety
Medication adherence for cholesterol (statins)	Percent of plan members with a prescription for a cholesterol medication (a statin drug) who fill their prescription often enough to achieve proportion of days covered (PDC) of 80% or more	Medicare Part D star rating	Drug pricing patient safety
Medication Therapy Management program completion rate for comprehensive medication review (CMR)	Some plan members are in a program (called a Medication Therapy Management program) to help them manage their drugs. The measure shows how many members in the program had a comprehensive medication review (vs. a targeted medication review) assessment of their medications from the plan. The assessment includes a discussion between the member and a pharmacist (or other health care professional) about all the member's medications. The member also receives a written summary of the discussion, including an action plan that recommends what the member can do to better understand and use his or her medications	Medicare Part D star rating	Drug pricing patient safety

continued

TABLE 18–2. EXAMPLE MEDICATION MEASURES AND EVALUATION (*CONTINUED*)

Measure Name	Measure Description	Setting[a]	Evaluation Domain[b]
Fibrinolytic therapy received within 30 minutes of hospital arrival	Acute myocardial infarction (AMI) patients receiving fibrinolytic therapy during the hospital stay and having a time from hospital arrival to fibrinolysis of 30 minutes or less	Hospital value-based purchasing	Clinical care process measures
Influenza immunization	This prevention measure addresses acute care hospitalized inpatients age 6 months and older who were screened for seasonal influenza immunization status and were vaccinated prior to discharge if appropriate	Hospital value-based purchasing	Clinical care process measures
Coronary artery disease (CAD) anti-platelet therapy	Percentage of patients aged 18 years and older with a diagnosis of coronary artery disease seen within a 12-month period who were prescribed aspirin or clopidogrel	Practices Merit-Based Incentive Payment System (MIPS), quality	Quality measures
Avoidance of antibiotic treatment in adults with acute bronchitis	The percentage of patients 18–64 years of age with a diagnosis of acute bronchitis who were not dispensed an antibiotic prescription	MIPS	Quality measures
Medication management for people with asthma	The percentage of patients 5–64 years of age during the measurement year who were identified as having persistent asthma and were dispensed appropriate medications that they remained on for at least 75% of their treatment period	MIPS	Quality measures
Atrial fibrillation (AF) and atrial flutter: chronic anticoagulation therapy	Percentage of patients aged 18 years and older with a diagnosis of nonvalvular atrial fibrillation or atrial flutter whose assessment of the specified thromboembolic risk factors indicate one or more high risk factors or more than one moderate risk, as determined by CHADS2 risk stratification, who are prescribed warfarin OR another oral anticoagulant drug that is U.S. Food and Drug Administration (FDA) approved for the prevention of thromboembolism	MIPS	Quality measures
Adherence to anti-psychotic medications for individuals with schizophrenia	Percentage of individuals at least 18 years of age as of the beginning of the measurement period with schizophrenia or schizoaffective disorder who had at least two prescriptions filled for any antipsychotic medications and who had a proportion of days covered (PDC) of at least 0.8 for antipsychotic medications during the measurement period (12 consecutive months)	MIPS	Quality measures

[a]Setting is the entity or area applied for the measure.
[b]Domain is the type or category the measure is attributed.

Multiple PQA-endorsed measures have been adopted by CMS for inclusion in their quality evaluation systems, including Medicare Part D five-star rating and the Quality Reporting System (QRS). For measurement year 2019, there were five PQA measures utilized in the Medicare Part D Star Ratings system which provides information on quality of part D plans that cover Medicare beneficiaries. The five measures include three proportion of days covered (PDC) measures for specified drug classes (diabetes medications, renin angiotensin system antagonists [RASA], and statins), statin use in persons with diabetes (SUPD), and completion rate for **comprehensive medication review (CMR)**. The QRS provides information on quality of health plans involved in health insurance exchanges (federal and state-based exchanges). Medication quality measures in the QRS include: the three previously addressed PDC measures for diabetes, RASA, and statins, in addition to international normalized ratio (INR) monitoring for individuals receiving warfarin. Data on performance for each of the measures is considered when calculating the overall quality rating of the plan.

Other programs include a myriad of different medication measures for specific disease states for quality-of-care assessment. One example is the hospital value-based purchasing program.[67] A process measure of clinical care, for the disease acute myocardial infarction, includes evaluation of receipt of fibrinolytic therapy within 30 minutes of hospital arrival and for another process, prevention management, receipt of an immunization (influenza vaccine). The hospital is evaluated based on a total performance score and the clinical care process measures constitute a percentage (in 2019–2021, 25%) of the total (100%) performance composite score. Weighted scoring changes occur over the years of the program.

In the MIPS program for eligible providers, there are four categories that are part of a composite performance score; each category contributes to the total performance score.[68] The total performance score is an overall assessment for the clinician for a performance period. The score is determined by assessing an MIPS eligible clinician's applicable measures and activities for each performance category. The MIPS eligible clinician's final score determines their payment adjustment. The four categories and the associated 2019 percentages contributions include: quality (45%), improvement activities (15%), promoting interoperability (formerly advancing care information or "meaningful use"; 25%), and cost (15%). Within the first three categories, there are multiple options for providers to select the measures they want to be assessed for performance, and many of these options include medication measures. Under the category quality, there are over 270 measures and a provider must select six. Many of quality measures are medication related, such as patients with chronic stable coronary artery disease (CAD) who were prescribed antiplatelet therapy, aspirin, or clopidogrel within a 12-month period; antibiotic avoidance in patients with bronchitis; or the percentage of asthma patients dispensed appropriate asthma controller medications. Overall provider performance will be determined by the performance within each category as part of the composite score. The interested reader should access the CMS website on MIPS categories "weights" and "payment adjustments" periodically as these change over time as required by law (https://qpp.cms.gov/mips/quality-measures).

Quality and Safety Monitoring: Adverse Drug Events (ADEs)

An adverse drug event (ADE) is defined by the National Academy of Medicine (formerly Institute of Medicine) as "an injury resulting from medical intervention related to a drug."[69] A large majority of ADEs are preventable. The Department of Health and Human Services (HHS) released the National Action Plan for Adverse Drug Event Prevention (ADE Action Plan) in 2014 identifying anticoagulants, opioids, and diabetes agents as high-priority drug class targets for ADE prevention efforts.[70] The ADE Action Plan suggests a four-pronged approach to reduce patient harms from these three drug classes: surveillance, prevention, incentives and oversight, and research. The initial challenge for organizing national efforts to prevent ADEs, noted in the report, is the lack of a public health surveillance system that measures outpatient ADE rates and reports in a timely fashion. The report also notes the complex array of factors contributing to ADEs that are important considerations for prevention strategies, including polypharmacy and associated patient misuse of medications.

Recently, the **Quality Innovation Network–Quality Improvement Organization (QIN-QIO)** program's 11th Scope of Work (SOW) set out to identify patients from the FFS Medicare population possessing an increased risk of ADEs.[71] Patients defined as high risk of ADEs were those identified via Part D claims as receiving at least three chronic medications, including at least one medication from a priority medication class (anticoagulants, diabetes agents, and opioids). This project applied the framework proposed by Budnitz *et al.*, which proposed applying principles of injury epidemiology to ADE reduction by focusing prevention efforts on potentially modifiable host characteristics.[72] Patients who were designated as being high risk were retrospectively evaluated for occurrences of ADE-related hospital utilization (including emergency department [ED] visits, observation stays, and inpatient admissions). The authors found that rates of ADEs in the high-risk group were more than double of that in the overall FFS Medicare population, demonstrating that claims data can be an effective tool for ADE surveillance and can assist in identifying areas to target quality improvement efforts.[71]

MEASURING HEALTH EQUITY

In determining quality and performance, the development of indicators, measurement, and collection of data must take into consideration the distinguishing characteristics of all people. Despite advances in health care, there are numerous reports of minority groups experiencing differences in care and worse outcomes; the CMS Office of Minority Health (CMS OMH) has a number of brief reports on health disparities by diseases from atrial fibrillation to osteoporosis to stroke available on their website.[73]

Definition of Health Equity

❽ *A commitment to health equity and the elimination of health disparities are necessary to achieve optimal health for all.* Healthy People 2020 defines **health equity** as the attainment of the highest level of health for all people. Health systems that are committed to a culture of equity must focus on valuing each patient or customer equally regardless of what demographic group(s) they are assigned. When measuring health equity, an identified health disparity may be associated with one or more social, economic, environmental, or other distinguishing factors. Health disparities indicate differences or gaps in care experienced by individuals due to systematic obstacles associated with conditions of their birth, or how they live, work, grow, and age. Factors such as race and/or ethnicity; religion; socioeconomic status; gender; age; mental health, cognitive, sensory, or physical disability; sexual orientation or gender identity; geographic location; or other characteristics of discrimination or exclusion can adversely affect the health care they receive.[74]

Measurement Standards

Our ability to measure and address health disparities is dependent on the standardized collection of data for vulnerable groups. The ACA authorized the implementation of national data collection standards for documenting patient information to better understand, respond to, and evaluate progress in eliminating health disparities.[75] Health care facilities use electronic health records, as part of Stage 2 Meaningful Use, to capture data elements such as race, ethnicity, gender, preferred language, and date of birth or REaL data (race, ethnicity, and language) to inform their understanding of how well they provide care to patients.[76] However, a lack of standardized procedures for data collection can result in inconsistencies in data captured, impeding the development of culturally appropriate data categories needed to identify disparities. To achieve health equity, the PDCA must include demographic data collection and assessment of all the populations that allow for the development of focus interventions to address differences in care.[77] The Institute of Healthcare Improvement (IHI) offers a guide to achieving health equity that outlines the business case for addressing disparities. The guide includes a case study, tools, and a description of measurement for different subpopulations. It identifies measures in two categories: summary or aggregated and **stratified** or **disaggregated**.[78] Pharmacy information systems and prescription drug claims will require consistent data element capture for vulnerable groups to identify disparities in medication prescribing and pharmacy services. Recently, CMS reported 2014 Medicare Advantage data that identified differences in two patient experience measures by race: obtaining needed prescription drugs and obtaining information about prescription drugs. Results for the two measures were highest in Whites at 91.1% and 82.2% and lowest in Asian or Pacific Islanders (API) 85.1% and 72.7%, respectively. In Blacks, results for the two measures were 90% and 77.7%, in American Indian or Alaska Native 87.3% and 79.9%, and in Hispanics 88% and 76.8%, respectively.[79] These results are similar to a study from 2008 of surveyed Medicare Part D beneficiaries of the same measures. Blacks, Hispanics, and API results were 2 to 11 points lower as compared with Whites.[80] The current Coronavirus Disease 2019 (COVID-19) pandemic is an example of how race ethnic socioeconomic equity concerns are relevant, as early data indicate the majority cases and deaths are in Blacks.[81] However, the ability to capture this data is hampered in the United States due to failure of information systems' data interoperability standards and requirements for collection and/or documentation of critical data elements. A report by Kaiser Health News stated that race ethnicity data is missing 85% of the time and home address is missing half the time in electronic health records.[82]

Case Study 18–3

In evaluating medication reconciliation at admission in a nursing home, the medical director believes that there are differences in medication discrepancies based on patient demographics and would like the nursing staff and consultant pharmacist to present data to refute or confirm. What steps should the nursing home take to assess the medication discrepancies by patient subgroups?

MEDICATION USE EVALUATION

Medication use evaluation (MUE) is often included in the overall performance improvement programs within institutional settings to provide in-depth assessment of the medication use process. MUE is an in-depth multidisciplinary assessment of the medication use process including prescribing, order verification, dispensing, administering, monitoring, with the overall goal to improve patient medication use-related outcomes. MUE programs should, over time, examine all aspects of medication use and require direct involvement of pharmacists.[83,84] ❾ *MUE is often part of an organization's overall performance improvement program that uses definitions of safe and effective use of medications to assess components of the medication use process.* These definitions are usually described as **criteria** and are endorsed by the organization within which they are to be applied. These criteria are developed by organizations' multidisciplinary team through an in-depth environmental scan of the medication(s) use data to identify critical points for the assessment of the effectiveness, quality, and safety of the medication(s) in a specific environment (hospital, clinic, infusion center, etc.). Criteria summarize an organization's definition of appropriate or acceptable use of the medication. Data collection of the way medications are used, administered, and monitored within the organization is compared with the criteria to determine if actual practice matches the best (or at least acceptable) practice as stated with the criteria. For example, based on the evidence that slowing the infusion rate of a specific intravenous medication reduces the risk of serious adverse events, the criteria may state that the medication should be infused over at least 60 minutes. However, when actual practice is accessed as part of an MUE, results indicate that the medication is infused over 30 minutes or less in 50% of cases, and adverse effects were noted in most of these cases. These results indicate that best practice is not followed.

Case Study 18–4

Opioid use and associated harm are an ongoing public health care crisis. Prescribers and pharmacists are responsible for appropriate opioid prescription management. The state Department of Health has identified steps each professional and organization shall take to improve prescription opioid use and decrease associated adverse events, up to and including death. Your organization is assessing their compliance with your state laws. What specific items will you review?

Endorsement of criteria is usually provided by a multidisciplinary group that includes medical staff (e.g., the pharmacy and therapeutics [P&T] committee—see Chapter 15). The goal of MUE is to provide all patients with the most rational, safe, and effective drug therapy through the assessment and improvement of specific medication use processes. MUE may focus on a specific medication (e.g., oxycodone), a class of medications (e.g., opioids), medications used in the management of a specific disease state or clinical setting (e.g., acute or chronic pain management), medications related to a clinical event (e.g., surgical or procedural intervention), a specific component of the medication use process (e.g., time to patient receipt of initial dose of analgesic), or can be based on specific outcomes (e.g., pain score and patient response pre- and postpain medication). MUE is not designed to address if-then questions (such as if one dose is used instead of another, then will outcomes be affected), but simply determines if the actual use of a medication is consistent with the standards established within the criteria. Although MUE is no longer explicitly addressed within TJC Standards, it remains an important component of broader requirements related to performance improvement within organizations. In order to be effective, challenges such as a lack of resources or authority, politics, difficulty in identifying issues (e.g., high-use, high-risk, or problematic medications or processes) or in acting upon data to improve performance, and cumbersome or ineffective reporting structure or processes must be addressed. For example, unless the organization has a functional process to use the information generated by MUE to improve patient care, outcomes are unlikely to improve. If a minority of prescribers or any single group (e.g., nursing, clinical laboratory, pharmacy, respiratory therapy) can unilaterally disagree with the recommendations from an MUE and successfully block efforts to implement process improvement initiatives, efforts will fail. For MUE to effectively improve patient care, the organization must have a commitment to improving medication use and a committee structure that facilitates multidisciplinary collaboration and cooperation.

The Medication Use Process

In 1989, a multidisciplinary task force was organized by TJC to describe the **medication use process** as a component of their effort to develop tools to assess medication use. The medication use process is the outline of the steps involved in providing medications to patients (e.g., prescribing, dispensing) and what happens after the medication is administered (e.g., monitoring). The original definition of the medication use process included prescribing, transcribing, dispensing, administering, monitoring, and systems and management control (see Table 18-2 for the full definition). This description serves as the basis for MUE.[85,86] The transcribing step has also been described as the order verification step, which includes ensuring the appropriate dosage of the medication, and identification of pertinent interactions. Transcription is less common today due to widespread adoption of electronic health records (EHRs); however, paper-based systems exist, especially in small provider practices and some nursing homes, where transcription is still in place and is associated with errors. Currently, systems and management control are often not included within the description of the medication use process as it applies to virtually all aspects of patient care. Medication acquisition, storage, distribution, and disposal may also be assessed if pertinent (Table 18-3).

It is important to note that this description outlines a process that is more multidisciplinary than the categories might imply. For example, while the prescribing category may imply a function of a prescriber (e.g., physician, nurse practitioner, physician assistant), pharmacists are often involved as they assist in drug selection and individualization of the therapeutic regimen.

TABLE 18–3. DESCRIPTION OF STEPS IN THE MEDICATION USE PROCESS

Function	Description
Prescribing	Assessing the need for/selecting the correct drug
	Individualizing the therapeutic regimen
	Defining the desired therapeutic response
Order verification	Processing the medication order
	Reviewing the order for correct dose and indication for use
	Reviewing the order for pertinent interactions (e.g., drug-drug, drug-disease, drug-herbal)
Dispensing	Compounding/preparing the drug
	Dispensing the drug in a timely manner
	Counseling the patient on new or changed prescription
Administering	Administering the right medication to the right patient
	Administering the medication at the right time
	Informing the patient about the medication
	Including the patient in administration (self-administered medications and appropriate technique and timing)
Monitoring	Monitoring and documenting the patient's response to the medication
	Identifying and reporting adverse drug reactions
	Re-evaluating the drug selection, drug regimen, frequency, and duration
Systems/ Management control	Collaborating and communicating among caregivers
	Reviewing and managing the patient's complete therapeutic drug regimen

Medication Use Evaluation and The Joint Commission

The terminology used to describe MUE has changed over time and can be confusing. MUE, drug usage evaluation (DUE), and drug utilization review (DUR) were often used interchangeably despite being different in their approach and application. DUE is similar to MUE with the same basic elements but does not include the focus of clinical outcome. DUR is a program related to outpatient pharmacy services designed to educate physicians and pharmacists in identifying and reducing the frequency and patterns of fraud, abuse, gross overuse, or inappropriate or medically unnecessary care. DUR frequently is retrospective in nature and utilizes claims data as its primary source of information; however, the process can be prospective or concurrent. The ASHP states "DUE and DUR generally refer to an ongoing, systematic, criteria-based, drug- or disease-specific assessment that ensures appropriate medication utilization at the individual patient level" whereas MUE can be differentiated by the emphasis on improving patient outcomes and quality of life through assessment of clinical outcomes via a multidisciplinary approach.[84] ADEs evaluation is generally included in MUE as they are an unintended outcome (Table 18-4). Greater consistency in terminology and standards were established with an initiative called the Agenda for Change from TJC in 1986.[87,88]

TABLE 18–4. ACRONYMS ASSOCIATED WITH THE EVALUATION OF MEDICATION USE

Term	Origin	Description
Drug Use Review (DUR)	1969 Task Force on Prescription Drugs	Retrospective evaluation to monitor medication use patterns. Usually quantitative and limited to trending
	1990 Medicaid Anti-Discriminatory Drug Price and Patient Benefit Restoration Act (*Pryor II*)	Usually retrospective evaluation based on claims data. Results used to direct education and to reduce fraud, abuse, overuse, and inappropriate or unnecessary care
	1990 Omnibus Budget Reconciliation Act of 1990 (OBRA 90)	Required pharmacy to provide to Medicaid beneficiaries (States could require of other patients): Prospective drug utilization review—is the drug necessary/appropriate; Patient counseling standards—offer the patient counseling by a pharmacist; Maintain patient records—accurate and up to date
Medication Use Evaluation (MUE)	1992 Joint Commission on Accreditation of Healthcare Organizations (JCAHO) Standards	Expansion of MUE to include all medications and all aspects of medication use including prescribing, dispensing, administering, monitoring, and outcome. Drug Use Evaluation (DUE) prior used term referred to the medication use processes and prescribing but did not include patient outcomes
Adverse Drug Event (ADE)	2007 Institute of Medicine (IoM), Preventing Medication Errors	An injury resulting from medical intervention related to a drug. This term encompasses harms that occur during medical care that are directly caused by the drug including, but are not limited to medication errors, adverse drug reactions, allergic reactions and overdoses
	National Action Plan for Adverse Drug Events (HHS)	

It was intended to improve standards by focusing on key functions of quality of care, to monitor the performance of health care organizations using indicators, to improve the relevance and quality of the survey process, and to enhance the accuracy and value of TJC accreditation. Indicators are quantitative measures of an aspect of patient care and are used to screen for potential problems; indicators will be discussed in detail later in the chapter. The revised process was to focus on actual performance versus the capability to perform well. An organization could no longer hide behind having well-designed processes or policies and procedures on paper; TJC surveyors would now be looking at how processes were carried out. Within this initiative, TJC endorsed the concept of CQI, whereby data would be used to uncover problems and use that information to correct issues and avoid problems in the future and included CQI within its standards beginning in 1994.

As part of this process, the Accreditation Manual for Hospitals (AMH) was significantly modified and much of the definition of expectations related to organization performance was deleted.[89] Multidisciplinary involvement in the evaluation of medication use was emphasized. Eventually, the standards were moved from the Medical Staff Chapter of the AMH to the Care of Patients and Performance Improvement Chapters. In 1992, the terminology was also changed from drug use evaluation to MUE to reflect that all medications and all medication-related functions are included in the standard. This change also broadened the scope to reflect TJC's expanded reach into nonacute care settings (such as clinics and intravenous infusion centers) and clarified that the process did not focus on illicit drug use. MUE standards first appeared in the 1992 AMH and were required of all institutions beginning in 1994.

Current standards focus on performance improvement, but no longer require that a specific approach be used. The organization can select, based on its characteristics and structure, a performance-improvement approach (e.g., FOCUS-PDCA, Six Sigma) that best meets their needs and that of its patients. Standards state that MUE should be a systematic, multidisciplinary process focusing on continual improvement in the medication use process and patient outcomes. The use of data for reappointment or recredentialing is still required, but the emphasis is on continuous performance improvement.

Priorities should be established based on:

- Effect on performance and improved patient outcomes
- Selected high-volume, high-risk, or problem-prone processes
- Resources and organizational priorities

Evaluation of the use of high-cost medications is often a priority within organizations hoping to optimize use of available financial resources. However, in the past, many organizations based their topic selection solely on cost-saving initiatives rather than on improving the quality of medication use. As a result, this category, when stated as a sole rationale for topic selection, is no longer considered to be consistent with the goals of MUE. High-cost medications continue to be a focus of evaluation, but organizations are careful to justify the evaluation based on other criteria, such as the use of the medication being problem-prone or its importance in determining patient outcome.

The pharmacist plays a key role within the multidisciplinary MUE process. Although not always involved in specific initiatives, all pharmacists should actively identify opportunities for improvement in processes.[90] Although many pharmacists within the organization will have some role in the MUE process, those responsible for coordination and implementation of MUE initiatives are often those with drug information or performance improvement responsibilities, as well as those with specialized knowledge or experience in the component of medication use under assessment. The American Society of Health-System Pharmacists (ASHP) has developed guidelines for pharmacist's participation in MUE.[84] These guidelines can serve as a resource to those developing or revising an MUE program or for practitioners new to the process.

The MUE Process

The process of medication use evaluation has often been implemented through a 10-step process described by TJC in 1989.[91] Although this specific process is no longer mandated by TJC, it does offer a reasonable model for MUE. The process is tied to the PDCA discussed earlier in this chapter and referred to in Figure 18-1. The 10 steps are:

1. Assign responsibility for monitoring and evaluation.
2. Delineate scope of care and service provided by the organization.
3. Identify important aspects of care and service provided by the organization.
4. Identify indicators, data sources, and collection methods to monitoring important aspects of care.
5. Establish means to trigger evaluation (e.g., trends or patterns of use, thresholds).
6. Collect and organize data.
7. Initiate evaluation of care (as indicated by triggers set in step 5).
8. Take actions to improve care and service.
9. Assess the effectiveness of actions and maintain the improvement; document improvements in care.
10. Communicate results to relevant individuals and groups.

Please note, as these steps are described below, they are often concurrent and overlapping. For example, the final step of communication is important throughout the other steps.

Responsibility for the Medication Use Evaluation Function

The 10-step process begins with the organization defining which group or groups will participate in and be responsible for the evaluation of medication use. These groups oversee the process, since everyone must provide effort toward performing or implementing quality assurance activities. Although TJC standards no longer assign the responsibility for MUE to the P&T committee, nor do they require a P&T committee at all, the function is well suited to this group as well as to a performance/quality improvement committee. Pharmacist responsibilities are well established for MUE leadership, responsibility, and data collection/evaluation.[92] Performance improvement committees are usually interprofessional but may lack medical staff participation due to time constraints and lack of funding for the work needed to achieve success. Their focus may be quite broad and may include oversight for a wide variety of performance improvement functions throughout the organization. Some organizations have formed an MUE subcommittee to the P&T group, while others have distributed the responsibility for MUE along patient population or product lines. Subcommittees are generally assigned responsibility for a specific set of responsibilities or information and report to the larger committee. They serve as a platform to work through the details of an issue or process and generate recommendations to the parent committee. A patient safety committee may also play a role in identification of topics, evaluation of findings, and implementation of corrective actions. The entire committee may participate in evaluations or working groups, consisting of committee members, may be established;

nonmembers may be appointed to address specific issues. The size, scope, and makeup of the health care organization and its approach to performance improvement should determine the approach to be used. The participants in the group charged with overseeing MUE must have a clear understanding that the purpose is that of improving the quality of the medication use process and that each member is expected to actively participate. Newly formed groups may benefit from an overview of the organization's overall approach to quality improvement and how MUE contributes to overall goals.

Topic Selection

Topic selection should be based on the mission and scope of care of the organization and should focus on high-volume, high-risk, or problem-prone medication-related processes. Topics may also focus on institutional priorities (e.g., initiation of new clinical programs or services). Several sources of information are commonly used to identify these agents and issues. They include medication error reports, adverse drug reactions (ADRs), advances in patient care modalities that involve changes in optimal pharmacotherapy, disease- or diagnosis-based length of stay or cost outliers within an organization, purchasing reports indicating a significant increase in the use of an agent (without a related shift in patient population), medications that are a key component of a process or procedure (e.g., $P2Y_{12}$ inhibitors, such as clopidogrel, and percutaneous coronary intervention), and more. It is essential that the topics selected reflect the overall scope of medication use throughout the organization, including inpatients, outpatients, emergency care, and short-stay settings, rather than always centering on a finite area.

The inclusion of specific requirements within TJC's Medication Management Standards and National Patient Safety Goals related to identification and monitoring of medications described as high risk or high alert within the organization provides another mechanism to target specific medications for additional assessment. High-risk or high-alert medications are those that are most likely to result in adverse outcomes if used inappropriately or if errors are made.

Ideally, the group charged with MUE should develop an annual plan that will establish goals for new topics to be assessed and provide for follow-up on previous evaluations. Priorities should be re-evaluated, and the scope and breadth of recent evaluations should be assessed relative to the scope of care provided within the organization. For example, if recent MUE efforts focused primarily on issues related to antibiotic use, the plan for the upcoming year should deemphasize assessment of this therapeutic class in favor of a more balanced topic selection. The planning process can identify follow-up assessments (used to assess and document that previous efforts were successful in improving performance) that remain to be performed. The failure to perform and document these follow-up evaluations is problematic in many organizations but is a key component of the quality improvement process. Development of an annual plan also allows an opportunity to discontinue activities that are no longer useful, such as an ongoing assessment that has demonstrated sustained improvement and can now be replaced by periodic rechecks to assure continued compliance.

Criteria, Standards, and Indicators

Criteria are statements of the activity to be measured and standards define the performance expectations. For example, criteria for the management of patients with pneumonia might state that the first dose of antibiotic must be administered within 2 hours. The standard for this criteria statement would be set at 100%, if there were no acceptable exceptions to this time frame. Criteria should be based on current best or at least accepted practice or available organization-based clinical care plans, appropriate for the target patient population(s), and be supported by current literature. Ideally, a multidisciplinary group develops the criteria. The membership of this group (e.g., prescribers, nurses, pharmacists, respiratory therapists, social workers, clinical laboratory and information systems personnel, discharge planners) should be determined by the nature of the process under evaluation. Inclusion of all involved disciplines initially will also facilitate implementation of corrective actions, if deficiencies are identified. However, criteria are most often developed by one or two of the involved disciplines and are subsequently approved by a multidisciplinary group with representation from all applicable practice groups (e.g., prescribers, pharmacists, nurses). Explicit (objective) criteria are preferred, in that they are clear cut, based on specific measurable parameters, and are better suited for automation. Implicit (subjective) criteria require that a judgment be made and require appropriate clinical expertise to be effective. They are often too subjective to be consistently evaluated (i.e., different people would interpret them differently). Table 18-5 compares implicit and explicit criteria statements. Appendix 18-2 provides an example of criteria. It is imperative that the appropriate oversight group approves the criteria prior to initiation of data collection.

TABLE 18–5. EXAMPLES OF IMPLICIT AND EXPLICIT CRITERIA STATEMENTS

Implicit Criteria Statements	Explicit Criteria Statements
Blood work ordered	Pretreatment white blood cell (WBC) with differential ordered and completed within 48 hours prior to the initiation of therapy
Renal function assessed routinely	Serum creatinine evaluated every 3 days during therapy
Neutropenic patients	Patients with WBC $< 1000/\text{mm}^3$

Case Study 18–5

An antibiotic was infused too rapidly, which is an agent recommended for use in prevention of surgical infections and for infections caused by gram-positive (+) organisms. There is some evidence of other issues with the use of this antibiotic and an MUE is planned. The preoperative dose is given in the surgical area and the postoperative doses and treatment doses are given throughout the health system and in-home care patients. Who would you invite to participate in an evaluation of the use of this antibiotic?

Criteria should be phrased in yes/no or true/false (along with *not applicable,* as appropriate) formats and should avoid interpretation on the part of data collectors. They should assess important aspects in the use of the medication or therapy under evaluation and focus on aspects most closely related to outcomes of the care provided. Definition of outcome should also be established within the criteria based on the scope of care provided by the organization. For example, in a truly acute care setting, the outcome assessment of antibiotic management of pneumonia may be limited to a decrease in clinical signs and symptoms indicating a response to therapy and the ability to be discharged on an oral antibiotic(s). However, in an integrated system that includes both acute and ambulatory or long-term care, the evaluation could continue through the entire treatment course and outcome could be assessed based on cure or control of the disease state at the conclusion of therapy.

As the criteria are finalized, it is helpful to consider how opportunities for improvement identified via a criteria statement could be addressed. For example, could the computer system be used as a tool to improve prescribing, would a double check by a nurse and a pharmacist help to prevent errors, or could the dispensing process be modified to improve delivery time? If the corrective action would involve participation of a group not represented in the development process, it may be wise to add them to the team at this point.

Validity should be assessed as part of the development process. Validity assessments consider how effective the criteria will be in providing the information necessary to obtain an actual comparison of what is happening to the expectations outlined in the criteria. Table 18-6 outlines several questions to test the validity of criteria or indicators.[93–96] A short pilot of data collection with an analysis of resulting information is often a good way to test the validity of criteria and its utility in assessing medication use.

Although general guidelines related to criteria are available, some texts providing example criteria are published, but may be dated.[50,51,97,98] Many group purchasing organizations and other networks have systems to facilitate sharing of MUE materials

TABLE 18-6. TESTS OF VALIDITY FOR CRITERIA OR INDICATORS

Types of Validity	Questions That Can be Used to Test Validity
Face validity	Are they important to patient outcome?
	Do they assess a problematic area?
	Do they have some utility in improving patient care?
	Do they reflect system-wide performance?
	Are they appropriate, based on current practice standards and literature?
External validity	Have they been thoroughly reviewed by practitioners with expertise in the use of the medication?
	Are they applicable within the organization?
	Has the review process clarified and improved the criteria/indicators without weakening their intent?
Feasibility of data collection and retrieval	Are they clear and not subject to interpretation?
	Are data available?
	How many cases will need to be evaluated in order to provide adequate data?
	How difficult or complex will the data collection process be?
	What benefits will be gained versus the effort for data collection?
	Will data collection methods be consistent?

(e.g., criteria, data collection forms) and methods of comparing results with those from similar organizations. The advantages to using predeveloped criteria include prior expert review and assessment, and time savings. However, criteria developed outside the organization must be adapted to the practice setting and patient population as appropriate and must be approved by the designated multidisciplinary group prior to data collection. For example, criteria intended for use in a general adult population may not be appropriate for geriatric patients without modification. Also, predeveloped criteria may include uses of a medication not applicable to certain settings or aspects of use that are not a priority for assessment within the organization. For example, criteria for the use of midazolam that address its use for conscious sedation in a setting where conscious sedation is not performed can be streamlined by eliminating criteria related to conscious sedation. Criteria related to the use of antibiotics to treat infection, when the concerns prompting the evaluation relate solely to perioperative use, should be streamlined to focus solely on perioperative use. Criteria may also be derived from guidelines for use developed or adopted within the organization. For example, the P&T committee may agree to add a medication to the formulary for specific indications and require that the use of the agent and patient outcomes be concurrently evaluated based on these guidelines. In this situation, the criteria for use of the medication would reflect the indications approved by the committee and the MUE would assess the desired outcomes as defined by the committee. Data collection would begin as the medication is first used with results reported to the P&T committee at specific intervals (e.g., quarterly) or after a defined period (e.g., for the first 6 months).

Case Study 18–6

Within your organization, anticoagulants are responsible for more adverse events than any other medication. Your MUE findings and the Joint Commission Sentinel event alert 61[126] with evidence guidelines from the American College of Cardiology[127] provide guidance to identify opportunities to reduce the number and severity of adverse effects associated with warfarin and direct oral anticoagulants (DOACs). What specifications and criteria from existing guidelines or standards and your MUE will improve anticoagulant use outcomes?

Performance indicators can also be used to evaluate medication use. As described previously, an indicator is a quantitative measure of an aspect of patient care that is used as a screening tool to detect potential problems in quality.[51] For example, the number of doses of naloxone administered to reverse the effects of opioids administered in a procedure area or in outpatient areas could serve as an indicator of the appropriateness of opioids in clinical management. While the criteria used in MUE are focused and assess specific important components of medication use, indicators measure symptoms of a medication use system that could indicate that something is not working well, but there is no assurance that there really is a problem when an indicator is not met. They can serve as a tool to identify potentially problematic aspects of care but require more focused assessment (such as an MUE) to identify the cause.

Within the MUE process, standards are used to define optimal performance and are usually set at 0% (should never happen) or 100% (should always happen). Thresholds are similar to standards, but they specify an acceptable level of compliance or performance and are usually set higher than 0% or lower than 100% based on acceptable variation, standards of practice, or benchmarks.[99] Thresholds are sometimes used instead of standards to allow limited noncompliance with the criteria when the clinical impact of noncompliance is felt to be of low risk. They should not be used to avoid intervention. Thresholds are useful when the group overseeing the MUE process is most interested in addressing performance that is clearly unacceptable, while allowing some variation from best practice.

Control limits can be used when measurements continue over an extended period (e.g., weeks or months). Unlike standards and thresholds, they are usually not applied in the initial MUE, but can be used to follow a process over time. For example, an MUE was conducted for the new requirements in a state for new opioid prescriptions for a duration of 3 days. Measurement for 1 month of averaging the duration of therapy each day of all new opioid prescriptions revealed the 3-day therapy duration exceeded the two standard deviations above the mean control limits on several days. These outlier results indicate the need for review for improvement. Remeasurement for several weeks is required to assess any intervention changes. Control limits are used to monitor the ongoing use of the medication to assure that the improvement was sustained over time. Control limits define the limits of allowable or **expected variation** or referred to as common-cause variation in performance (often within two to three times the standard deviation from the mean initially is acceptable) and may be used to assess the results on ongoing monitoring. If performance remains between the upper and lower control limits, action is not necessary to address the variations that occur over time. Performance outliers of unexpected or unusual events above or below the control limits is referred to as **special variation** and prompts assessment as to what factor(s) resulted in the special variation and should result in actions being taken to address the impact of these factors over time. For example, within an organization training medical residents, the number of pharmacists' interventions as documented on a control chart might spike upward around July 1, corresponding to the start date for the new residents. While the organization may have limited opportunity to stagger starting dates, specific aspects of their orientation process could be enhanced to improve initial performance. As actions are taken to address factors resulting in special variations and the overall variability is reduced, control limits should narrow.[100] An example of a control chart with limits is provided in Figure 18-6.

❿ *Performance, as demonstrated by data collected in the performance improvement process, not meeting the defined standard or threshold, or falling outside the control limits (for ongoing or follow-up assessments) indicates that intervention to improve performance is necessary.* This usually results from expectations being set too high (e.g., that the rate of adverse effects with any agent will be 0%) or when the criteria fail to include the appropriate exceptions. In some cases, performance outside the defined parameters may, upon review, be acceptable to the oversight group. There should be a criteria included to allow for efficient amendment or adjustment of criteria when changes occur in disease therapy or infectious diseases (organisms) to be included in a review. In some cases, "off-label" uses could be deemed appropriate for a change in a defined standard. For example, if a medication not previously determined to be efficacious has new study data to show benefit. Another case is the coronavirus where there are currently no approved effective therapies, but there may be new treatments or old medications to treat the virus, but not included in the FDA-approved package insert information. When this occurs, the multidisciplinary oversight group must agree that the level of performance is acceptable, and that intervention is not necessary. These decisions must be clearly documented in meeting minutes or summaries of results. If this is not done, regulatory bodies may infer that the organization chose to ignore the findings of the evaluation, thus failing to meet the quality improvement requirements. In some cases, it will be determined that the criteria are inappropriate in some manner, which needs to be corrected before further data is collected. In that case, the criteria may be altered and further data may be collected.

Data Collection

Prior to the initiation of data collection, the multidisciplinary oversight group must approve the topic selection, criteria, patient selection process, sample size, sampling method (e.g., all consecutive patients, intermittent sampling, random sampling), evaluation time frame, data collection method, and standards of performance.[84] It may be appropriate to distribute the approved criteria as an educational tool prior to data collection. Although this may address some performance issues prior to data collection and result in less dramatic results, it may support the goal of improving care and do so in a more expedient manner. In this situation, if there is a need to document the overall impact of an MUE effort, collection of baseline performance data even as criteria are being finalized and approved can provide a more accurate representation of before and after. If at any point problems are identified in the criteria or indicators or with any component of the evaluation, the issue should be brought back to the oversight group and modifications made as appropriate. Bringing necessary modifications back to the oversight group ensures that the MUE is conducted based on their guidance and approval and helps to assure their support of the results and recommendations resulting from the MUE. This step is not unusual but can often be avoided through careful preparation and review of criteria early in the MUE process.

The timing of data collection can be influenced by seasonal variations in the types of care provided (e.g., increased frequency of pneumonia in the winter months), systems issues (e.g., construction, implementation of new computer systems, initiation of new services), and personnel issues (e.g., the influx of new health professional graduates and medical house staff that occurs during the summer months, staff absences during vacation or flu seasons). Therefore, the time frame for data collection, both in duration and time of year, should be considered in the planning process. For example, an assessment of care provided to patients with pneumonia is usually best performed during the winter months when this diagnosis is more frequent, while an assessment of the management of near drowning may be more appropriate during the summer months. The longer the data collection period, the more likely various fluctuations in quality of care will be identified.

Retrospective data collection was used primarily in the era of DUR. This method involved reviewing the patient's medical record after discharge. It allowed data collection to be scheduled when convenient or when staff was available but was totally dependent on documentation in the medical record. If an opportunity for improvement was identified, there was no opportunity to improve that patient's care; it would only help future patients. It may still be necessary in some situations; however, concurrent or prospective data collection is considered superior, since the care of a current patient may be improved.

Concurrent data collection occurs while the patient is still actively receiving the medication, but after the first dose is dispensed or administered. Data sources other than the medical record are available (e.g., staff or patient interviews) and there is an opportunity to improve patient care while the patient is receiving it. Based on complete information, results may be more complete as well as more accurate.[101] However, the need for data collection is constant and must occur within a specific time frame, which is not always convenient. This often results in an increased number of personnel being involved in the data collection process and increased inconsistency.

Prospective evaluation occurs before the patient receives the first dose of medication and is initiated whenever an order for the medication is generated. Simple prospective evaluations can be at least partially automated and are likely to become more common. An example of this is a clinical information system that generates a warning to the pharmacist or prescriber if the dose of a drug is outside the normal limits based on a patient's organ function. Clinical judgment must also be applied in many of these settings.

In systems with computerized prescriber order entry, the system itself can drive prescribing to comply with guidelines and standards by limiting prescribing options or directing users to specific therapy, such as appropriate dosing, stop notices, and injectable to oral changes.[102] In some cases, the system can report instances where prescribers attempt to prescribe a medication outside established limits. These limits are usually developed by the P&T committee, optimally as the agent is being considered for addition to the formulary, and fall into three general categories: diagnosis, prescriber, and medication specific. Diagnosis-based limits may define the allowable indications for use or may drive the use of an agent under a specific protocol approved by the committee. Prescriber limits may restrict the use of an agent to a specific subset of prescribers (e.g., infectious disease or critical care specialists). Medication specific limits can designate approved dosage regimens (e.g., disallow intravenous push promethazine), frequency of administration (e.g., once-daily dosing of ceftriaxone), and duration of therapy (e.g., no more than ten doses or days of therapy).

Prospective evaluations that are not automated are the most cumbersome to implement because the evaluation must occur promptly every time an order is initiated to avoid therapy delays. This requires personnel to be available to collect data and always report results and force immediate interaction between practitioners. This approach not only offers the greatest opportunity for intervention and education, but also increases the risk for potentially negative interactions with prescribers and other health professionals and can result in therapy delays. Furthermore, it is essential that the interventions made as part of the prospective evaluation are documented in order to evaluate workload and effectiveness of the interventions, and that outcomes are assessed in some manner.

Limiting the number of data collectors or automating data collection is valuable in maintaining consistency. When multiple data collectors are involved, it becomes even more important to have clear, explicit criteria that are not subject to interpretation. For example, a data dictionary that defines each data element and identifies the location(s) in the record for gathering data should be developed and utilized to obtain consistent results.

The selection of patients or cases for inclusion in the evaluation should be determined and approved by the oversight group prior to data collection. It is essential that the selection be unbiased, consistent, and representative of the care provided. Sample size should be based on the size of the patient population. It has been suggested that, for frequently occurring events, a sample of at least 5% of cases be used, and for events occurring less frequently a minimum of 30 cases be assessed.[103]

Data Analysis

Reports should compare actual performance with expectations defined by the standards (or thresholds or control limits) established and approved prior to data collection. Performance not meeting standards (or threshold or control limits) may be considered opportunities for improvement. The multidisciplinary oversight group does not usually conduct the actual analysis but should be involved in interpreting the results. This group may determine that the standards were too rigorous, that unforeseen exceptions were encountered, and/or that actual performance falls within current acceptable standards of practice. Specific corrective actions should be recommended for all identified opportunities for improvement (e.g., for all criteria statements for which the standard of performance was not met) whenever possible. The need for and nature of follow-up should also be assessed based on the frequency, prevalence, and/or severity of the issue. For example, if an evaluation of the management of pneumonia identified no issues with drug selection, but did identify an unacceptable delay in time to first dose of antibiotic (e.g., greater than 2 hours after admission), the follow-up evaluation could focus on the time to first dose and not assess antibiotic selection. Furthermore, if this issue was identified in patients admitted to a specific unit, then the follow-up could focus on assessing and documenting improvement in only that unit.

Computer software programs (e.g., relational databases and spreadsheets) can be very helpful in collecting data, managing data, providing alerts, mitigating adverse events, and reporting results.[104–107] Handheld devices, barcode technology, and proprietary software products and computer systems used within the organization's clinical departments can be employed as tools to assist in patient identification, data collection and analysis, and documentation.[108,109]

The report to the oversight group should contain: (1) the rationale for the topic selection, (2) team members involved in the evaluation, (3) a description of the patient population evaluated, (4) any selection criteria used, (5) a copy of the criteria/indicators, (6) discussion of the results, (7) identification of likely causes for performance improvement opportunities identified, and (8) recommendations for corrective action and follow-up evaluation. An example is provided in Appendix 18-1. In most settings, delineation of results on a practitioner-specific basis is not appropriate at this level. The exception would be if a subset of practitioners consistently fell outside the criteria.

Interventions and Corrective Actions

The key to quality improvement is improving the process and outcomes whenever possible and not blaming an individual or group of individuals. Steps to improve performance or avoid similar outcomes in the future fall into three categories: educational, restrictive interventions, and process changes. Educational interventions are most appropriate when knowledge deficits contribute to performance outside the criteria. They are most effective when they are directed personally, take place soon after the problem occurs, the educator is a peer or superior of the person being educated, and when the education is supported in the literature or by practice standards.[110] In addition, improvement requires leadership to support and reinforce the initiatives through actions and behaviors, providing resources and addressing culture.[111] One-on-one or group discussion of results, letters, emails, newsletters, and presentation via quality improvement channels are examples of educational approaches. Generally, educational interventions incorporated into ongoing processes (e.g., education screens in computer order entry systems) are more effective while one-time efforts (e.g., newsletters, emails) may not have a sustained effect. In many situations, educational interventions are the most palatable.

Restrictive approaches may involve special ordering procedures, compliance with guidelines for use, consultation with a specialty service, or formulary restrictions. The impact of restrictive interventions often reverses when the restrictions are removed.[112,113] Restrictive interventions are perhaps most effective when used to establish appropriate practice patterns when an agent is first made available for use within the organization and as part of a medication safety program.[114]

Process changes incorporate the correction into routine practice. This approach may involve changes in policy or procedures, implementation of new services, acquisition of new equipment, changes in staffing, or generation of regular notifications, etc., when practice does not appear to meet standards. As clinical information and physician order entry systems become more sophisticated, process changes can be built directly into the prescribing, dispensing, and administering processes.

Disciplinary actions against individuals are not commonly employed as an intervention; however, when individuals refuse to modify their behavior, discipline may eventually be required. Discipline may include placing limits on an individual's activities and responsibilities or termination of employment. When possible, punitive actions should be avoided, since they can result in loss of acceptance of quality improvement efforts and fear of retribution.[115,116] Generally, the concept of Just Culture is useful to consider. Further information on Just Culture is found in Chapter 20.

Communication

Communication of MUE-related information is important and must be done carefully throughout the process. Communication of the purpose of the evaluation and the significance of its outcomes should be reported to all groups involved in or impacted by the process. If a process is changed based on MUE results, the reason for the change should be explained. If, as a result of an MUE, a prescriber will be required to change the way they prescribe a medication or a nurse will no longer be able to access a medication as they had in the past, the reason for the change should be communicated along with the announcement of the change. Confidentiality of patient information (e.g., names and other identifiers) must be maintained. The identity of practitioners (physicians, pharmacists, nurses) must be revealed only in information provided for use by managers or designated peer-practitioners for assessment of personal performance.

Follow-up

Follow-up evaluation should occur within a reasonable time frame after completion of the initial evaluation and completion of the corrective action. Follow-up is designed to assess the effectiveness of the intervention. The same criteria, standards, and sample should generally be used for the follow-up assessment as in the initial evaluation. Exceptions to this rule should be made if there was a problem with the initial criteria, standards, and sample, if the standard of practice changes in the interim, or if there is an opportunity to focus on a subset of the original data elements or patient population. For example, if issues were only found in the administration component of the use of a medication (and not in the prescribing, dispensing, or monitoring components) or only in a specific age group, follow-up evaluation could focus on these issues or populations rather than repeating the broader assessment performed initially.

MUE has been criticized as being heavy-handed, non-patient-focused, and for not addressing the issue of accountability for provision of care based on a unique body of knowledge. If MUE is utilized in its true spirit, many of these challenges are addressed. MUE is a truly multidisciplinary, process-oriented approach to evaluate the quality of medication use. The process goes beyond numbers and percentages to identify opportunities for improvement and more importantly, to improve the quality of care.

Quality in Drug Information

Quality standards for drug information practice have not been established to date, and quality assessment techniques used in drug information practice vary greatly among practice sites.[117-119] Several studies have found inconsistencies in the quality of drug information practice and have called for increased emphasis on quality and the development of practice standards.[120-123] Most drug information services conduct some form of quality assessment based on the scope of service provided by that center and preestablished levels of acceptable performance. Quality assessment is usually conducted on the responses provided to drug information requests, medical literature search and evaluation processes, availability, accuracy, and timeliness of drug information resources, and the quality of materials produced by the drug information service staff (e.g., monographs, newsletters, continuing education programs, and websites). Although some quality assessment processes are conducted concurrently, most assessments are done retrospectively, often by randomly sampling of drug information requests, monographs, and so forth. Furthermore, assessments may be performed via peer review or by the director of the service. Currently, no standards have been developed for this process.[124]

Assessment of the quality of responses to drug information inquiries may include components such as timeliness, completeness and appropriateness of response, and the method of communication of the response. Additionally, aspects such as documentation of search terms, references utilized, and the availability of appropriate background or patient-specific information may also be assessed. This assessment may be carried out internally based on standards of practice at the site. This usually offers the advantage of peer review by practitioners skilled in these functions. Another method is to poll those using the service about the quality of service and response received. This approach is hampered because consumers of the response are rarely able to assess the quality or appropriateness of the search strategy utilized to formulate the response that they received in lieu of performing the search themselves or being present while the search is performed. An example assessment tool is provided in Appendix 18-4. Questions that are often asked in the process of assessing drug information responses include:

- Is the response correct and appropriate to the situation presented?
- Is the response provided promptly?
- Does the response completely address the question posed?
- Is the response communicated appropriately?
- Are search terms and references appropriately documented?
- Is the response clear, concise, and appropriate for the clinical situation?
- If follow-up was warranted, was it provided?

The search process itself can be assessed by evaluation of the appropriate depth and breadth of resources used, the timeliness of the resources accessed, and the search strategy. This process can also assess documentation issues, the application of literature evaluation skills to the information, and resources used by the practitioner completing the search.

Drug information practitioners are often responsible for assessing and recommending drug information resources available within the organization. These resources may include printed references such as handbooks, textbooks, educational materials, or electronic resources such as large search engines or Internet websites. This process should assess whether the appropriate information resources are available based on the scope of care provided and expertise of the practitioners and whether the resources contain accurate and timely information that can be applied in clinical situations. Available primary, secondary, and tertiary resources should be evaluated based on established standards. The explosion of medical information on the Internet has created new challenges in evaluating drug and medical information resources. Because there are currently no regulations of content on Internet sites, caution must be used when utilizing these resources to support clinical decision-making. With the number of websites expanding faster than most practitioners can assess their content and editorial policies (if any), it has become increasingly difficult for drug information practitioners to stay abreast of those sites that offer legitimate and validated information compared to those offering only conjecture and opinion. Information obtained from other sources including manufacturer's drug information services should also be assessed. See Chapters 3 to 5 for further information on assessing information.

A final component of quality relates to material produced by the drug information service. This includes newsletters, websites, drug monographs, and clinical guidelines developed by the service. Most measure quality related to the accuracy, timeliness, and clinical applicability of such documents. Unfortunately, more time is often spent on assessing quality of grammar and writing style than is devoted to clinical content and interpretation. Once again, Chapters 4 and 5 provide further information on assessing the quality of the material itself.

Publication of Quality Improvement Studies

Individuals or organizations interested in reporting their quality improvement interventions and results should use the SQUIRE 2.0 (Standards for Quality Improvement Reporting Excellence). SQUIRE was developed to provide authors guidance in reliably and consistently reporting their improvement work and for contributing knowledge to the "science of improvement."[125] SQUIRE is for reporting of systematic efforts and qualitative and quantitative interventions involved in improving quality, safety, and value in health care. The guidance document includes the sections for the improvement documents, such as title, abstract, problem description, available knowledge, rational, specific aims, methods context, interventions, study of interventions, measures, analysis, ethical considerations, results, discussion summary, interpretation, limitations, conclusions, other information, and funding. Explanations and examples are also provided for each section. Peer-reviewed journals will request the SQUIRE format for quality improvement manuscripts. The question whether the organization's institutional review board (IRB) submission and approval is required should be addressed with your IRB prior to submission of reports; generally, quality improvement work, not intended for publication outside the organization, is provided an exemption. The importance of quality improvement publication is described by the SQUIRE authors as essential for others to learn about successes and failures in health care quality improvement work.[125] Refer to Chapter 5 for more information on SQUIRE 2.0.

Conclusion

The health care system continues to move toward greater transparency of quality as part of an overall shift toward value-driven health care. Government agencies and private purchasers of health care are demanding more evidence on quality and safety in the use of medications, and a growing number of accreditation programs are also scrutinizing performance indicators as a means for reaccreditation of organizations and providers. Thus, it is imperative that all practitioners involved in the medication use system understand how to measure and improve quality in the use of medications. As the American health care system continues to evolve, health care practitioners should maintain awareness and be ready to quickly adjust to the changes that will occur in measuring quality and performance for medication use.

Self-Assessment Questions

1. The major driver for quality measurement in U.S. health care today is:
   a. Federal government (e.g., CMS)
   b. State Marketplace Health Insurance Plans
   c. The International Organization for Standardization (ISO) 9000
   d. Consumers that purchase their own health insurance

2. The PDCA model of quality improvement stands for:
   a. Prepare, Develop, Calculate, Assess
   b. Produce, Design, Cost-control, Act
   c. Plan, Develop, Check, Assess
   d. Plan, Do, Check, Act
   e. None of the above

3. Which of the following is **NOT** a characteristic of continuous quality improvement?
   a. Systems oriented
   b. Data driven
   c. Team oriented
   d. Punitive
   e. a and d

4. Which of the following would be considered an adverse drug event (ADE)?
   a. Pharmacist inadvertently fills a prescription for levothyroxine 100 µg instead of 75 µg as prescribed.
   b. Nurse pulls lorazepam instead of azithromycin for administration.
   c. Patient presents with *C. difficile* after antibiotic exposure.
   d. Patient decides not to take their blood pressure medication.

5. What are the four approaches recommended by the U.S. Department of Health and Human Services National Action Plan to reduce patient harms from ADEs?
   a. Surveillance, Promotion, Sustainability, and Research
   b. Sustainability, Prevention, Oversight, and Publication
   c. Surveillance, Documentation, Publication, and Sustainability
   d. Surveillance, Prevention, Incentive and Oversight, and Research

6. When is it useful to directly measure aspects of the process of care?
   a. When the outcome is difficult to measure
   b. When the outcome is far removed in time from the process
   c. When the outcome is affected by many different processes
   d. All of the above
   e. None of the above since outcomes are the only valid indicator of quality

7. A sentinel indicator:
   a. Reflects the occurrence of a serious event that requires further investigation
   b. Can be subdivided into rate-based or aggregate indicators
   c. Could be a death from an adverse drug-related event
   d. Is typically expressed as a percentage
   e. a and c

8. Which of the following is **NOT** a quality measures developer?
   a. NCQA
   b. NABP
   c. CMS
   d. PQA

9. A rate-based indicator:
   a. Is typically expressed as a percentage
   b. Is a type of aggregate indicator
   c. Is typically expressed as a count of events over time
   d. Can only be used to track safety events in hospitals
   e. a and b

10. Value-based purchasing refers to purchase or payment of health care services based on performance. Which of the following is NOT a value-based program?
    a. Medicare Part D MTM program
    b. ESRD-quality incentive program
    c. Hospital value-based purchasing
    d. Skilled nursing facility value-based program

11. Medication measures (pharmacy) quality reporting occurs through which of the following:
    a. Medicare Part D insurance plans
    b. Pharmacy Compare
    c. Pharmacy Quality Alliance
    d. Pharmacy benefits managers

12. In the MIPS program for eligible providers there are four categories that are part of a composite performance score, which of the following is *NOT* part of the composite performance score?
    a. Quality
    b. Improvement activities
    c. Promoting interoperability (formerly advancing care information)
    d. Cost
    e. All of the above comprise the composite performance score

13. To ensure health equality, health care organizations will provide all the following except:
    a. Collect data using standard elements of groupings such as age, race, ethnicity, sex (gender), gender identity, payers, socioeconomic
    b. Health disparities awareness training for all staff

c. Inform stakeholder employers of services provided

d. Outcomes analysis of services by subgroups

14. Which of the following is **NOT** true about the "enhanced" medication therapy management (MTM) incentive payment program?

a. The program was conceived and initiated under the CMMI organization of CMS.

b. Any prescription drug plan may participate in the program.

c. Incentive payments are awarded to the plans meeting reductions in medical spending meeting the 2% goal.

d. CMRs and TMRs are identified as integral to the MTM services.

15. Medication reconciliation is a process intended to reduce patient harm related to medication use; which of the following is true?

a. Obtaining the best possible medication history is part of the process.

b. Medication reconciliation is a quality measure in several value-based programs.

c. The process is required in all care settings for all patients in the United States.

d. Pharmacists are the health professional responsible for the process.

e. All the answers are true.

f. Answers a and b are true

REFERENCES

1. Centers for Medicare & Medicaid Services. Roadmap for implementing value-driven health care in the traditional Medicare fee for service program [Internet]. Baltimore (MD): Centers for Medicare & Medicaid Services. 2012 Nov 25 [cited 2013 Oct 2]. Available from: http://www.cms.gov/Medicare/Quality-Initiatives-Patient-Assessment-Instruments/QualityInitiativesGenInfo/Downloads/VBPRoadmap_OEA_1-16_508.pdf

2. Chee TT, Ryan AM, Wasfy JH, Borden WB. Current state of value-based purchasing programs. Circulation. 2016;133:2197-205.

3. VanLare JM, Conway PH. Value-based purchasing—national programs to move from volume to value. New Engl J Med. 2012;367:292-5.

4. CMS.gov. CMS Quality Strategy 2016 [Internet]. Baltimore (MD): Centers for Medicare & Medicaid Services. [Cited 2016 Aug 15]. Available from: https://www.cms.gov/Medicare/Quality-Initiatives-Patient-Assessment-Instruments/QualityInitiativesGenInfo/Downloads/CMS-Quality-Strategy.pdf

5. CMS.gov Value-based programs [Internet]. Baltimore (MD): Centers for Medicare & Medicaid Services. [Cited 2019 Aug 5]. Available from: https://www.cms.gov/medicare/quality-initiatives-patient-assessment-instruments/value-based-programs/value-based-programs.html

6. CMS.gov. Hospital value-based purchasing—resources [Internet]. Baltimore (MD): Centers for Medicare & Medicaid Services. [Cited 2019 Aug 5]. Available from:

https://www.qualitynet.org/dcs/ContentServer?c=Page&pagename=QnetPublic%2FP age%2FQnetTier3&cid=1228772237202

7. CMS.gov. Skilled nursing facility quality reporting program (SNF QRP): requirements for the fiscal year (FY) 2021 program year. 2019 Apr [cited 2019 Aug 5]. Available from: https://www.cms.gov/Medicare/Quality-Initiatives-Patient-Assessment-Instruments/ NursingHomeQualityInits/Downloads/SNF-QRP-Requirements-for-the-Fiscal-Year-FY2021-Program-Year+.pdf

8. Federal Register. Medicare and Medicaid programs; CY 2019 home health prospective payment system rate update and CY 2020 case-mix adjustment methodology refinements; home health value-based purchasing model; home health quality reporting requirements; home infusion therapy requirement and training requirements for surveyors of national accrediting organizations [Internet]. [Cited 2019 Aug 5]. Available from: https://www. federalregister.gov/documents/2018/11/13/2018-24145/medicare-and-medicaid-pro-grams-cy-2019-home-health-prospective-payment-system-rate-update-and-cy

9. QPP.CMS.gov. Explore measures and activities [Internet]. Baltimore (MD): Department of Health and Human Services. 2018 Nov 13 [cited 2019 Aug 5]. Available from: https:// qpp.cms.gov/mips/explore-measures/quality-measures

10. Federal Register. Medicare program; merit-based incentive payment system (MIPS) and alternative payment model (APM) incentive under the physician fee schedule, and cri-teria for physician-focused payment models. 2016 May 9 [cited 2019 Aug 5]. Available from: https://www.federalregister.gov/articles/2016/05/09/2016-10032/medicare-program-merit-based-incentive-payment-system-mips-and-alternative-payment-model-apm

11. Medicare.gov. Hospital compare [Internet]. Baltimore (MD): Department of Health and Human Services. [Cited 2020 Mar 1]. Available from: https://www.medicare.gov/ hospitalcompare/search.html

12. Medicare.gov. Nursing home compare [Internet]. Baltimore (MD): Department of Health and Human Services [Cited 2020 Mar 1]. Available from: http://www.medicare. gov/NursingHomeCompare/search.aspx

13. Report cards [Internet]. National Committee for Quality Assurance (NCQA). [Cited 2019 Aug 5]. Available from: https://www.ncqa.org/report-cards/health-plans/

14. Medicare.gov. Medicare plan finder [Internet]. Baltimore (MD): Department of Health and Human Services. [Cited 2016 Jul 31]. Available from: https://www.medicare.gov/ find-a-plan/questions/home.aspx

15. Medicare.gov. Home health compare [Internet]. Baltimore (MD): Department of Health and Human Services. [Cited 2016 Jul 31]. Available from: https://www.medicare.gov/ homehealthcompare/search.html

16. Medicare.gov. Dialysis facility compare [Internet]. Baltimore (MD): Department of Health and Human Services. [Cited 2016 Jul 31]. Available from: https://www.medicare. gov/dialysisfacilitycompare/

17. Medicare.gov. Physicians compare [Internet]. Baltimore (MD): Department of Health and Human Services. [Cited 2016 Jul 31]. Available from: https://www.medicare.gov/ physiciancompare/search.html

18. Massachusetts Health Quality Partners [Internet]. Watertown (MA): Massachusetts Health Quality Partners. 2012 Nov 25 [cited 2013 Oct 2]. Available from: www.mhqp.org

19. The Leapfrog Group [Internet]. Washington (DC): The Leapfrog Group. 2012 Nov 25 [cited 2013 Oct 2]. Available from: www.leapfroggroup.org

20. Robert Woods Johnson Foundation Aligning forces for quality. How employers can improve value and quality in health care [Internet]. Princeton (NJ): Robert Woods Johnson Foundation. 2013 Jan 1 [cited 2016 Jul 31]. Available from: http://www.rwjf. org/content/dam/farm/reports/issue_briefs/2013/rwjf403361

21. HealthCare.gov. Quality ratings of health plans on Healthcare.gov [Internet]. Baltimore (MD): Department of Health and Human Services. 2013 Jun 21 [cited 2020 Apr 4]. Available from: https://www.healthcare.gov/quality-ratings/

22. CMS.gov. Health Insurance Exchange Quality Ratings System 101. CMS Bulletin on Display of Quality Reporting System (QRS) star ratings and Qualified Health Plan (QHP) Enrollee Survey results for QHPs offered through Exchanges [Internet]. Baltimore (MD). 2019 Aug 15 [cited 2020 Apr 4]. Available from: https://www.cms.gov/Medicare/ Quality-Initiatives-Patient-Assessment-Instruments/QualityInitiativesGenInfo/ Downloads/Quality-Rating-Information-Bulletin-for-Plan-Year-2020.pdf

23. Maryland Health Benefit Exchange [Internet]. Lanham (MD): Maryland Health Connections; c2019 [cited 2019 Aug 26]. Available from: https://www.marylandhealthconnection.gov/

24. PQA Pharmacy Quality Alliance. PQA performance measures [Internet]. Alexandria (VA). 2018 [cited 2019 Aug 5]. Available from: https://www.pqaalliance.org/pqa-measures

25. Pillittere-Dugan D, Nau DP, McDonough K, Zakiya P. Development and testing of performance measures for pharmacy services. J Am Pharm Assoc. 2009;49:212-9.

26. Doucette WR, Conklin M, Mott DA, Newland B, Plake KS, Nau DP. Pharmacy Quality Alliance phase I demonstration projects: descriptions and lessons learned. J Am Pharm Assoc. 2011;51:544-50.

27. PQA Pharmacy Quality Alliance. PQA pharmacy performance measures in development [Internet]. Alexandria (VA). [Cited 2021 Jan 15]. Available from: https://www.pqaalliance. org/pharmacy-measures

28. CMS.gov. Medicare 2019 Part C & D star ratings technical notes [Internet]. Baltimore (MD): Centers for Medicare & Medicaid Services. 2019 Mar 21 [cited 2019 Aug 5]. Available from: https://www.cms.gov/Medicare/Prescription-Drug-Coverage/PrescriptionDrug CovGenIn/Downloads/2019-Technical-Notes.pdf

29. Pharmacy Quality Alliance. Adherence measures [Internet]. Alexandria (VA). 2018 Aug 18 [cited 2020 Mar 30]. Available from: https://www.pqaalliance.org/adherence-measures

30. Reinke T. Preference for preferred networks grows along with community pharmacist anger. Managed Care. 2015 Mar [cited 2016 Aug 15]. Available from: http://www.managedcaremag.com/ archives/2015/3/preference-preferred-networks-grows-along-community-pharmacist-anger

31. How health plans and PBMs evaluate pharmacy performance. 2014 Mar 12 [cited 2016 Aug 15]. Available from: http://smartretailingrx.com/patient-care-counseling/health-plans-pbms-evaluate-pharmacy-performance/

32. Ferries E, Dyer JT, Hall B, Ndehi L, Schwab P, Vaccaro J. Comparison of medication therapy management services and their effect on health care utilization and medication adherence. J Manag Care Spec Pharm. 2019;25:688-95.

33. Department of Health and Human Services, Centers for Medicare & Medicaid Services. Part D enhanced medication therapy management model first year performance based payment results fact sheet [Internet]. Baltimore (MD): Centers for Medicare & Medicaid Services. [Cited 2019 Aug 26]. Available from: https://innovation.cms.gov/Files/x/mtm-firstyrresults-fs.pdf

34. McLaughlin CP, Kaluzny AD. Continuous quality improvement in health care. 2nd ed. Gaithersburg (MD): Aspen Publishers; 1999.

35. CMS.gov. Quality measures [Internet]. Baltimore (MD): Centers for Medicare & Medicaid Services. [Cited 2016 Aug 15]. Available from: https://www.cms.gov/Medicare/Quality-Initiatives-Patient-Assessment-Instruments/QualityMeasures/index.html

36. National Quality Forum. Measuring performance [Internet]. Washington (DC). [Cited 2016 Aug 15]. Available from: http://www.qualityforum.org/Measuring_Performance/Measuring_Performance.aspx

37. CMS.gov. Hospital quality initiative [Internet]. Baltimore (MD). Centers for Medicare & Medicaid Services. [Cited 2020 Mar 30]. Available from: https://www.cms.gov/Medicare/Quality-Initiatives-Patient-Assessment-Instruments/HospitalQualityInits

38. The Joint Commission. Measures: history of performance measures [Internet]. Oakbrook Terrace (IL). [Cited 2020 Mar 30]. Available from: https://www.jointcommission.org/en/measurement/measures/

39. AHRQ.gov. National Quality Measures Clearinghouse [Internet]. Rockville (MD). 2018 Jul [cited 2020 Mar 30]. Available from: https://www.ahrq.gov/gam/about/index.html

40. National Quality Forum. Measures, reports & tools [Internet]. Washington (DC). [Cited 2016 Aug 15]. Available from: http://www.qualityforum.org/measures_reports_tools.aspx

41. National Committee for Quality Assurance. HEDIS and performance measurement [Internet]. Washington (DC): National Committee for Quality Assurance. [Cited 2019 Aug 24]. Available from: https://www.ncqa.org/hedis/

42. National Committee for Quality Assurance. Immunizations for adolescents (IMA) [Internet]. Washington (DC): National Committee for Quality Assurance. [Cited 2019 Aug 24]. Available from: https://www.ncqa.org/hedis/measures/immunizations-for-adolescents/

43. Deming WE. Out of the crisis. Cambridge (MA): Massachusetts Institute of Technology, Center for Advanced Engineering Study; 1986.

44. Deming WE. The new economics for industry, education, government. Cambridge (MA): Massachusetts Institute of Technology, Center for Advanced Engineering Study; 1993.

45. Edmonds J, Zagami M. QI team shares ownership and gets results. J Health Qual. 1992;14:24-8.

46. Donabedian A. Explorations in quality assessment and monitoring. In: The definition of quality and approaches to its assessment. Ann Arbor (MI): Health Administration Press; 1980. p. 79-128.

47. Farris KB, Kirking DM. Assessing the quality of pharmaceutical care. II. Application of concepts of quality assessment from medical care. Ann Pharmacother. 1993;27:215-23.

48. Lohr KN. Outcomes measurement: concepts and questions. Inquiry. 1988;25:37-50.

49. Kozma CM, Reeder CE, Schulz RM. Economic, clinical and humanistic outcomes: a planning tool for pharmacoeconomic research. Clin Ther. 1993;15:1121-32.

50. Lipowski EE. Evaluating the outcomes of pharmaceutical care. J Am Pharm Assoc. 1996;NS36:726-34.

51. Angaran DM. Selecting, developing and evaluating indicators. Am J Hosp Pharm. 1991;48:1931-7.

52. Braithwaite J, Hibbert P, Blakely B, Plumb J, Hannaford N, Long JC, Marks D. Health systems frameworks and performance indicators in eight countries: a comparative international analysis. SAGE Open Med. 2017;5:1-10.

53. Institute of Medicine. Race, ethnicity, and language data: standardization for health care quality improvement. Washington (DC): The National Academies Press; 2009 [cited 2020 Apr 30]. Available from: https://www.ahrq.gov/sites/default/files/publications/files/iomracereport.pdf

54. Nadzam DM, Turpin R, Hanold LS, White RE. Data-driven performance improvement in health care: the Joint Commission's Indicator Measurement System (IMSystem). Jt Comm J Qual Improv. 1993;19:492-500.

55. Haller G, Stoelwinder J, Myles PS, McNeil J. Quality and safety indicators in anesthesia: a systematic review. Anesthesiology. 2009;110:1158-75.

56. Joint Commission on Accreditation of Healthcare Organizations. A guide to performance improvement for pharmacies. Oakbrook Terrace (IL): Joint Commission; 1997.

57. Hepler CD, Segal R. Preventing medication errors and improving drug therapy. Boca Raton (FL): CRC Press; 2003.

58. Kerr EA, Krein SL, Vijan S, Hofer TP, Hayward RA. Avoiding pitfalls in chronic disease quality measurement: a case for the next generation of technical quality measures. Am J Manag Care. 2001;7:1033-43.

59. Agency for Healthcare Research & Quality. Consumer Assessment of Healthcare Providers & Systems (CAHPS) [Internet]. Rockville (MD): Agency for Healthcare Research & Quality; 2012 Nov 25 [cited 2013 Oct 2]. Available from: http://cahps.ahrq.gov/

60. Blalock SJ, Keller S. Consumer assessment of pharmacy quality. In: Warholak T, Nau DP, eds. Quality & safety in pharmacy practice. New York: McGraw-Hill; 2010.

61. Kerr EA, Smith DM, Hogan MM, Krein SL, Pogach L, Hofer TP, Hayward RA. Comparing clinical automated, medical record, and hybrid data sources for diabetes quality measures. Jt Comm J Qual Improv. 2002;28:555-65.

62. Kerr EA, Smith DM, Hogan MM, Hofer TP, Krein SL, Bermann M, Hayward RA. Building a better quality measure: are some patients with 'poor quality' actually getting good care? Med Care. 2003;41:1173-82.

63. NLM.NIH.org. Overview of SNOMED CT [Internet]. Bethesda (MD): National Library of Medicine. Available from: https://www.nlm.nih.gov/healthit/snomedct/snomed_overview.html

64. Pharmacy Health Information Technology (HIT) Collaborative. Implementing SNOMED CT in practice: a beginner's guide. Assessing pharmacy value sets [Internet]. [Cited 2016 May 27]. Available from: https://www.pharmacyhit.org/pdfs/workshop-documents/VSC-Post-2016-01.pdf

65. Moczygemba LR, Holdford DA. Statistical process control. In: Warholak T, Nau DP, editors. Quality & safety in pharmacy practice. New York (NY): McGraw-Hill; 2010.

66. Nau DP. Measuring pharmacy quality. J Am Pharm Assoc. 2009;49:154-63.

67. QualityNet. HVBP measures [Internet]. Baltimore (MD): Centers for Medicare & Medicaid Services. [Cited 2020 Mar 1]. Available from: https://www.qualitynet.org/inpatient/hvbp/measures

68. Quality Payment Program [Internet]. Baltimore (MD): Centers for Medicare & Medicaid Services. 2017 Jan [cited 2017 Feb 19]. Available from: https://qpp.cms.gov/

69. Kohn LT, Corrigan JM, Donaldson MS; Institute of Medicine. To err is human: building safer health systems. Washington (DC): National Academy Press; 2000.

70. U.S. Department of Health and Human Services, Office of Disease Prevention and Health Promotion. National action plan for adverse drug event prevention [Internet]. Washington (DC): U.S. Department of Health and Human Services; 2014 [cited 2020 Mar 1]. Available from: https://health.gov/hcq/pdfs/ADE-Action-Plan-508c.pdf

71. Digmann R, Thomas A, Peppercorn S, Ryan A, Zhang L, Irby K, Brock J. Use of Medicare administrative claims to identify a population at high risk for adverse drug events and hospital use for quality improvement. J Manag Care Spec Pharm. 2019;25(3):402-10.

72. Budnitz DS, Lovegrove MC, Shehab N, Richards CL. Emergency hospitalizations for adverse drug events in older Americans. N Engl J Med. 2011;365(21):2002-12.

73. CMS.gov. CMS OMH data snapshots [Internet]. Baltimore (MD): Centers for Medicare & Medicaid Services Office of Minority Health. 2016 Jun 16 [cited 2019 Aug 27]. Available from: https://www.cms.gov/About-CMS/Agency-Information/OMH/research-and-data/information-products/data-snapshots/index.html

74. National Partnership for Action to End Health Disparities. National Stakeholder Strategy for Achieving Health Equity [Internet]. Rockville (MD): U.S. Department of Health and Human Services, Office of Minority Health; 2016 Mar 25 [cited 2016 Aug 25]. Available from: https://minorityhealth.hhs.gov/npa/templates/content.aspx?lvl=1&lvlid=33&ID=286

75. Data collection standards for race, ethnicity, primary language, sex, and disability status [Internet]. Rockville (MD): U.S. Department of Health and Human Services, Office of Minority Health. 2016 Jun 16 [cited 2016 Aug 25]. Available from: https://minorityhealth.hhs.gov/omh/browse.aspx?lvl=2&lvlid=23.

76. Health Research & Educational Trust. Reducing health care disparities: collection and use of race, ethnicity and language data. Chicago (IL): Health Research & Educational Trust. 2013 Aug [cited 2016 Aug 25]. Available from: http://www.hpoe.org/Reports-HPOE/Equity_Care_Report_August2013.PDF

77. HealthIT.gov. Meaningful use and the shift to the merit-based incentive program. advancing care information [Internet]. Washington (DC): Department of Health

and Human Services. 2019 Oct 22 [cited 2020 Apr 4]. Available from: https://www.healthit.gov/providers-professionals/achieve-meaningful-use/core-measures-2/record-demographics

78. Wyatt R, Laderman M, Botwinick L, Mate K, Whittington J. Achieving health equity: a guide for health care organizations. IHI White Paper. Cambridge (MA): Institute for Healthcare Improvement; 2016 [cited 2016 Aug 25]. Available from: http://www.ihi.org/resources/Pages/IHIWhitePapers/Achieving-Health-Equity.aspx

79. CMS.gov. Racial and ethnic disparities in health care in Medicare Advantage [Internet]. Baltimore (MD): Centers for Medicare & Medicaid Services Office of Minority Health; 2016 Apr [cited 2016 Aug 25]. Available from: https://www.cms.gov/About-CMS/Agency-Information/OMH/Downloads/National-Level-Results.pdf

80. Haviland AM, Elliott MN, Weech-Maldonado R, Hambarsoomian K, Orr N, Hays RD. Racial/ethnic disparities in Medicare Part D experiences. Med Care. 2012;50:S40-7.

81. CDC.gov. Coronavirus Disease 2019 (COVID-19): COVID-19 in racial and ethnic minority groups [Internet]. Atlanta (GA). 2020 Apr 22 [cited 2020 Apr 30]. Available from: https://www.cdc.gov/coronavirus/2019-ncov/need-extra-precautions/racial-ethnic-minorities.html

82. Shulte F. As coronavirus strikes crucial data in electronic health records hard to harvest. Kaiser Health News. 2020 Apr 30 [cited 2020 Apr 30]. Available from: https://khn.org/news/as-coronavirus-strikes-crucial-data-in-electronic-health-records-hard-to-harvest/

83. Stolar MH. Drug use review: Operational definitions. Am J Hosp Pharm. 1978;35:76-8.

84. American Society of Health-System Pharmacists. ASHP guidelines on medication-use evaluation [Internet]. Bethesda (MD): American Society of Health-System Pharmacists; 2020 [cited 2020 Nov 23]. Available from: https://www.ashp.org/-/media/assets/policy-guidelines/docs/guidelines/medication-use-evaluation.ashx

85. Nadzam DM. Development of medication-use indicators by The Joint Commission on Accreditation of Healthcare Organizations. Am J Hosp Pharm. 1991;48:1925-30.

86. Cousins DD. Medication use: a systems approach to reducing errors. Chicago (IL): Joint Commission on Accreditation of Healthcare Organizations; 1998.

87. New accreditation process model for 1994 and beyond. Am J Hosp Pharm. 1993;50:1111-2, 1121.

88. Ente BH. The Joint Commission's agenda for change. Curr Concepts Hosp Pharm Manage.1989 Summer;11(2):6-14.

89. The Joint Commission on Accreditation of Hospitals. 1990 AMH. Accreditation Manual for Hospitals. Chicago (IL): Joint Commission on Accreditation of Hospitals; 1989.

90. Flagstad MS, Williams RB. Assuming responsibility for improving quality. Am J Hosp Pharm. 1991;48:1898.

91. Covington TR, Alexander VL. Drug use evaluation: The fundamentals. Indianapolis: Eli Lilly & Co.; 1991.

92. Fanikos J, Jenkins KL, Piazza G, Connors J, Goldhaber SZ. Medication use evaluation: pharmacist rubric for performance improvement. Pharmacotherapy. 2014;5S-14S.

93. Schaff RL, Schumock GT, Nadzam DM. Development of The Joint Commission's indicators for monitoring the medication use system. Hosp Pharm. 1991;26:326-9, 350.

94. Bernstein SJ, Hilborne LH. Clinical indicators: the road to quality care? Jt Comm J Qual Improv. 1993;19(11):501-9.

95. Tully MP, Cantrill JA. The validity of explicit indicators of prescribing appropriateness. Int J Qual Health Care. 2006;18:87-94.

96. Wallerstedt SM, Belfrage B, Fastbom J. Association between drug specific indicators of prescribing quality and quality of drug treatment: a validation study. Pharmacoepidemiol Drug Saf. 2015;24:906-14.

97. Knapp DA. Development of criteria for drug utilization review. Clin Pharmacol Ther. 1991;50(Part 2):600-3.

98. Samilki JAE, Lau TTY, Elbe DHT, Aulach AK, Lun EMC. Drug use evaluation of moxifloxacin (Avelox) using a hand-held electronic device at a Canadian teaching hospital. P T. 2012;37:291-9.

99. Threshold vs. standards. QRC Advisor. 1988;5(2):5.

100. Neuhauser D, Provost L, Bergman B. The meaning of variation to healthcare managers, clinical and health-services researchers and individual patients. BMJ Qual Saf. 2011;20(Suppl 1);i36-40.

101. Makela EH, Davis SK, Piveral K, Miller WA, Pleasants RA, Gadsden RHSr, Leman RB. Effect of data collection method on results of serum digoxin concentration audit. Am J Hosp Pharm. 1988;45:126-30.

102. Forrest GN, Van Schooneveld TC, Kullar R, Schulz LT, Duong P, Postelnick M. Use of electronic health records and clinical decision support systems for antimicrobial stewardship. Clin Infec Dis. 2014;59:S122-33.

103. What is an adequate sample? QRC Advisor. 1985;1(Aug);4-5.

104. Grasela TH, Walawander CA, Kennedy, Jolson HM. Capability of hospital computer systems in performing drug-use evaluations and adverse event monitoring. Am J Hosp Pharm. 1993;50:1889-95.

105. Zarowitz BJ, Petitta A, Mlynarek M, Touchette M, Peters M, Long P, Patel R. Bar-code technology applied to drug-use evaluation. Am J Hosp Pharm. 1993;50:935-9.

106. Burnakis TG. Facilitating drug-use evaluation with spreadsheet software. Am J Hosp Pharm. 1989;46:84-88.

107. Jha AK, Laguette J, Seger A, Bates DW. Can surveillance systems identify and avert adverse drug events? A prospective evaluation of a commercial application. J Am Med Inform Assoc. 2008;15:647-53.

108. Libby D, Grove C, Adams M. Collaborative use of informatics among hospitals to benchmark medication use processes. Jt Comm J Qual Improv. 1997;23:626-52.

109. Strykowski J, Hadsall R, Sawchyn B, VanSickle S, Niznick D. Bar-code assisted medication administration: a method for predicting repackaging resource needs. Am J Health-Syst Pharm. 2013;70:154-60.

110. Soumerai SB, McLaughlin TJ, Avorn J. Improving drug prescribing in primary care: a critical analysis of the experimental literature. Milbank Q. 1989;67:268-317.

111. Singer SJ, Benzer JK, Hamdan SU. Improving health care quality and safety: the role of collective learning. J Healthc Leadersh. 2015;7:91-107.

112. Avorn J, Soumeri SB, Taylor W. Reduction of incorrect antibiotic prescribing through a structured educational order form. Arch Intern Med. 1991;151:1825-32.

113. Kowalsky SF, Echols RM, Peck F. Preprinted order sheet to enhance antibiotic prescribing and surveillance. Am J Hosp Pharm. 1982;39:1528-9.

114. American Society of Health-System Pharmacists. ASHP guidelines on preventing medication errors in hospitals. Am J Health-Syst Pharm. 2018; 75:1493-517.

115. Pierson JF, Alexander MR, Kirking DM, Solomon DK. Physician's attitudes toward drug-use evaluation interventions. Am J Hosp Pharm. 1990;47:388-90.

116. Himmelberg CJ, Pleasants RA, Weber DJ, Kessler JM, Samsa GP, Spivey JM, Morris TL. Use of antimicrobial drugs in adults before and after removal of a restriction policy. Am J Hosp Pharm. 1991;48:1220-7.

117. Restino MS, Knodel LC. Drug information quality assurance program used to appraise students' performance. Am J Hosp Pharm. 1992;49(6):1425-9.

118. Wheeler-Usher DH, Hermann FF, Wanke LA. Problems encountered in using written criteria to assess drug information responses. Am J Hosp Pharm. 1990;47(4):795-7.

119. Moody ML. Revising a drug information center quality assurance program to conform to Joint Commission standards. Am J Hosp Pharm. 1990;47(4):792-4.

120. Smith CH, Sylvia LM. External quality assurance committee for drug information services. Am J Hosp Pharm. 1990;47(4):787-91.

121. Halbert MR, Kelly WN, Miller DE. Drug information centers: lack of generic equivalence. Drug Intell Clin Pharm. 1977;11:728-35.

122. Beard SL, Coley RM, Blunt JR. Assessing the accuracy of drug information responses from drug information centers. Ann Pharmacother. 1994;28(6):707-11.

123. Calis KA, Anderson DW, Auth DA, Mays DA, Turcasso NM, Meyer CC, Young LR. Quality of pharmacotherapy consultations provided by drug information centers in the United States. Pharmacotherapy. 2002;20:830-6.

124. Ghaibi S, Ipema H, Gabay M. ASHP guidelines on the pharmacist's role in providing drug information. Am J Health-Syst Pharm. 2015;72:573-7.

125. Ogrinc G, Davies L, Goodman D, Batalden P, Davidoff F, Stevens D. SQUIRE 2.0 (Standards for QUality Improvement Reporting Excellence): revised publication guidelines from a detailed consensus process. BMJ Qual Saf. 2016 Dec;25(12):986-92.

126. The Joint Commission. Sentinel event alert 61 DOACs the joint commission requirements [Internet]. 2019 Jun 19 [cited 2019 Aug 5]. Available from: https://www.jointcommission.org/-/media/tjc/documents/resources/patient-safety-topics/sentinel-event/sea-61-doac-requirements.pdf

127. Dixon DL. Latest in cardiology: clinical monitoring of direct acting oral anticoagulants [Internet]. Washington (DC): American College of Cardiology; 2017 Mar 21 [cited 2019 Aug 12]. Available from: https://www.acc.org/latest-in-cardiology/ten-points-to-remember/2017/03/21/13/48/clinical-monitoring-of-direct-acting-oral-anticoagulants

SUGGESTED READINGS

1. Curtiss FR, Fry RN, Avey SG. Framework for pharmacy services quality improvement: a bridge to cross the quality chasm. J Manag Care Spec Pharm. 2020;26:798-816.

2. Warholak TL, Nau DP. Quality and safety in pharmacy practice. New York: McGraw-Hill Medical; 2010.

3. Mainz J. Developing evidence-based clinical indicators: a state-of-the-art methods primer. Int J Qual Health Care. 2003;15(Suppl 1):i5-11.

4. Damberg CL, Sorbero ME, Lovejoy SL, Lauderdale K, Wertheimer S, Smith A, Waxman DA, Schnyer C. An evaluation of the use of performance measures in health care [Internet]. Santa Monica (CA): RAND Corporation; 2011. Available from: https://www.rand.org/pubs/technical_reports/TR1148.html

5. Langley GL, Moen R, Nolan KM, Nolan TW, Norman CL, Provost LP. The improvement guide: a practical approach to enhancing organizational performance. 2nd ed. San Francisco (CA): Jossey-Bass Publishers; 2009.

6. Dreischulte T, Grant AM, McCowan C, McAnaw JJ, Guthrie B. Quality and safety of medication use in primary care: consensus validation of a new set of explicit medication assessment criteria and prioritization of topics for improvement. BMC Clin Pharmacol. 2012;12:1-17.

7. Thielemier B, Tu A. Pharmacists' impact on quality measures and opportunities for pharmacy enhanced services [Internet]. America's Pharmacist. 2017 May:45-53. Available from: http://www.ncpa.co/issues/APMAY17-CE.pdf

8. Pharmacy Quality Alliance. PQA performance measures [Internet]. Alexandria (VA): Pharmacy Quality Alliance. Available from: https://www.pqaalliance.org/pqa-measures

9. American Society of Health-System Pharmacists. ASHP statement on the health-system pharmacist's role in national health care quality initiatives. Am J Health-Syst Pharm. 2010;67:578-9.

10. U.S. Department of Health and Human Services, Office of Disease Prevention and Health Promotion. National action plan for adverse drug event prevention [Internet]. Washington (DC): U.S. Department of Health and Human Services; 2014. Available from: https://health.gov/hcq/pdfs/ADE-Action-Plan-508c.pdf

11. U. S. Department of Health and Human Services, Centers for Medicare and Medicaid Services. Center for clinical standards and quality/survey & certification group: medication-related adverse events in nursing homes [Internet]. Baltimore (MD): Centers for Medicare and Medicaid Services; 2015. Available from: https://www.cms.gov/Medicare/Provider-Enrollment-and-Certification/SurveyCertificationGenInfo/Downloads/Survey-and-Cert-Letter-15-47.pdf

19

Chapter Nineteen

Medication Safety I: Adverse Drug Reactions

Kelly Besco • Megan E. Keller

Learning Objectives

After completing this chapter, the reader will be able to:

- Define adverse drug reactions (ADRs).
- Discuss the impact of ADRs on health care systems and patients.
- Explain methods for determining causality and probability of an ADR.
- Identify specialty drug information resources that can be used to locate information related to ADRs.
- Classify ADRs based on type and severity.
- Use guidelines from national organizations to implement an ADR reporting program.
- Describe the use of technology in ADR monitoring and reporting.
- Explain when, where, and how to report an ADR to the U.S. Food and Drug Administration (FDA).
- Explain how to report adverse reactions related to dietary supplements, vaccines, and medical devices.

Key Concepts

❶ ADR refers to any unexpected, unintended, undesired, or excessive response to a medicine.

❷ One of the first steps in establishing an ADR program is to define what each facility or organization categorizes as ADRs.

❸ Several algorithms have been published that try to incorporate information about an ADR into a more objective form.

❹ Communication is a critical component throughout the ADR monitoring process.

❺ Technology plays an important role in monitoring, identifying, and minimizing ADRs.

❻ ADR surveillance serves as a means to primarily provide early signals about possible problems with a medication.

Introduction

The terminology surrounding ADRs is often confusing. All adverse drug events (ADEs), ADRs, and medication errors fall under the umbrella of medication misadventures. Medication misadventure is a very broad term, referring to any iatrogenic hazard or incident associated with medications. An ADE is the next broadest term, and refers to any injury caused by a medicine. An ADE encompasses all ADRs, including allergic and idiosyncratic reactions, as well as medication errors that result in harm to a patient.[1-5] ADRs and medication errors are the most specific terms. ❶ *Adverse drug reaction refers to any unexpected, unintended, undesired, or excessive response to a medicine.* A medication error is any preventable event that has the potential to lead to inappropriate medication use or patient harm.[1] Figure 19-1 shows one way of graphically classifying these terms. Many of these concepts will be explored in greater depth elsewhere in this text, including Chapter 20, "Medication Safety II: Medication Errors." The present chapter focuses on ADRs, highlighting the impact of ADRs, pertinent definitions and classifications, specialty drug information resources, ADR reporting systems, and future approaches to detecting and managing ADRs.

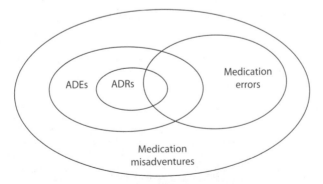

Figure 19–1. Relationship among medication misadventures, adverse drug events, medication errors, and adverse drug reactions.

Impact of Adverse Drug Reactions

All medications, including the inactive ingredients of a product, are capable of producing adverse reactions.[6] ADRs account for four emergency department visits per 1000 Americans annually, cause patients to lose confidence in their health care providers, and lead to a significant increase in morbidity and mortality.[7] In 2017, there were over 70,000 deaths in the United States that were attributed to ADRs.[8]

ADRs have economic consequences as well. ADRs result in an estimated annual cost of $30 billion in the United States.[9] These costs are attributable to the overall cost-of-illness generated by an ADR, including initial and prolonged hospitalization, loss of income from occupational absences, as well as utilization of new medication(s) for management of symptoms and conditions induced by the medication that initially caused the reaction. Direct hospital costs in the United States because of ADRs may be as high as $1.56 billion annually. After experiencing an ADR, patients spend an average of 8–12 days longer in the hospital, with potential to increase the cost of their hospitalization by $14,000 to $19,000.[9,10]

The incidence of ADRs for hospitalized patients has been reported to be as high as 16%.[10] Of course, ADRs do not affect hospitalized patients alone; however, there is limited data available regarding the incidence of ADRs that occur in the ambulatory care setting. An estimated 4.5 million ambulatory visits each year in the United States are related to ADRs. These outpatient events typically result in visits to physician office practices.[11] Health care professionals agree that these estimates may be conservative because many ADRs go undetected, unreported, and untreated.[12] One systematic review of 37 studies concluded that the level of underreporting is likely to be in excess of 90%.[13]

Several agencies and professional organizations have an active role in minimizing the occurrence and impact of ADRs. Some of the key organizations include the World Health Organization (WHO), the U.S. Food and Drug Administration (FDA), The Joint Commission (TJC), and the American Society of Health-System Pharmacists (ASHP) (see Table 19-1). Despite the numerous organizations involved, **pharmacovigilance**, the process of preventing and detecting adverse effect caused by medications, depends heavily on individual health care practitioners, including pharmacists, physicians, and nurses, to take measures to minimize ADRs and report events. Practitioners should understand the potential for ADRs and be prepared to recognize and prevent such occurrences in order to minimize adverse outcomes.

Pharmacists play a vital role in avoiding ADRs. One study published in Pharmaco therapy reviewed which inpatient-based, clinical pharmacy programs were associated with reduced ADR rates. Significant reductions occurred in hospitals offering pharmacist-obtained admission medication histories, drug protocol management, and ADR management programs.

TABLE 19-1. ORGANIZATIONS INVOLVED IN PREVENTING ADVERSE DRUG EVENTS

Food and Drug Administration (FDA)	http://www.fda.gov
The Joint Commission (TJC)	http://www.jointcommission.org
World Health Organization (WHO)	http://www.who.int
Institute for Safe Medication Practices (ISMP)	http://www.ismp.org
The United States Pharmacopeial Convention (USP)	http://www.usp.org
American Society of Health-System Pharmacists (ASHP)	http://www.ashp.org
National Coordinating Council for Medication Error Reporting and Prevention (NCC MERP)	http://www.nccmerp.org
Agency for Healthcare Research and Quality (AHRQ)	http://www.ahrq.gov

Facilities with these programs were found to have lower incidence of ADR rates as compared to hospitals without these services. Presence of these three services additionally translated to lower death rates, length of hospital stays, and inpatient drug charges. For example, patients admitted to hospitals without a pharmacist-led medication history service were found to have 86% increased likelihood of developing an ADR and $127,253 in additional Medicare patient charges.[14]

Definitions

After reading this chapter, the reader should be able to evaluate ADRs and, potentially, develop and implement an ADR surveillance program at their practice setting. ❷ *One of the first steps in establishing an ADR program is to define what each facility or organization categorizes as ADRs.* There are many definitions for ADRs that have been described in the literature, including guidance from national and international organizations, as well as individual facilities and practitioners. Several of these definitions are presented below. Rather than getting bogged down in the differences between these many definitions, use this information for guidance when starting to evaluate ADRs and when developing an ADR monitoring and reporting system. Remember that institutions, as well as clinicians, use different definitions depending on their practice needs. WHO defines an ADR as "a response to a medicine which is noxious and unintended, and which occurs at doses normally used in man" referring to harmful unexpected experiences related to medications.[15] Additionally, **side effect** is defined as an "expected, well-known reaction resulting in little or no change in patient management" referring to effects that are expected and predictable based on the dose of the medication.[16] For example, constipation could be considered a side effect of opioids. Note that, in clinical practice, side effect is a broad term that

• may be used synonymously with ADR, or may even refer to an ADE. Defined by the FDA, an ADE is any "undesirable experience" associated with the use of a drug in a patient.[17] This definition is fairly broad, as it includes events occurring from both preventable ADEs and non-preventable ADR causes. The FDA is particularly interested in reports of *unexpected* adverse reactions which are considered reactions that are not listed in the current labeling for a medication as having been reported or associated with the use of the drug. Reporting ADRs to the FDA will be discussed later in this chapter. Although common or expected ADRs are relevant and important to report, they do not provide the FDA with new or additional safety information. Unexpected drug reactions may be symptomatically or pathophysiologically related to an ADR listed in the current labeling, but may differ from the labeled ADR because of greater severity or specificity. For example, a medication may have abnormal liver function listed in its labeling as an adverse reaction. A health care practitioner should still report a case of hepatic necrosis following administration of the drug, because it represents an unexpected ADR of greater severity.[18]

• Edwards and Aronson propose another definition of an ADR: "An appreciably harmful or unpleasant reaction, resulting from an intervention related to the use of a medicinal product, which predicts hazard from future administration and warrants prevention or specific treatment, or alteration of the dosage regimen, or withdrawal of the product."[19] This is a very practical definition for health care practitioners, because it highlights the need to take action in order to manage the effects of the adverse reaction.

Finally, Karch and Lasagna,[20] two early researchers in the area of ADRs, define an ADR as

• any response to a drug which is noxious and unintended, and which occurs at doses used in man for prophylaxis, diagnosis, or therapy, excluding therapeutic failures.
Many institutions use Karch and Lasagna's definition because it excludes accidental poisonings as well as problems with drugs of abuse.

Remember, these definitions are intended to provide guidance and food for thought; in daily practice, the differences between these descriptions may not be relevant or clinically meaningful. What is important is that individuals find or develop a definition of ADRs that works for the needs of their practice setting.

Causality and Probability of Adverse Drug Reactions

One of the challenges in defining and managing ADRs is determining causality. How can it be determined whether or not a drug caused a patient's adverse reaction? A cause-and-effect relationship is difficult to prove in general, and ADRs are no exception. Many investigators have dealt with this problem by developing and publishing definitions, algorithms, and questionnaires that try to determine the probability of a reaction—that is, the likelihood that an ADR was caused by a particular drug or medication. There are over 30 different published methods for assessing adverse drug reaction causality. They fall into three broad categories[21]:

1. **Expert judgment/Global introspection**: This method involves the individual assessment of the event by a health care practitioner, based on his or her clinical knowledge and experience without using any form of standardized tool.
2. **Algorithm**: This method uses specific questions to assign a weighted score that helps determine the probability of causality in a given reaction.
3. **Probabilistic**: This method uses Bayesian approaches and epidemiological data to calculate and estimate the probability of causality with advanced statistical methods.

To date, none of these attempts have been able to prove actual causality. These tools, however, are used to determine the probability that a particular drug caused an adverse event and will be described further below.

These algorithms and definitions use several important key concepts.[17,22] Dechallenge and rechallenge are often discussed. **Dechallenge** occurs when the drug is discontinued and the patient is then monitored to determine whether the ADR abates or decreases in intensity. **Rechallenge** occurs when the drug is discontinued and, after the ADR abates, the same drug is administered in an attempt to elicit the response again. Dechallenge and rechallenge are effective means for establishing a strong case that the drug was responsible for the ADR. A dechallenge is often essential in clinical practice, but a rechallenge may not be practical and may be unethical due to the risk of further harm to the patient. Nevertheless, a rechallenge may be clinically necessary if the medication the patient is intolerant to is essential to sustain life (e.g., chemotherapy). Rechallenges are typically performed under medical supervision through use of a desensitization protocol. If successful, desensitization will allow a patient to tolerate exposure to a specific medication to which they are allergic. Desensitization protocols involve giving the medication to the patient in slowly increasing amounts, starting with small doses, and ending with the full dose prescribed by a physician. For example, desensitization can be performed for a patient with a confirmed penicillin allergy that has a diagnosis that requires treatment with penicillin or a closely related antimicrobial. Unfortunately, the lasting effects of desensitization are somewhat uncertain. For medications that are taken on a daily basis, the body remembers and retains a state of desensitization; however, if more than 2 days pass between doses, desensitization often needs to be performed again prior to rechallenging the patient to the medication.[23]

Another important concept to consider is the temporal relationship between the drug and the event. Does the timeframe for development of the ADR make sense? Did the patient's exposure to the drug precede the suspected ADR? If there are previous reports of the ADR in the literature, do these reports describe a temporal relationship between the drug and the event? Case reports, specialty drug information resources, and package inserts can be helpful in noting if a drug has been known to cause a certain type of reaction in a certain timeframe in the past. Unfortunately, the literature is not likely to be helpful for rare or new ADRs, but this does not discount the fact that a reaction may have occurred.

Naranjo and colleagues[22] developed the following definitions to assist in determining the probability of a suspected ADR:

"Definite ADR is a reaction that: (1) follows a reasonable temporal sequence from administration of the drug, or in which the drug level has been established in body fluids or tissue; (2) follows a known response pattern to the suspected drug; (3) is confirmed by dechallenge; and (4) could not be reasonably explained by the known characteristics of the patient's clinical state.

Conditional ADR is a reaction that: (1) follows a reasonable temporal sequence from administration of the drug; (2) does not follow a known response pattern to the suspected drug; and (3) could not be reasonably explained by the known characteristics of the patient's clinical state.

Doubtful ADR is any reaction that does not meet the criteria above." [22]

USING ALGORITHMS

❸ *Several algorithms have been published that try to incorporate information about an ADR into a more objective form.* As described above, these algorithms each use a set of specific questions to determine the likelihood that the drug was responsible for the reaction and establish a rational and scientific approach to what previously required strictly clinical judgment. Although algorithms are helpful in offering a systematic approach to assessing the probability of ADRs, they can be very time-consuming and the results vary significantly according to the interpretation of multiple observers.

In 1979, Kramer and colleagues published a questionnaire composed of 56 yes or no questions (Appendix 19-1).[24] This questionnaire includes sections about the patient's previous experience with the drug or related drugs, alternative etiologies, timing of events, drug concentrations, dechallenge, and rechallenge. Responses to each question are given a weighted value and these values are totaled. The total value then correlates to one of four categories: unlikely, possible, probable, or definite. One of the problems with the Kramer method (as well as other algorithms) is that clinicians can disagree on the weighted values because the user must make subjective judgments for some of the questions. Another problem inherent with this questionnaire is that an unexpected ADR may not score well because of lack of literature or previous experience with the ADR. If the reaction is not universally accepted or in the most recent edition of the Physicians' Desk Reference, the suspected reaction would score a 0 in this section. This makes the method devised by Kramer and associates less useful for new medications and for unexpected or emergent ADRs. Overall, however, the questionnaire provides health care professionals with the opportunity to use a standardized tool. Hutchinson and colleagues evaluated the reproducibility and validity of the Kramer questionnaire and concluded that, although the questionnaire was cumbersome to use, the method was superior to clinical judgment alone.[25]

Naranjo and colleagues developed an alternative algorithm in 1981 (Appendix 19-2).[22] This algorithm asks 10 questions involving the following areas: temporal relationship, the pattern of response, dechallenge or administration of an antagonist, rechallenge, alternative causes, placebo response, drug level in the body fluids or tissue, dose-response relationship, previous patient experience with the drug, and confirmation by any other objective evidence. Like the algorithm proposed by Kramer and associates, the answer to each question is assigned a score. The score is then totaled and placed into a category from definite to doubtful. In the initial published report of this algorithm, Naranjo and colleagues tested the reproducibility and validity of the algorithm and found that their tool was a valid means of assessing ADRs. Today, the Naranjo algorithm is one of the most commonly used methods to assess ADR causality, and has been considered the gold standard of assessing ADR causality. Compared to the method devised by Kramer and associates, the Naranjo tool is much quicker to administer. However, it is not without its faults. The tool emphasizes rechallenge and dechallenge, which may pose some problems in evaluating ADRs as described previously. The Naranjo algorithm also asks about a response to placebo, which is rarely (if ever) administered in clinical practice today.

In 1982, Jones published an algorithm that allows health care practitioners to answer a series of *yes* or *no* questions to determine the probability that an ADR occurred (Appendix 19-3).[26] The Jones algorithm asks similar questions as those used in the methods described above, but uses a dichotomous key design. Like the Naranjo algorithm, the tool developed by Jones is shorter and quicker to complete than Kramer's questionnaire. Unlike either Kramer or Naranjo's algorithms, the Jones method does not require summation of a score. Of note, the Jones algorithm was originally designed for use in a community health setting, illustrating that the assessment of ADRs is not limited to inpatient or institutional settings only.

All of the algorithms described above possess a certain degree of observer variability. However, each can be used to help determine whether an adverse event was precipitated by a certain drug or drug-drug combination. Michel and Knodel compared the three algorithms by Kramer, Jones, and Naranjo.[27] Their study found that the Naranjo algorithm was simpler and less time-consuming, and compared favorably to the 56 questions asked by Kramer. The highest correlation was found between the Naranjo algorithm and the Kramer questionnaire, and authors concluded that more data was needed to support the use of the algorithm developed by Jones and colleagues. These algorithms were the basis of ADR determination for over 20 years until a more modern approach was developed.

A newer approach to assessing the causality of ADRs has been developed by researchers at the University of Liverpool's Institute of Translational Medicine (Appendix 19-4).[28] Their algorithm, the Liverpool ADR Causality Assessment Tool (CAT), has been proposed as an alternative to traditional methods, and aims to improve the inter-rater reliability of ADR assessment techniques. The Liverpool CAT includes a sequence of questions that allow a user to arrive at a decision regarding whether the presence of an ADR was definite, probable, possible, or unlikely. The tool was developed while the originators were undertaking an observational study of ADRs in children and encountered concerns with the sensitivity of the Naranjo scale to predict ADR likelihood.[28] While studies have yet to demonstrate if the Liverpool ADE CAT is superior to alternative algorithms, the originators believe the tool to be practical for assessing the probability of ADRs in a clinical setting and its use in observational studies regarding ADRs had continued to grow.

At this time, no algorithm for assessing the causality or probability of an ADR has been proven superior.[21] Therefore, it is reasonable to select a method based on factors such as availability, speed, and ease of completing the tool, and clinician preference.

PROBABILISTIC METHODS

A Bayesian approach to assessing adverse reactions was developed by Lane.[29] Using the Bayesian approach, relevant information is collected and a quantitative measure of the odds that a particular drug caused a particular event is calculated. The Bayesian approach has the potential to be an outstanding tool for predicting populations that may be at higher risk for ADRs; however, this method requires complex calculations, significant time investments to develop the model, and the involvement of a statistician.[30] Due to these requirements, the Bayesian approach is likely not practical for implementation in individual clinics or hospitals, but WHO is using these methods to analyze data in their international drug monitoring network.

In addition to the methods for assessing adverse drug reaction causality and probability discussed above, there are also tools for assessing specific types of ADRs. For example, different methods exist for assessing drug-related liver toxicity.[31]

Case Study 19–1

A female patient presents to the Emergency Department with complaints of dizziness, shaking, and nausea. While interviewing the patient, you learn that she is taking a product called *Keto-gone* that is marketed as a weight loss dietary supplement. She started taking the product 4 weeks ago to help her lose weight. On physical exam, the patient is found to have increased blood pressure and rapid heartbeat. You research the product and find out that it contains raspberry ketones, which are known to have stimulant properties. The patient is admitted to the hospital and 2 days after she stopped taking *Keto-gone*, her symptoms resolve and she is discharged from the hospital.

- *In this case, was there a dechallenge? If so, what happened when the suspected product was dechallenged?*
- *Was there a temporal relationship between taking this product and the reaction the patient experienced?*
- *Based on what you know about this product, is the reaction consistent with its known pharmacology?*
- *What is the likelihood of this product causing the reaction?*

SPECIALTY RESOURCES FOR ADVERSE DRUG REACTIONS

Methods used to assess the causality of ADRs, including the Kramer and Naranjo algorithm, rely in part on previous documentation of the reaction occurring in response to administration of the suspected drug. For common or well-known ADRs, the prescribing information (also called the package insert) and major drug information compendia can be useful. However, for other suspected ADRs, specialty resources may be necessary.

Chapter 3 introduces ADR specialty resources, including gold standard references Meyler's Side Effects of Drugs and Side Effects of Drugs Annual. This section briefly describes a few additional specialty resources that may be useful.

FDA's MedWatch program for voluntary reporting of ADRs is discussed later in this chapter and Chapter 20. The results of this program are disseminated through a special section of the FDA website dedicated to ADRs and other medication safety topics (http://www.fda.gov/Safety/Medwatch). This online reference contains the FDA's latest safety alerts and recalls as well as resources for health care professionals. The site also provides monthly summaries of changes to drug labeling that the FDA has made in response to reports from health care providers and others involved in pharmacovigilance.[32] Users can sign up to receive safety alerts by email, or follow FDA MedWatch on Twitter using Internet-enabled mobile devices such as smartphones or tablet computers (http://www.twitter.com/FDAMedWatch).

Adverse event reports submitted to the FDA are compiled and made searchable to the public via the FDA Adverse Event Reporting System (FAERS) Public Dashboard and can be accessed at https://www.fda.gov/drugs/surveillance/questions-and-answers-fdas-adverse-event-reporting-system-faers. This database supports the FDA's post-marketing safety surveillance program through aggregation of reports received from manufacturers, health care providers, and consumers. The information has always been available to the public in different formats over the years; however, the new user-friendly dashboard has made the information more accessible and transparent. When utilizing the dashboard, it is important to remember there are limitations to the data (i.e., duplicate reports, missing information, reports not verified), and the existence of a report does not establish event causation. Despite these limitations, the dashboard is beneficial in identifying reported trends and events not previously seen in clinical trials.[33]

An alternative solution is VigiAccess™ (http://www.vigiaccess.org), WHO's global database of adverse reaction reports. The database is a user-friendly web application that allows the public to access information about adverse reactions with medicines and vaccines that have been reported to the WHO Programme for International Drug Monitoring (WHO PIDM) by its more than 110 members, including FDA's MedWatch. Although the depth of information provided by VigiAccess™ is minimal, the site can be used to determine whether an adverse reaction has been previously reported in response to a particular drug.[34]

Published case reports can also be useful in assessing and evaluating ADRs (see Chapter 5 for more information on evaluating case reports). Reactions Weekly is a weekly publication that indexes and abstracts ADR case reports and ADR-related news from around the world (see also Chapter 3). Because it pulls information from biomedical journals, scientific meetings, and the WHO PIDM, Reactions Weekly can be useful for efficiently searching the available information related to a suspected ADR.[35] Clin-Alert is a similar publication that summarizes reports of adverse clinical events from more than 100 key research journals, although its focus is primarily on reports of drug-drug interactions.[36]

Classification of Adverse Drug Reactions

Various definitions and terminology have been used to classify ADRs. As discussed above, algorithms such as those developed by Naranjo, Kramer, and Jones use the definite, probable, possible, and unlikely categories to classify ADRs by their probability. Other classification systems rank ADRs by severity or by their mechanism. When developing an ADR monitoring program, these various systems can be used to determine probability (cause and effect) and severity of ADRs and help describe and quantify data. The data may help identify severity of reactions that are occurring and which medications cause the most severe reactions. Classification systems can also help health care practitioners organize and present data, and facilitate monitoring of ADR trends and potential causative agents. These trends can be used to change prescribing habits or to alert institutions and organizations to potential problems with medications.

CLASSIFYING BY SEVERITY

Karch and Lasagna[20] developed a method of classifying ADRs by severity, from minor to severe, as defined below:

- **Minor**: No antidote, therapy, or prolongation of hospitalization is required in response to the ADR.
- **Moderate**: The management of the ADR requires a change in drug therapy, specific treatment, or an increase in hospitalization by at least 1 day.
- **Severe**: The ADR is potentially life threatening, causing permanent damage or requiring intensive medical care.
- **Lethal**: The ADR directly or indirectly contributes to the death of the patient.

The FDA also uses severity to classify ADRs. According to the FDA, an event is serious when it results in death, is life-threatening, causes or prolongs hospitalization, causes a significant persistent disability, results in a congenital anomaly, or requires intervention to prevent permanent damage.[17]

Another method of classifying ADRs by severity is the National Cancer Institute Common Terminology Criteria for Adverse Events (CTCAE). This system was developed by the National Cancer Institute (NCI) and formerly referred to as "common toxicity criteria" (CTC) as a way to grade the severity of adverse medication reactions or organ toxicity for patients receiving cancer therapy. This system utilizes five grades to define toxicity, with Grade 1 being Mild and Grade 5 referring to death as outlined below[37]:

- **Grade 1—Mild:** The adverse event was either asymptomatic or noted only via clinical observations; no intervention was required.
- **Grade 2—Moderate:** Adverse event was minimal and/or localized; any required interventions were noninvasive.
- **Grade 3—Severe:** The adverse event is medically significant but not immediately life-threatening and/or requires hospitalization.
- **Grade 4—Life-threatening consequences:** The adverse event requires urgent intervention.
- **Grade 5—Death:** Referring to death related to the adverse event.

CLASSIFYING BY MECHANISM

Karch and Lasagna also described various mechanisms by which ADRs occur.[20] These mechanisms are related to the pharmacologic or pharmacodynamic properties of drugs, and can be used to classify the type of reaction that occurs:

- **Idiosyncrasy:** an uncharacteristic response of a patient to a drug, usually not occurring on administration.
- **Hypersensitivity:** a reaction, not explained by the pharmacologic effects of the drug, caused by altered reactivity of the patient and generally considered to be an allergic manifestation.
- **Intolerance:** a characteristic pharmacologic effect of a drug produced by an unusually small dose, so that the usual dose tends to induce a massive overaction.
- **Drug interaction:** an unusual pharmacologic response that could not be explained by the action of a single drug, but was caused by two or more drugs.
- **Pharmacologic:** a known, inherent pharmacologic effect of a drug, directly related to dose.

Another mechanism-based reaction classification system from Edwards and Arson, with an easy-to-recall mneumonic is[38]:

- Dose-related (Augmented): Common adverse reaction with low mortality risk related to the expected actions of a drug such as toxic effects (e.g., digoxin) or side effects (e.g., sedation with benzodiazepines).
- Non-dose-related (Bizarre): Uncommon and unpredictable adverse reaction not related to the action of the drug. This category has a higher mortality risk and includes immunological reactions (e.g., drug allergies) and idiosyncratic reactions (e.g., malignant hyperthermia).
- Dose-related and time-related (Chronic): Uncommon adverse reactions related to the total dose over time such as renal failure with long-term use of nonsteroidal anti-inflammatory drugs (NSAIDs).
- Time-related (Delayed): Uncommon adverse reactions presenting after longer duration of use that are typically dose-related (e.g., tardive dyskinesia).
- Withdrawal (End of use): Uncommon adverse reactions occuring after the drug has been discontinued (e.g., opiate withdrawal syndrome).
- Unexpected failure of therapy (Failure): Common, dose-related adverse reactions which can be caused by drug interactions (e.g., CYP450 interactions).

Classifying the ADR by its mechanism may aid in identifying similar drugs that can be expected to cause a reaction, or may help explain patient-specific reactions to medications.

Implementing a Program

Well-designed programs that monitor and identify ADRs, as well as broadcast information to the medical community, are essential. Prior to implementing an ADR program, the health care facility must educate its staff on the importance and significance of the program. The pharmacy department is in an excellent position to provide this education because of its involvement in the pharmacy and therapeutics (P&T) committee, pharmacokinetic dosing, medication use evaluation (MUE), and drug distribution. The pharmacy department can be an excellent resource for developing an ADR program, as well as providing data about ADRs to the P&T committee and/or the institution's Medication Safety Committee.

STEPS FOR IMPLEMENTING A PROGRAM

Accrediting bodies like The Centers for Medicare & Medicaid Services (CMS)[39] and TJC[40] require that hospitals and health care organizations have an ADR reporting program. These programs are generally a function of the P&T committee (or other medical staff committee) and the department of pharmacy. ASHP also encourages pharmacists and health care practitioners to take an active role in monitoring adverse events. ASHP has published very specific guidelines on ADR monitoring and reporting as part of its practice standards.[41] TJC and ASHP standards can be used as a basis for starting an ADR monitoring program. In addition to the standards, the pharmacy and medical literature are rich with examples of successful programs, some of which will be reviewed in this chapter.

Steps for implementing an ADR monitoring program include the following:

1. Develop definitions and classifications of ADRs that work for the institution. The definitions and classifications in this chapter provide a good starting point for discussion.
2. Assign responsibility for the ADR program within the pharmacy and throughout other key departments. A multidisciplinary approach is an essential factor. This will improve awareness of the monitoring program and increase ADR reporting at all levels of patient care.
3. Develop a program with approval from the pharmacy department, risk management, the medical staff and nursing departments, as well as other appropriate areas within the facility. Cooperation is essential in initiation of a successful program.
4. Promote awareness of the program. Newsletters, emails, in-services, grand rounds presentations, and other educational programs are opportunities to increase awareness and garner support for the program.

TABLE 19–2. ADE INDICATOR DRUGS

Antidiarrheal agents
Atropine (except preoperatively)
Dextrose 50% (IV push)
Diphenhydramine (except at bedtime)
Epinephrine (IV push)
Flumazenil
Naloxone
Potassium supplement (diuretic or digoxin patients)
Protamine
Sodium polystyrene sulfonate (patients on potassium sparing diuretics or ACE inhibitors)
Topical steroids
Vitamin K

5. Promote awareness of ADRs and the importance of reporting such events in order to increase patient safety. Again, newsletters, emails, in-services, grand rounds presentations, and other educations programs can be utilized to increase awareness of specific ADRs.

6. Establish mechanisms for screening ADRs continuously. These mechanisms should include retrospective reviews and concurrent monitoring, as well as prospective planning for high-risk groups. It is worthwhile to educate pharmacists to check for ADRs when they see orders for certain indicator drugs that are often used in treating an ADR (see Table 19-2), orders to discontinue or hold drugs, and orders to decrease the dose or frequency of a drug.[42] Also, electronic screening methods (e.g., trigger tools) to check for laboratory tests (e.g., drug levels, *Clostridium difficile* toxin assays, elevated serum potassium, low white blood cell counts) that are indicative of ADEs or ADRs can be helpful.[43] Emergency box usage is another event that may trigger investigation by the pharmacist to determine if an ADR has occurred (e.g., use of epinephrine for anaphylaxis). The previous examples highlight specific approaches to monitor for ADRs continuously. Additionally, retrospective review of indicator drug orders, laboratory tests, and/ or emergency box usage may also bring to light previously unreported ADEs or ADRs.

7. Develop internal forms or other mechanisms for data collection and reporting of ADRs. A quick Internet search will identify a number of ADR report forms used at specific institutions across the country. Many institutions use computer reporting as well as hotline phone numbers.

8. Develop policies and procedures for handling ADR reports. Indicate who is responsible for sending them to the FDA and review current accrediting body criteria such

as CMS Conditions of Participation (CoPs)[39] and TJC Medication Management standards,[40] to ensure that the framework of the developed program meets expectations of regulatory agencies that regulate and certify the organization.

9. Establish procedures for evaluating the causality and probability of ADRs, usually based on one of the classification systems previously discussed.

10. Routinely review ADRs for trends.

11. Develop preventive interventions. Examples of these include flagging patients who are at high risk of developing ADRs, labeling reactions in the electronic health record in a standardized manner, and identifying specific drugs which are likely to cause ADRs. Monitoring these patients and drugs more closely will help prevent or reduce the severity of possible ADRs.

12. Report all findings to P&T, Medication Safety Committee, and/or other appropriate committee(s).

13. Develop strategies for decreasing the incidence of ADRs, depending on the opportunities presented by the ADRs reported. An example is developing a standard for providing a patient with a dose of a corticosteroid to prevent recurrent allergic reactions associated with iodinated contrast media. This vital step has often been ignored in the literature; however, for an ADR program to be part of the quality assurance process, it must be included wherever possible.

❹ *Communication is a critical component throughout the ADR monitoring process.* To ensure that the suspected drug is not administered again, and that patients receive necessary treatment and monitoring, reaction details and severity of an ADR should be documented thoroughly in the patient's medical record. However, this action alone is not sufficient, as the information is often poorly visible and may be difficult to access. The ISMP recommends that ADRs be communicated to members of the patient's health care team in a standardized manner, such as documenting the reaction on a standardized order form, either in paper or electronic form, just as if prescribing drug therapy or ordering lab draws.[44] This increases visibility of the information and facilitates a timely response by all individuals involved in the patient's care. In addition, ASHP recommends that patients and their caregivers be notified when a suspected ADR has occurred.[41] Well-informed patients can help prevent ADRs from recurring in the future.[44]

The Role of Technology in ADR Surveillance

❺ *Technology plays an important role in monitoring, identifying, and minimizing ADRs.* Information systems are available that can identify and alert practitioners to potential ADRs and detect potential drug-drug interactions that may contribute to ADRs. These systems search patient records and medical data to find drug names, drug levels, or drug-lab interactions (sometimes called triggers) that frequently indicate an ADR has occurred.[45] See Chapter 28 for more information on this topic. Sophisticated systems may also search through International Classification of Diseases, Tenth Revision (ICD-10) codes, nursing notes, or outpatient medical records. For example, a medication profile that includes an angiotensin-converting enzyme inhibitor and a note in the medical chart that mentions cough might trigger the ADR surveillance system. This information is then used to alert a pharmacist or prescriber who can investigate the suspected ADR and manage any adverse effects. [45]

INPATIENT ADR SURVEILLANCE PROGRAMS

At Duke University Health System (DUHS), a computerized adverse drug event surveillance program was developed that monitors medical records and automatically identifies hospitalized patients who may have experienced an ADR.[46] The system screens the DUHS electronic health record (EHR) platform for abnormal laboratory results, medication orders for antidotes, and drug-laboratory combinations to identify potential ADRs. Once one of the aforementioned triggers is identified, a notification is transmitted to a web-based queue that is reviewed by a pharmacist who can follow up to determine if an actual adverse event has truly occurred. The pharmacist reviews the patient's EHR and discusses the findings with clinicians involved in patient's care. Over a 1-year period for Duke University Hospital pediatric inpatients, the surveillance system was able to detect 1537 medication-related events for required investigation.[47]

AMBULATORY ADR SURVEILLANCE PROGRAMS

Because hospitals are required by accrediting bodies to have an ADR reporting system, the use of technology for identifying, reporting, and minimizing ADRs is very common in the inpatient setting. Unfortunately, this is quite different from the ambulatory care setting. In general, the reporting of ADRs and other drug-related events has experienced minimal uptake in the primary care setting. Reasons for this include busy physician schedules, high cost of implementation, and complexity of outpatient prescribing practices. Because of this, the Agency for Healthcare Research and Quality (AHRQ) initiated a project to develop and test a reporting system for use in ambulatory clinics nationwide. Called the Medication Error and Adverse Drug Event Reporting System (MEADERS), the system was intuitive, allowing health care professionals to report events using both simple data entry and open text boxes in order to capture the complete story regarding each medication error or adverse drug event. MEADERS also included the option of sending reports to the FDA's MedWatch program.[48] MEADERS was an Internet-based report viewing system that allowed users to browse reports from ambulatory settings across the country, providing capabilities for practitioners to compare their local or organizational reports to national data.[49] Initial field testing of MEADERS involved 24 practice sites who submitted a total of 507 reports during the pilot period. Of these reports, 70% involved medication errors and 27% described adverse drug events linked to medication therapy.

Unfortunately, MEADERS is no longer an active reporting database, and data supporting ADR monitoring and reporting programs in the outpatient setting remains limited. Traditionally, hospital-based pharmacists have been the health care professional to provide the greatest number of spontaneous ADR reports to the FDA.[50] However, community pharmacists are in a unique position to report on ADRs relating to nonprescription medications and dietary supplements. Community pharmacists can also report on reactions that patients are likely to detect themselves, such as ophthalmic and dermatological disorders. In fact, in countries such as the Netherlands, Japan, and Spain, most ADR reports originate from community, rather than hospital, pharmacists.[50]

One of the finest examples concerning the use of information technology for ADR monitoring and reporting comes from the Department of Veterans Affairs (VA). The VA refined its methods for collecting and reporting patient-specific ADR information by developing two distinct, yet complementary, databases. The first involves patient-specific information related to ADRs. Health care providers within the VA system are responsible for entering ADR information into a specific part of the patients' electronic medical record, called the Adverse Reaction Tracking (ART) package. This locally entered ADR information is then automatically extracted to construct a national ART database. Since its inception, the ART database has received over 50,000 entries per month. The second database, the VA Adverse Drug Event Reporting System (VA ADERS), is external to the electronic medical record and requires providers to report detailed information related to specific, preselected ADRs. VA ADERS also allows for direct submission to the FDA's reporting programs MedWatch and the Vaccine Adverse Event Reporting System (VAERS), discussed later in this chapter. The impact of VA ADERS on ADR reporting is demonstrated by the number of reports generated compared to the VA's previous system (the legacy Adverse Drug Event System). In the 5 years prior to the implementation of the VA ADERS, only 21,000 ADR reports were generated. In the 3 years after the implementation of the VA ADERS, nearly 150,000 ADR reports were generated.[51]

Reporting Adverse Drug Reactions

❻ *ADR surveillance serves as a means to primarily provide early signals about possible problems with a medication.* Because preapproval studies typically involve a limited number of patients and populations, it is not possible to anticipate all potential side effects a medication may produce once it is made available to the general public. Therefore, it is necessary to establish mechanisms to identify effects of a medication that did not appear during pre-approval studies. This monitoring process is referred to as **postmarketing surveillance**, or the process of continually monitoring and reviewing suspected adverse reactions associated with medications once they reach the market and are available to the public (see Chapter 24 for more about postmarketing surveillance). In order to detect an ADR that occurs once in every 10,000 patients exposed to the drug, at least 30,000 people would need to be treated with the medication.[12] Clinical trials that are required to approve a new drug may not enroll a sufficient number of patients, and often exclude special groups such as children, pregnant women, and the elderly. Due to the limited sample size and populations included in these trials, the FDA relies on postmarketing information to establish a better understanding of adverse events. In addition, the short duration of most clinical trials means that ADRs with a delayed onset may not be detected.[52] Pharmaceutical companies are required by the FDA to submit quarterly reports of all ADRs for the first 3 years that a drug is on the market, followed by annual reports thereafter, as part of the postmarketing surveillance system. However, the success of postmarketing surveillance is directly dependent on the active involvement of health care practitioners. Postmarketing ADR reports from health care providers have led to changes in prescribing habits, changes to drug labeling, and the withdrawal of various drugs from the market.

REPORTING ADRS TO THE FDA

With the passage of the Kefauver–Harris Amendment of 1962, the FDA was required to maintain a Spontaneous Reporting System (SRS). The structure of the SRS has changed over time. Today, all health care professionals and consumers can report ADRs and participate in the postmarketing surveillance process by submitting reports to the FDA's MedWatch. With MedWatch, the FDA receives reports via mailings, phone calls, faxes, and the Internet. From 2006 to 2014, the number of reports submitted annually through MedWatch grew from 470,261 to 1,289,133.[53]

The current MedWatch system allows health care providers, manufacturers, and consumers to report suspected ADRs for prescription medications and/or dietary supplements using FDA Form 3500 (Appendix 19-5), which can be submitted by mail, fax, phone, or online.[54] The MedWatch form asks for information related to the suspected ADR, the patient's relevant medical history and medication regimen, and pertinent laboratory tests, although this information does not need to be complete in order for an ADR report to be submitted. From start to finish, the FDA estimates that it takes 36 minutes to complete a MedWatch form, including gathering the patient's data, reviewing the instructions, and submitting the report.

Once submitted through the MedWatch system, ADR reports are received by a unit of the FDA called the Central Triage Unit. The Central Triage Unit screens reports and forwards them to the appropriate FDA program within 24 hours of receipt. The report becomes part of a database used by the FDA to identify signals or warnings related to drug safety which require further study or regulatory action (see Pharmacovigilance portion of chapter). As a reminder, MedWatch is interested in capturing reports of serious ADRs, which the FDA defines as death, life-threatening events, hospitalization, disability, congenital anomaly, or requiring intervention to prevent permanent impairment or damage, as well as unexpected ADRs. The MedWatch program asks individuals to report an event even if they are not certain that the drug product was the cause.[55]

Barriers to Reporting ADRs

The MedWatch program does not overcome the traditional lack of reporting seen with voluntary systems. It is important to recall that pharmaceutical manufacturers are required to report all adverse events to the FDA, whereas individual health care practitioners do so only voluntarily. Various explanations can account for the failure of practitioners to participate in the FDA program. Hoffman[55] elucidates several reasons that physicians do not voluntarily report ADRs, as follows:

1. Failure to detect the reaction due to a low level of suspicion.
2. Fear of potential legal implications.
3. Lack of training about drug therapy.
4. Uncertainty about whether the drug causes the reaction.
5. Lack of clear responsibility for reporting.
6. Paperwork and time involved.
7. No financial incentive to report.
8. Unaware of reporting procedure or little understanding of it.
9. Lack of readily available reporting forms.
10. Desire to publish the report.
11. Fear that a useful drug will be removed from the market or given a bad name.
12. Complacency and lethargy.
13. Guilty feelings because of patient harm.
14. Reaction not worth reporting.

In a systematic review of available evidence, Lopez-Gonzalez and colleagues identified additional reasons why ADRs are underreported, including the beliefs that a single ADR report cannot meaningfully contribute to medical knowledge and that only safe drugs are allowed on the market.[56] Another potential explanation for the lack of reporting is that medical record personnel, whose jobs might be to categorize and report data, are not familiar with ADRs and/or their method of documentation.[55]

Many of the reasons noted above also explain pharmacists' barriers to ADR reporting. A survey of Texas pharmacists investigated attitudes about voluntary reporting of serious adverse drug events in both community and hospital settings. While nearly 90% of respondents felt reporting could improve patient safety, 72.6% noted that the reporting process was time-consuming. Furthermore, 55.5% of respondents felt the reporting process disrupted their normal workflow. Some of the pharmacists in this survey also mentioned the reporting would increase the risk of malpractice, compromise relationships with physicians, and potentially break trust with their patients.[57] Ultimately, the benefit of increased patient safety should be enough to overcome the barriers to reporting faced by health care practitioners.

Reporting by Consumers

Historically, consumer reporting of adverse events has provided little data to MedWatch in comparison to the number of reports submitted by health care professionals. With the passage of the Food and Drug Administration Amendments Act (FDAAA) in 2007, however, consumer reports have been increasing. The FDAAA called for increased measures to assure the safety of marketed drugs. In an effort to increase consumer reporting of adverse events to the FDA, the act requires direct-to-consumer advertisements of prescription drugs to include the following statement: "You are encouraged to report negative side effects of prescription drugs to the FDA. Visit http://www.fda.gov/medwatch, or call 1-800-FDA-1088."[58]

In fact, in 2006, before the FDAAA was passed, consumers reported only 126,918 adverse event reports to MedWatch. In 2014, consumers were responsible for reporting 823,813 adverse event reports, bypassing the total provided by all health care providers that year.[59] While this trend is encouraging, there is still room for an increased rate of reporting by consumers. Efforts to educate the public on its role in ADR reporting could significantly impact public health.

Although consumers have the option of submitting ADR reports directly to the MedWatch program, FDA Form 3500 may be difficult for patients to navigate and complete. For example, they may not have ready access to their medical records, laboratory test results, and so on. Fortunately, a simplified, consumer-focused Form 3500B is available for patients to report ADRs to the FDA. A reporting mechanism is available for these individuals through the FDA's Consumer Complaint Coordinators. Available by telephone, these coordinators listen to consumer complaints, document the suspected problem, and follow up when needed. In the past, the FDA has recalled nonprescription products after just two or three reports of serious problems were received through the Consumer Complaint Coordinators.[60]

DIETARY SUPPLEMENT ADR REPORTING

Dietary supplements, including herbs, vitamins, minerals, and other so-called "nutraceu-ticals," can and do cause ADRs. Many of these products have powerful pharmacologi-cal effects and, therefore, can cause ADRs. The medical literature contains many case reports that describe ADRs related to dietary supplements. However, the exact incidence of ADRs with dietary supplements is not known. In one survey of 2743 adults, 4% who took a dietary supplement reported an adverse event in the previous 12 months.[61]

Dietary supplements are regulated much differently than pharmaceuticals. The most striking difference is that these supplements can reach pharmacies and grocery store shelves without FDA approval and without any proof of safety or effectiveness. In the past, manufacturers of these products were not required to monitor safety of their products through postmarketing surveillance, nor were they required to share informa-tion about safety with the FDA. However, the Dietary Supplement and Nonprescription Drug Consumer Protection Act of 2006 changed this. This legislation now requires that any manufacturer, packager, or distributor of a dietary supplement whose name appears on a product label must collect and report ADR information related to their product(s). Manufacturers or marketers of dietary supplements who receive reports or information about severe adverse reactions related to their products are now required to share these reports with the FDA.[62] Retailers who sell these products may report events upstream to the manufacturer, packer, or distributor.

In response to the growing dietary supplement industry, the FDA recently announced new efforts to strengthen the regulation of dietary supplements. In April 2019, the FDA created the Dietary Supplement Ingredient Advisory List as a means to quickly alert the public that a supplement may have the potential to cause serious side effects until final determinations are made. It is important to note that supplements on this list are not confirmed as harmful, but may have potential for harm based on preliminary assessments.[63] The public is able to subscribe to email updates via the FDA Subscription Management Center (https://updates.fda.gov/subscriptionmanagement). Another initia-tive to strengthen the regulation of dietary supplements was the enhancement of the New Dietary Ingredient (NDI) notification process. This process provides the FDA with an opportunity to review a new ingredient before it becomes available to consumers. The FDA continues to develop guidance documents around this process.[64]

An interesting case related to dietary supplements and ADRs involves the herb ephe-dra, also known as *ma huang*. This herb was marketed as a dietary supplement and pro-moted primarily for weight loss and enhancing athletic performance. It received negative media attention when a Minnesota football player died of heat exhaustion during a train-ing session. It turned out that the football player was using ephedra for weight loss. Over a period of several years, there were well over 100 reports to the FDA of life-threatening

ADRs linked to ephedra, including heart attacks, strokes, seizures, and death. In March 2004, the FDA banned the sale of dietary supplements containing ephedra,[65] although this ban was lifted by a judge in 2010.[66] Still, the FDA could not prove that ephedra was the cause of these numerous ADRs. Because there were no reporting standards or requirements for manufacturers to collect data on their products' safety at this time, the agency had to act based upon the best available evidence. The FDA's actions on ephedra will have long-lasting effects, and has ultimately set the precedent by which other cases against dietary supplements will be decided.

Currently, ADRs related to dietary supplements can be submitted by health care practitioners and consumers through the Department of Health and Human Services' Safety Reporting Portal. Previously, dietary supplement ADRs could be reported directly to FDA MedWatch program using the same approach that is used for prescription drugs. In 2014, the FDA transitioned the reporting process to the Safety Reporting portal to improve the efficiency and convenience of the reporting process. There are also third-party systems for collecting adverse event data such as Natural MedWatch (TRC Healthcare). Natural MedWatch (https://naturaldatabase.therapeuticresearch.com/nd/adverseevent.aspx?s=ND&cs=naturalstandard) allows consumers or health care professionals to complete an electronic form reporting an adverse event related to any dietary supplement. This system uses a database of around 90,000 commercially available dietary supplements that allows the user to select the specific commercial product used by the patient. Since many commercially available dietary supplements contain multiple ingredients, this system may improve the reliability of adverse reaction reporting for supplements. Natural MedWatch is integrated with the drug information resource Natural Medicines, which increases its accessibility for health care practitioners. Natural MedWatch asks similar questions to those on the FDA MedWatch Form 3500, and all reports submitted through this system are also simultaneously shared with the FDA.[67]

Just as with conventional drugs, reporting ADRs related to dietary supplements is voluntary for health care professionals. Practitioners and consumers have many options for reporting dietary supplement ADRs. As described above, they may submit them directly to the FDA via the Safety Reporting Portal, through a third-party system such as Natural MedWatch, or to the manufacturer or product distributor. Each of these avenues ultimately results in the information being provided to the FDA for evaluation and analysis. Within the FDA, these reports are sent to the Center for Food Safety and Applied Nutrition (CFSAN), which maintains a special group charged with evaluating these adverse events. The CFSAN Adverse Event Reporting System (CAERS) allows for a more efficient evaluation of reports specifically related to dietary supplements.[68]

Despite the availability of this reporting infrastructure, the number of adverse events submitted by health professionals is minimal. From 2004 to 2013 a total of 15,430 voluntary reports related to dietary supplement ADRs were submitted to the FDA.[69] Some of the reports were transmitted through mandatory mechanisms, such as manufacturer or distributor reporting. Most of these reports originate from consumers rather than health professionals.[68]

There may be a variety of reasons why few health professionals submit reports on dietary supplements to the FDA. Some of these may include:

- Patients often do not tell their providers about supplements use, or about the adverse effects they experience.
- Health professionals often do not ask about the use of dietary supplements.
- Consumers do not believe health professionals are able to answer questions about dietary supplements.
- Health professionals do not know where or how to submit reports of adverse reactions.
- There is a lack of information available to assess dietary supplement adverse reactions.
- Health care professionals may face a lack of time or support from management.
- Practitioners may have a fear of litigation.

ADRs related to dietary supplements can be assessed in much the same way as conventional drugs. However, there are some unique considerations. For example, when it comes to supplements, there is no such thing as generic equivalency. In other words, two supplement products made by different manufacturers cannot be considered equivalent. Different manufacturing practices and different extraction methods can dramatically change how a substance acts in the body, and this is especially true when it comes to herbal extracts. Because herbal extracts are made from plant material, variables such as extraction method, time of harvest, growing conditions, and so on can affect the chemical makeup of the extract. Therefore, two supplements containing Echinacea should not necessarily be considered equivalent. This may also mean that an ADR caused by one version of a supplement may not occur with another version.

VACCINE ADR REPORTING

While MedWatch accepts adverse event reports for all FDA-regulated drugs, biologics, and medical devices, a separate process has been established for the reporting of adverse reactions related to vaccinations. The Vaccine Adverse Event Reporting System (VAERS) is a postmarketing surveillance program supported by the FDA and the Centers for Disease Control and Prevention (CDC). It was established after the passage of the National Childhood Vaccine Injury Act in 1986. This act requires health care providers to report specific adverse events that follow vaccination. These events include those listed by the vaccine manufacturer as a contraindication to subsequent doses of the vaccine, as well as certain other reactions defined by the FDA and CDC. A list of these reportable reactions is available on the VAERS website (http://vaers.hhs.gov).[70] Around 30,000 reports are submitted to VAERS annually. Of these, approximately 13% are considered serious.[71]

Similar to the MedWatch program, patients and practitioners can submit reports of adverse reactions to VAERS online, by fax, or by mail. Detailed instructions regarding this process are also available on the VAERS website.

Case Study 19–2

A patient with a history of diabetes approaches you at the community pharmacy. She explains that she began taking a dietary supplement called *Kleanse Caps* 3 days ago as part of a detoxification and cleansing regimen. The patient reports that she has been feeling increasingly fatigued. You research the product and find out that it contains American Ginseng, which is known to lower blood glucose. The *Kleanse Caps* product labeling does not feature a warning about use in Diabetes. After interviewing the patient and evaluating the available information, you suggest that the patient measure her blood glucose on her glucometer and it results at a lower than normal value of 65 mg/dL. You advise the patient to stop taking *Kleanse Caps* and take 15–20 g of an oral glucose supplement. You determine that *Kleanse Caps* caused the patient's hypoglycemia.

- *As a health care professional, how can you report this suspected ADR to the FDA?*
- *Your patient decides she would like to take responsibility for reporting this ADR on her own. How can she accomplish this task?*

MEDICAL DEVICE ADR REPORTING

In addition to understanding medication, vaccine, and supplement reporting, one should also understand how to report serious issues related to medical devices. Medical devices are defined by the FDA as instruments or apparatuses intended for use in diagnosis, treatment, or prevention of disease and do not achieve their primary purpose through chemical action within the body.[72] Examples of medical devices include tongue depressors, glucometers, pacemakers, and x-ray machines.

Any events related to medical devices that may have caused or contributed to a death or serious injury should be reported to the FDA. Medical Device Reporting (MDR) is one of the FDA's postmarketing surveillance tools used to evaluate safety issues related to medical devices. Mandatory reporting requirements for manufacturers are outlined in the MDR regulations and typically utilize the MedWatch Form 3500A or electronic equivalent. Health care professionals, patients, and consumers also play a valuable role in reporting medical device problems voluntarily. Any device-related errors, issues with product quality, or therapeutic failures should be reported via MedWatch as it contributes vital information to improve patient safety.[73]

MDRs submitted to the FDA by both mandatory and voluntary reporters are compiled into the Manufacturer and User Facility Device Experience Database (MAUDE). The searchable database contains the last 10 years of data and is updated monthly. As with other FDA databases, it is important to note the data limitations. With MAUDE, keep in mind variations in trade, product, and company names will affect search results.[74]

The FDA also has a mobile app called MedWatcher, which can be used for voluntary reporting of medical device problems. The app also provides the option to upload photographs of medical devices which aids in identification of visible problems. Users can also receive MedWatch safety alerts and FDA safety communications via the app. In regard to confidentiality, the app does not store personal information or adverse event reports once submitted.[75]

Case Study 19-3

Using a point-of-care device used to monitor the effects of anticoagulants, you obtain a patient's blood sample to assess their warfarin therapy. To your surprise, the patient's International Normalized Ratio (INR) result is 6.0 which is above the 2.0–3.0 goal range for this patient. Many things can alter this number, such as diet or other medications, so you obtain a thorough history from the patient. The patient denies any changes and does not have any signs or symptoms of bleeding. After a thorough investigation, you conclude there are no patient factors contributing to this unexpected result. Furthermore, this patient has consistently been in range for the last year. All manufacturer guidelines were followed and the device passed the quality checks before use. You realize this is the first test you have done with the new box of test strips and send the patient to the lab for confirmation testing before making any treatment decisions. The INR result comes back in range, at 2.5, and you suspect the test strips are the cause of the inaccurately high readings.

- *As a health care professional, how can you report this suspected ADR to the FDA?*
- *Which adverse event reporting database would you search in order to find similar reports?*

Future Approaches to Pharmacovigilance

The FDA has recognized that voluntary postmarketing evaluations of drug safety data alone are not sufficient to identify serious ADRs. High-profile adverse events related to drugs, such as propoxyphene (Darvon®; Darvocet®) and isotretinoin (Accutane®), are prime examples of the insufficiency of the voluntary reporting system. In recent years, the FDA has grown more sophisticated in their approach to postmarketing surveillance through the development of an electronic data monitoring system, called Sentinel.[76] The program provides FDA access to claims data on nearly 200 million patients that are a part of the program's 18 data partners, which are predominately major health insurers. Since launching Sentinel, the FDA has completed a multitude of projects utilizing information obtained through these partners. For example, an older version of the rotavirus vaccine was removed from the market due to increased risk of intussusception (a life-threatening adverse event), but pre-market trials of newer rotavirus vaccines did not detect similar findings. Examination of data from Sentinel established a link between one of the newer vaccines and the adverse event. While incidence of intussusception cases was not overwhelming and the FDA deemed that the findings did not necessitate removal of the newer vaccine from the market, the labeling of the vaccine was updated with information about the risk of occurrence. As a targeted strategic initiative, the FDA aims to further advance the capabilities of the program to detect signals about the safety of approved products over the next decade.[76]

Hospitals have also invested in technologies and adopted pharmacovigilance methodologies for evaluating the safety profile of drugs at their institutions. The New York Presbyterian Hospital implemented a pharmacovigilance system that involved the electronic health record and used natural language computer processing. Various statistical techniques were used to establish associations between drugs and ADRs, as well as cutoff thresholds. In the hospital's feasibility study, seven drug classes were evaluated for novel adverse events. The researchers believed that the use of a comprehensive, unstructured data-monitoring program of electronic health records was a feasible option for computerized pharmacovigilance at the local health-system level. This study demonstrates that data mining and signal detection, even at the local level, provide an effective mechanism for ADR reporting.[77]

The traditional randomized controlled trial (RCT) is primarily designed to test the effectiveness of a drug or therapy and is not usually powered to detect relevant safety information. With this in mind, it is easy to see why ADRs may go undetected in these trials. As discussed previously, it is estimated that any ADR that occurs in fewer than 1 in 10,000 people will not be detected in most RCTs. Therefore, some experts have recommended the use of what is known as a large, simple trial (LST) to increase sample sizes and to monitor larger numbers of patients during clinical testing. LSTs have less stringent eligibility criteria than traditional RCTs, and subjects are typically studied for shorter periods of time. LST designs still use randomization techniques and continue to have important safety monitoring thresholds; they are not powered to determine efficacy. The larger sample sizes seen with the LST design provide more data for ADR monitoring methods like signal detection. In addition, the larger number of subjects increases the probability of picking up adverse events that are less common.[78] However, because LSTs are of relatively short duration, they do not overcome the challenge of detecting ADRs with a long latency.

Pharmacovigilance has traditionally relied on retrospective reports of ADRs, and relatively little information is available that helps health care professionals prospectively decide whether or not to use a drug in a particular patient. Pharmacogenomics may offer a solution for identifying characteristics and risk factors that predispose an individual to an ADR. Genetic variations in enzymes that metabolize and eliminate drugs can lead to a patient's increased exposure to a medication, potentially increasing their risk for adverse effects as well as reduced medication exposure and hence reduced effectiveness.[79] Genome-wide association studies scan for genetic markers across the DNA of many individuals to find variations that may be associated with serious ADRs.[80,81] A list of over 380 pharmacogenomic associations that have been identified and validated is available from the FDA and is regularly updated with label warnings of new medications found to have genomic biomarkers.[82]

Conclusion

ADRs are a serious problem in the U.S. health care system, causing significant morbidity and mortality as well as costing billions of dollars annually. Because of documented underreporting, these numbers represent only a small fraction of the ADRs occurring annually. Recognition of the problem is an important step in developing strategies to minimize the occurrence of ADRs. Reporting of these reactions by health care professionals is vital to gauging progress and directing the U.S.'s efforts in medication safety and patient care.

Health care practitioners play a vital role in developing, maintaining, and promoting ADR monitoring programs. Key steps in the development of these programs include identifying an institution-wide definition of ADRs, obtaining buy-in throughout the facility, establishing a mechanism to continuously screen for ADRs, and assigning responsibility for transmitting ADR reports. These programs provide valuable information about ADRs within the institution, as well as spontaneous reports of ADRs that can be forwarded to the FDA to aid in signal detection. ADR monitoring programs improve communication channels, generate additional education on adverse events, and positively impact patient care.

Technology is essential for monitoring, identifying, and minimizing ADRs, with most institutions and facilities utilizing computerized systems to screen for and alert practitioners to potential ADRs. The role of technology continues to expand as the FDA develops new approaches for signal detection and data mining. In addition, advances in pharmacogenetics may soon help practitioners proactively identify risk factors that predispose patients to an ADR, optimizing prescribing and medication management practices.

Despite the impact of ADRs and the tools available to assist in their management, ADRs remain underreported. Physicians and pharmacists report several barriers to reporting ADRs, including the time and hassle involved in reporting, as well as the belief that a single ADR report cannot contribute to medical knowledge to influence change in practice and regulations. ADR monitoring programs can only be successful if health care providers believe in their potential to improve patient safety and are willing to be active participants. Therefore, future efforts should focus on strategies for overcoming barriers to ADRs reporting in order to improve medication safety-related outcomes and improve patient care.

Self-Assessment Questions

1. Which of the following refers to an adverse drug reaction (ADR)?
   a. Any iatrogenic hazard or incident associated with a medication
   b. Any injury caused by a medication
   c. Any preventable event that leads to inappropriate medication use or patient harm
   d. Any unexpected, unintended, undesired, or excessive response to a medication
   e. Any reaction related to the intentional or unintentional overdose of a medication

2. Which of the following reactions is **NOT** an example of an ADR that the FDA would like health care professionals to report?
   a. A life-threatening reaction to a drug
   b. An ADR that is not currently listed in the drug's labeling
   c. A reaction that is a more severe form of a previously reported ADR
   d. A common or expected side effect
   e. An ADR of which the exact cause is not known

3. The first step in establishing an adverse drug reaction program at a facility is to:
    a. Determine the institution's definition of an adverse drug reaction
    b. Decide who is responsible for reporting adverse reactions to the FDA
    c. Develop an ADR reporting hotline
    d. Identify drugs most likely to cause adverse reactions
    e. Report findings of the ADR program to the P&T committee

4. Which of the following factors is **NOT** used to determine adverse reaction causality?
    a. Dechallenge
    b. Rechallenge
    c. Temporal relationship
    d. Patient gender
    e. Known response pattern

5. Which of the following has been cited as being superior for assessing the causality and probability of an ADR?
    a. Bayesian approach
    b. Kramer method
    c. Naranjo algorithm
    d. Liverpool ADR Causality Assessment Tool
    e. No algorithm has been proven superior

6. Which of the following statements is/are *true* regarding the Vaccine Adverse Event Reporting System (VAERS)?
    a. VAERS is a partnership between the FDA and the CDC.
    b. ADRs related to vaccine administration should be reported to VAERS instead of MedWatch.
    c. VAERS provides specific guidance on the kind of reactions that should be reported.
    d. Over 30,000 ADR reports are reported to VAERS annually.
    e. All of the above are true.

7. Which of the following best describes the role of technology in the management of ADRs?
    a. Technology can help identify and alert practitioners to potential ADRs.
    b. Technology eliminates the need for pharmacists to get involved in ADR management.
    c. Technology systems have not proven useful in the management of ADRs.
    d. Technology can only be used to report ADRs, not to aid in their detection.
    e. Technology has nearly eliminated fatalities due to ADRs.

8. Patients that experience an ADR typically encounter the following *except*:
   a. Loss of income from occupational absences
   b. Initial or prolonged hospitalization
   c. Increased visits to their primary care physician
   d. Lower cost of hospitalization
   e. Use of new medications to manage symptoms induced by the ADR

9. Which of the following are resources that can be used to assess and evaluate ADRs?
   a. Clin-Alert
   b. Reactions Weekly
   c. VigiAccess
   d. Meyler's Side Effects of Drugs
   e. All of the above

10. Which of the following is considered a barrier to reporting an ADR?
    a. Fear of litigation
    b. Guilt
    c. Paperwork and time involved
    d. Complacency
    e. All of the above

11. Which of the following statements about ADRs associated with dietary supplements is TRUE?
    a. Manufacturers of dietary supplements are not required to share ADR reports they receive with the FDA.
    b. The Dietary Supplement Ingredient Advisory List is a list of recommended ingredients that are safe for consumers.
    c. Dietary supplements are approved by the FDA and have a decreased chance of causing an ADR.
    d. Patients often do not tell their health care provider about supplement use or the ADRs they experience from them.
    e. The New Dietary Ingredients (NDI) Notification Process is only used for prescription medications.

12. The Sentinel System uses a data infrastructure that allows the FDA to rapidly access electronic health care data from data partners including:
    a. The World Health Organization
    b. Health insurers
    c. The Joint Commission
    d. a and b
    e. All of the above

13. All of the following are true regarding MAUDE *except*:
    a. MAUDE contains only device-related adverse event reports from manufacturers.
    b. Searchable data in MAUDE is limited to adverse events reported in the past 10 years.
    c. Variations in trade, product, and company names affect search results.
    d. MAUDE data is not intended to be used to evaluate rates of adverse events.
    e. All of the above.

14. Using the classification of ADR severity developed by Karch and Lasagna, an event that led to an additional length of stay in the hospital would be classified as:
    a. Minor
    b. Moderate
    c. Severe
    d. Lethal
    e. Event would NOT qualify as an ADR

15. Using the classification of ADR event type developed by Karch and Lasagna, an event where a patient developed unexpected, intractable nausea and vomiting from an unusually small dose of a medication would be labeled as:
    a. Idiosyncrasy
    b. Hypersensitivity
    c. Intolerance
    d. Drug interaction
    e. Pharmacologic

REFERENCES

1. American Society of Health-System Pharmacists. Suggested definitions and relationships among medication misadventures, medication errors, adverse drug events, and adverse drug reactions. Am J Health-Syst Pharm. 1998;55:165-6.
2. Rich DS. A process for interpreting data on adverse drug events: determining optimal target levels. Clin Ther. 1998;20(suppl C):C59-71.
3. Rich DS. The Joint Commission's revised sentinel event policy on medication errors. Hosp Pharm. 1998;33:881-5.
4. Kohn LT, Corrigan JM, Donaldson MS, editors. Institute of Medicine. To err is human: building a safer health system. Washington (DC): National Academy Press; 1999 Nov 1. p. 311.
5. White TJ, Arakelian A, Rho JP. Counting the costs of drug-related adverse events. Pharmacoeconomics. 1999;15:445-8.
6. Wong YL. Adverse effect of pharmaceutical recipients in drug therapy. Ann Acad Med. 1993;22:99-102.

7. Shehab N, Lovegrove MC, Geller AI, Rose KO, Weidle NJ, Budnitz DS. US emergency department visits for outpatient adverse drug events, 2013-2014. JAMA. 2016;316:2115–25.

8. Kochanek KD, Murphy SL, Xu J, Arias E. Deaths: final data for 2017. Natl Vital Stat Rep. 2019 Jun 24;68(9):1-77.

9. Sultana J, Cutroneo P, Trifiro G. Clinical and economic burden of adverse drug reactions. J Pharmacol Pharmacother. 2013 Dec;4(Suppl 1): S73–7.

10. Miguel A, Azevedo LF, Arajuo M, Pereira AC. Frequency of adverse drug reactions in hospitalized patients: a systematic review and meta-analysis. Pharmacoepidemiol Drug Saf. 2012;21(11):1139-54.

11. Sarkar U, Lopez A, Maselli JH, Gonzales R. Adverse drug events in U.S. adult ambulatory medical care. Health Serv Res. 2011 Oct;46(5):1517–33.

12. Fincham JE. An overview of adverse drug reactions. Am Pharm. 1991;NS31:435–41.

13. Hazell L, Shakir SA. Under-reporting of adverse drug reactions: a systematic review. Drug Saf. 2006;29(5):385-96.

14. Bond CA, Raehl CL. Clinical pharmacy services, pharmacy staffing, and adverse drug reactions in United States hospitals. Pharmacotherapy. 2006 Jun;26(6):735-47.

15. Lepakhin VK. Safety of medicines—a guide to detecting and reporting adverse drug reactions—why health professionals need to take action [Internet]. Geneva: World Health Organization; 2002. Available from: https://apps.who.int/iris/handle/10665/67378

16. American Society of Health-System Pharmacists. ASHP guidelines on adverse drug reaction monitoring and reporting. Am J Health-Syst Pharm. 1995;52(4):417-9

17. U.S. Food and Drug Administration. What is a serious adverse event? [Internet]. Silver Spring (MD): U.S. Food and Drug Administration; 2016 Feb 1 [cited 2019 Aug 26]. Available from: https://www.fda.gov/safety/reporting-serious-problems-fda/what-serious-adverse-event

18. U.S. Food and Drug Administration. Code of Federal Regulations Title 21 [Internet]. Silver Spring (MD): U.S. Food and Drug Administration; 2018 Apr 1 [cited 2019 Aug 26]. Available from: http://www.accessdata.fda.gov/scripts/cdrh/cfdocs/cfcfr/cfrsearch.cfm?fr=312.32

19. Edwards R, Aronson JK. Adverse drug reactions: definitions, diagnosis, and management. Lancet. 2000;356:1255-9.

20. Karch FE, Lasagna L. Toward the operational identification of adverse drug reactions. Clin Pharmacol Ther. 1977;21:247–54.

21. Agbabiaka TB, Savovic J, Ernst E. Methods for causality assessment of adverse drug reactions: a systematic review. Drug Safety. 2008;31:21-37.

22. Naranjo CA, Busto U, Sellers EM, Sandor P, Ruiz I, Roberts EA, Janecek E, Domecq C, Greenblatt DJ. A method of estimating the probability of adverse drug reactions. Clin Pharmacol Ther. 1981;30:239–45.

23. Castells MC, Solensky R. Rapid drug desensitization for immediate hypersensitivity reactions [Internet]. In: Adkinson NF, editor. UpToDate. Waltham (MA): UpToDate; 2017 [cited 2019 Aug 26]. Available from: www.uptodate.com

24. Kramer MS, Leventhal JM, Hutchinson TA, Feinstein AR. An algorithm for the operational assessment of adverse drug reactions: I. Background, description, and instructions for use. JAMA. 1979;242:623–32.

25. Hutchinson TA, Leventhal JM, Kramer MS, Karch FE, Lipman AG, Feinstein AR. An algorithm for the operational assessment of adverse drug reactions: II. Demonstration of reproducibility and validity. JAMA. 1979;242:633–8.

26. Jones JK. Adverse drug reactions in the community health setting: approaches to recognizing, counseling, and reporting. Fam Comm Health. 1982;5(2):58–67.

27. Michel DJ, Knodel LC. Comparison of three algorithms used to evaluate adverse drug reactions. Am J Hosp Pharm. 1986;43:1709–14.

28. Gallagher RM, Kirkham JJ, Mason JR, Bird KA, Williamson PR, Nunn AJ, Nunn AJ, Turner MA, Smyth RL, Pirmohamed M. Development and inter-rater reliability of the Liverpool Adverse Drug Reaction Causality Assessment Tool. PLoS ONE. 2011;6(12): e28096. doi:10.1371/journal.pone.0028096.

29. Lane DA. The Bayesian approach to causality assessment: an introduction. Drug Info J. 1986;20:455–61.

30. Lactot KL, Naranjo CA. Comparison of the Bayesian approach and a simple algorithm for assessment of adverse drug events. Clin Pharmacol Ther. 1995;58:692-8.

31. Garcia-Cortes M, Stephens C, Fernandez-Castaner A, Andrade RJ; Spanish Group for the Study of Drug-Induced Liver Disease. Causality assessment methods in drug induced liver injury: strengths and weaknesses. J Hepatol. 2011;55(3):683-91.

32. U.S. Food and Drug Administration. MedWatch: the FDA safety information and adverse event reporting program [Internet]. Silver Spring (MD): U.S. Food and Drug Administration; 2019 Jun 19 [cited 2019 Aug 26]. Available from: http://www.fda.gov/Safety/MedWatch/SafetyInformation/default.htm

33. U.S. Food and Drug Administration. FDA Adverse Event Reporting System (FAERS) Public Dashboard [Internet]. Silver Spring (MD): U.S. Food and Drug Administration; 2018 Jul 23 [cited 2019 Sep 11]. Available from: https://www.fda.gov/drugs/questions-and-answers-fdas-adverse-event-reporting-system-faers/fda-adverse-event-reporting-system-faers-public-dashboard

34. Vigiaccess. About [Internet]. [place unknown]: World Health Organization; [cited 2019 Sep 16]. Available from: http://www.vigiaccess.org/

35. Springer—International Publisher Science, Technology, Medicine. Reactions Weekly: About this journal [Internet]. Berlin (DE): Springer Science+Business Media; c2016 [cited 2019 Sep 16]. Available from: http://www.springer.com/adis/journal/40278

36. SAGE Journals. Clin-Alert [Internet]. Thousand Oaks (CA): SAGE Journals; c2016 [cited 2019 Sep 16]. Available from: http://cla.sagepub.com/

37. U.S. Department of Health and Human Services. Common Terminology Criteria for Adverse Events (CTCAE). Version 5.0. 2017 Nov 27 [cited 2020 Sep 25]. Available from: https://ctep.cancer.gov/protocolDevelopment/electronic_applications/docs/CTCAE_v5_Quick_Reference_5x7.pdf

38. Edwards R, Aronson JK. Adverse drug reactions: definitions, diagnosis, and management. Lancet. 2000;356:1255-9.

39. Centers for Medicare & Medicaid Services. Transmittal 72 Revised Appendix A: conditions of participation and interpretive guidelines for hospitals [Internet]. Baltimore (MD): Department of Health & Human Services and Centers for Medicare & Medicaid Services; 2011 Nov 18 [cited 2019 Aug 27]. Available from: https://www.cms.gov/Regulations-and-Guidance/Guidance/Transmittals/downloads/R72SOM.pdf

40. Joint Commission. Comprehensive Accreditation Manual for Hospitals (e-edition). Joint Commission Resources; c2019 [cited 2019 Aug 27]. Available from: https://e-dition.jcrinc.com/MainContent.aspx

41. ASHP guidelines on adverse drug reaction monitoring and reporting. Am J Health-Syst Pharm. 1995 Feb 15;52(4):417-9.

42. Saltiel E, Johnson E, Shane R. A team approach to adverse drug reaction surveillance: success at a tertiary care hospital. Hosp Form. 1995 Apr;30(4):226-8, 231-2.

43. Classen DC, Pestotnik SL, Evans RS, Burke JP. Computerized surveillance of adverse drug events in hospitalized patients. Qual Saf Health Care. 2005 June;14:221-6.

44. Institute for Safe Medication Practices. Adverse drug reactions: documentation is important but communication is critical. ISMP Medication Safety Alert Acute Care Newsletter. 2000 Sep 6;5(18):1.

45. AHRQ: Archive [Internet]. Rockville (MD): AHRQ; c2016. Making health care safer: a critical analysis of patient safety practices—Evidence report/technology assessment, No. 43. 2001 Jul [cited 2019 Aug 28]. Available from: http://archive.ahrq.gov/clinic/ptsafety/.

46. Cozart H, Horvath MM, Long A, Whitehurst J, Eckstrand J, Ferranti J. Culture counts—sustainable inpatient computerized surveillance across Duke University Health System. Q Manage Health Care. 2010 Oct-Dec;19(4):1-10.

47. Ferranti J, Horvath MM, Cozart H, Whitehurst J, Eckstrand J. Reevaluating the safety profile of pediatrics: a comparison of computerized adverse drug event surveillance and voluntary reporting in the pediatric environment. Pediatrics. 2008 May;121(5):e1201-7.

48. Hickner J, Zafar A, Kuo GM, Fagnan LJ, Forjuoh SN, Knox LM, Lynch JT, Stevens BK, Pace WD, Hamlin BN, Scherer H, Hudson BL, Oppenheimer CC, Tierney WM. Field test results of a new ambulatory care medication error and adverse drug event reporting system—MEADERS. Ann Fam Med. 2010 Nov-Dec;8(6):517-25.

49. Zafar A, Hickner J, Pace W, Tierney W. A medication error and adverse drug event reporting system for ambulatory care (MEADERS). AMIA Annu Symp Proc. 2008;6:839-43.

50. van Grootheest AC, de Jong-van den Berg LTW. The role of hospital and community pharmacists in pharmacovigilance. Res Soc Admin Pharm. 2005 Mar;1(1):126-33.

51. Emmendorfer T, Glassman PA, Moore V, Leadholm TC, Good CB, Cunningham F. Monitoring adverse drug reactions across a nationwide health care system using information technology. Am J Health-Syst Pharm. 2012 Feb 15;69(4):321-8.

52. Harmark L, van Grootheest AC. Pharmacovigilance: methods, recent developments and future perspectives. Eur J Clin Pharmacol. 2008 Aug;64:743-52.

53. FDA: Drugs [Internet]. Silver Spring (MD): FDA; c2019. Reports received and reports entered into FAERS by year. 2015 Nov 10 [cited 2019 Aug 29]. Available from: https://www.fda.gov/drugs/questions-and-answers-fdas-adverse-event-reporting-system-faers/reports-received-and-reports-entered-faers-year

54. FDA: Safety [Internet]. Silver Spring (MD): FDA; c2019. Reporting by health professionals. 2016 Mar 25 [cited 2019 Aug 29]. Available from: https://www.fda.gov/safety/reporting-serious-problems-fda/reporting-health-professionals

55. Hoffman RP. Adverse drug reaction reporting—problems and solutions. J Mich Pharm. 1989;27:400-3, 407-8.

56. Lopez-Gonzalez E, Herdeiro MT, Figueiras A. Determinants of under-reporting of adverse drug reactions: a systematic review. Drug Saf. 2009;32(1):19-31.

57. Gavaza P, Brown CM, Lawson KA, Rascati KL, Wilson JP, Steinhardt M. Influence of attitudes on pharmacists' intention to report serious adverse drug events to the Food and Drug Administration. Br J Clin Pharmacol. 2011 Jul;72(1):143-52.

58. Du DT, Goldsmith J, Aikin KJ, Encinosa WE, Nardinelli C. Despite 2007 law requiring FDA hotline to be included in print drug ads, reporting of adverse events by consumers still low. Health Aff (Millwood). 2012 May;31(5):1022-9.

59. FDA: Drugs [Internet]. Silver Spring (MD): FDA; c2016. AERS reporting by healthcare providers and consumers by year. 2015 Nov 24 [cited 2019 Sep 16]. Available from: http://www.fda.gov/Drugs/GuidanceComplianceRegulatoryInformation/Surveillance/AdverseDrugEffects/ucm070456.htm

60. FDA: For consumers [Internet]. Silver Spring (MD): FDA; c2016. FDA 101: How to use the Consumer Complaint System and MedWatch. 2016 Sep 9 [cited 2019 Sep 16]. Available from: http://www.fda.gov/ForConsumers/ConsumerUpdates/ucm049087.htm

61. Timbo BB, Ross MP, McCarthy PV, Lin CT. Dietary supplements in a nationwide survey: prevalence of use and reports of adverse events. J Am Diet Assoc. 2006;106:1966-74.

62. U.S. Food and Drug Administration. Select amendments to the FD&C Act: Dietary Supplement and Nonprescription Drug Consumer Protection Act [Internet]. Silver Spring (MD): U.S. Food and Drug Administration; 2009 May 20 [updated 2009 May 20; cited 2019 Sep 16]. Available from: https://www.fda.gov/regulatory-information/laws-enforced-fda/selected-amendments-fdc-act

63. U.S. Food and Drug Administration. Dietary Supplement Ingredient List [Internet]. Silver Spring (MD): U.S. Food and Drug Administration; 2019 Jun 24 [cited 2019 Sep 11]. Available from: https://www.fda.gov/food/dietary-supplement-products-ingredients/dietary-supplement-ingredient-advisory-list

64. U.S. Food and Drug Administration. New Dietary Ingredients (NDI) Notification Process [Internet]. Silver Spring (MD): U.S. Food and Drug Administration; 2019 Sep 6 [cited 2019 Sep 11]. Available from: https://www.fda.gov/food/dietary-supplements/new-dietary-ingredients-ndi-notification-process

65. U.S. Government Printing Office. Federal Register Volume 69, Number 28 [Internet]. Washington (DC): U.S. Government Printing Office; 2004 Feb 11 [cited 2019 Sep 16]. Available from: http://www.gpo.gov/fdsys/pkg/FR-2004-02-11/html/04-2912.htm

66. American Botanical Council. Federal court overturns FDA ban on ephedra at low doses [Internet]. Austin (TX): American Botanical Council; c2016 [cited 2019 Sep 16]. Available from: http://cms.herbalgram.org/press/FDAephedra.html

67. Natural Medicines Comprehensive Database. Natural MedWatch: Adverse event reporting form [Internet]. Stockton (CA): Therapeutic Research Center; c2019 [cited 2019 Sep 16]. Available from: https://naturaldatabase.therapeuticresearch.com/nd/adverseevent.aspx

68. Woo JJY. Adverse event monitoring and multivitamin-multimineral dietary supplements. Am J Clin Nutr. 2007;85:323S-324S.

69. Timbo BB, Chirtel SJ, Ihrie J, Oladipo T, Velez-Suarez L, Brewer V, Mozersky R. Dietary supplement adverse event report data from the FDA center for food safety and applied nutrition adverse event reporting system (CAERS), 2004-2013. Ann Pharmacother. 2018; 52(5):431-8.

70. Vaccine Adverse Event Reporting System. Information for healthcare professionals [Internet]. Rockville (MD): U.S. Department of Health and Human Services; [cited 2019 Sep 16]. Available from: http://vaers.hhs.gov/professionals/index

71. Centers for Disease Control and Prevention. Vaccine Adverse Events Reporting System (VAERS) [Internet]. Atlanta (GA): U.S. Department of Health and Human Services; 2015 Aug 28 [cited 2019 Sep 16]. Available from: https://www.cdc.gov/vaccinesafety/ensuringsafety/monitoring/vaers/index.html

72. U.S. Food and Drug Administration. Medical Device Overview; 2018 Sep 14 [cited 2019 Sep 11]. Available from: https://www.fda.gov/industry/regulated-products/medical-device-overview

73. U.S. Food and Drug Administration. Medical Device Reporting (MDR): how to report medical device problems [Internet]. Silver Spring (MD): U.S. Food and Drug Administration; 2019 Jul 8 [cited 2019 Sep 11]. Available from: https://www.fda.gov/medical-devices/medical-device-safety/medical-device-reporting-mdr-how-report-medical-device-problems

74. U.S. Food and Drug Administration. MAUDE—Manufacturer and User Facility Device Experience [Internet]. Silver Spring (MD): U.S. Food and Drug Administration; 2019 Aug 31 [cited 2019 Sep 11]. Available from: https://www.accessdata.fda.gov/scripts/cdrh/cfdocs/cfMAUDE/TextSearch.cfm

75. U.S. Food and Drug Administration. MedWatcher Mobile App [Internet]. Silver Spring (MD): U.S. Food and Drug Administration; 2018 Sep 25 [cited 2019 Sep 11]. Available from: https://www.fda.gov/medical-devices/medical-device-reporting-mdr-how-report-medical-device-problems/medwatcher-mobile-app

76. Kuehn BM. FDA's foray into big data still maturing. JAMA. 2016 May 10; 315(18):1934-6.

77. Want XY, Hripcsak G, Markatou M, Friedman C. Active computerized pharmacovigilance using natural language processing, statistics, and electronic health records: a feasibility study. J Am Med Inform Assoc. 2009;16:328-37.

78. Peto R, Collins R, Gray R. Large-scale randomized evidence: large, simple trials and overview of trials. J Clin Epidemiol. 1995;48:23-40.

79. National Human Genome Research Institute. Genome-wide association studies fact sheet [Internet]. Bethesda (MD): National Institutes of Health; 2015 Aug 15 [cited 2019 Sep 9]. Available from: http://www.genome.gov/20019523

80. Kacevska M, Ivanov M, Ingelman-Sundberg M. Perspectives on epigenetics and its relevance to adverse drug reactions. Clin Pharm Ther. 2011;89(6):902-7.

81. Daly AK. Using genome-wide association studies to identify genes important in serious adverse drug reactions. Ann Rev Pharmacol Toxicol. 2012;582:21-35.

82. U.S. Food and Drug Administration. Table of pharmacogenomic biomarkers in drug labeling [Internet]. Silver Spring (MD): U.S. Food and Drug Administration; 2019 Sep 3 [cited 2019 Sep 9]. Available from: https://www.fda.gov/drugs/science-research-drugs/table-pharmacogenomic-biomarkers-drug-labeling

SUGGESTED READINGS

1. Harmark L, van Grootheest AC. Pharmacovigilance: methods, recent developments and future perspectives. Eur J Clin Pharmacol. 2008;64:743-52.

2. Lepakhin VK. Safety of medicines—a guide to detecting and reporting adverse drug reactions—why health professionals need to take action [Internet]. Geneva: World Health Organization; 2002. Available from: https://apps.who.int/iris/handle/10665/67378

3. Naranjo CA, Busto U, Sellers EM, Sandor P, Ruiz I, Roberts EA, Janecek E, Domecq C, Greenblatt DJ. A method for estimating the probability of adverse drug reactions. Clin Pharmacol Ther. 1981;30:239-45.

4. U.S. Food and Drug Administration. FDA drug topics: FDA Adverse Events Reporting System (FAERS) public dashboard—Webinar presentation [Internet]. Silver Spring (MD): U.S. Food and Drug Administration; 2018 Feb 21 [cited 2019 Sep 6]. Available from: https://www.fda.gov/about-fda/fda-pharmacy-student-experiential-program/fda-drug-topics-fda-adverse-events-reporting-system-faers-public-dashboard-january-30-2018

20

Chapter Twenty

Medication Safety II: Medication Errors

Katie Johnson • Liz Hess

Learning Objectives

After completing this chapter, the reader will be able to:

- Define and compare the terms "medication errors," "adverse drug events," and "adverse drug reactions."
- Describe methods to identify medication errors and adverse drug events.
- Assign an event type and severity to reported events.
- Describe skill-based, rule-based, and knowledge-based errors.
- Explain a systems approach to error.
- Determine strategies health care practitioners and health systems can implement to reduce medication errors.
- List two common methods of analyzing medication errors and adverse drug events that are utilized to develop action plans for error prevention and harm reduction.
- Compare and contrast a Just Culture with a blame-free culture, and punitive culture.
- Identify resources promoting best practices in patient and medication safety.

Key Concepts

❶ The terms "medication error," "adverse drug event," and "adverse drug reaction" are similar and often confused. They are interrelated, yet distinct occurrences.

❷ Several methods of identifying errors are recommended to gain a more global understanding of the risks and errors occurring within an organization.

❸ Classification of errors by type is a common method to identify common themes of medication events.

④ Understanding the three modes of human performance (skill-based, rule-based, and knowledge-based) is important to understanding human errors.

⑤ Humans will commit errors despite their best efforts not to. Therefore, it is critical to design systems that account for human error and put processes and technology in place to intercept errors before they reach and harm patients. The system should make it hard to do the wrong thing and easy to do the right thing.

⑥ Poorly designed systems and processes are a significant contributor to error and subsequent patient harm. Errors rarely occur solely because of a mistake by a single health care professional, but rather in combination with one or more latent system failures.

⑦ Incorporation of human factors (HF) principles into process design and product selection can improve safety.

⑧ Failure modes and effects analysis (FMEA) is a prospective method of evaluating processes to identify how and why a process could fail, potential impacts of failure, and developing actions to prevent failure and mitigate harm.

⑨ Evaluation of safety events through root cause analysis (RCA) and other methods is key to learning from errors and preventing reoccurrence.

⑩ A Just Culture is a balance between accountability of organizations for the systems designed and the behaviors of employees within that system.

Introduction

Much attention has been focused on adverse outcomes in health care in the past 20 years. While pockets of research in medical errors were developing prior to 2000, the National Academy of Medicine's (NAM; previously named the Institute of Medicine [IOM] at the time) report, To Err is Human: Building a Safer Health System,[1] released in late 1999, served as a catalyst for additional research in the causes and methods to prevent adverse outcomes in health care. Based on two landmark trials, this report estimated 44,000–98,000 people die each year as a result of medical errors.[1-3] The report notes that medication errors, a subset of medical errors, whether occurring within or outside of the hospital, were estimated to account for over 7000 deaths annually. The majority of literature to date has focused on work in the hospital setting, as it is, for the most part, a closed and controlled environment. Other settings are less well researched, although early studies of nursing homes and ambulatory settings have shown significant opportunities for improvement.[1] Few have attempted to capture the prevalence of medication errors resulting in death since the first NAM report. In 2016, authors Makary and Daniel estimated medical errors to be the third leading cause of death in the United States, behind heart disease and cancer, by extrapolating reported death rates from medical error to total U.S.

hospital admissions per year.[4] It is clear that medical errors and medication safety still represent serious concerns for patients and health care providers.

While many health care professionals have responsibilities in the medication use process, pharmacists play a pivotal role in ensuring the safe use of medication. Pharmacists' provision of accurate drug information and identification of potential medication-related adverse effects to diverse health care providers is of vital importance. Throughout the medication use process, there are many opportunities for unexpected events, including errors in prescribing, dispensing, and administering medications, and other adverse effects. These events can all be described as medication errors.[5] All health care providers need a sound understanding of the risks for error and the ability to identify the underlying causes of medication errors and be responsible for taking steps to prevent such occurrences and minimize adverse outcomes. This usually involves collaborative work with interprofessional health care team members to ensure optimal outcomes. Pharmacists in particular are well positioned to lead these efforts in reducing harm to patients.

Definitions: Medication Errors, Adverse Drug Events (ADES), and Adverse Drug Reactions (ADRS)

❶ *The terms "medication error," "adverse drug event," and "adverse drug reaction" are similar and often confused. They are interrelated, yet distinct occurrences.* The terminology surrounding medication errors is often confusing; there are many definitions that are very similar. The term **adverse events** is an overarching term, which includes medication errors, **adverse drug events (ADEs)**, and **adverse drug reactions (ADRs)**. The National Coordinating Council for Medication Error Reporting and Prevention (NCC MERP) defines a **medication error** as a preventable event:

> Any preventable event that may cause or lead to inappropriate medication use or patient harm while the medication is in the control of the health care professional, patient, or consumer. Such events may be related to professional practice, health care products, procedures, and systems, including prescribing; order communication; product labeling, packaging, and nomenclature; compounding; dispensing; distribution; administration; education; monitoring; and use.[6]

Key points related to medication errors include:

- Medication errors are preventable.
- Medication errors can be caused by errors in the planning (deciding what to do—which drug and/or what dose) or execution stages (completing the task that was decided on—administering the drug to the wrong patient).

- Medication errors include errors of omission (missed dose or appropriate medication not prescribed) or commission (wrong drug given).
- Medication errors may or may not cause patient harm.

Based on the NCC MERP definition, an error may occur at any point in the medication use process, including as a result of not adequately counseling or educating a patient on proper use of medication. When, for example, a patient inappropriately uses a metered-dose inhaler for asthma and fails to receive the full amount of the medication, a medication error has occurred. The error may be secondary to a lack of education or may have occurred despite adequate counseling and education. Independent of the cause, based on the above definition, a medication error did occur.

Based on this definition, a medication error also occurs when a prescriber orders the incorrect dose of a medication. Even if the prescriber is called by a pharmacist to clarify and change the order and the patient eventually receives an appropriately dosed medication, an error did occur in the process. An adverse outcome is not necessary to classify an event as a medication error. This would be a near miss medication error since the wrong dose of the medication did not reach the patient.

An ADE involves harm to a patient. An ADE is defined as an injury from a medicine or lack of intended medicine.[7] An ADE refers to all ADRs, including allergic or idiosyncratic reactions, as well as medication errors that result in harm to a patient. It is estimated that 3–5% of medication errors result in harm to a patient and can also be classified as an ADE.

An ADR is defined by the World Health Organization (WHO) as "any response that is noxious, unintended, or undesired, which occurs at doses normally used in humans for prophylaxis, diagnosis, therapy of disease or modification of physiological function."[8]

The relationship between the terms is illustrated in Figure 19-1 (see previous chapter). While there are standard definitions for medication errors, there may be significant differences in the interpretation, reporting rates, and severity ranking between institutions. Common questions that arise are included in Table 20-1. For example, one institution may determine that an error has occurred when a dose is not received by a patient

TABLE 20–1. COMMON QUESTIONS THAT ARISE IN DEFINING MEDICATION ERRORS AND ADVERSE DRUG EVENTS

- Is it an error if it does not reach the patient?
- Is it an error if it does not cause harm?
- What constitutes minimal harm? Moderate? Severe?
- Is it an error or event if it is not clinically significant?
- Should health care professionals interventions related to inappropriate orders by prescribers be documented and counted as prescribing errors?
- What is considered preventable?

within 30 minutes of the scheduled time, where another may permit 60 minutes before or after the scheduled administration time. Some institutions may not report an inappropriately written prescription, if that error is caught by a clinician before the medication reaches the patient. Instead, a pharmacist or nurse may report it as a professional intervention. According to most definitions, this would count as an error and can provide valuable information to improve the system. These variations make it very difficult to compare data from one institution to another. Therefore, it is best for an institution to use its own data to monitor improvement, rather than benchmark.

The Impact of Errors on Patients and Health Care Systems

Patients depend on health care systems and health care professionals to help them stay healthy. As a result, patients frequently receive drug therapy with the notion that these medications will help them lead a healthier life. The initiation of drug therapy is the most common medical treatment received by patients.[9] According to the Centers for Disease Control and Prevention (CDC), 73.9% of physician office visits and 81.1% of emergency department (ED) visits are related to medication therapy.[10] In virtually all cases, patients and their health care providers understand that when medications are given, there are some known and some unknown risks. It is important that patients understand that they may experience unexpected drug-related morbidity and mortality which, although rare, may be significant.

Several landmark studies have identified the risk of medication errors and ADEs in varying populations and settings. The Harvard Medical Practice Study I was a landmark study that estimated that 3.7% of hospitalized patients experience adverse events.[2] The findings and extrapolated statistics from this study along with the Harvard Medical Practice Study II served as the grounds for the statement (from To Err is Human) that approximately 44,000–98,000 people are killed by medical errors every year. For medication errors specifically, the National Academy of Medicine in 2007 estimated that hospitalized patients experience one medication error per day during each admission.[11] In oncology patients, a 2018 systematic review reported one to four errors per 1000 chemotherapy orders and estimated that 1–3% of oncology patients experience at least one medication error during their treatment course.[12] Pediatric patients appear to be at an increased risk of medication errors and ADEs compared to adult patients, with studies suggesting three times the risk of error and 2.4 times the risk of ADE versus adults.[13] Wrong dose errors are common in pediatrics, often arising from weight-based dose calculations and use of nonstandard medication doses and preparations. Patients in EDs are another population at increased risk of error, with studies estimating medication error rates of 4–14%, and even up to 39% in pediatric ED patients.[14,15] Contributing factors to errors in the ED include limited access to past medical history, high patient acuity, use of verbal orders, limited pharmacist oversight, and double checks on medication preparation, among other factors. In the outpatient setting, Gurwitz and associates reported 50.1 ADEs per 1000 person-years in ambulatory patients[16] and 227 ADEs per 1000 resident-years in the nursing home setting.[17] The economic impact of medication errors and ADEs is staggering and adds unnecessarily to the health care cost burden. Several important studies documented the economic burden of these events.[18–21] A landmark study in 1995 estimated that ADE-related costs in the United States were $76.6 billion annually in ambulatory patients alone.[18] Drug expenditures in ambulatory patients at that time were $80 billion per year. This means that for every $1 spent for a drug, almost $1 was also being spent due to a drug-related problem. These costs exceed the total cost of managing patients with diabetes or cardiovascular diseases.[19] A subsequent study demonstrated that the cost of drug-related morbidity and mortality in the ambulatory setting exceeded $177 billion in 2000.[21] A study from 2011 found that inappropriate medication use resulted in $500 billion in annual avoidable costs worldwide.[22]

While it was initially thought that medication errors were caused by individual health care practitioners, including pharmacists, physicians, and nurses, now it is clear that our health care systems and processes often are causative or contributing factors in the majority of errors and events. Efforts to decrease adverse outcomes will not be successful if these system and process-related issues are not addressed. Multiple agencies and professional organizations across the country are now contributing efforts to minimize these events (Table 20-2), discussed later on in the chapter.

Identification and Reporting of Medication Errors and Adverse Drug Events

❷ *Several methods of identifying errors are recommended to gain a more global understanding of the risks and errors occurring within an organization.* It is important that a systematic approach to the identification and assessment of errors and adverse events be utilized in order to identify trends and opportunities for improvement based on events occurring at a location. This should involve several methods, and include prospective and retrospective methods of identifying errors and risks when possible. Many methods of identifying errors in health care exist, including voluntary reporting, direct observation, chart review, trigger identification, and computerized monitoring. These methods are described further here.

TABLE 20–2. ORGANIZATIONS INVOLVED IN PREVENTING MEDICATION ERRORS AND ADVERSE DRUG EVENTS

Organization	Website
Agency for Healthcare Research and Quality (AHRQ)	https:// www.ahrq.gov
AHRQ Patient Safety Network	https:// psnet.ahrq.gov
Alliance for Safe Online Pharmacies (ASOP)	https://buysaferx.pharmacy
American Society of Health-System Pharmacists (ASHP)	https:// www.ashp.org
Centers for Disease Control and Prevention (CDC)	https:// www.cdc.gov
Centers for Medicare and Medicaid Services (CMS)	https://www.cms.hhs.gov
Center for Safe Internet Pharmacies (CSIP)	https://safemedsonline.org
Global Enteral Device Supplier Association (GEDSA)	https:// www.gedsa.org
Institute for Healthcare Improvement (IHI)	https://www.ihi.org
Institute for Safe Medication Practices (ISMP)	https:// www.ismp.org
International Medication Safety Network (IMSN)	https:// www.intmedsafe.net
Massachusetts Coalition for the Prevention of Medical Errors	https:// www.macoalition.org
National Quality Forum (NQF)	https://www.qualityforum.org
Patient Safety and Quality Healthcare (PSQH)	https://www.psqh.com
The Advisory Board	https:// www.advisory.com
The Joint Commission (TJC)	https:// www.jointcommission.org
The Joint Commission International	https:// www.jointcommissioninternational.org
The Leapfrog Group	https:// www.leapfroggroup.org
United States Pharmacopeia (USP)	https://www.usp.org
U.S. Food and Drug Administration (FDA)	https://www.fda.gov
U.S. Health Resources and Services Administration (HRSA)	https:// www.hrsa.gov
World Health Organization (WHO)	https:// www.who.int

1. A voluntary reporting system (online, paper, or telephonic) is the most common method of identification of errors and events. Many institutions include an anonymous option for those who do not feel comfortable providing their name and contact information. Anyone detecting or committing an error can report it without associating their name with the error. It is essentially risk-free for the reporter and, therefore, it may increase the likelihood of having an error reported. While voluntary reporting is the least labor-intensive method, it is also the least-effective method of identifying errors and adverse events.[23] When compared with other methods of detection, voluntary reporting only identifies approximately 1 in 20 errors and 1 in 90 adverse events.[24,25] Therefore, it is important to utilize other methods of detection in addition to a voluntary reporting system.

2. The direct-observation method uses trained observers to watch the real-time delivery of medications. Notes from the observations are compared with prescribers'

orders to determine if an error has occurred. Results with this method are more valid and reliable than with voluntary reporting, but the impact of the observer on the subject being observed and interobserver agreement has been questioned.[26,27] This method is costly, time-consuming, and limited to the identification of errors that occur during the administration phase of the medication use process. It typically samples a selected time period on a selected unit, limiting the extrapolation to other time periods or patient care areas. On the positive side, errors are often identified that may never be discovered through other methods as they may go unrecognized.

3. Chart review identification of medication errors and ADEs is very labor intensive and is not generally practical outside of the research environment. Various trained staff review charts looking for particular cues or data elements that signify an error or event has occurred. This method relies on practitioners to document these events when identified during the patient care encounter, which may lead to an underestimation of the true occurrence.

4. A modified version of chart review can be performed with the use of trigger tools. Trigger tools involve searching patient charts for cues or triggers that signal a patient may have experienced an error and/or adverse event. There are several types of trigger tools promoted by the Institute for Healthcare Improvement (IHI); the tool specific to medications is called the **ADE Trigger Tool**.[28] Example triggers (See Table 20-3) include the use of reversal agents (e.g., flumazenil, naloxone, phytonadione) and abnormal lab values such as high international normalized ratio (INR) or low blood glucose value. When these triggers are identified in a patient's chart, the chart is reviewed for additional evidence of error and/or level of harm, and data is collected and collated to determine potential common causes. For example, reviewing the charts of patients who experience hypoglycemia may reveal errors, such as incorrect insulin dosing while patients are receiving nothing by mouth in preparation for a surgical procedure. Upon review of patients requiring the use of naloxone, it may be discovered that the dosing for hydromorphone and morphine are often confused during the prescribing, administration, and monitoring phases leading to oversedation. The advantage to using this trigger method is that these types of events are rarely reported as errors. Specific information on the use of this tool is available at http://www.ihi.org.

5. Health information technology (HIT) (see Chapter 28 for more information on this topic) is another important source of data on medication errors.[29-35] Electronic health records (EHRs), computerized provider order entry (CPOE), barcoded medication dispensing (e.g., carousels, sterile products workflow systems), automated dispensing cabinets (ADCs), barcoded medication administration

TABLE 20–3. ADVERSE DRUG EVENT TRIGGERS

Medications

Antidiarrheal agents

Atropine (exclude preoperative use)

Dextrose 50% (IV push)

Diphenhydramine (excluding orders for sleep)

Epinephrine (IV push)

Flumazenil

Naloxone

Droperidol

Sodium polystyrene sulfonate

Vitamin K

Conditions

PTT > 100 sec

INR > 6

WBC < 3 K/uL

Glucose < 50 mg/dL

Rising serum creatinine

Clostridium difficile-positive stool

Digoxin level > 2 ng/mL

Lidocaine level > 5 μg/mL

Gentamicin/tobramycin peak > 10 μg/mL or trough > 2 μg/mL

Amikacin peak > 30 μg/mL or trough > 10 μg/mL

Vancomycin level > 26 μg/mL

Theophylline level > 20 μg/mL

Oversedation, lethargy, fall, rash

Abrupt medication stop

Transfer to higher level of care

(BCMA), and smart infusion pumps are examples of HIT that can be leveraged for medication error detection and investigation. For example, every keystroke a nurse makes in programming a smart infusion pump is recorded. This data can be analyzed to detect potential unreported errors or in response to a known error to investigate the details and root causes. Examples of HIT data that can be reviewed to detect potential errors are barcode scan mismatches and overrides during medication dispensing and administration, medications overridden out of an ADC without an electronic order, and smart infusion pumps programmed over or under safety limits. Data might be reviewed as a set to derive common themes, or by searching for specific text or data points with a logic-based rule system.

Classification of Error Types

❸ *Classification of errors by type is a common method to identify common themes of medica-tion events.* The most common way to classify errors is to identify them by type of error. There have been many taxonomies of errors developed by various groups, including WHO, TJC, MEDMARX®, and others. The most commonly utilized event-type classifica-tion of medication errors is defined by NCC MERP taxonomy.[36]

- Wrong patient—A wrong patient error occurs when a medication is given to the wrong patient, usually caused by an error in patient identification and confirma-tion. Two identifiers should be used to identify the patient every time a patient is given a medication. Confirming patient identification is necessary whenever a pharmacist or physician writes or enters an order, or dispenses a medication in outpatient areas, or when a nurse administers a medication.
- Dose omission—This error occurs when a dose intended for a patient is not administered. This may occur when a decision is made to start a medication, but the first dose is missed. Another example is if the patient is off the unit and the medication is not administered when the patient arrives back on the floor. Patients who refuse a dose are excluded.
- Wrong time error—What constitutes a wrong time error may vary considerably among organizations. In general, this type of error occurs when a dose is not administered in accordance with a predetermined administration interval. Most organizations realize that it is often impossible to be totally accurate with the administration interval and typically allow 15–60 minutes outside that interval. Establishing a policy to indicate what constitutes an error in this category is needed for consistent reporting and data collection.
- Improper dose—An incorrect dose error can occur when a prescriber orders an inappropriate dose of a medication or when the dose administered is different than what was prescribed. An omission error occurs when a patient does not receive a scheduled dose of medication.
- Wrong dosage form—A wrong dosage form error can occur when the prescriber makes an error or when a patient receives a dosage form different from that pre-scribed, assuming the appropriate dosage form was originally ordered. An exam-ple is administration of an immediate-release medication when an extended-release version of the medication was ordered.
- Wrong strength/concentration—This is an error that can occur at several points in the medication use process, from prescribing to administration. The provider may choose the wrong strength when entering the order, a pharmacy technician may select the wrong drug for dispensing, or a nurse may choose the wrong drug

upon administration. The appropriate use of barcode administration of medications in the inpatient setting makes it harder for these errors to occur.

- Wrong drug—This error occurs when a medication is ordered, retrieved, or administered that was not intended for the patient. This may occur when a patient receives a medication intended for another patient, due to inadequate patient identification, or when a nurse obtains the incorrect medication for administration, perhaps from floor stock. Barcode scanning is designed to prevent these errors and others.

- Wrong route of administration—Some of the most harmful incorrect route errors have included administration of enteral tube feeding into an intravenous (IV) line or instillation of an IV medication intrathecally that is not designed to be given this route.[37,38] One significant cause is the fact that these varying types of tubing fit together, which is considered a systems problem. In an effort to reduce the chance of this occurrence, tubing designed to fit only based on the intended use would be optimal (e.g., IV, enteral feeding, intrathecal, dialysis).

- Wrong technique—When medications require some type of preparation, such as reconstitution, this type of error may occur. These kinds of errors may also occur in the compounding of various IV admixtures and other products and can occur when nurses, pharmacists, or technicians are preparing medications.

- Wrong rate (e.g., too fast, too slow, or unknown rate)—This category generally applies to IV infusions, but can also apply to an IV push medication if the drug is pushed too quickly or too slowly.

- Wrong duration—The patient receives the medication for a shorter or longer time period than prescribed. For example, a patient has an order for antibiotics without a defined stop date and the provider does not discontinue the order for several days after the intended course of therapy is already completed.

- Deteriorated drug error—This error occurs when a drug is administered after its expiration date or has deteriorated prematurely due to improper storage conditions.

- Monitoring error (subcategories drug-drug, drug-food, documented allergy, drug-disease, clinical)—These errors may occur due to lack of adequate interfaces between different computer or technology software programs, resulting in the appropriate information not being available to apprise health care providers of potential risks. Alternatively, the information may have been available in the electronic system but overridden without due consideration by the health care provider. An example of this is a medication known to be contraindicated for the patient due to the presence of a drug-drug interaction or drug-food interaction being administered to the patient without proper consideration of the interaction.

- Other medication error—Any other medication error that does not fit into one of the above categories.

As a result of the development of **Patient Safety Organizations** (PSOs), a common taxonomy and language was developed to enable health care providers to collect and submit standardized information related to safety events. These standard event reporting forms are called the Common Formats. The Common Formats define the standardized data elements associated with errors and events that are to be collected and reported to the PSO. The scope of Common Formats applies to all patient safety concerns including events reaching the patient (with or without harm), near miss events that do not reach the patient, and unsafe conditions that have the potential to cause an error or event.[39] The Common Formats most recently updated (V2.0) by the Agency for Healthcare Research and Quality (AHRQ) are likely to become the standard for reporting (https://www.psoppc.org/psoppc_web/publicpages/commonFormatsHV2.0). The common formats are similar to NCC MERP Event Types, with one additional category: Incorrect patient action (self-administration error). This type of error occurs when patients use medications inappropriately. Proper patient education and follow-up may play a significant role in minimizing this type of error. This type of error may be a direct result of insufficient patient counseling from a pharmacist, a prescriber, or both.

The second classification section of the medication Common Formats report asks at what part of the medication use process the incorrect action originated (regardless of where or when the incorrect action was discovered). The medication use process begins when a drug is purchased. It then follows the medication through storage, prescribing, transcribing if applicable, order verification, preparation and dispensing, administration, and finally monitoring.

Prescribing errors generally focus on inappropriate drug selection, dose, dosage form, or route of administration. Examples may include ordering duplicate therapies for a single indication, prescribing a dose that is too high or too low for a patient based on age or organ function, writing a prescription illegibly, prescribing an inappropriate dosage interval, or ordering a drug to which the patient is allergic.

In one study, the most common type of prescribing error (56.1%) was related to an inappropriate dose (either too high or too low).[9] The second most common prescribing error was related to prescribing an agent to which the patient was allergic (14.4%). Prescribing inappropriate dosage forms was the third most common error (11.2%). Other relatively common prescribing errors have included failing to monitor for side effects and serum drug levels, prescribing an inappropriate medication for a particular indication, and inappropriate duration of therapy.

Monitoring errors occur when patients are not monitored appropriately either before or after they have received a drug. For example, if a patient is placed on warfarin therapy and adequate blood tests (baseline and ongoing) are not performed to assess the patient's response, a monitoring error has occurred and has the potential to result in a life-threatening hemorrhage. TJC recognized this as a significant safety risk and developed a National Patient Safety Goal in 2015 in an effort to encourage organizations to improve and standardize this process.[40] In July 2019, this National Patient Safety Goal was updated to include direct oral anticoagulants, and TJC published a Sentinel Event Alert (SEA) on managing the risks of direct oral anticoagulants.[41]

These types of medication errors are not mutually exclusive. Multiple types of errors may occur during a single administration of a drug and a single adverse patient outcome may be the result of more than one type of error.

Additional information is gathered in the PSO reporting process. As the use of Common Formats grows, individual health care organizations will need to adopt these classifications, likely developing a standard taxonomy over time. Visit the PSO website for updated versions of the Common Formats at https://pso.ahrq.gov/common-formats.

Classifying Patient Outcomes

Although the classification of errors or events frequently is based on type, they are also classified by the patient outcome related to the error or event. When an error occurs, there is not always an adverse outcome. It is important for institutions to monitor both the types of errors that occur and the outcomes associated with them. Most reporting systems request information regarding event type and outcome of a medication error.

The NCC MERP developed a medication error index that serves to categorize errors based on the severity of harm or outcome of the error. This index is divided into four main categories and nine subcategories as follows.[42] See the index for event classification and corresponding algorithm at http://www.nccmerp.org/types-medication-errors.

1. No error
   - **Category A:** Circumstances or events that have the capacity to cause error.
2. Error, no harm
   - **Category B:** An error occurred, but the medication did not reach the patient.
   - **Category C:** An error occurred that reached the patient, but did not cause the patient harm.
   - **Category D:** An error occurred that resulted in the need for increased patient monitoring, but caused no patient harm.
3. Error, harm
   - **Category E:** An error occurred that resulted in the need for treatment or intervention and caused temporary patient harm.
   - **Category F:** An error occurred that resulted in initial or prolonged hospitalization and caused temporary patient harm.
   - **Category G:** An error occurred that resulted in permanent patient harm.

- **Category H:** An error occurred that required intervention necessary to sustain life (e.g., CPR, defibrillation, intubation and cardiac arrest).

4. Error, death

- **Category I:** An error occurred that may have contributed to or resulted in patient's death.

Oftentimes, the initial staff member(s) reporting the error has an opportunity to indicate their interpretation of the level of harm to the patient. In follow-up, a medication safety pharmacist and the unit/department manager may investigate further details and assign a final severity classification based on the ultimate outcome to the patient.

Institutions may use information about outcomes to focus their error prevention efforts on the types of errors resulting in the most serious outcomes. It is important to remember that examining near miss events (those that do not reach the patient) can be as valuable in preventing future errors as focusing on serious outcomes. These near miss events are often clues to the underlying process issues that require attention before they cause harm to a patient.

External Reporting

Reporting of medication errors is important for every practitioner without regard to their practice setting. However, institutional internal reporting is often emphasized above external reporting. Drug information specialists or medication safety officers are in an ideal position to encourage the importance of medication error and adverse drug reaction reporting to all health professionals, especially when they are consulted to answer questions related to potential cases. In an effort to share institutional experiences and avoid the same errors being repeated at several institutions, external reporting systems for institutions have evolved.

- **MedWatch:** This program was developed by the FDA Medical Products Reporting Program for the purpose of monitoring problems with medical products. MedWatch monitors quality, performance, and safety of medical products, devices, and medications. This program contributes to surveillance of medication errors that may be associated with product labeling and names.[43] MedWatch also collects reports about faulty products (e.g., improperly functioning devices). Significant reports may result in distribution of email and safety alerts to health care professionals. These announcements can also be viewed on the Internet at http://www.fda.gov/Safety/ MedWatch/default.htm. Health care professionals and consumers can report ADEs and product problems by completing an FDA Form 3500 form online, by mailing a form to the FDA, or by calling 1-800-FDA-1088. It is recommended to report serious adverse events online: https://www.accessdata.fda.gov/scripts/medwatch/.

- **Manufacturer:** ADEs may also be reported to the manufacturer of the product, in which case the manufacturer is then required to submit a MedWatch report. Sometimes this is more useful to the reporter than submitting a MedWatch directly, because the manufacturer may be able to provide additional information about the incidence or management of these ADEs that is not available upon directly reporting to the FDA.
- **ISMP Medication Errors Reporting Program (MERP):** This program provides a venue for voluntary medication error reporting to the Institute for Safe Medication Practices (ISMP). Reports can be submitted online at https://www.ismp.org/report-medication-error. ISMP is a federally certified PSO which collates errors and provides summary information of multiple cases in an effort to identify risk and support prevention strategies.
- **Subscription-based reporting systems:** One example of a subscription-based reporting system is Quantros®, which took over the prior USP-MEDMARX® reporting system. This program, and others, is an anonymous, subscription-based, voluntary reporting system that enables facilities to collect and report medication error, ADE, and ADR data. Subscribing organizations utilize the system to report and monitor organization-specific errors online, as well as compares their error rates with other subscribing organizations of similar type. These products differ from the ISMP MERP program, in that they are fee-based services that enable comparison to data within the database.

Managing an Event Reporting System

The 1999 NAM report spotlighted a serious need to capture data that would help to reduce harm to patients. Congress subsequently passed The Patient Safety and Quality Improvement Act of 2005 (Patient Safety Act). The act authorized the creation of a nation-wide network of PSOs to improve safety and quality through the collection and analysis of data on patient events.[44] The act provides a venue for institutions to report information related to errors and events with the goal of collating the information and learning the underlying risks across similar types of events. The act provides confidentiality and privilege protection to organizations. The fear of legal action related to reported event information has prevented many organizations from voluntarily reporting errors and events to external agencies. The privilege protections limit or forbid the use of protected information in criminal, civil, and other proceedings. Specifically, the information will not be subject to subpoena, discovery, or disclosure to any federal, state, or local criminal, civil, or administrative proceeding. The information may not be used in a professional disciplinary hearing, nor be admitted as evidence.

One example, the Pennsylvania Patient Safety Reporting System, has been collating error data since 2004 and publishes regular advisories with the goal of improving health care delivery systems and educating providers about safe practices. For example, in December 2009, the advisory reviewed errors with neuromuscular blocking agents.[45] In a 5-year span, 154 reports related to neuromuscular blocking agents were submitted. The advisory provides specific information related to the contributing factors (unsafe storage, look-alike drug names, similar packaging, and unlabeled syringes) that increase the risk for a fatal error. Specific risk reduction strategies are outlined. The same errors tend to recur in facilities across the United States. There was a series of errors in the administration of heparin to premature infants that occurred at least three times in different states with similar causes.[46] It is imperative that health care professionals commit to learn from others and critically self-assess the processes within their own institution to assure their process is as safe as possible. Being a learning organization is essential to prevent errors within an organization. A **learning organization** is one in which the leadership supports organizational learning, creating an environment where structured processes are developed to support this. Examples include communication of performance data to the staff level, formal training in performance improvement and problem solving at the unit or department level, and active engagement of staff in local problem-solving. It is recommended that hospitals, ambulatory centers, and other organizations join a PSO and commit to forwarding data related to adverse outcomes, enabling the collation of larger quantities of data, which the PSO can analyze and feedback recommendations to member organizations. This enables local- and broad-scale learning from errors and events.

TJC and American Society of Health-System Pharmacists (ASHP) standards can be used as a basis for starting an error reporting program. In addition to the standards, the pharmacy and medical literature contain abundant examples of successful programs. The following steps are a compilation of several of these references.

1. Develop and utilize standardized definitions and classifications for errors and events. The definitions and classifications in the literature and this chapter provide a good starting point for discussion. It is anticipated that the Common Formats developed in preparation for external reporting to PSOs will eventually become the standard.
2. Assign responsibility for the error review program within the pharmacy and throughout other key departments. A multidisciplinary approach is an essential factor. The program needs a medication safety leader and an advocate. It also needs the involvement of nursing, physicians, quality, and risk management departments in order to function as a collaborative team to work toward improved processes.

3. Develop forms or online methods for data collection and reporting (see #1 above). Other mechanisms for reporting (hotline phone numbers) may be used as well. Electronic reporting can often be designed such that medication errors are reviewed by a medication safety pharmacist to confirm severity of the event and gather additional information as needed in order to determine whether further analysis is appropriate. It is important to develop internal processes to assure awareness of key staff and leaders while maintaining protection from discovery. Protections vary from state to state making it important to work with legal and risk management. This serves as the voluntary reporting component of the program.

4. Promote awareness of the program and the importance of reporting errors and adverse events. Provide feedback to reporters and individual units to discuss their errors as well as those of others, along with steps taken to prevent them. Providing feedback is very important to assure that those reporting feel that the identified errors are reviewed and methods to prevent recurrence are developed and implemented.

5. Develop policies and procedures for determining which errors, events, and ADRs are reported to the FDA. The responsibility for this reporting should be defined and usually resides with someone in the pharmacy department.

6. Establish mechanisms for regular screening and identification of potential medication errors and ADEs to supplement voluntary reporting. These mechanisms should include retrospective reviews, concurrent monitoring, as well as prospective planning for high-risk groups. Additionally, electronic screening methods to check for laboratory tests that are indicative of potential events (e.g., drug levels, *Clostridium difficile* toxin assays, elevated serum potassium, and low white blood cell counts) can be helpful.[31]

7. Routinely review medication errors, ADEs, and ADRs for trends. Report all findings to the pharmacy and therapeutics committee and other hospital or organization quality and safety committees. It is beneficial to present facility-specific data, nationally reported errors of significance, as well as incorporate storytelling into various presentations. Oftentimes, telling a de-identified story that engages one's emotions, followed by data specific to the event, engages clinicians in the efforts to work toward safer processes.

8. Develop strategies for decreasing the incidence of medication errors and adverse events utilizing the data collected through the various identification and reporting systems. Use caution in aggregating data by error types or other surface-level classifications. The key is getting to the causes of the errors—not just the fact that the majority of errors are omitted doses. Why are the doses omitted? Is the automated dispensing cabinet filled at inappropriate intervals, is there not a clear and standardized process for delivering medications where they are easily located, or

do the batteries on the computers-on-wheels drain too quickly and the doses just are not charted? Seek to discover why the doses are omitted, as these are the issues that need to be resolved.

9. Review national resources that identify errors in other organizations such as the ISMP, the FDA, and the USP. It is likely that a local institution is experiencing risks similar to other institutions. Learn what risk reduction strategies are recommended, take a close look at your local processes, and implement additional risk reduction strategies where warranted. There is no need to repeat errors at every institution to learn what steps need to be taken for prevention.

Human Error or System Error?

HUMAN PERFORMANCE MODES AND ERRORS

Human error occurs when there is a failure in mental or physical actions to achieve their intended outcome—either actions do not go as intended or the actions are not correct for the situation at hand.[47] It is important to note that implicating human error in a safety event is not the same as assigning blame to an individual. To better understand why health care professionals make errors, it is necessary to look at the cognitive processes that occur at the time of the error.

❹ *Understanding the three modes of human performance (skill-based, rule-based, and knowledge-based) is important to understanding human errors.*

Skill-based human performance occurs when carrying out routine tasks that are practiced and automatic, like eating or driving a car to work. These activities are effortless, unconscious, and do not require much thought or attention. Skill-based errors are termed slips, lapses, or fumbles.[47] Slips are usually associated with attention or perception failures, while lapses generally involve memory failures. For example, a slip is placing the cereal box in the refrigerator instead of the milk. An example of a lapse is walking into the kitchen only to say, "Why did I come in here?" A fumble might be accidentally knocking over the milk in the process of putting it back into the refrigerator.

Rule-based human performance occurs when problem solving and making decisions. Perhaps a road is closed on the usual route to school or work and it is necessary to problem-solve to find an alternate route. People are trained to deal with many situations, perhaps by learning a policy or procedure, so it is possible to determine which rule to apply to the situation encountered. A wrong rule may be chosen because one misperceives the situation and applies the wrong rule. If one misapplies a rule, a rule-based error has occurred. It is possible to unconsciously pull the wrong pattern or rule from memory.

This is not the same as intentional rule-based noncompliance with defined policies and procedures, in which an individual chooses an action despite the knowledge that they should take a different action (e.g., a nurse administers a medication without scanning the patient's arm band or medication because the patient is sleeping).[47]

Finally, **knowledge-based human performance** relies on a person's prior knowledge, understanding, and experience with a situation or task. Knowledge-based errors can occur when an individual is in a situation to which he or she has never been exposed, or has no preprogrammed rules to apply. The person has a lack of required knowledge to complete the task, or has possibly misinterpreted the problem. When in knowledge-based mode, people are much more likely to make an error than when in skill-based or rule-based mode. The best scenario is that the person recognizes that he or she is lacking the information needed and takes the time to consult with colleagues or other resources to determine the appropriate course of action. Oftentimes, humans feel pressured to proceed in the face of uncertainty, because of perceived time constraints, to avoid acknowledging lack of knowledge to complete the task, or because of overconfidence. The worst-case scenario is that an individual does not realize he or she is in knowledge-based mode, has misinterpreted the situation, and proceeds without any question.

Confirmation bias is another common type of human error. It occurs when individuals select what is familiar to them or what they expect to see, rather than what is actually there. **Inattentional blindness** is similar and occurs when a person is so focused on performing the assigned task that he or she fails to see an error or change right in front of his or her eyes. It is human nature for people to associate items by certain characteristics, for example, color of vial, cap, or text. It is very important for the health care community to recognize the role that confirmation bias may play in medication errors and to work to develop systems with the understanding that this phenomenon exists and is part of natural human behavior. These types of accidents are common, even with intelligent, vigilant, and attentive people.[47]

THE SYSTEMS APPROACH TO ERROR

The historical response to error has focused on humans and human actions, attributing events to carelessness or negligence. Strategies to prevent error recurrence focused mostly on human behavior, including urging staff to be more careful, writing policies, educational campaigns, retraining, shaming, and even legal action.[48] This approach often puts the blame on the last person involved with the patient and does not acknowledge other factors contributing to the error. Conversely, the systems approach to error views human error as inevitable and attributes errors to a combination of human behavior and one or multiple failures in the system. Humans may be led to commit errors because the way the system is designed shapes their behaviors. Accordingly, the focus of error response is on the failure of the system design rather than on the human failure.

❺ *Humans will commit errors despite their best efforts not to. Therefore, it is critical to design systems that account for human error and put processes and technology in place to intercept errors before they reach and harm patients. The system should make it hard to do the wrong thing and easy to do the right thing.*

Norman and Reason have written extensively on the topics of human error and the systems approach.[47,49,50] Weaknesses and error-prone conditions in a system are referred to as latent failures which arise from decisions made by organizations, management, software design, and building design, among others. Mistakes committed by individuals are termed "active failures." This concept is often depicted with Reason's Swiss Cheese Model of Accident Causation, where the slices of Swiss cheese represent layers of safe guards in the system while the holes in the cheese represent the latent and active failures. A hole in one layer does not result in an error as long as the other layers are intact, but errors occur when holes in multiple layers align.

❻ *Poorly designed systems and processes are a significant contributor to error and subsequent patient harm. Errors rarely occur solely because of a mistake by a single health care professional, but rather in combination with one or more latent system failures.*

HUMAN FACTORS ENGINEERING

Human factors engineering (HFE) incorporates human behavior, strengths, and limitations into the design of equipment, environments, and activities to increase ease of use and reduce the risk of error.[51] Tools, software, workspaces, and processes designed with human factors (HF) in mind can make it easier for humans to do work the right way, while design without consideration of HF can result in products and processes prone to confusion, inefficiency, and errors. Some examples are design of medication packaging and labeling, infusion pump software user interfaces (UIs), and workflows within EHR software. ❼ *Incorporation of HF principles into process design and product selection can improve safety.*

Core principles of HF design include the following:

- Simplify and standardize—A process that requires a policy and procedure of 20 pages is one that is much too complex.
- Reduce reliance on memory—The human mind can only hold a limited number of things (four to seven items) in short-term memory. Formulating other methods of prioritization or reminders is likely to be more effective than relying on recall.
- Improve information access—Insufficient drug information and patient information are common contributing factors to medication errors.[52] Electronic access to patient data via EHRs and drug information resources can save clinicians time and reduce errors. Integrating patient and drug information together with clinical decision

support (CDS) tools in EHRs can provide the necessary information at the right time in a process to enhance human performance; for example, including medication administration instructions for the nurse on the medication order and label.

- Use constraints and forcing functions—Mistake proofing is the use of process or design features to prevent errors.[53] The next section explains this concept more in depth.

SYSTEM DESIGN AS ERROR PREVENTION

When implementing a new process or developing an action plan in response to an error, system design should be considered to identify risk points and build effective error reduction strategies into the system or process. ISMP's Hierarchy of Interventions (also known as Hierarchy of Intervention Effectiveness or Hierarchy of Safety Interventions) can assist with selecting effective error prevention strategies.[54-56] The hierarchy ranks strategies from least to most effective on a continuum of how much the strategy relies on system design (more effective) to how much it relies on human initiative (less effective).

Actions such as re-educating the department, asking staff to be more careful, and developing a policy or procedure have been the norm for years. However, these strategies alone cannot compensate for poorly designed systems. Each strategy has a role in error prevention, but emphasis should be placed on systems strategies in order to detect and stop errors before they reach the patient or eliminate the error from occurring entirely. See Figure 20-1 for visualization of the hierarchy. Strategies and examples are described below:

- **Forcing functions and constraints** – Designing the system so it is virtually error-proof. Example: institutional closed drug formularies eliminate the risk of errors with non-formulary drugs.
- **Automation, computerization, and technology** – Reduce reliance on human memory and human error. Example: machine-readable barcodes used in medication preparation and administration may identify incorrect drug products that humans may not pick up on.
- **Simplification and standardization** – Decrease variation and reduce the number of steps needed to carry out a process. Example: using standard medication-use protocols and order sets.
- **Checklists and double checks** – Build redundancies into a process. This does not prevent error but may intercept an error already made. Example: pharmacist verification of provider orders; pharmacist double check of products prepared by a pharmacy technician.
- **Policies and rules** – May control human actions but does not error-proof the system. Use in combination with other more effective strategies.

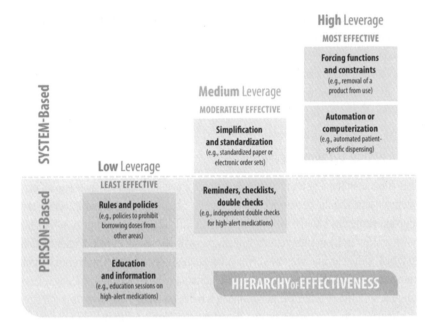

Figure 20–1.   Hierarchy of Effectiveness. Reprinted with permission from ISMP Canada. Available from: https://www.ismp-canada.org/download/ocil/ISMPCONCIL2013-4_EffectiveRecommendations.pdf.

- **Education, information, and personal vigilance** – Effective training and education are important but will not prevent errors if used alone, must be combined with higher-level strategies. Example: "Be more careful".

Case Study 20–1

A physician is ordering oxycodone 5 mg–acetaminophen 325 mg, a combination product for their patient's pain. Since this is a combination product, the order entry screen provides an option of tablets instead of milligrams. The physician orders five tablets. The pharmacist verifies this order, not recognizing the overdose. Upon obtaining this product from the automated dispensing cabinet, the nurse questions the order and calls the pharmacist. The pharmacist realizes the error and instructs the nurse not to administer the medication. The pharmacist clarifies the order with the physician, who intended oxycodone 5 mg–acetaminophen 325 mg, or one tablet. The error does not reach the patient, harm is averted, and the pharmacist submits a near miss event to the internal reporting system.

Discussion Question: Debate and discussion often ensues over whether it is possible to eliminate all errors, eliminate all harm events, or eliminate preventable harm events. Think about human nature and system design.

Is it possible to eliminate all errors? What should be the goal? No errors? No events of harm? No preventable harm?

- *What questions would you like to ask the pharmacist involved in the error as part of an interview?*
- *Would you classify this error as human-error only, system-error only, or a combination of both and why?*

Risk Factors for Errors and Events

The ultimate purpose for defining, classifying, analyzing, and reporting medication errors is to enable individuals and organizations to implement better systems that prevent medication errors. ASHP has identified a multitude of risk factors associated with the occurrence of medication errors as outlined below.[5,57]

- Shift work—switching from days to nights or vice versa
- Inexperienced or inadequately trained staff
- Medical services with special needs (e.g., pediatrics and oncology)
- Higher number of medications per patient
- Environmental factors such as high levels of noise, poor lighting, and frequent interruptions
- High workload for staff
- Poor communication among health care providers
- Dosage form—more errors with injectable drugs
- Drug category—more errors with certain classes of drugs (e.g., antibiotics)
- Type of drug distribution systems—unit dose system is associated with fewer errors; high levels of floor stock are associated with increased errors
- Improper drug storage
- Calculations—increased errors with increased complexity and frequency of amount of calculations required
- Poor handwriting
- Verbal orders
- Lack of effective policies and procedures
- Poorly functioning oversight committees

Personal and environmental factors are thought to interact to influence cognitive function that may lead to slips. There are several factors specific to the professional involved and their working environment that may contribute to their risk of committing an error. Grasha and O'Neill[58] have outlined some of the factors that may affect cognitive processes, resulting in lapses of performance.

1. **Excessive task demand:** Many clinicians attribute their errors to this situation, complaining that their workload is so heavy and they are overloaded with tasks, making it difficult to work error free. Pharmacists have noted workload, workflow, and environment (e.g., lighting, noise, interruptions) as contributing factors to dispensing errors.[59] Similarly, nurses also noted increased workload, in terms of task demand, also contributes to medication errors.[60] The authors concluded reducing workload during medication administration in the form of minimizing interruptions, concomitant demands, and time pressure would reduce medication errors. Most pharmacists and experts in medication errors agree that work overload may be the most significant factor contributing to medication errors. Re-evaluation of the workload distribution, with an eye for streamlining processes, may be valuable. Developing a detailed map of all the steps required to accomplish a task is one way to discover the complexity of a task. This is called **process mapping**.

2. **Personal characteristics:** Personal factors, such as age, sensory deficits, or state of health, may contribute to performance lapses. Personal levels of stress or fatigue may also have an impact. Someone who is bored at work may be more error prone.

3. **Extra-organizational factors:** Similar product names or packaging from pharmaceutical companies may have an extensive impact on the commission of errors with particular drugs. In one study, look-alike or sound-alike drugs were involved in 37% of medication errors.[61] As an example, this issue is currently being addressed for the sound-alike drugs celecoxib (Celebrex®), fosphenytoin (Cerebyx®), and citalopram (Celexa®). Drug manufacturer changes, supply interruptions, and shortages also influence errors and patient outcomes; a 2019 systematic review of 40 studies found increased medication errors, ADRs, and mortality during times of drug shortages.[62] Complex insurance plans are also extra-organizational factors that may serve to complicate the medication use process and contribute to slips. The profession of pharmacy has been referred to as the most heavily regulated of all professions. Legal mandates for policing illegal prescriptions and other regulatory requirements are also good examples of extra-organizational factors.

4. **Work environment:** Poor working conditions may influence the rate of error committal. Poor illumination and high noise levels have been shown to affect the dispensing error rate in pharmacies.[63] Other factors in this category may include high ambient temperatures and frequent interruptions from the telephone or patients.

5. **Intra-organizational factors:** There is a significant emphasis on other factors besides the quality and safety of medication use within health care systems. Concerns related to finances, throughput, customer service, and quality of employee work life are often competing priorities and major areas of focus in many institutions. Policies and procedures demanding high output or mandating long working hours may significantly affect cognition and the ability to prevent error occurrence.

6. **Interpersonal factors:** Conflicts among coworkers or with patients may distract professionals from the tasks at hand and contribute to error commission. General interruptions from people may also fall into this category.

Some factors that may contribute to cognitive lapses and the commission of medication errors may fall into more than one of these categories. Furthermore, factors from multiple categories may occur simultaneously to contribute to error commission.

Health care professionals have indicated that other factors may also contribute to medication errors. Some of those factors are as follows:

1. **Lack of effective communication:** This factor may also fall under interpersonal factors listed above. Failure to communicate effectively among fellow employees or among health care professionals has frequently been named as contributing to medical and medication errors. For example, an error may be more likely to occur if a pharmacist chooses not to clarify physician orders, or if the pharmacist does not communicate all the pertinent information so the physician can make an informed decision. Poor physician handwriting and verbal orders are also significant contributing factors.[64]

2. **Failure to comply with policy:** This is a common factor in dispensing and administering drugs. In one survey, 42–46% of pharmacists said that failing to check drugs before dispensing was a significant factor in dispensing errors.[58] Noncompliance with policy has also been associated with drug administration errors and is the result of several factors: perceived burden of the task, perceived risk of a bad outcome, and the perceived risk of being observed. Often, nurses develop specific personal routines for administration of certain agents, which they perceive to be an improvement in the medication administration process, despite contrary policy.[64] It is important to understand the challenges that make work difficult. Assure that processes have been designed with safety in mind.

3. **Lack of knowledge:** This is a frequently cited factor in the committal of medication errors. Mistakes, rather than slips, are typically committed because of inadequate knowledge. Placing inexperienced recent graduates in positions where they cannot interact with more experienced practitioners may increase medication errors. Nonspecialists covering a service that is normally staffed by a specialist may also lead to errors.[61] Nurses with less exposure to pharmacology may be less likely to

recognize potential inconsistencies in disease state and medication usage and doses, resulting in the increased possibility of medication errors reaching the patient.[64]

4. **Lack of patient counseling:** The last safety check prior to dispensing medication should be counseling the patient. Talking to the patient allows the pharmacist to correlate the medication and dose with the patient's condition and helps the pharmacist to detect any errors that may have occurred in the medication use process. In one study, 89% of errors committed in a community pharmacy were detected during patient counseling.[65] However, errors may occur not only from a lack of counseling, but also from providing incorrect information during patient counseling.[66] Providing incorrect information may also fall in the lack of knowledge category. One additional factor that plays a major part in understanding the patient is health care literacy. All professionals should assess the level of patient literacy to assure that appropriate language and teaching methods are used in our interactions with patients.

The examples provided above are a partial list of contributory factors at the level of the health care practitioner. These factors influence the occurrence of slips or performance lapses and mistakes committed by individuals. They do not address failure of a system or failure of a safety net as a whole process. The medication use process involves multiple health care professionals, nonprofessional staff, patients, and multiple physical environments. To adequately address the causes of errors, failures in the system must be addressed. Although, it is important to address the problem of individuals committing errors (e.g., increasing training if a knowledge deficit was identified and enforcing policy), adequately developed safety systems should be in place to significantly minimize the number of errors reaching patients.

Types of Safety Analyses

PROSPECTIVE RISK ANALYSIS

❽ *Failure modes and effects analysis (FMEA) is a prospective method of evaluating processes to identify how and why a process could fail, potential impacts of failure, and developing actions to prevent failure and mitigate harm.* Prospective risk evaluations place emphasis on prevention of errors and patient harm rather than reactive analysis after the error has already occurred. One example of a prospective risk evaluation is FMEA, which is commonly used to evaluate a new process before implementation or to evaluate changes to an already existing process. Conducting an FMEA involves reviewing each step in a process for what could go wrong (the "failure mode"), why the failure could happen, and the effect or harm caused by the failure. Each failure mode should be assessed for likelihood of occurrence (O), likelihood of detection (D), and severity of harm (S), with each being ranked from 1 to 10 (1 = low occurrence/high detection/low harm and 10 = high occurrence/low detection/high harm). Multiplying these numbers together yields a score of 1 to 1000, called a criticality index or risk profile number (RPN). After calculating the RPN for each failure mode, sort from highest to lowest RPN in order to prioritize actions to take to avoid failures and reduce risk.[67] Alternatively, the action priority (AP) method can be used instead of the RPN calculation.[68] In the AP method, failure modes are sorted into high, medium, or low action priority based on their O, D, and S values. High priority items must be addressed, medium priority should be addressed, and low priority items can but do not need to be addressed.

RETROSPECTIVE EVENT ANALYSIS

❾ *Evaluation of safety events through root cause analysis (RCA) and other methods is key to learning from errors and preventing recurrence.* RCAs are evaluations carried out after an error has already occurred to better understand why the error happened by identifying underlying vulnerabilities in the system. It is also sometimes called root cause analysis and actions (RCA^2 or "RCA squared") to emphasize that the analysis itself is not enough—actions must be taken to improve the system, reduce risk, and prevent errors with similar root causes from occurring again in the future.[69] Typical steps to conducting an RCA are as follows.

1. **Determine what happened** by reviewing medical records, visiting the location of the error, interviewing staff involved, and other methods of information-gathering. Output of this step could be a description of the events surrounding the error, a timeline, or a flowchart.
2. **Establish what should have happened** by reviewing policies, procedures, evidence-based practices, regulatory requirements, etc. RCAs should not focus on staff performance as a primary cause of error, but assessing barriers to compliance by individuals and the organization as a whole is an important consideration.
3. **Identify the direct and contributing factors of the error.** Direct factors are the most apparent causes of error but are usually just symptoms of larger problems rather than the root causes. "Human error" and procedural violation cannot be root causes—there must be a preceding cause that influenced them to occur.[70] Asking "why" at least five times is one strategy to see past the direct factors to the deeper contributing factors and root causes. It can also be helpful to organize factors into seven categories: environment, task and technology, team, individual staff members, patient characteristics, organization and management, and institutional context. Output of this step is usually a graphical representation of all the possible factors that led toward the error known as a fishbone, Ishikawa, or cause-and-effect diagram.

4. **Identify actionable root causes and implement measures to prevent recurrence.** Recommended actions should be clear, specific, and measurable to ensure that changes made have improved safety of the system. See previous section on "System Design as Error Prevention" for examples of error prevention strategies that can be used in an RCA action plan.

Conducting an RCA on any event can be a valuable learning experience for an organization. Errors do not necessarily need to cause harm to be evaluated with an RCA, as the root causes of near-miss events and errors causing minimal harm are often the same as the root causes that can lead to serious harm. For example, a nurse administers an antibiotic, rather than an antiemetic, to a patient. Fortunately, there is no adverse outcome. If the same error occurred with a different drug, such as a paralytic agent, the outcome could be fatal. Contributing factors to errors can be reviewed in aggregate to determine if there are common themes that may warrant further investigation and process changes.

It is often not feasible for organizations to conduct RCAs on every error, so some may only conduct them on sentinel events. A **sentinel event** is defined by TJC as "an unexpected occurrence involving death or serious physical or psychological injury, or the risk thereof [including] any process variation for which a recurrence would carry a significant chance of a serious adverse outcome."[71] TJC is an accrediting body that is focused on continuously improving health care for the public by evaluating health care organizations. The goal of TJC is to ensure each organization meets designated standards for quality and safety. The expectation is that the organization will conduct a timely, thorough, and credible RCA in response to a sentinel event, develop and implement an action plan to reduce the risk of recurrence, and monitor the effectiveness of the plan and its implementation.

Case Study 20–2

A hospitalized patient experienced irritation and swelling in his arm after infusion of an IV medication. The nurse submitted this event to the hospital's online incident reporting system and it was investigated by the hospital's medication safety pharmacist. Investigation revealed the rate on the order and pharmacy bag label was incorrect, causing the nurse to run the bag too quickly. The physician who ordered the medication intended an infusion time of "120 minutes," but instead typed "12 minutes." The pharmacist who verified the order stated she did not remember seeing any rates that looked too fast or inappropriate to her on that day, but also noted the laptop she normally brings on rounds was broken and there were no back-up computers available, so she used her personal laptop that day. Further investigation revealed the laptop had a small screen resolution, and infusion rate could not be seen on the order verification screen without scrolling down.

No disciplinary action was taken against the physician, pharmacist, or nurse for being involved in this event.

- *How would you classify this error, by event type and harm score?*
- *What tool could be used to investigate underlying system factors that contributed to the error?*
- *What are latent and active failures that contributed to this scenario?*
- *What actions would be **most** effective to prevent this event from occurring again?*

Just Culture

In some instances, reporting medication errors, particularly severe or life-threatening errors, have had adverse consequences for both individuals and the organizations involved. Health care professionals have lost their jobs or voluntarily resigned from their jobs and, at times, have left their profession entirely. Consequently, health care professionals and health systems have been reluctant to open themselves up to repercussions associated with reporting medication errors.[72] For example, in one hospital there were only 36 incident reports regarding medication errors over a yearlong reporting period. At the same institution, an observational study revealed that as many as 51,200 errors were likely to have occurred during that same reporting period.[73]

Hindsight bias often plays a role in the way people react to an error. Hindsight bias is the inclination to see events that have occurred as being more predictable than they were before the event took place. In other words, the person should have known that this would be the outcome. It is very easy to examine the information after the event and conclude that, of course, this bad outcome was going to occur. What investigators and facilitators do not have the benefit of is the vast number of exact circumstances and choices that the individual was facing, along with their thought processes that led them to their conclusions.

In Nevada, a pharmacy was fined 2 weeks' net profit for a dispensing error that resulted from understaffing.[65] A medical center in New Jersey was successfully sued for $12 million and fined by the state board of pharmacy after a medication error killed an infant.[74] In 1996, a medication error occurred in a hospital in Colorado that resulted in the death of a newborn infant. Three nurses involved in the infant's care were indicted on charges of criminally negligent homicide.[75] District attorneys in Colorado pressed criminal charges that could have resulted in 3–5 years imprisonment. A pharmacist in Ohio was indicted and jailed for a chemotherapy error resulting in the death of a young patient.[76] In 2019, a nurse in Tennessee was prosecuted by the state for a medication error resulting in the death of a patient.[77] In these cases, there were underlying system concerns that likely contributed to the event. Without resolution of these system issues, a similar event may occur with a different clinician. These cases reiterate the need to identify root causes to prevent recurrence.

Learning from errors, events, and near misses is vital to improvement. Despite the negative actions that have been taken against individuals and organizations in the past, the health care culture is evolving toward a culture of safety. Leaders are learning more about **Just Culture**. Just culture is a balance between accountability of institutions for the systems designed and the behaviors of employees within that system. Employees are responsible for the quality of their behavioral choices in addition to reporting errors and system susceptibilities.[78] The outcome of the error should not determine the fate of the individual. One must understand the circumstances (including poorly designed systems) in which errors occur before decisions related to discipline are made. If a system sets up one individual to fail, the next person in the same situation is also likely to fail in the same manner as the first. If the system is not specifically designed to avert likely human errors (no double-check of a high-risk calculation, such as chemotherapy), human errors will continue to reach patients with significant potential for harm.

Action plans to prevent recurrence of an event should be designed according to the type of error(s) made. It does not make sense to retrain someone in a procedure if they are very skilled, were distracted by a colleague, and made a skill-based error. Similarly, if a knowledge-based error is identified, working to decrease distractions and interruptions will have little impact on decreasing future repeat errors with the activity. When interviewing individuals involved in errors, it is important to ask them to describe what happened and what else was going on at the time, ask them to walk through their decision-making process, and find out why they think the event occurred. It is also important to understand the options presented to them at the time.

Recall those headlines again—Child Dies from Medication Error, Journalist Dies of Chemotherapy Error…. The rest of the story usually involves details about what happened (on the surface) and who was fired or reprimanded. What disciplinary action should be taken in these cases—if any? It depends on the circumstances entirely. It is important to have a thorough understanding of exactly what happened and the "whys" behind the decisions and actions taken. If an individual did not consciously make an unsafe decision, how does discipline help one learn from mistakes? Will not staff be less willing to report and discuss them without fear of retribution? Retraining, counseling, and discipline have been hallmark actions taken to prevent error and have failed to substantially improve patient care. There may be circumstances where discipline is appropriate. While uncommon, reckless behavior, in which there is intent to cause harm, warrants swift disciplinary action. Reckless behavior occurs when the risk is unjustifiable and knowingly disregarded. The actions of Dr. Christopher Duntsch are described in a podcast called

"Dr. Death."[79] Dr. Duntsch knowingly harmed patients by performing inadequate spinal surgeries, leaving patients paralyzed or dead. Another example of reckless behavior was identified when there was a fungal meningitis outbreak in 2012.[80] These infections were traced back to a compounding facility, the New England Compounding Center (NECC). There were 753 patients diagnosed with fungal meningitis, and 64 of these patients died from the infection, due to inappropriate sterility practices at the NECC. The pharmacist in charge was found guilty of misbranding drugs, with the intent to defraud and mislead, sentencing them to 8 years in prison.

The culture of blame shifted in the 1990s in the health care industry when it was recognized that the punitive nature of discipline was not the best way to encourage staff to talk about risks and errors, and assist in the process of decreasing errors. The culture then shifted to a blame-free culture in an effort to promote reporting. This culture recognized that humans will err, that most unsafe acts are slips or lapses, and that weaknesses in systems and environments contribute significantly to errors in medicine.[81] What was not recognized at the time was that a solely blame-free culture (also termed nonpunitive) failed to attend to those few who knowingly ignore designated safety procedures and those who are unreasonably reckless or negligent. This undermines those who work hard at providing safe care.

⑩ *A Just Culture is a balance between accountability of organizations for the systems designed and the behaviors of employees within that system.* It is unacceptable to discipline all errors regardless of their circumstances, and is just as unacceptable to be nonpunitive in the face of individuals who are intentionally ignoring safe operating principles.

The hard part is distinguishing between those who make a conscious decision to complete an unsafe action, despite knowledge that it is unsafe (i.e., reckless behavior), and those who usually work in a safe manner and experienced a slip or lapse (i.e., human error). In between is the choice to complete an unsafe action, but the risk is not recognized (i.e., at-risk behavior). The use of a substitution test has proven to be useful in these instances.[47] When dealing with a serious event and a person is implicated in an unsafe act, describe the scenario to several other individuals (at least three) of the same qualifications and experience (optimally, who are not aware of the actual incident) and ask them in the circumstances at the time, what decisions they would have made. If they would have made the same decision and completed the same actions, then blaming the individual is not likely appropriate, as there is evidence that this issue has a larger scope. Another option is to observe individuals in the same situations, if possible, to determine how others behave in similar instances. This helps one determine whether the problem may lie with an individual, an expanded group (perhaps a unit or department), or is a more global problem. This also helps in the development of an action plan. There is no need to re-educate an entire department on a process, if there is only one individual that needs coaching.

The use of a series of questions helps determine the culpability and accountability of a person's actions and are taken from the Decision Tree for determining the Culpability of Unsafe Acts.[47] Appropriate discipline, when warranted, should be taken when unsafe behaviors are identified, regardless of the outcome.[82]

1. Were the actions as intended?
2. Was the person under the influence of unauthorized substances?
3. Did he or she knowingly violate a safe operating procedure? If so, was the procedure available, workable, intelligible, and correct? This gets at those procedures that staff feel make no sense and are not value-added in their workflow. Perhaps they have a point and there is a component of system-induced error.
4. Do they pass the substitution test described above? Would others have made the same decisions and, if so, less likely to be culpable? If not, were there deficiencies in training or experience?
5. Does the individual have a history of unsafe acts? If not, again less likely to be culpable.

The use of these questions should be used to assist in determining the level of culpability of an individual. The actions in the first few questions bear more culpability than those that occur in the last several questions. Therefore, disciplinary actions are more likely to be appropriate for those acts that are intended and/or undertaken while under the influence of unauthorized substances.

There are always a few outliers within any profession; those who intentionally do not follow the processes as designed, feeling that they are immune from human error and/or believing their process is better. There is a difference between unintentional human error, at-risk behavior, and reckless behavior. Intentionally unsafe behavior is identified by the first question and is generally dealt with through disciplinary action. At-risk behavior may be amenable to coaching about the reason for the process as designed and a request to commit to better choices.

Establishing a Just Culture is one part of an institution's culture of safety. Culture of safety is not one specific item, but many actions by individuals or an organization that define it. Along with the application of Just Culture, increased event reporting, increased employee engagement scores, and improved patient outcomes are just a few items that define an organization's culture of safety. An organization that has a positive culture of safety is one that supports a learning culture, i.e., learning from errors to improve the system and coach the human.

Case Study 20-3

A patient received an overdose of a hydromorphone drip, requiring naloxone reversal, but recovered without permanent harm. Drips are programmed into the infusion pump by entering the total amount of drug in the bag, the volume of the bag, and the drip rate. Upon investigation, it was discovered the nurse programmed the pump incorrectly by entering the concentration of the drip into the total drug amount field, resulting in the pump calculating a falsely low concentration which resulted in overdelivery of the drug. The pump gave a low concentration alert, but it was only a soft limit alert which was overridden by the nurse; no hard limits were set. This is the first error identified for this nurse who has practiced here for over a year. It was also discovered that the manufacturer of the hydromorphone drips recently changed and labels appeared differently than the previous drip bags; the concentration appeared on the label more prominently than the total drug amount and volume in the bag which does not conform to USP <7> drug label design principles.

- *What system issues contributed to the error?*
- *Discuss how to apply Just Culture to this situation.*
- *What potential system fixes can you identify?*

Key Organizations for Safety Best Practices

There are many resources that identify best practice error prevention strategies. Listed here are various resources as well as strategies to assure medication use processes are as safe as they can be. See Table 20-2 for a list of resources and organizations. Commit to be a learning organization by constantly reviewing local and national information and taking proactive steps to prevent error. Do not wait until it happens to you.

The **Institute for Safe Medication Practices** publishes a "Quarterly Action Agenda" that describes known risks and errors and describes recommendations for risk reduction strategy implementation. These can be found on the website at http://www.ismp.org.

The **Institute for Healthcare Improvement (IHI)** has sponsored several campaigns (e.g., The 100,000 Lives Campaign and the 5 Million Lives Campaign) to save lives and protect patients from harm. At least half of the 12 recommended interventions within the two campaigns involve improving the safe use of medications. See Table 20-4. In addition to

TABLE 20–4. SELECTED INTERVENTIONS RECOMMENDED BY THE INSTITUTE FOR HEALTHCARE IMPROVEMENT (IHI) TO SAVE LIVES AND REDUCE PATIENT INJURIES[83]

Strategies from the 100,000 Lives Campaign
- **Prevent Adverse Drug Events (ADEs)**...by implementing medication reconciliation
- **Prevent Surgical Site Infections**...by reliably delivering the correct perioperative antibiotics at the proper time

Strategies from the 5 Million Lives Campaign
- **Prevent Harm from High-Alert Medications**...starting with a focus on anticoagulants, sedatives, narcotics, and insulin

these two campaigns, the IHI offers many programs, conferences, Action Community networks, best practice postings, the IHI Open School, and much more. The IHI Open School provides a mechanism by which students and their mentors in nursing, medicine, pharmacy, dentistry, health care administration, and other health care professions can interact and learn in an interdisciplinary fashion. There are online courses in quality and safety, basic and advanced certifications in quality improvement and patient safety, case studies, podcasts, videos, and feature articles. Visit http://www.ihi.org for more information.

TJC's National Patient Safety Goals can serve as a guide to improving the safety of health care. Many of TJC's National Patient Safety Goals released each year are related to safe medication use and pharmacists should be involved in assuring that the facility meets these goals. They are divided into the type of health care provided—hospital, home care, ambulatory care, behavioral health care, etc. There are other goals aside from those listed, some of which indirectly relate to pharmacy. These goals change frequently. A partial list includes the following:

- Accurately and completely reconcile medications during transitions within and across organizations (e.g., inpatient to outpatient).
- Improve the effectiveness of communication between caregivers.
- Label all medications, medication containers (e.g., syringes, medicine cups, basins), or other solutions on and off the sterile field.
- Reduce the likelihood of patient harm associated with the use of anticoagulant therapy.
  ○ Includes an anticoagulation management program, approved protocols for initiation and maintenance, individualized care, appropriate baseline, and ongoing lab monitoring.
- Implement best practices for preventing surgical site infections, including timely administration of appropriately chosen antibiotics. Consult the TJC website for the most up-to-date standards (https://www.jointcommission.org/standards/).

The National Quality Forum (NQF)'s "Safe Practices for Better Healthcare" identifies 34 practices with demonstrated effectiveness in reducing the occurrence of adverse events in health care. The Safe Practices related to medication use are as follows:

- Medication reconciliation—Many adverse events are the result of patients presenting to an acute care facility such as a hospital, identifying a list of the medications that they are taking at home, yet somewhere during the admission, transfer, or discharge process, these medications are inadvertently omitted or duplicate therapy occurs due to therapeutic substitution at discharge. The organization must develop a process to identify, reconcile (compare and confirm which medications are appropriate for the patient to take during the hospitalization or outpatient visit), and communicate an accurate patient medication list throughout the continuum of care (to other primary care and specialist providers).

- Pharmacist leadership structure—Pharmacy leaders should have an active role on the administrative leadership team that identifies their accountability for the performance of the medication management systems across the institution.
- Improving patient safety by creating and sustaining a culture of safety.
  - ° The elements of this safe practice include leadership structures and systems, culture measurement and intervention, teamwork training, and identification and mitigation of risks and hazards.
- Improving patient safety by facilitating information transfer and clear communication.
  - ° Elements of this chapter include communication of critical information, order read-back, safe adoption of CPOE, and avoiding unapproved abbreviations. Each organization must define a list of unapproved abbreviations, monitor the frequency of use, and develop strategies to reduce the use of these abbreviations. Several high-risk abbreviations have been identified (by ISMP and other organizations) such as MSO_4 and $MgSO_4$ which may be inadvertently misread and administered causing harm to patients and U (for units) which has been misinterpreted as a zero, causing 10-fold overdoses of insulin. The FDA and TJC support this recommendation from ISMP (https://www.ismp.org/recommendations/error-prone-abbreviations-list).
- Improving patient safety through condition and site-specific practices.
  - ° This grouping includes perioperative myocardial infarction and ischemia prevention, venous thromboembolism prevention, anticoagulation therapy, and contrast media-induced renal failure prevention. Visit the NQF website for the latest version (https://www.qualityforum.org/Publications/2010/04/Safe_Practices_for_Better_Healthcare_%E2%80%93_2010_Update.aspx).

Case Study 20–4

A nurse caring for a birthing mother removed a bag of bupivacaine from the automated dispensing machine prior to the arrival of the anesthesiologist in order to have everything readily available when needed. The anesthesiology department had requested a preparation checklist with other supplies and the epidural. The same patient required prophylactic penicillin for coverage of Group B streptococcus. Both bags of similar size were in the patient's room. The nurse administered what was thought to be the penicillin bag, but did not use the bar-coding system. The patient immediately decompensated and expired. It was discovered that the epidural bupivacaine was administered IV instead of the penicillin bag. Upon further investigation, it was identified that the bar-coding system had been implemented in the majority of the hospital, but was not fully implemented in the Labor and Delivery area due to several technologic and cultural issues.

Read the related article cited below to identify additional information about the case. Lead a discussion related to system errors and their impact on health care professional's behaviors and the potential impact to patients. Smetzer J, Baker C, Byrne FD, Cohen MR. Shaping systems for better behavioral choices: lessons learned from a fatal medication error. Jt Comm J Qual Patient Saf. 2010 Apr;36(4):152–63.

- *What system or process issues can you identify?*
- *What are the two types of technology that could have helped prevent this error?*
- *Discuss challenges with implementation of new technology.*
- *Discuss challenges in culture and prioritization of safety principles.*
- *Discuss confirmation bias and look-alike packaging.*

Conclusion: Safety as a Priority

Providing safe medication use is paramount to the safety of all patients. Diligent efforts to identify errors (utilizing several methods), understand human capability and propensity to commit errors in everyday life, analyze and determine the root causes and contributing factors, and devise systems that support humans and prevent expected errors are all a part of developing a culture of safety. Involving staff on the front line when reviewing safety events and developing action plans to prevent recurrence is important. It is important not only to the development of an appropriate action plan, but also to garner support and confidence that once errors are identified, leadership is committed to improving the processes in which staff have to work every day.

In 1998, the NAM formed the Quality of Healthcare in America Committee that was charged with developing a strategy to improve quality in health care. In their published report, To Err is Human: Building a Safer Health System,[1] the committee highlighted what was currently known about the extent of medical errors, what contributes to medical errors, and recommendations to minimize errors and improve the quality of health care in the United States. Many of the goals set forth in this report are becoming closer to reality. The many other reports by the NAM have provided additional detail and insight into what is necessary to optimize the safety of the health care system in the United States.

Medication errors continue to be a serious problem in the U.S. health care system, both in the hospital and the ambulatory care setting. Working to provide safe care is a journey or, rather, a marathon. Changing a culture is not something that is accomplished in a few years; it may take 10 or more years. Much of that is dependent on the leadership of executives and staff. Those with a passion for safety may need to help enlighten those in higher leadership positions. Learn from others. It is an important method of preventing errors from occurring within your institution/facility. Take a close look at processes when reading a local or national headline about an error. There continues to be ongoing research aimed at increasing the safety and quality of health care. Health care will continue to be complex and require effective coordination and communication. Technology will continue to evolve. Safety truly needs to be a core value that is held by all. Teamwork and mutual respect are vital parts to success. Only through collaboration and a shared, dedicated commitment will patient safety truly become a reality.

Self-Assessment Questions

1. As the medications safety pharmacist, you review the weekly barcode medication administration mismatch report. The report indicates that clindamycin 900 mg was scanned instead of the ordered dose of 300 mg. The nurse documented on electronic medication administration record (eMAR) as task performed with override reason as "dose appropriate." Inventory showed that the post-anesthesia care unit (PACU) ADC only carries clindamycin 900 mg. The ADC report showed that nurse pulled clindamycin 900 mg dose on override with reason as "Urgent for patient discomfort or distress." Patient may have been overdosed. What is the appropriate event type classification?
   a. Wrong patient
   b. Wrong drug
   c. Wrong dose
   d. Wrong route

2. Which of the following is **NOT** an example of a trigger tool to detect potential ADEs?
   a. Voluntary reporting of an error
   b. Administration of dextrose 50% IV
   c. INR > 6
   d. Abrupt medication stop

3. Congress passed the Patient Safety and Quality Improvement Act of 2005, from which Patient Safety Organizations (PSOs) were created. Which of the following is **NOT** a true statement?

   a. This act provides two types of protections: confidentiality and privilege protections.
   b. One of the goals of the PSOs is to collate and analyze data related to safety errors and events.
   c. PSOs will forward information about facility-specific reported events to The Joint Commission and the media.
   d. PSOs will require the use of Common Formats (standardized reporting and terminology) for reporting errors and events.

4. Patient A is given a low dose of regular insulin intended for Patient B. The patient became hypoglycemic and required two doses of dextrose 50% to reverse the effects but did become symptomatic and did not require further treatment. Which of the following NCC MERP classification is most appropriate?
   a. Category A
   b. Category B
   c. Category C
   d. Category E
   e. Category F

5. You are a hospital pharmacist working on the medical-surgical unit. You receive an electronic order for a medication that you are not familiar with. Before verifying the order, you reference the drug package insert, an online drug information database, and double-check with another pharmacist. If you had proceeded to verify the order without consulting additional resources, what type of human error could you have made?
   a. Skill-based error
   b. Rule-based error
   c. Knowledge-based error
   d. Interruption-based error

6. A Just Culture exists when there is a punitive environment, where staff are disciplined based on errors, to assure events will not recur.
   a. True
   b. False

7. Which of the following methods utilizes observation of drug administration and comparison with physician orders in order to identify medication errors and is considered very time consuming, rarely used on an ongoing basis?
   a. ADE Trigger Tool
   b. Observation method
   c. Voluntary reporting method
   d. None of the above

8. Which of the following is a thorough and deliberate retrospective analysis of an error or event in an effort to design risk reduction strategies to prevent a recurrence?
   a. Root cause analysis (RCA)
   b. Interview people involved in previous errors
   c. Failure mode and effects analysis (FMEA)
   d. Trending of error and event reports

9. A wrong dose medication error occurred that could have been intercepted by the use of barcode medication administration (BCMA). When investigating the error it is discovered the nurse who administered the drug did not use the BCMA system. Which of the following is *NOT* a latent failure in this scenario?
   a. Docking stations for charging BCMA scanners often malfunction.
   b. Network connectivity issues on the unit where this nurse works.
   c. The nurse did not pay close enough attention to the dose.
   d. Interface issues between the EHR and ADCs that allowed the nurse to remove the wrong dose.

10. Which of the following statements are true?
    a. All adverse drug events involve harm.
    b. All medication errors cause harm.
    c. There is no harm involved in an adverse drug reaction.
    d. All of the above are true.

11. Which of the following is/are example(s) of using data collected by health information technology (HIT) to detect medication errors?
    a. Barcode scan override report from the BCMA system.
    b. Infusions programmed over safety limits from the smart infusion pump.
    c. Logic-based report of medication orders entered via CPOE on one patient then cancelled and reentered on a second patient.
    d. All of the above.

12. Which of these strategies are generally the **LEAST** effective or less reliable than other strategies?
    a. Change a policy or procedure.
    b. Re-educate everyone (especially when it was an individual failure).
    c. Coach associate(s) to be more careful (vigilant).
    d. All of the above are examples of less reliable strategies.

13. Which organization publishes national patient safety goals?
    a. Institution for Safe Medication Practices
    b. The Joint Commission

c. National Quality Forum

d. Institute for Healthcare Improvement

14. A pharmacist is alone in the pharmacy, entering a physician order, when she receives a call about a patient. In order to answer the question, she must exit the current patient's profile to pull up another patient's profile. Once the question has been answered, she hangs up and proceeds to finish entering the order on the patient's profile (the wrong patient). Which error prevention strategy would most likely be the **LEAST** effective at preventing a recurrence of this error?

a. Discipline the pharmacist and remind her to be more careful—do patient identification correctly on every order.

b. Purchase (or develop) technology that automatically links a physician order to the patient's profile in the pharmacy system—a forcing function.

c. Alter the practice such that there are minimal to no interruptions for pharmacists entering orders (route calls to one area and responsible staff, segregate order-entry staff to decrease interruptions).

d. All of the above will be effective and prevent the recurrence.

15. Your hospital is adding a new drug to formulary. Which of the following could be used to evaluate the new drug for potential safety issues and develop and prioritize actions to prevent failure and mitigate harm.

a. Root cause analysis (RCA)

b. Failure modes and effects analysis (FMEA)

c. Swiss cheese model

d. Fishbone diagram

REFERENCES

1. Institute of Medicine. To err is human: building a safer health system. Washington (DC): National Academy Press; 1999.
2. Brennan TA, Leape LL, Laird NM, Hebert L, Localio R, Lawthers AG, Newhouse JP, Weiler PC, Hiatt HH. Incidence of adverse events and negligence in hospitalized patients: results of the Harvard Medical Practice Study I. N Engl J Med. 1991;324:370-6.
3. Leape LL, Brennan TA, Laird NM, Lawthers AG, Localio AR, Barnes BA, Hebert L, Newhouse JP, Weiler PC, Hiatt H. The nature of adverse events in hospitalized patients: results of the Harvard Medical Practice Study II. N Engl J Med. 1991;324(6):377-84.
4. Makary MA, Daniel M. Medical error: the third leading cause of death in the US. BMJ. 2016 May 3;353:i2139.
5. Billstein-Leber M, Carrillo CJ, Cassano AT, Moline K, Robertson JJ. ASHP guidelines on preventing medication errors in hospitals. Am J Health-Syst Pharm. 2018;75(19):1493-1517.
6. National Coordinating Council for Medication Error Reporting and Prevention. Contemporary view of medication-related harm. A new paradigm [Internet]. 2019 [cited

2019 Sep 8]. Available from: https://www.nccmerp.org/sites/default/files/nccmerp_fact_sheet_2015-02-v91.pdf

7. Bates DW, Cullen DJ, Laird N, Peterson LA, Small HD, Servi D, Laffel G, Sweitzer BJ, Shea BF, Hallisey R, Vander Vliet M, Nemeskal R, Leape LL for the ADE Prevention Study Group. Incidence of adverse drug events and potential adverse drug events. JAMA. 1995;274:29-34.

8. Lamy PP. Adverse drug effects. Clin Ger Med. 1990;6:293-307.

9. Lesar TS, Lomaestro BM, Pohl H. Medication-prescribing errors in a teaching hospital: a 9-year experience. Arch Intern Med. 1997;157:1569–76.

10. National Center for Health Statistics. Therapeutic drug use [Internet]. Atlanta (GA): Centers for Disease Control and Prevention; [cited 2020 Dec 19]. Available from: https://www.cdc.gov/nchs/fastats/drug-use-therapeutic.htm

11. Institute of Medicine. Preventing medication errors. Washington (DC): The National Academies Press; 2007.

12. Weingart SN, Zhang L, Sweeney M, Hassett M. Chemotherapy medication errors. Lancet Oncol. 2018;19(4):e191-9.

13. Kennedy AR, Massey LR. Pediatric medication safety considerations for pharmacists in an adult hospital setting. Am J Health-Syst Pharm. 2019;76(19):1481-91.

14. Croskerry P, Shapiro M, Campbell S, LeBlanc C, Sinclair D, Wren P, Marcoux M. Profiles in patient safety: medication errors in the emergency department. Acad Emerg Med. 2004;11(3):289-99.

15. Weant KA, Bailey AM, Baker SN. Strategies for reducing medication errors in the emergency department. Open Access Emerg Med. 2014;6:45-55.

16. Gurwitz JH, Field TS, Harrold LR, Rothschild J, Debellis K, Seger AC, Cadoret C, Fish LS, Garber L, Kelleher M, Bates DW. Incidence and preventability of adverse drug events among older persons in the ambulatory setting. JAMA. 2003;289:1107-16.

17. Gurwitz JH, Field TS, Avorn J, McCormick D, Jain S, Eckler M, Benser M, Edmondson AC, Bates DW. Incidence and preventability of adverse drug events in nursing homes. Am J Med. 2000;109:87-94.

18. White TJ, Arakelian A, Rho JP. Counting the costs of drug-related adverse events. Pharmacoeconomics. 1999;15:445-58.

19. Johnson JA, Bootman JL. Drug-related morbidity and mortality. Arch Intern Med. 1995;155:1949-56.

20. Classen DC, Pestotnik SL, Evans S, Loyd JF, Burke JP. Adverse drug events in hospitalized patients. JAMA. 1997;277:301-16.

21. Ernst FR, Grizzle AJ. Drug-related morbidity and mortality: updating the cost-of-illness model. J Am Pharm Assoc. 2001;41:192-9.

22. Aitken M, Gorokhovich L. Advancing the responsible use of medicines: applying levers for change. Parsippany (NJ): IMS Institute for Healthcare Informatics; 2012.

23. Meyer-Massetti C, Cheng CM, Schwappach DL, Paulsen L, Ide B, Meier CR, Guglielmo BJ. Systematic review of medication safety assessment methods. Am J Health-Syst Pharm. 2011;68(3):227-40.

24. Classen DC, Resar R, Griffin F, Federico F, Frankel T, Kimmel N, Whittington JC, Frankel A, Seger A, James BC. "Global trigger tool" shows that adverse events in hospitals may be ten times greater than previously measured. Health Aff. 2011;30(4):581-9.

25. Phillips MA. Voluntary reporting of medication errors. Am J Health-Syst Pharm. 2002;59:2326-8.

26. Barker KN, Flynn EA, Pepper GA. Observation method of detecting medication errors. Am J Health-Syst Pharm. 2002;59:2314-6.

27. Barker KN, Mikeal RI, Pearson RE, Illig NA, Morse ML. Medication errors in nursing homes and small hospitals. Am J Hosp Pharm. 1982;39:987-91.

28. Rozich JD, Haraden CR, Resar RK. Adverse drug event trigger tool: a practical methodology for measuring medication related harm. Qual Saf Health Care. 2008;12:194-200.

29. Jha AK, Kuperman GJ, Teich JM, Leape L, Shea B, Rittenberg E, Burdick E, Seger DL, Vander Vliet M, Bates DW. Identifying adverse drug events: development of a computer-based monitor and comparison with chart review and stimulated voluntary reporting. J Am Med Inform Assoc. 1998;3:305-14.

30. Classen DC, Pestotnik SL, Evans RS, Burke JP. Description of a computerized adverse drug event monitor using a hospital information system. Hosp Pharm. 1992;27:774, 776-9, 783.

31. Classen DC, Pestotnik SL, Evans RS, Burke JP. Computerized surveillance of adverse drug events in hospital patients (published erratum appears in JAMA. 1992;267:1992). JAMA. 1991;266:2847-51.

32. Raschke RA, Gollihare B, Wunderlich TA, Guidry J, Leibowitz A, Peirce, J, Lemelson L, Heisler MA, Susong C. A computer alert system to prevent injury from adverse drug events: development and evaluation in a community teaching hospital (published erratum appears in JAMA 1999;281:420). JAMA. 1998;280:1317-20.

33. Bates DW, Evans RS, Murff H, Stetson PD, Pizziferri L, Hripcsak G. Detecting adverse events using information technology. J Am Med Inform Assoc. 2003;10:115-28.

34. Bates DW. Using information technology to screen for adverse drug events. Am J Health-Syst Pharm. 2002;59:2317-9.

35. Schneider PJ. Using technology to enhance measurement of drug-use safety. Am J Health-Syst Pharm. 2002;59:2330-2.

36. National Coordinating Council for Medication Error Reporting and Prevention. Taxonomy of medication errors now available [Internet]. National Coordinating Council for Medication Error Reporting and Prevention; c2001 [cited 2019 Sep 8]. Available from: https://www.nccmerp.org/taxonomy-medication-errors-now-available

37. Institute for Safe Medication Practices. ENFit enteral devices are on their way...important safety considerations for hospitals [Internet]. Horsham (PA): Institute for Safe Medication Practices; 2015 Apr 9 [cited 2020 Dec 20]. Available from: https://www.ismp.org/resources/enfit-enteral-devices-are-their-wayimportant-safety-considerations-hospitals

38. Institute for Safe Medication Practices. NRFit: A global "fit" for neuraxial medication safety [Internet]. Horsham (PA): Institute for Safe Medication Practices; 2020 Jul 16 [cited 2020 Dec 20]. Available from: https://www.ismp.org/resources/nrfit-global-fit-neuraxial-medication-safety

39. Patient Safety Organization Privacy Protection Center (PSO PPC). Available from: https://www.psoppc.org/psoppc_web/publicpages/commonFormatsOverview

40. The Joint Commission. Hospital National Patient Safety Goals 2015 [Internet]. Available from: https://www.jointcommission.org/-/media/deprecated-unorganized/imported-assets/tjc/system-folders/assetmanager/2015_hap_npsg_erpdf.pdf

41. Sentinel Event Alert: Managing the risks of direct oral anticoagulants [Internet]. The Joint Commission; 2019 Jul 30 [cited 2019 Sep 8]. Available from: https://www.jointcommission.org/assets/1/18/SEA_61_DOACs_FINAL.pdf

42. Dunn EB, Wolfe JJ. Medication error classification and avoidance. Hosp Pharm. 1997;32:860-5.

43. Kessler DA for the working group. Introducing MedWatch: a new approach to reporting medication and device adverse effects and product problems. JAMA. 1993;269(21):2765-8.

44. The Patient Safety Act and Quality Improvement Act of 2005. Public Law 109-41, 109th Congress, July 29, 2005.

45. Pennsylvania Patient Safety Authority. Vol 6(4), December 2009.

46. Institute for Safe Medication Practices. Heparin errors continue despite prior, high-profile fatal events [Internet]. Horsham (PA): Institute for Safe Medication Practices; 2008 Jul 17 [cited 2020 Dec 20]. Available from: https://www.ismp.org/resources/heparin-errors-continue-despite-prior-high-profile-fatal-events

47. Reason J. Human error. Cambridge (England): Cambridge University Press; 1990.

48. Bogner MS. Human error in medicine. Hillsdale (NJ): Lawrence Erlbaum Associates; 1994.

49. Norman DA. The design of everyday things. New York: Basic Books; 1988.

50. Reason J. Managing the risks of organizational accidents. Burlington (VT): Ashgate; 1997.

51. Henriksen K, Dayton E, Keyes MA, Carayon P, Hughes R, Hughes RG. Understanding adverse events: a human factors framework. In: Hughes RG, editor. Patient safety and quality: an evidence-based handbook for nurses. Rockville (MD): Agency for Healthcare Research and Quality; 2008: 67-83.

52. Vaida AJ, Zipperer L. Safe medication information delivery: the role of the medical librarian. Patient Saf Qual Healthc. 2006 Nov/Dec;3(6):42-5.

53. Grout J. Mistake-proofing the design of health care processes. Rockville (MD): AHRQ Publication No. 07-0020; 2007.

54. Institute for Safe Medication Practices. Medication error prevention "toolbox". Medication Safety Alert! 1999;4(11):1.

55. ISMP Canada. Designing effective recommendations [Internet]. 2013 [cited 2019 Sep 8]. Available from: https://www.ismp-canada.org/download/ocil/ISMPCONCIL2013-4_EffectiveRecommendations.pdf

56. Woods DM, Holl JL, Angst D, Echiverri S, Johnson D, Soglin D, Srinivasa G, Barnathan J, Amsden L, Lamkin L, Weiss K. Improving clinical communication and patient safety: clinician-recommended solutions. In: Henriksen K, Battles JB, Keyes MA, Grady ML, editors. Advances in patient safety: new directions and alternative approaches. Vol. 3. Rockville (MD): Agency for Healthcare Research and Quality; 2008: 4-13.

57. American Society of Hospital Pharmacists. ASHP guidelines on preventing medication errors in hospitals. Am J Hosp Pharm. 1993;50:305-14.

58. Grasha AF, O'Neill M. Cognitive processes in medication errors. US Pharm. 1996;21:96-109.

59. Abel SR, Intrevado P, Ozsen L. Literature review of interprofessional research on inpatient pharmacy operations. Am J Health-Syst Pharm. 2013 Jun 1;70(11):989-96.

60. Holden RJ, Scanlon MC, Patel NR, Kaushal R, Escoto KH, Brown RL, Alper SJ, Arnold JM, Shalaby TM, Murkowski K, Karsh BT. A human factors framework and study of the effect of nursing workload on patient safety and employee quality of working life. BMJ Qual Saf. 2011 Jan;20(1):15-24.

61. DeMichele D. Preventing medication errors. US Pharm. 1995;20:69-75.

62. Phuong JM, Penm J, Chaar B, Oldfield LD, Moles R. The impacts of medication shortages on patient outcomes: a scoping review. PLoS One. 2019;14(5):e0215837.

63. Davis NM. Lack of knowledge as a cause of medication errors. Hosp Pharm. 1997;32:16-25.

64. Pepper GA. Errors in drug administration by nurses. Am J Health-Syst Pharm. 1995 Feb 15;52(4):390-5.

65. The Joint Commission (TJC). (2007). Sentinel Events Statistics, Mar 31, 2007. Available from: http://www.jointcommission.org/Sentinel_event_data_general/

66. Fitzgerald WL, Wilson DB. Medication errors: lessons in law. Drug Top. 1998;142:84-93.

67. Institute for Healthcare Improvement. Quality improvement essentials toolkit: failure modes and effects analysis [Internet]. 2017 [cited 2019 Sep 8]. Available from: http://www.ihi.org/resources/Pages/Tools/FailureModesandEffectsAnalysisTool.aspx

68. Automotive Industry Group (AIAG) and the Verband der Automobilindustrie (VDA). Failure mode and effects analysis (FMEA) handbook. Southfield (MI): AIAG; 2019.

69. National Patient Safety Foundation. RCA2: Improving root cause analyses and actions to prevent harm [Internet]. 2015 [cited 2019 Sep 8]. Available from: http://www.ihi.org/resources/Pages/Tools/RCA2-Improving-Root-Cause-Analyses-and-Actions-to-Prevent-Harm.aspx

70. University of Michigan Center for Healthcare Engineering and Patient Safety. Root cause contributing factor statements: applying the five rules of causation [Internet]. 2015. Available from: https://cheps.engin.umich.edu/wp-content/uploads/sites/118/2015/04/Five-Rules-of-Causation.pdf

71. The Joint Commission Sentinel Event Policy and Procedure. Available from: http://www.jointcommission.org/Sentinel_Event_policy_and_procedures/

72. Abood RR. Errors in pharmacy practice. US Pharm. 1996;21:122-32.

73. Coleman IC. Medication errors: picking up the pieces. Drug Top. 1999;143:83-92.

74. Glut of medication errors focuses pharmacists on event reporting. Drug Util Rev. 1998:201-6.

75. Cohen MR. ISMP medication error report analysis: the mistake of blaming people and not the process. Hosp Pharm. 1997;32:1106-11.

76. ISMP Newsletter. An injustice has been done: jail time given to pharmacist who made an error. 2009 Aug 21. Available from: https://www.ismp.org/resources/injustice-has-been-done-jail-time-given-pharmacist-who-made-error

77. Marx D. Reckless homicide at Vanderbilt? A Just Culture analysis [Internet]. Outcome Engenuity; 2019 [cited 2019 Aug 24]. Available from: https://www.outcome-eng.com/wp-content/uploads/2019/03/Vanderbilt-Homicide-A-Just-Culture-Analysis_David-Marx.pdf

78. Introduction to Just Culture. In: Just Culture training for managers, healthcare edition. Plano (TX): Outcome Engenuity; 2008. p. 7-10.

79. Beil, L. Wondery [Internet]. West Hollywood (CA): Wondery, Inc.; c2020. [Podcast], Dr. Death; 2018. Available from: https://wondery.com/shows/dr-death/.

80. U.S. Food and Drug Administration. New England Compounding Center pharmacist sentenced for role in nationwide fungal meningitis outbreak [Internet]. Silver Spring (MD): U.S. Food and Drug Administration; c2020 [2019 Jan 31, cited 2020 Dec 20]. Available from: https://www.fda.gov/inspections-compliance-enforcement-and-criminal-investigations/press-releases/january-31-2018-new-england-compounding-center-pharmacist-sentenced-role-nationwide-fungal

81. ISMP Newsletter: Our long journey towards safety-minded just culture. Part I: Where we've been. 2006 Sep 7. Available from: https://www.ismp.org/resources/our-long-journey-towards-safety-minded-just-culture-part-i-where-weve-been

82. GAIN Working group E, Flight Ops/ATC Ops Safety Information Sharing. A roadmap to a Just Culture: enhancing the safety environment. Available from: http://flightsafety.org/files/just_culture.pdf

83. Berwick DM, Calkins DR, McCannon CJ, Hackbarth AD. The 100,000 Lives Campaign: setting a goal and a deadline for improving health care quality. JAMA. Jan 2006;295(3):324-7.

SUGGESTED READINGS

1. Gandhi TK, Weingart SN, Borus J, Seger A, Peterson J, Burdick E, Seger D, Shu K, Federico F, Leape L, Bates D. Adverse drug events in ambulatory care. N Engl J Med. 2003;348:1556-64.

2. Rozich JD, Haraden CR, Resar RK. Adverse drug event trigger tool: a practical methodology for measuring medication related harm. Qual Saf Health Care. 2008;12:194-200.

3. Howard R, Avery A, Bissell P. Causes of preventable drug-related hospital admissions: a qualitative study. Qual Saf Health Care. 2008;17:109-16.

4. Kale A, Keohane CA, Maviglia S, Gandhi TK, Poon EG. Adverse drug events caused by serious medication administration errors. BMJ Qual Saf. 2012;21:933-8.

5. Bagian JP, Gosbee J, Lee CZ, Williams L, McKnight SD, Mannos DM. The Veterans Affairs root cause analysis system in action. Jt Comm J Qual Improv. 2002;28:531-45.

6. Smetzer J, Baker C, Byrne FD, Cohen MR. Shaping systems for better behavioral choices: lessons learned from a fatal medication error. Jt Comm J Qual Patient Saf. 2010 Apr;36(4):152-63.

7. National Patient Safety Foundation. RCA^2: Improving root cause analyses and actions to prevent harm. 2015. Available from: http://www.ihi.org/resources/Pages/Tools/RCA2-Improving-Root-Cause-Analyses-and-Actions-to-Prevent-Harm.aspx

8. Norman D. The design of everyday things. New York: Basic Books; 1988.

9. Wachter R. The digital doctor: hope, hype, and harm at the dawn of medicine's computer age. New York: McGraw-Hill; 2015.

10. Institute of Medicine. Health IT and patient safety: building safer systems for better care. Washington (DC): The National Academies Press; 2012.

11. Larson C, Saine D. Medication safety officer's handbook. Bethesda (MD): American Society of Health-System Pharmacists; 2013.

12. Cohen M. Medication errors. 2nd ed. Washington (DC): American Pharmacists Association; 2007.

13. The Case for Medication Safety Officers (MSO). Horsham (PA): Institute for Safe Medication Practices; 2018.

14. Marx D. Whack-a-mole: the price we pay for expecting perfection. Plano (TX): By Your Side Studios; 2009.

15. Marx D. Dave's subs: a novel story about workplace accountability. Plano (TX): By Your Side Studios; 2015.

Chapter Twenty-One

Policy, Procedure, and Guideline Development

Whitney Mortensen • Gregory Heindel • Conor Hanrahan

Learning Objectives

● *After completing this chapter, the reader will be able to:*

- Differentiate between types of practice documents (e.g., policy, procedure) and approaches for managing those documents.
- Discuss the roles and responsibilities of individuals/groups involved in the practice document development and review process (e.g., document owner, stakeholders, and consultants).
- Identify factors that influence document development (e.g., regulations, scope, and review periods).
- Describe the systematic methodology to develop and revise practice documents.

Key Concepts

❶ Documents should ultimately meet the need of employees who are responsible to adhere to the policy, procedure, or guideline. Thus, implementation of practice documents should result in perpetual compliance and safe medication practices.

❷ The first step to understanding the practice document development requirements is to evaluate the process for the organization.

❸ Review periods for documents vary depending on the organization (typically a biennial or triennial review) or as defined by a regulatory agency or accrediting body.

❹ The first step in developing practice documents is to identify the need for the document.

⑤ It is important to gather relevant data to the practice document topic.

⑥ Practice documents should be evidence based and reflect standard of care or best practice.

⑦ Ensure the format, ease of use, and reading level are appropriate for the intended audience and end users.

⑧ After composition, the draft document must be disseminated for review and comments.

⑨ After approval, publication and education are essential to the success of any practice document.

⑩ The last step in the development and maintenance of practice documents is to ensure compliance with any changes.

Introduction

Health care professionals in health systems and other settings are often asked to develop **practice documents** (e.g., **policies, procedures**, and **guidelines**) that not only apply to their department, but also pertain to other parts of the organization or even the organization in its entirety. Given the breadth of knowledge that pharmacists possess regarding medication use, they are poised to contribute to development of practice documents affecting each aspect of the medication-use cycle (e.g., prescribing, preparation, inventory management, dispensing, and administration). These types of practice documents are appropriate for various reasons and are often created to establish best practices, ensure safe and reliable operational practices, and meet regulatory requirements. Further explanation of these various document types and justifications for document development is included throughout this chapter.

The nuances of document development are unfamiliar to many clinicians, particularly outside of clinical guidelines. Literature available to help the health care professional on document development is limited and often directed toward more general application of evidence-based medicine (EBM) and use of outcomes research in the medication-use policy development process.[1-3] Selected resources are also available in the nursing literature.[4] Much of what the individual is exposed to in these areas is on-the-job training. This skill set should be taught early in the educational process for pharmacists, with a specific recommendation from the Center for the Advancement of Pharmacy Education to engage pharmacy students in the development of professional documents that are relevant to needs of various organizations, specifically formulary monographs and policy development.[5] This may be accomplished in the drug information curriculum. The information presented in this chapter is derived from the literature and other available resources and designed to assist with the development of policies, procedures, guidelines, and other documents.[6] For more in-depth training, professional certificate programs or relevant Masters programs (e.g., Master of Business Administration [MBA], Master of Healthcare Administration [MHA], and Master of Science [MS] program) may be of interest.

Regulatory Considerations

Health care is a highly regulated field, with clinical and operational regulations from many organizations, including **The Joint Commission (TJC)** (https://www.joint commission.org/), state regulators, boards of pharmacy, the United States Food and Drug Administration (FDA) (https://www.fda.gov), **URAC®** (https://www.urac.org/), and the Drug Enforcement Administration (DEA) (https://www.dea.gov/), among others. Hospitals and health systems often employ compliance programs to manage these regulations and ensure safe and appropriate practice in all areas of the organization. Health care professionals and leaders should understand regulatory requirements and the level of detail or documentation that is expected to meet the requirements of these accrediting or regulatory bodies. As a result, clinicians often are responsible to develop, review, and revise practice documents on a routine basis. It is important to note that while practice documents should be compliant to all regulatory requirements, the ❶ *documents should ultimately meet the need of employees who are responsible to adhere to the policy, procedure, or guideline. Thus, implementation of practice documents should result in perpetual compliance and safe medication practices.* Additional considerations to ensure regulatory compliance are detailed in the systematic approach to practice documents later in this chapter.

Practice Document Design and Organization

Practice document design and organization is institution- or organization-specific. Appendix 21-1 provides an example policy. ❷ *The first step to understanding the practice document development requirements is to evaluate the process for the organization.* While some organizations still manage practice documents, including policies and procedures, manually, some employ **workflow software solutions** for document management. However, there is not a standard approach to designing and organizing the documents themselves. The organizational standards and requirements of each individual document must be understood. For example, some organizations may have a standard glossary of terms to be used for all policies and procedures, while others may define terms separately in each document. Additionally, the types of documents employed by the organization must be considered. Some organizations solely use policies and procedures, while others supplement policies and procedures with additional guidance documents, such as practice guidelines, standard operating procedures, or protocols. Policies are documents that set a minimum standard, whereas procedures describe the steps or tasks required to meet those standards. What is considered a policy or a procedure is relatively consistent between organizations; however, there is significant variability around how other practice documents are defined. For example, the content of some practice documents (e.g., manual, job aide, protocol) may be considered a mandate by one organization but a suggestion by another organization. Thus, it is critical to understand the organization's expectations for each type of document.

Organizations generally adopt one of two standard methods for document management. In the consolidated approach, both policy statements and procedural steps are combined in a single document focused on a given topic (e.g., controlled substances). Alternatively, in the separated approach, individual, but related, documents are created. A policy is written separately from other supporting documents (e.g., procedure, manual) which provide additional detail on the same topic to implement the policy. When selecting the type of supporting document, the intent of the document and the organization's approach to document selection should be considered.

Factors Influencing Practice Document Development

A stepwise approach to document development is presented in the following section. However, an understanding of factors that may influence the development of practice documents is warranted. To begin, it is necessary to look at the time frame in which these documents need to be approved and reapproved. Some documents need regular review. ❸ *Review periods for documents vary depending on the organization (typically a biennial or triennial review) or as defined by a regulatory agency or accrediting body* (e.g., URAC® requires a review of documents every 2 years). Attention is required to ensure adequate time for all stakeholders to review and edit the documents prior to approval in the required review cycle. Documents should have a defined **scope statement** that may include location, practice area, patient versus nonpatient care areas, or other considerations. It is important to identify the scope statements for the organization and indicate the most appropriate statement for the document created. The subject matter of the document varies. Table 21-1 details common health system policy classifications.

Appropriate time should be allowed for document review and workflow processes. It is sometimes beneficial and efficient to collect feedback from all stakeholders

TABLE 21–1. HEALTH SYSTEM POLICY SAMPLE CLASSIFICATIONS

Administrative: Policies that address organizational operations

Department specific: Policies that address an individual department or work area (e.g., pharmacy, nursing, laboratory, food, and nutrition)

Human resources: Policies that address the work environment and employee rights

Patient care: Policies that affect patient care directly or indirectly and cross more than one department or work area

Procurement: Policies that address purchasing and inventory management

Safety policies and emergency operations plans: Policies that address backup operational practices in the event of emergent situations (e.g., loss of power, system downtime, natural disaster)

TABLE 21–2. SEQUENTIAL DOCUMENT REVIEW PROCESS EXAMPLE

1. Document owner identifies need for revision (e.g., scheduled review, new information)
2. Document owner identifies content experts and coordinates a review and update by these stakeholders
3. Document owner incorporates stakeholder feedback and submits review document to pharmacy document coordinator (e.g., drug information service) for review of content, format, consistency with other documents
4. Pharmacy document coordinator facilitates approval and publication of the revised document with the organizational department responsible for all practice documents (e.g., compliance department)

concurrently or have a single virtual or in-person discussion with all stakeholders. In many situations, though, a sequential feedback and approval process is preferred. This is especially true if the organization has divided responsibilities among several groups. For example, if multiple groups or disciplines need to review the document, the sequence of the review should be considered. It would be prudent for those reviewing for clinical or operational content to provide feedback prior to a group who reviews the final draft to ensure regulatory compliance and alignment with organizational document standards. A sequential review process should eliminate the risk of duplicative work among stakeholders. Table 21-2 provides an example for a sequential review process. A continuous quality improvement process should be applied to practice document development. A thorough discussion on continuous quality improvement is found in Chapter 18.

There are several critical skills that are beneficial when overseeing document development and management. Attention to detail, strong written communication skills, and a system or population perspective to patient care are needed. Pharmacists with additional training in drug information are often involved with policy development, given their involvement with medication safety and formulary management.[7] Additionally, a pharmacist with a strong drug information skill set is an ideal candidate to participate in policy development since it requires thorough and accurate analysis of EBM (see Chapter 8) and quality improvement initiatives, as well as strong written communication skills (see Chapter 13).

TABLE 21–3. SYSTEMATIC METHOD FOR PRACTICE DOCUMENT DEVELOPMENT AND MAINTENANCE

Before beginning: evaluate and understand institution-specific process

1. Identify need and determine purpose
2. Gather data
3. Research regulations, standard of care, best practices, and published evidence
4. Synthesize practice document and incorporate stakeholder input
5. Gain document approval
6. Publication, education, and implementation
7. Continual evaluation of practice document compliance

Systematic Method for Practice Document Development and Maintenance

Before undertaking the task of practice document development or maintenance, it is important to appreciate the approval process at an institution. The approving bodies, time needed for approval, and relevant stakeholders may vary greatly from one institution or practice document to the next. Fully understanding the process at an individual institution in the context of the document topic will help determine the timeline, urgency for review, and prioritization for development of different documents. While individual practice documents, institutions, and scenarios may require unique considerations, the overall approach will generally consist of many similar steps. Table 21-3 describes the systematic method for development and maintenance of practice documents. This framework may be followed for both new documents and revisions of existing documents. It is important to note that some aspects of this framework may need slight adjustment based upon culture, manpower, and stakeholders at different institutions. The necessary steps are described below.

STEP 1: IDENTIFY THE NEED

❹ *The first step in developing practice documents is to identify the need for the document.* A wide spectrum exists for the need of practice documents. Accrediting bodies (e.g., TJC, URAC®, American Society of Health-System Pharmacists [ASHP]) may require up-to-date practice documents. Internal groups, such as the human resources department, may require other departments to maintain specific practice documents to establish clear expectations within the workplace (e.g., paid time off, dress codes). Practice documents may also be utilized to limit the variability in a process through standardization (e.g., the patient identifiers used prior to dispensing a prescription, the appropriate steps to unit-dose packaging tablets). Established practice documents also enable managers to hold workers accountable to the clear standards for practice and, if needed, discipline violators of those standards. Finally, clinical guidelines and best practice recommendations (e.g., from the Institute for Safe Medication Practices [ISMP] or the Infectious Diseases Society of America [IDSA]) can be executed through practice document development, approval, and implementation.

STEP 2: GATHER RELEVANT DATA

Next, ❺ *it is important to gather relevant data to the practice document topic.* Internal data, such as medication error reports or TJC findings, may help inform decisions or identify gaps that the practice document should address. Data may also be helpful in defining the scope of the practice document and identifying relevant institutions, departments, or practice areas. A search for other similar or related practice documents should also be completed to ensure the content is not duplicative or contradictory. For example, the institution-wide document describing paid time-off requests may be adequate for a pharmacy department to adopt and a new, pharmacy-specific document may not be required. Similarly, storage and temperature monitoring standards for medication refrigerators may be within pharmacy, nursing, and environmental department-specific documents. The defined expectations should, at minimum, not conflict and the need for duplicative documents certainly warrants discussion. Understanding the purpose and the need (or lack thereof) for a practice document in context of internal data is an important step to help prioritize work and direct research efforts in the next step.

STEP 3: FOLLOW BEST-PRACTICE RECOMMENDATIONS

Whenever possible, ❻ *practice documents should be evidence based and reflect standard of care or best practice.* The appropriate sources for information related to practice documents may vary depending on subject matter but will likely include a combination of tertiary and primary literature. Clinical practice guidelines should be informed heavily by professional organizations' recommendations. For example, a clinical practice guideline on pulmonary arterial hypertension should consider published recommendations from the American College of Chest Physicians. For more detailed information on evidence-based practice guidelines, see Chapter 8. Professional organizations' position papers and other recommendations are also available for nonclinical topics and should be incorporated when relevant. Regulatory guidelines and requirements should also be reviewed to ensure that the practice document meets appropriate accreditation and legal standards. Subject-matter experts should also be consulted to identify unpublished considerations; for example, an industrial hygienist would lend valuable expertise to documents pertaining to hazardous substances. Lastly, a survey of other institutions may help identify solutions, safeguards, or overlooked considerations.

Case Study 21–1

As a clinical pharmacist at a large academic medical center, you participate in formulary management to support the efforts of the pharmacy department and the health system to provide safe, effective, and cost-effective medications for use within the system. Currently, intravenous acetaminophen is on formulary but restricted to use in patients who are strictly NPO (nothing by mouth). A medication-use evaluation of this product found significant nonadherence to the restriction. You are asked to develop an IV-to-PO (intravenous-to-oral) conversion policy for the health system to decrease the amount of inappropriate prescribing of this agent.

- *List the steps used to approach this assignment.*
- *Discuss the resources used when gathering background information.*
- *Explain the process to summarize the information collected for development of the policy.*
- *Define stakeholder and identify key stakeholders for this policy.*

STEP 4: DRAFT THE DOCUMENT

After gathering all pertinent background information, recommendations, and literature, the information should be synthesized into a working draft. Most organizations or departments have specific templates that should be followed for each of the different types of practice documents. Depending on the complexity and content of the document, the document owner may individually draft the document, or the owner may assemble a work group to jointly develop the document. Involving key stakeholders in a work group early in the process can be an efficient way of preventing significant revisions later. Regardless of the method, an evidence-based approach to the review of information and development of documents is preferred. ❼ *Ensure the format, ease of use, and reading level are appropriate for the intended audience and end users.* Relevant key words and links to supporting documents should also be incorporated. It is important to follow any standard terminology or definitions used at the organization to ensure consistency between documents. Educational efforts and tools addressing potential practice changes for affected individuals are also important to consider.

STEP 5: DISSEMINATE FOR REVIEW AND COMMENTS

❽ *After composition, the draft document must be disseminated for review and comments.* Stakeholder and experts' review and input are probably most important at this stage of the systematic method but would also be valuable in both previous steps and later steps, depending on the scenario. See Chapter 22 on project management for details on how to best identify appropriate stakeholders. Typically, the document owner will compile comments and make edits as needed. The finalized document should integrate an evidence-based practice with clinical, regulatory, and stakeholder expertise. It is important to acknowledge that this review, comment, and edit cycle may be repeated many times before the documents are ready for approval.

STEP 6: RECEIVE APPROVAL

The approving bodies for practice documents will fluctuate immensely between different institutions, subject matters, and types of practice documents. Table 21-4 provides common types of practice documents, approval bodies, and relevant stakeholders. In general, departmental specific documents may be reviewed by a process manager or relevant committee. Interdisciplinary and interdepartmental documents will often require approval through one or more interdisciplinary committees. The **pharmacy and therapeutics committee** (see Chapter 15) is probably the most common interdisciplinary body that regularly approves pharmacy-related documents. Notably, in some instances an individual (e.g., vice president of clinical operations) may have ultimate approval rights for a practice document. The approval of documents, the stakeholders included, and any relevant discussion points should always be recorded, regardless of the approving body. This information is important not only to implementation and enforcement of the document, but a powerful reference tool during future reviews of the document.

STEP 7: PUBLISH, EDUCATE, AND IMPLEMENT

❾ *After approval, publication and education are essential to the success of any practice document.* In general, the document should be readily accessible to end users as a point-of-care reference or guide. In most cases, current versions are available in an online document repository. Some institutions provide printed copies within relevant areas, while others

TABLE 21-4. COMMON EXAMPLES OF PRACTICE DOCUMENTS, APPROVAL BODIES, AND IMPORTANT STAKEHOLDERS

Practice Document	Approval Bodies	Important Stakeholders
Medication Storage Policy	Pharmacy and Therapeutics Committee	Pharmacy operations managers
		Nurse unit managers
		Environmental services
		Infection control
		Legal/risk management
Patient Identification Before Dispensing Medications Procedure	Legal/Risk Management	Pharmacists
		Technicians
		Medication safety pharmacist
		Nurses
		Legal/risk management
Antibiotic Desensitization Guideline	Pharmacy and Therapeutics Committee	Infectious disease specialists
		Allergy/immunology specialist
		Infectious disease pharmacists
		IV pharmacists
		Nurses
Intravenous (IV) Batch Procedure	Pharmacy Operations Committee, IV Room Manager	IV pharmacists
		IV technicians
Central Venous Catheter Assessment Policy	Nurse Practice Council	Infection control
		Nurses
		Pharmacists
		Infectious disease specialists

actively restrict the ability to print or save digital copies. Documents for an entire health system, institution, or department may also be stored in one physical or virtual location or may be spread into separate and secluded sections. Links within electronic health records and/or electronic formularies may also be considered. Each of these strategies presents different advantages and disadvantages regarding the effort required to access documents, the ease of end users to find relevant documents, and the energy required to update all copies of a document. Regardless of the method used to disseminate the documents, a historical record of previous versions should be maintained. Clinical policies, procedures, and guidelines are often implemented into practice using standard order sets, order templates, or other clinical decision support tools in the electronic medical record. These strategies help ensure that institutional best practices are applied by frontline clinicians. Nonetheless, robust education (e.g., computer-based training modules, attestations, continuing education programs) about document changes is crucial to successful adoption of new practice documents. A plan for education and communication regarding practice documents should be carefully considered throughout the process.

STEP 8: MONITOR COMPLIANCE

❿ *The last step in the development and maintenance of practice documents is to ensure compliance with any changes.* This often-overlooked step is arguably the most important. The value of a practice document lies in the intent and purpose (identified in Step 1), and compliance audits represent an evaluation of the successful execution of that intent or purpose. A compliance audit ensures specific requirements of the policy or procedure were adopted into practice. Poor compliance may indicate the need for re-evaluation of the stakeholder input, publication, or education process. Finally, document management strategies should be assessed by compliance with the established review periods and adjusted as indicated, and a process should be implemented to ensure the change is successfully maintained. Chapter 18 details continuous quality improvement methodology which may be useful in monitoring document compliance.

Conclusion

Pharmacists, with their expertise in pharmacotherapy, medication safety, operations, and formulary management, are uniquely situated to be involved in and lead policy development. The tools that health care professionals use for these activities are gradually being introduced via health care literature and professional societies. Pharmacists with additional training in drug information are often involved with policy development, given their involvement with medication safety and formulary management. Additionally, a pharmacist with a strong drug information skill set is an ideal candidate to participate in policy development since it requires thorough and accurate analysis of EBM and quality improvement initiatives.

Case Study 21-2

The IV-to-PO conversion policy you developed was approved. You are now tasked with implementing this new policy.

- *Discuss options for disseminating the document.*
- *List which staff/groups require education on this policy.*
- *Identify strategies to ensure compliance with the policy.*

Self-Assessment Questions

1. The following health-system policies require a pharmacist's participation, **EXCEPT:**
   a. Hazardous Substances Policy
   b. Sterile Compounding Policy
   c. Time and Attendance Policy
   d. Antimicrobial Stewardship Policy
   e. Drug Shortages Policy

2. When gathering information for inclusion in a health system policy, what is the initial step:
   a. Conduct a literature search using CINAHL Information Systems.
   b. Ask for a meeting with the director of pharmacy.
   c. Contact colleagues who work at other health systems.
   d. Gather background information including the justification of the policy.
   e. Conduct a literature search using PubMed®.

3. Which of the following ensures consistency, establishes expectations, and sets minimum standards?
   a. Policy
   b. Guideline
   c. Project description
   d. Purpose statement
   e. Project activities

4. Which of the following resources may be used to research the standard of care before engaging in writing a policy?
   a. Tertiary references
   b. Clinical treatment guidelines
   c. Primary literature
   d. Colleagues and coworkers
   e. All of the above

5. Which of the following is/are a type(s) of health-system policy classification?
   a. Patient care
   b. Procurement
   c. Administrative
   d. Human resource
   e. All of the above

6. The frequency with which practice documents are reviewed is solely determined by the organization.
   a. True
   b. False

7. Which of the following represents the correct sequence of the systematic approach for practice document development?
   a. Gather relevant data, identify the need, draft document, ensure compliance with the policy/procedure, provide education to end users.
   b. Identify the need, gather relevant data, draft document, provide education to end users, ensure compliance with the policy/procedure.
   c. Ensure compliance with the policy/procedure, identify the need, gather relevant data, draft document, provide education to end users.
   d. Provide education to end users, identify the need, gather relevant data, draft document, ensure compliance with the policy/procedure.
   e. Draft document, identify the need, gather relevant data, ensure compliance with the policy/procedure, provide education to end users.

8. Additional resources to build a skill set in practice document development:
   a. Professional pharmacy organization programs
   b. Business programs (e.g., MBA program)
   c. Tertiary references (e.g., textbooks)
   d. Agency for Healthcare Research and Quality (AHRQ)
   e. All of the above

9. The following stakeholders would be *MOST* appropriate to involve in the policy development of anticoagulation management within the organization:
   a. Pharmacist, cardiologist, human resources director
   b. Cardiologist, pharmacist, pharmacy and therapeutics committee chairperson
   c. Legal/risk manager, cardiologist, chief operating officer
   d. Environmental services, nurse practice council, cardiologist
   e. Quality officer, cardiologist, pharmacist

10. Which of the following is an accurate description of a procedure?
    a. A document that outlines the steps or specific actions to implement a policy
    b. A document that provides suggestions or advice for a particular activity
    c. A document that changes infrequently and addresses "what," "who," and "why"
    d. A general term referring collectively to multiple types of documents
    e. A document that sets minimum standards

11. Policies are prescriptive in their direction.
    a. True
    b. False

12. Poor compliance with practice documents may indicate which of the following?
    a. Need for additional education
    b. Re-evaluation of stakeholder input
    c. Re-evaluation of the formatting and reading level
    d. Re-evaluation of standard of care or best practice
    e. All of the above

13. Practice documents should always be in compliance with all related regulatory requirements.
    a. True
    b. False

14. A scope statement of the policy is a step-by-step description of how the issue addressed in the policy should be managed.
    a. True
    b. False

15. Hospital policies should consider accreditation standards from The Joint Commission.
    a. True
    b. False

REFERENCES

1. Gray T, Bertch K, Galt K, Gonyeau M, Karpiuk E, Oyen L, Sudekum MJ, Vermeulen LC. Guidelines for therapeutic interchange—2004. Pharmacotherapy. 2005;25(11):1666–80.
2. Vermeulen LC, Beis SJ, Cano SB. Applying outcomes research in improving the medication-use process. Am J Health-Syst Pharm. 2000;57:2277–82.
3. Vermeulen LC, Rough SS, Thielke TS, Shane RR, Ivey MF, Woodward BW, Pierpaoli PG, Thomley SM, Borr CA, Zilz DA. Strategic approach for improving the medication-use process in health systems: the high-performance pharmacy practice framework. Am J Health-Syst Pharm. 2007;64:1699–1710.
4. Oman KS, Duran C, Fink R. Evidence-based policy and procedures: an algorithm for success. JONA. 2008;38(1):47–51.
5. Medina MS, Plaza CM, Stowe CD, Robinson ET, DeLander G, Beck DE, Melchert RB, SupernawRB, Roche VF, Gleason BL, Strong MN, Bain A, Meyer GE, Dong BJ, Rochon J, Johnston P. Center for theAdvancement of Pharmacy Education (CAPE) Educational Outcomes 2013. Am J Pharm Educ. 2013;77(8):article 162.

6. AHRQ: Agency for Healthcare Research and Quality [Internet]. Rockville (MD): U.S. Department of Health and Human Services [cited 2019 Aug 24]. Available from: https://www.ahrq.gov

7. Tyler LS, Cole SW, May JR, Millares M, Valentino MA, Vermeulen LC, Wilson AL. ASHP guidelines on the pharmacy and therapeutics committee and the formulary system. Am J Health-Syst Pharm. 2008;65:1272–83.

22

Chapter Twenty-Two

Project Management

Conor Hanrahan • Candice Burns Wood

Learning Objectives

After completing this chapter, the reader will be able to:

- Differentiate between a project, program, and portfolio.
- Assess the viability and value of projects.
- Describe the key components of a project charter, including scope, goals, success criteria, and stakeholders.
- Discuss tools used for planning projects, including a work breakdown structure, requirements matrix, risk management plan, communication management plan, and change management plan.
- Explain factors important for the successful execution of a project.
- List key activities to complete when closing a project.

Key Concepts

❶ Understanding programs and portfolios is critical to successful project management.

❷ Knowing the success criteria provides a measurable way to define when the project is finished and the goal has been achieved.

❸ Knowing the stakeholders involved is a key step because many times the success of the project depends on their buy-in and input.

❹ It is extremely important to define the scope in order to put boundaries on the project and define its endpoint.

❺ After identifying tasks and the resources needed to accomplish those tasks, a project timeline can be developed.

Introduction

Health care today is perhaps more complex than it has ever been in history. Instead of the autonomous, physician-centric model of medicine practiced for decades, more organizations are recognizing the value of an interdisciplinary, patient-centric, and population-health approach. Furthermore, integrated health care delivery systems, as opposed to independently owned and disparate entities, are becoming the norm. Standardization and quality improvement processes are now core to many organizations wanting to reduce costs, improve safety, and increase their overall ability to care for patients. Government agencies are further propelling this transformation through changes in payment models and new regulations, adding another layer of complexity.

As a result, health care professionals are increasingly inundated with projects and responsibilities, often without being given more time or resources. Furthermore, most health care workers have historically not applied project management frameworks to these complex tasks. It is little surprise, therefore, that many projects in health care fail to succeed. Imagine, for instance, that a surgeon is about to perform a complex cardiac operation. However, instead of reading through the patient's chart, talking with the surgical team, prescheduling time in the operating room, and working through the step-by-step techniques needed to perform the operation, the physician decides to just begin the surgery without a plan. It should be clear that this patient's outcome would likely not be good, or at least that the surgery itself would not go smoothly. The same principle is also true with projects. Although a well thought out plan and systematic approach cannot guarantee success, it can certainly help increase the likelihood of success, improve productivity, reduce unnecessary stress and waste, and increase quality.

The practice of pharmacy is no exception. Drug information specialists and other pharmacy specialties develop, manage, and execute projects every day—everything from policy and guideline development to sweeping standardization efforts and patient care initiatives. As such, strong project management skills are paramount to success. In many ways, project management can be thought of as an extension of the existing drug information skillset by helping work get done quicker and more efficiently, as well as ensuring that best practices are implemented correctly.

Thus, the goal of this chapter is to provide readers with a meaningful framework for managing projects, which includes selection, project initiation, planning, execution, monitoring, and closing (see Figure 22-1). While several tools and strategies will be discussed, it is important to recognize that the level of project planning rigor should be proportional to the project at hand. For instance, the effort that goes into planning a 6-week long project should be much less than the planning needed for a 2-year long endeavor. As such, it is incredibly important to balance the planning of the project in relation to its urgency and complexity.

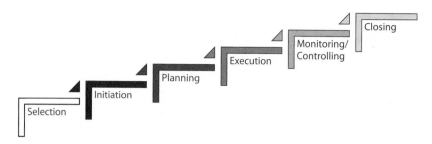

Figure 22–1. Overarching steps in project management.

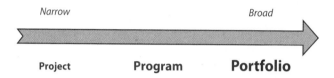

Figure 22–2. Relationship between projects, programs, and portfolios.

Projects, Programs, and Portfolios

Understanding the relationship between a project, program, and portfolio is also important (see Figure 22-2). At the highest level is a **portfolio**, which encompasses various plans to meet an overall strategic objective. Within a portfolio are **programs**, which involve a group of related projects that are managed in a coordinated way. Programs have their own goals and objectives that ultimately support the main strategic objective of the portfolio. For instance, the Pharmacy Services Department of a hospital might be considered a portfolio, while the subdivisions within Pharmacy Services (e.g., hospital, community, specialty) would be considered programs.

Projects are finite endeavors with a distinct beginning and end that ultimately support the overall efforts within a program or portfolio. Projects are also considered to be progressively elaborate, meaning that at the beginning there is relatively little information or detail; however, as the project evolves, a greater level of detail and planning is achieved. In contrast, **operations** encompass more routine day-to-day activities, are not progressively elaborate, and do not have a finite beginning and end. For example, designing a new car would be considered a project, whereas the ongoing manufacturing of the car after it has been designed would be considered an operation. Another example related to health care could be that of intravenous medication compounding. Implementing a technical solution to ensure safe and accurate compounding would be considered a project, whereas the ongoing use of that technology to compound medications would be considered an operation.

❶ *Understanding programs and portfolios is critical to successful project management.* Perhaps most importantly, a project that is aligned with portfolio and program goals will help ensure that the organization is achieving what it wants to accomplish. In such cases, it is also much easier to obtain project buy-in and approval from leaders and stakeholders within the organization. Alignment with organizational goals will also help in the prioritization of projects—especially in situations where there are many good ideas, but limited resources. For instance, the informatics departments of many organizations may have limited bandwidth or resources to work on all requests submitted by employees. Thus, one way they may prioritize work is to preferentially focus on projects that support major organizational needs.

Selecting Projects

PROJECT VIABILITY AND VALUE

One of the most challenging aspects of project management can be that of selecting and prioritizing projects. As mentioned above, successful projects are often those that are aligned with organizational priorities and can add value when completed. Value can be provided in different ways depending on the culture and objectives of the organization. Value might be demonstrated as the ability to execute on the organization's strategy and bring goals to fruition. It may also be shown in the ability to enable and bring forth change—particularly in rigid environments that lack the ability to change and adapt. Process improvement, or the idea that existing processes could become more efficient, safer, and higher quality, is also a common way of providing value. Additionally, improved regulatory compliance and avoidance of legal risk are sometimes used as a value proposition. Lastly, and perhaps most commonly, value is demonstrated through financial means (e.g., saving money, increasing revenue, better reimbursement).

In all cases, the added value should be measurable and quantifiable. For instance, if the value of implementing a new compounding system is reducing medication errors or gaining efficiencies, then one should be able to estimate how many medication errors may be avoided or define how much more efficient work would become. Ideally, an unbiased and evidence-based assessment should be done when determining value—especially with measures that are more malleable or harder to quantify. For instance, in the above example the published literature could be searched to identify medication error rates, or an internal time study could be conducted looking at workflow efficiency with and without the software. In addition to being quantifiable, it is important to ensure that the added value is meaningful and relevant in the eyes of those approving the project. This nuance is particularly helpful when multiple projects are competing for the same pool of limited resources. Those projects where the return-on-investment and the value proposition are high will often be prioritized above projects that show less value to the organization.

CREATING A BUSINESS CASE

Once the added value has been determined, it is often necessary to develop a compelling business case that can be presented to those approving the project. Without a cogent case or argument for the project, there may not be a convincing reason to move forward. While each organization may have their own requirements for a business case, it should typically include an overview of the current landscape or issue to be addressed, what will be accomplished, and a description of the value proposition. Details regarding business case development are beyond the scope of this chapter; however, several useful resources have been written on this topic if more information is desired.[1-3]

Initiating a Project

After a project has been selected, two key deliverables related to initiation can be developed: the **project charter** and the **stakeholder matrix**. The charter is a written document that serves as the guidepost for the project and helps outline the overall vision. Although project charters can vary, they typically contain several key elements including goals and success criteria, final deliverables, stakeholders, budgets, as well as any obvious assumptions, risks, and dependencies. An example of a project charter and its components is outlined in Appendix 22-1. The concept of the stakeholder matrix will be discussed more below.

GOALS, SUCCESS CRITERIA, AND DELIVERABLES

Project goals refer to the desired outcome of the project, whereas **success criteria** are quantifiable measures that define when the goal is accomplished. For example, if a goal is to regain a lost market segment of specialty pharmaceuticals, a success criterion might be a 30% increase in sales. ❷ *Knowing the success criteria is critical because they provide a measurable way to define when the project is finished and the goal has been achieved.* Importantly, it should be noted that success criteria might be easier or harder to measure depending on the goal. A goal to improve the reliability of the compounding process, for instance, will have markedly different success criteria than a goal to reduce deaths associated with errors in compounding. Thus, a thoughtful and realistic approach is required when developing goals and success criteria. Lastly, a **deliverable** refers to the tangible component that will be produced as a result of the project in order to achieve the success criteria. For example, if a criterion for success is a 30% improvement in sales, a deliverable might include a real-time dashboard that tracks sales over time.

STAKEHOLDERS

The other key deliverable during project initiation involves the identification of stakeholders. A **stakeholder** refers to anyone (internal or external to the organization) involved in, interested in, or impacted by the project. For instance, stakeholders for a project to install a new robot for filling prescriptions in a community pharmacy might include the pharmacists and technicians who would use the robot, the pharmacy manager or director who has oversight of the pharmacy and budget, patients whose prescriptions will be filled by the machine; environmental or maintenance services who install the robot, as well as information technology specialists who must integrate the robot with existing pharmacy dispensing software. ❸ *Knowing the stakeholders involved is a key step because many times the success of the project depends on their buy-in and input.* Stakeholders can be identified in many ways. A **stakeholder impact analysis** could be conducted to help recognize people affected by the project. This is a simple process whereby the project team brainstorms possible stakeholders and then estimates each stakeholder's corresponding impact on the project. Similarly, evaluating past projects could provide insight regarding individuals who might be interested or involved in the current endeavor. Those with responsibility for project approval and budgeting are also likely going to be key stakeholders. Consultation with the project sponsor or senior leaders may also be helpful.

Stakeholder Matrix

Once the stakeholders have been identified, it is important to understand their needs and manage them appropriately. One way to do this is to develop a stakeholder matrix or registry, which outlines who they are, their involvement in the project, their expectations from the project, their interest in the project, and how to engage them (see Appendix 22-2 for an example). Regarding stakeholder interest level, it can vary considerably and can often be classified into one of five categories:

1. Unaware: refers to those who are not aware of the project or its impact.
2. Resistant: refers to those who are aware of the project, but resistant to the change.
3. Neutral: refers to those who are aware of the project, but have low interest.
4. Supportive: refers to those who are aware and supportive with the project.
5. Leading: refers to those who are aware and actively engaged in the project.

Once the interest level of a stakeholder is known, it can be combined with their power/influence over the project to determine how they should be managed and engaged

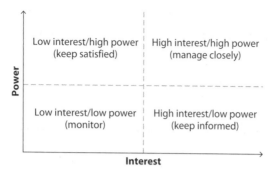

Figure 22–3. Stakeholder power/interest grid.

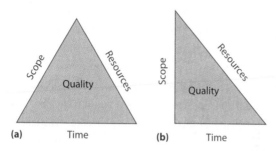

Figure 22–4. Influence of project constraints on quality. **(a)** Quality is a function of the project constraints (such as scope, available resources, and time), which are balanced in this part. **(b)** In this part, however, notice that if the time constraint is decreased, either the resources needed increases or scope must decrease in order to maintain the same level of quality.

(see Figure 22-3). For instance, a stakeholder with low interest and low power would not require as much attention as someone with both high interest and high power. Such analyses are helpful to determine how often each stakeholder should receive communication about the project or how they should be strategically engaged (e.g., weekly emails, monthly in-person meetings).

PROJECT CONSTRAINTS

In addition to analyzing stakeholders, it is also helpful to assess **project constraints**— namely scope, time, and available resources, with resources encompassing aspects such as funding, staff, available technology, etc. (see Figure 22-4). Knowing the constraints of the project and managing them effectively are critical to success and the ultimate outcome. For instance, if the staff resources that are needed to complete a project are limited, then either the time needed to complete the project must be increased or the scope must be decreased to compensate. Similarly, if the allotted timeline for the project is shortened, this means that either the scope must decrease or the available resources must increase to maintain the quality of the work being completed and ultimately the project's success.

ENVIRONMENTAL AND SWOT ANALYSES

Aside from the charter and stakeholder matrix, it is also important to understand the operating environment and all external aspects that may impact a potential project. As such, it may be useful to conduct a **PESTLE analysis**, which encompasses political, economic, social, technological, legal, and environmental factors that may influence the project (see Appendix 22-3).[4] The probability, severity, and potential response to the event can then be determined as a means to help mitigate risk. These analyses are helpful in projects related to the health care field. For instance, a wholesaler who wants to implement a new software program for shipping medications must be aware of regulatory requirements with the Drug Supply Chain and Security Act (DSCSA), which could alter the software and reporting needs.

Another common tool is a **SWOT analysis**, which evaluates strengths, weaknesses, opportunities, and threats. In particular, such analyses are helpful to capitalize on strengths and opportunities, while minimizing weaknesses and threats.[5] For instance, a potential strength within an organization might be the high level of engagement from colleagues about the project, while a weakness that should be minimized may include a reduction in funding due to budget cuts. It should be noted that it is typically more useful and efficient to focus on minimizing threats and weaknesses, rather than improving strengths and opportunities.

Planning a Project

After completing the assessments and components associated with project initiation, the next part of the project management process is to develop the project plan. This planning typically involves defining scope, identifying resources and deliverables, creating a timeline, and other various management plans, which are reviewed below.

SCOPE

Project **scope** refers to the amount of work to be done, as well as what the project will and will not entail. ❹ *It is extremely important to define the scope because it puts boundaries on the project and defines what the endpoint is* (recall that projects must have a clearly defined end). Without a clearly defined scope, it is nearly impossible to know when the project is finished. In fact, the project may continue to grow and encompass aspects not originally intended at the outset (a concept referred to as "scope creep"). A clear scope also helps to set expectations with those impacted by the project and helps in the determination of timeline and budget considerations.

WORK BREAKDOWN STRUCTURE AND PROJECT TIMELINE

One of the key elements used when planning a project is a **work breakdown structure (WBS)**. As the name implies, a WBS is essentially a large task list that encompasses all the deliverables for the project (see Appendix 22-4 for an example). Each deliverable is then broken down into the other deliverables or inputs that are required for completion. For example, one major deliverable when building a new house is the exterior finishes. Exterior finishes can be further broken down to include shutters, driveway, mailbox, etc. Another example might be that of adding a new sterile compounding hood in a pharmacy clean room. A major deliverable would include a document detailing a modification to the pharmacy's workflow, which could be further broken down into the following inputs: a description of the current pharmacy workflow before the hood, the future state of the new workflow after installation of the hood, and a workflow **gap analysis** to identify the difference between expected performance and how things are performed currently. Doing so helps visualize and identify all the tasks involved in a project and ensures that important deliverables are not missed.

Additionally, the WBS can also be used to elucidate the number of resources needed. For instance, after completing the WBS for the new sterile compounding hood, it is estimated that 30 days' worth of pharmacist effort is required. Knowing that only one pharmacist is available to work on this project, and that only a few hours per day of this pharmacist's time can be spent completing the work, it is possible to estimate the total time needed to complete the hood installation project. However, if the compounding hood must be installed and functioning by a certain date, one could estimate the number of additional pharmacist resources needed to meet the project deadline.

❺ *After identifying tasks and the resources needed to accomplish those tasks, a project timeline can be developed.* A project timeline is useful for assigning a timeframe to each task and, ultimately, determining an overall project schedule. For example, installation of the driveway for the new house might be assigned to the pavers and require 2 days' worth of work, while installation of the mailbox might be assigned to the general contractor and take 3 hours. Once all the required times are known, a clearer understanding of the total project time can be elucidated. Another useful byproduct of a project timeline is the identification of dependencies between tasks and inputs. For instance, in the sterile compounding hood example, the gap analysis is dependent on the current and future workflow evaluation (i.e., it cannot be completed before those other activities are finished). However, in the new home example, installation of the exterior shutters is not dependent on installation of the mailbox (i.e., it can be completed either before or after).

Estimating how long a task will take can be challenging and highly nuanced. In general, it is helpful to think of time in terms of effort (the time actively involved in doing the work) and duration (the length of time it will actually take to complete). In the sterile compounding hood scenario, for example, the overall effort time to conduct the gap analysis might be 2 days; however, because the person responsible also has to attend meetings, care for patients during rounds, teach learners, etc., the total time in terms of duration might be 14 days. In many cases, it is not always clear exactly how long a task may take to complete. In these scenarios, it is often helpful to compare the activity to one that has already been completed. Alternatively, it may be useful to consider the best-case scenario (the soonest it could be completed) and the worst-case scenario (the longest it might take), and then use an average. Achieving a balance will help avoid developing timelines that are either too aggressive or too lax. Regardless, it is important to be realistic about the time required and understand that people usually have other responsibilities and cannot dedicate all their time to the project.

Gantt Chart

Once all the dependencies and durations of the tasks are known, a **Gantt chart** can be created. Gantt charts are used to show a visual progression and overall timeline for the project (see Figure 22-5).[5] Depending on the complexity of the project and the needs of the project owner, a Gantt chart can be quite intricate (including every task and associated dependencies) or more global (only including the major deliverables or milestones). These charts can often be developed using common software, such as Microsoft® Excel®, although more nuanced charts may require dedicated project management software, such as Microsoft® Project® (an in-depth discussion of project management software is

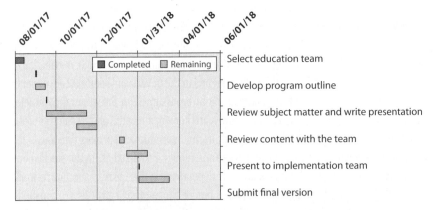

Figure 22–5. Gantt chart for a simple project using Microsoft® Excel® software.

beyond the scope of this chapter). Although not every project will need a Gantt chart, such visuals are often useful as a communication and tracking tool for stakeholders and leaders supporting the project.

Case Study 22–1

You are a clinical pharmacist practicing in an inpatient care unit of a large, academic medical center. As part of your job responsibilities, you periodically participate in formulary management activities designed to ensure that evidence-based, safe, and cost-effective medications are used within your facility. One of your assignments for this year is to evaluate the formulary status of a new biosimilar medication for the treatment of breast cancer.

- *What other information would you want to know before starting this assignment or outlining a charter?*
- *Discuss potential success criteria and deliverables for this project.*
- *List potential stakeholder groups relevant to this project.*
- *Describe potential constraints for this project.*
- *Identify some important tasks that should be included in a work breakdown structure that informs the project timeline.*

OTHER COMPONENTS OF A PROJECT PLAN

Requirements Matrix

A **requirements matrix** is a tool used to align the requirements of a project with the goals in the charter. Defining the relationship between goals and requirements at the onset of the project clarifies scope and stakeholder expectations. Within the requirements matrix, each requirement is assigned a person responsible for its completion, a way to track whether it has been completed, and some type of quality assessment metric. Documenting and tracking these details helps ensure that the day-to-day activities are executed in a manner that supports the vision for the project. It is also a useful means of monitoring goal completion and can serve as the documentation used for closing the project (discussed further below).

Risk Management Plan

Risk can be thought of as uncertainty during a project that can impact the ability to meet overall goals. In a risk management plan, each potential risk is identified and then analyzed in terms of the probability (or likelihood) of it occurring and impact it would have if it did occur. Impact is typically described using a continuum that includes no impact, minimal impact, moderate impact, severe impact, and project failure. Risks with both a high probability of occurrence and high impact require a thoughtful response plan. Although some types of risks are unavoidable, most can usually be mitigated or even avoided. For instance, one risk during the implementation of a new electronic health record (EHR) system might be a hospital-wide power outage. Having identified this risk, a response plan that includes clear downtime procedures could be developed in order to mitigate the impact of any outages that occur.

Communication Management Plan

Another important aspect of the project plan involves communication. Having an upfront strategy for clear and regular communication with stakeholders helps to create transparency, avoid uncertainty, and maintain engagement. These plans are typically based on the results of the stakeholder matrix analysis conducted during the initiation phase. For instance, stakeholders who are highly interested and have a great amount of power over the project may require more frequent and detailed status reports, whereas someone with low interest and power may only want a brief monthly email. When thinking about a communication plan it is also important to understand the organization's culture and how receptive it is to the change. Project implementation may not succeed unless people within the organization have had time to adjust and buy-in to the concept. Thus, the communication plan may also need to be designed to communicate benefits and advantages of the project to facilitate acceptance.

Change Management Plan

Change, whether expected or not, is likely to happen at some point during a project. Without a well-defined change management process, the scope of the project may expand beyond the initial commitment. Such scope creep can lead to unanticipated delays in implementation, strained resources, budget overruns, unmet expectations, and failed projects. Thus, changes to the project should usually go through a formal and objective review process to fully understand the impact. Depending on the complexity of the project, formal approval or vetting through a change management advisory board may be needed.

Executing a Project

Once the project has been planned, it can then be executed. Following the previously defined strategy for the project will make the work more straightforward and increase the likelihood of accomplishing it successfully. Along the way, it is important to keep team members engaged and maximize their efforts. It is also important to track the planned work versus the work accomplished and communicate this information to relevant stakeholders. Not only does this help track if the project is on schedule, but it is also useful to estimate what additional resources are needed in the event work must be accelerated. For instance, knowing that only 30% of the planned work has been completed allows the project coordinator to estimate how much additional time or resources are needed to finish the project.

Monitoring and Controlling a Project

It is important to be able to navigate unanticipated obstacles that may occur during project execution. While most challenges can be prepared for ahead of time using tools such as a risk management plan, many projects fail because of unanticipated issues. As such, continuously evaluating and managing quality throughout the project is crucial. **Project quality** essentially refers to how good the end result or accomplishment will be. To achieve the highest quality, an appropriate balance of time, scope, and resources are needed. It may also be a measure of stakeholder expectations and how well the deliverables conform to their requirements.

Measuring quality is typically done through quality assurance and quality control mechanisms. **Quality assurance** refers to activities that ensure the value of the final product/deliverable itself, whereas **quality control** refers to activities that prevent deficiencies along the process. For example, quality control would include checks put in place during the sterile compounding process (e.g., routine use of isopropyl alcohol, garbing requirements). Quality assurance would include quarantining the final compounded product and conducting a sterility test. Usually it is best to strike a balance between prevention techniques and detection techniques; however, this choice will depend on the nature of the project. As alluded to above, it is also useful to conduct and document quality checks as the project goals or deliverables are completed. It is important to remember that it is the project coordinator's responsibility to keep the project plan up-to-date and stakeholders involved when quality issues my impact the project.

Closing a Project

After all the work has been completed, several key steps should be taken to close the project. One of the most important activities is to ensure all the predetermined requirements have been met and accepted by the project sponsor and key stakeholders. Recall that the success criteria developed during project initiation and the requirements matrix developed during project planning are useful tools in this endeavor. Additionally, it is very important to celebrate with the project team and evaluate lessons learned. Depending on the scope and nature of the project, a fun group lunch or social outing could be a great way to congratulate the team and show appreciation for their work. It also provides an opportunity for open discussion about how the project went—evaluating what went well and what could be done differently for next time. Such iterative learning is invaluable for future projects and is often referred to as an **after-action review** (AAR). An AAR provides a structured framework, often using a facilitator, for the project team to reflect on strengths, weaknesses, and opportunities for improvement. It also provides guidance for future teams who may engage in similar work. While a complete guide to conducting an AAR is beyond the scope of this chapter, readers can refer to several useful articles on the topic.[6-8] Lastly, it is important to finish any project documentation (budgets, completed requirements matrix, etc.) and store it in a readily accessible place. Past project materials often serve as useful templates for the future and having them easily available can save time and work.

Conclusion

Projects are a part of daily life in today's health care environment. Knowing how to manage them appropriately is not only vital to personal success, but can also help improve project outcomes and quality; increase overall efficiency; reduce stress and uncertainty; and lower costs. Although several key concepts to project management were discussed throughout this chapter, it is important to remember that the rigor involved should be proportional to the project at hand. For example, smaller projects or those that need to be completed within a limited timeframe may not benefit from a detailed WBS. Nevertheless, the critical components of effective project management should still be considered, including defining the scope, goals, and success criteria, developing a stakeholder matrix and risk mitigation strategy, and outlining a realistic timeline for the major tasks involved. Various project management programs, such as Microsoft Project®, can also be leveraged. Again, however, routine use of these tools is often unnecessary for the average health care professional who deals with projects. General workplace productivity software and resources are often sufficient (e.g., Microsoft Excel®, Microsoft Word®, Microsoft

Teams®, white boards). The key is to use a routine, organized, and systematic process that can be followed from project selection through completion.

Self-Assessment Questions

1. Which one of the following best describes a project?
   a. Ongoing, day-to-day activities that support an organization
   b. A finite, progressively elaborate endeavor with a beginning and end
   c. A group of plans that support an overall strategic organizational objective
   d. An endeavor with a larger scope than either a program or portfolio
   e. None of the above

2. Which one of the following is a quantifiable measure that defines when a goal is accomplished?
   a. Deliverables
   b. Success criteria
   c. Work breakdown structure (WBS)
   d. Scope
   e. Constraints

3. Which of the following considerations is important when determining the value proposition of a project?
   a. Measurable and quantifiable
   b. Aligned with the priorities of the organization
   c. Primarily related to financial incentives or profits
   d. Both a and b
   e. All of the above

Please use the following case for questions 4 through 6:
A pharmacist wants to conduct a project to standardize how Pharmacy Services works with other clinical staff to collect medication histories in the emergency department.

4. Which individuals would be considered a stakeholder for this project (select all that apply)?
   a. Pharmacist team lead over the emergency department
   b. Medication Safety Officer for the hospital
   c. Nurse Manager in the emergency department

   d. Pharmacists and pharmacy technicians who work in the emergency department

   e. Physician Chair of Internal Medicine for the hospital

5. Why would it be useful for the team to develop a stakeholder matrix as part of the project planning process?

   a. It is a helpful tool to understand stakeholder needs and manage them appropriately.

   b. It is useful for identifying new stakeholders who have a vested interest in the work.

   c. It is a helpful tool to gather and organize feedback from stakeholders about the project.

   d. A stakeholder matrix would not be helpful for this project.

6. Which of the following might be considered a constraint of this project?

   a. Lack of 24-hour pharmacy coverage in the emergency department.

   b. Limited medication reconciliation functionality in the electronic health record system.

   c. Lack of dedicated time away from patient care duties to conduct team meetings.

   d. All of the above

7. A PESTLE analysis is used to evaluate political, economic, social, technological, legal, and environmental factors that may influence a project.

   a. True

   b. False

8. Which one of the following is used to put boundaries on the project?

   a. Deliverables

   b. Success criteria

   c. Work breakdown structure (WBS)

   d. Scope

   e. Constraints

9. _____ is a tangible component of a project needed to achieve predefined success criteria?

   a. Deliverable

   b. Success criteria

   c. Work breakdown structure

   d. Scope

   e. Constraint

10. _____ is a useful tool for visualizing the progression and timeline of a project.
    a. Gantt chart
    b. Work breakdown structure
    c. PESTLE analysis
    d. SWOT analysis
    e. Charter

11. Which of the following correctly outlines the progression of a project?
    a. Initiation, selection, planning, execution, monitoring, closing
    b. Selection, initiation, planning, execution, monitoring, closing
    c. Selection, planning, initiation, execution, monitoring, closing
    d. Selection, initiation, planning, monitoring, execution, closing

12. When monitoring and controlling a project, which of the following is usually considered the most important?
    a. Review the Gantt chart and work breakdown structure daily.
    b. Conduct regular SWOT and PESTLE analyses.
    c. Continually assess and manage the quality of the project.
    d. Routinely update the project charter.
    e. Document daily status reports for leadership.

13. Quality assurance refers to which of the following?
    a. Activities that prevent deficiencies throughout a project
    b. Activities that ensure the value of the final product or deliverable
    c. The balance between time, scope, and resources
    d. Activities used to navigate unanticipated obstacles that may occur during project execution

14. _____ is a framework used by a project team to reflect on strengths, weaknesses, and opportunities for improvement after the project has been completed.
    a. Stakeholder matrix
    b. Action register
    c. Work breakdown structure
    d. After action review (AAR)
    e. Quality assurance review

15. Smaller projects, or projects with short timelines, should still use a detailed work breakdown structure, charter, change management strategy, and all other components of a project plan.
    a. True
    b. False

REFERENCES

1. Schumock GT, Stubbings J. How to develop a business plan for pharmacy services. 2nd rev. ed. Lenexa: American College of Clinical Pharmacy; 2013.
2. Sahlman WA. How to write a great business plan. Harv Bus Rev. 1997 Jul–Aug;75(4):98–108.
3. Chisholm-Burns MA, Vaillancourt AM, Shepherd M, editors. Pharmacy management, leadership, marketing, and finance. Burlington: Jones & Bartlett Learning, LLC; 2014.
4. What is PESTLE analysis? A tool for business analysis [Internet]. Newark (DE): Weberience LLC; [cited 2017 Apr 3]. Available from: http://pestleanalysis.com/what-is-pestle-analysis/
5. Project Management Institute. A guide to the project management body of knowledge (PMBOK®). 6th rev. ed. Newtown Square: Project Management Institute, Inc.; 2017.
6. Salem-Schatz S, Ordin D, Mittman B. Guide to the after action review [Internet]. Center for Evidence-Based Management; 2010 Oct. Available from: https://www.cebma.org/wp-content/uploads/Guide-to-the-after_action_review.pdf
7. World Health Organization. Guidance for after action review (AAR) [Internet]. Geneva, Switzerland: World Health Organization; 2019. Available from: https://apps.who.int/iris/handle/10665/311537
8. Darling M, Parry C, Moore J. Learning in the thick of it. Harv Bus Rev. 2005 Jul–Aug; 83(7):84–92, 192.

SUGGESTED READINGS

Kerzner H. Project management: a systems approach to planning, scheduling, and controlling. 12th rev. ed. Hoboken: John Wiley & Sons, Inc.; 2017.

Project Management Institute homepage [Internet]. Newtown Square (PA): Project Management Institute; [cited 2016 Sept 22]. Available from: https://www.pmi.org/

Project Management Institute. A guide to the project management body of knowledge (PMBOK®). 6th rev. ed. Newtown Square: Project Management Institute, Inc.; 2017.

Schwalbe K, Furlong D. Healthcare project management. 2nd rev. Minneapolis (MN): Schwalbe Publishing; 2017.

23

Chapter Twenty-Three

Investigational Drugs

Bambi J. Grilley

Learning Objectives

After completing this chapter, the reader will be able to:

- List the major legislative acts that led to the current system of drug evaluation, approval, and regulation used in the United States.
- List the steps in the drug approval process.
- List the components of an Investigational New Drug Application (IND).
- Describe the difference between commercial, treatment, emergency use, and individual investigator INDs.
- Define orphan drug status and list the advantages of classifying a drug as an orphan drug.
- List all of the requirements (as specified by the Office of Human Research Protections [OHRP]) for an institutional review board (IRB).
- Prepare appropriate protocol assessments for use by the IRB or other review committees when they evaluate new human subject protocols.
- Describe the type of support that is necessary for clinical research, including (but not limited to) the following:
  a. Ordering drug supplies for ongoing clinical trials
  b. Maintaining drug accountability records as required by the Food and Drug Administration (FDA)
  c. Preparing drug and protocol data sheets for use by health care personnel in the hospital
  d. Preparing pharmacy budgets for sponsored clinical research
  e. Aiding investigators in designing and conducting clinical trials in their institution
  f. Assisting investigators in initiating and conducting clinical trials (including emergency use INDs)

Key Concepts

1 The FDA is the federal agency that decides which drugs, biologics, and medical devices are safe and effective, determinations upon which the agency decides if a product can be marketed in the United States.

2 In addition to review by the FDA, research protocols are also reviewed for ethical appropriateness by IRBs.

3 The drug approval process in the United States is standardized by FDA review. It consists of preclinical testing and Phases I through IV of clinical testing.

4 The Investigational New Drug Application (IND) is the application submitted by the study sponsor to the FDA to begin clinical trials in humans.

5 The IND should be amended as necessary. There are four types of documents used to amend the IND:

   a. Protocol amendments
   b. Information amendments
   c. IND Safety Reports
   d. IND Annual Reports

6 After sufficient evidence is obtained regarding the drug's safety and effectiveness, the sponsor will submit a New Drug Application/Biologics Licensing Application to the FDA requesting approval of the agent for marketing.

7 An orphan drug is one that is used for the treatment of a rare disease, affecting fewer than 200,000 people in the United States, or one that will not generate enough revenue to justify the cost of research and development.

8 Drug accountability records are mandated by law. They can be electronic or in paper form. Necessary components include the following:

   a. The date of the transaction
   b. The type of the transaction
   c. The receiving party of the transaction (if this is a drug dispensation, the subject initials and an identifying number are required)
   d. The number of units being used or received (for patient dispensation this should include the actual dose the patient will receive)
   e. The lot number of the drug (if multiple lot numbers were used, each one should be documented)
   f. The initials of the individual who performed the transaction

Introduction

It is now estimated that approximately $2.6 billion is spent to get a new **drug product** to market in the United States.[1,2] Although there is some controversy surrounding these estimates, there is no doubt that the costs of drug development continue to escalate.[3] Currently, there are more than 8000 medicines in clinical development globally, with 74% of those having the potential to be first-in-class treatments.[4,5] This should be compared to 59 novel drugs approved by the **Food and Drug Administration (FDA)** in 2018.[6] In fact, the FDA monitors the manufacture, import, transport, storage, and sale of 25% of all goods purchased in the United States annually.[7] The centers of the FDA involved in regulating biologics, drugs, and medical devices used in humans are as follows:

- Center for Biologics Evaluation and Research (CBER)
- Center for Drug Evaluation and Research (CDER)
- Center for Devices and Radiological Health (CDRH)[8]

Since this book only includes drug-related information, this chapter will concentrate only on the regulations associated with CBER and CDER.

Since 1940, more than 10,000 new **drug applications (NDAs)** have been approved in the United States.[9] An NDA is the application to the FDA requesting approval to market a new drug for human use. The NDA contains data supporting the safety and efficacy of the drug for its intended use.[10] It is very important that the clinical trials upon which the FDA will base their decisions be both scientifically accurate and complete. Health care professionals can play an important role in ensuring that the clinical trials conducted at their institutions meet the goals set forth by the study sponsor, the local investigator, and ultimately the FDA.

Currently, most research conducted on investigational drugs is performed in medical schools, hospitals, and organizations specifically designed to conduct clinical research trials. In some institutions, a pharmacist will be hired specifically to handle investigational drugs. More frequently, however, this role falls to staff pharmacists and occasionally to other health care providers. To successfully manage investigational drugs, this individual or team of individuals must be a bookkeeper, inventory control manager, and, most importantly, an information disseminator.

History of Drug Development Regulation in the United States[11]

For more than a century after the Declaration of Independence, drug products were not regulated in the United States. Available drugs were often ineffective, addictive, toxic, or even lethal. During this same period, physicians were not licensed and nearly anyone could practice medicine. The public was, for the most part, responsible for using common sense when evaluating which products they would use.

The evolution of drug regulations in this country is a study in human tragedy. Crises have instigated the development of many of the laws regulating drug development, preparation, and distribution.

- The first federal law developed to deal with drug quality and safety was the Import Drug Act of 1848. This law was passed after it was discovered that American troops involved in the Mexican-American War had been supplied with substandard imported drugs. The act provided for the inspection, detention, and destruction or reexport of imported drug shipments that failed to meet prescribed standards.

- The Pure Food and Drugs Act was passed in 1906. This law required that drugs not be mislabeled or adulterated, and stated that they must meet recognized standards for strength and purity. Mislabeling in this context only referred to the identity or composition of drugs (not false therapeutic claims). False therapeutic claims were prohibited with the passing of the Sherley Amendment in 1912.

In 1937, the drug sulfanilamide was released. This drug showed promise as an antiinfective agent and was prepared as an oral liquid. The vehicle used for this preparation was diethylene glycol (a sweet-tasting solvent similar to ethylene glycol (automobile antifreeze). A total of 107 people died after taking this preparation. Within a year of this tragedy, the Food, Drug, and Cosmetic Act of 1938 was enacted. This law required that the safety of drugs, when used in accordance with the labeled instructions, be proven through testing before they could be marketed. It was in this law that the submission of an NDA to the FDA was first described. The NDA was required to list the drug's intended uses and provide scientific evidence that the drug was safe. If, after 60 days, the FDA had not responded to the manufacturer regarding the NDA, the manufacturer was free to proceed with marketing of the product.

- In 1951, the Durham–Humphrey Amendment was passed. This law divided pharmaceuticals into two distinct classes:

1. Over-the-counter (OTC) medications that could be safely self-administered
2. Prescription (Rx) medications that had potentially dangerous side effects and therefore required expert medical supervision

This law required the following statement be added to the labels for all prescription medications: "Caution: Federal Law prohibits dispensing without a prescription."

In 1962, another drug tragedy occurred that resulted in additional regulations. In that year, an inordinate number of pregnant women in Western Europe gave birth to children with severe deformities related to the use of the drug thalidomide. Although U.S. consumers were not directly affected by this tragedy, because thalidomide had not been released in the U.S. market, it was a compelling reason for the legislature to develop stronger laws regarding the testing of new drug products. The Kefauver–Harris Drug Amendment was passed the same year. This law specified that the manufacturer had to demonstrate proof of efficacy, as well as safety, prior to marketing any new drug. Additionally, this law required that drug manufacturers operate in conformity with Current Good Manufacturing Practices (CGMP). Finally, it stated that the FDA had to formally approve an NDA before the drug could be marketed.

There are numerous other laws and regulations that affect drug products in the United States, but those mentioned above provide the legal foundation for the current regulation of drug products in the United States. Based on these laws, the FDA has assumed a large role in assessing the safety and efficacy of drug products prior to their distribution in the United States.

EVOLUTION OF FDA'S DRUG APPROVAL PROCESS

❶ *The FDA is the federal agency that decides which drugs, biologics, and medical devices are safe and effective, determinations upon which the agency decides if a product can be marketed in the United States.* The goal of the FDA is to provide American consumers with safe and effective drugs, biologics, and devices.[5] Extensive debate regarding the need to reform the FDA has been ongoing in the United States for years. Critics of the FDA have long claimed that the approval process for drugs in the United States is too costly and time consuming.[12,13] Interestingly, however, data shows that the FDA leads the world in the first introduction of new active substances and that the majority of novel therapeutic agents are approved in the United States first. In 2017, 15 new products were approved only in the European Union, 52 were approved only in the United States, and 36 were approved in both regions.[14] Additionally, approval times in the United States are on average 2 months faster than in the European Union and Canada.[15] Nevertheless, over the past two decades, the FDA and the federal government have initiated many reforms and initiatives designed to address these criticisms. Included in these reform acts are the Prescription Drug User Fee Act of 1992 (PDUFA), which was reauthorized every 5 years, with the most recent reauthorization occurring in 2017, and the Food and Drug Administration Modernization Act of 1997 (FDAMA). PDUFA redefined the timeframes for NDA reviews and established revenues to fund the increased demands created by the new timeframes.[16] The FDAMA, which reauthorized PDUFA in 1997, was much broader in scope and impacted not only the drug approval process, but also other aspects of the practices of pharmacy and medicine.[17] The Food and Drug Administration Amendments Act (FDAAA), which was signed into law in 2007, further expanded PDUFA to provide the FDA with additional resources to conduct timely and comprehensive reviews of new drugs in the United States.[18] Most recently, the Food and Drug Administration Safety and

Innovation Act of 2012 (FDASIA) signed into law on July 9, 2012, not only reauthorized PDUFA, but also gave the FDA a new product designation known as the "breakthrough therapy" designation, which will be discussed in more detail later in this chapter.[19] Finally, the 21st Century Cures Act, signed into law in December 2016, provided an even more expedited review option, by establishing the Regenerative Medicine Advanced Therapy (RMAT) designation and the Breakthrough Devices Program. RMAT will also be discussed later in this chapter.[20]

Aside from looking at review times, the FDA has also been concerned about the increasing difficulty in drug and biologic development. To attempt to address this issue, the FDA launched a new initiative in March 2004 called the Critical Path Initiative. Having identified an increasingly large gap between laboratory discoveries and new treatments for patients with serious diseases such as diabetes, cancer, and Alzheimer disease, the Critical Path Initiative is the FDA's attempt to facilitate modernization of the sciences and improve regulatory decision-making. The FDA has been working with the public, the pharmaceutical industry, other regulatory agencies, and academia to identify projects that they feel are most likely to help the drug development process from test tube to bedside.[21]

More recently, as a result of FDASIA, the FDA has increased their focus on patient engagement.[19] A notable example of this initiative is a patient advocacy-initiated draft guidance submitted to the FDA to help accelerate development and review of potential therapies for Duchenne syndrome. A major point of emphasis was that the parents of children affected by Duchenne syndrome were willing to accept a higher risk profile for potential therapies even those that may improve patient's quality of life without prolonging life.[22,23]

Finally, the FDA has undertaken many information technology initiatives to facilitate the regulatory review process. Included in these initiatives is the development of systems allowing for electronic submission, management, and review of regulatory information.[24] The FDA mandated that all NDA, **Biologics Licensing Applications (BLA)**, **Abbreviated New Drug Application (ANDA)**, and **Drug Master Files (DMF)** be in the Electronic Common Technical Document (eCTD) format by May 2017 and all commercial **Investigational New Drug Applications (INDs)** be in eCTD format by May 2018.[2,25,26]

Overall, the goal of all of the above-mentioned initiatives is to review priority drugs in 6 months and standard drugs within 10 months, with an emphasis on improving consistency and transparency of the review process.[27] Other attempts by the FDA to increase availability of investigational drugs to patients will be discussed later in this chapter.

TRANSPARENCY AND HARMONIZATION OF DRUG DEVELOPMENT

First initiated in response to components of FDAMA, the National Institutes of Health (NIH) developed a web-based system that offers information about ongoing clinical trials for a wide range of diseases and conditions. The site is available at http://clinicaltrials. gov. Initially intended as a system to provide a registry of clinical trials, it allows potential study **subjects** to search for studies for particular diseases and identify treatment centers that offer enrollment into those studies. The FDA requires that, for studies being conducted under an IND, the **sponsor** verify that the study is posted to the system through submission of Form 3674 to the IND.[28] Requirements for postings have become increasingly more stringent over time. In 2016, both the FDA and NIH implemented initiatives intended to further enhance the availability of clinical trial information. Both entities require registration of all applicable studies in the system no later than 21 days after enrollment of the first participant. The difference in the scope being related to the definition of an applicable study. The FDA defines an applicable study as any clinical trial, including an FDA-regulated product, but excludes Phase 1 or small feasibility device studies. In contrast, NIH defines an applicable study as all clinical trials funded by NIH, including only behavioral interventions. Both the NIH and the FDA require reporting of results from applicable studies no later than 12 months after the primary completion date (the date that the last participant reached the primary objective). Results reporting includes not only information about the subjects (demographics and participant flow), but also information about adverse events, outcomes, and statistical analyses.[29,30]

Drug development has become an increasingly global process. Historically, the regulatory requirements for drug approval varied from country to country, resulting in a significant amount of time and money being spent to receive multiple approvals. For this reason, the International Conference on Harmonization (ICH), established in 1990, has brought together officials from Europe, the United States, and Japan to develop common guidelines for ensuring the quality, safety, and efficacy of drugs. The ICH now includes 16 members and 32 observers. The FDA has been very involved in the development of the ICH guidelines. The ultimate goal of these guidelines is to provide a method to ensure simultaneous submission and rapid regulatory approval in the world's major markets, thus minimizing duplication of effort, improving efficiency, and increasing the quality and consistency of medical treatments available to patients worldwide.[31] In fact, the FDA and other world health agencies are making strides in providing concurrent review. Project Orbis is an initiative of the FDA Oncology Center of Excellence and provides a framework for concurrent submission and review of oncology products among international partners. In September 2019, the FDA, Health Canada, and the Australian Therapeutic Goods Administration took their first action by releasing simultaneous decisions regarding two oncology products.[32]

Clinical trials utilizing gene therapy products have had a slightly more complicated history of regulation. At this time, the only remaining difference between review of gene therapy products and other drug and biological products is the requirement for review and approval by the local Institutional Biosafety Committee(s) in addition to review and approval by the FDA and **Institutional Review Board (IRB)** (discussed below).[33] Individuals interested in this history of regulatory requirements of gene therapy products can refer to other references such as the book chapter entitled "Regulations governing clinical trials in gene therapy" included in the book Cancer Gene Therapy by Viral and Non-viral Vectors.[34]

THE HISTORY OF PROTECTION OF HUMAN SUBJECTS

❷ *In addition to the regulatory review of investigational drugs by the FDA, research protocols are also reviewed for ethical appropriateness by IRBs.* The formalized process for protecting human subjects began with the Nuremberg Code. This code was used to judge the human experimentation conducted by the Nazis around the middle of the twentieth century. The Nuremberg Code states that "the voluntary consent of the human subjects is absolutely essential." The code goes on to specify that the subject must have the capacity to consent, must be free from coercion, and must comprehend the risks and benefits involved in the research.[35] The Declaration of Helsinki reemphasized the above points and distinguished between therapeutic and nontherapeutic research. This document was first developed in 1964 and has been revised multiple times, most recently in 2013.[36]

The NIH, as part of the DHHS, used these two documents to develop its own policies for the Protection of Human Subjects in 1966. These policies were raised to regulatory status in 1974 and established the IRB as a mechanism through which human subjects would be protected. The Belmont Report, released in 1978, further delineates the basic ethical principles underlying medical research on human subjects.[37] Title 45 Part 46 of the Code of Federal Regulations (CFR), which was released in 1981, was designed to make uniform the protection of human subjects in all federal agencies.[38] Title 21 Part 50 (approved in 1980) of the CFR sets forth guidelines for appropriate informed consent and Title 21 Part 56 (approved in 1981) of the CFR sets forth guidelines for the IRB.[39,40] Copies of these regulations can be obtained on the Internet at http://www.ecfr.gov/cgi-bin/ECFR?page=browse. These two documents are used by the FDA and the DHHS to evaluate the ethical conduct of clinical trials in the United States. Further information regarding the role of the IRB will be presented later in this chapter.

The Drug Approval Process

❸ *The drug approval process in the United States is standardized by FDA review. It consists of preclinical testing and Phase I through IV of clinical testing.* The first step in the drug approval process is preclinical testing. This testing is conducted either *in vitro* or in animals. Before filing an **IND** for an **Investigational New Drug**, the sponsor must have developed a pharmacologic profile of the drug, determined its acute and subacute toxicity, and have sufficient information regarding chronic toxicity to support the drug's use in humans.[41]

INVESTIGATIONAL NEW DRUG APPLICATION

After the preclinical testing is completed, the sponsor will file an IND with the FDA. **❹** *The IND is the application by the study sponsor to the FDA to begin clinical trials in humans.* Most often, the sponsor is a pharmaceutical company, but occasionally an individual **investigator** will file an IND and serve as a **sponsor-investigator**.[2] A commercial IND is one for which the sponsor is usually either a corporate entity or one of the institutes of the NIH.[42] In addition, the FDA may designate any other IND as commercial, if it is clear that the sponsor intends the product to be commercialized at a later date. An investigator IND is submitted when an investigator plans to use an approved drug for a new indication (i.e., one that is outside the package labeling), or on occasion, for an unapproved product or for a **New Molecular Entity (NME)**.[2] The IND requirements for the sponsor-investigator are the same as those for any other sponsor. For that reason, no differentiation will be made in the following discussion of the drug approval process.

An IND is not required if the drug to be studied is marketed in the United States and all of the following requirements are met:

1. The study is not to be reported to the FDA in support of a new indication.
2. The study does not involve a different dose, route, or patient population that increases the risk to patients.
3. IRB approval and informed consent are secured.
4. The study will not be used to promote the drug's effectiveness for a new indication (see Chapter 25 for more discussion on drug promotion regulations).

The FDA has developed a guidance document specifically to assist in determining whether or not an IND is required. However, in situations where it is unclear whether an IND is required or not, a call to the FDA is the best way to determine the appropriate way to proceed.[43]

In recent years, there have been several therapeutic products developed that depend on the use of an *in vitro* companion diagnostic device (or test) for their safe and effective use. It is important to note that in this situation, the in vitro device should be approved or cleared concurrently by the FDA for the use indicated in the therapeutic **product labeling**. To be clear, this might require the study of the diagnostic device under an **Investigational Device Exemption (IDE)** while the therapeutic product is being studied under an IND. If the diagnostic device and therapeutic product are to be studied together to support their respective approvals (or clearance in the case of a device), both products can be studied in the same investigational study if the study has been developed and conducted in a manner that meets both IND and IDE regulations.[44] One other interesting issue related to devices is the use of a mobile app (i.e., a software application on a mobile platform such as an iPhone or Android) for the diagnosis, cure, mitigation, treatment or prevention of disease, or to affect the structure or function of the body. In these situations, the mobile app can be considered to be a medical device subject to IDE regulations.[45] IDE regulations and components will not be further discussed in this chapter; however, the applicable regulations can be found in 21CFR812 and the FDA has extensive guidance regarding these products and their development.[46]

Contents of IND

As specified in 21CFR212.23 an IND application needs to contain the following information:

1. **Cover sheet:** Form 1571 (available at the FDA website under Forms, http://www. fda.gov/AboutFDA/ReportsManualsForms/Forms/default.htm). This form identifies the sponsor, documents that the sponsor agrees to follow appropriate regulations, and identifies any involved **Contract Research Organization (CRO).**[2] This is a legal document.

2. **Table of contents**

3. **Introductory statement:** States the name, structure, pharmacologic class, dosage form, and all active ingredients in the investigational drug; the objectives and planned duration of the investigation should be stated here.

4. **General investigational plan:** Describes the rationale, indications, and general approach for evaluating the drug, the types of trials to be conducted, the projected number of patients that will be treated, and any potential safety concerns; the purpose of this section is to give FDA reviewers a general overview of the plan to study the drug.

5. **Investigator's brochure:** An information packet containing all available information on the drug including its formula, pharmacologic and toxicologic effects, pharmacokinetics, and any information regarding the safety and risks associated with the drug. It is important that this brochure be kept current and comprehensive; therefore, it should be amended as necessary. The investigator's brochure may be used by the investigator or other health care professionals as a reference during the conduct of the research study.

6. **Clinical protocol**
   - *Objectives and purpose:* A description of the purpose of the trial (a typical Phase I objective would be to determine the maximum tolerated dose of the investigational drug, whereas a typical Phase III objective would be to compare the safety and efficacy of the investigational drug to placebo or standard therapy).

- *Investigator data:* Provides qualifications and demographic data of the investigators involved in the clinical trial (may be presented on form 1572 (available at the FDA website under Forms, http://www.fda.gov/AboutFDA/ReportsManuals Forms/Forms/default.htm).
- *Patient selection:* Describes the characteristics of patients that are eligible for enrollment in the trial and states factors that would exclude the patient.
- *Study design:* Describes how the study will be completed; if the study is to be randomized, this will be described here with a description of the alternate therapy including a description of the **control group.**[47]
- *Dose determination:* Describes the dose (with possible adjustments) and route of administration of the investigational drug; if retreatment or maintenance therapy of patients is allowed, it will be detailed in this section.
- *Observations:* Describes how the objectives stated earlier in the protocol are to be assessed.
- *Clinical procedures:* Describes all laboratory tests or clinical procedures that will be used to monitor the effects of the drug in the patient; the collection of this data is intended to minimize the risk to the patients.
- *IRB approval for protocol:* Documentation of this approval is not required as part of the IND application process; however, form 1571 does state that an IRB will review and approve each study in the proposed **clinical investigation** before allowing initiation of those studies.[2]

7. **Chemistry, manufacturing, and control data**
   - **Drug substance:** Describes the drug substance including its name, bio- logical, physical, and chemical characteristics; the address of the manufac- turer; the method of synthesis or preparation; and the analytical methods used to assure purity, identity, and the substance's stability.[48]
   - *Drug product:* Describes the drug product, including all of its components; the address of the manufacturer; the analytical methods used to ensure identity, quality, purity, and strength of the product; and the product's stability.
   - *Composition, manufacture, and control of any placebo used in the trial:* The FDA does not require that the placebo be identical to the investigational drug; how- ever, it wants to ensure that the lack of similarity does not jeopardize the trial.
   - *Labeling:* Copies of all labels and labeling used for the drug substance or prod- uct or packaging as it will be provided to each investigator. Labels in this context mean the information affixed to the product and used to identify the contents while labeling in this context relates to product information including prescrib- ing information.
   - *Environmental assessment:* Presents a claim for categorical exclusion from the requirement for an environmental assessment (a statement that the amount of

waste expected to reach the environment may reasonably be expected to be nontoxic).

8. **Pharmacology and toxicology data**
   - *Pharmacology and drug disposition:* Describes the pharmacology, mechanism of action, absorption, distribution, metabolism, and excretion of the drug in animals and *in vitro*.
   - *Toxicology:* Describes the toxicology in animals and *in vitro*.
   - A statement that all nonclinical laboratories involved in the research adhered to Good Laboratory Practice (GLP) regulations.
9. **Previous human experience:** Summary of human experiences, which includes data from the United States and, where applicable, foreign markets. Known safety and efficacy data should be presented (especially if the drug was withdrawn from foreign markets for reasons of safety or efficacy).
10. **Additional information:** Other information that would help the reviewer evaluate the proposed clinical trial should be included here. For example, if a drug has the potential for abuse, data on the drug's dependence and abuse potential should be discussed in this section.[41]

The Letter of Authorization (LOA) to cross reference a DMF, IND, or NDA (referred to in item 9 on page 1 of Form 1571) is required when the investigational product (or some component of the investigational product) being used in the research is being supplied by a manufacturer other than the study sponsor. The original holder of the IND/NDA/DMF prepares the LOA. An LOA is frequently required when two companies are working together toward development of a product.[26]

Finally, proof of compliance with the requirements of ClinicalTrials.gov through submission of Form 3674 (available at the FDA website under Forms: http://www.fda.gov/AboutFDA/ReportsManualsForms/Forms/default.htm) is required as part of the IND.[28]

Amendment of IND

⑤ *The IND should be amended as necessary. There are four types of documents used to amend the IND:*

1. **Protocol amendments**: Submitted when a sponsor wants to change a previously submitted protocol or add a new study protocol to an existing IND.[49]
2. **Information amendments**: Submitted when information becomes available that would not be presented using a protocol amendment, IND safety report, or annual report (example: new chemistry data).[50]
3. **IND safety reports**: Reports clinical and animal adverse reactions; reporting requirements depend on the nature, severity, and frequency of the experience. The following definitions are used to help evaluate adverse reactions.

- *Suspected adverse reaction:* An adverse reaction for which there is evidence to suggest a causal relationship between the drug and the adverse event.
- *Serious adverse event or serious suspected adverse reaction:* An event that results in any of the following outcomes: death, a life-threatening adverse drug experience, inpatient hospitalization or prolongation of existing hospitalization, a persistent or significant disability/incapacity, or a congenital anomaly/birth defect. Important medical events that may not result in death, be life-threatening, or require hospitalization may be considered serious adverse drug experiences when, based on appropriate medical judgment, they may jeopardize the patient or subject and may require medical or surgical intervention to prevent one of the outcomes listed in this definition.
- *Unexpected adverse event or unexpected suspected adverse reaction:* An adverse reaction that is not listed in the current labeling for the drug product. This includes events that may be symptomatically and pathophysiologically related to an event listed in the labeling, but differs from the event because of greater severity or specificity.
- For serious and unexpected suspected adverse reactions, the sponsor must report the event to the FDA in writing within 15 calendar days. Those events that are serious and unexpected as well as require notification of the FDA within 7 calendar days. The written reports should describe the current adverse event and identify all previously filed safety reports concerning similar adverse events. The written report may be submitted as a narrative or as Form 3500A (available at http://www.fda.gov/safety/medwatch/howtoreport/downloadforms/default.htm).[51,52]

4. **IND annual reports**: Submitted within 60 days of the annual effective date of an IND; it should describe the progress of the investigation including information on the individual studies, summary information of the IND (summary of adverse experiences, IND safety reports, preclinical studies completed in the last year), relevant developments in foreign markets, and changes in the investigator's brochure.[53]

Each submission to a specific IND is required to be numbered sequentially (starting with 000). A total of three sets (the original and two copies) of all submissions to an IND file (whether a new IND or revisions to an existing IND) are sent to the FDA.[41]

Once submitted to the FDA, the IND will be forwarded to the appropriate review division based on the therapeutic category of the product. Examples of the different divisions include oncology products, hematology products, anti-infective products, and medical imaging products. Following submission, the IND and clinical trial will be assigned to a review team that includes the following individuals:

- The Regulatory Project Manager (RPM): Contact information for the RPM is provided in the letter sent to the applicant acknowledging receipt of the application.

This will be the sponsor's (see below) primary FDA contact person. Each application that is submitted is assigned an RPM. If the RPM is changed during the course of the review, the applicant is notified by the new RPM.

- A Chemistry, Manufacturing, and Controls (CMC) reviewer.
- A nonclinical Pharmacology/Toxicology reviewer.
- A Clinical reviewer.
- Other reviewers as needed (e.g., statisticians, epidemiologists, site inspectors, patient representatives).[54]

The FDA has 30 days after receipt of an IND to respond to the sponsor. The sponsor may begin clinical trials if there is no response from the FDA within 30 days.[55] The FDA delays initiation of a new study or discontinues an ongoing study by issuing a clinical hold. Clinical holds are most often used when the FDA identifies an issue (through initial review or through later submissions) that the agency feels poses a significant risk to the subjects. After this issue has been satisfactorily resolved, the clinical hold can be removed and the investigations can be initiated or resumed.[56]

PHASES OF CLINICAL TRIAL

There are four phases of clinical trials. Clinical studies generally begin cautiously. As experience with the agent grows, the dose and duration of exposure to the agent may also increase. The number of patients treated at each phase of study and the duration of the studies can vary significantly depending on statistical considerations, the prevalence of patients affected by the disease, and the importance of the new drug. However, some general guidelines regarding the four phases of clinical testing are presented below.

Phase I

A Phase I trial is the first use of the agent in humans. As such, these studies are usually initiated with cautious (low) doses and in a small numbers of subjects. Doses may be increased as safety is established. A Phase I study will usually include 20–80 subjects who receive the investigational product. Phase I trials last an average of 6 months to 1 year. The purpose of a Phase I trial is to determine the safety and toxicity of the agent. Frequently, these trials include a pharmacokinetic portion. These trials assist in identifying the preferred route of administration and a safe dosage range. When possible, these trials are initiated in normal, healthy volunteers. This allows for evaluation of the effect of the drug on a subject who does not have any preexisting conditions. In situations in which this is not practical, such as oncology drugs, in which the drug itself can be highly toxic, these drugs are usually reserved for patients who have exhausted all conventional options.

Phase II

A Phase II trial is one in which the drug is used in a small number of subjects who suffer from the disease or condition that the drug is proposed to treat. The purpose of a Phase II trial is to evaluate the efficacy of the agent. Data from the Phase I trial, *in vitro* testing, and animal testing may be used to identify which group of patients is most likely to benefit from therapy with this agent. Phase II trials usually treat between 100 and 200 patients and will average about 2 years in duration. Following Phase II trials, study sponsors will frequently assess these preliminary results and predicted marketability of the product prior to initiating the larger and more expensive Phase III trials.

Phase III

Phase III trials build on the experience gained during the Phase II trials. The purpose of a Phase III study is to further define the efficacy and safety of the agent. Frequently, in Phase III studies, the new agent is compared to current therapy. These trials are usually multicenter studies, generally treat from several hundred to 3000 patients, and the study will usually last about 3 years (although an individual subject's participation may be significantly shorter). Usually, some of the Phase III trials will be considered pivotal studies and will serve as the basis for the NDA/BLA for a medicinal product's marketing approval.[57]

Pharmacogenomics

One interesting scientific advance in the area of drug development has been the impact of pharmacogenomics (PGx) on the field. PGx is the study of variations of DNA and RNA characteristics as related to drug response, including effectiveness and adverse effects. As such, PGx can contribute to evaluation of interindividual differences in the response to drugs. While pharmacogenomic studies can occur in any phase of drug development, the FDA is encouraging study sponsors to include PGx in early stage studies to assist in areas such as identifying populations that should receive a lower or higher dose of a drug; identify potential responder populations; and identify groups at risk of serious adverse effects. An important prerequisite to using PGx in drug development is collection and storage of DNA samples from all clinical trials. Ideally, sample collection should be collected at the time of study enrollment or at baseline in order to avoid bias related to subjects who do not complete the study. At the time of drug approval, information gained from PGx studies would be included in the product labeling to inform prescribers of the impact of a certain genotype or phenotype relative to response or adverse events. Similar approaches should be considered for proteomic (scientific analysis of proteins) and metabolomic evaluations (scientific analysis of the chemical processes involving metabolites).[58] PGx studies bring interesting challenges to obtaining informed consent from prospective subjects on clinical trials. First and foremost is identifying and potentially sharing sensitive genetic information that may not have been the intended purpose of the research. This issue requires careful consideration before the research is initiated and the research team should have a plan for what data they would share with a subject and their family and how that data would be shared. Another challenge relates to the fact that samples or DNA may be archived and/or immortalized cell lines may be created to facilitate future, as yet unidentified, research. Additionally, data or genetic materials may be shared with secondary users or used for purposes beyond that of the initially proposed clinical trial. Data may be pooled in the laboratory or it may be anonymized for sharing in databases, making the ability for the subject to withdraw the sample impossible. Some clinical trials are developed to allow participation in pharmacogenetic studies as optional, while in other studies it is an inherent component of the trial. For those studies where participation is optional or the subject is allowed a choice regarding the use of the samples and data, there should be a clear way of documenting their decisions. Subjects should be provided with detailed plans regarding timelines for use of the samples as well as for sample destruction. Finally, the subject should be given detailed information regarding the confidentiality of the data obtained during the research, methods used to ensure such confidentiality, the right to withdraw from the research (inclusive of detailed instructions on the method of asking to be withdrawn), and as mentioned above the fact that if their data is pooled or anonymized and shared they will not be able to withdraw.[59]

Case Study 23–1

Company CaCure (not a real company) has developed a drug called ALLCure. The product is FDA approved as an intravenous product used to treat severe headaches. Dr. Smith has conducted preclinical laboratory work that indicates that when given intrahepatically, the product can cause shrinkage of liver metastases.

Dr. Smith wants to try to use this ALLCure in 10 patients with cancer that is metastatic to the liver and see if the results hold true in humans.

- *Does Dr. Smith or ALLCure need approval from the FDA to transition this work into patients?*

NEW DRUG APPLICATION

❻ *After sufficient evidence is obtained regarding the drug's safety and effectiveness, the sponsor will submit an NDA/BLA to the FDA requesting approval of the medicinal product for marketing.* Except as noted for products being developed using accelerated approval pathways, the FDA requires the completion of two well-designed, well-controlled clinical trials prior to submission to the FDA. However, the sponsor will include information gathered from all of the clinical trials to show that the medicinal product is safe and effective and to describe the pharmacology and pharmacokinetics of the drug. The NDA/BLA will include all preclinical data, clinical data, manufacturing methods, product quality assurance, relevant foreign clinical testing (or marketing experience), and all published reports of experience with the medicinal agent (whether sponsored by the company or not). A proposed package insert will be supplied as well.[60]

Review of New Drug Application

The NDA/BLA will be distributed to the same FDA review division assigned while the product was under IND status. As noted, these divisions are based on the therapeutic group of the medicinal agent. The same reviewer may be assigned to review the IND and the NDA/BLA.[54]

The speed at which the NDA will be processed is to some extent determined by the classification the drug receives during its initial review. Each agent is rated with a number–letter designation that evaluates two separate aspects of the agent. The number portion of the rating is associated with the uniqueness of the drug product (ranging from 1 for an NME to 10 for new indications submitted as a separate NDA—see Table 16-1). The letter portion of the rating is associated with the therapeutic potential of the medicinal agent. The P (priority review) designation is given to drugs that represent a therapeutic advance with respect to available therapy, whereas an S (standard review) is given to drugs that have little or no therapeutic gain over previously available drugs—see Table 16-2. BLA prioritization is slightly simplified but similar.[61]

During the review process, the FDA may utilize one of its prescription drug advisory committees to help review the NDA. These committees are composed of experts who provide the agency with independent, nonbinding advice and recommendations regarding the NDA. Currently the FDA has 31 advisory committees, many of which are composed of various panels. Examples of such committees include the allergenic products' advisory committee and the cellular, tissue, and gene therapies' advisory committee.[61,62] Within 180 days of receipt of an NDA, the FDA will review the application and send the applicant an approval letter or a complete response letter.[63] When an approval letter is sent, the drug is considered approved as of the date of the letter.[64] A complete response letter is issued to let the sponsor know that the review period for the drug is complete, but that the application is not yet ready for approval. It will describe specific deficiencies, and when possible, identify recommended actions that the sponsor might take to address those deficiencies. In response to the complete response letter, the sponsor amends the NDA, withdraws the NDA, or requests a hearing with the FDA to clarify whether grounds exist for denying approval of the application.[65]

Expanded Access to Investigational Drugs for Treatment Use

As mentioned previously in this chapter, the FDA has been under considerable criticism relative to the time taken for drug review. They have implemented many initiatives to address these criticisms. The most recent initiative implemented by the FDA is referred to as "Expanded Access to Investigational Drugs for Treatment Use." The expanded access rule clarifies existing regulations and adds new types of expanded access for treatment use. Specifically, the rule allows for investigational drugs to be used for treatment in patients with serious or life-threatening diseases where there is no other comparable or satisfactory alternative therapy. The FDA defines immediately life-threatening conditions as those where death is likely to occur within a matter of months or in which premature death is likely without early treatment. Serious conditions are defined as those associated with morbidity that has substantial impact on day-to-day functioning.[66] The rules specify different requirements for expanded access for individual patients in emergencies; intermediate-size patient populations; and larger populations under a treatment protocol or treatment IND.[67]

The FDA must determine that in addition to the patient having a serious or immediately life-threatening disease for which there is no satisfactory alternative therapy, the potential patient benefit must outweigh the risk and that the requested use will not interfere with clinical investigations that could support marketing approval of the expanded access use. In all cases, an expanded access submission to the FDA is required. The submission may be a new IND or a protocol amendment to an existing IND (see the above explanation). Except as justified by emergency use guidelines further discussed in this chapter, all other regulations governing new INDs and protocol amendments, including regulations regarding study initiation, adverse reaction reporting, and annual reports, are identical to that described for standard INDs and described elsewhere in this chapter.[68]

For individual patients, submission requirements must include information adequate for the FDA to determine that the risk to the person from the investigational drug is not greater than the probable risk from the disease and that the patient cannot obtain the drug under another type of IND. Treatment is generally limited to a single course of therapy for a specified duration unless the FDA expressly authorizes multiple courses or chronic therapy. Individual patient expanded access submissions can be made in accordance with the standard submission requirements for an IND as outlined elsewhere in this chapter or they may be submitted utilizing Form 3926. In this type of submission, the FDA does allow for emergency procedures if the patient must be treated before a written submission can be made. In that situation, the FDA may authorize the emergency use by telephone. The sponsor must agree to submit an expanded access submission within 15 business days of the FDA's authorization of the use.[69] In addition, although the FDA must authorize emergency use of a test article (investigational drug), 21CFR56.104 allows for treatment to occur without prospective IRB approval in situations where there is insufficient time to obtain such review. In such situations, the emergency use must be reported to the IRB within 5 days after the treatment. Newer guidance from the FDA allows an investigator submitting an individual patient expanded access IND to request a waiver from full IRB review under 21CFR56.105 when the investigator obtains concurrence by the IRB chairperson or another designated IRB member before treatment use begins.[70]

For intermediate patient populations, there must be sufficient evidence that the drug is safe at the dose and duration proposed for treatment, and that there is at least preliminary clinical evidence of effectiveness of the drug. The sponsor must also indicate whether the drug is being developed and define the patient population. If the drug is being studied in a clinical trial, the sponsor must explain why the expanded access patient population cannot be enrolled in the clinical trial and under what circumstances the sponsor would conduct a clinical trial in those patients.[71]

The treatment IND, or treatment protocol, is a way the FDA has allowed for increased accessibility of experimental drugs for widespread treatment use. The drug must be investigated in a clinical trial under an IND designed to support a marketing application for the expanded access use, or if all clinical trials have been completed, the sponsor must be actively pursuing marketing approval of the drug for the expanded access use. When the expanded access use is for an immediately life-threatening disease, the available scientific evidence (usually clinical data from Phase II or Phase III trials) must provide reasonable assurance that the drug may be effective for the expanded access use and would not expose patients to significant risk.[72]

Right to Try

The Right to Try Act was signed into law on May 30, 2018. This law is another way for patients with life-threatening conditions without other alternatives, and unable to participate in a clinical trial, to obtain access to certain unapproved treatments. Right to Try treatments are those that are defined as eligible investigational drugs according to the following criteria:

- A Phase I trial has been completed.
- The product is not FDA approved for any use.
- An application has been filed with the FDA that will form the basis for a claim of effectiveness and an IND has been submitted to the FDA.
- Active development of the product is ongoing and has not been discontinued by the manufacturer or placed on hold by the FDA.

Neither the FDA nor an IRB review Right to Try Act uses. A physician working with a patient will contact the sponsor of the investigational product to determine if it is an eligible investigational drug under the Right to Try Act. The Right to Try Act does not require a sponsor to provide an eligible investigational drug to an eligible patient.[73,74]

Cost of Using Investigational Drugs

The FDA allows for the manufacturer to charge for an investigational drug under certain conditions. The sponsor must obtain prior written authorization from the FDA to charge for an investigational drug. In order to charge for an investigational drug, the sponsor must provide evidence that the drug has a potential clinical benefit that would provide a significant advantage over available products, demonstrate that the data to be obtained from the clinical trial would be essential to establishing that the drug is effective or safe, and demonstrate that the clinical trial could not be conducted without charging because the cost of the drug is extraordinary to the sponsor. The sponsor may only charge recovery costs for direct cost attributable to making the investigational drug, including raw materials, labor, nonreusable supplies, and equipment used to manufacture the drug or costs to acquire the drug from another manufacturer or to ship and handle the drug. In addition, for expanded access studies for intermediate-size patient populations or treatment IND/protocols, a sponsor may recover the cost of monitoring the expanded access IND or protocol, complying with IND reporting requirements, and other administrative costs directly associated with the expanded access IND.[75–77]

Expedited Review for New Drugs

The FDA has also attempted to expedite the review process for new drugs in several ways:

1. Priority review: The FDA determines a drug will potentially provide a significant advance in medical care and sets a target to review the drug within 6 months instead of the standard 10 months.
2. Fast Track review: The FDA determines that a drug can treat unmet medical needs. Fast Track speeds new drug reviews, for instance, by increasing the level of communication the FDA allocates to developers and by enabling developers to use a rolling review process such that portions of an application can be reviewed ahead of the submission of the full application.
3. Accelerated Approval program: The FDA determines that a drug is intended for use in serious or life-threatening illness and offers a benefit over current treatments. This approval is based on a surrogate endpoint (e.g., a laboratory measure) or other clinical measure that the FDA considers reasonably likely to predict clinical benefit. After this approval, the drug must undergo additional testing to confirm the benefit.
4. Breakthrough Therapy: Allows for expedited development and review of drugs which are intended to treat serious conditions and which may demonstrate a substantial improvement over available therapy.
5. Regenerative Medicine Advanced Therapy (RMAT) Designation: CBER gives this designation to certain human gene therapies and xenogeneic cell products if it

determines that the product is intended for use in serious or life-threatening illness and preliminary clinical evidence indicates that the drug has the potential to address an unmet medical need for such disease or condition. RMAT designation includes all the benefits of the fast track and breakthrough therapy designation programs.[78]

These designations relate directly to an IND and become an integral part of the review of the product being studied under the IND.

PHASE IV POSTMARKETING SURVEILLANCE

After the drug has been approved, postmarketing studies may be initiated. They are conducted for the approved indication, but may evaluate different doses, the effects of extended therapy, or the drug's safety in patient populations that were not represented in premarketing clinical trials. The final phase of clinical study is referred to as Phase IV trials. These Phase IV trials may be requested by the FDA or they may be initiated by the sponsor in an attempt to gather more data on the safety and efficacy of the drug or to identify a competitive advantage of the drug over other available therapies.

Risk Evaluation and Mitigation Strategies (REMS)

In some situations, the FDA may actually approve a product with restrictions limiting use to certain facilities or providers, or limiting the patient population to only those who have demonstrated certain performance on specified medical procedures.[79,80] Specifically, the FDA has started to utilize risk evaluation and mitigation strategies (REMS) when they determine that safety measures are needed beyond the labeling to ensure that a drug's benefits outweigh its risks. REMS can be required before or after a drug is approved. REMS are developed by drug sponsors; however, the FDA reviews and approves them. Factors that are considered in determining the need for a REMS include the following[81]:

- The seriousness of any known or potential adverse events that may be related to the drug and the background incidence of such events in the population likely to use the drug
- The expected benefit of the drug with respect to the disease or condition
- The seriousness of the disease or condition that is to be treated with the drug
- Whether the drug is an NME
- The expected or actual duration of treatment with the drug
- The estimated size of the population likely to use the drug.

The REMS may include the following components: a medication guide (patient package insert) and a communication plan (for providing key information to health care providers). The FDA may also require Elements to Assure Safe Use (ETASU) if the drug has been shown to be effective, but is associated with a specific serious risk. Sample ETASU components include required training or certifications for health care providers, limitations on health care settings where the drug can be infused, dispensing the drug only with evidence of safe conditions (e.g., specific laboratory results), monitoring of drug use by the patient, and enrollment of the patient on a registry. The REMS must be assessed for adequacy at least by 18 months, 3 years, and 7 years after approval.[82] As an example, the drug bexanolone (trade name Zulresso) was approved to treat postpartum depression. It is provided as a 60-hour IV infusion. It can cause sedation and loss of consciousness. Due to these risks the drug was approved with a requirement for a REMS. The approved REMS calls for:

- Ensuring that Zulresso is administered only to patients in a medically supervised setting that provides monitoring while Zulresso is administered
- Ensuring that pharmacies and health care settings that dispense ZULRESSO are certified
- Ensuring that each patient is informed of the adverse events of excessive sedation and loss of consciousness and the need for monitoring while ZULRESSO is administered
- Enrollment of all patients in a registry to characterize the risks and support safe use.[83]

Case Study 23–2

CaCure (refer to Case Study 21-1) decided to help develop ALLCure for this indication. They successfully submitted an IND and have now completed not only Phase I and Phase II studies, but have completed two positive Phase III studies in patients with metastatic disease to the liver. The company can now apply for an NDA for this new application. Unfortunately, during the studies they became aware that some patients developed cirrhosis months or even years after treatment.

- *Assuming that the cirrhosis is related to this new route of administration, what would be an important component of the submission to the FDA as they seek licensing approval?*
- *What will be appropriate components of the REMS?*

The Orphan Drug Act

The Orphan Drug Act was passed in 1983 and provides incentives for manufacturers to develop orphan drugs. ❼ *An orphan drug is one used for the treatment of a rare disease, affecting fewer than 200,000 people in the United States, or one that will not generate enough revenue to justify the cost of research and development.* There are currently more than 7000 rare diseases impacting approximately 30 million Americans. [84]

The Orphan Drug Act is administered by the FDA's Office of Orphan Products and the related program has enabled the development and marketing of over 600 drugs and biologic products for rare diseases since its inception in 1983.[85] Of note, although to qualify for consideration as an orphan drug a product must be under evaluation as part of an IND, the review and approval process for an orphan drug designation is separate from that of the IND. The orphan drug designation (also known as the orphan status) is awarded only if both the drug and the disease meet certain qualifications.

The orphan drug designation provides the following incentives:

- **Tax incentives**: The sponsor is eligible to receive a tax credit for money spent on research and development of an orphan drug.
- **Waive filing fees**: The sponsor is eligible to file for a waiver from the application fee associated with the review of an NDA.
- **Protocol assistance**: If a sponsor can show that a drug will be used for a rare disease, the FDA will provide assistance developing the preclinical and clinical plan for the product.
- **Grants and contracts**: The FDA budget may allot money for grants and contracts to be used in developing orphan drugs. The current annual budget for orphan drug grants is $15 million with $10 million for ongoing noncompete renewals and $5 million to fund new projects annually. The orphan grants process has been used to bring more than 60 products to marketing approval.[86]
- **Marketing exclusivity**: The first sponsor to obtain marketing approval for a designated orphan drug is allowed 7 years of marketing exclusivity for that indication, but identical versions of the same product marketed by another manufacturer may be approved for other indications.

The Orphan Drug Act does not provide advantages for the drug approval process. Sponsors seeking approval for drugs that will be designated as orphan drugs must still provide the same safety and efficacy data as all other drugs evaluated by the FDA. Exceptions to the rules governing the number of patients that should be treated in the clinical trials may be made based on the scarcity of patients with the condition. Additionally, because in many cases there are no alternative therapies for the disease, the drug may be given a high review priority during the NDA process.[87,88]

Institutional Review Board/Institutional Ethics Committee

The institutional review board (IRB) known outside of the United States as the institutional ethics committee is a committee formed to review proposed clinical trials and the progress of such studies to ensure that the rights and welfare of human subjects are protected. The IRB must contain at least one member who has specialized in a scientific area (in situations where drugs and biologics are being reviewed this is usually a physician) and at least one board member who has a specialty in a nonscientific area such as law, ethics, or religion. Additionally, the IRB must contain at least one individual who is not affiliated with the institution where the research is being conducted. Membership of the IRB varies between institutions. Common members of IRBs include physicians, pharmacists, nurses, lawyers, clergy, and laypeople. The IRB is also responsible for ensuring that the proposed clinical trial is not in conflict with the institution's research policies or philosophy. The IRB and the study sponsor will have little, if any, direct contact. The primary investigator generally acts as the liaison between these two parties.

Cumulatively the rules governing IRBs are known as human subject protections. The FDA has their own policies regarding human subjects enrolled in clinical trials that utilize products that they regulate. More globally, however, human subject protections are overseen by a number of federal agencies, most notably the Office of Human Research Subject Protections (OHRP) as part of the DHHS through oversight and enforcement of Federal Policy for the Protection of Human Subjects, also known as the Common Rule. A major revision of the Common Rule was implemented in 2018 replacing a version that had been in effect with only minor revisions since 1991. The revised Common Rule impacts the content of informed consent forms but does not more globally impact the oversight of human subject protections in the setting of investigational products, so this chapter will not further discuss changes made to the Common Rule.[89]

REVIEW OF CLINICAL RESEARCH PROTOCOL

The IRB should evaluate the research proposal to ensure that the following requirements are met:

- The risks to subjects are minimal.
- The expected risk/anticipated benefit ratio must be reasonable.

- Equitable subject selection is used.
- Informed consent must be received from each participant (or his or her legally authorized representative).
- Informed consent must be documented in writing.
- Data must be monitored to ensure subject safety.
- Patient confidentiality must be maintained.
- If appropriate, additional safeguards against coercion must be included in studies that include vulnerable subjects (children, prisoners, pregnant women, mentally disabled people, or economically or educationally disadvantaged persons).

A notable exception to the requirements for written informed consent, as described above, has been provided for research done in emergency circumstances involving human subjects who cannot give informed consent because of their emerging, life-threatening medical condition (for which available treatments are unproven or unsatisfactory), and where the intervention must be administered before informed consent from the subject's legally authorized representative is feasible. In these situations, the exception from informed consent requirements may proceed only after the sponsor has received prior written permission from the FDA (via IND approval) and from the IRB. In this type of research, both community consultation and public disclosure must be provided for the protocol.[90]

RESPONSIBILITIES OF IRB

The IRB must, at a minimum, perform annual reviews of all ongoing clinical trials and evaluate adverse experiences to ensure that the criteria listed above continue to be met.[91,92]

The IRB must maintain documentation of all IRB activities including copies of all research proposals reviewed, minutes of IRB meetings, records of continuing review activities, copies of all correspondence between the IRB and the investigators, a list of IRB members, written procedures of the IRB, and statements of significant new findings provided to subjects. This documentation and records that pertain to research should be retained for 3 years after the research is completed.[93,94]

Some institutions divide their review of proposed clinical research into two separate processes. One of these is the review of the protocol for scientific worth (scientific review), and the other is the review of the protocol for ethical considerations (IRB review). For many years, the role of the IRB and the effectiveness of the informed consent process have been questioned.[95,96] In some institutions, the IRB is also responsible for evaluating research misconduct. Research misconduct means fabrication, falsification, or plagiarism in proposing, performing, or reviewing research, or in reporting research results.[97] Research misconduct is an issue of increasing concern to study sponsors, institutions, and the government as the pressure on investigators and their associates to produce results has increased. In most institutions, as the emphasis on identifying and handling research misconduct has increased, the institutions have developed separate review processes and policies to deal with the issue.

IRBs are also involved in evaluating conflict of interest (COI). As with research misconduct, evaluation and control of COI is a shared responsibility for the institution, the IRB, and the investigator (and staff). Of specific concern to the IRB is whether or not financial interests may impact the protection of human subjects. The IRB should identify a mechanism for reporting such COI, develop a mechanism for managing or eliminating such COI, and as deemed necessary require that such conflicts be provided to potential study subjects as part of the informed consent process.[98]

Training of investigators and staff in human subject protections, Good Clinical Practice (GCP), and COI is an institutional responsibility that is sometimes enforced by the IRB.[99] Many institutions use the Collaborative Institutional Training Initiative (CITI) to provide and track such training of investigators and staff.[100]

Case Study 23–3

The FDA has mandated that before ALLCure (refer to Case Study 21-1) can be approved, further clinical trials will be required to determine the mechanism of action of developing cirrhosis and whether there are clinical or genetic factors that can define the at-risk population. The lawyers at CaCure do not want the cirrhosis information provided in the consent form, as the relationship between the toxicity and the drug is not yet definitely proven.

- *What is a likely IRB determination?*
- *What special issues need to be considered if children are to be included in this study to further define the risk of cirrhosis?*
- *What is required if a child reaches their legal age of majority (as defined by state law) while enrolled in this study?*

Next the role of health care professionals in clinical research will be discussed.

Role of the Health Care Professional

The health care professional can play a vital role in the clinical research process by:

- Being the primary investigator (PI) on a study

- Completing case report forms and reporting adverse events
- Preparing the IND
- Serving on the IRB and, where applicable, on the Scientific Review Committee
- Providing financial evaluations of investigational protocols
- Disseminating information regarding both the protocol and the investigational drug to other health care personnel
- Maintaining drug accountability records
- Ordering, maintaining, and, when necessary, returning drug supplies for ongoing clinical trials
- Randomizing and, when necessary, blinding drug supplies for a clinical trial

GETTING INVOLVED IN CLINICAL RESEARCH

The American Society of Health-System Pharmacists (ASHP) released guidelines for managing investigational products in 2018.[101] Some of the guidelines are not specific to pharmacists, while others are more closely linked to the pharmacist training and expertise. The health care professional can serve as the Principal Investigator (PI) on clinical research studies. The type of study for which an individual can serve as a PI varies based on their expertise and experience. Common types of studies for which nonphysicians serve as PIs include pharmacoeconomic, pharmacology/pharmacokinetic, quality of life, and other nontherapeutic and minimal risk studies. For some of these trials, an IRB may insist that a physician be a coinvestigator.

The health care professional can assist the investigator by completing **case report forms (CRFs)** and reporting clinical trial adverse reactions to the FDA. A discussion of the types of adverse reactions and the applicable reporting requirements was presented in the section of this chapter referred to as the drug approval process. Further information about the concept of adverse drug reaction reporting, including identification and classification of adverse events, can be found in the adverse drug reaction section of Chapter 19. CRFs are completed using source documents such as the medical record. Traditionally, source documents were paper based and generally part of the patient's medical record; however, as the medical record in many institutions has transitioned to the use of electronic systems, these require some focused attention. While these electronic systems provide opportunities to improve data accuracy and clinical trial efficiency inclusive of improved long-term follow-up, the health care professional should be cognizant of the system being used. In general, electronic systems that comply with the ONC Health IT Certification program are in compliance with regulatory expectations. Electronic systems that do not comply with the program may need additional documentation and analysis regarding data privacy and security protection to ensure the quality and integrity of data being used in a clinical protocol.[102-104]

The health care professional can assist in preparing the IND by following the guidelines presented earlier in this chapter. Equally important, the health care professional can assist in writing the protocol. One issue that should be considered when writing a protocol is the issue of potential drug shortages of commercially available products. As discussed in Chapter 17 of this book, drug shortages are an increasingly common problem in the United States. In the context of clinical trials if a drug that is included in a protocol is unavailable for any portion of the study, the impact on study conduct and outcome evaluations can be significant. In such a situation, the following options are available:

- Temporary or permanent study hold/termination
- Drug substitution

If drug substitution is selected, there are two possible options to consider, including a specific drug (as specified by the sponsor) or allowing for drug substitution by individual investigators without specification by the sponsor. While the second option may allow for better personalized clinical decision-making, it is likely to yield study outcomes that are difficult to interpret. In any event, the decision about how to proceed at the time of a drug shortage will be driven by the length of time the drug is anticipated to be in short supply, the role (pivotal or not) of the drug in the study and study questions, and the rapidity at which drug substitutions need to be made. In general, drug substitutions will need to be made in the body of the protocol as an amendment. However, for a drug with therapeutic purposes where the suspected duration of drug shortage may be prolonged, the treatment may need to be altered prior to approval of the amendment. This type of rapid modification of treatment is allowed for in situations where the subjects are considered to be at immediate risk of harm.[105] More generally, the impact of drug shortages on protocols can be avoided by only specifying drugs that are critical to study outcomes, allowing for institutional preferences in drug selection, and referencing institutional treatment Standard Operating Procedures (SOPs) rather than specific drugs.

Preferably, nonphysician, health care professionals will be included as voting members of the IRB and as such may have some control over clinical trials initiated at the institution. While it is important that they recuse themselves from voting on studies which they are involved with, their knowledge can be quite valuable to the IRB. First and foremost, they can aid in the scientific review of the protocol, whether this occurs as part of the scientific review committee or as part of the IRB. When reviewing a protocol for scientific purposes, they should help verify that the information in the protocol is complete and that it is logistically possible for the protocol to be conducted as presented. In addition, the health care professional should confirm that any potential toxicities specified in the protocol are detailed for the patient in the informed consent of the protocol.

The health care professional can play a crucial role in implementing protocols within the institution. The preparation of protocol-specific order templates and protocol information summaries help to ensure compliance with the protocol. The protocol information summary will likely be a key resource not only for individuals directly involved in the research study but also nonresearch staff and physicians who may be involved in patient care. Components of a protocol information sheet include the following:

- Protocol number (as assigned by the institution)
- Protocol title
- Agent name(s) (synonym[s])
- Protocol description
  1. Objectives
  2. Study design
     a. Registration requirements
     b. Primary location of patients
     c. Type of study
  3. Treatment course (including retreatment criteria)
- Availability
  1. Supplier
  2. Status
  3. How supplied
- Storage, stability, and compatibility
  1. Intact drug
  2. Prepared drug (for injectables this should include both reconstitution and dilution guidelines)
- Dosage range
- Dose preparation guidelines (this portion should be written or confirmed by a pharmacist)
- Administration guidelines
- Special notes or handling guidelines for the investigational agent
- Primary investigator
- Key study staff including the research nurse

Training of hospital staff (again including providers who may not be investigators) is important to ensure the safety of study subjects as well as protocol compliance. Training materials should be developed, and training sessions for identified key individuals should be scheduled. Different training materials may be required for different individuals. Documentation of training is important and should be properly recorded and stored.

To ensure accuracy, the primary investigator and study sponsor should approve training materials, the protocol summary, and drug data sheet (described below) before dissemination.

ROLE OF THE PHARMACIST

Reviewing the Research Protocol

The pharmacist should verify that the protocol or associated documents such as the investigator's brochure contain the following information:

- The name and synonyms of the study agent
- The chemical structure of the study agent
- The mechanism of action of the study agent
- The dosage range of the study agent (with appropriate rationale)
- Animal toxicologic and pharmacologic information (when available, any known human toxicologic and pharmacologic information should also be presented)
- How the agent will be supplied (dosage form and size)
- The preparation guidelines for the agent (including stability and compatibility information when appropriate)
- The storage requirements of the agent (both before and, when appropriate, after preparation)
- The route of administration (and, if applicable, the rate of administration)

The pharmacist should also review the protocol for other potential problems (such as incompatibilities and inappropriate infusion devices). The pharmacist can review the protocol for clinical and scientific issues appropriate to his or her knowledge level and experience. Those pharmacists with research experience or a strong clinical background may, and probably should, comment on the study design or scientific merit of a particular protocol.

Managing Drug Costs

With the central role of financial considerations in today's research environment, pharmacists can also provide valuable insight into the costs associated with clinical research. Traditionally, the study sponsors would provide the investigational drug free of charge to the hospital (and to the patient) and the patient (or the third-party payer) would be responsible for paying for all other charges associated with therapy. These charges could include hospitalization charges, laboratory tests, and examinations to name a few. Some third-party payers are reluctant to pay for such charges unless they can be considered to be standard of care. Effective in September 2000, Medicare began to cover the costs of qualifying clinical trials (QCTs) inclusive of items and services that are generally available to Medicare recipients, excluding only the investigational agent, evaluations being done only for research purposes, and other items and services customarily provided by research sponsors.[106] Hospitals and other health care institutions and providers are increasingly using the QCT determination system to evaluate the costs and financial risks of the research protocol. Many (but not all) insurers will agree to cover similar costs for subjects not enrolled on research studies. However, uninsured, underinsured, and patients whose insurance will not accept the QCT assessment are left in a financially risky situation. This leaves the patient, and subsequently the health care institution, in a financially risky situation. Developing cost assessments and QCT evaluations can assist the investigator, the institution, and the review boards with important information regarding the potential cost of the research, allowing all parties to make a more educated decision regarding appropriation of resources for research purposes. In situations where there is no study sponsor, an economic review of the study can be even more extensive and look at key components of the study, such as:

- Can the therapy be converted from inpatient to outpatient?
- Can the method of infusion or the infusion device be changed to one that is more cost effective?
- Does the treatment plan call for administration of compatible medications that could be mixed in the same container?
- Is the supportive care adequate and not excessive (this is especially important with high-cost drugs, such as growth factors)?

More recently, some sponsors have started to implement programs for cost recovery for investigational drugs. As discussed earlier, the sponsor applies to, and receives approval from, the FDA for a specific dollar amount that can be charged. FDA approval of this charge must be in place before cost recovery can begin.[75-77] The institution will need to have procedures in place for billing properly for investigational drugs.

Disseminating Research Information

Following approval of the research project, the investigational drug pharmacist should assist in disseminating information about the investigational agent by preparing an investigational agent data sheet that may be used by pharmacy and nursing personnel (and in some situations by practitioners who may be unfamiliar with the research). This information can be distributed using various methods including paper, web-based systems, and the electronic medical record. The investigational agent data sheet should include the following elements:

- Agent name (synonyms)
- Therapeutic classification
- Pharmaceutical data
- Stability and storage data
- Dose preparation guidelines (where applicable)
- Usual dosage range

- Route of administration
- Known side effects and toxicities
- Mechanism of action
- Status (phase of study)
- Date effective (and dates of revision)
- References

Securing Drug Supplies for Research

The pharmacist can assume primary responsibility for ordering and maintaining adequate drug supplies for conducting the clinical trial. All investigational drugs should be stored in a locked area, preferably a pharmacy. Investigational drugs that are also controlled substances will have increased requirements for ordering, storing, and shipping and must comply with Drug Enforcement Administration (DEA) regulations.[107] Shipment and receipt of any investigational drug can vary from one day to several weeks (or sometimes months for very specialized drug products). The individual responsible for ordering drug must be sufficiently knowledgeable regarding the rate of patient enrollment in the protocol and subsequent drug usage to ensure that the institution does not run out of drug. The same individual(s) should also assume responsibility for returning unused drug supplies at the completion of the study. The sponsor may authorize on-site destruction of unused supplies, provided this will not increase the risk to humans (or to the environment). Many study sponsors will attempt to have the site save and return all used drug supplies as well. This is not an FDA requirement and for safety and space reasons should be discouraged. Additionally, if the investigational drug is considered to be hazardous, the shipment must comply with U.S. Department of Transportation regulations for shipping hazardous materials.[108]

Implementing the Study

As appropriate, the pharmacist should ensure that the investigational product is entered into the pharmacy computer dispensing system and the hospital's electronic medical record system. A dispensing label for the investigational drug product will need to be prepared. The label will need to comply with all state and federal laws. The label must include the statement "Caution: New Drug—Limited by Federal (or United States) Law to Investigational Use."[109]

Maintaining Drug Accountability Records

Related to the activities above, the same individuals (or team) should assume responsibility for maintaining drug accountability records. ❽ *Drug accountability records are mandated by law. They can be electronic or in paper form.* The records must document all drug shipments, returns, and dispensing to patients. *Necessary components include:*

- *The date of the transaction*
- *The type of the transaction*

- *The receiving party of the transaction (if this is a drug dispensation, the subject initials and an identifying number are required)*
- *The number of units being used or received (for patient dispensing this should include the actual dose the patient will receive)*
- *The lot number of the drug (if multiple lot numbers were used, each one should be documented)*
- *The initials of the individual who performed the transaction*

An audit trail is required. The National Cancer Institute (NCI) has prepared a sample drug accountability form that may be used as a guide (available at https://ctep.cancer. gov/forms/docs/agent_accountability.pdf).

Computer systems that will maintain drug accountability records are available commercially. These systems are generally standalone, but can interface with other systems. Some of these systems will also provide drug labels, bar codes, drug and protocol information, summaries of investigational drug dispensing (useful in the preparation of productivity reports), and even monthly billing summaries to be used for posting charges to the study budget. The development of a personalized system that meets the specific needs of the institution or pharmacy is another possibility; however, this can be costly, laborious, and time consuming. If a personalized system is developed, it is important to remember that the system must be able to maintain the integrity of the records and that a clear audit trail needs to be maintained. Ultimately, the decision to computerize drug accountability records and the selection of which system to use is one that should be made only after evaluating the needs of the institution/pharmacy and the available budget.[109-111]

Drug accountability records and drug supplies may be inspected at any time by the sponsor. The frequency of these inspections may vary according to the wishes of the sponsor. They may be monthly, quarterly, or annually. The FDA also has the right to inspect these records. The investigational drug pharmacist should play a key role in providing drug accountability information to either the FDA or the sponsor during an audit. If proper records are not being maintained, the sponsor or the FDA may discontinue the investigator's participation in the clinical investigation.

After the clinical trial is complete, records must be maintained at the study site for the following time periods:

- Two years after approval of the NDA *or*
- Two years after the FDA received notification that the investigation was discontinued[112]

Maintaining Adequate Control of Drug Supplies for Randomized and Blinded Interventions

Randomization and blinding are two important ways to reduce or eliminate the bias of a clinical trial (see Chapter 4). A randomized study is one in which patients are randomly assigned (similar to flipping a coin) to different therapies. More details regarding the statistical basis for randomized studies are included in Chapter 6 of this book. Usually the assignment is done using a computer-generated randomization list; however, a manual list may be used as well. The randomization groups may include a number of different therapy options as well as variations in the number of subjects enrolled to each arm of a study. Similarly, how the drug will be dispensed may vary dependent on the policies of the study sponsor. In some cases, a study sponsor may provide drug to the site ready to allocate to a specific patient. In other cases, the sponsor may provide supplies for the different therapy options in bulk, thus requiring the pharmacist to dispense drug according to the arm to which the patient was assigned. In either case, the importance of the pharmacist in dispensing the proper drug to the proper patient and maintaining the blind (if the study is blinded) cannot be overemphasized.

Establishing an Investigational Drug Pharmacy

The staffing and space needs for an investigational pharmacy will be driven by the volume and complexity of the protocols that are supported. Funding can come from a variety of sources:

- Direct cost recovery
- Indirect funding from overhead collected by the institution from grants and contracts negotiated by the institution
- Philanthropic or foundation funding
- Direct funding of the institution by absorbing the costs of the program

Many institutions use a combination of these approaches to support the investigational drug pharmacy.

Direct Cost Recovery for an Investigational Drug Pharmacy Service

Investigational drug pharmacies should negotiate funds for these services from the study sponsor before initiation of the protocol. The majority of pharmacies charge a base fee for each protocol initiated at the institution. This base fee may be fixed or it may vary based on the size of the patient population, the complexity of the protocol, or the number of doses to be prepared. Some institutions also charge an annual renewal fee for ongoing clinical trials. Most pharmacies will charge a separate fee for randomizing and blinding a clinical trial. This fee can be a one-time (per study) fee or it can be a per-patient fee. Some hospitals also charge dispensing fees per dose or per amount of time required to prepare a dose. Pharmacies can also charge a monthly fee for drug storage and inventory. This fee varies based on the amount of space and type of storage (freezer, room temperature, or refrigerator) required. The pharmacist can also charge a professional fee for services that exceed the standard services provided for in the base fee. Examples of pharmacy-specific additional services include special compounding, ordering and handling controlled substances, and completing sponsor-specific drug accountability records. These services are usually charged using an hourly rate. More general clinical research services that should be considered and charged for include regulatory submissions, coordination of protocol-driven care, monitoring of patients, and completing case report forms.

Conclusion

Assisting in the implementation and conduct of clinical trials can be a satisfying role for the health care professional. Clinical trials that utilize drugs, biologics, and devices in the United States are largely controlled by the FDA and by local IRBs. A thorough under-standing of the regulations governing those entities is extremely helpful when conducting clinical trials. The health care professional can use that knowledge to help investigators develop clinical trials, obtain and maintain proper approvals for those clinical trials, and assist in the conduct of clinical trials. Related to the conduct of clinical trials, health care professionals (and specifically pharmacists) are frequently involved in obtaining, storing, and dispensing the agents being utilized in the clinical trial. In addition, the health care professional (and specifically pharmacists) can be quite involved in providing protocol and drug information to the investigators, other study personnel, and equally importantly to the study subjects. Health care professionals can and should play an integral role in the conduct of clinical trials at their institution.

Self-Assessment Questions

1. What is the primary role of the FDA related to drugs, biologics, and medical devices in the United States?
   a. Evaluating the safety and efficacy of the products
   b. Determining that the rights and welfare of human subjects are protected
   c. Evaluating prescribing trends of physicians among similar products
   d. Determining the price of the products

2. What is the primary purpose of IRB review of research?
   a. Evaluating the safety and efficacy of products used in an investigational protocol
   b. Determining that the rights and welfare of human subjects are protected

   c. Evaluating the risk-benefit ratio of an investigational protocol

   d. Determining that the consent form is written at an appropriate reading level

3. The drug approval process in the United States is:
   a. Codified by the NIH
   b. Inclusive of usage analysis
   c. Based on preclinical and clinical studies
   d. Initiated by submission of an IDE to the FDA

4. A sponsor-investigator IND:
   a. Has the same requirements as a commercial IND
   b. Allows for treatment of patients even when consent cannot be obtained
   c. Automatically receives fast track review
   d. Allows for increase in accessibility of the product for widespread use

5. IND safety reports:
   a. Are submitted annually to describe the progress of the investigation
   b. Should be submitted if a manufacturing change may impact product safety
   c. Are only required when there is proof that an adverse event is related to the product
   d. Should be submitted for new safety data obtained from humans or animals

6. What would be an appropriate example of a REMS and the associated requirements to mitigate those risks?
   a. Liver damage—counseling patients on signs of liver failure
   b. Serious infection—sending patients home with antibiotics
   c. Severe birth defects—requiring a negative pregnancy test prior to dispensing each dose of medication
   d. Leukemia—meeting with an oncologist prior to initiating treatment

7. An Orphan Drug designation:
   a. Can be given to any product affecting less than 500,000 people worldwide
   b. Provides funding to all manufacturers of products used to treat rare diseases
   c. Encourages the development of products with limited potential profit
   d. Allows approval of products with limited safety and efficacy data

8. A manufacturer can charge for an investigational product:
   a. If it is part of a QCT
   b. When they demonstrate that the cost of the drug is extraordinary
   c. When Phase III protocols are initiated
   d. If it is part of a Treatment IND

9. What does an IND allow a sponsor to do?
   a. Market the product
   b. Charge for the product
   c. Initiate a clinical trial
   d. Name the product

10. Who is the sponsor's primary contact at the FDA?
    a. Medical reviewer
    b. Pharmacology/Toxicology reviewer
    c. Regulatory Project Manager
    d. CMC reviewer

11. ClinicalTrials.gov:
    a. Is a mechanism of distributing information among investigators
    b. Is only required for studies funded by the NIH
    c. Only requires posting of clinical trials used to treat serious diseases
    d. Only requires reporting of results for certain trials

12. Right to Try access:
    a. Must be requested directly from the sponsor by the patient
    b. Must be provided by the sponsor upon request
    c. Can only be provided in association with an active IND
    d. Can only be provided following approval by an IRB

13. The investigational agent data sheet should include the following elements:
    a. Dose preparation guidelines
    b. Principal investigator name
    c. Indications for use
    d. The lot numbers of the product to be dispensed

14. Drug accountability records:
    a. Must be manually generated
    b. Must include the full name of the patient
    c. Are optional dependent on the needs of the sponsor
    d. Must include the dose to be administered to the patient

15. Which of the expedited review mechanisms utilized by the FDA is based on a different evaluation of the outcome measure as opposed to targeting a more rapid review process:
    a. Fast Track review
    b. Priority review
    c. Accelerated Approval Program
    d. Regenerative Medicine Advanced Therapy

REFERENCES

1. DiMasi JA, Grabowski HG, Hansen RW. Innovation in the pharmaceutical industry: new estimates of R&D costs. JHE. May 2016;47:20-33.

2. Food and Drug Administration [Internet]. Drugs@FDA glossary of terms. Updated through 2017 Nov [cited 2019 Oct]; [11 p.]. Available from: http://www.fda.gov/drugs/informationondrugs/ucm079436.htm

3. Carroll A. $2.6 billion to develop a drug? New estimate makes questionable assumptions. NYT [Internet]. 2014 Nov 18 [cited 2019 Oct]; [4 p.]. Available from: http://www.nytimes.com/2014/11/19/upshot/calculating-the-real-costs-of-developing-a-new-drug.html?_r=0

4. ADIS R&D Insight Database [Internet]. [Cited 2019 Jun].

5. Analysis Group. The biopharmaceutical pipeline: innovative therapies in clinical development [Internet]. 2017 Jul [cited 2019 Oct]; [1 p.]. Available from: https://www.analysisgroup.com/Insights/publishing/the-biopharmaceutical-pipeline--innovative-therapies-in-clinical-development/

6. Food and Drug Administration. Novel Drug Approvals for 2018 [Internet]. [Updated through 2019 Sep; cited 2019 Oct]; [16 p.]. Available from: https://www.fda.gov/drugs/new-drugs-fda-cders-new-molecular-entities-and-new-therapeutic-biological-products/novel-drug-approvals-2018

7. Food and Drug Administration. Executive summary: strategic plan for regulatory science [Internet]. [Updated through 2018 Mar; cited 2019 Oct]; [3 p.]. Available from: https://www.fda.gov/science-research/advancing-regulatory-science/executive-summary-strategic-plan-regulatory-science

8. Food and Drug Administration. FDA organization chart [Internet]. [Updated through 2019 Oct; cited 2019 Oct]; [2 p.]. Available from: https://www.fda.gov/about-fda/fda-organization-charts/fda-overview-organization-chart

9. Food and Drug Administration [Internet]. Summary of NDA approvals and receipts, 1938 to the present. [Updated 2018 Jan; cited 2019 Oct]; [3 p.]. Available from: https://www.fda.gov/about-fda/histories-product-regulation/summary-nda-approvals-receipts-1938-present

10. United States Federal Government Code of Federal Regulations. 21CFR314. [Updated 2018 Apr].

11. Meadows M. Promoting safe and effective drugs for 100 years. FDA consumer [Internet]. [Last updated 2019 Apr; cited 2019 Oct]; [9 p.]. Available from: https://www.fda.gov/about-fda/histories-product-regulation/promoting-safe-effective-drugs-100-years

12. Bruderle TP. Reforming the Food and Drug Administration: legislative solution or self-improvement. Am J Health-Syst Pharm. 1996;53:2083-90.

13. Reichert J. A guide to drug discovery: trends in development and approval times for new therapeutics in the Unites States. Nat Rev Drug Discov. 2003;2(9):695-702.

14. Terese Johansson PhD. Europe vs USA: new drug product approvals in 2017. NDA [Internet]. 2017 [cited 2019 Oct]; [6 p.]. Available from: https://www.ndareg.com/europe-vs-usa-new-drug-product-approvals-in-2017/

15. Eastlake Research Group. Canadian, European and United States new drug approval times now relatively similar (abstract). Regul Toxicol Pharmacol. 2018 July [cited 2019 Oct]; [1 p.]. Available from: https://www.ncbi.nlm.nih.gov/pubmed/29730446

16. Food and Drug Administration [Internet]. PDUFA VI: fiscal years 2018-2022. [Last updated 2019 May; cited 2019 Oct]. Available from: https://www.fda.gov/industry/prescription-drug-user-fee-amendments/pdufa-vi-fiscal-years-2018-2022

17. Food and Drug Administration [Internet]. Milestones in U.S. Food and Drug law history. [Updated 2018 Jan; cited 2019 Oct]. Available from: https://www.fda.gov/about-fda/fdas-evolving-regulatory-powers/milestones-us-food-and-drug-law-history

18. Food and Drug Administration [Internet]. Food and Drug Administration Amendments Act of 2007. [Updated 2018 Mar; cited 2019 Oct]. Available from: https://www.fda.gov/regulatory-information/selected-amendments-fdc-act/food-and-drug-administration-amendments-act-fdaaa-2007

19. Food and Drug Administration [Internet]. Food and Drug Administration Safety and Innovation Act (FDASIA). [Updated 2018 Mar; cited 2019 Oct]. Available from: https://www.fda.gov/regulatory-information/selected-amendments-fdc-act/food-and-drug-administration-safety-and-innovation-act-fdasia

20. Food and Drug Administration [Internet]. 21st Century Cures Act. [Updated 2018 Mar; cited 2019 Oct]. Available from: https://www.fda.gov/regulatory-information/selected-amendments-fdc-act/21st-century-cures-act

21. Food and Drug Administration [Internet]. Critical path initiative. [Updated 2018 Apr; cited 2019 Oct]. Available from: https://www.fda.gov/science-research/science-and-research-special-topics/critical-path-initiative

22. CDER; Food and Drug Administration [Internet]. Duchenne muscular dystrophy and related dystrophinopathies: developing drugs for treatment: guidance for industry. 2018 Apr [cited 2019 Oct]. Available from: http://www.fda.gov/downloads/drugs/guidancecomplianceregulatoryinformation/guidances/UCM450229.pdf

23. FDA draft guidance on Duchenne. EndDuchenne.org [Internet]. 2019 Jun [cited 2019 Oct]. Available from: http://www.parentprojectmd.org/site/PageServer?pagename=Advocate_fdaguidance

24. Food and Drug Administration [Internet]. Electronic regulatory submissions and review. [Updated 2019 Aug; cited 2019 Oct]. Available from: http://www.fda.gov/Drugs/DevelopmentApprovalProcess/FormsSubmissionRequirements/ElectronicSubmissions/default.htm

25. Food and Drug Administration [Internet]. Electronic Common Technical Document (eCTD). [Updated 2019 Sep; cited 2019 Oct]. Available from: http://www.fda.gov/Drugs/DevelopmentApprovalProcess/FormsSubmissionRequirements/ElectronicSubmissions/ucm153574.htm

26. CDER; Food and Drug Administration [Internet]. Guideline for Drug Master Files. [Updated 2015 Nov; cited 2019 Oct]. Available from: http://www.fda.gov/Drugs/DevelopmentApprovalProcess/FormsSubmissionRequirements/DrugMasterFilesDMFs/ucm073164.htm

27. Food and Drug Administration. Assessment of the program for enhanced review transparency and communication for NME NDAs and Original BLAs in PDUFA V [Internet]. 2016 Nov [cited 2019 Oct]. Available from: https://www.fda.gov/media/104487/download

28. Food and Drug Administration [Internet]. FDA's role: ClinicalTrials.gov information. 2019 Sep [cited 2019 Oct]. Available from: http://www.fda.gov/scienceresearch/special topics/runningclinicaltrials/fdasroleclinicaltrials.govinformation/default.htm

29. ClinicalTrials.gov. History, policies, and law [Internet]. Last reviewed 2018 Aug [cited 2019 Oct]. Available from: https://clinicaltrials.gov/ct2/about-site/history

30. NIH.gov [Internet]. Summary table of HHS/NIH initiatives to enhance availability of clinical trial information. [Updated 2016 Sep; cited 2019 Oct]. Available from: https://www.nih.gov/news-events/summary-table-hhs-nih-initiatives-enhance-availability-clinical-trial-information

31. International Conference on Harmonization. History of ICH [Internet]. [Updated 2019; cited 2019 Oct]. Available from: http://www.ich.org/about/history.html

32. Food and Drug Administration. Project Orbis [Internet]. [Updated 2019 Sep; cited 2020 Jan]. Available from: https://www.fda.gov/about-fda/oncology-center-excellence/project-orbis

33. Office of Science Policy. NIH guidelines for research involving recombinant or synthetic nucleic acid molecules (NIH guidelines) Section IV-B [Internet]. 2019 Apr [cited 2020 Jun]. Available from: https://osp.od.nih.gov/wp-content/uploads/2019_NIH_Guidelines.htm#_APPENDIX_Q._PHYSICAL

34. Grilley BJ. Regulations governing clinical trials in gene therapy. In: Brenner M, Hung M, editors. Cancer gene therapy by viral and non-viral Vectors. Wiley & Sons, Inc.; 2014:131-49.

35. Office of NIH History. The Nuremberg code: trials of war criminals before the Nuremberg Military Tribunals under Control Council Law [Internet]. 1949 [cited 2019 Oct]. Available from: https://history.nih.gov/research/downloads/nuremberg.pdf

36. The World Medical Association. Declaration of Helsinki [Internet]. Updated 2013 version. [Updated 2018 Jul; cited 2019 Oct]. Available from: https://www.wma.net/policies-post/wma-declaration-of-helsinki-ethical-principles-for-medical-research-involving-human-subjects/

37. The Belmont Report: ethical principles and guidelines for the protection of human subjects of research [Internet]. 1979 Apr 18 [cited 2019 Oct]. Available from: https://www.hhs.gov/ohrp/regulations-and-policy/belmont-report/read-the-belmont-report/index.html

38. United States Federal Government Code of Federal Regulations. 45CFR46. Updated 2018 Jul.

39. United States Federal Government Code of Federal Regulations. 21CFR50. Updated 2018 Apr.

40. United States Federal Government Code of Federal Regulations. 21CFR56. Updated 2018 Apr.

41. United States Federal Government Code of Federal Regulations. 21CFR312.23. Updated 2018 Apr.

42. CDER; Food and Drug Administration. MAPP 6030.1: IND process and review procedures [Internet]. [Updated 2018 Feb; cited 2019 Oct]; [9 p.]. Available from: https://www.fda.gov/media/72751/download

43. CDER/CBER; Food and Drug Administration. Guidance for industry: investigational New Drug Applications (INDs)—determining whether human research studies can be conducted without an IND [Internet]. 2013 Sep [cited 2019 Oct]. Available from: http://www.fda.gov/downloads/drugs/guidancecomplianceregulatoryinformation/guidances/ucm229175.pdf

44. CDER/CBER/CDRH; Food and Drug Administration. Guidance for industry and Food and Drug Administration staff: in vitro companion diagnostic devices [Internet]. 2014 Aug [cited 2019 Oct]. Available from: http://www.fda.gov/downloads/medicaldevices/deviceregulationandguidance/guidancedocuments/ucm262327.pdf

45. CBER/CDRH; Food and Drug Administration. Policy for device software functions and mobile medical applications [Internet]. 2019 Sep [cited 2019 Oct]. Available from: http://www.fda.gov/downloads/medicaldevices/deviceregulationandguidance/guidancedocuments/ucm263366.pdf

46. United States Federal Government Code of Federal Regulations. 21CFR812. Updated 2018 Apr.

47. International Conference on Harmonization (ICH). Guidance for Industry: E10 Choice of Control Group and Related Issues in Clinical Trials [Internet]. 2001 Jan [cited 2019 Oct]; [29 p.]. Available from: https://www.ema.europa.eu/en/documents/scientific-guideline/ich-e-10-choice-control-group-clinical-trials-step-5_en.pdf

48. United States Federal Government Code of Federal Regulations. 21CFR314.3. Updated 2018 Apr.

49. United States Federal Government Code of Federal Regulations 21CFR312.30. Updated 2018 Apr.

50. United States Federal Government Code of Federal Regulations. 21CFR312.31. Updated 2018 Apr.

51. United States Federal Government Code of Federal Regulations. 21CFR312.32. Updated 2018 Apr.

52. CDER/CBER; Food and Drug Administration. Guidance for industry and investigators: safety reporting requirements for INDs and BA/BE studies [Internet]. 2012 Dec [cited 2019 Oct]. Available from: http://www.fda.gov/downloads/Drugs/GuidanceComplianceRegulatoryInformation/Guidances/UCM227351.pdf

53. United States Federal Government Code of Federal Regulations. 21CFR312.33. Updated 2018 Apr.

54. Yager JA, Kallgren DL. Roles of regulatory project managers in the U.S. Food and Drug Administration's Center for Drug Evaluation and Research. Drug Inf J. 2000;34:289-93.

55. United States Federal Government Code of Federal Regulations. 21CFR312.40. Updated 2018 Apr.

56. United States Federal Government Code of Federal Regulations. 21CFR312.42. Updated 2018 Apr.

57. Food and Drug Administration. The FDA's drug review process: ensuring drugs are safe and effective [Internet]. [Updated 2014 Nov; cited 2019 Oct]. Available from: http://www.fda.gov/Drugs/ResourcesForYou/Consumers/ucm143534.htm

58. CDER/CBER/CDRH; Food and Drug Administration. Clinical pharmacogenomics: premarket evaluation in early-phase clinical studies and recommendations for labeling [Internet]. 2013 Jan [cited 2016 Sep]. Available from: http://www.fda.gov/downloads/Drugs/GuidanceComplianceRegulatoryInformation/Guidances/UCM337169.pdf

59. Anderson DC, Gomez-Mancilla B, Spear BB, Barnes DM, Cheeseman K, Shaw PM, Friedman J, McCarthy A, Brazell, Ray SC, McHale D, Sandbrink R, Watson ML, Salerno RA, Cohen N, Lister CD on behalf of the Pharmacogenetics Working Group. Elements of informed consent for pharmacogenetic research; perspective of the pharmacogenetics working group. Nature Pharmacogenom J. 2002;2:284-92.

60. United States Federal Government Code of Federal Regulations. 21CFR314.50 Updated 2018 Apr.

61. Food and Drug Administration. Drug development and review definitions [Internet]. 2015 Aug [cited 2019 Oct]. Available from: http://www.fda.gov/Drugs/DevelopmentApprovalProcess/HowDrugsareDevelopedandApproved/ApprovalApplications/InvestigationalNewDrugINDApplication/ucm176522.htm

62. Food and Drug Administration. 21CFR14: Public Hearing before a public advisory committee. Updated 2018 Apr.

63. United States Federal Government Code of Federal Regulations. 21CFR314.100. Updated 2018 Apr.

64. United States Federal Government Code of Federal Regulations. 21CFR314.105. Updated 2018 Apr.

65. United States Federal Government Code of Federal Regulations. 21CFR314.110. Updated 2018 Apr.

66. United States Federal Government Code of Federal Regulations. 21CFR312.300. Updated 2018 Apr.

67. CDER/CBER; Food and Drug Administration. Expanded access to investigational drugs for treatment use—questions and answers. 2017 Oct [cited 2019 Oct]. Available from: http://www.fda.gov/downloads/drugs/guidancecomplianceregulatoryinformation/guidances/ucm351261.pdf

68. United States Federal Government Code of Federal Regulations. 21CFR312.305. Updated 2018 Apr.

69. United States Federal Government Code of Federal Regulations. 21CFR312.310. Updated 2018 Apr.

70. United States Federal Government Code of Federal Regulations. 21CFR56.105. Updated 2018 Apr.

71. United States Federal Government Code of Federal Regulations. 21CFR312.315. Updated 2018 Apr.

72. United States Federal Government Code of Federal Regulations. 21CFR312.320. Updated 2018 Apr.

73. Food and Drug Administration. Right to Try [Internet]. 2019 May [cited 2019 Oct]. Available from: https://www.fda.gov/patients/learn-about-expanded-access-and-other-treatment-options/right-try

74. United States Congress. Right to try act, public law 115-176 [Internet]. 2018 Jan [cited 2019 Oct]. Available from: https://www.congress.gov/115/bills/s204/BILLS-115s204enr.pdf

75. CDER/CBER; Food and Drug Administration. Charging for investigational drugs under an IND—questions and answers [Internet]. 2019 Apr [cited 2019 Oct]. Available from: https://www.fda.gov/regulatory-information/search-fda-guidance-documents/charging-investigational-drugs-under-ind-questions-and-answers

76. United States Federal Government Code of Federal Regulations. 21CFR312.7. Updated 2018 Apr.

77. United States Federal Government Code of Federal Regulations. 21CFR312.8. Updated 2018 Apr.

78. Food and Drug Administration. Guidance for industry: expedited programs for serious conditions [Internet]. 2019 Feb [cited 2019 Oct]. Available from: https://www.fda.gov/media/120267/download

79. Food and Drug Administration. Phase IV commitment category [Internet]. 2014 Dec [cited 2019 Oct]. Available from: http://www.fda.gov/drugs/developmentapprovalprocess/formssubmissionrequirements/electronicsubmissions/datastandardsmanualmonographs/ucm071716.htm

80. United States Federal Government Code of Federal Regulations. 21CFR314.520. Updated 2018 Apr.

81. Food and Drug Administration. Guidance for industry: REMS: FDA's application of statutory factors in determining when a REMS is necessary [Internet]. 2019 Apr [cited 2019 Oct]. Available from: https://www.fda.gov/media/100307/download

82. Food and Drug Administration. Draft guidance for industry: format and content of a REMS document [Internet]. 2018 Feb [cited 2019 Oct]. Available from: https://www.fda.gov/media/77846/download

83. Food and Drug Administration. Approved risk evaluation and mitigation strategies (REMS); Zulresso (brexanolone) [Internet]. 2019 Dec [cited 2020 Jan]. Available from: https://www.accessdata.fda.gov/scripts/cder/rems/index.cfm?event=IndvRemsDetails.page

84. Food and Drug Administration. About orphan products natural history grants [Internet]. 2018 Oct [cited 2020 Jan]. Available from: https://www.fda.gov/industry/orphan-products-natural-history-grants/about-orphan-products-natural-history-grants

85. Food and Drug Administration. Developing products for rare diseases & conditions [Internet]. 2018 Dec [cited 2019 Oct]. Available from: https://www.fda.gov/industry/developing-products-rare-diseases-conditions

86. Food and Drug Administration. FAQ concerning the orphan products clinical trials grants program [Internet]. 2017 Dec [cited 2019 Oct]. Available from:

https://www.fda.gov/industry/orphan-products-clinical-trials-grants-program/faq-concerning-orphan-products-clinical-trials-grants-program

87. United States Federal Government Code of Federal Regulations. 21CFR316. Updated 2018 Apr.

88. Food and Drug Administration. Draft guidance for industry: rare diseases: common issues in drug development [Internet]. 2019 Feb [cited 2019 Oct]. Available from: https://www.fda.gov/media/120091/download

89. Office of Human Research Protections. Revised common rule educational materials. 2018 Jun [cited 2019 Oct]. Available from: https://www.hhs.gov/ohrp/education-and-outreach/revised-common-rule

90. United States Federal Government Code of Federal Regulations. 21CFR50.24. Updated 2018 Apr.

91. United States Federal Government Code of Federal Regulations. 45CFR46.109 Updated 2018 Jul.

92. United States Federal Government Code of Federal Regulations. 21CFR56.109. Updated 2018 Apr.

93. United States Federal Government Code of Federal Regulations. 21CFR56.115. Updated 2018 Apr.

94. United States Federal Government Code of Federal Regulations. 45CFR46.115. Updated 2018 Jul.

95. Laurence DJ. The therapeutic misconception: not just for patients [Internet]. J Can Chiropr Assoc. 2008 Aug [cited 2016 Sep]. Available from: http://www.ncbi.nlm.nih.gov/pmc/articles/PMC2528258/

96. Hochhauser M. "Therapeutic misconception" and "recruiting doublespeak" in the informed consent process. IRB Ethics Human Res. 2002 Jan-Feb; 240-1.

97. Office of Research Integrity. Research misconduct [Internet]. [Cited 2016 Sep]. Available from: http://ori.hhs.gov/research-misconduct-0

98. Department of Health and Human Services. Financial conflict of interest: HHS guidance [Internet]. 2004 May [cited 2016 Sep]. Available from: http://www.hhs.gov/ohrp/regulations-and-policy/guidance/financial-conflict-of-interest/#

99. International Conference for Harmonization (ICH). E6 guideline for good clinical practice: glossary [Internet]. 2016 Dec [cited 2019 Oct]; [4 p.]. Available from: https://ichgcp.net/1-glossary/

100. Collaborative Institutional Training Initiative (CITI) Program [Internet]. [Cited 2019 Oct]. Available from: https://about.citiprogram.org/en/

101. Kay SC, Luke DG, Tamer HR. ASHP guidelines for the management of investigational drug products. Am J Health-Syst Pharm. 2018;75:561-73.

102. Food and Drug Administration. Use of electronic health record data in clinical investigations. 2018 Jul [cited 2019 Oct]. Available from: https://www.fda.gov/regulatory-information/search-fda-guidance-documents/use-electronic-health-record-data-clinical-investigations-guidance-industry

103. ONC. About ONC: What we do [Internet]. 2019 Feb [cited 2019 Oct]. Available from: https://www.healthit.gov/topic/about-onc

104. United States Federal Government Code of Federal Regulations. 45CFR170. 2016 Oct.

105. OHRP guidance: unanticipated problems involving risks & adverse events guidance (2007). [Updated 2016 Mar; cited 2020 Jun]. Available from: https://www.hhs.gov/ohrp/regulations-and-policy/guidance/reviewing-unanticipated-problems/index.html

106. Medicare coverage~clinical trials: final national coverage decision [Internet]. [Cited 2016 Sep]. Available from: https://www.cms.gov/medicare/coverage/clinicaltrialpolicies/downloads/finalnationalcoverage.pdf

107. United States Federal Government Code of Federal Regulations. 21CFR1300. Updated 2019 Apr.

108. United States Federal Government Code of Federal Regulations. 49CFR172. Updated 2011 Oct.

109. United States Federal Government Code of Federal Regulations. 21CFR312.6. Updated 2019 Apr.

110. Burnham NL, Elcombe SA, Skorlinski CR, Kosanke L, Kovach JS. Computer program for handling investigational oncology drugs. Am J Hosp Pharm. 1989;46:1821-4.

111. Grilley BJ, Trissel LA, Bluml BM. Design and implementation of an electronic investigational drug accountability system. Am J Hosp Pharm. 1991;48:2816.

112. United States Federal Government Code of Federal Regulations. 21CFR312.57. Updated 2019 Apr.

SUGGESTED READINGS

1. FDA. Available from: http://www.fda.gov/

2. FDA clinical trial forms. Available from: https://www.fda.gov/science-research/clinical-trials-and-human-subject-protection/clinical-trial-forms

3. Code of Federal Regulations. Available from: http://www.ecfr.gov

4. FDA Dockets Management Page. Available from: http://www.fda.gov/ohrms/dockets/default.htm

5. ICH. Available from: www.ich.org

6. NIH/OHRP. Available from: http://www.hhs.gov/ohrp/

7. CenterWatch. Available from: http://centerwatch.com/

Chapter Twenty-Four

Regulatory Affairs and Pharmaceutical Industry

Jennifer L. Dill • Daniel A. Kapp

Learning Objectives

After completing this chapter, the reader will be able to:

- Compare and contrast the missions of the Department of Health and Human Services (DHHS), the Food and Drug Administration (FDA), and Center for Drug Evaluation and Research (CDER).
- Describe the methods the FDA uses to communicate important safety information.
- Describe the role of the CDER Division of Drug Information (DDI).
- List the main services provided by the CDER DDI.
- Categorize the different clinical and regulatory resources provided by the FDA.
- Identify the FDA and DDI resources for small business and the pharmaceutical industry.
- Discuss student and professional opportunities within the FDA and the pharmaceutical industry.
- Describe how health care professionals (HCPs) are regulated in the pharmaceutical industry.
- Determine acceptable interactions between pharmaceutical companies and practitioners.
- Explain the importance of collecting adverse event and product complaint information.

Key Concepts

❶ The mission of the FDA is "to protect the public health by ensuring the safety, efficacy, and security of human and veterinary drugs, biological products, and medical devices; and by ensuring the safety of our nation's food supply, cosmetics, and products that emit radiation."

❷ Accurate, clear, and timely communication of important safety information is necessary for health care providers, patients, and the public to make informed decisions on the risks and benefits of a therapy.

❸ The FDA uses an array of methods and tools to communicate drug, biologic, and medical device safety information to the public.

❹ The mission of the CDER Division of Drug Information (DDI) is to provide accurate, timely, and relevant information about human drug products through traditional and social media channels.

❺ Publicly available resources and databases developed by the FDA serve as authoritative references for pharmacists and HCPs across a variety of disciplines.

❻ The FDA offers a broad range of training, professional development, and employment opportunities for both current and future health professionals. Participation in an FDA scientific internship, fellowship, or training program allows one to gain direct practical experience in regulatory and clinical sciences.

❼ Pharmaceutical companies' medical information practices are highly regulated by the FDA.

❽ Unsolicited requests are those initiated by persons or entities completely independent of influence by the relevant pharmaceutical company.

❾ To ensure ongoing safety of medications available to the American public, the FDA has established postmarketing surveillance programs to identify serious adverse events that may not have appeared during drug development or an increased incidence of known adverse events that may require changes in a product's prescribing information and, rarely, reconsideration of the product's approval status.

❿ Pharmaceutical companies' scientific or medical departments are staffed with highly trained HCPs working in a multitude of specialized fields.

Introduction

Behind every medication available to treat patients in the United States is a critical network of individuals, teams, and organizations within the government responsible for protecting the health of citizens, and within the pharmaceutical industry who bring innovative treatments to the market. In public health agencies, such as the DHHS, HCPs support the organization's mission to protect public health and provide essential human services, especially for those who are least able to help themselves. The FDA, an agency of the U.S. Public Health Service (USPHS) under the DHHS, supports the pharmaceutical industry by providing expert regulatory and scientific advice during the drug development process and throughout the life cycle of a marketed drug. For example, the FDA provides oversight of medical information practices within the pharmaceutical industry to ensure that information provided to HCPs and consumers about a marketed product is objective, fair-balanced, and scientifically rigorous in order to promote the safe and effective use of medications for optimal patient care.

The first portion of this chapter will provide an overview of the structure and function of groups within select public health agencies and drug information resources available from the FDA. Later in chapter, the reader will become familiar with medical information practices within the pharmaceutical industry and gain an understanding of expectations that HCPs may have when receiving medical information from a pharmaceutical company about a marketed product. The roles and responsibilities of HCPs employed by these entities will be discussed, and opportunities for students, graduates, and HCPs are highlighted for those interested in pursuing a career within a regulatory agency or the pharmaceutical industry.

Anatomy of the Department of Health and Human Services and the Food and Drug Administration

In the United States, a multidisciplinary group of specialized individuals is designated to provide essential human services to populations through a variety of government-sponsored programs, forming the DHHS. The principle mission of the DHHS is to enhance the health of Americans and to promote scientific advances in medicine, public health, and social services.[1] The work of the DHHS also crosses U.S. borders, where teams engage in international leadership initiatives and provide expertise in global health diplomacy.

To achieve its mission, the DHHS is responsible for a spectrum of programs, initiatives, and activities with wide-ranging effects on public health and welfare. The complexity of these services requires focused efforts by several offices, divisions, and agencies within DHHS. Eight USPHS agencies and three human services agencies form the 11 operating divisions of the DHHS, each responsible for a specific area of focus (Table 24-1).[2] Overall, oversight of the organization and programs is by the Office of the Secretary, with the Secretary of Health and Human Services acting as the general manager and chief policy officer.[3,4] The FDA, one of the eight agencies of the USPHS, serves as the primary regulatory body of drugs and biologic products intended for use in humans.

MISSION OF THE FOOD AND DRUG ADMINISTRATION

❶ *The mission of the FDA is "to protect the public health by ensuring the safety, efficacy, and security of human and veterinary drugs, biological products, and medical devices; and by ensuring the safety of our nation's food supply, cosmetics, and products that emit radiation."*[5]

TABLE 24–1. LIST OF HEALTH AND HUMAN SERVICES AGENCIES AND OFFICES[1,2]

Agency or Office	Purpose (or Mission)
Office of the Secretary (OS)	"To enhance the health and well-being of all Americans, by providing for effective health and human services and by fostering sound, sustained advances in the sciences underlying medicine, public health, and social services."
Administration for Children and Families (ACF)	"…to provide family assistance (welfare), child support, childcare, Head Start, child welfare, and other programs relating to children and families."
Administration on Aging (AoA)	"…to develop a comprehensive, coordinated and cost-effective system of home and community-based services that helps elderly individuals maintain their health and independence in their homes and communities."
Agency for Healthcare Research and Quality (AHRQ)	"…to improve the quality, safety, efficiency, and effectiveness of health care for all Americans. Information from AHRQ's research helps people make more informed decisions and improve the quality of health care services."
Agency for Toxic Substances and Disease (ATSDR)	"… serves the public by using the best science, taking responsive public health actions, and providing trusted health information to prevent harmful exposures and diseases related to toxic substances."
Centers for Disease Control and Prevention (CDC)	"…serves as the national focus for developing and applying disease prevention and control, environmental health, and health promotion and health education activities designed to improve the health of the people of the United States."
Centers for Medicare and Medicaid Services (CMS)	"… to ensure effective, up-to-date health care coverage and to promote quality care for beneficiaries."
Food and Drug Administration (FDA)	"…to protect the public health by assuring the safety, efficacy, and security of human and veterinary drugs, biological products, medical devices, our nation's food supply, cosmetics, and products that emit radiation."
Health Resources and Services Administration (HRSA)	"… to improve health and achieve health equity through access to quality services, a skilled health workforce and innovative programs."
Indian Health Service (IHS)	"…to raise the physical, mental, social, and spiritual health of American Indians and Alaska Natives to the highest level."
National Institutes of Health (NIH)	"…to seek fundamental knowledge about the nature and behavior of living systems and the application of that knowledge to enhance health, lengthen life, and reduce the burdens of illness and disability."
Office of Inspector General (OIG)	"…to protect the integrity of Department of Health and Human Services (HHS) programs, as well as the health and welfare of the beneficiaries of those programs."
Substance Abuse and Mental Health Services Administration (SAMHSA)	"…to reduce the impact of substance abuse and mental illness on America's communities."

Additionally, the FDA is responsible for accelerating drug and biologic therapy innovation, and providing information to the public about medication therapy and food products (Table 24-2).[6] Within the FDA, there are six centers and 12 offices (Figure 24-1).[7] The three centers, overseeing biologics, drugs, and medical devices, are the Center for Biologics Evaluation and Research (CBER), Center for Drug Evaluation and Research (CDER), and the Center for Devices and Radiological Health (CDRH) (see Chapter 21).[7]

TABLE 24–2. INNOVATION AT FDA[8–19]

Initiative	Goals	Established	Website	Relevant Legislation	Recent Advancements
Artificial Intelligence and Machine Learning					
	"To develop an approval framework for artificial intelligence and machine learning technologies to allow modifications to be made from real-world learning and adaptation, while still ensuring that the safety and effectiveness of the software as a medical device is maintained."	2019	https://www.fda.gov/medical-devices/software-medical-device-samd/artificial-intelligence-and-machine-learning-software-medical-device	21st Century Cures Act	- Draft framework proposed April 2019 - Artificial intelligence in clinical decision support included in FDA guidance September 2019
Biosimilars Action Plan					
	"To provide more treatment options, increase access to care by patients, and to potentially lower health care costs due to competition."	2009	FDA Biosimilar Hub: https://www.fda.gov/drugs/therapeutic-biologics-applications-bla/biosimilars	Biologics Price Competition and Innovation Act (BPCI Act) of 2009, 351(k) of the Public Health Service Act (PHS Act) (42 U.S.C. 262(k)) Patient Protection and Affordable Care Act (Affordable Care Act)	- 23 approved biosimilar products; No products approved as "interchangeable" as of September 2019 - Final FDA guidance on pathway for "interchangeable" biologics published May 2019 - Patient education website made available by FDA September 2019
Digital Health Innovation Action Plan					
	"To ensure all Americans have timely access to high-quality, safe and effective digital health products."	2017	https://www.fda.gov/medical-devices/digital-health	21st Century Cures Act	- Digital Health Precertification (Pre-Cert) Program pilot launched 2017 - Clinical Decision Support Software guidance and Changes to Existing Medical Software Policies Resulting from Section 3060 of the 21st Century Cures Act guidances published September 2019

continued

TABLE 24-2. INNOVATION AT FDA[8-19] (CONTINUED)

Initiative	Goals	Established	Website	Relevant Legislation	Recent Advancements
FDA Advanced Manufacturing Programs					
	CDER: "To promote the adoption of innovative approaches to pharmaceutical product design and manufacturing." CBER: "To promote dialogue, education, and input among CBER staff and between CBER and prospective innovators/developers of advanced manufacturing technologies that are intended to be implemented in CBER-regulated products."	2017	https://www.fda.gov/emergency-preparedness-and-response/mcm-issues/advanced-manufacturing	21st Century Cures Act	- Two new drug approvals based on advanced continuous manufacturing processes in 2018 - Eight grants awarded to academic programs in 2018 - CBER Advanced Technologies Program established 2019
FDA Complex Innovative Trials Designs Pilot Program					
	"To support the goal of facilitating and advancing the use of complex adaptive, Bayesian, and other novel clinical trial designs."	2018	https://www.fda.gov/drugs/development-resources/complex-innovative-trial-designs-pilot-program	FDA Reauthorization Act of 2017	- Meetings with drug sponsors to occur between 2019 and 2022 - Complex innovative trial designed used in trial to test potential Ebola therapies
Framework for the Regulation of Regenerative Medicine Products					
	"To address how the agency plans to support and expedite the development of regenerative medicine products, including human cells, tissues, and cellular and tissue-based products."	2017	https://www.fda.gov/vaccines-blood-biologics/cellular-gene-therapy-products/framework-regulation-regenerative-medicine-products	21st Century Cures Act	- Expedited Programs for Regenerative Medicine Therapies for Serious Conditions and Evaluation of Devices Used with Regenerative Medicine Advanced Therapies guidances published May 2019

TABLE 24–2. INNOVATION AT FDA[8-19]

Initiative	Goals	Established	Website	Relevant Legislation	Recent Advancements
Modernizing New Drugs Regulatory Program					
	"To better serve patients and better support staff in their work to carry out the center's mission – to protect and promote health by making sure that human drugs are safe and effective for their intended use, that they meet established quality standards, and that they are available to patients."	2017	https://www.fda.gov/ drugs/regulatory-science- research-and-education/ modernizing-fdas-new- drugs-regulatory-program	–	- Increased the number of OND offices from six to eight and increases the number of OND clinical divisions from 19 divisions to 27, plus six nonclinical review divisions in September 2019 - Began implementation of new integrated review for drug marketing applications, new IND review management, and postmarket safety management
Project Facilitate					
	"To assist oncology health care professionals in requesting access to unapproved therapies for patients with cancer."	2019	https://www.fda.gov/ about-fda/oncology- center-excellence/ project-facilitate	21 CFR 312 Subpart I	- Established a call center to act as a single point of contact for physicians seeking assistance with FDA's Expanded Access program
Real World Evidence Program					
	"To evaluate the potential use of RWD to generate RWE of product effectiveness to help support approval of new indications for drugs approved or to satisfy post-approval study requirements."	2016	https://www.fda. gov/science-research/ science-and-research- special-topics/ real-world-evidence	21st Century Cures Act	- RWE Subcommittee of the Medical Policy Program and Review Committee established 2017 - Framework for FDA's RWE program published December 2018 - Goal to complete 30 demonstration trials by 2020

continued

TABLE 24–2. INNOVATION AT FDA[8-19] (*CONTINUED*)

Initiative	Goals	Established	Website	Relevant Legislation	Recent Advancements
Regenerative Medicine Advanced Therapy Designation					
	"To expedite the development and review of regenerative medicines intended to treat, modify, reverse, or cure a serious condition has the potential to address unmet medical needs for such disease or condition."	2016	https://www.fda.gov/vaccines-blood-biologics/cellular-gene-therapy-products	21st Century Cures Act	- FDA published Expedited Programs for Regenerative Medicine Therapies for Serious Conditions guidance February 2019 - Since 2017, 108 requests made from sponsor for RMAT designation and 40 RMAT designations granted
Sentinel Initiative					
	"To achieve a sustainable national resource to monitor the safety of marketed medical products and expand real-world data (RWD) sources use to evaluate medical product performance."	2008	https://www.fda.gov/safety/fdas-sentinel-initiative	FDA Amendments Act (FDAAA) of 2007	- Mini-Sentinel System pilot program transitioned to full Sentinel System February 2016 - FDA collaborating with 23 institutions as of September 2019 - Sentinel expands to three distinct coordinating centers: Sentinel Operations Center, Innovation Center, and Community Building and Outreach Center September 2019

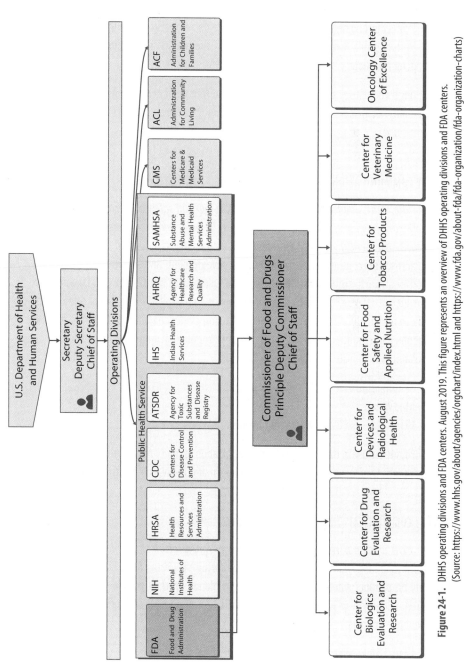

Figure 24-1. DHHS operating divisions and FDA centers. August 2019. This figure represents an overview of DHHS operating divisions and FDA centers. (Source: https://www.hhs.gov/about/agencies/orgchart/index.html and https://www.fda.gov/about-fda/fda-organization/fda-organization-charts)

The mission of CDER, the primary center involved with the review of drugs, is to:

- Promote public health by helping to ensure the availability of safe and effective drugs.
- Protect public health by promoting the safe use of marketed drugs.
- Protect public health by helping to ensure the quality and integrity of marketed drug products.

Though regulatory oversight and structure differ, each center shares the common responsibility for protecting the public by ensuring these products and devices are safe for human use.

SAFETY COMMUNICATION BY THE FOOD AND DRUG ADMINISTRATION

❷ *Accurate, clear, and timely communication of important safety information is necessary for health care providers, patients, and the public to make informed decisions on the risks and benefits of a therapy.*[20] Safety assessment of a medicine or medical device by the FDA occurs across the continuum of the product's development, and includes an increasing focus on **postmarketing surveillance** and the use of real-world data (RWD) and real-world evidence (RWE).[21,22] Since the conditions of a controlled clinical trial often differ from those in daily life, the FDA is tasked with using evidence collected from the diverse populations and conditions a drug is used in after regulatory approval.[23] The FDA initiatives related to drug safety include the following:

- Sentinel Initiative[24]
- MedWatch[25]
- FDA's Adverse Event Reporting System (FAERS)[26]

Through the use of these methods, communication of safety-related information occurs through a variety of means to ensure the right information is available to the right audience.

SAFETY COMMUNICATION METHODS AND TOOLS

❸ *The FDA uses an array of methods and tools to communicate drug, biologic, and medical device safety information to the public.* Monitoring programs used by the FDA focus not only on product safety, but also product problems, product recalls, and postmarket event reporting. These programs use a combination of important communication tools and mediums such as:

- Drug Safety-related Labeling Changes (SrLC)
- **Medication Guides**

- Drug Safety Communications (DSCs)
- **Risk Evaluation and Mitigation Strategies (REMS)**
- MedWatch Safety Alerts
- FDA Drug Safety Podcasts
- Potential Signals of Serious Risks/New Safety Information Identified from FAERS

To ensure simple and timely access to this safety information, the FDA has centralized information related to its numerous safety programs, methods, and communications to an online safety hub (https://www.fda.gov/safety). It is essential for a health care practitioner to be familiar with these methods and tools; use of up-to-date information is needed to adequately discuss and weigh the risks and benefits of a particular therapy with a patient.

LABELING UPDATES

The prescription drug labeling (i.e., prescribing information, medication guide, patient package insert) is the primary official source of information related to safety, efficacy, and use of an approved drug.[27,28] Throughout a product's life cycle, new safety information may emerge, such as long-term adverse side effects, drug interactions, or identification of populations at high risk for adverse events (AEs). For this reason, regulations require the prescribing information to be updated by the manufacturer when new information leads the labeling to become false, inaccurate, or misleading.[29] If necessary, a formal process may be initiated where the FDA is authorized to require and order a manufacturer to make labeling changes based on this new safety information.[30] While not all new safety data will lead to labeling changes in this special process, new information about a serious unexpected or previously known risk will likely lead to formal assessment by the FDA. Whether initiated by the FDA or the manufacturer, this new safety information is added by the manufacturer to the drug's labeling. The FDA's SrLC database provides all FDA reviewed and approved safety-related labeling changes.[31]

Risk Evaluation and Mitigation Strategies

The creation of REMS is one of several methods to communicate drug safety information and reinforce safe medication use behaviors.[32] REMS is a plan to mitigate specific and serious risks associated with a particular drug or drug class. Not all drugs will require REMS.[33] The authority of FDA to require REMS, if needed, was established by the Food and Drug Administration Amendments Act of 2007 (FDAAA).[34] REMS may be implemented at any time during a product's life cycle. The FDA may require or a manufacturer may voluntarily submit a REMS plan as part of the New Drug Application (NDA) process, or the FDA may require REMS after a drug receives approval. Multiple factors are assessed by the FDA when determining the need for REMS, including the severity of the treated disease, intended population, expected benefits of the drug, duration of drug therapy, and ultimately the degree of the drug's risk compared with the overall benefit of treatment.[35] An abbreviated REMS plan template is provided (Appendix 24-1).

Medication Guides and Patient Package Inserts

• Medications Guides, established as a method of communication by the FDA in 1998, contain important patient information on the safe and effective use of a drug or biologic product associated with serious AEs or special use requirements (e.g., strict adherence to prescribed instructions).[36] Not all drugs or biologics require a Medication Guide; the FDA may require the creation of a Medication Guide for a specific medication if additional information beyond the package insert is needed for the medication to be used safely. If a medication has a Medication Guide, the dispenser is required to provide the Medication Guide directly to the patient or patient's agent each time the product is dispensed; however, the FDA offers guidance on exemptions to this requirement in specific scenarios (e.g., use in inpatients) and issues related to inclusion of Medication Guides in REMS.[36] Similar to Medication Guides, patient package inserts (PPIs) are required to be included as part of the FDA-approved drug labeling for specific drugs or drug classes (e.g., oral contraceptives). The PPI is intended to inform patients of the potential risks and benefits of the product's use.[37,38]

Drug Safety Communications

• Introduced in 2010, the DSC is the FDA's primary and standardized safety communication tool for important postmarketing drug safety issues, though additional online resources are available on FDA's online safety hub.[39,40] Previously, safety communications were issued by the FDA in a variety of formats, under different titles, and directed to different audiences (e.g., Early Communications about Ongoing Safety Reviews, Public Health Advisory, Patient Information Sheet, Healthcare Professional Sheet). DSCs are intended for HCPs, patients, and the public. Generally, DSCs communicate the following information and format:

- A summary of the safety issue and the nature of the risk being communicated
- The established benefit or benefits of the drug being discussed
- Recommended actions for HCPs and patients, when appropriate
- A summary of the data reviewed or being reviewed by the FDA

It is important to note that while a DSC communicates important safety issues about marketed drugs, it is not intended to be a crisis communication method. If a drug product is defective, tainted, or poses some other form of immediate danger, the FDA uses other communication tools (e.g., Public Health Alerts, press releases, stakeholder calls) to inform the public rapidly.

ADVISORY COMMITTEES

FDA advisory committees play an important role in regulatory activities.[41,42] An advisory committee provides independent advice from outside experts and public stakeholders including consumer, sponsor, and patient representatives.[43] Advisory committees may be involved in the approval of a drug product, premarket approval of medical devices, trial design specifications, or policy-related issues. While these committees provide valuable input to the FDA on the above issues, final decisions are made by the FDA.

Division of Drug Information

❹ *The mission of the CDER Division of Drug Information (DDI) is to provide accurate, timely, and relevant information about human drug products through traditional and social media channels.*[44] The information provided by the CDER DDI, whether as a general communication or in response to a specific inquiry, is developed for a broad range of audiences including HCPs, industry, small business, government agencies, and the general public. The division is staffed by pharmacists and HCPs with clinical and regulatory expertise to perform a variety of critical and innovative services:

- Engage and interact with the public on all aspects of CDER's activities.
- Communicate drug information through the Drug Safety, CDER SBIA Chronicles, and Drug Information Soundcast in Clinical Oncology (DISCO) podcasts.
- Support CDER activities by collaborating with internal staff.
- Provide education through the FDA Drug Info Rounds media series.
- Manage the Drug Safety-Related Labeling Changes (SrLC) database.
- Collaborate with the Global Alliance of Drug Information Specialists (GADIS) online community.
- Train the next generation of drug information and regulatory specialists through the FDA Pharmacy Student Experiential Program and Regulatory Pharmaceutical Fellowship.
- Provide leadership to the CDER Small Business and Industry Assistance (SBIA) program.

At its core, DDI is comprised of highly trained individuals in drug information, communication, and management. These specialists utilize a variety of external and internal resources to provide DDI services, including publicly available FDA databases and information from subject matter experts within CDER.

SCOPE OF THE DIVISION OF DRUG INFORMATION SERVICES

While the content of each service provided by the DDI varies greatly, the purpose of each service can generally be categorized as the provision of information to:

(1) An individual (e.g., correspondence related to a specific inquiry)
(2) A group or population (e.g., general dissemination of knowledge)
(3) Peers and trainees (e.g., professional development)

On average, the DDI responds to 1300 emails, 4000 telephone calls, and over 60 letters each month. The most common inquiries are related to regulatory issues, such as the drug review and approval process. Often, the same question will be asked from different perspectives (e.g., patient and HCP). In these instances, the drug information specialist must accurately translate complex medical information into meaningful information within a specific context, an essential skill relied upon by both CDER and the public.

FDA DRUG INFORMATION RESOURCES

❺ *Publicly available resources and databases developed by the FDA serve as authoritative references for pharmacists and health care professionals across a variety of disciplines.*

Table 24-3 lists pertinent FDA topic sites (i.e., collection of related websites and content) and the intended purpose of each. In order to select the most appropriate resources, practitioners must have a basic understanding of the available content and its context (e.g., clinical information, guidance on regulations). It is important to note that these resources are updated frequently in order to accommodate the dynamic nature of medical information and consumer needs.

In addition to dedicated DSC channels, DDI has several proactive and innovative tools to communicate information about human drug products to the public. Information is frequently disseminated through digital and social media via as-delivered (e.g., email) or on-demand (e.g., continuing education webinars) methods. Table 24-4 highlights the innovative approaches to communicate safe and effective use of human drug products use by DDI.

CDER SMALL BUSINESS AND INDUSTRY ASSISTANCE

One important and unique relationship maintained by DDI is with the pharmaceutical industry through its CDER SBIA program. SBIA assists domestic and international

TABLE 24–3. FDA-SPONSORED DRUG INFORMATION LINKS

Website URL	Website Name and Purpose
https://www.fda.gov/aboutddi	**Division of Drug Information (DDI)** Provides background, mission, and purpose of DDI Also maintains several helpful links for finding information relating to: • Student and fellowship opportunities • Small business and industry assistance • CE programs, webinars, trainings, audio podcasts, videos, Twitter, and listserv • Drug identification
https://www.fda.gov/drugs	CDER DDI's first resource for responding to questions from the public and where most questions pertaining to regulations can be answered Site maintains sections dedicated to the following topics: • Drug approvals and databases • Drug safety and availability • Drug development and approval process • Guidances, compliance, and regulatory information • Drug science and research • Consumer, health professional, and industry resources • Recalls and alerts • Approvals and clearances
http://www.fda.gov/Drugs/DrugSafety/PostmarketDrugSafety InformationforPatientsand Providers/ucm111085.htm	Index to Drug-Specific Information This page provides a list of drugs that have been the subject of postmarketing drug safety communication efforts
https://www.fda.gov/drugs/tools-keep-you-informed	Tools to Keep You Informed This page provides information on apps, email alerts, news feeds, podcasts, webinars, and other resources to keep up-to-date on FDA-related news
https://www.accessdata.fda.gov/scripts/cder/drugsatfda/index.cfm	Drugs@FDA Searchable FDA database containing official information about FDA-approved brand and generic drugs and therapeutic biological products. This database also contains: • Labels for approved drug products • Medication guides • Consumer information for drugs approved after 1998 • Approval history for drug products (including FDA review documents)

continued

TABLE 24–3. FDA-SPONSORED DRUG INFORMATION LINKS (*CONTINUED*)

Website URL	Website Name and Purpose
https://www.fda.gov/cder/ob	Orange Book: Approved Drug Products with Therapeutic Equivalence Evaluations Free electronic access to the Approved Drug Products with Therapeutic Equivalence Evaluations list Can search by active ingredient, proprietary name, patent, applicant holder, or application number
https://www.fda.gov/drugs/drug-approvals-and-databases/national-drug-code-directory	National Drug Code Directory Searchable list of universal product identifiers for human drugs. OLD and NEW NDC Directories available, background page provides overview of differences between the two databases
http://www.fda.gov/Training/ForHealthProfessionals/default.htm	CDERLearn Web page for CDER-sponsored educational tutorials, some of which have CE credit available
https://www.accessdata.fda.gov/scripts/cder/rems/index.cfm	REMS@FDA Database of approved Risk Evaluation and Mitigation Strategies (REMS) Historical information about past REMS also available
https://www.fda.gov/MedWatch	MedWatch Homepage for the FDA's safety information and adverse event reporting program Contains a searchable list of safety labeling changes and updated safety information. Also, it contains links to online and downloadable forms to report serious problems to the FDA
http://www.fda.gov/DrugSafetyPodcasts	Drug Safety Podcasts Podcasts broadcast in conjunction with the release of new Drug Safety Communication. Also available on iTunes under Drug Safety Podcasts
https://www.fda.gov/drugs/information-healthcare-professionals-drugs/fda-drug-info-rounds-video	FDA Drug Info Rounds Series of training videos for practicing clinical and community pharmacists. Also available on YouTube
https://www.fda.gov/drugs/development-approval-process-drugs/cder-small-business-industry-assistance-sbia	CDER's Small Business & Industry Assistance Interacts with regulated industry by assisting regulated domestic and international small pharmaceutical businesses seeking timely and accurate information relating to development and regulation of human drug products. Information about outreach activities including workshops and webinars available
https://www.fda.gov/gadis	Global Alliance of Drug Information Specialists (GADIS): A Partnership among Pharmacists for the Advancement of Public Health GADIS provides a network among drug information pharmacists and the FDA to support collaborative strategies on critical trends and transformations for addressing FDA regulatory actions

pharmaceutical companies seeking timely and accurate information about the development and regulation of drug products.[45] While targeted for industry use, SBIA resources and outreach activities are available to anyone interested in gaining an understanding of FDA drug regulation. Example educational and outreach programs include the Small Business and Industry Education Series, Small Business Chronicles, and Regulatory Education for Industry conferences.

CDER TRADE PRESS

The CDER Trade Press within the Office of Communications is dedicated to the dissemination of accurate and timely information regarding CDER initiatives, policies, and programs to members of the trade press.[46] They foster and maintain relationships with members of the trade press, coordinate interviews with CDER officials, and provide assistance to the FDA's Field Office Public Affairs Specialists. The CDER Trade Press team is also responsible for alerting FDA leadership and staff to relevant coverage of the FDA in the trade media.

SOCIAL MEDIA OUTREACH

The DDI uses social media to provide up-to-date, interactive, and engaging information to the public through a variety of formats.[44] The use of social media allows the DDI and other divisions of the FDA to increase interaction and disseminate real-time information to a broad audience. Social media services are highlighted in Table 24-4.

GLOBAL ALLIANCE OF DRUG INFORMATION SPECIALISTS

The DDI collaborates with fellow drug information specialists across the globe through GADIS to advance public health by promoting partnerships among drug information pharmacists in academia, hospitals, and federal government.[47] GADIS brings together a community of drug information specialists to support collaborative strategies, exchange evidence-based best practices, and provide an opportunity to gain insight and feedback from peers. Insights into the real-world implementation and outcomes of FDA regulation are also discussed among members, making GADIS an important resource for advancing innovation in the regulatory sciences. GADIS offers an array of useful resources for drug information specialists and other HCPs, including free continuing education webinars, safety and shortage alerts, and press announcements.

TABLE 24–4. DRUG INFORMATION SERVICES PROVIDED BY THE DDI

Audience: individuals (i.e., correspondence related to a specific inquiry)	Audience: groups and populations (i.e., general dissemination of knowledge)	Audience: peers and trainees (i.e., professional development)
Phone calls • Drug Information 1-855-543–DRUG • MedWatch Adverse Event Reporting (1-800-FDA-1088) • CDER Small Business & Industry Assistance (1-866-405-5367) **Emails** • Drug Information and MedWatch (DrugInfo@fda.hhs.gov) • CDER Small Business Assistance (CDERSBIA@fda.hhs.gov) • GDUFA (AskGDUFA@fda.hhs.gov) • GADIS (GADIS@fda.hhs.gov) **Mail:** • Division of Drug Information (CDER) or CDER SBIA • Office of Communications • 10001 New Hampshire Avenue Hillandale Building, 4th Floor • Silver Spring, MD 20993	• **DDI Website** • **Listservs** • DDI, CDER Small Business Assistance, GADIS • **Social Media** • Twitter: @FDA_Drug_Info • Facebook: U.S. Food and Drug Administration (@FDA) • LinkedIn: CDER Small Business and Industry Assistance (SBIA), Global Alliance of Drug Information Specialists (GADIS) • **Publications, Posters, Presentations** • **Exhibits** • **CDERLearn** • **CDER Small Business Workshops** • **CDER Trade Press**	• **FDA Pharmacy Student Experiential Program** • **Regulatory Pharmaceutical Fellowship** • **Global Alliance of Drug Information Specialists** • **Student Webinars** • **CDERLearn** • **CDER Small Business Workshops and Webinars** • **CDER Trade Press**

Case Study 24–1

In December 2016, the 21st Century Cures Act (Cures Act) was signed into law to bring new medical innovations to patients more rapidly and efficiently. As a result, many new initiatives and programs have been introduced to modernize FDA's drug, biologic, and medical device review process, improve collaboration across the agency, and incorporate the patient's voice in the decision-making process. Due to the wide-reaching effects of the Cures Act, an increasing number of inquiries from patients, providers, and manufacturers related to these initiatives are being received by CDER's DDI.

Discussion Questions:

• *A pharmacy student on rotation with DDI asks where to find general information about the Cures Act to be prepared for potential questions. What resources are available on FDA's website?*

- *A manufacturer has an inquiry about the new expedited development programs created as a result of the Cures Act. How do you respond?*
- *A patient calls after seeing a press release about the patient-centered drug development initiatives for cancer patients, and would like to know more about the Oncology Center of Excellence (OCE). How would you describe OCE's mission and vision?*
- *A health professional involved with formulary evaluation of new drug products for a hospital calls about the use of "real-world evidence" in FDA's review of new drug applications. Specifically, the caller asks about the difference between real-world evidence (RWE) and real-world data (RWD). How would you explain the difference between RWE and RWD?*

Opportunities within the FDA

❻ *The FDA offers a broad range of training, professional development, and employment opportunities for both current and future health professionals. Participation in an FDA scientific internship, fellowship, or training program allows one to gain direct practical experience in regulatory and clinical sciences.*

FOR THE STUDENT

The FDA Pharmacy Student Experiential Program offers many opportunities for health professional students to gain a broad understanding of the FDA's mission and organizational structure.[48] Students will learn about the multidisciplinary processes involved in the regulation of drugs, biologics, and medical devices and gain an appreciation for the FDA's collaboration with pertinent associations (e.g., American Pharmacists Association, American Society of Health-System Pharmacists). Training sites are numerous and encompass most areas of practice relevant to pharmacists (e.g., CDER, CBER, Office of New Drugs, Office of the Commissioner). Most of the program opportunities are available in Silver Spring, MD, and rotations occur during the last year of pharmacy school.

The USPHS Commissioned Officer Student Training and Extern Program (COSTEP) is also available for students in the health professions.[49] The COSTEP program allows students to train in the environment where active duty Commission Corps officers are assigned. There are two programs in COSTEP: the Junior COSTEP and Senior COSTEP. Students in selected health care fields can apply to the Junior COSTEP program if they have completed at least 1–2 years of their professional program. The Junior COSTEP program is scheduled during official school breaks and typical assignments are 31–120 days. There is no obligation to commit to working for the Commissioned Corps after graduation, as this opportunity is focused on allowing students to experience the program before joining. Students are exposed to the diverse career opportunities available after completion of the COSTEP program. Prior students have entered careers with the Indian Health Service, labs at the National Institutes of Health, Bureau of Prisons, or have joined agencies within the FDA or CDC.[50] The Senior COSTEP program is available to students entering their final year of graduate school or professional training. Trainees in the program are paid while in school in exchange for a commitment to enroll in the USPHS Commissioned Corps after graduation (students are guaranteed a spot in the USPHS Commissioned Corps upon graduation). The service obligation after graduation is equal to twice the time sponsored by the program.

FOR THE GRADUATE

The FDA offers postgraduate fellowships in research, regulatory review, and pharmaceutical regulation.[51] The Regulatory Pharmaceutical Fellowship offers advanced training opportunities over 2 years in one of three tracks: medical and regulatory aspects of drug information, advertising and promotion, or medication safety.[52] The fellow is expected to develop advanced skills relevant to his or her selected track through direct application of skills and multidisciplinary collaboration with members of the FDA, academia, and the pharmaceutical industry. There are several opportunities for health professional students and graduates interested in regulatory affairs beyond what is described here, and interested readers are encouraged to contact programs directly for further information.

FOR THE PROFESSIONAL

HCPs have a variety of opportunities to further the mission of the FDA under civil service or as a member of the U.S. Commissioned Corps. The "Jobs and Training at FDA" website is a central hub for job information: https://www.fda.gov/about-fda/jobs-and-training-fda. Job responsibilities for positions within the FDA mirror those of the larger public and private sectors and are based on the employee's training and skills. For example, responsibilities related to review of an NDA include the following[53,54]:

- Physicians participate in the overall evaluation of safety and efficacy based on the interpretation of submitted trial data.
- Pharmacists participate in the review of clinical pharmacology, toxicology, and submitted trial data.

- Pharmacologists participate in the comprehensive clinical pharmacology review.
- Biologists participate in the evaluation of nonclinical pharmacology, toxicity, and bioanalytical methods.
- Statisticians review and evaluate scientific data, and mathematical and statistical methods used to evaluate the efficacy and safety of the product.

Consumer safety officers are vital to managing and monitoring regulatory teams in certain divisions.[55] They may be referred to as project managers or division liaisons, and are typically held by biologists, chemists, pharmacists, nurses, physicians, engineers, and others. The team of HCPs working at the FDA is diverse and so are the opportunities to fulfill the mission of assuring the quality, safety, and efficacy of drugs available to the public.

The Food and Drug Administration and the Pharmaceutical Industry

As the gatekeeper for drug availability on the U.S. market, the FDA's CDER is instrumental in ensuring that Americans have access to the safest and most advanced pharmaceutical system in the world. Before a drug can be sold in the United States, it must earn the stamp of FDA approval. A pharmaceutical company must conduct extensive research and provide data to support the drug's safety and efficacy for its intended use. A team of CDER scientists, statisticians, and HCPs conducts a comprehensive, independent, and unbiased review of the data to ensure that the known risks of the drug do not outweigh its potential health benefits.[56]

Generally, FDA review involves analysis of currently available treatments for the target condition or illness to establish context compared to drugs that are currently available to treat the disease. Within that context, data from well-designed clinical trials comparing the safety and efficacy of the drug to placebo and/or a comparator drug in the target population is evaluated to determine risk-to-benefit ratio of the drug. As all drugs involve risk, an essential element of review is development of the drug's FDA-required labeling (e.g., prescribing information, package insert) which is to be a fair-balanced representation of the drug's benefits and risks and include strategies to detect, mitigate, and manage risk to patients.[44] If the FDA review concludes that the drug's health benefits outweigh its known risks, the pharmaceutical company may sell the drug on the U.S. market.

Prescribing information becomes the foundation for communication of essential information about a drug and all information provided by the pharmaceutical company must be consistent with this FDA-required labeling. The primary source of drug information, otherwise known as medical information, provided by a pharmaceutical company is from the company's medical communications department. The FDA provides oversight of medical information practices within the pharmaceutical industry to ensure that information provided to HCPs and consumers about a marketed drug is objective, fair-balanced, and scientifically rigorous in order to promote the safe and effective use of medications for optimal patient care. The remainder of this chapter will provide an overview of medical information practices in the pharmaceutical industry.

Medical Communications in the Pharmaceutical Industry

In the pharmaceutical industry, medical communications refers to departments or individuals who provide product-related medical information to HCPs, consumers, and health care organizations (e.g. health systems, managed care) to support their ability to make decisions that improve patient care. Medical communications may also be referred to as drug information, product information, or medical information and is both a headquarters-based and field-based discipline.[57] In contrast to nonindustry-based drug information practices, the provision of medical information by the pharmaceutical industry requires a unique perspective on regulatory issues.

FDA Regulatory Oversight

❼ *Pharmaceutical companies' medical information practices are highly regulated by the FDA.* The FDA regulates the U.S. pharmaceutical industry in all aspects of the manufacture, sale, and distribution of drugs and devices under the authority of the Federal Food, Drug and Cosmetic Act (FD&C Act) and the Public Health Service Act (PHSA), which along with subsequent amendments and implementing regulations are codified into the Code of Federal Regulations (CFR) Title 21. This includes oversight of labeling, advertising, and other types of medical communications for prescription drugs and restricted devices.[58,59]

FDA GUIDANCE DOCUMENTS

The FDA publishes hundreds of guidance documents each year on a wide variety of topics which may be general (e.g., Demonstrating Substantial Evidence of Effectiveness for Human Drug and Biological Products) or very specific (e.g., Development and

Licensure of Vaccines to Prevent COVID-19) and can be accessed through a search-able database at https://www.fda.gov/regulatory-information/search-fda-guidance-documents#guidancesearch. Guidance documents represent the FDA's current thinking on a topic and are very useful because they expand upon and provide clarification of the regulations. Guidance documents are published in draft form and are posted for open comment. They often remain in draft form for a long period of time or are never finalized. Even when final, they do not establish legally enforceable rights or responsibilities for any person, the public, or the FDA. Unless specific statutory or regulatory requirements are cited, guidance documents are to be interpreted as recommendations.[59] HCPs working for a U.S. pharmaceutical company must achieve a thorough understanding of relevant regulations and guidance documents to ensure compliance as they carry out their daily duties. To assist in this understanding, several important key concepts and definitions with examples are provided.

LABELED VS. OFF-LABEL INFORMATION

As previously discussed, a drug's FDA-required labeling (e.g., prescribing information, package insert) is reviewed and approved by the FDA to ensure that the stated indications and conditions for use are supported by the required level of evidence, and the benefits outweigh the risks of using the drug in the manner described. Any information that is contained in the prescribing information is considered "labeled" and by default, any other information is referred to as "off-label." The prescribing information must be distributed with the drug itself as well as with communications provided by or on behalf of a pharmaceutical company and it governs how a drug can be marketed and what medical information can be communicated by various personnel within a pharmaceutical company.[59]

As pharmaceutical companies are prohibited from marketing a drug for an unapproved use (see Chapter 25 for additional information), sales representatives are limited to providing only labeled information in their promotional activities and must refer requests for off-label information to medical communications. However, prescribing information is not intended to communicate all that is known about a drug for its approved use. The FDA does not consider information that is consistent with, although not specifically stated in, the prescribing information as a new intended use, but does require that the information be truthful and non-misleading. The FDA's Guidance for Industry: Medical Product Communications That Are Consistent With the FDA-Required Labeling—Questions and Answers describes the FDA's current thinking about how they evaluate whether medical information provided by a pharmaceutical company about a drug's approved use is consistent with the FDA-required labeling.[59]

The FDA acknowledges that off-label use of a drug may be a beneficial treatment option for patients. HCPs may lawfully use or prescribe FDA-approved drugs for uses not included in the drug's labeling, which may lead to the request for off-label information. The FDA has long taken the position that pharmaceutical companies' medical communications departments can provide off-label information as long as it is a truthful, balanced, non-misleading, non-promotional response to a specific **unsolicited request**.[60,61]

UNSOLICITED REQUESTS

❽ *Unsolicited requests are those initiated by persons or entities completely independent of influence by the relevant pharmaceutical company.* FDA's draft Guidance for Industry: Responding to Unsolicited Requests for Off-Label Information About Prescription Drugs and Medical Devices describes the FDA's current thinking about how pharmaceutical companies can respond to unsolicited requests for off-label information related to their FDA-approved drugs. An important portion of this guidance document addresses how a pharmaceutical company should respond to unsolicited requests that are encountered through emerging electronic media.[62] Requestors may include HCPs, managed care organizations, formulary committees, patients, and caregivers. Requests that are prompted in any way by a pharmaceutical company or its representatives are not unsolicited requests.[60–62]

Types of Unsolicited Requests

Nonpublic unsolicited requests: A nonpublic unsolicited request is one that is directed privately from a requestor to a pharmaceutical company where the request would not be visible to the public. For example, a patient calls the medical communications department to request information about off-label use of a drug. Medical communications would respond directly to that individual and the response would not be visible to the public.[50]

Public unsolicited requests: A public unsolicited request is one that is directed from a requestor to a pharmaceutical company or a forum at large where the request would be visible to the public. For example, a patient posts a question about off-label use of a drug on a discussion forum that is visible to the public. Medical communications may post a response to the discussion forum that would be visible to the public.[62]

SOLICITED REQUESTS

The FDA considers any request for off-label information prompted by a pharmaceutical company or its representatives to be a solicited request. For example, a pharmaceutical company announces results of a study via Twitter and suggests that the drug is safe and effective for an off-label use. Any requests received in response would be considered solicited requests. Furthermore, the FDA may consider off-label information provided in response to a solicited request to be promotion of an unapproved use, which would constitute a violation of the FD&C Act.[62]

STANDARD OPERATING PROCEDURES

Pharmaceutical companies develop standard operating procedures (SOPs) to help employees establish a consistent methodological approach to conducting business and to comply with the regulations governing their duties. SOPs are intended to define expected practices and supplement regulations to make them applicable to employees and their everyday job functions. They are mandated by state and federal regulations, including the CFR, and are the legally binding first line of defense in any inspection. Furthermore, strict adherence to SOPs may help minimize legal exposure and protect the inadvertent distribution of proprietary information. Well-written SOPs are clear, concise, up-to-date, and do not conflict with one another.[63-65] A pharmaceutical company's regulatory department is responsible for ensuring that SOPs provide employees proper guidance for complying with all applicable regulations. Example SOPs include the process to respond to unsolicited requests and the development of standard response letters.

Fulfillment of Medical Information Requests

A typical process for responding to medical information requests (MIRs) is described in Figure 24-2.[60] When HCPs and consumers contact a pharmaceutical company with questions regarding a medication, the answer may be readily available from the prescribing information or standard response letters. If an answer is not readily available, the development of a custom response may be required.

RESPONSE LETTERS

Clinical response letters, also known as standard responses, are written correspondence that are internally reviewed and contain content in response to unsolicited requests for medical information. Response letters are created from source documents (e.g., prescribing information, published literature, internal proprietary information) and drafted in anticipation of, or in response to, frequently asked questions. The application

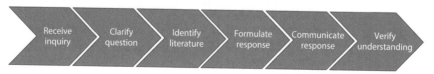

Figure 24–2. Process for responding to medical information requests.

of evidence-based medicine (EBM) in response letters is imperative to ensure the provision of objective, fair-balanced, and scientifically rigorous information. While many EBM processes exist, a practical, time-saving, five-step EBM process that can be applied by medical communications professionals in their day-to-day activities has been proposed.[66] Response letters are usually created according to a company-specific template and style manual to ensure consistency in content and format.

Standard response letters developed by companies may be either proactive or reactive. For example, if the evening news reports that Drug A causes yellow stripes to appear on patients' skin, the company that makes Drug A should react immediately by developing a response letter to address questions from HCPs and patients on this AE (i.e., reactive). In another example, a company launching Drug B, a drug with a similar mechanism of action to Drug A, may wish to proactively develop a response letter in anticipation that the likelihood of experiencing yellow stripes with Drug B will be frequently asked, based on the report of this reaction with Drug A (Appendix 24-2).

CUSTOM RESPONSES FOR NONFREQUENTLY ASKED QUESTIONS

Patient variability, clinician expertise, and previously unaddressed questions may require personalized responses that cannot be fulfilled with a standard response letter. Medical communications professionals use their literature searching and evaluation skills to determine if relevant information has been published or is available through internal company data on file. If no information is identified, the requestor is informed that the company cannot provide any information. If relevant information is identified, a custom response is drafted and peer reviewed to ensure the accuracy of the information and that the response adequately answers the original inquiry. The custom response is then provided to the requestor along with a verbal conversation (if possible) to discuss the findings and applicability to the requestor's situation. Requestors expect their inquiry to be addressed in a timely manner and for the response to be succinct and individualized to their specific request, often preferring a verbal answer and follow-up with written information.[67]

Assessment of MIRs received by a medical communications department is a valuable method for the company to gain insight as to the current state of the drug in clinical practice. The type and frequency of MIRs are typically compiled and analyzed by product to identify patterns and trends, which are published internally in the form of periodic reports. Periodic reports may highlight gaps in the medical information needs of practitioners related to a drug, signal that a standard response letter is needed for a frequently asked question, or lead to the development of a new drug formulation. Periodic reports may also signal that previous "hot topics" are no longer of interest to practitioners which may lead to the archival of outdated standard responses.

Case Study 24-2

DRUG A is a FDA-approved medication for the treatment of moderate to severe hiccups, manufactured by the pharmaceutical company Amazing Drugs LP. Since approval, Amazing Drugs LP has received multiple MIRs from HCPs who are interested in using DRUG A for the off-label use to treat uncontrollable laughter. A competitor, More Amazing Drugs LP, has successfully completed Phase III studies for DRUG B in the treatment of uncontrollable laughter and has filed a New Drug Application (NDA) with the FDA. DRUG B is in the same pharmacologic class as DRUG A. If approved, it is suspected that DRUG B will have a REMS program and restricted distribution program approved by the FDA along with the drug because it is known to occasionally cause yellow stripes to appear on the skin.

Discussion Questions:

- *What should Amazing Drugs LP do to prepare for inquiries regarding product comparisons to DRUG B and other investigational compounds?*
- *What questions should Amazing Drugs LP anticipate receiving due to their similar indication to DRUG B?*

Required Safety Reporting to FDA

Pharmaceutical companies are required to submit reports to the FDA as part of postmarketing safety surveillance. To illustrate, the ADVERSE REACTIONS section of a drug's prescribing information contains a profile of clinically relevant adverse reactions known about the drug to assist health care providers in making treatment decisions, and monitoring and counseling patients. This information is largely derived from premarketing clinical trials which are conducted in a controlled manner and include a limited patient population.[68] Following FDA approval, medications are often used in a more diverse patient population for a wider variety of indications, which may lead to the emergence of unexpected AEs. For example, a Drug Safety Communication was published regarding mental health side effects including suicidal thoughts or actions with use of montelukast based upon submitted case reports. The FDA required the pharmaceutical company to strengthen the warning in the prescribing information with the addition of a boxed warning and advised that it should not be used first-line for the treatment of allergic rhinitis in favor of alternative drugs with a long history of safe and effective use.[69]

❾ *To ensure ongoing safety of medications available to the American public, the FDA has established postmarketing surveillance programs to identify serious AEs that may not have appeared during drug development or an increased incidence of known AEs that may require changes in a product's prescribing information and, rarely, reconsideration of the product's approval status.*[70,71]

ADVERSE EVENT REPORTING

An adverse drug experience (AE) is defined by the FDA as, "Any AE associated with the use of a drug in humans, whether or not considered drug related, including the following: an AE occurring in the course of the use of a drug product in professional practice; an AE occurring from drug overdose whether accidental or intentional; an AE occurring from drug abuse; an AE occurring from drug withdrawal; and any failure of expected pharmacological action."[72]

All pharmaceutical company employees are responsible for ensuring that AEs related to the use of a medication marketed by their company are promptly reported to the FDA. Pharmaceutical company employees may become aware of AEs in a variety of ways, including sales calls, postmarketing trials, publications, news reports, or even overhearing a personal conversation. While pharmaceutical companies should review websites they sponsor for AEs, they are not required to review websites they do not sponsor, although they should report any AEs they become aware of whether it was reported on a sponsored or nonsponsored website. Medical communications professionals are often the first to become aware of AEs during interactions with HCPs or consumers. Depending on company policy, they may be responsible for capturing the AE information and/or referring the reporter to the company's safety department for AE reporting. Pharmaceutical company employees should not assume their responsibilities are fulfilled by suggesting that the reporter submit a safety report directly to the FDA.[73]

Pharmaceutical companies must submit postmarketing safety reports to the FDA for the following types of events: (1) serious and unexpected AEs (domestic and foreign) and (2) spontaneous, unsolicited AEs (domestic only) that are serious and expected, nonserious and unexpected, or nonserious and expected. Unexpected AEs are those not listed in the product's prescribing information. As defined by the FDA, a serious AE must involve at least one of the following criteria: (1) death, (2) life-threatening, (3) initial hospitalization or prolonged hospitalization, (4) persistent or significant incapacity/disability, (5) birth defect/congenital anomaly (including fetal), and/or (6) important medical event that may require surgical or medical intervention to prevent one of the previous criteria. For an AE to be reportable to the FDA, the four basic elements must be known, including: (1) identifiable patient, (2) identifiable reporter, (3) suspect drug or biologic product, and (4) AE or fatal outcome suspected to be due to the suspect drug or biologic product. If one of these elements or the outcome as described above is unknown, the pharmaceutical company should continue to actively pursue this information and document their efforts to do so.[73]

Pharmaceutical companies must submit AEs related to human drug and biologic products electronically using mandatory FDA Form 3500A, with the exception of vaccine products which should be reported on a Vaccine Adverse Event Reporting System (VAERS) form. HCPs and consumers are encouraged to voluntarily report AEs using FDA Form 3500 and FDA Form 3500B, respectively, which can be accessed for download or online reporting from the MedWatch page on the FDA website.[74] Further information on voluntary reporting of AEs can be found in Chapter 19.

Case Study 24–3

Use information from Case Study 24-2.

The company that manufactures DRUG A begins receiving reports of patients noting yellow stripes on their skin.

Discussion Questions:

- *How must Amazing Drugs LP document patient reports of yellow stripes?*
- *Does Amazing Drugs LP need to send the reports of yellow stripes to any additional agency or organization?*

PRODUCT COMPLAINT REPORTING

A product complaint (PC), or product quality problem, is a problem concerning the quality, performance, or safety of a product. Some examples include: suspected counterfeit product, therapeutic failure, or confusing labeling or packaging. As part of an early warning system to identify quality defects in distributed products and protect the American public, pharmaceutical companies are required to submit a Field Alert Report (FAR) via Form FDA 3331a within 3 business days of becoming aware of certain types of product quality problems related to a medication marketed by their company. These include the following event types: (1) an incident causing the product to be mistaken for or its labeling to be applied to another product, (2) microbiological contamination, (3) any significant physical, chemical, or other deterioration or change in the distributed product, or (4) one or more distributed lots of the product fail to meet specifications established in its application. PCs can also be voluntarily submitted by HCPs and consumers via FDA MedWatch as described for AE reporting. While PCs may be reported to the FDA and/or to the pharmaceutical company, reporting these events to the pharmaceutical company directly may allow the HCP to take advantage of a refund or replacement product. PC reports may prompt a product recall or modification in product design to improve patient safety.[74,75]

Code on Interactions with Healthcare Professionals

Interactions between pharmaceutical companies and HCPs are defined, but not regulated, by the Code on Interactions with Healthcare Professionals established by the Pharmaceutical Research and Manufacturers of America (PhRMA). The code sets forth best practices for HCPs in the pharmaceutical industry to ensure that their interactions with HCPs are highly ethical, meet legal requirements, and are intended solely to promote treatment that is in the best interest of the patient as determined by the HCPs clinical judgment. Promotional materials provided by pharmaceutical representatives should be accurate, appropriately substantiated by scientific evidence, provide a fair-balanced perspective of risk versus benefit, and meet all FDA requirements governing such interactions.[76]

Opportunities for Health Professionals within Industry

There are several opportunities for both current and future HCPs within the pharmaceutical industry. The sections that follow address some of these opportunities.

FOR THE STUDENT

There are many opportunities for HCP students in training to gain exposure to the roles and responsibilities within the pharmaceutical industry. Many pharmaceutical companies offer internships in various departments, which allow students to learn the skills required for these positions, network with industry professional, and understand the work environment. Additionally, many companies host students in different health professions during advanced rotational experiences. Some companies allow their HCPs to visit school campuses to share and promote their upcoming internship opportunities.

FOR THE GRADUATE

• Many postgraduate opportunities are available upon completion of school and training. This includes postdoctoral fellowships which are structured for graduates to gain in-depth knowledge of the industry, advances professional development, and allows HCPs to utilize their clinical knowledge to help patients and providers better manage their health. Pharmaceutical industry fellowships vary in curriculum, structure, and objectives. Fellowships can be focused in one specific department or multiple departments in a rotational fashion (e.g., medical information, regulatory affairs, medical education). Many programs offer rotational opportunities within regulatory agencies or partner with an agency for a more regulatory focused experience. Additionally, some programs include academic opportunities, such as serving as a preceptor to students, working within a clinical environment and providing direct patient care, researching and publishing articles or conference posters, or teaching in a didactic nature and obtaining a teaching certificate. Upon completion of the fellowship, individuals have a wide breadth and depth of experience that allows them to successfully contribute to the pharmaceutical industry.

FOR THE PROFESSIONAL

• ⑩ *Pharmaceutical companies' scientific or medical departments are staffed with highly trained health care professionals working in a multitude of specialized fields* (Figure 24-3).[57] The various roles in the pharmaceutical industry allow HCPs to incorporate their expertise and experience to complex medical conditions and corporate environments. HCPs have the ability to interpret scientific literature and guidelines, understand the nuances of complex health care systems and formulary plans, and provide advice regarding patient

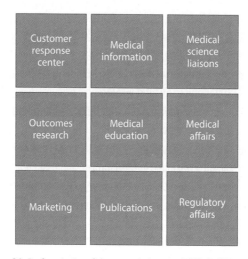

Figure 24–3. Organization of pharmaceutical companies' Medical Department.

therapy management, all of which influence strategic decisions made about a drug product. HCPs are able to utilize their clinical skills to collaborate with other professionals in an effort to develop new medications to bring to patients. Job titles and descriptions may vary slightly from company to company, but the importance of HCPs within each area is constant. The following section will highlight specific opportunities within the pharmaceutical industry for HCPs.

Customer Response Center

Customer response center representatives are the first-line response team for unsolicited requests for medical information from patients and providers. HCPs serving in this capacity often have direct patient care experience from previous roles (e.g., nurses, pharmacists, nurse practitioners, physician assistants) and must be efficient in searching for information and have excellent verbal communication skills. While many companies hire HCPs in this role, some companies rely on non-HCPs to address nonclinical questions (e.g., product availability) or to triage MIRs to an appropriate HCP to address.

HCPs in customer response centers are faced with a variety of responsibilities which include triaging nonmedical and MIRs and capturing reported AEs or PCs. They are provided with a variety of tools to assist in answering unsolicited requests for medical information, such as product labeling (or package inserts), standard response letters, question & answer (Q&A) documents, and clinical topic overviews which are typically drafted by peers in the medical information department. Some MIRs may require additional research or analysis resulting in the customer response center HCPs escalating the request to a medical information specialist for further investigation.

Medical Information

Medical information specialists respond to inquiries, provide training, and draft materials for a variety of internal and external audiences. Medical information specialists have a variety of education and training, including health professionals (e.g., pharmacists, nurses) and other scientific degrees (PhD). The skills required for this position include knowledge of disease states and medications, literature evaluation, medical writing ability, and communication of scientific information, which makes them invaluable resources for analyzing and synthesizing information.

Medical information specialists support the customer response center by creating and maintaining the standard response letter database and responding to escalated MIRs as they often have access to additional resources (e.g., comprehensive reports from clinical trials, posters and abstracts, marketing materials, and contacts in other departments). In addition, medical information specialists provide support to external customers through the development of Academy of Managed Care Pharmacy (AMCP)-formatted dossiers[77] for formulary consideration by health systems and managed care organizations

TABLE 24–5. MEDICAL INFORMATION ACTIVITIES TO SUPPORT INTERNAL BUSINESS PARTNERS

Promotional review
Scientific meeting support
Publication planning
Training for sales representatives and medical science liaisons
Adverse event and product complaint reporting
Product labeling support
Medical education
Website support

TABLE 24–6. RESPONSIBILITIES OF MEDICAL SCIENCE LIAISONS

Building and maintaining relationships with key opinion leaders
Recruiting investigators for clinical trial research
Supporting advisory boards
Providing peer-to-peer exchange of information
Presenting at meetings with formulary decision makers
Training for speakers' bureau, medical residents, sales representatives, etc.
Performing and overseeing clinical trial and health outcomes research
Providing continuing education and branded product presentations

and they may provide information and review product monographs for compendia publishers (e.g., Lexicomp®, IBM® Micromedex® Micromedex, Clinical Pharmacology). While the primary role of medical information specialists is to provide fair-and-balanced medical information to HCPs and consumers, they are increasingly looked upon to lend their therapeutic knowledge, mastery of the literature, and role as product experts to support other departments within the company through a variety of activities (Table 24-5).[78–80]

Medical Science Liaisons

The position of **medical science liaison** (MSL) originated as a highly specialized pharmaceutical sales representative.[81] MSLs support, and are supported by, the medical information team. They aim to contribute to improved patient outcomes through timely provision of medical information, facilitating professional education, and collaborating with **key opinion leaders** to identify mutual clinical and scientific interests including unmet needs within therapeutic areas for future research.[82] Their responsibilities differ from company to company and may involve a wide variety of activities (Table 24-6).[81–82] They may focus on one product or therapeutic area, so there may be overlapping MSLs working for the same company in one location, supporting different products and specialty areas, or vice versa, there may be one MSL in a remote location responsible for multiple products and therapeutic areas.

Managed Markets

Managed market specialists are known in some companies as field-based outcomes liaisons or FBOLs.[83] This position is similar to that of an MSL, except the focus of FBOLs may be to demonstrate the value of a product to managed care organizations (e.g., accountable care organizations), pharmacy benefit managers (PBMs), or other HCPs in similar decision-making roles through the generation of outcomes data. Outcomes data typically provides studies focused on identifying, measuring, and evaluating the end result of a health care service or treatment. For example, a company that is marketing an antiplatelet medication might request their FBOLs demonstrate to customers the value of the product through quality-life years gained or may request the FBOLs create a risk stratification tool to assist clinicians in determining appropriate therapy options for their patients.

Outcomes Research

Health economics and outcomes research (HEOR) compares a product's effectiveness to other interventions, evaluates the efficacy of a product or service, and assesses the cost efficiency compared to incremental benefit. These studies may be retrospective or prospective and utilize electronic medical records (EMR), data collected from physicians, and patient-reported outcomes to provide real-world evidence. Studies can assess drug utilization, medication adherence and compliance, quality of life, patient-reported outcomes, burden of illness, and health care utilization and costs. The HEOR department can work with key experts in a certain field, including academicians, to generate new evidence. For example, clinical studies published in the literature may have insufficient data or inconsistent conclusions regarding cost and resource utilization (e.g., physician office visits, pharmacy claims, hospitalizations) for a specific disease state. To address this lack of information, individuals in HEOR design a study using a national claims database, which contains data from thousands of individuals with the same private insurance. These researchers conduct a retrospective analysis that provides information on the burden of the specific disease state on the health care industry and areas that may require improvement. Data generated from the HEOR department supports the conversations driven by liaisons in the managed markets field-based positions.

Medical Education

HCPs in medical education evaluate funding requests for continuing medical education (CME), continuing education (CE), and other programs submitted by qualified organizations. Grants are reviewed by medical education to ensure the program outlined in the grant addresses specific needs of clinicians in clinical practice and is consistent with the company's educational goals and objectives for a specific therapeutic area.[57] Additionally, the pharmaceutical industry collaborates with CE companies to provide education to various HCPs. These programs may include various topics, such as disease state overviews, changes to clinical practice, and medication therapy management. CE programs must meet standards set by the corresponding accrediting body for the audience (e.g., Accreditation Council for Continuing Medical Education [ACCME])[84] and should follow guidance documents published by regulatory bodies.[85]

Medical Affairs

Medical affairs HCPs have strategic oversight of marketed products, and typically manage Phase IV clinical trial programs. They may also be involved with preclinical studies through Phase IV or postmarketing studies. These HCPs are primarily conducting research on marketed pharmaceuticals in areas of high therapeutic demands or information need. Medical affairs HCPs play a key role in shaping the direction of future clinical development including where to focus resources on specific disease states, what drug candidates to support in human clinical studies, and what marketed drugs to develop with new indications or to study through the investigator-initiated study process. In addition, medical affairs staff is involved in a variety of tasks with peers in medical information, marketing, and with key opinion leaders in the field. These tasks include reviewing promotional and marketing materials, supporting Phase IV clinical trial sites and maintaining communication with trial investigators, reviewing product labeling, formulary dossiers, training materials for promotional and education purposes, and developing and presenting original research in the form of posters, abstracts, and manuscripts. Medical affairs HCPs are responsible for reviewing these materials for accuracy of medical information and to ensure that the final products (e.g., promotional materials, package inserts) are unbiased, fair-balanced, and not misleading.[57]

Marketing

HCPs in the marketing department of a pharmaceutical company are responsible for developing the branded messages for a product. The tag lines and main selling points seen in journal advertisements, on web pages, and on printed materials are created by the marketing department. It is important for HCPs in marketing to understand the clinical practice environment of their peers, so they can provide useful and valuable tools and materials. Marketing drafts a plethora of promotional materials ranging from journal and television advertisements to functional educational tools such as dose conversion guides. These materials are then reviewed by peers in medical information and medical affairs, and other internal business partners in regulatory and legal departments.[57]

Direct to consumer advertising (DTCA) is a source of information for patients and care-givers, which is allowed in a limited number of countries (e.g., the United States, New Zealand) and is regulated by various government agencies. DTCA can impact multiple factors, including patient education and awareness of treatments and enhanced discussion between physician and patient. However, DTCA may also be associated with medication utilization, health care costs, and misinformation. For additional information on DTCA, please refer to Chapter 25.

Publications

The team of HCPs in the publications department has the important task of ensuring the appropriate information reaches the appropriate audience. The publication process includes planning the dissemination of preclinical studies, clinical trials, and review articles for therapeutic areas of interest and company-sponsored studies through scientific channels. For example, a company coming to market with a new antihypertensive medication would want its publications department to create a plan that would publish trial data (preclinical through posthoc and review data) concurrently with major meetings of prescribers treating hypertension or to coincide with FDA approval of the medication so that prescribers and formulary decision makers have published data to base their decisions upon.

The publications department ensures that reprints of posters, abstracts, and manuscripts are readily available for dissemination to HCPs in the field. HCPs in this department are also responsible for reviewing the final content of publications and drafting comments if necessary, often through a partnered review process with medical affairs and medical information, to make certain accurate information is available for practitioners in clinical practice.[57]

Regulatory Affairs

Many HCPs work within the regulatory affairs role, which combines the clinical expertise of an HCP with regulatory knowledge. The responsibilities of individuals in regulatory affairs are to interact with regulatory governing bodies, including the FDA, develop strategies for submission documents (e.g., new drug applications, investigational new drug applications), and prepare product labeling. Regulatory interactions within the FDA include contacts with various offices, including the Office of New Drugs, and the Office of Drug Evaluation, among others. The regulatory affairs department also understands and interprets the changes in the regulatory environment to the company's standard procedures. Personnel in regulatory affairs work closely with the drug development process to ensure that the company adheres to regulatory requirements and may rely upon guidance documents to gain a more in-depth understanding into the FDA's interpretation of those regulations.

Conclusion

Regulatory agencies and the pharmaceutical industry provide important services to the public and have many professional opportunities for HCPs. Just as pharmaceutical companies have detailed and structured processes for responding to clinician's questions, DDI uses effective internal and external interactions to provide timely, accurate, and useful responses to individual inquiries. Efforts are currently ongoing to make the business of drug development more transparent, with regulatory agencies focusing on ways to improve communication of risk versus benefit and pharmaceutical companies focusing on fair and balanced marketing of medications. An informed HCP is one who is aware of the valuable information available from the FDA and industry, can effectively communicate safety and risk information, and dedicates his or her career to positively impacting public health.

Self-Assessment Questions

1. Which of the following is NOT a service offered by CDER's DDI?
   a. Provide education through the FDA Drug Info Rounds media series.
   b. Act as an independent FDA advisory committee.
   c. Engage and communicate with the public through social media.
   d. Manage the Drug Safety Labeling Changes database.

2. Which of the following is NOT a tool used by the FDA to communicate drug safety information?
   a. Drug safety communication
   b. Medication guide
   c. Standard response letters
   d. Risk Evaluation and Mitigation Strategies
   e. Product labeling

3. A pharmaceutical company's Customer Response Center representative speaks to a patient regarding the proper way to take her medication. What would be the best resource for the representative to use to answer this question?
   a. Package insert
   b. Medication guide
   c. Drug safety communication
   d. a and b
   e. b and c

4. A small business calls DDI with questions regarding the drug approval and regulatory pathways available in the United States. When DDI responds, which of the following resources is best to highlight for this caller?
   a. CDER Trade Press
   b. Global Alliance of Drug Information Specialists (GADIS) online community
   c. CDER Small Business & Industry Assistance program
   d. The COSTEP program

5. A pharmacist contacts DDI and asks if they can assist in identifying the exclusivity for a specific medication. Which website would be the best place to refer the requestor for this information?
   a. CDER homepage
   b. Federal Register
   c. Electronic Orange Book
   d. National Drug Code Directory online
   e. CDER Small Business & Industry Assistance homepage

6. Which of the following is NOT a student opportunity within the FDA?
   a. Junior COSTEP Program
   b. Senior COSTEP Program
   c. FDA Pharmacy Student Experiential Program
   d. FDA/CDER Academic Collaboration Program
   e. Commissioned Corps Officer Student Training and Extern Program

7. Which of the following statements is TRUE regarding FDA guidance documents?
   a. They are intended to replace regulations that are codified in the CFR.
   b. They are legally binding for the pharmaceutical industry but not for the FDA.
   c. They reflect the FDA's current thinking on a topic and are subject to change.
   d. They are published in final form and not subject to public comment.

8. Which of the following is FALSE regarding a product's FDA-required labeling?
   a. It is required to be distributed with any labeling provided by the manufacturer.
   b. It contains information about off-label uses.
   c. It is written by the pharmaceutical company without input from the FDA.
   d. b and c.
   e. All of the above.

9. Which of the following representatives of pharmaceutical companies are authorized to provide information about off-label use of an FDA-approved medication?
   a. Customer Response Center Representative
   b. Sales Representative

    c. Marketing Specialist

    d. Medical Information Specialist

10. Which of the following parties can initiate an unsolicited MIR (select all that apply)?

    a. Patient

    b. Health care provider

    c. Key opinion leader speaking on behalf of a pharmaceutical company

    d. Caregiver

    e. Sales representative

11. Which of the following is the correct sequence in responding to an MIR?

    a. Receive inquiry, clarify question, identify literature, formulate response, communicate response, verify understanding

    b. Clarify question, receive inquiry, identify literature, formulate response, communicate response, verify understanding

    c. Receive inquiry, clarify question, formulate response, identify literature, communicate response, verify understanding

    d. Clarify question, receive inquiry, clarify question, identify literature, formulate response, verify understanding, communicate response

12. Which of the following documents CANNOT be used to create a clinical response letter?

    a. Data on file

    b. Published literature sponsored by the pharmaceutical company

    c. Published literature sponsored by a competitor

    d. Prescribing information

    e. None of the above

13. A pharmaceutical company employee is required to report which of the following to the FDA?

    a. AE that is not considered related to the company's drug

    b. AE that has already been reported by the patient's physician to the FDA

    c. PC not related to an AE

    d. AE already listed in the prescribing information

    e. All of the above

14. Which of the following is FALSE regarding the Code of Interactions with Healthcare Professionals (select all that apply)?

    a. It is a legally binding agreement between the Pharmaceutical Research and Manufacturers of America (PhRMA) and FDA.

b. It sets forth best practices for pharmaceutical company representatives as they interact with HCPs.

c. It is intended to ensure that patients are prescribed medications that provide financial benefit to both the patient's physician and the pharmaceutical company.

d. It indicates that promotional materials provided by pharmaceutical representatives should provide a fair-balanced perspective of risk versus benefit.

15. Responsibilities of Medical Science Liaisons may include:
    a. Building relationships with key opinion leaders
    b. Recruiting investigators for clinical trial research
    c. Supporting advisory boards
    d. Training for sales representatives
    e. All of the above

REFERENCES

1. Assistant Secretary for Planning and Evaluation (ASPE). Introduction: about HHS [Internet]. Washington (DC): U.S. Department of Health & Human Services; c2019 [cited 2019 Aug 13]. Available from: https://www.hhs.gov/about/strategic-plan/introduction/index.html

2. Assistant Secretary for Planning and Evaluation (ASPE). HHS agencies and offices [Internet]. Washington (DC): U.S. Department of Health & Human Services; c2019 [cited 2019 Aug 13]. Available from: https://www.hhs.gov/about/strategic-plan/introduction/index.html

3. Assistant Secretary for Planning and Evaluation (ASPE). HHS family of agencies [Internet]. Washington (DC): U.S. Department of Health & Human Services; c2019 [cited 2019 Aug 13]. Available from: https://www.hhs.gov/about/agencies/index.html

4. Assistant Secretary for Planning and Evaluation (ASPE). HHS leadership [Internet]. Washington (DC): U.S. Department of Health & Human Services; c2019 [cited 2019 Aug 13]. Available from: https://www.hhs.gov/about/leadership/index.html

5. U.S. Food and Drug Administration. What we do [Internet]. Silver Spring (MD): U.S. Department of Health and Human Services; c2018 [cited 2019 Aug 12]. Available from: https://www.fda.gov/about-fda/what-we-do

6. U.S. Food and Drug Administration. Innovation at FDA [Internet]. Silver Spring (MD): U.S. Department of Health and Human Services; c2017 [cited 2019 Sep 16]. Available from: https://www.fda.gov/about-fda/innovation-fda

7. U.S. Food and Drug Administration. FDA overview (text version) [Internet]. Silver Spring (MD): U.S. Department of Health and Human Services; c2019 [cited 2019 Sep 16]. Available from: https://www.fda.gov/about-fda/fda-organization-charts/fda-overview-text-version

8. U.S. Food and Drug Administration. Statement from FDA Commissioner Scott Gottlieb, M.D. on steps toward a new, tailored review framework for artificial intelligence-based

medical devices [Internet]. Silver Spring (MD): U.S. Department of Health and Human Services; c2019 [cited 2019 Aug 21]. Available from: https://www.fda.gov/news-events/press-announcements/statement-fda-commissioner-scott-gottlieb-md-steps-toward-new-tailored-review-framework-artificial

9. U.S Food and Drug Administration. Artificial intelligence and machine learning in software as a medical device [Internet]. 2020 [cited 2020 Sep 4]. Available from: https://www.fda.gov/medical-devices/software-medical-device-samd/artificial-intelligence-and-machine-learning-software-medical-device

10. U.S. Food and Drug Administration. Biosimilars [Internet]. 2020 [cited 2020 Sep 4]. Available from: https://www.fda.gov/drugs/therapeutic-biologics-applications-bla/biosimilars

11. U.S. Food and Drug Administration. Digital Health Action Plan [Internet]. 2020 [cited 2020 Sep 4]. Available from: https://www.fda.gov/medical-devices/digital-health

12. U.S. Food and Drug Administration. Advanced Manufacturing [Internet]. Silver Spring (MD): U.S. Department of Health and Human Services; 2020 [cited 2020 Sep 4]. Available from: https://www.fda.gov/emergency-preparedness-and-response/mcm-issues/advanced-manufacturing

13. U.S. Food and Drug Administration. Complex Innovative Trial Designs Pilot Program. Silver Spring (MD): U.S. Department of Health and Human Services; 2020 [cited 2020 Sep 4]. Available from: https://www.fda.gov/drugs/development-resources/complex-innovative-trial-designs-pilot-program

14. U.S. Food and Drug Administration. Framework for the regulation of regenerative medicine products [Internet]. Silver Spring (MD): U.S. Department of Health and Human Services; 2020 [cited 2020 Sep 4]. Available from: https://www.fda.gov/vaccines-blood-biologics/cellular-gene-therapy-products/framework-regulation-regenerative-medicine-products

15. U.S. Food and Drug Administration. Modernizing FDA's New Drugs Regulatory Program. Silver Spring (MD): U.S. Department of Health and Human Services; 2020 [cited 2020 Sep 4]. Available from: https://www.fda.gov/drugs/regulatory-science-research-and-education/modernizing-fdas-new-drugs-regulatory-program

16. U.S. Food and Drug Administration. Project facilitate. Silver Spring (MD): U.S. Department of Health and Human Services; 2020 [cited 2020 Sep 4]. Available from: https://www.fda.gov/about-fda/oncology-center-excellence/project-facilitate

17. U.S. Food and Drug Administration. Real-world evidence. Silver Spring (MD): U.S. Department of Health and Human Services; 2020 [cited 2020 Sep 4]. Available from: https://www.fda.gov/science-research/science-and-research-special-topics/real-world-evidence

18. U.S. Food and Drug Administration. Cellular & gene therapy products [Internet]. 2020 [cited 2020 Sep 4]. Available from: https://www.fda.gov/vaccines-blood-biologics/cellular-gene-therapy-products

19. U.S. Food and Drug Administration. FDA's sentinel initiative [Internet]. Silver Spring (MD): U.S. Department of Health and Human Services; 2020 [cited 2020 Sep 4]. Available from: https://www.fda.gov/safety/fdas-sentinel-initiative

20. U.S. Food and Drug Administration. FDA guidance: drug safety information—FDA's communication to the public [Internet]. Silver Spring (MD): U.S. Department of Health

and Human Services; c2012 [cited 2019 Aug 13]. Available from: http://www.fda.gov/downloads/Drugs/GuidanceComplianceRegulatoryInformation/Guidances/UCM295217.pdf

21. U.S. Food and Drug Administration. Postmarketing surveillance programs [Internet]. Silver Spring (MD): U.S. Department of Health and Human Services; c2016 [cited 2019 Aug 13]. Available from: https://www.fda.gov/drugs/surveillance/postmarketing-surveillance-programs

22. U.S. Food and Drug Administration. Real-world evidence [Internet]. Silver Spring (MD): U.S. Department of Health and Human Services; c2019 [cited 2019 Aug 12]. Available from: https://www.fda.gov/science-research/science-and-research-special-topics/real-world-evidence

23. U.S. Food and Drug Administration. Regulations and policies and procedures for postmarketing surveillance programs [Internet]. Silver Spring (MD): U.S. Department of Health and Human Services; c2015 [cited 2019 Aug 13]. Available from: https://www.fda.gov/drugs/surveillance/regulations-and-policies-and-procedures-postmarketing-surveillance-programs

24. U.S. Food and Drug Administration. FDA's sentinel initiative [Internet]. Silver Spring (MD): U.S. Department of Health and Human Services; c2019 [cited 2019 Sep 26]. Available from: https://www.fda.gov/safety/fdas-sentinel-initiative

25. U.S. Food and Drug Administration. MedWatch: The FDA Safety Information and Adverse Event Reporting Program [Internet]. Silver Spring (MD): U.S. Department of Health and Human Services; c2019 [cited 2019 Sep 26]. Available from: https://www.fda.gov/safety/medwatch-fda-safety-information-and-adverse-event-reporting-program

26. U.S. Food and Drug Administration. Questions and answers on FDA's Adverse Event Reporting System (FAERS) [Internet]. Silver Spring (MD): U.S. Department of Health and Human Services; c2019 [cited 2019 Sep 26]. Available from: https://www.fda.gov/drugs/surveillance/questions-and-answers-fdas-adverse-event-reporting-system-faers

27. 21 CFR 201.57; 21 CFR 201.56(a)(1) and (2): Specific requirements on content and format of PLR format labeling for human prescription drugs, including biological products. Available from: https://www.ecfr.gov/cgi-bin/text-idx?SID=467396391e8b4b96742e806bf1c0b8e7&mc=true&node=se21.4.201_157&rgn=div8

28. U.S. Food and Drug Administration. PLR requirements for prescribing information [Internet]. Silver Spring (MD): U.S. Department of Health and Human Services; c2019 [cited 2019 Aug 21]. Available from: https://www.fda.gov/drugs/laws-acts-and-rules/plr-requirements-prescribing-information

29. Section 505(o)(4) of the Federal Food, Drug, and Cosmetic Act (FD&C Act) (21 U.S.C. 355(o)(4)) (added by section 901 of the Food and Drug Administration Amendments Act of 2007 [FDAAA]).

30. U.S. Food and Drug Administration. FDA guidance: safety labeling changes—implementation of Section 505(o)(4) of the FD&C Act [Internet]. Silver Spring (MD): U.S. Department of Health and Human Services; c2012 [cited 2019 Aug 21]. Available from: https://www.fda.gov/media/116594/download

31. U.S. Food and Drug Administration. Drug safety-related labeling changes (SrLC) [Internet]. Silver Spring (MD): U.S. Department of Health and Human Services; c2019 [cited 2019 Aug 21]. Available from: https://www.accessdata.fda.gov/scripts/cder/safetylabelingchanges/

32. U.S. Food and Drug Administration. Risk evaluation and mitigation strategies (REMS) [Internet]. Silver Spring (MD): U.S. Department of Health and Human Services; c2019 [cited 2019 Aug 22]. Available from: https://www.fda.gov/drugs/drug-safety-and-availability/risk-evaluation-and-mitigation-strategies-rems

33. U.S. Food and Drug Administration. What's in a REMS? [Internet]. Silver Spring (MD): U.S. Department of Health and Human Services; c2018 [cited 2019 Aug 22]. Available from: https://www.fda.gov/drugs/risk-evaluation-and-mitigation-strategies-rems/whats-rems

34. U.S. Food and Drug Administration. FDA's role in managing medication risks [Internet]. Silver Spring (MD): U.S. Department of Health and Human Services; c2018 [cited 2019 Aug 23]. Available from: https://www.fda.gov/drugs/risk-evaluation-and-mitigation-strategies-rems/fdas-role-managing-medication-risks

35. U.S. Food and Drug Administration. FDA guidance: REMS: FDA's application of statutory factors in determining when a REMS is necessary [Internet]. Silver Spring (MD): U.S. Department of Health and Human Services; c2019 [cited 2019 Aug 21]. Available from: https://www.fda.gov/media/100307/download

36. U.S. Food and Drug Administration. FDA guidance: Medication guides—distribution requirements and inclusion in risk evaluation and mitigation strategies (REMS) [Internet]. Silver Spring (MD): U.S. Department of Health and Human Services; c2019 [cited 2019 Aug 21]. Available from: https://www.fda.gov/media/79776/download

37. Patient package inserts for oral contraceptives, 21 C.F.R. Sec. 310.501 (2012). Available from: https://www.accessdata.fda.gov/scripts/cdrh/cfdocs/cfcfr/cfrsearch.cfm?fr=310.501

38. U.S. Food and Drug Administration. Learn about your medicines [Internet]. Silver Spring (MD): U.S. Department of Health and Human Services; c2018 [cited 2019 Aug 23]. Available from: https://www.fda.gov/patients/learn-about-your-medicines

39. U.S. Food and Drug Administration. FDA guidance: drug safety information—FDA's communication to the public (withdrawn) [Internet]. Silver Spring (MD): U.S. Department of Health and Human Services; c2012 [cited 2019 Aug 17]. Available from: https://www.fda.gov/media/83097/download

40. U.S. Food and Drug Administration. Drug safety and availability [Internet]. Silver Spring (MD): U.S. Department of Health and Human Services; c2018 [cited 2019 Aug 21]. Available from: https://www.fda.gov/drugs/drug-safety-and-availability

41. U.S. Food and Drug Administration. Advisory committee laws, regulations and guidance [Internet]. Silver Spring (MD): U.S. Department of Health and Human Services; c2018 [cited 2019 Aug 22]. Available from: https://www.fda.gov/advisory-committees/about-advisory-committees/advisory-committee-laws-regulations-and-guidance

42. U.S. Food and Drug Administration. FDA-TRACK—advisory committees dashboard [Internet]. Silver Spring (MD): U.S. Department of Health and Human Services; c2018 [cited 2019 Aug 22]. Available from: https://www.fda.gov/about-fda/fda-track-agency-wide-program-performance/fda-track-advisory-committees-dashboard

43. U.S. Food and Drug Administration. Advisory committee membership [Internet]. Silver Spring (MD): U.S. Department of Health and Human Services; c2019 [cited 2019 Aug 22]. Available from: https://www.fda.gov/advisory-committees/about-advisory-committees/advisory-committee-membership

44. U.S. Food and Drug Administration. CDER Division of drug information [Internet]. Silver Spring (MD): U.S. Department of Health and Human Services; c2019 [cited 2019 Aug 24]. Available from: https://www.fda.gov/about-fda/center-drug-evaluation-and-research-cder/cder-division-drug-information

45. U.S. Food and Drug Administration. About CDER small business and industry assistance (SBIA) [Internet]. Silver Spring (MD): U.S. Department of Health and Human Services; c2018 [cited 2019 Aug 21]. Available from: https://www.fda.gov/drugs/cder-small-business-industry-assistance-sbia/about-cder-small-business-and-industry-assistance-sbia

46. U.S. Food and Drug Administration. CDER Trade Press [Internet]. Silver Spring (MD): U.S. Department of Health and Human Services; c2018 [cited 2019 Aug 21]. Available from: https://www.fda.gov/about-fda/center-drug-evaluation-and-research-cder/cder-trade-press

47. U.S. Food and Drug Administration. Global alliance of drug information specialists (GADIS) [Internet]. Silver Spring (MD): U.S. Department of Health and Human Services; c2018 [cited 2019 Aug 19]. Available from: https://www.fda.gov/drugs/information-healthcare-professionals-drugs/global-alliance-drug-information-specialists-gadis

48. U.S. Food and Drug Administration. FDA Pharmacy student experiential program [Internet]. Silver Spring (MD): U.S. Department of Health and Human Services; c2019 [cited 2019 Aug 24]. Available from: https://www.fda.gov/about-fda/scientific-internships-fellowships-trainees-and-non-us-citizens/fda-pharmacy-student-experiential-program

49. Commissioned Corps of the U.S. Public Health Service. Student opportunities and training [Internet]. Washington (DC): U.S. Department of Health and Human Services; c2019 [cited 2019 Aug 28]. Available from: https://www.usphs.gov/student/

50. Commissioned Corps of the U.S. Public Health Service. Internship/externship program [Internet]. Washington (DC): U.S. Department of Health and Human Services; c2019 [cited 2019 Aug 28]. Available from: https://www.usphs.gov/student/jrcostep.aspx

51. U.S. Food and Drug Administration. Scientific internships, fellowships / trainees and non-U.S. citizens [Internet]. Silver Spring (MD): U.S. Department of Health and Human Services; c2019 [cited 2019 Aug 28]. Available from: https://www.fda.gov/about-fda/jobs-and-training-fda/scientific-internships-fellowships-trainees-and-non-us-citizens

52. U.S. Food and Drug Administration. Regulatory pharmaceutical fellowship [Internet]. Silver Spring (MD): U.S. Department of Health and Human Services; c2019 [cited 2019 Aug 28]. Available from: https://www.fda.gov/about-fda/center-drug-evaluation-and-research-cder/regulatory-pharmaceutical-fellowship

53. U.S. Food and Drug Administration. Good review practices [Internet]. Silver Spring (MD): U.S. Department of Health and Human Services; c2019 [cited 2019 Aug 28]. Available from: https://www.fda.gov/drugs/guidance-compliance-regulatory-information/good-review-practices-grps

54. U.S. Food and Drug Administration. Career descriptions [Internet]. Silver Spring (MD): U.S. Department of Health and Human Services; c2019 [cited 2019 Aug 28]. Available from: https://www.fda.gov/about-fda/career-descriptions/pharmacist-positions-fda

55. U.S. Food and Drug Administration. Consumer safety officer positions at FDA [Internet]. Silver Spring (MD): U.S. Department of Health and Human Services; c2019 [cited 2019 Aug 28]. Available from: https://www.fda.gov/about-fda/career-descriptions/consumer-safety-officer-positions-fda

56. U.S. Food and Drug Administration. Development & approval process drugs [Internet]. Silver Spring (MD): U.S. Department of Health and Human Services; c2020 [cited 2020 Aug 31]. Available from: https://www.fda.gov/drugs/development-approval-process-drugs#Developing

57. Cadogan AA, Fung SM. The changing roles of medical communications professionals: evolution of the core curriculum. Drug Inf J. 2009 Nov;43(6):673–84.

58. U.S. Food and Drug Administration. Federal food, drug, and cosmetic act [Internet]. Silver Spring (MD): U.S. Department of Health and Human Services; c2018 [cited 2019 Aug 25]. Available from: https://www.fda.gov/regulatory-information/laws-enforced-fda/federal-food-drug-and-cosmetic-act-fdc-act

59. U.S. Food and Drug Administration. Guidance for industry: medical product communications that are consistent with the FDA-required labeling—questions and answers [Internet]. Silver Spring (MD): U.S. Department of Health and Human Services; c2018 [cited 2019 Aug 25]. Available from: https://www.fda.gov/regulatory-information/search-fda-guidance-documents/medical-product-communications-are-consistent-fda-required-labeling-questions-and-answers

60. Graves DA, Baker RP. The core curriculum for medical communications professionals practicing in the pharmaceutical industry. Drug Inf J. 2000 Oct-Dec;34(4):995–1008.

61. Salter FJ, Kramer PF, Palmer-Shevlin NL. Pharmaceutical industry medical communications departments: regulatory and legal perils and pitfalls. Drug Inf J. 2000 Oct-Dec;34(4):1009–15.

62. U.S. Food and Drug Administration. Guidance for industry: responding to unsolicited requests for off-label information about prescription drugs and medical devices [Internet]. Silver Spring (MD): U.S. Department of Health and Human Services; c2011 [cited 2019 Sep 1]. Available from: https://www.fda.gov/regulatory-information/search-fda-guidance-documents/responding-unsolicited-requests-label-information-about-prescription-drugs-and-medical-devices

63. Gough J, Hamrell M. Standard operating procedures (SOPs): why companies must have them, and why they need them. Drug Inf J. 2009 Jan;43(1):49–54.

64. Gough J Hamrell M. Standard operating procedures (SOPs): how companies can determine which documents they must put in place. Drug Inf J. 2010 Jan;44(1):463–8.

65. Gough J, Hamrell M. Standard operating procedures (SOPs): how to write them to be effective tools. Drug Inf J. 2010 Jul;44(4):463–8.

66. Bryant PJ, Steinberg MJ, Marrone CM. A practical approach to evidence-based medicine for the medical communications professional. Drug Inf J. 2009 Nov;43(6):663–72.

67. Fett R, Bruns K, Lischka-Wittmann S. Results of a qualitative market research study evaluating the quality of medical letters. Drug Inf J. 2009 Nov;43(6):697–703.

68. U.S. Food and Drug Administration. FDA guidance for industry: adverse reactions section of labeling for human prescription drug and biological products—content and format [Internet]. Silver Spring (MD): U.S. Department of Health and Human Services; c2006 [cited 2019 Sep 28]. Available from: https://www.fda.gov/regulatory-information/search-fda-guidance-documents/adverse-reactions-section-labeling-human-prescription-drug-and-biological-products-content-and

69. U.S. Food and Drug Administration. FDA requires Boxed Warning about serious mental health side effects for asthma and allergy drug montelukast (Singulair); advises restricting use for allergic rhinitis [Internet]. Silver Spring (MD): U.S. Department of Health and Human Services; c2020 [cited 2020 Aug 31]. Available from: https://www.fda.gov/drugs/drug-safety-and-availability/fda-requires-boxed-warning-about-serious-mental-health-side-effects-asthma-and-allergy-drug

70. U.S. Food and Drug Administration. Surveillance: postmarket drug and biologic safety evaluations [Internet]. Silver Spring (MD): U.S. Department of Health and Human Services; c2018 [cited 2019 Sep 28]. Available from: https://www.fda.gov/drugs/surveillance/postmarket-drug-and-biologic-safety-evaluations

71. U.S. Food and Drug Administration. Surveillance: post drug-approval activities [Internet]. Silver Spring (MD): U.S. Department of Health and Human Services; c2018 [cited 2019 Sep 28]. Available from: https://www.fda.gov/drugs/guidance-compliance-regulatory-information/surveillance

72. Postmarketing reporting of adverse drug experiences, 21 C.F.R. Sec. 314.80 (2018).

73. U.S. Food and Drug Administration. FDA guidance for industry: postmarketing safety reporting for human drug and biological products including vaccines [Internet]. Silver Spring (MD): U.S. Department of Health and Human Services; c2001 [cited 2019 Sep 28]. Available from: https://www.fda.gov/regulatory-information/search-fda-guidance-documents/adverse-reactions-section-labeling-human-prescription-drug-and-biological-products-content-and

74. U.S. Food and Drug Administration. Reporting serious problems to FDA [Internet]. Silver Spring (MD): U.S. Department of Health and Human Services; c2018 [cited 2019 Sep 30]. Available from: https://www.fda.gov/safety/medwatch-fda-safety-information-and-adverse-event-reporting-program/reporting-serious-problems-fda

75. U.S. Food and Drug Administration. FDA guidance for industry: field alert report submission questions and answers [Internet]. Silver Spring (MD): U.S. Department of Health and Human Services; c2018 [cited 2019 Sep 29]. Available from: https://www.fda.gov/regulatory-information/search-fda-guidance-documents/field-alert-report-submission-questions-and-answers-guidance-industry

76. Pharmaceutical Research and Manufacturers of America. Code on interactions with healthcare professionals [Internet]. Washington (DC): Pharmaceutical Researchers and Manufacturers of America; c2008 [cited 2016 Aug 26]. Available from: https://www.phrma.org/-/media/Project/PhRMA/PhRMA-Org/PhRMA-Org/PDF/Code-of-Interaction_FINAL21.pdf

77. Academy of Managed Care Pharmacy (AMCP). The AMCP format for formulary submissions; a format for submissions of clinical and economic evidence in support of formulary consideration. Version 4.0. Alexandria (VA): Academy of Managed Care Pharmacy; c2016 [cited 2010 Sep 30]. Available from: http://www.amcp.org/sites/default/files/2019-03/AMCP-Format-V4.pdf

78. Soares SC, March C. Metrics implementation in an industry-based medical information department and comparison to metrics tracked within other industry-based medical information departments. Drug Inf J. 2008 Mar;42(2):175–82.

79. Werner AL, Poe TE, Graham JA. Expanding medical communications services to internal customers. Drug Inf J. 2000 Oct-Dec;34(4):1053–61.

80. Wu K, Schmelz LS, Doshi SM. Medical information specialists: benchmarks in practice. Ther Innov Regul Sci. 2013 Mar;47(2):190–7.

81. Morgan DK, Domann DE, Collins GE, Massey KL, Moss RJ. History and evolution of field-based medical programs. Drug Inf J. 2000 Oct-Dec;34(4):1049–52.

82. Marrone CM, Bass JL, Klinger CJ. Survey of medical liaison practices across the pharmaceutical industry. Drug Inf J. 2007 Jul;41(4):457–70.

83. Bass JL, Marrone CM, Klinger C. Survey of medical liaison practices 3: assessing practice trends across the pharmaceutical industry. Drug Inf J. 2010 Sep;44(5):535–49.

84. Accreditation Council for Continuing Medical Education. Standards for commercial support: standards to ensure independence in CME activities. Chicago (IL): Accreditation Council for Continuing Medical Education; c2014 [cited 2019 Sep 30]. Available from: https://www.accme.org/sites/default/files/2019-01/174_20190118_ACCME_Standards_for_Commercial_Support.pdf

85. U.S. Food and Drug Administration. FDA guidance for industry: industry-supported scientific and educational activities [Internet]. Silver Spring (MD): U.S. Department of Health and Human Services; c1997 [cited 2019 Sep 30]. Available from: https://www.fda.gov/media/75334/download

SUGGESTED READINGS

1. U.S. Food and Drug Administration Drug Guidance Database. Available from: https://www.fda.gov/drugs/guidance-compliance-regulatory-information/guidances-drugs Updated daily with draft and final guidance from FDA on drug-related topics

25

Chapter Twenty-Five

Assessing Drug Promotions

Genevieve Lynn Ness • Robert D. Beckett

Learning Objectives

• *After completing this chapter, the reader will be able to:*

- Define drug promotions.
- List recommendations by the World Health Organization (WHO) for appropriate drug promotions.
- Describe the role of the U.S. Food and Drug Administration (FDA) Office of Prescription Drug Promotion (OPDP).
- Determine whether a piece of direct-to-consumer advertising (DTCA) has been cited in FDA warning letters to companies.
- Describe the allowed content for a specific type of DTCA.
- Evaluate a given piece of DTCA based on FDA and Pharmaceutical Manufacturer's Association (PhRMA) guidelines.
- Report a drug promotion concern using the Bad Ad Program.
- Evaluate the appropriateness of a piece of drug promotion designed for a health care professional.
- List systematic and individual strategies that may be used to combat proliferation of misinformation in drug promotions.
- Identify logical fallacies used in drug promotion, when given an interaction with a pharmaceutical industry representative.
- Describe the goals and design of academic detailing programs.
- Describe the clinical, economic, and humanistic effects of academic detailing.

Key Concepts

① Drug promotion is defined by the WHO as material or information provided by drug manufacturers with the ultimate goal of increasing prescribing or purchasing of medications.

② The FDA currently recognizes and outlines appropriate content for three types of direct-to-consumer advertising (DTCA): help-seeking advertisements, reminder advertisements, and product claim advertisements/full product promotions.

③ The following information should be considered when validating appropriateness of DTCA: (1) balance of risk and benefit information and inclusion of a brief summary of the risks listed in the labeling, (2) a statement encouraging patients to seek information from their physician, and (3) references to other sources to find the full prescribing information.

④ Drug promotion to health care professionals makes up the majority of drug promotions activity in terms of financial expenditure on the part of pharmaceutical industry; this information can be effective in eliciting changes in prescribing behavior.

⑤ All health care professionals, including pharmacists, should arm themselves using strategies of information mastery and vigilance for potentially flawed reasoning when interacting with pharmaceutical sales representatives.

⑥ Health care professionals are encouraged to report drug promotion violations to the FDA's Bad Ad Program.

⑦ Academic detailing programs, often led by pharmacists, are designed to combat pharmaceutical industry detailing by providing evidence-based information in the form of one-on-one or small-group interactions between a clinician and prescribers.

Introduction

❶ **Drug promotion** is defined by the WHO as material or information provided by drug manufacturers with the ultimate goal of increasing prescribing or purchasing of medications. Each year, the pharmaceutical industry spends billions of dollars on advertising their medications to the public and to health care professionals.[1-10] Annual spending on marketing of prescription drugs, health services, disease awareness campaigns, and laboratory testing increased from $17.7 billion in 1997 to $29.9 billion in 2016.[11] In 2017, AbbVie's Humira®, Pfizer's Lyrica®, and Pfizer's Xeljanz® spent the most on measured media advertising ($410 million, $346 million, and $267 million, respectively).[12] Companies use medical journals, newspapers, radio, television, magazines, websites, social media, search engine marketing, distributed promotional materials, billboards, direct mailings, medication samples, and sales representatives to advertise their products.[6,8,13,14] A report assessing drug advertising submissions to the FDA by pharmaceutical companies from 2001 to 2014 found that there were three times more non-Internet advertisements targeting health care professionals than consumers.[15]

Health care professionals and consumers may not recognize the impact that drug promotion can have on individual behavior.[6] The literature has reported increased prescribing patterns, rapid implementation of new medications, and an increase in inappropriate prescribing among physicians who utilize promotional materials to obtain drug information.[6] The effect of medication promotion on overall public health remains controversial. WHO suggests clinical trials be conducted to assess the correlation of drug promotion with inappropriate prescribing and the occurrence of adverse events, to identify the public health outcomes of drug promotion.[6] For these reasons, health care professionals must be prepared to critically interpret and evaluate verbal and written drug promotions. In particular, because pharmacists directly counsel patients on medications promoted in advertisements, they play an important role as interpreters of drug advertisements for patients. The following section describes the full scope of drug promotion according to WHO.

Ethical Criteria for Medicinal Drug Promotion

In 1988, WHO published criteria for the ethical promotion of medications.[16] The guidelines state the promotion of drugs should comply with the national standards established by the country where the drugs are being promoted. These guidelines apply to both domestic and exported drug products. Overall, information presented for the purposes of promotion should be balanced, accurate, and current. Advertisements targeted specifically to health care professionals should follow the approved product labeling and all writing should be clear and readable.

HEALTH CARE PROFESSIONALS

A scientific summary is required when product claims are made within an advertisement directed toward health care professionals.[16] These advertisements should include: (1) generic name, (2) brand name, (3) amount of active ingredient per dosage form, (4) other ingredients that can lead to allergies or adverse effects, (5) indications, (6) dosage form, (7) adverse reactions, (8) warnings and precautions, (9) contraindications, (10) drug interactions, (11) additional notable interactions, (12) manufacturer/distributor name and address, and (13) scientific literature references. Detailed information about the scientific properties of a medication should be made available to health care professionals as appropriate.

CONSUMERS

The WHO criteria also provide information about **direct-to-consumer advertising** (DTCA).[16] According to WHO, DTCA should assist consumers in making decisions about nonprescription medications; however, the use of DTCA for prescription medications is not recommended. Scientific evidence must support all factual information provided. DTC advertisements should not use fearful language or tactics, but use only information available in the approved labeling, including the following: (1) generic name, (2) brand name, (3) indications, (4) major warnings and precautions, (5) contraindications, and (6) the manufacturer/distributor name and address.

PHARMACEUTICAL REPRESENTATIVES

WHO also outlines guidelines for pharmaceutical representatives.[16] It is important to note that these guidelines specifically address medical representatives and not medical science liaisons, the former being more focused on sales, unlike the latter. These personnel should be properly trained and retain adequate technical and medical knowledge. The information presented should only discuss the material from the approved labeling. The pharmaceutical industry is responsible for the statements made by their sales representatives and the salary of those representatives should not be influenced by the number of prescriptions written for the product they are promoting. WHO recognizes that free samples of prescription medications can be given to prescribers in small quantities upon request.

The WHO guidelines outline the proper features of drug promotion that are required to produce beneficial and accurate materials. These criteria provide the basis of drug promotion regulations and evaluative strategies that will be discussed in more detail later in this chapter.

Direct-to-Consumer Advertising (DTCA)

DEFINITION OF DTCA

The FDA defines DTCA as advising created by a pharmaceutical company to promote products to consumers.[14] The goal of such advertising is to encourage patients to discuss a medication with their prescriber, ultimately leading to a prescription.[10]

The number of prescription drug direct-to-consumer (DTC) advertisements has increased dramatically from 79,000 in 1997 to 4.6 million in 2016.[11]

There are many methods that pharmaceutical companies use to present DTC advertisements to patients. The three most well-known are (1) print, through magazines or newspapers, (2) broadcast through television, and (3) electronic, in online banners, videos, search engine advertisements, and websites.[17] The Pharmaceutical Research and Manufacturers of America (PhRMA) defines DTC print advertisements as "space that is bought by a company in newspaper or magazine publications targeted to patients or consumers, or a direct mail communication paid for and disseminated by a company to patients or consumers, for the purpose of presenting information about one or more of the company's medicines."[18] PhRMA also defines DTC television advertisements as a "portion of television air time on broadcast or cable television that is bought by a company for the purpose of presenting information about one or more of the company's medicines."[18]

The most common form of DTC advertisements submitted to the FDA in 2014 was Internet materials (12,136 submissions).[15] This increase in the use of the Internet for DTCA may be because this type of advertising can focus on specific patient populations, exposes a larger number of consumers to medications, and is more cost effective than television or print advertisements.[17] This approach seems to be effective at reaching consumers, in that a 2018 study conducted in 626 college students found that 81.9% watched television advertisements online, with 63.9% specifically watching on YouTube.[19] Additionally, it has been reported that when a patient trusts drug information presented online, they are more likely to talk with their physician about the medication.[20]

Pharmaceutical companies have also increased their presence on social media. In a study assessing 15 pharmaceutical companies, 14 had links to social media sites on their websites, with Twitter being the most common (93%, 14/15).[21] Facebook followed behind with 66% of the companies linking to this social media site.[21] The 2018 study discussed above found that approximately 75% of college students read print advertisements on the Internet, with 44.4% reading on Facebook.[19] These students also reported higher trust for videos and print advertisements posted on Twitter.[19] Lower trust was reported in students that watched advertisements on conventional television.[19]

EFFECTS OF DTCA ON PRESCRIPTIONS

DTCA has been correlated to increased prescription drug profit for the pharmaceutical industry.[22] Specifically, for each dollar spent on DTCA, the company makes about $4.20 in sales.[10,22] A study assessing DTCA and statin prescription data from 2005 through 2009 found that DTCA resulted in an increase of 58,516 total statin prescriptions during the study period.[23] A study assessing the DTCA of Advair®, Singular®, Symbicort®, and Asmanex® found that the average number of doses dispensed per 100,000 patients

TABLE 25–1. DTCA AND PHARMACEUTICAL INDUSTRY PROFIT

Medication(s)	Investment	Result
Aromatase inhibitors[213]	For every $1 million on DTCA	0.15% increase in new prescriptions after 3 months
Crestor® and Lipitor®[23]	For each 100-unit increase in DTC ad viewing	2.22% increase in doses dispensed[a]
Chantix®[214]	After one exposure to a DTC ad	1.5% increase in the rate of new prescriptions
Zelnorm®[5,22]	For every $1 million on DTCA	1796 prescriptions were written
Advair®, Singular®, Symbicort®, and Asmanex®[24]	For every additional DTC ad to which the household was exposed	2% higher rate of prescriptions were dispensed[a]
Testosterone[215]	DTCA exposure	Increase monthly: • Testosterone testing (rate ratio=1.006) • Initiation of testosterone treatment (rate ratio=1.007) • Initiation of testosterone treatment without testing (rate ratio=1.008)

[a]After controlling for confounders.

increased from 392,000 in 2005 to 483,000 in 2009 per designated marketed area.[24] The DTCA for these drugs was moderately correlated with total sales ($r = 0.28$, $p < 0.001$).

In 2002, the U.S. General Accounting Office (GAO) projected that eight million Americans requested and received prescriptions due to DTCA each year.[5] In 2009, there were 1-million extra physician visits and 397,025 additional irritable bowel syndrome (IBS) diagnoses during the first quarter of tegaserod (Zelnorm®) DTCA compared to 17,105 extra physician visits and 2266 additional diagnoses in the quarter just prior to DTCA.[22] A study conducted in 2013 assessed 2057 survey respondents in New Zealand and found that after viewing DTC advertisements 11.4% of the respondents requested a prescription from their physician.[25] Additional statistics regarding the benefit of DTCA for the pharmaceutical industry can be found in Table 25-1.

COST OF DTCA

Based on these reports, it is not surprising that DTCA spending peaked in 2006 to $5.4 billion; however, spending decreased in 2007, 2010, and 2013 to $4.8 billion, $4.3 billion, and $3.83 billion, respectively.[7,8,9,26] Since then, DTCA has made a comeback with an increase in spending to $4.53 billion in 2014, followed by a new peak of $5.6 billion in 2016.[11,26,27]

Today, most of the DTCA spending is allotted for television advertisements, which results in the average American watching about 16 hours of televised drug advertisements per year.[5,8,28] In 2018, AbbVie spent the most on televised DTC advertisements for their product Humira® ($375 million) followed by Pfizer's Lyrica® ($213 million) and Xeljanz® ($209 million).[29]

TYPES OF DTCA

❷ *The FDA currently recognizes and outlines appropriate content for three types of DTCA: help-seeking advertisements, reminder advertisements, and product claim advertisements/ full product promotions.* The following statements describe each of these types of advertisements in detail, including evaluative criteria.[14]

- **Help-seeking advertisements** do not recommend a particular medication but provide information about a disease state or condition.[5,8,14,22,30] The advertisement can describe particular symptoms, point patients to discuss their symptoms with their physician, and offer a phone number for more information about the disease state.[30,31] These advertisements are regulated by the Federal Trade Commission (FTC) since a specific drug product is not mentioned.[30,31] In a study assessing pharmaceutical companies' use of social media for DTCA, help-seeking advertisements were found to be the most common form (40%, 301/740).[21] These were found mostly on YouTube and Twitter as opposed to Facebook. Recently, PhRMA companies have gotten creative in regard to the distribution of help-seeking advertisements. Incyte Corporation, the manufacturer of Jakafi® (ruxolitinib), partnered with producers of the daytime soap opera *General Hospital* to create a plot in which one of the characters was diagnosed with polycythemia vera (PV), a myeloproliferative neoplasm (MPN), and a blood clot.[32] The storyline included an overview of the disease state and the physician recommending treatment with phlebotomy and anticoagulation. The patient expressed concerns with this form of treatment and asked if there were other options available. Since Jakafi® was not specifically mentioned in the scene, this was considered a disease awareness promotion or a help-seeking advertisement. However, at the time, Jakafi® was the only FDA-approved kinase inhibitor indicated for the treatment of PV.[32,33]
- **Reminder advertisements** do not describe the indication of a medication but do present the brand name.[5,8,14,22,34] These particular advertisements are created with the assumption that patients are already familiar with the drug's indication.[30] Risk information is not included in these advertisements, and therefore, reminder advertisements of drugs with boxed warnings are illegal.[5,8,30,35] Any information or even implied information (through images or text) about a product's benefits or

TABLE 25-2. INFORMATION NOT REQUIRED FOR INCLUSION IN DTCA[37]

Generic availability

Availability of similar drugs that have the same indication with less adverse effects

Whether lifestyle changes could help the condition (this is only required if it is listed in the prescribing information for the product)

Incidence of the disease that the medication treats

Mechanism of action:

    Onset of action (if the product states that it works quickly it must define the meaning of quickly)

    How many people have experienced benefit from the drug

risks are not permitted in reminder advertisements.[30] For example, a medication for osteoporosis would not have an image of bones in the reminder advertisement as this implies the product's indication.

- **Product claim advertisements or full product promotions** require more detail and should contain the drug name, the indication, as well as a balance between the risks and benefits associated with the product.[5,8,14,22,30,34] Specifically, printed product claim advertisements should include a brief summary that provides details about all of the risk information listed in the FDA-approved labeling.[8,30] Printed advertisements must also include a reference to the FDA MedWatch program (http://www.fda.gov/Safety/MedWatch/) for patients to report medication side effects.[30] Product claim advertisements that are broadcasted by either television, radio, or phone are not required to include the brief summary of risk information.[30] Instead, television advertisements are required to contain a **major statement** of the main risks associated with the product, which can be presented verbally.[7,8,30,34,36] In addition, when broadcast advertisements do not include all risk information listed in the labeling, the advertisement is expected to provide resources that patients can consult to obtain the full prescribing information.[30] For example, the advertisement can refer a patient to consult with their health care professional, call a toll-free number, visit the product website, or refer to a printed advertisement that contains information that is more detailed.[30,36] This is known as the adequate provision requirement.[2,8,30] Information that does not need to be included in DTCA is listed in Table 25-2.[37]

Tone and themes of DTC advertisements can vary.[34,36] Many advertisements portray patients after successfully taking the product (i.e., healthy patients); similarly, advertisements tend to portray the product as a facilitator of healthy or recreational activities.[34] Most advertisements rely on emotional, rather than logical appeals; these emotional appeals could be positive, negative, or both. A study assessing the use of "expectation violations" such as "Do you sometimes feel lonely and vulnerable? Scientists may know why,"

TABLE 25–3. DTCA TECHNIQUES UTILIZED BY PHARMACEUTICAL COMPANIES WHEN CREATING DTCA[20]

Technique	Description
Disease mongering	Companies create a new disease state as part of the marketing plan to promote their medication.
Medicalization of drugs	Nonmedical problems become treated and defined as medical problems.
Normalization	Normalizing a disease state by utilizing prevalence statistics to motivate readers to purchase the medication through emotional reactions versus logic.
Identification	Prompt readers to have a personal connection or emotional reaction to the advertisement message.
Self-diagnosis	Encourages self-awareness for patients to take action and discuss conditions with their physicians.
Drug efficacy information	Increasing patient understanding of the medicine through the presentation of efficacy information in direct numerical formats or visual aids.
Comparative drug claims	Advertisements that include a direct comparison of at least two medications. The comparator product can be named or unnamed.
Nonbranded (Help-seeking advertisements)	These advertisements describe the disease state and symptoms without mentioning a treatment.
Format	Using large fonts, colors, and disclosure formatting devices, to increase patients' ability to recall medication benefits.
The ego segment	Advertisements that appeal to the patient's ego or self-image.
The ration segment	Highlight the quality and competitiveness of the medication to encourage patients to choose the advertised medication.
Endorsers	The use of expert, celebrity, or noncelebrity endorsers to promote the product.
Website factors	Website "trust cues" are positively correlated with consumers' trust of DTCA websites, which in turn increased their likelihood of seeking a drug consultation with their physician.

found that adults that viewed this type of ad experienced more psychological disequilibrium, had more positive evaluations of the ad as well as the drug, had positive outcome expectations, and increased intentions of medication use.[38]

Another study performed a content analysis to describe major themes present in advertisements and found that promotion, prevention, individualism, collectivism, cheerfulness, quiescence, dejection, agitation, fear, and affection were all prevalent.[36] In addition, a study found that patients prefer human spokes-characters versus animated spokes-characters in advertisements.[39] Further techniques identified as used by pharmaceutical companies when developing DTCA can be found in Table 25-3.[20]

DTCA LEGISLATION

Currently, among developed countries, DTCA is only permitted in the United States and New Zealand.[5,8,14,22,34] DTCA is banned in Canada; however, in the mid-1990s and early 2000s, Health Canada permitted the dissemination of unbranded "help-seeking" advertisements and branded prescription "reminder advisements" to consumers.[40] New Zealand relies on self-regulation of DTCA by the pharmaceutical companies; however, in the United States, the FDA is responsible for overseeing DTCA (except help-seeking advertisements as described above).[5]

● FDA's Oversight on DTCA

The FDA's authority over prescription drug advertising targeted to health care professionals was established in 1962 by the Kefauver-Harris Amendment.[2,8,41] Shortly after, in 1969, the FDA released regulations requiring health care professional drug advertisements to: (1) be accurate and not misleading; (2) contain a brief summary of indications, adverse effects, warnings, and contraindications; (3) be **fair balanced**; and (4) include only factual information about the product's advertised uses.[6,8,36,42,43]

The FDA first allowed companies to promote their products directly to consumers in 1985.[2,8,9] However, the "brief summary" requirement was still in place.[44] This regulation would have made television advertisements too lengthy for broadcast.[44] In 1997, the FDA released a draft guidance stating that television advertisements no longer required the brief summary; however, the guidance did require a **major statement** of the main safety risks and referral to a source for detailed information about the product.[1,7,8,36] This guidance was finalized in 1999.[2,8] In addition, printed product claim advertisements were required to include the entire prescribing information prior to the release of 2004 regulations stating that only a simplified brief summary is required.[8] However, patient mailings, brochures, and other drug company materials that promote a drug product are still required to include the full FDA-approved prescribing information if any such materials mention the benefits of the medication.[30] In 2007, the FDA Amendments Act (FDAAA) required the MedWatch reporting statement to be added to all printed advertisements, which states: "You are encouraged to report negative side effects of prescription drugs to the FDA. Visit MedWatch, or call 1-800-FDA-1088."[30,45] Today, prescription drug advertising regulations can be found in title 21, part 202 of the Code of Federal Regulations (CFR).[43]

In August 2017, the FDA released a Federal Register notice seeking comments regarding risk information in DTC broadcast advertisements.[46] The FDA expressed concerns that the **major statement** is not clear to patients, can minimize risks by not including all important information, and increase noncompliance due to fear of side effects. The FDA is considering limiting the risks to only life-threatening or serious risks with a disclosure statement that other risks are not included in the advertisement. All advertisements would still be required to have a "fair balance" of risk and benefit information. A study testing the use of this revised risk statement (only including serious and actionable risks) in television advertisements found that patients viewing the revised statement recalled and recognized more risks than patients that viewed the unedited statement.[47] Comments regarding this notice were accepted until November 20, 2017; however, at the time of this writing, risk statement changes have not been implemented.[46]

Enforcement of the DTCA Legislation

To ensure that DTCA follows FDA guidelines and to protect consumers from false information, the FDA maintains a surveillance and enforcement program through their Office of Prescription Drug Promotion (OPDP) division.[48] It is important to remember that the FDA has the authority only over DTCA for prescription medications.[37] DTCA for nonprescription medications and help-seeking advertisements are regulated by the FTC.[30,31,37] In addition, the FDA does not require pharmaceutical companies to submit DTC advertisements prior to its distribution or being aired.[37] This has been reported as a misconception among patients (i.e., 68.8% of patients surveyed believed that the FDA must approve DTC advertisements prior to publication).[5,8,49] However, the FDA does require advertisements to be submitted for review as soon as they are released to the public.[5,10,37]

If the FDA discovers a DTC ad is not in compliance with the set of laws in place, warning letters can be issued to the pharmaceutical company, requesting the removal of the advertisement, and addressing the material that violates the law.[10,37] These letters are publicly available on the FDA's Warning Letters website.[37,50] If the advertisement has created a severe threat on public health, the FDA can also request the company to correct the advertisement and publish or broadcast the corrected version.[37] A study by Aikin *et al.*, found that corrected versions of broadcasted advertisements are effective in correcting patients' perceptions of the drug's efficacy and risk.[51] In addition, the timing in which the patients viewed the corrective advertisement did not affect the patients' drug benefit and risk recall (i.e., no exposure delay up to a 6-month exposure delay). In rare cases, the FDA may bring criminal charges against the company in court and seize the company's drug supply.[37] The FDA does not have authority to levy fines on pharmaceutical companies for DTCA violations.[10]

One study stated that there has been a decrease in the number of DTCA regulatory actions by the FDA.[8] The author explains that this could be the result of decreased FDA supervision, but it could also be due to better compliance with DTCA laws.[8] Another added factor is that all warning letters must be reviewed and approved by the FDA's Office of Chief Counsel, which was mandated by the Secretary of Health and Human Services (HHS) in 2002.[8] This action alone may have resulted in a decline in the number of promotional related warning letters issued between 2001 and 2002, which were 68 and 28, respectively.[8] In recent years, the number of warning letters sent to pharmaceutical companies by OPDP has remained low (Year-number of letters: 2015-9, 2016-11, 2017-5, 2018-7, and 2019-10).[52-56] In addition, the FDA has limited staff to review DTC advertisements. Fewer than six FDA employees were assigned to review greater than 15,000 brochures and DTC advertisements in 2006.[8] Since then, the OPDP staff has increased to accommodate the growing number of advertisements to review.

Recently, the issue of FDA regulation has sparked controversy in reference to the First Amendment, free speech.[57] Amarin Corporation, the manufacturer of Vascepa® (icosapent ethyl), sued the FDA in 2015, stating that the First Amendment permits the promotion of their product for a broader patient population (off-label) without adequate evidence to support its use. Amarin stated that a judge should be responsible for determining if promotional claims are misleading or false. The judge ruled in favor of the pharmaceutical company, finding the FDA's threat to prosecute the company based on truthful, non-misleading speech to be unconstitutional. Unsurprisingly, a recent study published in Circulation found that physicians were more likely to prescribe Vascepa® off-label if they received off-label product information from the manufacturer (38%) compared to those that received on-label information (7%, $p < 0.001$).[58] However, physicians that received off-label information with evidence context (discussed three clinical trials that did not demonstrate cardiovascular effectiveness) were less likely to endorse the medication for off-label use.

This ruling is extremely concerning to health care professionals on several levels. First, judges do not have the expertise or the access to clinical data to be able to assess drug promotions effectively.[57] The ruling similarly could put the onus on the pharmaceutical industry to determine what information is "truthful," as opposed to the FDA. Second, this could discourage pharmaceutical companies from producing superior clinical evidence to support their medications. Third, off-label promotion of medications could put patients at increased risk, as these indications may not be supported by clinical evidence. Overall, health care professionals should be extremely concerned about the patient safety issues this type of ruling creates, and increased off-label promotion will necessitate pharmacists to take an even more active role in promoting rational, evidence-based drug therapy.

Monitoring Online Promotion

After warning letters were issued from the FDA in 2009 stating that online search engine results need to include risk information since both the drug name and indication are mentioned, the pharmaceutical companies now only include either the name of the drug or the indication in search engine links.[8] A study assessing 73 FDA notices of violations and warning letters for online DTC advertisements from 2004 to 2014 found that 47.9% were in reference to advertisements on drug websites, 24.7% for links on search engines and banner advertisements, 21.9% for videos, 2.7% for emails, and 2.7% for social media widgets.[17] The main violation reported in the warning letters for online DTCA was omission or minimization of risk (32.4%).[17] This continues to be an issue with online promotion. In February 2020, Outlook Pharmaceuticals, Inc. received a warning letter from the FDA in reference to the Procentra® link listed on Google.[59] The link was considered false and misleading because risk information about the product was not included with the benefits.

Strategies that pharmaceutical companies have used to promote their products on social media include "one clicks," which provide risk information "one click away," and human interest stories with branded medication information excluded, which do not fall under FDA DTCA regulations.[60] A study conducted in 2017 found that patients were able to recall and recognize more risk information if the risks were presented just below the benefits on a website's homepage or if the webpage included a red banner above the benefits that read, "Please see Important Safety Information below."[61]

The FDA released a draft guidance in June 2014 regarding the presentation of risk and benefit information on Internet and social media platforms with character space limitations.[62] Essentially, if a company includes product benefit information, risk information (at a minimum the most serious risks) should also be included. In addition, a reference (i.e., hyperlink) to more complete risk information should be included. If this is not possible with the character limitations, the company should avoid promoting their products through this platform.

PhRMA'S GUIDING PRINCIPLES FOR DTCA

With the increasing role of DTCA in health care, PhRMA established guiding principles for DTCA of prescription medications.[18] These principles are voluntary, but do serve as guidance for pharmaceutical companies to create accurate, educational, and encouraging DTC advertisements that follow FDA regulations. See Table 25-4 for an overview of the PhRMA principles. A commitment to follow the PhRMA guiding principles, and completion of an annual certification, entitles the company to be identifiable as a signatory company and be recognized by PhRMA online.

SUPPORT FOR DTCA

Supporters of DTCA believe these advertisements serve a public health need.[5,18] Through DTCA, patients become educated about different disease states, which can assist them in making better treatment decisions and create more knowledgeable patients in the health care environment.[1,5,8,9,18,42,63,64] However, a study assessing seniors' ($n = 626$) knowledge of disease found that DTCA was positively correlated with seniors' *subjective* knowledge ($\beta = 0.11$, $p < 0.05$) but negatively correlated their *objective* knowledge ($\beta = -0.004$, $p > 0.095$).[65] This means that DTCA may not have as much of an impact on patient's disease state knowledge as originally thought.

Additionally, DTCA is considered to help improve the quality of patient-professional interactions and help patients identify meaningful questions to ask of their health care

TABLE 25–4. PHRMA GUIDING PRINCIPLES FOR DTCA[18]

1. Information presented in DTCA should be accurate, not misleading, align with the FDA approved labeling, and exclude off-label information.

2. The company should obtain insight from patients and health care professionals to identify what educational information should be included in DTCA.

3. Prescription medications should be clearly identified as such in DTC advertisements.

4. The ad should encourage patients to discuss the risks and benefits of the advertised medication with their prescriber.

5. Health care professionals should be educated about new prescription medications prior to the release of DTCA in order to be able to accurately respond to patient questions.

6. Once unknown safety risks about an advertised product are discovered, companies should edit or remove DTC advertisements while continuing collaboration with the FDA.

7. All new DTC advertisements should be submitted to the FDA prior to public release.

8. All printed DTC advertisements should contain the FDA's MedWatch number or website to report adverse events. Television DTC advertisements should point patients to print advertisements with the FDA's MedWatch information and/or present the organization's toll-free number.

9. The ad should clearly identify the use of actors portraying health care professionals and disclose any financial compensation if actual health care professionals are utilized.

10. If a celebrity advocate is used in the DTC ad, the claims made by the celebrity should reflect their factual views and experiences while taking the medication.

11. When applicable, the DTC ad should also highlight alternatives to treat the condition being advertised such as diet and lifestyle changes.

12. Television DTC advertisements that discuss a particular product should present the major risks and the approved indications.

13. Medication benefit and risk information should be balanced, including information about boxed warnings (presented in plain language). Television DTC advertisements should point patients to where they can obtain additional information about product risks and benefits.

14. The disease state should be presented seriously and reverently throughout the DTC advertisements.

15. DTCA that may be inappropriate for children should not be aired or published in mediums where children could witness the advertisement.

16. Information about the disease and health awareness should be presented in DTCA.

17. Patient assistance programs for the uninsured and underinsured population should be mentioned in DTCA when applicable.

18. Television DTC advertisements should provide information about where patients can locate typical out-of-pocket or potential costs of the medication.

providers.[5,8,18] This has also been disputed in the literature, where only 33% of 366 survey respondents stated that DTCA resulted in seeking additional information about a drug or condition; of which only 31% indicated that their physicians were the source of this information (44% searched for additional information on the Internet).[66] Additionally, a study assessing the association between statin DTCA and outpatient visits related to high cholesterol found that each 100-unit increase in ad viewing was associated with only a 1.44% increase in visits.[23]

DTCA provides patients with information about treatment options available early on, which can result in lower health care costs.[8] It has been asserted that health care costs can be saved if medication therapy is started sooner because of DTCA for a disease that could eventually lead to surgery if not treated.[8] However, there is limited data to support this claim. Supporters mention that DTCA can also lower drug prices due to increased competition between products.[8]

DTCA may increase appropriate care for underdiagnosed diseases and encourage the implementation of healthy activities.[1,5,8,18,64] DTCA also has been credited with reducing the stigma of certain diseases, making them acceptable for discussion (e.g., psychiatric disorders).[5,8,9,67] A study found that college students viewing televised DTC advertisements containing images of discrimination, cognitive separation, and stereotyping reported lower social distance (stigma) scores for depression and anxiety patients compared to students not exposed to DTC advertisements.[68]

Lastly, supporters claim DTCA improves adherence to prescribed medications.[5,8] A 2015 study credited depression-related DTCA for assisting patients to remember to take their depression medication, which can improve medication adherence.[69]

OPPOSITION TO DTCA

In contrast, many who oppose DTCA express its potential threat to public health. Several critiques of DTCA are addressed below.

Imbalance Between Benefits and Risks

Sixty-five percent of physicians reported that patients tend to underestimate the risks and overemphasize the benefits of a drug, mostly after viewing a television advertisement.[10] A study analyzing television drug advertisements found that patients remembered the benefits of a drug more easily than the risks. This may be due to the dominance of visual messages over audio when presented jointly and the fact that much of the safety information is presented verbally in television advertisements.[8] A study assessing 97 television advertisements found that 100% presented risk information alongside distracting visuals and 78% presented the risk information as audio instead of running text.[70] In addition, a lack of consistency has been reported in the relative percentages of risk and benefit information presented in television advertisements for medications within the same class.[71] This study also found that none of the advertisements assessed ($n = 18$) included over 80% of the warnings listed in the corresponding package insert.

Patients have been reported to overemphasize a product's benefits and develop misconceptions regarding a drug's toxic effects because DTCA exaggerates the happiness achieved with a medication.[8,72] This is especially concerning in vulnerable patient populations, such as oncology patients.[73] An article in the New York Times quoted a cancer

patient referring to the pharmaceutical industry as shameful for releasing DTC advertisements promoting a "chance to live longer" with nivolumab when, in reality, only a
2.8-month increase in overall survival was reported in clinical trials.[85] In addition, a study
assessing social media advertising found that drug product claim posts mentioned only
benefits (44.8%, 216/482) more often than both risks and benefits (28%, 135/482) or risks
alone (27.2%, 131/482).[21] The study discussed above assessing the 97 television advertisements found that only 33% included all contraindications/limitations for use and 13%
marketed off-label indications.[70]

Opponents of DTCA state that FDA regulations are too lenient because pharmaceutical companies are only held responsible for the information presented in DTCA if there is
a violation.[8] As a result, some advertisements include inappropriate information. PhRMA
released DTCA guidelines that suggest companies should submit DTC advertisements
to the FDA for review prior to distribution; however, these guidelines are optional and
unenforceable.[8]

The content of DTCA is usually not written in lay person language (i.e., an eighth
grade reading level), making it challenging for consumers to understand.[8] Along these
lines the use of words, such as usually, mild, and may, to describe safety information could
lead to consumer confusion about the exact meaning of these terms.

In contrast, critics mention that the safety information required in DTCA could cause
patients to have concerns and may lead to issues with patient compliance.[8] A 2017 study
assessing medication adherence in 246 patients with serious mental disorders found that
DTCA exposure increased the odds of nonadherence by five times compared to patients
not exposed.[74] This study also found that 64% of respondents discussed side effect concerns with their doctor after seeing a DTC ad; however, 61% of these patients made
changes to their medication regimen before discussing concerns with their physician.
This could lead to serious health issues for patients.

Statistical Inaccuracy

There have been multiple reports of statistical exaggeration of product benefits in advertisements.[75] One study of DTCA reported that only two of 67 advertisements found in
U.S. magazines presented results of the clinical trials assessing the promoted drug versus
placebo as absolute rates of clinical outcomes (e.g., absolute risk reduction [ARR]), which
is considered the most appropriate method to represent data.[75] Other advertisements
only presented data in the form of relative risk reduction (RRR) (see Chapter 6 for further
information about RRR and ARR).[75] Some provided references to clinical studies but did
not provide any data from the studies in the advertisements.[75] One additional advertisement claimed that the promoted drug provided a clinical cure compared with competitors
but did not explain exactly what was defined as a clinical cure.[75] In a study assessing
16 advertisements, only one provided frequency of adverse events using quantitative

methods, two presented using comparative language, and the majority used a qualitative approach.[75] An additional study published in 2018 found that only 25 out of 97 (26%) television advertisements included quantitative data for reporting efficacy.[70] Prevalence of the disease state that the product is treating is also rarely reported in advertisements. In a study from 2004, only three of 31 advertisements provided information on disease prevalence.[75]

Potential for Inappropriate Prescribing

DTCA increases patient requests for advertised medications during their provider visits.[6] This can lead to the undermining of health care professional authority and hinder provider-patient relationships.[2,5,8,9] This interference in the provider-patient relationship has been reported in the literature by 30% of patients and 39% of physicians who participated in a national survey.[8] Additionally, 16% of advanced practice nurse prescribers (APNP) believed that patients were challenging their prescriptive authority during conversations about DTC advertisements.[76] If a prescriber refuses to provide a medication that the patient is requesting, the patient is more likely to switch prescribers.[8] This pressure from patients can increase the risk of inappropriate prescribing.[2,3,5,8,9] An FDA study reported about 8% of physicians felt some pressure to prescribe a particular medication after a patient reported seeing DTC advertisements for the product.[42] One study found that during physician visits, 40% of patients requested a medication that they saw in DTC advertisements and about 50% of the requests were granted by the prescriber.[8] However, a study conducted in 2006 reported that, of the patients who requested a medication due to DTCA, only about 2% to 7% received a prescription for the product in the end.[8] In contrast, a more recent study reported a 53% physician-prescribing rate in response to depression patients' DTC ad requests for brand-specific medications.[77]

Another concern is that patients may try to fit the type of patient that is presented in the DTC ad, which can also lead to inappropriate prescribing, diagnosis, and ultimately unnecessary side effects.[5,8] A study found that about half of physicians participating in a focus-group discussion presumed that patients diagnosed themselves accurately based on DTCA.[5] In addition, physicians may simply treat the symptoms using the advertised medication versus screening the patient for other medical conditions that may be causing the symptoms.[78]

The added time for providers and patients to discuss DTC advertisements during scheduled appointments could take away from other important aspects of the appointment and lead to negative patient outcomes.[9] Along the same lines, DTCA can lead to unnecessary physician visits and make patients believe that they have a particular disease.[1,7,8] For example, critics blame DTCA for converting the perception of menopause from a normal life process into an insufficient hormone disease.[8]

This increase in unnecessary prescribing can lead to an increase in prescription drug spending.[7] An article referencing unnecessary prescribing stated that physicians must serve as the intermediary between the patient and the drug.[79] Prescribers should not be afraid to say "no" when necessary. Additionally, health care professionals need to be sure to treat their patients as patients and not consumers.[80]

Increased Health Care Costs

The use of DTCA to advertise "me too" drugs (drugs that are structurally similar to other available medications)[81] can increase health care costs since many patients will request the brand name drug when there may be inexpensive generic options available.[3,8] A study found that patients were more likely to switch from lansoprazole to omeprazole in areas that were more exposed to DTCA since omeprazole was advertised via DTCA and lansoprazole was not.[5,82] This switch cost the patient on average an extra $400 per year in total expenditures.

The expense of DTCA may also drive up consumer costs for the product as pharmaceutical companies increase prices to compensate for advertising costs.[4] For example, one study found that the cost of clopidogrel increased by $0.40 (12%) per unit after the launch of the DTCA campaign.[4,5] In a study assessing television DTC advertisements, the high-cost medications had longer airtime for the advertisements (60 seconds) compared with medium-cost medications (47.9 seconds).[1]

Due to concerns regarding the increasing cost of medications, the American Medical Association (AMA), the American Society of Health-System Pharmacists (ASHP), and the American Public Health Association (APHA) called for a ban on DTCA.[83–85] The AMA criticized these advertisements for causing increased demand for novel and expensive treatment options when generic alternatives were available.[83] A ban on DTCA is viewed by some as unlikely due to the constitutional right of free speech.[72,73]

Insufficient Safety Data with DTCA

Most of the time, DTC advertisements are released to the public before the majority of the safety information is collected (i.e., postmarketing surveillance).[8] For example, rofecoxib (Vioxx®), which was one of the most promoted medications in the United States ($100 million/year spent on promotion), was not discovered to cause myocardial infarction (80,000–140,000 cases) or stroke until after the DTCA campaign.[5,8] This additional safety information led to its voluntary recall in 2004.[5,8]

Another example of a highly marketed product whose side effects were not fully discovered until after DTCA was Belviq® (lorcaserin), which was later withdrawn from the market due to increased risk of cancer.[86,87]

For the many reasons described above, information included in DTC advertisements should be closely scrutinized for errors, promotional violations, and other misleading information.

SUGGESTIONS FOR IMPROVEMENT

Suggestions for the improvement of DTCA have been reported in the literature. One suggestion would eliminate the need for DTCA altogether. A group of representatives from industry, government, and academia would be tasked with creating public service announcements that discuss appropriate treatment for conditions known to cause morbidity or mortality, have effective and safe treatments available, and are identified as being undertreated and underdiagnosed.[7,8] This solution has not been implemented in the United States at this time; however, unbranded advertisements about disease states and public relations campaigns have been used in countries where DTCA is banned.[88,89]

The U.S. Institute of Medicine (IOM—now referred to as the National Academy of Medicine [NAM]) proposed enforcing a 2-year delay from the time a drug product is released to launching DTCA.[5,8] This can ensure that adequate time has passed for collection of postmarketing data and allow physicians to become educated about the product.[8] However, in 2011, the U.S. Congressional Budget Office stated that the benefits of providing information about new medications outweighed the risks and, therefore, the proposal was not supported.[5]

Having the FDA review all DTC advertisements before they are released to the public is another recommendation.[8] However, this would only be achievable assuming additional user fees were paid to the FDA by the pharmaceutical industry. There was a proposal for such a program in 2008, but it was not funded by Congress, and therefore could not be enforced by the FDA.

There have also been debates about the most appropriate DTC ad format.[90] A study assessing consumer preferences found that more patients preferred the drug-facts-box format, which is similar to the nonprescription labeling.[90] In addition, more patients were able to recall risk information when presented in this manner compared to the traditional brief summary format. Schwartz *et al.* published an article detailing the components of the one-page drug-facts box, which included balanced drug information.[91] This suggestion was submitted to the FDA for consideration but was determined to be difficult to implement.[72,73]

Other suggestions include listing adverse effects on drug advertisements in bullet form from highest to lowest possibility of occurance.[9] Additionally, modifying DTCA to incorporate health literacy principles can significantly increase comprehension and information retention.[92] In August 2015, the FDA proposed new changes to print DTC advertisements, which would include a new "consumer brief summary" that would include "the most important risk information" that can easily be comprehended by patients.[93,94] This guidance is still in draft status.

Requiring quantitative data in DTC advertisements has also been suggested.[8] A study assessing 2504 cholesterol patients found that patients were more likely to report *correct* efficacy information if the data was presented in a bar chart or table on a print advertisement.[95] For televised advertisements, patients that viewed an ad with any visual aid (pie chart, bar chart, table, or pictograph) were more likely to report *correct* efficacy information.[95]

Including definitions of certain statistical concepts may help improve patient comprehension of DTC advertisements. O'Donoghue *et al.*[49] conducted focus groups with 38 patients and found that only a few were familiar with the term **"composite score."** Additionally, of 2957 patients surveyed, 45.3% did not know the meaning of "composite score." A follow-up study assessed whether including the definition of a "composite score" in print advertisements would affect patient's understanding and recognition of drug effectiveness.[96] Patients were more likely to recognize that an advertisement reported a medication's effectiveness based on a "composite score" if the composite score definition was included versus simply listing the symptoms. Additionally, patients displayed increased symptom comprehension when the definition was present versus the general indication. However, patients that viewed the composite score definition expressed that they were not as confident in the medication's benefits compared to patients that viewed the general indication or the list of symptoms. This could discourage drug manufacturers from including "composite score" information in advertisements.

Mentioning if a generic alternative is available for the product has also been described as a method to improve DTCA.[8] This suggestion may not be well accepted by the pharmaceutical industry. Another study suggested requirements to include specific information about the population at risk for the advertised condition, describe **nonpharmacologic treatment**, and discuss the effectiveness of other therapies in the advertisements.[34]

Technology-based suggestions involve the use of television control devices which would give the patient or consumer the option to watch TV with or without DTC advertisements.[97] Additionally, a publicly available database that includes information regarding the following: (1) the monetary amount spent on the DTCA, (2) type of DTC advertisements, (3) marketing channel, (4) language, (5) demographic location in which the DTC ad is presented, (6) time when the DTC ad will be available, (7) type of product being marketed, (8) therapeutic category of the product, (9) disease that the medication treats, and (10) branded name of the product has been proposed.[98]

Improvement Progress

In order to combat the rising health care costs, the U.S. government issued a requirement that, by July 2019, medications priced at greater than $35 for a 1-month supply must include the list price on *televised* advertisements.[99] This requirement could pose a problem for some companies with high-priced medications. A study was conducted in which patients were asked to view a DTC ad that included a high drug price, low drug price, or no pricing information.[100] Patients then indicated on a scale of 1 (highly unlikely) to 7 (highly likely) if they would ask their physician about the medication. Unsurprisingly, patients stated that they would be less likely to ask their physician about the medication if the price included was high (mean score [SD] = 2.90[2.21]) compared to no price included (mean score [SD] = 5.12[1.73] $p < 0.001$).

The pharmaceutical industry responded to the pricing requirement by suing the Department of Health and Human Services, claiming that it would be a violation of "free speech" and harmful to health care.[101] Specifically, the pharmaceutical companies claim that the drug prices listed on the advertisement would not be accurate, as they do not consider discounts or insurance coverage. However, patients that pay cash or cash percentage copayments could benefit from this requirement.

In July 2019, a U.S. District Court Judge ruled in favor of the pharmaceutical companies, stating that the Department of Health and Human Services does not have the authority to enforce the pricing rule.[102] The court did not address the companies' claim that including drug prices would violate the First Amendment.

In spite of this ruling, some pharmaceutical companies started including websites on their advertisements that provide information regarding pricing and payments.[102] This was a PhRMA supported proposal.

With the solutions, suggestions, and continued evolution, the hope for future DTCA will be a greater emphasis on using medications appropriately, sustained use of medications, and increased medication adherence.[44]

EVALUATING DTCA

❸ *The following information should be considered when validating appropriateness of DTCA: (1) balance of risk and benefit information and inclusion of a brief summary of the risks listed in the labeling, (2) a statement encouraging patients to seek information from their physician, and (3) references to other sources to find the full prescribing information.*

In general, DTCA must present only accurate statements, maintain a balance of risk versus benefit information throughout, align with the information presented in the FDA approved labeling, and only present content that is supported by robust evidence.[18,103] Common violations found in advertisements include (1) omitting or softening risk, (2) overstating effectiveness, and (3) misleading drug comparisons.[104] When evaluating DTCA, consider using the process outlined in Table 25-5.[105]

TABLE 25–5. EVALUATING DTC ADVERTISEMENTS[75]

Issues that health care professionals should consider:

- Identify what condition or disease state the advertised product treats.
- Determine the reasoning behind why the patient believes that they have the advertised condition.
- Decide if the patient would be considered an appropriate candidate for the drug based on the information.
- Recognize if the patient is permitted to take the medication with their current comorbidities.
- Identify if the patient is taking any other medications that could interact with the advertised medication.
- Determine which adverse effects may concern the patient.
- Decide if the drug could be affected by certain foods, dietary supplements, vitamins, or alcohol.
- Pinpoint any other medications (including generic products) that could treat the patient's current condition.
- Determine if other medications to treat this condition have different or less serious side effects.
- Identify if diet and exercise could help the patient with their condition.
- Locate additional information about the disease state and the drug described in the advertisement.
- Determine if absolute risk reduction (ARR) or number needed to treat (NNT) was used to present results (e.g., "Three out of five patients benefit from Drug X").
- Assess the appropriateness of the use of confidence intervals.
- Identify if statistical power has been adequately explained in the advertisement if referenced.
- Determine if the referenced literature is from the main journal in which the data were published and not from a supplement or symposia.
- Evaluate the appropriateness of presented graphs and tables.
- Recognize if claims are being supported by emotional reports rather than numerical data.

The FDA also provides information for patients and health care professionals on how to determine if an advertisement is false or misleading based on the type.[106] FDA guidance for evaluating specific types of advertisements is provided in Table 25-6. The FDA encourages patients to report promotional violations to the OPDP by calling 855-RX-BADAD or mailing a written complaint directly to the division.[37,104] Health care professionals are encouraged to report promotional violations using the Bad Ad Program, described below.

Case Study 25–1

While browsing Twitter, you identify a help-seeking advertisement regarding hypertension. Since this advertisement is visible to many members of the public, you decide to evaluate if it is appropriate.

- *What information should this help-seeking advertisement include?*
- *What information should this help-seeking advertisement not include?*

TABLE 25−6. FDA GUIDANCE FOR EVALUATING SPECIFIC TYPES OF ADVERTISEMENTS[31,35,45]

A product claim ad should:

- Identify the product's brand and generic name.
- State the product's FDA-approved indication (all claims made in the ad must be backed by clinical experience or evidence).
- Include a statement that the product is only available by prescription.
- Contain balanced amounts of drug's risk and benefit information.
- Clearly state that the product is intended for adults or children (this includes the use of pictures, such as children being featured for pediatric medications).
- Include the FDA MedWatch statement about reporting serious adverse effects to the FDA.
- Contain a brief summary of the product's risks listed in the FDA-approved labeling.
- Encourage patients to ask their physician about the medication, signifying that the patient cannot make the decision to prescribe.
- Include references to other resources to obtain detailed product information including a website or toll-free telephone number.

A reminder ad should:

- Include a product's brand and generic name.
- Not list the product's indication.

A help-seeking ad should:

- Include appropriate images of individuals who may be experiencing the discussed symptoms, but not include images of drug products.
- List possible symptoms but does not mention a treatment for these symptoms.
- Encourage patients to discuss their symptoms and seek medical advice from their prescriber.
- Provide company information and references to a telephone number or website for more information.

- *If you were to identify a violation, could you report this advertisement to the FDA? If so, how would you go about reporting to the FDA?*

Promotions to Health Care Professionals

❹ *Drug promotion to health care professionals makes up the majority of drug promotions activity in terms of financial expenditure on the part of pharmaceutical industry; this information can be effective in eliciting changes in prescribing behavior.*[107] The following sections describe the scope and response to this issue.

DETAILING

Marketing of prescription medications differs from typical consumer products, in that one individual—the prescriber—directly controls, to a large extent, purchasing decisions on behalf of the ultimate patient.[107] For this reason, in addition to the very high expenditures of pharmaceutical industry on DTCA, even greater financial resources are dedicated to promotions made directly to health care professionals, which is referred to as **detailing**.[107]

In 2016, an estimated $29.9 billion was spent in pharmaceutical promotions (up from $27.7 billion in 2010): $9.6 billion (32%) on DTCA and $20.3 billion (68%) on promotions to providers or health care professionals.[11] Of the $20.3 billion directed toward professionals, $13.5 billion was spent on samples, $5.6 billion on office visits, and $979 million on direct payments to physicians.[11] Visits to offices accounted for substantially more spending than hospital visits. Similarly, in an assessment of the promotional pieces submitted to the FDA, there were 58,142 professional pieces compared with 27,322 pieces intended for patients (i.e., DTCA).[15] Detailing, like any type of marketing, combines use of scientific knowledge, logic, and reason with appeals to emotions through techniques such as slogans and use of wishful thinking.[107] Detailing may be defined as a one-on-one or group interaction in which a pharmaceutical industry representative, who might or might not have a clinical background, provides drug information and marketing materials to a prescriber or health care professional.[107,108] The most commonly provided types of non-Internet materials include direct mailings, exhibits, sales aids, and presentation slides.[15] These activities could involve provision of product samples and continuing education. At its core, detailing is designed to produce a change in prescribing behavior.

Some aspects of detailing, such as education, funding, and availability of samples from pharmaceutical industry representatives may be viewed positively by some health care professionals; however, evidence suggests cause for concern as well.[109] Promotional activities, including detailing, have been found to decrease use of generic drugs in favor of unnecessary, more expensive brand name products.[110] One study suggested that the majority of participants from a sample of primary care physicians and endocrinologists had low to moderate understanding of basic terms that may be used during detailing, such as intent-to-treat analysis, noninferiority margin, and randomization[111]; lack of familiarity with key terms may make individuals more likely to be impacted by persuasive argument. Pharmaceutical industry representatives may overstate their product's effectiveness by attributing clinical outcomes improvement to drugs only approved based on surrogate markers; in one study this was done in nearly half of cases.[112] Drugs that are heavily promoted may not carry the highest value.[113] A recent study found that top promoted drugs were less likely to be innovative than top selling drugs (relative risk [RR] 0.46, 95% CI 0.25–0.86) and offered less advantage compared to top prescribed drugs (RR 0.25, 95% CI 0.10–0.62).[113] The extraordinary expenditures on detailing and related activities, as well as cases of illegal and unsupported drug promotion to health care professionals, suggest that critically assessing the information delivered in these interactions is of vital importance.

LEGAL ISSUES

● The same criteria described earlier for DTCA also apply to formal advertisements intended for health care professionals and information promotions such as detailing.[114] Briefly, the information provided must provide fair balance in addressing safety risks and efficacy benefits, describe factual information, and not be misleading. Additionally, information must be consistent with the FDA-approved product labeling (i.e., the package insert), including indications for which the medication may be used.[115] As discussed earlier, off-label information may be provided in scientific exchanges and at the request of a health care professional, but its role in drug promotion, even to health care professionals, is evolving.[116] Even prior to the previously discussed legal challenges,[57] pharmaceutical companies were allowed to provide off-label information in response to an unsolicited request from a health care professional, as well as peer-reviewed articles, clinical practice guidelines, and reference books that discuss off-label information. They may also support continuing education that addresses off-label uses.[117] However, recent cases suggest that the FDA may be willing to allow pharmaceutical companies to provide non-misleading, truthful off-label promotion; at the time of writing, the FDA has committed to update its guidance to industry regarding communication practices, including off-label promotion.[117] Given the recent Amarin case, such clarification would be even more valuable.

● FDA advertising rules also apply to industry-sponsored education programs that are, in actuality, promotional activities.[114] For a program to be considered independent and nonpromotional (and, thus, qualify as continuing education), the program must be conducted by a third party who controls the educational content. Additionally, all relevant financial relationships must be disclosed. PhRMA members adhere to voluntary standards that prohibit direct speaker honorariums, entertainment (e.g., sporting-event tickets), gifts, and noneducational practice-related items (e.g., coffee mugs, pens) at continuing education events and during detailing.[118] All programs must be conducted through an independent continuing-education provider.

PROMOTION EFFECTIVENESS

The majority of scientific literature assessing health care professionals' interactions with pharmaceutical industry centers around medical students, physicians, and nurse practitioners, and finds success on the part of industry in achieving their desired changes in attitudes and behaviors.[3,119–128] Little information is available regarding promotions targeted toward pharmacists. Two studies have attempted to quantify exposure to pharmaceutical promotion during medical training, with high proportions of medical students (mean of one gift or exposure per week) and residents (median of one personal representative meeting and 10 marketing lunches per year) reporting attending sponsored events.[119] Similar studies have not been repeated since the PhRMA Code on Interactions with Health Care Professionals took effect in 2009; however, in 2013, it was found that approximately 62% of medical students had been exposed to drug promotions, even prior to medical school.[129]

Studies vary in the degree to which medical residents and students value industry-sponsored information; however, survey responders generally perceive that they do not feel prepared to manage these types of interactions, but that drug promotions would not influence their prescribing habits.[120] One survey of nurse practitioners not only found that this group does not prefer to receive drug information from pharmaceutical-industry sources, but also found that approximately 36% have been offered paybacks in return for changes to prescribing habits.[121] Limited research describes which prescribers are more likely to meet with pharmaceutical industry representatives. One cross-sectional study found that factors of higher prescription volume (coefficient beta [CB] 0.286), rural practice (CB 0.069), and specialization in primary care (CB 0.132) were positively associated with this risk, and having a restrictive policy for representative interactions (CB −0.327), larger practice setting size (CB −0.95), and academic affiliation (CB −0.082) were inversely associated with this risk.[122]

Several studies have assessed effects of detailing and related activities on prescribing patterns. Two studies found increased prescribing and loyalty to brand name prescription medications when physicians were exposed to detailing.[3,22] Similar results were found in a study assessing effectiveness of industry-sponsored continuing education for physicians,[123] although it should be noted that it was conducted prior to publication of current industry guidelines. One systematic review noted that 17 of 29 assessed articles found increased prescribing of a target medication as a result of one-on-one detailing; the remaining studies found no difference in practice.[124] Similarly, five out of eight articles assessing effectiveness of sponsored education events found the expected changes in practice (i.e., increased prescribing of the target medication). A more recent review highlights that most prescribers do not believe that interactions with pharmaceutical industry alter their own prescribing behaviors, but that these interactions alter the prescribing behaviors of others.[109] Finally, a 24-month study of nearly 150,000 physicians confirmed previous findings from smaller studies that detailing, specifically visits from pharmaceutical industry representatives, is very effective at increasing probability of prescribing the marketed brand name drug.[130]

In the inpatient setting, one study found that physicians who request addition of a medication to a formulary are more likely to have accepted payment from industry to attend or lead symposia or to have personally met with industry representatives from the company producing the medication.[125] Payments have been associated with increased prescribing of branded medications in several recent studies involving commonly prescribed classes such as antidiabetic agents, antihypertensive agents, combinations of nonsteroidal anti-inflammatory drugs (NSAIDs) and proton pump inhibitors (PPIs), opioids, and statins,[131–134] although one study of anticancer agents did not detect a relationship between payment and prescribing.[135] Gifts provided by pharmaceutical industry may also influence prescribing.[136] A recent study of Medicare Part D prescribers found increased cost of claims across six medical specialties (dermatology, family medicine, internal medicine, obstetrics/gynecology, ophthalmology, urology), nurse practitioners, and physician assistants and more branded claims for family medicine, ophthalmology, and physician assistants associated with gifts. The value of the gift appeared to be related to the effect. Attendance at industry-sponsored meals has been shown to be related to increased prescribing of the drug of interest over comparable generic medications.[137] Coupons and samples have also been suggested to have significant impact on prescribing habits in theoretical models and experimental studies,[126–128] and have even been proposed as contributing factors in the ongoing opioid epidemic.[138] Overall, evidence suggests that even when pharmaceutical representatives are providing valued services, health care professionals should be wary that samples, payments, and gifts have generally been found to be effective ways to alter medication use practices.

The preponderance of data on the effectiveness of detailing and related activities suggests that all health care professionals should be mindful of their interactions with pharmaceutical industry and critically self-assess how these interactions have impacted their practice, and the role these interactions will be allowed to have on their practice in the future.

COMBATTING MISINFORMATION

⑤ *All health care professionals, including pharmacists, should arm themselves using strategies of information mastery and vigilance for potentially flawed reasoning when interacting with pharmaceutical sales representatives.* Systematic and individual strategies for combatting potential misinformation provided by pharmaceutical industry are discussed in the following sections.

Systematic and individual approaches are needed to ensure that undesired effects of drug promotions to health care professionals are minimized. This need is illustrated by several cases in which the pharmaceutical industry was fined for inappropriate promotion to health care professionals, including cases brought against the manufacturers of olanzapine (Zyprexa®), gabapentin (Neurontin®), and valdecoxib (Bextra®) for off-label promotion and/or lack of fair balance.[139]

A number of systematic strategies are active or have been proposed to decrease the potentially significant effect of promotions on prescribers and pharmacists at local, institutional, and national levels. Several of these strategies are described below:

- **Academic Detailing:** Research has demonstrated the value of structured one–on–one visits between traveling clinicians, or academic detailers, and prescribers in terms of evidence–based prescribing habits and increased use of generic medications.[108] Applications of academic detailing are described later in the chapter.

- Conflict of Interest Policies: Conflict of interest policies have been used in residency programs, colleges of medicine, and health systems in order to decrease the effect of pharmaceutical promotions.[140,141] Many health systems have very specific policies regarding the allowed interactions with industry representatives. The policy may even prohibit such meetings. A major analysis of 19 academic medical centers found that such policies can be effective at reducing prescribing of promoted drugs in favor of nonpromoted drugs (presumably generic medications).[142] Policy areas included restricting gifts and representative access along with active enforcement; eight out of eleven sites that implemented all three elements realized a significant prescribing change.

- Education: Several studies have assessed effectiveness of educational sessions focusing on pharmaceutical industry interactions with medical students and residents.[143-145] Study participants have generally expressed improved knowledge of the pharmaceutical industry and a greater ability to critically assess promotions, and identified potential behaviors they will change as a result of the program (e.g., stop seeing industry representatives).

- National Initiatives: In the United States, OPDP is responsible for reviewing submitted promotional materials, monitoring at professional meetings for inappropriate promotion, and reviewing Internet sites related to prescription medications.[48]

- Representative Tracking: Health systems often use industry credentialing programs to enforce institutional policies regarding content, frequency, and length of meetings between clinicians and industry representatives.[146] These programs allow health systems administrators to know when representatives are on campus and with whom they are meeting.

Additionally, several professional organizations provide guidelines regarding information provided by the pharmaceutical industry. ASHP guides members that a third party should control educational content of all industry-sponsored continuing education.[147] Similarly, AMA recommends physicians select continuing education that is accredited and fair-balanced. Promotional continuing education should be clearly denoted as such.[148] Both organizations counsel members to limit interactions with pharmaceutical industry to professional, scientific exchange of information and to avoid situations in which professional judgment is at risk and impropriety may be perceived.[147,148]

Even in the presence of systematic approaches to preventing misinformation in drug promotions, the need for health care professionals to critically evaluate specific information provided in drug promotions is clear. Considering the volume of medical information emerging every day, the task of analyzing, retaining, and synthesizing this information

TABLE 25–7. EXAMPLE LOGICAL FALLACIES USED IN PHARMACEUTICAL PROMOTION[107]

Fallacy	Description	Example
Appeal to Authority	Appeal to knowledge of a known expert with or without conferring with that expert	"I just spoke with the Head of Surgery who says he used Drug X in nearly every case."
Appeal to Pity	Appeal to the inner desire to "do good" without focusing on evidence	"Patients whom my other prescribers work with have benefited so much from Drug X. It's really been life-changing for them."
Bandwagon Effect	Appeal to popularity with or without confirming if that popularity is true or false	"All the other tertiary medical centers in the city have added Drug X to their formulary."
Red Herring	Including extraneous, irrelevant details in an argument	"In clinical studies, Drug X had a lower rate of headache (2%) compared with Drug Y (3%)."

can be monumental.[149] For this reason, health care professionals must develop skills and confidence in searching the medical literature and practicing evidence-based medicine (i.e., information mastery) using both patient-specific and general approaches (i.e., top down versus bottom up, see Chapter 8). It is recommended that health care professionals preferentially use tertiary drug information resources that are either FDA approved (i.e., the prescribing information) or prepared and published by unbiased sources (e.g., AHFS® Drug Information, IBM Micromedex 2.0). If health care professionals do meet with pharmaceutical industry representatives or use other promotional materials, they should be prepared to rigorously assess pharmaceutical promotions in the same way they would any tertiary resource (see Chapter 3), with extra vigilance considering heightened financial conflict of interest. Additionally, health care professionals should evaluate any print pharmaceutical promotions distributed by industry representatives using strategies similar to DTCA, outlined in Tables 25-4 to 25-6.

Many pharmaceutical industry representatives use flawed logic in order to persuade prescribers and pharmacists that their product is the ideal choice for their patients.[107] Errors in reasoning can introduce self-doubt on the part of the health care professional and increase likelihood of a behavior change. It is important to identify when arguments are logical and when they are irrational. In particular, pharmacists who manage pharmacy and therapeutics committee initiatives should be vigilant in their awareness of flawed logic and misleading messages. One of the best methods for combating logical fallacies is reviewing relevant information prior to interacting with an industry representative. See Table 25-7 for examples of misleading strategies that industry representatives might use. See Table 25-8 for general recommendations for interacting with pharmaceutical industry representatives.

TABLE 25–8. RECOMMENDED PRACTICES FOR INTERACTIONS WITH PHARMACEUTICAL INDUSTRY[148]

- Conduct visits politely and professionally.
- Determine the content of meetings ahead of time.
- Clearly communicate expectations for content and duration of meetings with the representative.
- Prepare for meetings using unbiased tertiary resources and review of primary literature.
- Come prepared with specific questions in mind.
- Use active listening skills.
- Use critical thinking to catch potential errors in reasoning.

Case Study 25–2

As part of your work with the pharmacy and therapeutics committee at an academic, tertiary care hospital, you are asked to conduct monthly meetings with pharmaceutical industry representatives. Your goal for these meetings is to get information about pipeline drugs that are not yet FDA approved.

- *What systems should you ensure are in place prior to scheduling such visits?*
- *What strategies should you use to prepare for visits once you know which representatives will be attending?*
- *What strategies can you use to remain objective during the visits?*

REPORTING INAPPROPRIATE PROMOTIONS

❻ *Health care professionals are encouraged to report advertising and other promotional violations to the FDA's Bad Ad Program.* All health care professionals have a responsibility to report inappropriate drug promotions using the process described below.

Health care professionals, particularly prescribers, are also targets of drug promotion in the form of print advertisements in medical journals.[150,151] One study found that approximately 16% of the pages in one oncology journal were devoted to drug promotion.[150] Advertisements appearing in medical journals are subject to the same standards as other print advertisements discussed earlier in the chapter, as well as ideally be in compliance with a journal's advertising policy. Advertising policies should be robust and available to the reader. Advertisements in these journals should be assessed using the same methods described for DTCA.

The FDA's Bad Ad Program encourages prescribers to report misinforming or incorrect prescription drug advertising and promotion to the FDA.[104] This assists OPDP in identifying and ceasing such advertisements. Advertisements for products such as dietary supplements, medical devices, and nonprescription drugs should not be reported through the Bad Ad Program since OPDP does not regulate the promotion of these products; rather, they should be submitted to the FTC. Due to the inability of FDA employees to be present at all dinner programs, promotional speaker events, and prescribers' offices, the FDA seeks the help of health care professionals to report promotional violations through this program.[152]

If an ad is found to be in violation, the FDA can take enforcement action or continue to monitor additional advertisement activities.[104] Advertising methods that are assessed and can be reported through the Bad Ad Program include: information presented in printed or written drug promotional materials or by sales representatives, presentations by program speakers, as well as advertisements on radio or television.[103,152]

Common violations identified in drug advertisements include: (1) inadequate risk information, including downplaying potential risks; (2) exaggeration of benefits; and (3) false or deceiving comparisons with other medications.[104] Comments to the FDA through the Bad Ad Program can be submitted anonymously; once received, they are analyzed by a member of the OPDP team.[103] The FDA accepts comments from health care professionals via email: BadAd@FDA.gov or by phone: 855-RX-BADAD (855-792-2323).

Case Study 25-3

You have been asked to attend a dinner program sponsored by the pharmaceutical industry. The main goal for you attending the program is to learn about new indications under study for an approved medication.

- *How do you interpret the information being presented at the program?*
- *What are the common violations that can occur in this setting?*
- *How do you report a violation to the FDA?*

ACADEMIC DETAILING

❼ *Academic detailing programs, often led by pharmacists, are designed to combat pharmaceutical industry detailing by providing evidence-based information in the form of one-on-one or small-group interactions between a clinician and prescribers.* The following sections address the design, effectiveness, and roles for pharmacists in academic detailing.

TABLE 25–9.   CORE FUNCTIONS OF AN ACADEMIC DETAILING PROGRAM[108]

- Identify a target therapeutic issue based on local trends (e.g., demographics, endemic disease states, prescriber preference, prescribing patterns).
- Identify a target prescriber population based on specific criteria (e.g., level of experience, prescribing patterns, need for management of drug cost).
- Synthesize the available evidence using strategies discussed in Chapters 2 and 8.
- Provide the synthesized evidence in an engaging small group or one-on-one format using a concise message that can be easily implemented into practice.
- Monitor program using identified metrics related to scope (e.g., quantity and quality of visits) and effectiveness (e.g., generic vs. brand prescribing, therapeutic area-specific issues).
- Develop relationships with prescribers by increasing communication and face time.

Definition

Academic detailing, also known as counterdetailing, prescriber outreach, and prescriber support and education, is a proactive approach developed to combat proliferation of potentially biased information provided by pharmaceutical sales representatives in prescriber workplaces.[108,153] The goal of academic detailing is to provide objective, scientific evidence to prescribers in order to improve patient outcomes. While originally focused on increasing use of generic medications when the practice emerged in the 1980s, today's academic detailing programs have expanded clinical roles including promotion of evidence-based medicine and dissemination of comparative effectiveness research. Although most commonly associated with outpatient settings, academic detailing programs have also been reported in inpatient and long-term care practices.[154,155] Pharmaceutical and academic detailing are similar, in that both are designed to change prescribing behavior.[108,153,156]

Designing an Academic Detailing Program

The core process of an academic detailing program is outlined in Table 25-9.[153,154] At its heart is a one-on-one, face-to-face interaction between a traveling health care professional (e.g., physician, pharmacist, nurse) and a prescriber.[108,153,156] The academic detailer may also have a concurrent academic or clinical appointment.[153] While the original format for these interactions—intended to be engaging and interpersonal—was inspired by the success of pharmaceutical detailing, a key difference is that academic detailing is intended to focus purely on evidence-based information without a promotional perspective.[108,153,156] Individuals providing academic detailing should have knowledge of clinical and information sciences as well as experience in providing direct patient care.[153] Interactions between the detailer and prescriber should be nonjudgmental, empathetic, and professional. Although there are examples of peer academic detailing, where fellow prescribers lead the initiative and provide the information,[157,158] most programs are led by or largely rely on pharmacists.

The most accepted goal of academic detailing is promotion of rational prescribing and increasing transparency by providing scientific information regarding medication efficacy, safety, and effectiveness.[108,153] One somewhat controversial aspect of academic detailing is whether improving cost-savings-related outcomes should also be a core function of these initiatives.[153] Programs are occasionally accused of allowing pursuit of cost savings to supersede promotion of evidence-based medicine. While simply encouraging use of generic medications in place of branded product is a generally accepted aim, therapeutic substitution of a different medication in the same class is a more divisive issue. Differences in philosophy may vary depending on the organization sponsoring the program; for-profit, third party, and government organizations may be more likely than academic groups to acknowledge a cost-savings goal.[108,153,156] As the field of academic detailing continues to evolve, new audiences such as community pharmacists have been proposed as potential recipients of this outreach.[159]

Key elements have been agreed upon by experts as critical for success of an academic detailing program.[160] Preferred detailers include physicians and pharmacists, and these individuals should be well trained in topics related to adult education, behavior change, and communication skills, as well as the clinical content. Providers should be selected based on geographic area and, ideally, their own practice patterns, with the patient population and setting important as well. The educational content, including best practices and input from opinion leaders, is the foundation of a program, but interventions should also provide specific feedback and recommendations for practice change as well as provide decision support tools and follow-up. The provided information should address the challenges of implementing the targeted behavior. Patient outcomes and clinician metrics should be used to evaluate success of the program.

Examples of Academic Detailing Program

For-profit, nonprofit, government, and academic organizations are all known to sponsor academic detailing programs.[108,153–156,161,162] Many of the most successful programs are collaborations among multiple groups. Large-scale academic detailing has been conducted by several Canadian provinces and at a national level in Australia; several states in the United States are considering or have developed programs modeled after the success of programs in these countries (where large-scale academic detailing has a much longer history).[153] One of the most well-known academic detailing programs in the United States is the Independent Drug Information Service (iDiS), a program of Alosa Health that is supported by the Pennsylvania Department of Aging's Pharmaceutical Contract for the Elderly (PACE) program and The Vermont Health Care Association and Vermont Department of Disabilities, Aging, and Independent Living.[163] This program spends approximately $600 million annually to provide medication to over 300,000 elderly patients who are ineligible for Medicaid.[153,161,163] PACE reports that cost savings generated from improving prescribing of common chronic medications (e.g., antihypertensives, anti-inflammatories) more than cover the costs of this program.[153] The content for iDiS visits is developed by an independent group of physicians, the National Resource Center for Academic Detailing (NaRCAD), located at Harvard Medical School and Brigham and Women's Hospital.[108]

Another example of an American academic detailing collaboration is the South Carolina Medicaid Academic Detailing Program (SCORxE), a collaboration of the South Carolina Department of Health and Human Services and the South Carolina College of Pharmacy.[153,162] This program focuses on providing pharmacist-led academic detailing with prescribers who provide care for rural and urban Medicaid patients, primarily on mental health topics.[164] The programming is provided by full-time pharmacists across 18 counties, with support from the Medical University of South Carolina Drug Information Center.

The U.S. Veterans Administration (VA) piloted and fully implemented an academic detailing program led by pharmacists.[165] Although the program was originally designed to focus on improving evidence-based treatment of mental illness, it has since expanded into other areas. Key components of this service include identification of focused areas for prescribing improvement based on evidence from medical records, development of educational materials and programming centered on key messages, use of informatics tools, such as clinical decision support, to further promote the key messages, and collaboration with prescribers to remove barriers to best practices.

Nationally, leadership in the area of academic detailing comes from NaRCAD, an Agency for Healthcare Research and Quality (AHRQ)-supported initiative.[108] NaRCAD collaborates with states and private organizations to determine their specific needs in an academic detailing program, based on local medication use.[108,153] Additionally, the service translates important comparative effectiveness research into usable tools, conducts education on academic detailing best practices and implementation, and helps organizations develop an assessment plan for their programs.[108] A final key role of NaRCAD is enlarging the network of organizations providing academic detailing in order to encourage information exchange.

Case Study 25–4

As part of your work in a managed care setting, you are asked to develop an academic detailing program designed to improve safety, efficacy, and cost-effectiveness of prescribing in an area of psychiatry.

- *How would you go about determining on which class of medications or disease state to focus?*

- *How would you develop your clinical materials? With which external organizations could you partner?*

- *Would you take a one-on-one or group approach to academic detailing? Discuss why you selected the strategy you did.*

- *What metrics could you assess to determine the effectiveness of your program?*

Effectiveness of Academic Detailing

The effectiveness of academic detailing was first established in a seminal randomized, controlled trial, published in 1983, that identified a 14% improvement in achieving the specific prescribing goals of reducing use of propoxyphene, cerebral and peripheral vasodilators, and cephalexin in favor of more appropriate alternatives.[166] While theoretical and observational data suggest huge potential for improvement in clinical and economic outcomes from academic detailing programs,[167,168] results from prospective, interventional studies assessing effectiveness of academic detailing programs have been mixed.[153,155,166,169–173] The nationwide academic detailing program in Australia demonstrated significant cost-effectiveness; however, less public information is available regarding tangible cost savings of such programs in the United States.[168] One early analysis (published in 1986) suggests that academic detailing provided by a pharmacist to small groups of physicians would result in average annual net savings of approximately $1,000,000 per 10,000 physicians.[168] From a clinical perspective, some individual programs have demonstrated both improved prescribing practices in addition to some cost savings in areas such as control of vasodilator use, adherence to hypertension clinical practice guidelines, statin prescribing, smoking cessation, oral diabetic selection, reducing inappropriate antibiotic prescribing, and evidence-based treatment of gastrointestinal reflux disease (GERD) and related disorders.[155,166,169,170,174–178] Conversely, some studies have had only marginal clinical and economic results.[171,172] Academic detailing has also been impactful for improving benzodiazepine use[179,180] and avoiding specific drug-drug interactions.[181]

In recent years, the focus of published academic detailing evaluations has largely shifted from specific, single-medication interventions only (although such initiatives still exist) to more disease or population-based initiatives. A large number of studies have been recently published suggesting academic detailing can meaningfully improve geriatric prescribing in accordance with Beers Criteria and other standards.[182–185] Antimicrobial agents have also been increasingly studied, with academic detailing found to be effective in improving management of specific infectious diseases or as a component of antimicrobial stewardship.[186–189] Clinical practice guideline-based programs in diverse areas such as alcohol use disorder, pain management, and acute kidney injury have also been found to be impactful.[190–192]

Recent years have also seen academic detailing proposed as a solution to public health challenges, including the opioid epidemic and improving vaccination rates. Academic detailing has been found to be effective for improving naloxone awareness (by both prescribers and patients), distribution, and use.[193–196] It also has been shown to impact opioid use by improving concordance with evidence-based best practices for dosing, duration, and drug selection[197]; promoting judicious use in the postpartum setting[198]; and improving awareness and use of a state prescription drug monitoring program.[199] Academic detailing has been shown to improve nurses' perceptions of vaccinations[200] and rates of pneumococcal vaccination.[201]

Most published studies of academic detailing have limited generalizability due to conduct within a specific HMO or institution, and interventions performed by a low number of individuals; however, these same limitations could signal good internal validity of individual programs and customizing based on local need, a key principle of academic detailing.[108,155,166,169–175,177,178] Another concern regarding effectiveness of academic detailing is that the resources dedicated to these programs are much less than the resources dedicated toward pharmaceutical detailing on the part of industry.[153,167] Meta-analyses of academic detailing studies found a consistent, small-to-moderate benefit in terms of changes in targeted practice behavior, but did not assess pharmacoeconomic outcomes.[202,203]

Viewpoints

Recent studies have evaluated physician and nurse practitioner viewpoints and impressions of the role of academic detailing in their practice.[204–211] In general, academic detailing provided by pharmacists and other personnel (e.g., physicians, nurses, scientists) appears to be generally (although not universally) well-received by prescriber audiences.[205,206,208,209,211] In particular, academic detailing appears to be well-viewed in related practice areas that include geriatrics, long-term care, and psychiatry, as well as by general practitioners. Peer academic detailing from colleague prescribers was also highly regarded in one evaluation.[204] Qualitative research has suggested challenges to academic detailing may include higher complexity in practice compared to guideline-based recommendations as well as conflict between individual experience and recommended best practices.[210] Prescribers may also perceive academic detailing and related initiatives as a challenge to practice autonomy. Academic detailing is best perceived when it is delivered in a constructive, positive manner[205] and is accompanied by high-quality, evidence-based materials distributed to prescribers.[204]

Pharmacist's Role in Academic Detailing

With their strong academic background in drug information and drug literature evaluation, pharmacists can be ideally positioned to engage in academic detailing.[108,153] Indeed, many of the academic detailing programs described in clinical literature and the media are centered around a team of pharmacists.[153,156,166,172,173] Pharmacists with postgraduate training in drug information may be particularly well-equipped for these types of positions as a result of their special skills in drug information service management, evidence-based medicine, and communications.[212] Pharmacists seeking to engage in academic detailing should critically assess local demographics and prescribing patterns in order to identify a specific detailing target, network and collaborate with established programs through organizations such as NaRCAD and local key stakeholders, and strive to build strong interpersonal relationships with target prescribers. Finally, as with any novel clinical service, identifying and monitoring key metrics is vital to justify direct and indirect costs of the program.

Conclusion

Drug promotion, including DTCA and promotion to health care professionals, represents significant expenditure on the part of pharmaceutical industry. The controversial issues surrounding DTCA and off-label promotion, in particular, continue to raise concerns about the benefits and harms of providing this type of information to patients. Detailing and direct advertisement to health care professionals continues to be an effective method of promotion. FDA calls on health care professionals to play a key role in reporting drug promotion violations related to advertising, detailing, and continuing education. As drug promotional methods evolve, pharmacists will continue to serve both health care professionals and the public as a valuable source in deciphering and evaluating materials distributed by pharmaceutical industry. Academic detailing may be one avenue for drug information specialists and other health care professionals to combat the influence of drug promotions on prescribing.

Self-Assessment Questions

1. Which of the following has been reported as a result of drug promotions?
   a. Increased generic drug usage
   b. Decreased pharmaceutical company profits

  c. Decreased inappropriate prescribing

  d. Increased brand drug usage

2. World Health Organization (WHO) recommendations for DTCA include which of the following?

  a. Utilizing fearful language or tactics

  b. Marketing nonprescription treatments

  c. Marketing prescription treatments

  d. Incorporating off-label indications

3. The Food and Drug Administration Amendments Act (FDAAA):

  a. Required the MedWatch reporting statement to be included on printed advertisements

  b. Eliminated the requirement for the brief summary on television advertisements

  c. Gave the FDA authority over prescription drug advertising

  d. Required printed advertisements to include the entire prescribing information

4. Which government agency regulates reminder advertisements?

  a. FTC

  b. FDA

  c. DEA

  d. USP

5. Which of the following advertisements are created with the assumption that patients are already familiar with the drug's indication?

  a. Reminder

  b. Help-seeking

  c. Product claim

  d. Academic detailing

6. For which of the following is the FDA considering changing the requirements to limit presented risk information to only serious or life-threatening risks accompanied by a disclosure statement?

  a. Substantial evidence

  b. Fair balance

  c. Brief summary

  d. Major statement

7. Which of the following was to be incorporated into television advertisements as of July 2019, prior to a court ruling?

  a. Onset of action

  b. Generic availability

    c. List price

    d. Mechanism of action

8. Which of the following advertisements are acceptable according to the PhRMA Guiding Principles for DTCA?

    a. A new cholesterol drug television advertisement that refers patients to a website detailing the potential cost

    b. A Tourette's syndrome drug television advertisement that portrays patients as little monsters

    c. An obesity drug printed advertisement that excludes diet and exercise as adjunctive therapy

    d. An erectile dysfunction drug television advertisement being aired during Saturday morning cartoons

9. If a DTCA has created a severe threat to public health, the FDA has the authority to:

    a. Ban the company from producing DTCA

    b. Levy fines against the company

    c. Request the company to publish a correction

    d. The FDA does not have the authority to act against the company

10. Due to concerns regarding increased health care costs, which of the following organizations called for a ban of DTCA?

    a. American Society of Health System Pharmacists (ASHP) House of Delegates

    b. American Public Health Association

    c. American Medical Association (AMA)

    d. All of the above

11. A pharmaceutical representative is permitted to provide off-label information regarding use of prescription medications when responding to an unsolicited request from a health care professional.

    a. True

    b. False

12. The primary goal of pharmaceutical detailing is to:

    a. Decrease use of brand medications.

    b. Promote evidence-based prescribing.

    c. Provide cost savings to third-party payers.

    d. Sell a product.

13. The strawman logical fallacy refers to:

    a. Bandwagon effect

b. Making the discussion personal

c. Providing distracting, unrelated detail

d. Referencing local content experts

14. The primary goal of academic detailing is to:
    a. Decrease use of brand medications.
    b. Promote evidence-based prescribing.
    c. Provide cost savings to third-party payers.
    d. Sell a product.

15. Academic detailing programs in the United States have been shown to do each of the following EXCEPT:
    a. Achieve the desired change in prescribing behavior
    b. Achieve national improvements in economic outcomes
    c. Improve the rate of evidence-based prescribing
    d. Increase generic drug utilization

REFERENCES

1. Brownfield ED, Bernhardt JM, Phan JL, Williams MV, Parker RM. Direct-to-consumer drug advertisements on network television: an exploration of quantity, frequency, and placement. J Health Commun. 2004;9(6):491-7.

2. Greene JA, Herzberg D. Hidden in plain sight marketing prescription drugs to consumers in the twentieth century. Am J Public Health. 2010;100(5):793-803. doi:10.2105/AJPH.2009.181255.

3. Hansen RA, Chen S-Y, Gaynes BN, Maciejewski ML. Relationship of pharmaceutical promotion to antidepressant switching and adherence: a retrospective cohort study. Psychiatr Serv. 2010;61(12):1232-8. doi:10.1176/appi.ps.61.12.1232.

4. Law MR, Soumerai SB, Adams AS, Majumdar SR. Costs and consequences of direct-to-consumer advertising for clopidogrel in medicaid. Arch Intern Med. 2009;169(21):1969-74. doi:10.1001/archinternmed.2009.320.

5. Mintzes B. Advertising of prescription-only medicines to the public: does evidence of benefit counterbalance harm? Annu Rev Public Health. 2012;33:259-77. doi:10.1146/annurev-publhealth-031811-124540.

6. Norris P HA, Lexchin J, Mansfield P. Drug promotion—what we know, what we have yet to learn—reviews of materials in the WHO/HAI database on drug promotion. EDM research series no. 032 [Internet]. World Health Organization and Health Action International; 2005 [cited 2020 Mar 12]. Available from: http://apps.who.int/medicinedocs/pdf/s8109e/s8109e.pdf

7. Ross JS, Kravitz RL. Direct-to-consumer television advertising: time to turn off the tube? J Gen Intern Med. 2013;28(7):862-4. doi:10.1007/s11606-013-2424-2. PubMed PMID: 23539285.

8. Ventola CL. Direct-to-consumer pharmaceutical advertising: therapeutic or toxic? P T. 2011;36(10):669-84.

9. Womack CA. Ethical and epistemic issues in direct-to-consumer drug advertising: where is patient agency? Med Health Care Philos. 2013;16(2):275-80. doi:10.1007/s11019-012-9386-8.

10. Vastag B. FDA considers tightening regulations for direct-to-consumer advertising. J Natl Cancer Inst. 2005;97(24):1806-7.

11. Schwartz LM, Woloshin S. Medical marketing in the United States, 1997-2016. JAMA. 2019;321(1):80-96. doi:10.1001/jama.2018.19320.

12. Marketing Fact Pack 2019 [Internet]. AdAge; 2018 Dec 17 [cited 2020 Mar 6]. Available from: http://adage.com/d/resources/resources/whitepaper/marketing-fact-pack-2019?utm_source=AA1&utm_medium=AA&utm_campaign=AA

13. Othman N, Vitry A, Roughead EE. Quality of pharmaceutical advertisements in medical journals: a systematic review. PLoS One. 2009;4(7):e6350. doi:10.1371/journal.pone.0006350.

14. From the manufacturers' mouth to your ears: direct to consumer advertising [Internet]. Silver Spring (MD): U.S. Food and Drug Administration; [updated 2015 Dec 23; cited 2020 Mar 12]. Available from: https://www.fda.gov/drugs/special-features/manufacturers-mouth-your-ears-direct-consumer-advertising

15. Sullivan HW, Aikin KJ, Chung-Davies E, Wade M. Prescription drug promotion from 2001-2014: data from the U.S. Food and Drug Administration. PLoS One. 2016;11(5):e0155035. doi:10.1371/journal.pone.0155035.

16. Ethical criteria for medical drug promotion [Internet]. Geneva: World Health Organization; 1988 [cited 2020 Mar 12]. Available from: http://apps.who.int/medicinedocs/documents/whozip08e/whozip08e.pdf

17. Kim H. Trouble spots in online direct-to-consumer prescription drug promotion: a content analysis of FDA warning letters. Int J Health Policy Manag. 2015;4(12):813-21. doi:10.15171/ijhpm.2015.157.

18. PhRMA guiding principles direct to consumer advertisements about prescription medicines [Internet]. Washington (DC): Pharmaceutical Research and Manufacturers of America (PhRMA); [updated 2018 Dec; cited 2020 Mar 12]. Available from: http://phrma-docs.phrma.org/files/dmfile/PhRMA_Guiding_Principles_2018.pdf

19. Fogel J, Adnan M. Trust for pharmaceutical company direct-to-consumer prescription medication advertisements. Health Policy Technol. 2018;7(1):26-34. doi:10.1016/j.hlpt.2018.01.002.

20. Babar Z-U-D, Siraj AM, Curley L. A review of DTCA techniques: appraising their success and potential impact on medication users. Res Social Adm Pharm. 2018;14(3):218-27. doi:10.1016/j.sapharm.2017.04.005.

21. Tyrawski J, DeAndrea DC. Pharmaceutical companies and their drugs on social media: a content analysis of drug information on popular social media sites. J Med Internet Res. 2015;17(6):e130. doi:10.2196/jmir.4357.

22. Dorn SD, Farley JF, Hansen RA, Shah ND, Sandler RS. Direct-to-consumer and physician promotion of tegaserod correlated with physician visits, diagnoses, and prescriptions. Gastroenterology. 2009;137(2):518. doi:10.1053/j.gastro.2009.05.005.

23. Chang H-Y, Murimi I, Daubresse M, Qato DM, Emery SL, Alexander GC. Effect of direct-to-consumer advertising on statin use in the United States. Med Care. 2017;55(8):759-64. doi:10.1097/MLR.0000000000000752.

24. Daubresse M, Hutfless S, Kim Y, Kornfield R, Qato DM, Huang J, Miller K, Emery SL, Alexander GC. Effect of direct-to-consumer advertising on asthma medication sales and health-care use. Am J Respir Crit Care Med. 2015;192(1):40-6. doi:10.1164/rccm.201409-1585OC.

25. Khalil Zadeh N, Robertson K, Green JA. "At-risk" individuals' responses to direct to consumer advertising of prescription drugs: a nationally representative cross-sectional study. BMJ Open. 2017;7(12):e017865. doi:10.1136/bmjopen-2017-017865.

26. Staton T. Pharma's ad spend vaults to $4.5b, with big spender Pfizer leading the way [Internet]. Framingham (MA): FiercePharma; 2015 Mar 25 [cited 2020 Mar 12]. Available from: https://www.fiercepharma.com/dtc-advertising/pharma-s-ad-spend-vaults-to-4-5b-big-spender-pfizer-leading-way

27. DeFrank JT, Berkman ND, Kahwati L, Cullen K, Aikin KJ, Sullivan HW. Direct-to-consumer advertising of prescription drugs and the patient-prescriber encounter: a systematic review. Health Commun. 2019:1-8. doi:10.1080/10410236.2019.1584781.

28. Mackey TK, Cuomo RE, Liang BA. The rise of digital direct-to-consumer advertising?: Comparison of direct-to-consumer advertising expenditure trends from publicly available data sources and global policy implications. BMC Health Serv Res. 2015;15:236. doi:10.1186/s12913-015-0885-1.

29. Bulik BS. In another record year for pharma TV advertisements, spending soars to $3.7B in 2018 [Internet]. Framingham (MA): FiercePharma; 2019 Jan 2 [cited 2020 Mar 12]. Available from: https://www.fiercepharma.com/marketing/another-record-year-for-pharma-tv-ads-spending-tops-3-7-billion-2018

30. Basics of drug ads [Internet]. Silver Spring (MD): U.S. Food and Drug Administration; [updated 2015 Jun 19; cited 2020 Mar 12]. Available from: https://www.fda.gov/drugs/prescription-drug-advertising/basics-drug-ads

31. Correct help-seeking ad [Internet]. Silver Spring (MD): U.S. Food and Drug Administration; [updated 2015 Dec 23; cited 2020 Mar 12]. Available from: https://www.fda.gov/drugs/prescription-drug-advertising/correct-help-seeking-ad

32. Mailankody S, Prasad V. Pharmaceutical marketing for rare diseases: regulating drug company promotion in an era of unprecedented advertisement. JAMA. 2017;317(24):2479-80. doi:10.1001/jama.2017.5784.

33. Jakafi. Wilmington (DE): Incyte Corporation; 2019 May. Package insert. NDC 50881-005-60, 50881-010-60, 50881-015-60, 50881-020-60, 50881-025-60.

34. Frosch DL, Krueger PM, Hornik RC, Cronholm PF, Barg FK. Creating demand for prescription drugs: a content analysis of television direct-to-consumer advertising. Ann Fam Med. 2007;5(1):6-13.

35. Reminder ad (correct) [Internet]. Silver Spring (MD): U.S. Food and Drug Administration; [updated 2015 Dec 23; cited 2020 Mar 12]. Available from: https://www.fda.gov/drugs/prescription-drug-advertising/reminder-ad-correct

36. Sumpradit N, Ascione FJ, Bagozzi RP. A cross-media content analysis of motivational themes in direct-to-consumer prescription drug advertising. Clin Ther. 2004;26(1):135-54.

37. Prescription drug advertising: questions and answers [Internet]. Silver Spring (MD): U.S. Food and Drug Administration; [updated 2015 Jun 19; cited 2020 Mar 12]. Available from: https://www.fda.gov/drugs/prescription-drug-advertising/prescription-drug-advertising-questions-and-answers

38. Rosenberg BD, Siegel JT. The effect of inconsistency appeals on the influence of direct-to-consumer prescription drug advertisements: an application of goal disruption theory. J Health Commun. 2016;21(2):217-27. doi:10.1080/10810730.2015.1058439.

39. Bhutada NS, Rollins BL, Perri M3rd. Impact of animated spokes-characters in print direct-to-consumer prescription drug advertising: an elaboration likelihood model approach. Health Commun. 2017;32(4):391-400. doi:10.1080/10410236.2016.1138382.

40. Lexchin J, Mintzes B. A compromise too far: a review of Canadian cases of direct-to-consumer advertising regulation. Int J Risk Saf Med. 2014;26(4):213-25. doi:10.3233/JRS-140635.

41. Kefauver-Harris Amendments revolutionized drug development [Internet]. Silver Spring (MD): U.S. Food and Drug Administration; [updated 2012 Sep 10; cited 2020 Mar 12]. Available from: https://www.fda.gov/consumers/consumer-updates/kefauver-harris-amendments-revolutionized-drug-development?source=govdelivery

42. The impact of direct-to-consumer advertising [Internet]. Silver Spring (MD): U.S. Food and Drug Administration; [updated 2015 Oct 23; cited 2020 Mar 12]. Available from: https://www.fda.gov/drugs/drug-information-consumers/impact-direct-consumer-advertising

43. e-CFR-code of federal regulations title 21: Part 202—prescription drug advertising [Internet]. Washington (DC): U.S. Government Publishing Office; [updated 2020 Mar 10; cited 2020 Mar 12]. Available from: https://www.ecfr.gov/cgi-bin/text-idx?SID=e03ec42d255dc5f1f9eb7eaf605bca2f&mc=true&node=pt21.4.202&rgn=div5

44. Bulik B. Pharmaceutical marketing [Internet]. Chicago (IL): Ad Age; 2011 Oct 17 [cited 2020 Mar 12]. Available from: https://adage.com/trend-reports/report.php?id=55

45. Product claim ad (correct) [Internet]. Silver Spring (MD): U.S. Food and Drug Administration; [updated 2015 Dec 23; cited 2020 Mar 12]. Available from: https://www.fda.gov/drugs/prescription-drug-advertising/product-claim-ad-correct

46. Kux L. Content of risk information in the major statement in prescription drug direct-to-consumer broadcast advertisements; establishment of a public docket; request for information and comments. Silver Spring (MD): Food and Drug Administration, Department of Health and Human Services; 2017 Aug 15. FR Doc. 2017-17563.

47. Betts KR, Boudewyns V, Aikin KJ, Squire C, Dolina S, Hayes JJ, Southwell BG. Serious and actionable risks, plus disclosure: investigating an alternative approach for presenting risk information in prescription drug television advertisements. Res Social Adm Pharm. 2018;14(10):951-63. doi:10.1016/j.sapharm.2017.07.015.

48. The Office of Prescription Drug Promotion (OPDP) [Internet]. Silver Spring (MD): U.S. Food and Drug Administration; [updated 2020 Feb 3; cited 2020 Mar 12]. Available from: https://www.fda.gov/about-fda/center-drug-evaluation-and-research/office-prescription-drug-promotion-opdp

49. O'Donoghue AC, Sullivan HW, Williams PA, Squire C, Betts KR, Fitts Willoughby J, Parvanta S. Consumers' understanding of FDA approval requirements and composite scores in direct-to-consumer prescription drug print ads. J Health Commun. 2016;21(8):927-34. doi:10.1080/10810730.2016.1179367.

50. Warning letters and notice of violation letters to pharmaceutical companies [Internet]. Silver Spring (MD): U.S. Food and Drug Administration; [updated 2019 May 10; cited 2020 Mar 12]. Available from: https://www.fda.gov/drugs/enforcement-activities-fda/warning-letters-and-notice-violation-letters-pharmaceutical-companies

51. Aikin KJ, Southwell BG, Paquin RS, Rupert DJ, O'Donoghue AC, Betts KR, Lee PK. Correction of misleading information in prescription drug television advertising: the roles of advertisement similarity and time delay. Res Social Adm Pharm. 2017;13(2):378-88. doi:10.1016/j.sapharm.2016.04.004.

52. Warning Letters 2015 [Internet]. Silver Spring (MD): U.S. Food and Drug Administration; [updated 2018 Jan 30; cited 2020 Mar 9]. Available from: https://www.fda.gov/drugs/warning-letters-and-notice-violation-letters-pharmaceutical-companies/warning-letters-2015

53. Warning Letters 2016 [Internet]. Silver Spring (MD): U.S. Food and Drug Administration; [updated 2018 Jan 30; cited 2020 Mar 9]. Available from: https://www.fda.gov/drugs/warning-letters-and-notice-violation-letters-pharmaceutical-companies/warning-letters-2016

54. Warning Letters 2017 [Internet]. Silver Spring (MD): U.S. Food and Drug Administration; [updated 2019 Jun 7; cited 2020 Mar 9]. Available from: https://www.fda.gov/drugs/warning-letters-and-notice-violation-letters-pharmaceutical-companies/warning-letters-2017

55. Warning Letters 2018 [Internet]. Silver Spring (MD): U.S. Food and Drug Administration; [updated 2020 Jan 8; cited 2020 Mar 9]. Available from: https://www.fda.gov/drugs/warning-letters-and-notice-violation-letters-pharmaceutical-companies/warning-letters-2018

56. Warning Letters 2019 [Internet]. Silver Spring (MD): U.S. Food and Drug Administration; [updated 2020 Feb 10; cited 2020 Mar 9]. Available from: https://www.fda.gov/drugs/warning-letters-and-notice-violation-letters-pharmaceutical-companies/warning-letters-2019

57. Kapczynski A. Free speech and pharmaceutical regulation—fishy business. JAMA Intern Med. 2016;176(3):295-6. doi:10.1001/jamainternmed.2015.8155.

58. Schwartz LM, Woloshin S, Lu Z, Ross KM, Tessema FA, Peter D, Kesselheim AS. Randomized study of providing evidence context to mitigate physician misinterpretation arising from off-label drug promotion. Circ Cardiovasc Qual Outcomes. 2019;12(11):e006073. doi:10.1161/CIRCOUTCOMES.119.006073.

59. Warning Letter ANDA 040776 Procentra [Internet]. Silver Spring (MD): U.S. Food and Drug Administration; 2020 Feb 21 [cited 2020 Mar 10]. Available from: https://www.fda.gov/media/135684/download

60. Yang YT, Chen B. Legal considerations for social media marketing by pharmaceutical industry. Food Drug Law J. 2014;69(1):39.

61. Sullivan HW, O'Donoghue AC, Rupert DJ, Willoughby JF, Aikin KJ. Placement and format of risk information on direct-to-consumer prescription drug websites. J Health Commun. 2017;22(2):171-81. doi:10.1080/10810730.2016.1258745.

62. Guidance for industry internet/social media platforms with character space limitations—presenting risk and benefit information for prescription drugs and medical devices [Internet]. Silver Spring (MD): U.S. Food and Drug Administration; 2014 Jun [cited 202 Mar 12]. Available from: https://www.fda.gov/media/88551/download

63. Tan ASL. Potential spillover educational effects of cancer-related direct-to-consumer advertising on cancer patients' increased information seeking behaviors: results from a cohort study. J Cancer Educ. 2014;29(2):258-65. doi:10.1007/s13187-013-0588-4.

64. Adams C. Direct-to-consumer advertising of prescription drugs can inform the public and improve health. JAMA Oncol. 2016;2(11):1395-6. doi:10.1001/jamaoncol.2016.2443.

65. Park JS. Direct-to-consumer prescription medicine advertising and seniors' knowledge of Alzheimer's Disease. Am J Alzheimers Dis Other Demen. 2016;31(1):40-47. doi:10.1177/1533317514550330.

66. Jiang P. Asking a doctor versus referring to the Internet: a comparison study on consumers' reactions to DTC (direct-to-consumer) prescription drug advertising. Health Mark Q. 2018;35(3):209-26. doi:10.1080/07359683.2018.1514735.

67. Corrigan PW, Kosyluk KA, Fokuo JK, Park JH. How does direct to consumer advertising affect the stigma of mental illness? Community Ment Health J. 2014;50(7):792-9. doi:10.1007/s10597-014-9698-7.

68. Rainone N, Oodal R, Niederdeppe J. The (surprising) impact of televised antidepressant direct-to-consumer advertising on the stigmatization of mental illness. Community Ment Health J. 2018;54(3):267-75. doi:10.1007/s10597-017-0164-1.

69. Bhutada NS, Rollins BL. Disease-specific direct-to-consumer advertising for reminding consumers to take medications. J Am Pharm Assoc. 2015;55(4):434-7. doi:10.1331/JAPhA.2015.14234.

70. Klara K, Kim J, Ross JS. Direct-to-consumer broadcast advertisements for pharmaceuticals: off-label promotion and adherence to FDA guidelines. J Gen Intern Med. 2018;33(5):651-8. doi:10.1007/s11606-017-4274-9.

71. Fahim G, Toscani M, Barone JA, Wang C, Gandhi S. Evaluation of risk versus benefit information in direct-to-consumer (DTC) prescription drug television advertisements. Ther Innov Regul Sci. 2018;52(1):114-7. doi:10.1177/2168479017716719.

72. Schnipper LE, Abel GA. Direct-to-consumer drug advertising in oncology is not beneficial to patients or public health. JAMA Oncol. 2016;2(11):1397-8. doi:10.1001/jamaoncol.2016.2463.

73. Schnipper LE. Direct-to-consumer advertising of cancer treatments. Clin Adv Hematol Oncol. 2017;15(10):748-50.

74. Green CE, Mojtabai R, Cullen BA, Spivak A, Mitchell M, Spivak S. Exposure to direct-to-consumer pharmaceutical advertising and medication nonadherence among patients

with serious mental illness. Psychiatr Ser. 2017;68(12):1299-1302. doi:10.1176/appi. ps.201700035.

75. Lexchin J. Statistics in drug advertising: what they reveal is suggestive what they hide is vital. Int J Clin Pract. 2010;64(8):1015-8. doi:10.1111/j.1742-1241.2010.02398.x.

76. Filipova AA. Direct-to-consumer advertising effects on nurse-patient relationship, authority, and prescribing appropriateness. Nurs Ethics. 2018;25(7):823-40. doi:10.1177/ 0969733016679469.

77. Becker SJ, Midoun MM. Effects of direct-to-consumer advertising on patient prescription requests and physician prescribing: a systematic review of psychiatry-relevant studies. J Clin Psychiatry. 2016;77(10):e1293-1300. doi:10.4088/JCP.15r10325.

78. Brown JL. Physician exposure to direct-to-consumer pharmaceutical marketing: potential for creating prescribing bias. Am J Med. 2017;130(6):e247-8. doi:10.1016/j. amjmed.2016.12.023.

79. Collier R. Pushback on drug ads. CMAJ. 2016;188(3):176. doi:10.1503/cmaj.109-5223.

80. Jue JS, Ramasamy R. Re: Association between direct-to-consumer advertising and testosterone testing and initiation in the United States, 2009-2013. Eur Urol. 2017;72(5):853. doi:10.1016/j.eururo.2017.08.032.

81. Shiel WC. Medical definition of me-too drug [Internet]. MedicineNet; 2018 Dec 21 [cited 2020 Mar 10]. Available from: https://www.medicinenet.com/what_not_to_eat_when_ pregnant_pictures_slideshow/article.htm

82. Hansen RA, Shaheen NJ, Schommer JC. Factors influencing the shift of patients from one proton pump inhibitor to another: the effect of direct-to-consumer advertising. Clin Ther. 2005;27(9):1478-87. doi:10.1016/j.clinthera.2005.09.006.

83. AMA calls for ban on DTC ads of prescription drugs and medical devices [Internet]. American Medical Association; 2015 Nov 17 [cited 2020 Mar 12]. Available from: https:// www.ama-assn.org/press-center/press-releases/ama-calls-ban-dtc-ads-prescription- drugs-and-medical-devices

84. Press release: pharmacist association calls for ban on prescription drug advertising [Internet]. Bethesda (MD): American Society of Health-System Pharmacists; 2016 Jun 14 [cited 2020 Mar 12]. Available from: https://www.ashp.org/news/2016/06/14/ pharmacist_association_calls_for_ban_on_prescription_drug_advertising#

85. Kuzucan A, Doshi P, Zito JM. Pharmacists can help to end direct-to-consumer advertising. Am J Health-Syst Pharm. 2017;74(10):640-2. doi:10.2146/ajhp160927.

86. Eisai Inc. Launches National Television Advertising Campaign for BELVIQ® (lorcaserin HCl) CIV [Internet]. BioSpace; 2014 Apr 14 [cited 2020 Mar 10]. Available from: https:// www.biospace.com/article/releases/eisai-inc-launches-national-television-advertising- campaign-for-belviq-and-0174-lorcaserin-hcl-civ-/

87. FDA requests the withdrawal of the weight-loss drug Belviq, Belviq XR (lorcaserin) from the market [Internet]. Silver Spring (MD): U.S. Food and Drug Administration; 2020 Feb 13 [cited 2020 Mar 10]. Available from: https://www.fda.gov/drugs/drug-safety-and- availability/fda-requests-withdrawal-weight-loss-drug-belviq-belviq-xr-lorcaserin-market

88. Leonardo Alves T, Poplavska E, Mezinska S, Salmane-Kulikovska I, Andersone L, Mantel-Teeuwisse AK, Mintzes B. Disease awareness campaigns in printed and online media in Latvia: cross-sectional study on consistency with WHO ethical criteria for medicinal drug promotion and European standards. BMC Public Health. 2018;18(1):1322. doi:10.1186/s12889-018-6202-2.

89. Zaitsu M, Yoo B-K, Tomio J, Nakamura F, Toyokawa S, Kobayashi Y. Impact of a direct-to-consumer information campaign on prescription patterns for overactive bladder. BMC Health Serv Res. 2018;18(1):325. doi:10.1186/s12913-018-3147-1.

90. Aikin KJ, O'Donoghue AC, Swasy JL, Sullivan HW. Randomized trial of risk information formats in direct-to-consumer prescription drug advertisements. Med Decis Making. 2011;31(6):E23-33. doi:10.1177/0272989X11413289.

91. Schwartz LM, Woloshin S. The Drug Facts Box: improving the communication of prescription drug information. Proc Natl Acad Sci U S A. 2013;110(Suppl 3):14069-74. doi:10.1073/pnas.1214646110.

92. Hwang MJ, Young HN. Enhancing the educational value of direct-to-consumer advertising of prescription drugs. J Am Pharm Assoc. 2017;57(5):571-8. doi:10.1016/j.japh.2017.05.008.

93. Greene JA, Watkins ES. The vernacular of risk-rethinking direct-to-consumer advertising of pharmaceuticals. N Engl J Med. 2015;373(12):1087-9. doi:10.1056/NEJMp1507924.

94. Brief summary and adequate directions for use: disclosing risk information in consumer-directed print advertisements and promotional labeling for prescription drugs: guidance for industry [Internet]. Silver Spring (MD): U.S. Food and Drug Administration; 2015 Aug [updated 2019 Jan 3; cited 2020 Mar 12]. Available from: https://www.fda.gov/regulatory-information/search-fda-guidance-documents/brief-summary-and-adequate-directions-use-disclosing-risk-information-consumer-directed-print

95. Sullivan HW, O'Donoghue AC, Aikin KJ, Chowdhury D, Moultrie RR, Rupert DJ. Visual presentations of efficacy data in direct-to-consumer prescription drug print and television advertisements: a randomized study. Patient Educ Couns. 2016;99(5):790-9. doi:10.1016/j.pec.2015.12.015.

96. Williams PA, O'Donoghue AC, Sullivan HW, Willoughby JF, Squire C, Parvanta S, Betts KR. Communicating efficacy information based on composite scores in direct-to-consumer prescription drug advertising. Patient Educ Couns. 2016;99(4):583-90. doi:10.1016/j.pec.2015.10.019.

97. Guessous I, Dash C. Direct to consumer advertising: the case for greater consumer control. J Gen Intern Med. 2015;30(4):392-4. doi:10.1007/s11606-015-3187-8.

98. Mackey TK, Liang BA. It's time to shine the light on direct-to-consumer advertising. Ann Fam Med. 2015;13(1):82-5. doi:10.1370/afm.1711.

99. Humer C, Erman M. U.S. government to require drugmakers to show prices in TV ads [Internet]. Reuters. 2019 May 8 [cited 2020 Mar 12]. Available from: https://www.reuters.com/article/us-usa-drugpricing-advertisement/u-s-government-to-require-drugmakers-to-show-prices-in-tv-ads-idUSKCN1SE1L1

100. Garrett JB, Tayler WB, Bai G, Socal MP, Trujillo AJ, Anderson GF. Consumer responses to price disclosure in direct-to-consumer pharmaceutical advertising. JAMA Intern Med. 2019. doi:10.1001/jamainternmed.2018.5976.

101. Rowland C. Drugmakers fight rule to disclose prices in TV ads [Internet]. Washington Post. 2019 Jun 14 [cited 2020 Mar 12]. Available from: https://wapo.st/2WLB5GR?tid=ss_mail&utm_term=.90d6d7b42288

102. Bulik BS. Drug prices in ads? Not so fast: Court strikes down HHS rule at 11th hour [Internet]. Framingham (MA): FiercePharma; 2019 July 9 [cited 2020 Mar 12]. Available from: https://www.fiercepharma.com/marketing/court-strikes-down-hhs-rule-drug-prices-tv-ad-one-day-before-implementation

103. Reporting misleading rx drug promotion [Internet]. Silver Spring (MD): U.S. Food and Drug Administration; [cited 2020 Mar 12]. Available from: https://www.fda.gov/media/78443/download

104. Truthful prescription drug advertising and promotion [Internet]. Silver Spring (MD): U.S. Food and Drug Administration; [updated 2018 Jun 21; cited 2020 Mar 12]. Available from: https://www.fda.gov/drugs/office-prescription-drug-promotion/truthful-prescription-drug-advertising-and-promotion

105. Prescription drug advertising: questions to ask yourself [Internet]. Silver Spring (MD): U.S. Food and Drug Administration; [updated 2015 Jun 19; cited 2020 Mar 12]. Available from: https://www.fda.gov/drugs/prescription-drug-advertising/prescription-drug-advertising-questions-ask-yourself

106. Prescription drug advertising [Internet]. Silver Spring (MD): U.S. Food and Drug Administration; [updated 2019 Jul 8; cited 2020 Mar 3]. Available from: https://www.fda.gov/drugs/drug-information-consumers/prescription-drug-advertising

107. Shaughnessy AF, Slawson DC, Bennett JH. Separating the wheat from the chaff: identifying fallacies in pharmaceutical promotion. J Gen Intern Med. 1994;9(10):563-8. doi:10.1007/bf02599283.

108. Improving care via 1:1 dialogue [Internet]. Boston (MA): Brigham and Women's Hospital and Harvard Medical School, Department of Medicine, Division of Pharmacoepidemiology and Pharmacoeconomics, National Resource Center for Academic Detailing; [cited 2020 Mar 12]. Available from: https://www.narcad.org/about-us.html

109. Fickweiler F, Fickweiler W, Urbach E. Interactions between physicians and the pharmaceutical industry generally and sales representatives specifically and their association with physicians' attitudes and prescribing habits: a systematic review. BMJ Open. 2017;7:e016408.

110. Howard JN, Harris I, Frank G, Kiptanui Z, Qian J, Hansen R. Influencers of generic drug utilization: a systematic review. Res Social Adm Pharm. 2018;14(7):619-27. doi:10.1016/j.sapharm.2017.08.001.

111. Moynihan CK, Burke PA, Evans SA, O'Donoghue AC, Sullivan HW. Physicians' understanding of clinical trial data in professional prescription drug promotion. J Am Board Fam Med. 2018;31(4):645-9. doi:10.3122/jabfm.2018.04.170242.

112. Habibi R, Lexchin J, Mintzes B, Holbrook A. Unwarranted claims of drug efficacy in pharmaceutical sales visits: are drugs approved on the basis of surrogate outcomes promoted appropriately? Br J Clin Pharmacol. 2017;83:2549-56. doi:10.1111/bcp.13360.

113. Greenway T, Ross JS. US drug marketing: how does promotion correspond with health value? BMJ. 2017;357:j1855. doi:10.1136/bmj.j1855.

114. Abood R. Pharmacy practice and the law. 7th ed. Burlington, MA: Jones & Bartlett Learning; 2014.

115. Greenwood K. The ban on "off-label" pharmaceutical promotion: constitutionally permissible prophylaxis against false or misleading commercial speech? Am J Law Med. 2011;37(2-3):278-98. doi:10.1177/009885881103700204.

116. Kesselheim AS, Avorn J. Pharmaceutical promotion to physicians and first amendment rights. N Engl J Med. 2008;358(16):1727-32. doi:10.1056/NEJMsb0708920

117. Richardson E. Health policy brief: off-label drug promotion [Internet]. Bethesda (MD): Health Affairs; 2016 Jun 30 [cited 2020 Mar 12]. Available from: https://www.healthaffairs.org/do/10.1377/hpb20160630.920075/full/

118. Code on interactions with health care professionals [Internet]. Washington (DC): Pharmaceutical Research and Manufacturers of America; 2019 Oct 2 [updated 2019 Oct; cited 2020 Mar 12]. Available from: https://www.phrma.org/codes-and-guidelines/code-on-interactions-with-health-care-professionals

119. Sierles FS, Brodkey AC, Cleary LM, McCurdy FA, Mintz M, Frank J, Lynn DJ, Chao J, Morgenstern BZ, Shore W, Woodard JL. Medical students' exposure to and attitudes about drug company interactions: a national survey. JAMA. 2005;294(9):1034-42. doi:10.1001/jama.294.9.1034.

120. Hodges B. Interactions with the pharmaceutical industry: experiences and attitudes of psychiatry residents, interns and clerks. CMAJ. 1995;153(5):553-9.

121. Clauson KA, Khanfar NM, Polen HH, Gibson F. Nurse prescribers' interactions with and perceptions of pharmaceutical sales representatives. J Clin Nurs. 2009;18(2):228-33. doi:10.1111/j.1365-2702.2008.02536.x.

122. Alkhateeb FM, Khanfar NM, Clauson KA. Characteristics of physicians who frequently see pharmaceutical sales representatives. J Hosp Mark Public Relations. 2009;19(1):2-14. doi:10.1080/15390940802581374.

123. Bowman MA, Pearle DL. Changes in drug prescribing patterns related to commercial company funding of continuing medical education. J Contin Educ Health Prof. 1988;8(1):13-20. doi:10.1002/chp.4750080104.

124. Spurling GK, Mansfield PR, Montgomery BD, Lexchin J, Doust J, Othman N, Vitry AI. Information from pharmaceutical companies and the quality, quantity, and cost of physicians' prescribing: a systematic review. PloS Med. 2010;7(10):e1000352. doi:10.1371/journal.pmed.1000352.

125. Chren MM, Landefeld CS. Physicians' behavior and their interactions with drug companies: a controlled study of physicians who requested additions to a hospital drug formulary. JAMA. 1994;271(9):684-9.

126. Mackey TK, Yagi N, Liang BA. Prescription drug coupons: evolution and need for regulation in direct-to-consumer advertising. Res Social Adm Pharm. 2014;10(3):588-94. doi:10.1016/j.sapharm.2013.08.002.

127. Hurley MP, Stafford RS, Lane AT. Characterizing the relationship between free drug samples and prescription patterns for acne vulgaris and rosacea. JAMA Dermatol. 2014;150(5):487-93. doi:10.1001/jamadermatol.2013.9715.

128. Daugherty JB, Maciejewski ML, Farley JF. The impact of manufacturer coupon use in the statin market. J Manag Care Pharm. 2013;19(9):765-72. doi:10.18553/jmcp.2013.19.9.765.

129. Hodges LE, Arora VM, Humphrey HJ, Reddy ST. Premedical students' exposure to the pharmaceutical industry's marketing practices. Acad Med. 2013;88(2):265-8. doi:10.1097/ACM.0b013e31827bfbce.

130. Datta A, Dave DM. Effects of physician-directed pharmaceutical promotion on prescription behaviors: longitudinal evidence Working paper 19592 [Internet]. Cambridge (MA): The National Bureau of Economic Research; 2013 Nov [updated 2014 Jan; cited 2020 Mar 12]. Available from: http://www.nber.org/papers/w19592

131. McCarthy M. Doctors who take company cash are more likely to prescribe brand name drugs, analysis finds. BMJ. 2016;352:i1645. doi:10.1136/bmj.i1645.

132. Sharma M, Vadhariya A, Johnson ML, Marcum ZA, Holmes HM. Association between industry payments and prescribing costly medications: an observational study using open payments and Medicare part D data. BMC Health Services Res. 2018;18:236. doi:10.1186/s12913-018-3043-8.

133. Yeh JS, Franklin JM, Avorn J, Landon J, Kesselheim AS. Association of industry payments to physicians with the prescribing of brand-name statins in Massachusetts. JAMA Intern Med. 2016;176(6):763-8. doi:10.1001/jamainternmed.2016.1709.

134. Zezza MA, Bachhuber MA. Payments from drug companies to physicians are associated with higher volume and more expensive opioid analgesic prescribing. PLoS One. 2018;13(12):e0209383. doi:10.1371/journal.pone.0209383.

135. Bandari J, Ayyash OM, Turner RM, Jacobs BL, Davies BJ. The lack of a relationship between physician payments from drug manufacturers and Medicare claims for abiraterone and enzalutamide. Cancer. 2017;123:4356-62. doi:10.1002/cncr.30914.

136. Wood SF, Podrasky J, McMonagle MA, Raveendran J, Bysshe T, Hogenmiller A, Fugh-Berman A. Influence of pharmaceutical marketing on Medicare prescriptions in the District of Columbia. PLoS One. 2017;12(1):e0186060. doi:10.1371/journal.pone.0186060.

137. DeJong D, Aguilar T, Tseng C-W, Lin GA, Boscardin WJ, Dudley RA. Pharmaceutical industry-sponsored meals and physician prescribing patterns for Medicare beneficiaries. JAMA Intern Med. 2016;176(8):114-22. doi:10.1001/jamainternmed.2016.2765.

138. Dewatripont M, Goldman M. Free drug samples and the opioid crisis. N Engl J Med. 2018;379(8):793-4. doi:10.1056/NEJMc1805809.

139. Lexchin J. Models for financing the regulation of pharmaceutical promotion. Global Health. 2012;8:24. doi:10.1186/1744-8603-8-24.

140. Epstein AJ, Busch SH, Busch AB, Asch DA, Barry CL. Does exposure to conflict of interest policies in psychiatry residency affect antidepressant prescribing? Med Care. 2013;51(2):199-203. doi:10.1097/MLR.0b013e318277eb19.

141. Grande D, Frosch DL, Perkins AW, Kahn BE. Effect of exposure to small pharmaceutical promotional items on treatment preferences. Arch Intern Med. 2009;169(9):887-93. doi:10.1001/archinternmed.2009.64.

142. Larkin I, Ang D, Steinhart J, Chao M, Patterson M, Sah S, Wu T, Schoenbaum M, Hutchins D, Brennan T, Loewenstein G. Association between academic medical center pharmaceutical detailing policies and physician prescribing. JAMA. 2017;317(17):1785-95. doi:10.1001/jama.2017.4039.

143. Fugh-Berman AJ, Scialli AR, Bell AM. Why lunch matters: assessing physicians' perceptions about industry relationships. J Contin Educ Health Prof. 2010;30(3):197-204. doi:10.1002/chp.20081.

144. Shankar PR, Singh KK, Piryani RM. Knowledge, attitude and skills before and after a module on pharmaceutical promotion in a Nepalese medical school. BMC Res Notes. 2012;5:8. doi:10.1186/1756-0500-5-8.

145. Shankar PR, Singh KK, Piryani RM. Student feedback about the skeptic doctor, a module on pharmaceutical promotion. J Educ Eval Health Prof. 2011;8:11. doi:10.3352/jeehp.2011.8.11.

146. About IntelliCentrics [Internet]. Flower Mound (TX): IntelliCentrics, Inc.; [cited 2020 Mar 12]. Available from: https://intellicentrics.com/who-we-are/.

147. ASHP guidelines on pharmacists' relationships with industry [Internet]. Bethesda (MD): American Society of Health-System Pharmacists, ASHP Council on Legal and Public Affairs; 1992 [updated 2001; cited 2020 Mar 12]. Available from: https://www.ashp.org/-/media/assets/policy-guidelines/docs/guidelines/pharmacists-relationships-industry.ashx

148. AMA's code of medical ethics opinion 9.2.7: financial relationships with industry in continuing medical education [Internet]. Chicago (IL): American Medical Association, Council Ethical and Judicial Affairs; [cited 2020 Mar 12]. Available from: https://www.ama-assn.org/delivering-care/ethics/financial-relationships-industry-continuing-medical-education

149. Slawson DC, Shaughnessy AF, Bennett JH. Becoming a medical information master: feeling good about not knowing everything. J Fam Pract. 1994;38(5):505-14.

150. Yonemori K, Hirakawa A, Ando M, Hirata T, Yunokawa M, Shimizu C, Tamura K, Fujiwara Y. Content analysis of oncology-related pharmaceutical advertising in a peer-reviewed medical journal. PLoS One. 2012;7(8):e44393. doi:10.1371/journal.pone.0044393.

151. Kesselheim AS. Covert pharmaceutical promotion in free medical journals. CMAJ. 2011;183(5):534-5. doi:10.1503/cmaj.110156.

152. Key points of the Bad Ad Program [Internet]. Silver Spring (MD): U.S. Food and Drug Administration; [updated 2014 Oct 9; cited 2020 Mar 12]. Available from: https://www.fda.gov/drugs/drug-marketing-advertising-and-communications/key-points-bad-ad-program

153. Academic detailing: a review of the literature and states' approaches [Internet]. Baltimore (MD): The Hilltop Institute; [updated 2009 Jan 18; cited 2020 Mar 12]. Available from: https://hilltopinstitute.org/publication/academic-detailing-a-review-of-the-literature/

154. Levinson W, Dunn PM. Counter-detailing. JAMA. 1984;251(16):2084. doi:10.1001/jama.1984.03340400020012.

155. Avorn J, Soumerai SB, Everitt DE, Ross-Degnan D, Beers MH, Sherman D, Salem S. A randomized trial of a program to reduce the use of psychoactive drugs in nursing homes. N Engl J Med. 1992;327(3):168-73. doi:10.1056/NEJM199207163270306.

156. Greg M. Confessions of a pharmacy counter-detailer [Internet]. Cranbury (NJ): Drug Topics; 2011 Apr 15 [cited 2020 Mar 12]. Available from: https://www.drugtopics.com/hse-business-management/confessions-pharmacy-counter-detailer

157. Grover ML, Nordrum JT, Mookadam M, Engle RL, Moats CC, Noble BN. Addressing antibiotic use for acute respiratory tract infections in an academic family medicine practice. Am J Med Qual. 2013;28(6):485-91. doi:10.1177/1062860613476133.

158. Rognstad S, Brekke M, Fetveit A, Dalen I, Straand J. Prescription peer academic detailing to reduce inappropriate prescribing for older patients: a cluster randomised controlled trial. Br J Gen Pract. 2013;63(613):e554-62. doi:10.3399/bjgp13X670688.

159. Watkins K, Trevenen M, Murray K, Kendall PA, Schneider CR, Clifford R. Implementation of asthma guidelines to West Australian community pharmacies: an exploratory, quasi-experimental study. BMJ Open. 2016;6:e012369. doi:10.1136/bmjopen-2016-012369.

160. Yeh JS, van Hoof TJ, Fischer MA. Key features of academic detailing: development of an expert consensus using the Delphi method. Am Health Drug Benefits. 2016;9(1):42-50.

161. Aging services: prescriptions [Internet]. Harrisburg (PA): Pennsylvania Department of Aging; [cited 2020 Mar 12]. Available from: https://www.aging.pa.gov/aging-services/prescriptions/Pages/default.aspx

162. SCORxE. [Internet] Columbia (SC): South Carolina College of Pharmacy, SCORxE; [cited 2020 Mar 12]. Available from: https://education.musc.edu/colleges/pharmacy/resources/scorxe

163. About Alosa Health [Internet]. Boston (MA): Alosa Health; [updated 2018; cited 2020 Mar 12]. Available from: https://alosahealth.org/about-us/.

164. Wisniewski CS, Robert S, Ball S. Collaboration between a drug information center and an academic detailing program. Am J Health-Syst Pharm. 2014;71(2):128-33. doi:10.2146/ajhp130225.

165. Wells DL, Popish S, Kay C, Torrise V, Christopher MLD. VA academic detailing service: implementation and lessons learned. Fed Pract. 2016;33(5):38-42.

166. Avorn J, Soumerai SB. Improving drug-therapy decisions through educational outreach. A randomized controlled trial of academically based "detailing". N Engl J Med. 1983;308(24):1457-63. doi:10.1056/NEJM198306163082406.

167. Archived Project Pew Prescription Project [Internet]. Boston (MA): Pew Prescription Project; [cited 2020 Mar 12]. Available from: https://www.pewtrusts.org/en/projects/archived-projects/pew-prescription-project

168. Soumerai SB, Avorn J. Economic and policy analysis of university-based drug "detailing". Med Care. 1986;24(4):313-31. doi:10.1097/00005650-198604000-00003.

169. Simon SR, Rodriguez HP, Majumdar SR, Kleinman K, Warner C, Salem-Schatz S, Miroshnik I, Soumerai SB, Prosser LA. Economic analysis of a randomized trial of academic detailing interventions to improve use of antihypertensive medications. J Clin Hypertens. 2007;9(1):15-20. doi:10.1111/j.1524-6175.2006.05684.x.

170. Ofman JJ, Segal R, Russell WL, Cook DJ, Sandhu M, Maue SK, Lowenstein EH, Pourfarzib R, Blanchette E, Ellrodt G, Weingarten SR. A randomized trial of an acid-peptic disease management program in a managed care environment. Am J Manag Care. 2003;9(6):425-33.

171. Franzini L, Boom J, Nelson C. Cost-effectiveness analysis of a practice-based immunization education intervention. Ambul Pediatr. 2007;7(2):167-75. doi:10.1016/j.ambp.2006.12.001.

172. Farris KB, Kirking DM, Shimp LA, Opdycke RAC. Design and results of a group counter-detailing DUR educational program. Pharm Res. 1996;13(10):1445-52. doi:10.1023/a:1016007024394.

173. Wall GC, Smith HL, Craig SR, Yost WJ. Structured pharmaceutical representative interactions and counterdetailing sessions as components of medical resident education. J Pharm Pract. 2013;26(2):151-6. doi:10.1177/0897190012465988.

174. Clyne B, Smith SM, Hughes CM, Boland F, Bradley MC, Cooper JA, Fahey T, OPTI-SCRIPT study team. Effectiveness of a multifaceted intervention for potentially inappropriate prescribing in older patients in primary care: a cluster-randomized controlled trial (opti-script study). Ann Fam Med. 2015;13(6):545-53. doi:10.1370/afm.1838.

175. Vinnard C, Linkin DR, Localio AR, Leonard CE, Teal VL, Fishman NO, Leonard CE, Teal VL, Fishman NO, Hennessy S. Effectiveness of interventions in reducing antibiotic use for upper respiratory infections in ambulatory care practices. Popul Health Manag. 2013;16(1):22-7. doi:10.1089/pop.2012.0025.

176. Ho K, Nguyen A, Jarvis-Selinger S, Novak Lauscher H, Cressman C, Zibrik L. Technology-enabled academic detailing: computer-mediated education between pharmacists and physicians for evidence-based prescribing. Int J Med Inform. 2013;82(9):762-71. doi:10.1016/j.ijmedinf.2013.04.011.

177. Jin M, Gagnon A, Levine M, Thabane L, Rodriguez C, Dolovich L. Patient-specific academic detailing for smoking cessation: Feasibility study. Can Fam Physician. 2014;60(1):e16-23.

178. Lowrie R, Lloyd SM, McConnachie A, Morrison J. A cluster randomised controlled trial of a pharmacist-led collaborative intervention to improve statin prescribing and attainment of cholesterol targets in primary care. PLoS One. 2014;9(11):e113370. doi:10.1371/journal.pone.0113370.

179. Bounthavong M, Lau MK, Popish SJ, Kay CL, Wells DL, Himstreet JE, Harvey MA, Christopher MLD. Impact of academic detailing on benzodiazepine use among veterans with posttraumatic stress disorder. Subst Abus. 2019. doi:10.1080/08897077.2019.1573777.

180. Montano M, Bernardy NC, Sherrieb K. Cultivating change door to door: educational outreach to improve prescribing practices in rural veterans with posttraumatic stress disorder. Subst Abus. 2017;38(2):129-34. doi:10.1080/08897077.2017.1303423.

181. Lamprecht DG, Todd BA, Denham AM, Ruppe LK, Stadler SL. Clinical pharmacist patient-safety initiative to reduce against-label prescribing of statins with cyclosporine. Ann Pharmacother. 2017;51(2):140-5. doi:10.1177/1060028016675352.

182. Moss JM, Bryan WE, Wilkerson LM, Jackson GL, Owenby RK, Van Houtven C, Stevens MB, Powers JS, Vaughan CP, Hung WW, Hwang U, Markland AD, McGwin G, Hastings SN. Impact of clinical pharmacy specialists on the design and implementation of a quality improvement initiative to decrease inappropriate medications in a veterans affairs emergency department. J Manag Care Spec Pharm. 2016;22(1):74-80. doi:10.18553/jmcp.2016.22.1.74.

183. Moss JM, Bryan WE, Wilkerson LM, King HA, Jackson GL, Owenby RK, Van Houtven CH, Stevens MB, Powers J, Vaughan CP, Hung WW, Hwang U, Markland AD, Sloane R, Knaack W, Hastings SN. An interdisciplinary academic detailing approach to decrease inappropriate medication prescribing by physician residents for older veterans treated in the emergency department. J Pharm Pract. 2019;32(2):167-74. doi:10.1177/0897190017747424.

184. Pond D, Mate K, Stocks N, Gunn J, Disler P, Magin P, Marley J, Paterson N, Horton G, Goode S, Weaver N, Brodaty H. Effectiveness of a peer-mediated educational intervention in improving general practitioner diagnostic assessment and management of dementia: a cluster randomised controlled trial. BMJ Open. 2018;8:e021125. doi:10.1136/bmjopen-2017-021125.

185. Rognstad S, Brekke M, Gjelstad S, Straand J, Fetveit A. Potentially inappropriate prescribing to older patients: criteria, prevalence and an intervention to reduce it. Basic Clin Pharmacol Toxicol. 2018;123:380-91. doi:10.1111/bcpt.13040.

186. Dyrkorn R, Gjelstad S, Espnes KA, Lindbaek M. Peer academic detailing on use of antibiotics in acute respiratory tract infections: a controlled study in an urban Norwegian out-of-hours service. Scand J Primary Health Care. 2016;34(2):179-84. doi:10.3109/02813432.2016.1163035.

187. Keller SC, Tamma PD, Cosgrove SE, Miller MA, Sateia H, Szymczak J, Gurses AP, Linder JA. Ambulatory antibiotic stewardship through a human factors engineering approach: a systematic review. J Am Board Fam Med. 2018;31(3):417-30. doi:10.3122/jabfm.2018.03.170225.

188. Ndefo UA, Norman R, Henry A. Academic detailing has a positive effect on prescribing and decreasing prescription drug costs: a health plan's perspective. Am Health Drug Benefits. 2017;10(2):129-33.

189. Saha SK, Hawes L, Mazza D. Effectiveness of interventions involving pharmacists on antibiotic prescribing by general practitioners: a systematic review and meta-analysis. J Antimicrob Chemother. 2019;74:1173-81. doi:10.1093/jac/dky572.

190. Harris AHS, Bowe T, Hagedorn H, Nevedal A, Finlay AK, Gidwani R, Rosen C, Kay C, Christopher M. Multifaceted academic detailing program to increase pharmacotherapy for alcohol use disorder: interrupted time series evaluation of effectiveness. Addict Sci Clin Pract. 2016;11:15. doi:10.1186/s13722-016-0063-8.

191. Noble RA, McKinnell JC, Shaw S, Bassett S, Woods L, Asrar M, Kolhe NV, Selby NM. Evaluating a process of academic detailing in primary care: an educational programme for acute kidney injury. BMC Med Educ. 2019;19:253. doi:10.1186/s12909-019-1659-y.

192. Bruyndonckx R, Verhoeven V, Anthierens S, Cornelis K, Ackaert K, Gielen B, Coenen S. The implementation of academic detailing and its effectiveness on appropriate prescribing of pain relief medication: a real-world cluster randomized trial in Belgian general practices. Implement Sci. 2018;13:6. doi:10.1186/s13012-017-0703-8.

193. Bounthavong M, Harvey MA, Wells DL, Popish SJ, Himstreet J, Oliva EM, Kay CL, Lau MK, Randeria-Noor PP, Phillips AG, Christopher MLD. Trends in naloxone prescriptions prescribed after implementation of a National Academic Detailing Service in the Veterans Health Administration: a preliminary analysis. J Am Pharm Assoc. 2017;57:S68-72. doi:10.1016/j.japh.2016.11.003.

194. Oliva EM, Christopher MLD, Wells D, Bounthavong M, Harvey M, Himstreet J, Emmendorfer T, Valentino M, Franchi M, Goodman F, Trafton JA. Opioid overdose education and naloxone distribution: development of the Veterans Health Administration's national program. J Am Pharm Assoc. 2017;S168-79. doi:10.1016/j.japh.2017.01.022.

195. Behar E, Rowe C, Santos G-M, Santos N, Coffin PO. Academic detailing pilot for naloxone prescribing among primary care providers in San Francisco. Fam Med. 2017;49(2):122-26.

196. Abd-Elsayed, Albert CA, Fischer M, Anderson B. Naloxone academic detailing: role of community outreach teaching. Curr Pain Headache Rep. 2018;22:72. doi:10.1007/211916-018-0730-4.

197. Larson MJ, Browne C, Nikitin RV, Wooten NR, Ball S, Adams RS, Barth K. Physicians report adopting safer opioid prescribing behaviors after academic detailing intervention. Subst Abus. 2018;39(2):218-24. doi:10.1080/08897077.2018.1449175.

198. Voelker KA, Schauberger C. Academic detailing for postpartum opioid prescribing. J Am Board Fam Med. 2018;31:944-6. doi:10.3122/jabfm.2018.06.180071.

199. Barth KS, Ball S, Adams RS, Nikitin R, Wooten NR, Qureshi ZP, Larson MJ. Development and feasibility of an academic detailing intervention to improve prescription drug monitoring program use among physicians. J Contin Educ Health Prof. 2017;37(2):98-105. doi:10.1097/CEH.0000000000000149.

200. Tamburrano A, Mellucci C, Galletti C, Vitale D, Vallone D, Barbara A, Sguera A, Zega M, Damiani G, Laurenti P. Improving nursing staff attitudes toward vaccinations through academic detailing: the HProImmune questionnaire as a tool for medical management. Int J Environ Res Public Health. 2019;16:2006. doi:10.3390/ijerph16112006.

201. Caffrey AR, DeAngelis JM, Ward KE, Orr KK, Morril HJ, Gosciminski M, LaPlante KL. A pharmacist-driven academic detailing program to increase adult pneumococcal vaccination. J Am Pharm Assoc. 2018;58:303-10. doi:10.1016/j.japh.2017.08.010.

202. O'Brien MA, Rogers S, Jamtvedt G, Oxman AD, Odgaard-Jensen J, Kristoffersen DT, Forsetlund L, Bainbridge D, Freemantle N, Davis DA, Haynes RB, Harvey EL. Educational outreach visits: effects on professional practice and health care outcomes. Cochrane Database Syst Rev. 2007(4):CD000409. doi:10.1002/14651858.CD000409.pub2.

203. Chhina HK, Bhole VM, Goldsmith C, Hall W, Kaczorowski J, Lacaille D. Effectiveness of academic detailing to optimize medication prescribing behaviour of family physicians. J Pharm Pharm Sci. 2013;16(4):511-29. doi:10.18433/j3kk6c.

204. Morrow RW, Tattelman E, Purcell JM, King J, Fordis M. Academic peer detailing—the preparation and experience of detailers involved in a project to disseminate a comparative effectiveness module. J Contin Educ Health Prof. 2016;36(2):123-6. doi:10.1097/CEH.0000000000000067.

205. Anthierens S, Verhoeven V, Schmitz O, Coenen S. Academic detailers' and general practitioners' views and experiences of their academic detailing visits to improve the quality of analgesic use: process evaluation alongside a pragmatic cluster randomized controlled trial. BMC Health Serv Res. 2017;17:841. doi:10.1186/s12913-017-279-8.

206. Clyne B, Cooper JA, Hughes CM, Fahey T, Smith SM. A process evaluation of a cluster randomised trial to reduce potentially inappropriate prescribing in older people in primary care (OPTI-SCRIPT study). Trials. 2016;17:386. doi:10.1186/s13063-016-1513-z.

207. Desveaux L, Saragosa M, Rogers J, Bevan L, Loshak H, Moser A, Feldman S, Regier L, Jeffs L, Ivers NM. Improving the appropriateness of antipsychotic prescribing in nursing homes: a mixed-methods process evaluation of an academic detailing intervention. Implement Sci. 2017;12:71. doi:10.1186/s13012-017-0602-z.

208. Kane-Gill SL, Hanlon JT, Fine MJ, Perera S, Culley CM, Studenski SA, Nace DA, Boyce RD, Castle Ng, Handler SM. Physician perceptions of the performance and importance of consultant pharmacist services associated with an intervention for the detection and management of adverse drug events in the nursing home. Consult Pharm. 2016;31(12):708-20. doi:10.4140/TCP.n.2016.708.

209. Riordan DO, Byrne S, Fleming A, Kearney PM, Galvin R, Sinnott C. GPs' perspectives on prescribing for older people in primary care: a qualitative study. Br J Clin Pharmacol. 2017;83(7):1521-31. doi:10.1111/bcp.13233.

210. Schmidt-Mende K, Hasselstrom J, Wettermark B, Andersen M, Bastholm-Rahmner P. General practitioners' and nurses' views on medication reviews and potentially inappropriate medicines in elderly patients—a qualitative study of reports by educating pharmacists. Scand J Primary Health Care. 2018;36(3):329-41. doi:10.1080/02813432.2018.1487458.

211. Vasudev K, Lamoure J, Beyaert M, Dua V, Dixon D, Eadie J, Husarewych L, Dhir R, Takhar J. Academic detailing among psychiatrists—feasibility and acceptability. Int J Health Care Qual Assur. 2017;30(1): 79-88. doi:10.1108/IJHCQA-04-2016-0047.

212. Educational outcomes, goals, and objectives for postgraduate year two (PGY2) pharmacy residencies in drug information [Internet]. Bethesda (MD): American Society of Health-System Pharmacists; 2008 [cited 2020 Mar 12]. Available from: https://www.ashp.org/-/media/assets/professional-development/residencies/docs/pgy2-drug-information.ashx

213. Abel GA, Chen K, Taback N, Hassett MJ, Schrag D, Weeks JC. Impact of oncology-related direct-to-consumer advertising. Cancer. 2013;119(5):1065-72. doi:10.1002/cncr.27814.

214. Kim Y, Kornfield R, Shi Y, Vera L, Daubresse M, Alexander GC, Emery S. Effects of televised direct-to-consumer advertising for varenicline on prescription dispensing in the United States, 2006-2009. Nicotine Tob Res. 2016;18(5):1180-7. doi:10.1093/ntr/ntv198.

215. Layton JB, Kim Y, Alexander GC, Emery SL. Association between direct-to-consumer advertising and testosterone testing and initiation in the United States, 2009-2013. JAMA. 2017;317(11):1159-66. doi:10.1001/jama.2016.21041.

26

Chapter Twenty-Six

Drug Information in Ambulatory Care

Suzanne M. Surowiec

Learning Objectives

● *After completing this chapter, the reader will be able to:*

- Describe the importance of drug information provided by the health care professional in the ambulatory care setting.
- Discuss the importance of access to up-to-date formulary information in the provision of care in the ambulatory setting.
- Identify sources with links to full-text evidence-based practice guidelines.
- Describe desired characteristics of drug information resources specific to the ambulatory care environment.
- Describe reputable drug information resources geared toward the health care professional that are also useful in providing drug information to patients.
- List ways in which practitioners may address concerns regarding access to information.
- Discuss the importance of providing drug information regarding disposal of unused, unwanted, or expired medications.
- Identify appropriate resources to obtain immunization information.
- Identify resources providing quality assurance indicators for optimal provision of ambulatory care.

Key Concepts

❶ The clinician in the ambulatory care setting routinely utilizes multiple drug information skills on a daily basis to not only provide drug information to patients and other health care providers, but to function competently and efficiently within this practice setting.

❷ Ambulatory care and community practitioners have the greatest opportunity to fill the role of medication information provider and interpreter to the lay public.

❸ Knowledge of formulary status of medications is only one part of the prescription decision-making process. Whenever they exist, evidence-based clinical practice guidelines should guide prescriptive decision-making.

❹ Ambulatory care practitioners have the responsibility to remain up-to-date regarding current practice guidelines.

❺ Increasingly more medical literature, including tertiary references, is being provided in the electronic or Internet-based format, and such references are attractive to utilize in ambulatory care for multiple reasons.

❻ Ambulatory care clinicians bear a responsibility to educate patients on the proper disposal of unused and unwanted medications and should therefore be aware of pertinent sites for information.

❼ While ambulatory care clinicians (in particular, pharmacists) typically recommend and/or dispense most medications, immunizations are medications that are *administered* in the ambulatory care setting. Those practitioners immunizing in this setting have the obligation to not only provide these services safely, but also serve as immediate sources of information (i.e., drug information) regarding the medications they are administering.

❽ Health care professionals involved in providing patient care in the ambulatory care setting should familiarize themselves with pertinent, established quality measures.

Introduction

This chapter covers a long list of drug information topics and skills specific to the ambulatory care setting, although not every clinician will use all of these skills on a daily basis. ❶ *The clinician in the ambulatory care setting routinely utilizes multiple drug information skills on a daily basis to not only provide drug information to patients and other health care providers, but to function competently and efficiently within this practice setting.*

The ambulatory care practitioner is required to use a variety of drug information skills and resources during routine encounters with patients to provide information at a personalized and appropriate level. Before doing so, the practitioner must know where to look for pertinent information, and how to interpret and practically apply this information to a specific patient or population.

Many patients are technologically savvy and utilize the Internet and news media to provide self-care in the outpatient setting. The quality of the medical and drug information that patients obtain themselves varies widely, depending on the source (see Chapter 3 for drug information resources). Even when quality information is obtained by a patient or family member, it is often necessary to have someone with clinical expertise and drug information training explain the medical information and provide guidance for decision-making.

Moreover, with increasing numbers of team-based patient care models, such as the **patient-centered medical home** (e.g., PCMH), the provision of accurate, comprehensive drug information in the ambulatory setting is growing exponentially. Thus, it is crucial to (a) research appropriate medical treatment, especially of chronic conditions, (b) bridge the gap between data provided from health information technology and how to most effectively use this data to treat patients on an individual and a population-based basis, and (c) educate patients about their treatments.

This chapter will discuss the resources commonly needed by the ambulatory care practitioner to provide appropriate drug information. Topics covered will include (a) commonly used references for accessing prescription formularies and evidence-based guidelines, (b) desired characteristics of drug information resources and examples of those particularly useful to the ambulatory care clinician, (c) information resources pertinent to the current trends in ambulatory care, such as the proper disposal of unused, unwanted, or expired medications, (d) preventive health information (specifically regarding immunizations), and (e) quality assurance measures in ambulatory care.

Ambulatory care encompasses a variety of settings. For example, an ambulatory care practitioner may be a clinician who practices in a community pharmacy (including persons in medication-dispensing roles), a clinic or physician's office, an outpatient setting of an institutional care facility, a transitions of care role in an inpatient setting, or someone who provides onsite services within an employer-provided wellness and disease management program. Further information on drug information in the community setting is available in Chapter 27. While ambulatory care pharmacy continues to grow exponentially, the drug information resources and skills remain steadfast tools clinicians will need to utilize to improve patient care.

Providing Drug Information in the Ambulatory Care Setting

"I CAN JUST GOOGLE® IT MYSELF."

Given the name of a medication, the average layperson may well be able to Google® the name of the drug, and would very likely find general information regarding its use and side effects. Blogs detailing the experiences of other people taking that medication may also be easily found, as well as anecdotal comments about the drug and the condition being treated, including outdated and incorrect information. The average patient is, in fact, able to access a plethora of information via websites and blogs; however, the reliability, accuracy, and timeliness of this information can vary widely, as discussed in Chapter 3. While some of these sources of drug information may be reputable, they are impersonal and can only offer general information to the reader. Such sites typically advise patients to talk with their practitioner for specific personal questions. Clinicians have extensive real-world experience that assist in the interpretation and application of drug information. For example, a clinician may be able to address a patient's concerns about a medication adverse effect listed online by providing information that they have never encountered it with any of their patients taking that medication. In contrast, practitioners may be able to identify an adverse effect caused by a medication that is not commonly listed online based on their experience of seeing that adverse effect in other patients taking that medication. As one can see, Google® cannot always provide the patient-specific information or clinical judgment needed for optimal medical care.

WHAT SHOULD THE PUBLIC (OR OTHER HEALTH CARE PROVIDERS) KNOW ABOUT UTILIZING CLINICIANS TRAINED IN DRUG INFORMATION VERSUS PERFORMING THEIR OWN SEARCHES?

In today's environment, with direct-to-consumer advertising (see Chapter 25) and increasing numbers of over-the-counter (OTC) products, the decision to use a medication is not made solely by prescribers, but also by patients themselves. It is evident that all decision-makers need guidance. Who guides these decision-makers?

Health care providers fill an important role in the provision and interpretation of drug information. While there is an ever-increasing trend toward patient empowerment, self-care, and self-education, the lay public is often unaware that health care providers have access to professional literature and databases (see Chapter 3) that expand upon and often provide critical analysis of the information available to the public. The layperson is usually unable to access or is poorly equipped to interpret such information. Depending on their clinical training, even certain health care providers may lack knowledge regarding available resources and how to best interpret health information data, making it necessary to improve clinical training in this area.

❷ *Ambulatory care and community practitioners have the greatest opportunity to fill the role of medication information provider and interpreter to the lay public.*

Although individuals may be able to personally access secondary or even primary literature in some cases, interpreting this information and putting it into context with their personal health conditions, as well as with current evidence-based guidelines (see Chapter 8) requires a health care professional trained in drug information. Understanding and evaluating primary literature (see Chapters 4 and 5) as well as locating and interpreting evidence-based guidelines are skills that require training and practice. Locating and evaluating primary literature (covered in Chapters 3–6) is a skill that the ambulatory care practitioner will need to utilize. For example, patients commonly inquire about new medication data that emerges as a result of a study, and this information will need to be accessed and interpreted by the practitioner prior to the release of an official guideline. Pharmacists receive more training in this area than any other health care provider during their professional education. As such, this profession bears the responsibility to educate both the public and fellow health care professionals. The following are examples of this type of educational opportunity in the ambulatory setting:

- Ensuring that biased sources such as pharmaceutical representatives are not the main source of new product education for prescribers
- Leading or facilitating discussions with prescribers regarding newly published studies, meta-analyses, and clinical guidelines, with emphasis on understanding limitations of these publications and how they apply specifically to their patient populations
- Researching and answering drug information questions (which may or may not be patient-specific)
- Disseminating information regarding pertinent media topics or specific to the conditions treated in the clinic(s) in which the pharmacist works
- "Debunking" misperceptions that may arise from direct-to-consumer advertising regarding exaggerated efficacy or risk associated with treatments
- Providing basic literature evaluation and statistical training, including concepts such as relative risk versus absolute risk of a treatment outcome, and how to calculate them (see Chapter 6)

In order to provide patient-specific drug information, complete medication profiles, past medical history, vital signs, labs, and other patient-specific information must be obtained. This often requires communication not only with outpatient/ambulatory care clinics, but also with one or more pharmacies to obtain all necessary information.

In today's busy society, pharmacist-provided drug information needs to be concise and accessible. To assist in improving quality of life and health outcomes for patients, pharmacists are taking on expanded roles that increase clinical responsibilities and collaboration with other providers. Studies and practice-based experiences have shown that when pharmacists are involved as members of the health care team, patient outcomes improve and health care costs are reduced.[1] The following section discusses drug information roles in ambulatory care as well as resources integral to the provision of drug information in this setting.

Drug Information Responsibilities in Ambulatory Care

Integral drug information-related responsibilities of the ambulatory care clinician are many. Several key responsibilities include but are not limited to the following:

- Assisting prescribers and consumers in selecting the most effective, safe, and cost-effective drug to treat a given condition
- Verifying that a prescribed medication is appropriate and follows current evidence-based guidelines (see Chapter 8)
- Ensuring a patient's understanding of the appropriate use of, and adherence to, their medications
- Guiding others regarding the proper disposal of unused or unwanted medications
- Delivering preventive health information
- Incorporating quality assurance indicators into daily practice

Practitioners who may not be the initial prescribers of medications (e.g., those who work under consult or collaborative practice agreements or who work with supervisory physicians or collaborating physicians) must be familiar with the key responsibilities listed above. Regardless of the degree (e.g., Doctor of Pharmacy, Bachelor of Science in Pharmacy, Physician Assistant, Certified Registered Nurse Practitioner) or location in which a clinician practices, sound recommendations regarding modifications in drug therapy, drug therapy renewal, and initial drug therapy recommendations all hinge upon a solid understanding of drug formularies, appropriate practice guidelines, and drug information database considerations.

DRUG FORMULARY INFORMATION

A major key to assisting prescribers and consumers in finding the most cost-effective treatment is familiarity with drug **formularies**. Whether a clinician is prescribing or filling a prescription order, formulary restrictions influence **medication usage patterns**. With a prescription insurance plan, a formulary is typically a list of medications that are covered by the plan and determines how much a patient will pay for the medication. It is important to note that even if a medication is not included on a formulary (i.e., is considered "nonformulary"), or is not listed as a preferred option by the payer for a patient's prescription drugs, the prescriber is *not* bound to this when deciding whether to prescribe the medication, and nothing prohibits the pharmacist from filling an appropriate medication for a patient, ***regardless*** of its formulary status (refer to Chapter 15 for more information about drug formularies).

One method for obtaining formulary information via the Internet is by typing the name of the prescription insurance provider + formulary + the calendar year you desire (e.g., 2019) in the Internet search engine (e.g., Google®, Bing™). Most prescription providers will have webpages that include (1) a full formulary guide, (2) a list of covered medications organized by drug name or by drug class, (3) **medication tier status** in which participants are subject to varying levels of copayment options for a given medication depending on its formulary status, (4) links to suggested alternatives to a medication if it is not covered, and (5) links for forms necessary for prior authorization, appeals, and exceptions. An advantage to using these websites is immediate access to information and necessary forms. Each insurance provider, however, will have a different webpage design and there is often inconsistency as to where the user will find such information.

Additionally, there are some medications that, while on formulary, may require prior authorization from the insurance company before they will be paid for. That does not mean it cannot be dispensed—it only means that the insurance company requires submission of information regarding medical need prior to covering a medication. The pharmacist plays an integral role in working with the prescriber on a patient's behalf to obtain an insurance company's authorization to fill a prescription for such a medication.

Formulary status contributes to the amount a patient will personally pay for a medication, and this may affect adherence if cost is a major concern. For example, a tier 1 medication would be preferred (i.e., lower patient responsibility for payment) over a tier 3 medication (i.e., higher patient responsibility for payment). Several useful resources exist to assist in determining formulary restrictions and then making decisions as to risks versus benefits of abiding by these restrictions.

A health care provider in an ambulatory care practice can play a tremendous role in helping patients afford their medications. Various companies such as GoodRx and NeedyMeds offer discounted pricing options such as coupon cards; these coupon cards can be accessed online, printed (by either the patient or health care professional), and taken to the dispensing retail pharmacy (see Chapter 27 for more information). Practitioners can also assist patients in finding manufacturer assistance programs or locating copay cards.

Centers for Medicare & Medicaid Services (CMS)

The Centers for Medicare & Medicaid Services (CMS) is a government agency within the U.S. Department of Health and Human Services (HHS) that is responsible for the administration of the U.S. Medicare and Medicaid services, through which medical and prescription benefits are available for some individuals, *traditionally* for the poor, elderly, and disabled. Historically, private insurances have modeled reimbursement structures for medical and medicine-related costs after the CMS model. The Affordable Care Act (ACA) has resulted in increasing numbers of persons who in the past were either uninsured or underinsured (without adequate prescription insurance to cover medical-related costs) to now being insured through either Medicaid or other government-mandated programs, although it is uncertain whether even further changes are coming.

The largest proportion of the population taking prescription medications are Medicare recipients.[2] Prescription drug coverage is provided to these individuals through an optional component of Medicare called Medicare Part D. Through this program, various insurance companies provide government-funded prescription coverage for Medicare recipients. Each insurance company has a different formulary or list of drugs that the plan will cover at a certain amount based on the tier, providing less cost to the Medicare recipient. As such, understanding formularies and their restrictions as well as the ability to access Medicare Part D formulary information is paramount. Although many patients may select their own Medicare drug provider and plan, others often look to a health care professional to assist them in this decision. Drug plan selection is done largely online and is based on a patient's prescription profile as well as geographic location. The State Health Insurance Assistance Program (SHIP) offers free counseling services on Medicare plan selection (available at https://www. shiptacenter.org/), which is a great resource for patients. A pharmacist can also assist with this process, as the health care professional is likely to be most familiar with various drug classes listed on drug plan formularies as well as acceptable over-the-counter and generic alternatives to specific medications.

Information to guide selection is available at http://www.medicare.gov by clicking on the link to "Find health and drug plans" (https://www.medicare.gov/find-a-plan/questions/home.aspx). Users choose their state of residence by using a drop-down menu, and then must enter an email address. Next, the user enters his/her prescription drug profile (i.e., the list of prescriptions the patient takes). The program will then provide a list of Medicare Part D plans that include some or all of the medications the patient takes, as well as information regarding the tier of each medication in a particular plan, and the number of pharmacies that participate with a plan in a given state. Although not required to prescribe for medications on a patient's specific drug plan, providers may use the site to determine if a drug will be paid for, and if not, if there are acceptable therapeutic alternatives that will be covered. Users, including prescribers, can also download complete formularies, as well as appeals and exceptions forms from this site. These are forms that may be completed, usually by the prescriber on behalf of the patient, asking for consideration of payment for a drug due to extenuating circumstances or a situation specific to that patient. This website can be used by patients alone or may be used by a provider on behalf of the patient. In contrast, Medicaid formularies vary by state. In some states, there is just one formulary for Medicaid but in others that have managed care Medicaid, the formulary can differ for each managed care provider.

Electronic Prescribing (e-prescribing) Platforms

Electronic prescribing (e-prescribing) is a provider's ability to electronically send a prescription directly to a pharmacy from the point of care.[3] E-prescribing can help improve accuracy, decrease errors of prescribing, and improve efficiency in the ambulatory care setting.[4] Clinicians with prescribing privileges should note that e-prescribing platforms provide drug and formulary information at the point of care. In a study conducted by the Agency for Healthcare Research and Quality (AHRQ) and published in the Archives of Internal Medicine, prescribers utilizing e-prescribing platforms with **formulary decision supports** (FDS) were significantly more likely to prescribe tier 1 medications, with resulting significant potential cost savings.[5] Chang and associates evaluated over 21,000 prescriptions for just over 1 year, and reported that generic drug use was 6% higher, formulary drug use was 3% higher, and cost savings for the payer and prescription drug member was over 17% higher for those prescriptions electronically prescribed.[6] It is important to note that e-prescribing is now required to avoid penalty fees from CMS for Medicare patients, so the majority of health care practitioners should have access to an e-prescribing platform in their practice. While FDS can be beneficial, it is not always accurate; insurance information for medical coverage is often included in the electronic medical record, but prescription coverage/insurance can be missing.

Some pharmacy apps/databases also contain formulary information. See the section entitled "A Review of Selected Drug Information Resources for the Ambulatory Care Clinician" for further details.

❸ *Knowledge of formulary status of medications is only one part of the prescription decision-making process. Whenever they exist, evidence-based clinical practice guidelines should guide prescriptive decision-making.*

CURRENT PRACTICE GUIDELINE INFORMATION

It is beyond the scope of this chapter to discuss in depth the development and the interpretation of evidence-based clinical practice guideline recommendations (see Chapter 8). It is important to note, however, that ❹ *ambulatory care practitioners have the responsibility to remain up-to-date regarding current practice guidelines.* No individual can be expected to know the current treatment guidelines for every condition; however, clinicians can and should be expected to be able to retrieve and apply this information quickly and efficiently. The following outlines several sources for guideline retrieval.

Open-Access Databases

Typically, government-sponsored organizations such as the Centers for Disease Control and Prevention (CDC), the National Heart, Lung, and Blood Institute (NHLBI), and the National Comprehensive Cancer Network (NCCN) publish clinical practice guidelines on their websites for free. Some of these guidelines are also available in mobile applications (apps), which may be especially useful to ambulatory care practitioners. The CDC website includes free mobile apps (compatible with Apple® and Android®) for a variety of medical conditions, available at http://www.cdc.gov/mobile/mobileapp.html.

At this time, the National Guideline Clearinghouse (a site that once indexed numerous treatment guidelines and included full-text links to many of these guidelines) is no longer available. Instead, practitioners may refer to the ECRI Institute website (https://guidelines.ecri.org/) for links to current treatment guidelines, although many of these documents require a subscription in order to access full text.[7]

- Health Services Technology Assessment Texts (HSTAT), available via the National Library of Medicine (http://www.ncbi.nlm.nih.gov/books/NBK16710/), is a useful source for locating several evidence-based summaries and reports.

- The Turning Research into Practice (TRIP) Database (http://www.tripdatabase.com) and PubMed® (https://www.ncbi.nlm.nih.gov/pubmed/) are great resources for locating pertinent and current practice guidelines; they allow the user to establish (for free) a user account, and the viewer can apply filters to assist in identifying guidelines. However, the guidelines may or may not be accessible in full text, depending on the specific subscription available at the practitioner's institution. Those that do not provide full-text article links provide full citations.[8]

Professional Association Websites

- Many health professions' organizations publish links to their affiliated practice guidelines in full text on their websites. For example, the American Diabetes Association (ADA) guidelines, the 2018 American College of Cardiology/American Heart Association (ACC/AHA) guideline on the management of blood cholesterol, and the 2017 ACC/AHA guideline for the prevention, detection, evaluation, and management of high blood pressure in adults are available on the organization websites without any subscription. Clinicians searching for current practice guidelines may wish to visit the websites of the guideline developers and affiliate organizations (e.g., American Academy of Dermatology, American Academy of Family Physicians). The American Society of Health-System Pharmacists (ASHP) website provides links to the organization's Best Practice Policies and Guidelines (http://www.ashp.org/bestpractices). The American Pharmacists Association (APhA) also provides links from its website to select practice guidelines (http://www.pharmacist.com).

Subscription-Based Databases

- UpToDate® (https://www.uptodate.com/home), available with a subscription, is a useful tool that can be used to access current practice guidelines. Each topic includes a section entitled "Society Guideline Links," which contains relevant international and country-specific guidelines. Other subscription databases that include links to pertinent practice guidelines include DynaMed® (https://www.dynamed.com/) and Lexicomp® (http://www.wolterskluwercdi.com/lexicomp-online/). Embase® and the Cochrane Database of Systematic Reviews indexing systems are other excellent subscription resources for retrieving clinical practice guidelines. The reader should refer to Chapters 3 and 8 for a more detailed description of these resources and others that may be utilized when searching for clinical practice guidelines. Of note, the most effective search term may be *practice guideline* in the publication type field of various search pages. An additional useful search term may be *treatment guideline*.

Case Study 26–1

Dr. Miller, an internal medicine physician who works with you, the clinical ambulatory care pharmacist, approaches you with a drug information question. "Can you help me? I am trying to find updated guidelines for the treatment of psoriasis for one of my patients. I don't treat this condition very often, so I want to know what my drug therapy options are?"

- *Where would you direct Dr. Miller to look to obtain current treatment guidelines?*

DESIRED CHARACTERISTICS OF DRUG INFORMATION RESOURCES IN THE AMBULATORY SETTING

❺ *Increasingly more medical literature, including tertiary references, is being provided in the electronic or Internet-based format, and such databases are attractive to utilize in ambulatory care for multiple reasons.*

- Easy access: Electronic databases are easily accessible, which is of utmost importance, as ambulatory care may take place in clinics or pharmacies that are part of the same health system, but located in multiple locations.
- Frequent updates: Electronic databases tend to be updated more easily and frequently, with new drug updates and pertinent changes in patient and disease management versus print copies of drug information that may outdate quickly.

- Efficient retrieval: Electronic drug information databases are more quickly and easily searched for specific topics pertinent to a given patient, and often utilize hyperlinks or search functions.

Examples of particularly useful databases are provided below.

A REVIEW OF SELECTED DRUG INFORMATION RESOURCES FOR THE AMBULATORY CARE CLINICIAN

The following is a brief overview of selected resources that (a) are available electronically, (b) are primarily geared toward the health care professional and are also particularly useful to the ambulatory care practitioner, (c) provide in-depth drug and alternative product monographs, and (d) provide useful patient-oriented material. More detailed information on these resources can be found in Chapter 3.

Clinical Pharmacology®

Available as an online subscription through Elsevier Gold Standard (http://www.clinicalpharmacology.com), this database includes clinical calculators, manufacturer contact information, normal laboratory reference values, drug class overviews, clinical comparison reports, and convenience charts (e.g., medications that should not be split, medications that interact with grapefruit juice). Information on complementary and alternative medicine (CAM) is also found in this database. This may be of particular value in the ambulatory setting as these patients are most likely to be concurrently taking or inquiring about CAM in addition to their prescription medications. This database has an app for Android® and Apple® devices.

Furthermore, MedCounselor® Consumer Drug Information Sheets that are available in both English and Spanish can be found here and include the date of last revision of any given patient education sheet. MedCounselor® Sheets are available via hyperlinks from drug monographs or by searching by drug product under a patient education tab within the site. This product includes patient education materials written at a 6th–8th grade reading level regarding prescription, nonprescription, and some herbal medications.

DailyMed

DailyMed (https://dailymed.nlm.nih.gov/dailymed/) is a U.S. government source where package inserts can be found for almost all available medications. Clinicians can access this free online resource for comprehensive and up-to-date Food and Drug Administration (FDA) label information.

Facts and Comparisons® eAnswers

Available through Wolters Kluwer (http://online.factsandcomparisons.com), the ambulatory care clinician can find several useful tools within this database: clinical calculators, comparative data tables and comparative efficacy tables within drug classes, a "do not crush/chew" list of medications, a drug identifier tool, drug interactions tool, immunization schedules, and even information regarding patient assistance programs for those patients experiencing difficulty affording their medication(s). Additional information on medication use during pregnancy and lactation, natural medicines, and toxicology treatment guidelines (e.g., for overdose treatment or for reversal of effects of medications) are also available. This database has an app for Android® and Apple® devices.

Facts and Comparisons® eAnswers also houses MedFacts Patient Information®, which provides customizable patient information in both English and Spanish for over 4000 brand and generic drugs, and includes some herbal medication patient education materials. The reading level is written at the 8th grade level or below, with the date of last issue clearly provided on each education sheet.

DynaMed®

- DynaMed® is an online subscription database (http://dynamed.com) available from EBSCO Industries. It includes information on disease states and medications, as well as a variety of medical calculators, and links to current guidelines. Continuing education credit is offered, and an app for Android® and Apple® devices.

Epocrates®

- Many clinicians may be familiar with Epocrates® software programs (http://www.epocrates.com/). Epocrates® markets programs with a variety of content areas including calculations, continuing medical education, diagnostics, a medical dictionary, disease state information, drugs, drug identification, medical news, and tables. These content areas are bundled into various data packages, some of which are free. All Epocrates® programs, including those that are available at no cost, include both national and regional formulary information, including Medicare Part D. Users can access formulary status and restrictions for over 3300 brand and generic medications. Users of these programs select the formulary or formularies they desire to include in their searches. Epocrates® updates formulary information at least once per week.[9]

Epocrates® has an app for Android® and Apple® devices. This program may prove to be a practical solution for providers who require timely formulary information and who operate without full Internet access.

GlobalRPh

- This online reference, available at https://globalrph.com/, is a helpful resource that includes clinical calculators (i.e., CrCl, vancomycin dosing, etc.), medical abbreviations, conversion of units, normal laboratory values, dosing nomograms, and many other practical clinical references. Additionally, one can choose a specific disease area of focus (e.g., cardiology), which will lead the user to many references and resources for that disease state. Ambulatory clinicians will find this free resource of great importance for many aspects of their work.

Lexicomp® Online

● Available as an online subscription through Wolters Kluwer (http://www.wolterskluwercdi. com/lexicomp-online/), Lexicomp® Online incorporates an Internet-based platform to provide not only the electronic version of information found in Lexicomp's Drug Information Handbook, but, depending on the subscription purchased, may also include information from the AHFS® Clinical Drug Information reference and prescription drug plans, including information regarding pricing, formulary status, and prior authorization status. Of particular interest to the ambulatory clinician, Lexicomp® includes links within drug monographs to both adult and pediatric patient education leaflets.

The patient education material delivers patient-specific education regarding a particular medication, disease, condition, or procedure. Condition and procedure information is available in either English or Spanish, with medication leaflets available in up to 19 different languages. Information is also available for select natural products. Patient information is written at a 5th–7th grade reading level, and may be personalized and printed for distribution to the patient.[10] This database has an app for Android® and Apple® devices.

MedlinePlus

● Available online from the U.S. National Library of Medicine (https://medlineplus.gov/), MedlinePlus is a reputable patient education resource written in layman's terms, and available free of charge. Information on prescription and over-the-counter medications is included as well as a medical encyclopedia and an explanation of medical tests. This information can be accessed in a multitude of different patient languages. Links to the CDC and NIH websites, for the most current public health information, are readily available on this site.

IBM Micromedex®

● Available as an online subscription through Truven Health Analytics (https://www. micromedex.com), Micromedex is a large database of information for health care professionals. The information is evidence-based and covers FDA-approved and off-label indications for medications. Drug interactions, drug identification, clinical calculators, and toxicology management are all included in this database.[11] This database has an app for Android® and Apple® devices.

IBM Micromedex® Health Care Series' Detailed Drug Information for the Consumer™

● Available as a subset of Micromedex (https://www.micromedex.com), the Micromedex Patient Connect Suite® includes educational resources written at a 3rd–7th grade reading level in up to 15 languages that may be delivered in multiple media formats (e.g., written, video, interactive tools, and more). This suite of resources is intended for use by not only retail and hospital pharmacists, physicians and nurses, but also patient education program coordinators.[12]

CareNotes™ System

● Also available as a subset of Micromedex (https://www.micromedex.com), the CareNotes® System enables the clinician to provide customizable patient education documents in 15 different languages (confirmed to be written at a 6th–8th grade reading level in English and Spanish). These documents may address general health condition information, pre-procedure or presurgical information, education regarding inpatient and discharge care for patients, laboratory test information, and a section titled DrugNotes, which includes patient-directed drug information for both prescription and nonprescription medications.[13]

Medscape®

● Medscape® (https://www.medscape.com) provides a very comprehensive set of tools to assist clinicians in practice. This database contains a drug reference, drug interaction checker, medical calculators, disease and condition reference, procedure reference, as well as formulary information. There are almost 2000 insurance plans, covering all 50 states, included to assist with comparison of tier drug status for patients. Medscape® also includes medical news, continuing education to support professional development for medical providers, and links to the MEDLINE® database to review journal articles and clinical evidence. Users can subscribe to free email updates addressing breaking medical and health news. This database has an app for Android® and Apple® devices.

Natural Medicines®, Pharmacist's Letter®, and Prescriber's Letter®

● All published by Therapeutic Research Center, subscriptions to each of these publications are available electronically, may be downloaded to electronic handheld devices, and may be of great value, especially in the ambulatory care setting. These databases have an app for Android® and Apple® devices.

Natural Medicines®

● Natural Medicines® (https://naturalmedicines.therapeuticresearch.com) is a paid subscription database providing evidence-based information regarding complementary, alternative, integrative, and natural medicines. The database, which combined former Natural Standard® with Natural Medicines Comprehensive Database®, provides detailed monographs with evidence-based ratings, safety ratings, and interaction ratings based on currently available literature. Natural Medicines® includes a useful natural product/drug interaction checker, and patient handouts written in both English and Spanish.[13]

An "efficacy" rating, which rates each natural medication on the likelihood of its being effective for a given condition, coined the NMBER (Natural Medicines Brand Evidence-based Rating), is provided in this reference. The NMBER is of particular use to the ambulatory clinician, enabling frank discussion of the risk versus benefit of complementary or natural medicines. Information regarding perioperative use of natural medications is also available.

Pharmacist's Letter® and Prescriber's Letter®

Pharmacist's Letter® (http://pharmacistsletter.com) and Prescriber's Letter® (http://prescribersletter.com) are paid subscription newsletters that provide detailed information regarding prescription and nonprescription medications, including full monographs with evidence-based ratings, safety rating, and interactions based on currently available literature. The main difference between these two databases is the target audience. Both publications cover new developments in drug therapy and trends in practice, concise updates, and advice regarding current therapeutic issues with links to a detailed document with a more in-depth explanation of the topic. These publications also include very useful comprehensive disease-, medication-, and practice-related charts. For example, ambulatory care clinicians may find comparison charts for statins, insulin products, injectable anticoagulants, and anticipated availability of first-time generics. Links to treatment guidelines for a variety of commonly treated conditions are also available (e.g., cardiology, diabetes, gastroenterological conditions, asthma, COPD). A "Rumor vs. Truth" section may also be of use for quick reference when fielding questions from the public on misstated facts or exaggerated efficacy claims in the media.

UpToDate®

UpToDate® (https://www.uptodate.com/home) can be used to access current practice guidelines, full-text articles, medication information, patient education, and much more. UpToDate® is particularly useful for finding information about disease states. Continuing education credit for health care professionals is also available. This database has an app for Android® and Apple® devices.

ACCESS CONSIDERATIONS

Because of increasing amounts of current drug information available exclusively online, or for which online access provides regularly updated information not otherwise available, it is strongly recommended that all providers of drug information and direct patient care have access to reputable Internet-based information in order to ethically, accurately, and competently perform their responsibilities. Health care professionals and employers should ensure that this is available to those providing medical information to others. Some colleges of pharmacy or medicine may provide access to subscription electronic resources for health care professionals who regularly precept or provide other educational opportunities for students from the college.

PATIENT EDUCATION

While the preceding section focused on patient education components of individual resources, this section further discusses the importance of educating patients on the appropriate use of their medications. Certainly, documents generated from the databases described above, manufacturer-provided patient information leaflets, and direct patient counseling at the pharmacy all serve to educate patients on intended use(s), cautions, possible side effects, and required monitoring for each medication, but this is not enough. Ambulatory care clinicians fill an important role in educating patients regarding the proper *administration* of certain medications (e.g., insulin, inhalers, injectable anticoagulants), the *management* of adverse reactions (e.g., hypoglycemia, bleeding), and dosing adjustments that may be required such as during perioperative periods or during periods of illness. While most of this information may be found within the individual drug information databases (e.g., how to reverse the effects of hypoglycemia caused by excess insulin or how to reverse the effects of warfarin), it is not always included in patient education materials, and must be *taught to the patient*. Additionally, for those medications that require specific administration technique, providing patients with written instructions is not enough.

Hands-on demonstration and teach-back communication are vital to ensuring medications are used optimally. Manufacturers of drug products that require special administration typically provide patient handouts for this purpose, and may provide practice devices for demonstration purposes. The CDC website (http://www.cdc.gov) also has useful videos, as well as tutorial sheets (e.g., asthma inhaler use, how to check blood glucose), which may be modified or used "as-is." Finally, for the condition of interest, there are often topic-specific patient education materials available from a national website for the disorder being treated. For example, http://www.diabetes.org includes links for recognizing and treating hypoglycemia, for testing blood glucose, and for "sick-day" management. Information obtained from any of these places, however, must be explained, tailored to the patient and the situation, and even demonstrated (e.g., glucose monitor, insulin pen) for the patient; ambulatory clinicians fill an important role in the provision of this type of drug information.

Case Study 26–2

Consider the following scenario:

Claire Collins, PharmD, is working in an outpatient anticoagulation clinic at a local physician's office, when PP, a Hispanic man in his mid-60s who takes warfarin for atrial fibrillation stops by to report a new medication and to confirm it is "okay" to take with his warfarin. PP states that "I'm always nervous about taking any new medication! I just filled the prescription and it was really expensive—they told me it 'wasn't on formulary,' whatever that means." After some discussion, Dr. Collins discovers that PP has been experiencing arthritis pain for the last month and saw his family doctor today who prescribed him celecoxib.

- *In addition to asking Dr. Collins to check for a drug interaction between warfarin and celecoxib, what drug information questions has PP either requested or implied he needs to know?*
- *How might Dr. Collins begin to answer each of these questions?*

    The patient (PP) requires the ambulatory care pharmacist to assist with several drug information queries. Before leaving the clinic, PP now asks for any information available (in addition to the leaflet stapled to the prescription bag he picked up at the pharmacy) regarding his new prescription. PP further requests that, if possible, he would like information in Spanish, as it is easier for him to read health-related information in his first language.

- *What resource database(s) could Dr. Collins refer to with patient information written at an appropriate level? Are there databases that are useful for traditional drug information geared toward the health care professional and that also have information geared toward patient education?*
- *Do any of these databases provide patient information in multiple languages?*

PATIENT DISPOSAL OF UNUSED MEDICATIONS

For the past several years, the Drug Enforcement Agency (DEA) has allowed community pharmacies in some states to voluntarily take part in drug take-back programs; this allows pharmacies to collect and appropriately dispose of unused medications from patients. This ruling affords patients the option of mailing their unused medications or placing them in pharmacy-maintained collection containers at a pharmacy. These containers can also be found at several local law enforcement agencies.[14] Health care providers can also take the next step and provide drug information to the inquirer regarding the safe and appropriate disposal of medications. For sharps disposal, few resources exist; the patient/provider should contact their local disposal company for additional information.

More often than in any other setting, ambulatory care practitioners are asked about disposal of unused or unwanted medications. While there are no specific laws regarding *personal* disposal of medications by patients, disposal of unused or unwanted pharmaceuticals (both prescription and nonprescription) is becoming an emerging and complex environmental issue. A nationally representative survey of 1006 adults completed by

Consumer Reports in 2017 found that about one-third of Americans haven't cleaned out the medicine cabinet in the past year; nearly one-fifth haven't done so in the past 3 years.[15] Drug information is often considered the provision of information to patients or health care providers about safe and appropriate use of medications, but it also includes serving as a resource for information about the proper storage and disposal of medications when they are not in use. ❻ *Ambulatory care clinicians bear a responsibility to educate patients on the proper disposal of unused and unwanted medications and should therefore be aware of pertinent sites for finding this information.*

The FDA (http://www.fda.gov) provides consumer health information regarding the disposal of unused medicines (https://www.fda.gov/drugs/safe-disposal-medicines/ disposal-unused-medicines-what-you-should-know) and has worked with the White House Office of National Drug Control Policy (ONDCP) to develop consumer guidance regarding this topic. Documents developed by these organizations are available online at the FDA and the ONDCP website.[16,17]

In addition, disposal information for some, but not all, medications may be found on DailyMed (http://dailymed.nlm.nih.gov/dailymed/about.cfm) by searching within prescription drug labels in one or more of the following fields: Information for Patients and Caregivers, Patient Information, Patient Counseling Information, Safety and Handling Instructions, or Medication Guide.

Additional useful online resources with information on the safe disposal of medications include those of the Pharmacist's Letter (http://www.pharmacistsletter.com) and the Institute for Safe Medical Practice (ISMP; http://www.ismp.org). The DEA also has an interactive database for locating drug take-back locations (https://apps2.deadiversion. usdoj.gov/pubdispsearch/spring/main?execution=e1s1). Finally, the Community Medical Foundation for Patient Safety (http://www.comofcom.com/) has developed a very useful document, the National Directory of Drug Take-Back and Disposal Programs.[18] Local and state drug take-back initiative sites may be listed on a case-by-case basis online; however, one site attempts to centralize drug take-back information on a national basis. The Product Stewardship Institute (PSI) addresses appropriate disposal of multiple types of products, including pharmaceuticals, and visitors to the PSI website may research take-back efforts and activities on a state-by-state basis.[19]

If no drug take-back locations are available and there are no specific disposal instructions in the medication guide, the following steps can be followed to dispose of most medicines in the trash[20]:

1. Mix medicines (liquid or tablets/capsules; do not crush) with an unappealing substance such as dirt, cat litter, or used coffee grounds.
2. Place the mixture in a container (e.g., a sealed plastic bag).
3. Throw away the container in the trash at home.

4. Delete all personal information on the prescription label of empty bottles or packaging, then trash or recycle.

There are a select few medications for which flushing *is* the FDA-recommended method of disposal. For these medications, the sentiment of FDA officials is that in order to best protect persons and animals that could inappropriately use these medications, prompt flushing of unused or unwanted medication is the preferred method of disposal.[21] The drugs are listed in Table 26-1.

Case Study 26–3

Abby P., who works in a diabetes and cardiology clinic, is approached by the widower of a former patient. The man is carrying a grocery bag which appears to be full of prescription bottles, insulin pens, and vials. "Can you take these, and perhaps donate or give them to someone who could use them? My wife passed away last month, and I probably have hundreds of dollars' worth of medication in this bag! If you can't use them, can you tell me where I should take them? I also have some used pen needles and syringes from her in this bag that I need to figure out how to get rid of."

- *Where can unused, unwanted, or expired medications be taken?*
- *If a patient wishes to dispose of medications, are there any associated legal requirements or guidelines?*

DRUG REPOSITORY PROGRAMS

Drug repository programs, which allow nursing homes, long-term care pharmacies, and wholesalers to donate unused medication for redistribution to those patients who meet prespecified criteria, may exist in certain states. While patients understandably may be reluctant to throw away their personal unused or unwanted medications, these medications, once dispensed and in patients' homes, are not eligible for donation to drug repository programs, as these drugs have left the custody and controlled environment of a pharmacy or institution. Practitioners should refer to their respective state's Board of Pharmacy website for information regarding drug repository programs.

PROVIDING IMMUNIZATION INFORMATION

Formerly provided primarily in the traditional clinician's office or in county or city health departments, immunizations are increasingly being delivered by pharmacists and other

TABLE 26–1. MEDICATIONS FORWHICH FLUSHING REMAINS THE FDA-RECOMMENDED METHOD OF DISPOSAL[17]

Medicine	Active Ingredient
Abstral, tablets (sublingual)	Fentanyl
Actiq, oral transmucosal lozenge[a]	Fentanyl citrate
Avinza, capsule (extended release)	Morphine sulfate
Belbuca, soluble film (buccal)	Buprenorphine hydrochloride
Buprenorphine hydrochloride, tablets (sublingual)[a]	Buprenorphine hydrochloride
Buprenorphine hydrochloride; Naloxone hydrochloride, tablets (sublingual)[a]	Buprenorphine hydrochloride; Naloxone hydrochloride
Butrans, transdermal patch system	Buprenorphine
Daytrana, transdermal patch system	Methylphenidate
Demerol, tablets[a]	Meperidine hydrochloride
Demerol, oral solution[a]	Meperidine hydrochloride
Diastat/Diastat AcuDial, rectal gel	Diazepam
Dilaudid, tablets[a]	Hydromorphone hydrochloride
Dilaudid, oral liquid[a]	Hydromorphone hydrochloride
Dolophine hydrochloride, tablets[a]	Methadone hydrochloride
Duragesic, patch (extended release)[a]	Fentanyl
Embeda, capsules (extended release)	Morphine sulfate; Naltrexone hydrochloride
Exalgo, tablets (extended release)	Hydromorphone hydrochloride
Fentora, tablets (buccal)	Fentanyl citrate
Hysingla ER, tablets (extended release)	Hydrocodone bitartrate
Kadian, capsules (extended release)	Morphine sulfate
Methadone hydrochloride, oral solution[a]	Methadone hydrochloride
Methadose, tablets[a]	Methadone hydrochloride
Morphabond, tablets (extended release)	Morphine sulfate
Morphine sulfate, tablets (immediate release)[a]	Morphine sulfate
Morphine sulfate, oral solution[a]	Morphine sulfate
MS Contin, tablets (extended release)[a]	Morphine sulfate
Nucynta ER, tablets (extended release)	Tapentadol
Onsolis, soluble film (buccal)	Fentanyl citrate
Opana, tablets (immediate release)	Oxymorphone hydrochloride
Oxecta, tablets (immediate release)	Oxycodone hydrochloride
Oxycodone hydrochloride, capsules	Oxycodone hydrochloride
Oxycodone hydrochloride, oral solution	Oxycodone hydrochloride
Oxycontin, tablets (extended release)[a]	Oxycodone hydrochloride
Percocet, tablets[a]	Acetaminophen; Oxycodone hydrochloride
Percodan, tablets[a]	Aspirin; Oxycodone hydrochloride
Suboxone, film (sublingual)	Buprenorphine hydrochloride; Naloxone hydrochloride

continued

TABLE 26–1. MEDICATIONS FOR WHICH FLUSHING REMAINS THE FDA-RECOMMENDED METHOD OF DISPOSAL[17] *(CONTINUED)*

Medicine	Active Ingredient
Targiniq ER, tablets (extended release)	Oxycodone hydrochloride; Naloxone hydrochloride
Xartemis XR, tablets	Oxycodone hydrochloride; Acetaminophen
Xtampza ER, capsules (extended release)	Oxycodone
Xyrem, oral solution	Sodium oxybate
Zohydro ER, capsules (extended release)	Hydrocodone bitartrate
Zubsolv, tablets (sublingual)	Buprenorphine hydrochloride; Naloxone hydrochloride

[a]These medications have a generic version or are only available as a generic.
Updated February 2019.

health care professionals in ambulatory care settings, including pharmacies and retail grocery stores. ❼ *While ambulatory care clinicians (in particular, pharmacists) typically recommend and/or dispense most medications, immunizations are medications that are administered in the ambulatory care setting. Those practitioners immunizing in this setting have the obligation to not only provide these services safely, but also serve as immediate sources of information (i.e., drug information) regarding the medications they are administering.*

Sources of Immunization Information
Centers for Disease Control and Prevention

While multiple texts exist regarding immunization and vaccine-preventable disease, The HHS, CDC website (http://www.cdc.gov) provides the most comprehensive, regularly updated information regarding immunizations. Links are available from the CDC webpage entitled Vaccines and Immunizations (http://www.cdc.gov/vaccines), for both the health care provider and for patients, providing up-to-date information regarding vaccine-preventable disease, as well as safety, adverse events, administration schedule, and dosing recommendations for immunizations. Also available from this site are Vaccine Information Statements (VISs), which must be distributed with their respective immunizations. Moreover, ambulatory care providers should engage in nonjudgmental discussions with patients/caregivers opposed to vaccinations (now termed "anti-vaxxers"), and provide information about where reputable information about vaccines can be found, such as the CDC website.

Epidemiology and Prevention of Vaccine-Preventable Disease

The textbook, commonly referred to as the Pink Book, is published annually by the Public Health Foundation.[22] It provides health care professionals, such as physicians, nurses, nurse practitioners, physician assistants, and pharmacists, comprehensive information regarding vaccine-preventable diseases. The textbook is available for purchase in print; however, PDFs of each chapter are available fully formatted for download from the CDC website at https://www.cdc.gov/vaccines/pubs/pinkbook/chapters.html. While this text does not provide vaccine-specific information, it provides detailed information regarding respective vaccine-preventable disease, including epidemiology, prevalence, and prevention recommendations.

Immunization Training for the Pharmacist

The prerequisites for pharmacists to administer immunizations vary from state to state, and pharmacists are advised to refer to their state's laws and confer with their state board of pharmacy regarding specific questions; however, in each state that allows for pharmacist-administered vaccines, a training program approved by the state pharmacy board is required. The most widely recognized training program, Pharmacy-Based Immunization Delivery, is offered nationally by APhA (http://www.pharmacist.com). Other programs do exist that may be recognized nationally or within specific states only. Pharmacists may wish to inquire with their specific state board of pharmacy regarding recognized and approved training programs. Regardless of the training program initially utilized, it is expected that pharmacists, as well as all other providers of health care, maintain and document appropriate continuing education for the immunizations and the associated drug information they deliver.

QUALITY ASSURANCE CONSIDERATIONS IN AMBULATORY CARE

Quality assurance is one of the key responsibilities of ambulatory care practitioners. While institutions that are under the umbrella of a health care facility generally consider the standards set forth by The Joint Commission (TJC) as a primary source of quality assurance guidelines, several other organizations provide quality assurance guidelines that may be applied to a variety of care settings.

Via a variety of initiatives, including the **Accountable Care Organizations** (ACOs) model, CMS has specified 33 required **quality measures** that are evaluated to determine payment structure for patient care networks, which are inclusive of ambulatory care settings. The quality measures themselves are standards set forth that evaluate efficiency (or resource use), structure, process, intermediate outcome, long-term outcome, and patient centeredness (which includes patient reports of satisfaction).[23] CMS has also contracted with Florida Medical Quality Assurance, Inc. (FMQAI) in a project particularly pertinent to quality assurance in the ambulatory care setting. The project, Medication Measure Special Innovation Project, is tasked with maintaining the current 33 quality measures and expanding them to include new measures focused on medication-related patient safety (e.g., detecting/preventing medication errors, adverse drug reactions). The project specifically includes a portfolio of six National Quality Forum (NQF)-endorsed measures for the ambulatory care setting, including measures related to patient adherence to specific medication classes, adherence to regular monitoring for warfarin (both routine and when on antibiotics), and adherence of patients with schizophrenia to antipsychotic therapy.

❽ *Health care professionals involved in providing patient care in the ambulatory care setting should familiarize themselves with the pertinent, established quality measures.*

Assuring patient safety is a crucial component of quality care and ISMP is an important resource for health care providers in any setting. ISMP publishes four distinct newsletters, each geared toward practitioners in a different health care setting. The ISMP Medication Safety Alert! Community/Ambulatory Care edition is targeted toward pharmacists, pharmacy technicians, nurses, physicians, and other community health professionals. This newsletter is sent monthly as an email, and provides up-to-date information about medication-related errors, adverse drug reactions, and their implications for community practice sites. Finally, the newsletter includes recommendations on how to improve medication safety within the community setting (http://www.ismp.org/Newsletters/default.asp). A subscription to this newsletter is recommended for all ambulatory care providers (ISMP Medication Safety Alert! Community/Ambulatory Care edition), but there is a cost associated with subscribing. More information regarding ISMP as well as its newsletters can be found at http://www.ismp.org.[24]

Finally, the tracking, reporting, and prevention of not only medication errors, but also "near misses," is paramount to assuring quality in any health care setting, including ambulatory care. ISMP and the National Coordinating Council for Medication Error Reporting and Prevention (NCC MERP) are two organizations dedicated to this task. The reader should refer to Chapter 20 for a complete discussion on organizations and programs devoted to assuring quality by reporting and prevention of medication errors.

The APhA website (https://www.pharmacist.com) has a Patient Safety and Quality Assurance page that provides links to AHRQ, ISMP, the National Patient Safety Foundation (NPSF), the United States Pharmacopeia (USP) Medication Errors Reporting Form, and the PSPC Collaborative.

Case Study 26–4

Paul, a recent graduate from a college of pharmacy, is working in a private practice ambulatory care clinic where he provides medication recommendations to prescribers and counsels patients regarding disease state management. The manager of the clinic approaches Paul and asks him to become involved in measuring quality assurance indicators for all health care providers in the clinic, including patient satisfaction with the care that has been provided.

- *What type of quality assurance indicators/metrics are utilized by outside organizations?*
- *Is patient satisfaction with care a recognized quality indicator?*
- *Are there published guidelines for quality indicators in ambulatory care?*

Conclusion

As health professionals committed to optimal patient care, the provision of drug information goes far beyond providing patient information leaflets with medications. Application of drug information is performed routinely in the ambulatory care setting in a variety of manners, and it is in this setting that the clinician pulls it all together and takes the most important step—imparting this information not only to patients and their caregivers, but to other health care providers in an understandable, personalized, and practical format that will serve to improve health care.

Self-Assessment Questions

1. Which of the following statements support the need for the skilled provision of drug information in ambulatory care? Select all that apply.
    a. There is not a consistent level of drug information education in the curricula of various health care professions.
    b. There is a lack of drug information freely available to the public.
    c. The ambulatory care clinician is able to access databases that may not be available to the public.
    d. A significant number of emergency room visits and hospital admissions each year are attributed to pharmaceuticals.

2. Which of the following best describes the drug information responsibilities of an ambulatory care clinician?
    a. Assisting prescribers and patients find the most cost-effective drug therapy for a given condition

b. Ensuring a prescribed medication is appropriate and follows current treatment guidelines
c. Ensuring a patient's understanding of the appropriate use of his/her medications
d. Guiding individuals regarding the proper disposal of unused or unwanted medications
e. All of the above

3. Which of the following statements is true regarding prescription formularies?
   a. A prescriber may not prescribe a medication if it is not on a patient's drug insurance formulary.
   b. Electronic prescribing has not been shown to affect the likelihood of prescribing tier 1 medications.
   c. Programs such as Lexicomp®, Epocrates®, and Medscape® include formulary information.
   d. Medicare Part D participants cannot perform side-by-side comparisons of prescription plans that are available to them and that cover some or all of their medications.

4. A Tier 1 medication will result in a lower patient responsibility for payment than a Tier 3 medication.
   a. True
   b. False
   c. Depends on the insurance company

5. Where can evidence-based clinical practice guidelines be found?
   a. Centers for Disease Control and Prevention (CDC)
   b. National Heart, Lung, and Blood Institute (NHLBI)
   c. American Society of Health-System Pharmacist (ASHP)
   d. PubMed
   e. All of the above

6. A physician would like to know which sources he can utilize to find current practice guidelines for his patient with hyperlipidemia. All of the following are appropriate to recommend EXCEPT:
   a. American College of Cardiology
   b. American Heart Association
   c. ECRI Institute
   d. Institute for Safe Medical Practice (ISMP)
   e. Centers for Disease Control and Prevention (CDC)

7. Which of the following characteristics are desirable for electronic drug information resources in the ambulatory care setting?
   a. Access is easy and readily available.
   b. Updates are frequent.
   c. An appropriate level of information is provided.
   d. All of the above.

8. A patient brings to her wellness appointment a variety of herbal supplements that she wants to know more about prior to taking. She requests information about the supplements' efficacy as well as safety. Which of the following databases would *best* assist the ambulatory practitioner in answering this patient's inquiries?
   a. Clinical Pharmacology®
   b. Drug Facts and Comparisons®
   c. Natural Medicines®
   d. Micromedex®
   e. Prescriber's Letter

9. The Pharmacist's Letter website provides all of the following *except*:
   a. Comparison tables for drug classes
   b. Links to medication error reporting databases
   c. Developments in drug therapy
   d. Downloadable documents for handheld devices

10. Which of the following are potential options to increase access to drug information when resources are limited?
   a. Encourage employers to ensure Internet access is available to all those providing medical information to others.
   b. Consider partnering resources with a local college of medicine or pharmacy.
   c. Utilize the services of a drug information center.
   d. All of the above.

11. The Food and Drug Administration (FDA) classifies each of the following as an inappropriate method for disposal of unwanted medications EXCEPT:
   a. Flushing unused liquid medications
   b. Mixing medications with cat litter
   c. Burning with other trash
   d. Using a community dumpster

12. Which of the following statements is true regarding immunizations? Select all that apply.
   a. They are not considered medications.

b. They may be administered by pharmacists.

c. They must be accompanied by a vaccine information statement (VIS) upon administration.

d. They are only available in physicians' offices.

13. Which of the following organizations utilizes reports which include quality indicators as rated by consumers of health care?
   a. Institute for Safe Medical Practice (ISMP)
   b. Centers for Medicare and Medicaid Services (CMS)
   c. Patient Safety Clinical Pharmacy Services (PSPC)
   d. Food and Drug Administration (FDA)

14. Which of the following organizations provides recent drug-related news, drug approvals, recalls and safety warnings, therapeutic equivalency codes, and MedWatch adverse event reporting data?
   a. Centers for Disease Control and Prevention (CDC)
   b. Food and Drug Administration (FDA)
   c. Medscape
   d. White House Office of National Drug Control Policy (ONDCP)

15. A care delivery model, led by a physician or other primary care provider that includes other types of providers including pharmacists, which coordinates patient treatment to ensure necessary care and optimized patient outcomes is called:
   a. Patient Centered Medical Home (PCMH)
   b. Accountable Care Organization (ACO)
   c. Agency for Healthcare Research and Quality (AHRQ)
   d. Electronic Health Record (EHR)

REFERENCES

1. Drug Topics. On the road to provider status [Internet]. 2019 Jun 13 [cited 2019 Sep 24]. Available from: https://www.drugtopics.com/clinical-news/road-provider-status.

2. MarketWatch. Almost half of Americans have used prescription drugs in the past month [Internet]. [Updated 2019 May 8; cited 2020 May 2]. Available from: https://www.marketwatch.com/story/almost-half-of-americans-have-used-a-prescription-drug-in-the-past-month-2019-05-08

3. Centers for Medicare and Medicaid Services. E-prescribing [Internet]. [Updated 2014 Feb 26; cited 2019 Sep 24]. Available from: https://www.cms.gov/Medicare/E-Health/Eprescribing/index.html?redirect=/eprescribing/.

4. Porterfield A, Engelbert K, Coustasse A. Electronic prescribing: improving the efficiency and accuracy of prescribing in the ambulatory care setting. Perspect Health Inf Manag. 2014.

5. Fischer MA, Vogeli C, Stedman M, Ferris T, Brookhart A, Weissman JS. Effect of electronic prescribing with formulary decision support on medication use and cost. Arch Intern Med. 2008;168(22):2433–9.

6. Chang C, Nguyen N, Smith A, Huynh D. Electronic prescribing increases generic and formulary drug use [Internet]. [Updated 2010 Jun 7; cited 2019 Sep 24]. Available from: http://www.physicianspractice.com/articles/electronic-prescribing-increases-generic-and-formulary-drug-use

7. ECRI Institute [Internet]. Plymouth Meeting (PA). [Cited 2019 Sep 30]. Available from: https://www.ecri.org

8. National Center for Biotechnology Information, U.S. National Library of Medicine, National Institutes of Health. PubMed.gov [Internet]. [Cited 2019 Sep 24]. Available from: http://www.ncbi.nlm.nih.gov/pubmed/.

9. Epocrates® [Internet]. San Mateo (CA). [Updated 2011; cited 2019 Sep 24]. Available from: http://www.epocrates.com./products/comparison_table.html

10. Lexicomp ONLINE User Guide [Internet]. Hudson (OH). [Cited 2019 Sep 24]. Available from: http://online.lexi.com

11. Micromedex DRUGDEX [Internet]. Truven Health Analytics, Inc. Ann Arbor (MI). [Cited 2020 May 2]. Available from: https://www.micromedexsolutions.com/micromedex2/4.85.0/WebHelp/Document_help/Drug_Eval_document.htm

12. Micromedex Consumer Health Information [Internet]. Truven Health Analytics, Inc. Ann Arbor (MI). [Cited 2019 Sep 24]. Available from: http://www.truvenhealth.com/your_healthcare_focus/hospital_patient_care_decisions/consumer_engagement.aspx

13. Natural Medicines [Internet]. Therapeutic Research Center. Somerville (MA). [Cited 2019 Sep 24]. Available from: https://naturalmedicines.therapeuticresearch.com/.

14. DEA: Pharmacies can voluntarily participate in take-back programs [Internet]. American Pharmacists Association. [Updated 2014 Oct 1; cited 2019 Sep 24]. Available from: http://www.pharmacist.com/dea-pharmacies-can-voluntarily-participate-take-back-programs

15. Consumer Reports. Many people fail to get rid of unneeded and expired drugs [Internet]. [Updated 2018 Jul 23; cited 2019 Sep 24]. Available from: https://www.washingtonpost.com/national/health-science/many-people-fail-to-get-rid-of-unneeded-and-expired-drugs/2018/07/20/0c87e024-65d6-11e8-a768-ed043e33f1dc_story.html

16. FDA Consumer Health Information. How to dispose of unused medications [Internet]. [Updated 2013 Dec; cited 2019 Sep 24]. Available from: http://www.fda.gov/downloads/Drugs/ResourcesForYou/Consumers/BuyingUsingMedicineSafely/UnderstandingOver-the-CounterMedicines/ucm107163.pdf.

17. Disposal of unused medications: what you should know [Internet]. [Cited 2019 Sep 24]. Available from: http://www.fda.gov/Drugs/ResourcesForYou/Consumers/BuyingUsingMedicineSafely/EnsuringSafeUseofMedicine/SafeDisposalofMedicines/ucm186187.htm.

18. Communities now has a resource to get rid of unused and expired medicines from home [Internet]. [Updated 2011 Sep 16; cited 2019 Sep 24]. Available from: http://www.comofcom.com/News%20Release_National%20Directory%20091611.pdf

19. Product Stewardship Institute. The drug take-back network [Internet]. [Cited 2019 Sep 24]. Available from: https://www.productstewardship.us/page/Pharmaceuticals

20. U.S. Food and Drug Administration. Disposal of unused medicines: what you should know [Internet]. [Updated 2019 Feb 1; cited 2020 May 2]. Available from: https://www.fda.gov/drugs/safe-disposal-medicines/disposal-unused-medicines-what-you-should-know

21. Medicines recommended for disposal by flushing [Internet]. [Updated 2016 Apr; cited 2019 Sep 24]. Available from: http://www.fda.gov/downloads/Drugs/ResourcesForYou/Consumers/BuyingUsingMedicineSafely/EnsuringSafeUseofMedicine/SafeDisposalofMedicines/UCM337803.pdf

22. Hamborsky J, Kroger A, Wolfe S. Centers for Disease Control and Prevention. Epidemiology and prevention of vaccine-preventable diseases [Internet]. 13th ed. Washington (DC). [Updated 2015; cited 2019 Sep 24]. Available from: http://www.cdc.gov/vaccines/pubs/pinkbook/index.html

23. Centers for Medicaid and Medicare Services. Quality measures and performance standards [Internet]. [Updated 2015 Mar 2; cited 2019 Sep 24]. Available from: https://www.cms.gov/Medicare/Quality-Initiatives-Patient-Assessment-Instruments/QualityMeasures/index.html

24. ISMP Medication Safety Alert®! Newsletters. Institute for Safe Medical Practice [Internet]. [Cited 2019 Sep 24]. Available from: http://www.ismp.org/Newsletters/default.asp

SUGGESTED READINGS

1. American Society of Health-System Pharmacists. ASHP Guidelines: minimum standard for ambulatory care pharmacy practice. Am J Health-Syst Pharm. 2015;72:1221–36.

2. Centers for Medicare and Medicaid Services. Accountable care organizations (ACO). [Updated 2019 Mar 8; cited 2019 Sep 3]. Available from: http://www.cms.gov/Medicare/Medicare-Fee-for-Service-Payment/ACO/index.html

Chapter Twenty-Seven

Drug Information and Contemporary Community Pharmacy Practice

Morgan L. Sperry • Heather A. Pace

Learning Objectives

After completing this chapter, the reader will be able to:

- Discuss limitations of the current approaches pharmacists use to deliver drug information to their patients.
- Compare and contrast patient education and consumer health information (CHI) as drug information sources for patients.
- Define social networking and describe how patients use this tool as a drug information source.
- Discuss mobile health information technology and its impact on how consumers are obtaining information.
- Describe the model for drug information services delivered by pharmacists.
- Design three strategies using electronic media to assist patients in receiving and applying high-quality drug information.
- Identify characteristics of a high-quality health literate Internet site.
- Define participatory medicine and describe how this model changes the dynamic of the patient and the health care professional.

Key Concepts

❶ The trend for patients to obtain their health information from sources disconnected from health care professionals continues to grow, contributing to shifted relationships between patients and their traditional touchstones in health care, namely physicians, nurses, and pharmacists.

② Answering drug information questions is a routine part of a pharmacist's day, but it is often a passive process that hinges upon the patient's initiative to ask important questions regarding their health.

③ Patient education delivers written or verbal drug information initiated by a health care provider. Potential goals include changing behavior, improving adherence, and ultimately improving patient health.

④ CHI is often sought by the patient in response to their desire or need for more information about their health. Importantly, CHI is not individualized for a specific patient.

⑤ Social media sites allow patients to create content and share information about their health on the Internet.

⑥ Wisdom of crowds is a belief that when patients share information about their common conditions through social networking, their collective wisdom is more beneficial than the expert opinion of just one individual.

⑦ The use of mobile technology to obtain CHI has continued to expand.

⑧ Pharmacists should discuss with their patients why they remain an important source of drug information. Patients should be encouraged not to see CHI as a replacement for personal interaction with a health care provider, but as an extension of care and a way to improve communication.

⑨ Patients often have difficulty finding accurate information in response to their specific health concerns on the Internet.

⑩ Once patients identify or are given quality health information, they still may face barriers in being able to use it to improve their health.

⑪ Participatory medicine is a model of cooperative health care. In this model, patients no longer play a passive part when it comes to their health care but an active role alongside the health care provider. Patients are seen as valuable health care resources, and providers are encouraged to view them as equal partners.

Introduction

Pharmacists' roles and responsibilities continue to evolve in response to changing pharmacy practice acts and a dynamic health care environment. One constant is the pharmacist's key function as a provider of quality, evidence-based drug information. However, pharmacists are not the only source of drug information. Use of the Internet, including social networking sites and mobile technology, has made information from sources other than health care professionals exponentially more accessible. The move toward patient-centered care and consumerism increases the desire for patients to be in control of their health care and be an active part of the decision-making process. ❶ *The trend for patients to obtain their health information from sources disconnected from health care professionals continues to grow and it has shifted relationships between patients and their traditional touchstones in health care, namely physicians, nurses, and pharmacists.*[1] According to the most recent Pew Internet and American Life Project national survey, 72% of Internet users went online to search for some type of health or wellness information within the past year. In fact, one-third of adults in the United States report going online to self-diagnose their illnesses. This group of people is often referred to as "online diagnosers."[2] The pharmacist's role as the drug information expert may also be changing in the eyes of the patient. The clinician still remains a central health information resource for a majority of patients, but the role that friends, family, and peers are playing both offline and online is ever expanding.[3]

Pharmacy practice is moving away from its emphasis on the hands-on drug distribution model toward an emphasis on system management and patient care services.[4,5] It is important for pharmacists to enhance patient care services for a multitude of reasons, one of which being the significant expenditures seen with unresolved drug-related problems. In the United States, the estimated annual cost of prescription drug-related morbidity and mortality resulting from nonoptimized medication therapy was $528 billion in 2016.[6,7] A key strategy to optimize medication therapy and adherence is to improve patients' understanding of their disease and its management, and includes individual needs in the treatment planning. This strategy requires individualized care that is not available from the Internet and other information sources. Pharmacists can remain a valuable drug information source for patients because they are one of the most accessible health care practitioners. Pharmacists can help patients customize and interpret information they find on the Internet and from other sources such as social media and mobile health applications. Project Destiny, an initiative aimed to validate community pharmacy's future role as a valuable and integral component in the delivery of health care, encouraged pharmacists to "embrace community pharmacy health care beyond dispensing," and paved the way for improved medication therapy management (MTM) services.[8] Within the MTM model, a pharmacist's role is not narrowed to just providing health care services related to medications, but includes providing comprehensive health care that optimizes patient outcomes, which can contribute to the overall lowering of health care costs.[9] In addition, pharmacists must step up and add drug information services beyond what a patient can find on their own, as well as develop demand for these services. Pharmacists are well positioned to address these drug information needs as they are medication experts and trusted professionals. Patients should view pharmacists as key medication advisors. Patients will often see results from clinical research on the news or through the Internet. They may not understand how these results relate directly to them and may reconsider continuing their medication. Pharmacists, with understanding of both the medical literature and the patient's medical history, can help the patient understand whether these new findings are clinically relevant to their individual situation. For example, in recent years the role aspirin plays for primary prevention of cardiovascular events has gotten a lot of media and press attention. This leaves those patients reading the headlines and watching the news stories on this topic confused and unsure of whether they should start, stop, or continue taking aspirin for this purpose. This is where pharmacists can step in and help patients make a decision that is right for them based on their individual circumstances and the evidence.

According to a recent survey, 94% of patients selected a specific pharmacy based on location and convenience. When price is not a factor, accuracy and trust provided by the pharmacists were cited as a reason for going to a pharmacy only 9% and 4% of the time, respectively. These results further support the need to develop consumer demand for pharmacy patient care services.[10] The purpose of this chapter is to shed light on how increased patient demand for autonomy and responsibility over their own health care and use of information sources beyond health professionals impacts pharmacy. With this move away from traditional health care models, it is essential that pharmacists create new services that will encourage patients to engage and view the pharmacist as an essential member of their health care team. Additionally, new models for pharmacists delivering drug information will be addressed.

Pharmacists as Drug Information Providers

Pharmacists are ideally equipped to provide health information to their patients regarding medications and disease states because of the variety of health care settings in which they practice. Whether it is a long-term care facility, an ambulatory care clinic, a patient's hospital room, or the local pharmacy, pharmacists have the access and ability to be a patient's primary drug information provider.

In the community setting, pharmacists are required by the Omnibus Budget Reconciliation Act of 1990 (OBRA '90) to deliver patient counseling when they dispense a Medicaid prescription.[11] Some individual states also mandate that counseling be extended to all patients, irrespective of their insurance. While some pharmacists are diligent in providing important information to their patients when they pick up a prescription, others only give information if specifically asked. In fact, although unacceptable and in violation of many state board regulations, patients may be asked by pharmacy staff to electronically sign to decline counseling without being asked whether they want it or not. Some patients do not even know what they are signing. ❷ *Answering drug information questions is a routine part of a pharmacist's day, but it is often a passive process that hinges upon the patient's initiative to ask important questions regarding their health.* A variety of reasons may preclude patients from using their pharmacist as a primary health information resource. One reason being that many patients do not understand the role their community pharmacists have in collaborative patient care. Some patients feel they can only get health information from their doctor. Additionally, although the most accessible health care professional to patients, pharmacists often may appear too busy and unavailable within the sometimes hectic pharmacy. As a result, technicians or cashiers may be the only staff who speak directly to the patient. Simply asking whether or not a patient has questions is the wrong way to initiate counseling. Patients may not be sure what they need to know, or feel embarrassed to admit their lack of knowledge. In some cases, patients are unaware they should be asking questions. Some simply do not understand the impact of pharmacotherapy to their long-term health and well-being and are not invested in learning about the appropriate use of their medication.

Patient leaflets are just one example why patients may not seek out their pharmacist as a primary health information resource. Instead of direct patient communication, patient leaflets are commonly stapled to the prescription as a substitute for actual patient education. Additionally, many of these leaflets are not properly written to accommodate those patients with poor health literacy. In fact, research has shown that the majority of patients do not even bother reading through the leaflet due to the complex language, small typeface, narrow spacing, and poor design.[12] Additional information on the importance of good health literacy will be discussed later in this chapter.

Some pharmacies have developed websites to direct patients to quality drug information and offer an additional path for patients to ask questions. Many large chain pharmacies and mail-order pharmacies have begun to post answers to the most frequently asked drug information questions for their consumers on their websites and some allow for even more interaction online by giving patients the opportunity to ask their questions to a pharmacist. It is important to note that while these pharmacies are headed in the right direction in terms of giving patients more readily available access to quality health information online, these websites still have many limitations. Patients enrolled in disease state management and MTM programs require the pharmacist to be engaged in focused and directed patient education as part of a comprehensive treatment plan; something that cannot be done by passive answering of questions or interfacing with a website alone.

Opportunities to provide quality health information to patients also exist for pharmacists working in many settings other than the community. From counseling that occurs during a clinic visit to discharge counseling done at the end of a hospital stay, pharmacists should have face-time with patients in order to ensure the patient understands how to best manage their medications and disease state(s). Pharmacists also play an important role within the emerging movement toward more effective transitions of care for patients. Moving patients around between various health care settings as their condition and care needs change is often a barrier to providing quality health information. The Joint Commission (TJC) names ineffective patient education as one of the root causes for why breakdown occurs during the transition of care process. Patients and caregivers often are given conflicting recommendations, complex medication regimens, and confusing instructions on how to follow up with their care. This is an area where pharmacists can provide an extremely beneficial service within the transitions of care multidisciplinary team.[13]

Patient Sources of Drug Information

The practice of collecting and disseminating drug information continues to evolve along with the profession. Drug information can be as simple as obtaining information from references, or as complex as an interactive experience between a specific patient and the pharmacist.[14] Drug information can be as active as counseling a patient on all of his or her medications and disease states or as passive as a pharmacy technician dispensing a medication leaflet with a prescription. Regardless of how drug information is delivered, patients need a more connected experience when receiving drug information, not only from health care professionals, but from peers as well.[1]

PATIENT EDUCATION VERSUS CONSUMER HEALTH INFORMATION

Patient education and **consumer health information (CHI)** are two distinct ways patients receive information about medications, although the two may merge when pharmacists truly engage their patients. ❸ *Patient education delivers written or verbal drug information initiated by a health care provider. Potential goals include changing patient behavior, improving adherence and ultimately improving patient health.*[15] Pharmacist-driven patient education formats include brief counseling when a patient picks up their medication, education to patients when administering immunizations, more comprehensive education as a part of MTM, point-of-care testing (e.g., blood glucose or cholesterol testing), and health screenings. Patient education can be delivered face-to-face or through a variety of technologies. The key is that pharmacists interact with individual patients to customize the information to their specific situation.

❹ *CHI is actively sought by the patient in response to their desire or need for more information about their health. Importantly, CHI is not individualized for a specific patient.* Unlike patient education, which is typically initiated by the pharmacist, CHI is completely patient-driven and has evolved out of the patient's need to be their own advocate. CHI has long been available to patients, but the rise of the Internet along with social media and mobile applications has accelerated both the access to and the volume of information; the choices are endless for patients seeking their own information. In 2013, at least 72% of U.S. adults had looked online for health information within the past year.[16] For either patient education or CHI to be of any value to the patient, it is crucial that information presented to the patient be of high quality. Controlling quality during a patient education encounter is easier because the health care professional filters information distributed to patients. In contrast, the quality and reliability of CHI is variable.[17] CHI may be of excellent quality and beneficial to the patient, or it may be of high quality but dangerous because it lacks relevance to their situation, be incomplete, or simply be wrong. Table 27-1 lists examples of popular CHI sites.

TABLE 27-1.   EXAMPLES OF CONSUMER HEALTH INFORMATION AND SOCIAL MEDIA SITES[18-28]

Consumer Health Platform	Description
American Cancer Society® (https://www.cancer.org/)	Supports and conducts research as well as is a source for patients. This site promotes healthy living to help prevent cancer, emotional support for patients, the latest cancer information for those who have been touched by cancer and much more. Resources are available 24 hours a day, 7 days a week.
Cleveland Clinic Health Library (https://my.clevelandclinic.org/health)	Provides patients access to thousands of health articles, videos, and tools in order to better manage their health.
Drugs.com (https://www.drugs.com/)	Aims to be the Internet's most trusted resource for drug and related health information. Provides patients with a variety information on over 24,000 prescription and over-the-counter drugs. A pill identifier, drug interaction checker, new drug approvals, and health-related news articles are all available to consumers as well.
Consumer Reports® (https://www.consumerreports.org/health/) (https://www.consumerreports.org/drugs/ consumer-reports-best-buy-drugs/)	Requiring a monthly or annual subscription, this online resource provides patients with information and unbiased ratings on topics such as healthy living, conditions and treatments, physicians, insurance companies, natural health, and prescription drugs. Health expert blogs are also provided for subscribers on an array of health topics. The Best Buy Drugs feature of this website was created in 2004 to help patients compare brand prescription drugs against generics and provide consumers with the best medicine to treat their disease state for their money.
Everyday Health® (http://www.everydayhealth.com)	Consumer-centric health company founded to empower and encourage patients to put themselves at the center of their health care. Claims to be a site for comprehensive health and medical information. Free to consumers, the site gears information toward the person they consider the family's chief medical officer (CMO), women or other caregivers. Blogs, forums, and online communities are available so patients can talk to people similar to themselves.

continued

TABLE 27–1. EXAMPLES OF CONSUMER HEALTH INFORMATION AND SOCIAL MEDIA SITES[18-28] (*CONTINUED*)

Consumer Health Platform	Description
GoodRx® (https://www.goodrx.com/)	A site available to consumers and health care professionals that gathers current prices and discounts to help users find the lowest cost pharmacy prescription medications.
Healthfinder (http://www.healthfinder.gov)	A site operated by the Department of Health and Human Services that serves as a gateway to consumer information. The major goal of this site is to improve consumer access to health information via government agencies, their partner organizations, and other trustworthy sources that serve the public interest.
Mayo Clinic (https://www.mayoclinic.org/)	A nonprofit organization committed to clinical practice, education and research, and providing expert whole-person care to everyone who needs healing. Among the many offerings this organization provides, health information regarding symptoms, disease states, medications, medical tests, and best healthy lifestyle practices can be found through this website.
MedlinePlus® (https://medlineplus.gov/)	An online health information resource for patients and their families and friends. A service of the National Library of Medicine, MedlinePlus® has a mission to present high-quality, relevant health and wellness information that is trusted, easy to understand, free of advertising, and free of cost.
PatientsLikeMe® (http://www.patientslikeme.com)	Privately funded social media site that was founded in 2004 with the intent of positively impacting patients diagnosed with life-changing diseases. This site is the world's largest personalized health network and welcomes patients living with any health condition. Through an online community of physicians, organizations, and patients, patients are encouraged to share information about their disease states, treatments, and overall experiences. The hope is that through this online platform patients will feel more connected to others going through similar circumstances as well as empowered and in more control of their disease state.
WebMD® (http://www.webmd.com)	Health website allowing patients to obtain their health information via a variety of different ways. Health information is available on a wealth of different topics such as drugs and treatments, disease states, and prevention. Online communities for patients seeking support or desiring to share their experiences are also set up in the form of blogs, video, and message boards. Additionally, patients have access to slide shows, newsletters, Food and Drug Administration (FDA) consumer updates, symptom checkers, drug identifiers, and ask the expert feature. WebMD has established an Independent Medical Review Board to ensure all health information made available to the public is accurate and timely.

SOCIAL MEDIA

Patients have long used friends, family, co-workers, and support groups as sources of medical information. The Internet adds to these traditional sources through **social media** as described in Table 27-2.[1] ⑤ *Social media sites allow patients to create content and share information about their health on the Internet.* Through the power of social media, the Internet goes beyond being merely a search engine and a source of information to a platform to create, share, and collaborate in developing new knowledge and opinions. Social networking is the phenomenon of online communities in which people share interests and/or activities with one another and has become an essential part of why patients are flocking to these sites. With the number of U.S. adults using social media climbing from 8% to 72% since 2005, it is clear this trend will likely continue to be a major factor.[29,30] With respect to CHI, patients no longer passively read about their health information online, but can have an active role in controlling content, creating new information, and sharing their experiences with others. This is often described as peer-to-peer health care. Patients realize that health care professionals provide a wealth of information but believe the wealth of information they can obtain from their peers with similar illnesses

TABLE 27-2. SOCIAL MEDIA DEFINITIONS AND PLATFORMS USED TO OBTAIN HEALTH INFORMATION[1,18]

Social Media	Definition	Platform Examples	URLs
Wikis	Allows user editing and adding of content via a collaborative website	Wikipedia Flu Wiki	http://www.wikipedia.org http://flu.wikia.com/wiki/Flu_Wiki
Social networks	A website where those with special interests in common can connect and share with one another	Angie's List® PatientsLikeMe® Everyday Health® Facebook Twitter	http://www.angieslist.com http://www.patientslikeme.com http://www.everydayhealth.com http://www.facebook.com http://www.twitter.com
Blogs	An online diary; one can log their personal thoughts on various topics and post to a web page	WebMD® Sharing Mayo Clinic	https://blogs.webmd.com/default.htm https://sharing.mayoclinic.org/
Online forums	Thoughts and ideas are shared and open discussion takes place via various mediums such as websites	Everyday Health® Google Health Yahoo! Groups	http://www.everydayhealth.com http://groups.google.com http://groups.yahoo.com
Video-sharing	A medium where information, ideas, and opinions can be shared via videos accessible to many	Instagram YouTube	www.instagram.com http://www.youtube.com

can be a significant supplement.[31] For example, PatientsLikeMe® (http://www.patients likeme.com/) is a privately funded company with the purpose of creating a community of patients with neurologic, neuroendocrine, psychiatric, and immune conditions. It quickly expanded and has become the world's largest personalized health network, welcoming all patients with any condition to connect with others. Site content is posted by actual patients and includes anything from treatments they have tried, what works and what does not work for them, and what side effects they have experienced. Discussions often include the quality of the care delivered by their providers.

❻ *Wisdom of crowds is a belief that when patients share information about their common conditions through social networking, their collective wisdom is more beneficial than the expert opinion of just one individual.* Some patients do not completely resist the advice of health professionals, but are just not as willing to rely on a single expert opinion for their information.[1] Health information received via social media is greatly valued by many consumers, especially the "net generation" as described by Don Tapscott in Grown Up Digital.[32] This "net generation" made up of consumers born in the early 1980s or after has grown up online and prefer to engage and collaborate via technology. Extremely used to the digital world, they often trust a search engine on the Internet to provide answers or an online peer review over an expert. Opinions, stories, successes and failures, treatment options, and adverse effects are just some of what this "net generation" of patients share on social media. This feeling of camaraderie and support obtained via networks is something patients may feel they cannot attain from health care professionals. Some patients may even have reservations when it comes to trusting their health care professional. According to the Edelman Trust Barometer, people are inclined more than ever to trust social media as a source for information.[33] In fact, almost one in five adult Internet users state they have gone online to connect with other people who have health conditions similar to themselves.[20] The concern with social media is that posts made by patients are a reflection of their unique experience and may be incorrect or inappropriate for another individual. It is imperative patients keep in mind that the information retrieved from peers should be used only to supplement the information provided by practitioners and that the Internet does not replace health care professionals.[34] Information found on social media can often lack quality and reliability, and be unreferenced and incomplete. Evidence-based medicine minimizes the importance of anecdotal reports where social media tends to affirm them, combining several different patient experiences into collective medical knowledge.[18] Most social media outlets that give consumers the ability to post opinions, recommendations, and health information state that they are not a substitute for advice of a qualified health professional. While the provision of these disclaimers can be a sign of a quality site, unfortunately, they are not always posted in the most visible place for many consumers on these websites, nor do consumers often heed these disclaimers' warning.

As health care professionals, it is also important to recognize the positive role social media can play in health care. Social media creates an additional opportunity for health care professionals to connect with their patients. Forty percent of consumers report that health information found via social media influences the way they approach their health.[35] In fact, 90% of patients 18–24 years old would engage in health activities or trust information found via social media versus 45% of patients aged 45–64.[36] This means that health care professionals have a duty to be a part of that discussion. By creating educational content as well as providing health information via social media platforms, health care professionals are able to reach a much larger audience all the while correcting misinformation and providing accurate information. Moreover, pharmacists can function as rumor control for incorrect information on the Internet, mainstream media, or from family and friends. Many physicians are already using social media to bolster patient health care education. By tweeting, making blog posts, recording videos, and participating in disease-specific discussions focused on patient education, some health care professionals are doing all they can to ensure evidence-based health information is getting to patients rather than inaccurate data that can be found on the Internet.[18] Patients appreciate interacting with their health care professionals online and a majority say they trust social media posts and activity by health care professionals over any other group.[24] In fact, recent studies have shown that social media interventions made by health care professionals affect patients in a variety of different ways such as weight loss, smoking cessation, reducing risky sexual behaviors, and increasing physical activity.[18]

While strides made by health care professionals to further connect with their patients via social media are a step in the right direction, it is still important to acknowledge that health information delivered over this medium also has barriers and drawbacks. Even when accurate information is shared, it is difficult to individualize to specific patients. Disclaimer made by health care professionals stating that patients should discuss any advice with their health care professional helps set this advice apart from CHI resources not run by health experts.

Case Study 27–1

You are the only pharmacist on duty at a local community pharmacy. You are short staffed, the phone is ringing, and you have 75+ prescriptions yet to verify. You are doing your best to make the wait as short as possible. In the midst of all this, one of your regular patients comes up to the counter and announces that she will no longer be taking her medication for her severe depression. She describes how lately she has been feeling strange and feels certain it is due to her Zoloft®. She then explains to you how she has recently gone online to find more information about the specific medication she is taking. "You wouldn't believe all the good information that is out there," she says, "I was able to talk to other patients and they were so helpful!" She then goes on to talk about the many patient testimonials she read telling her to discontinue her medication.

The patient seems adamant that she is going to stop taking her medication. As a pharmacist, this concerns you. The pharmacy technician calls you to resume verifying prescriptions because the pharmacy is quickly getting out of control.

- *Do you take the time to counsel this patient or do you get back to filling prescriptions before patients start complaining about the wait time?*
- *If you decide to counsel this patient, how would you educate her on the appropriate use of online resources to find health information?*
- *After counseling your patient, she still is determined to stop her Zoloft®. What is the most important advice you can give her at this point?*

MOBILE HEALTH (mHealth)

❼ *The use of mobile technology to obtain CHI has continued to expand.*

Smartphones have made obtaining health information online or via mobile software applications (also referred to as apps) much easier. In 2019, a total of 81% of U.S. adults owned a smartphone, up from 35% in 2011. Data from the Pew Research Center in 2015 showed that 62% of those smartphone owners have accessed health information with their smartphone within the past year. Among 18–29 year olds, 75% have gone online with their smartphone to look up a health condition.[37,38] With the vast majority of Americans owning a smartphone, retrieving health information is as simple as the touch of a fingertip. Nearly half of health care consumers are using mobile health apps (mHealth apps) to manage their health, with exercise, weight, pregnancy, and diet apps being among the most popular.[39,40] By 2023, the global mHealth app market is expected to reach US$102.35 billion. There were more than 318,000 mHealth apps available through the top app stores as of 2017, and this market continues to grow.[41] Consumers who download these mHealth apps may have a high trust in the accuracy of the information they provide.[28] It is clear smartphone use is here to stay for the foreseeable future, which means that U.S. adults are not only going on the Internet to find health information, but are also tracking and managing their own health data. Table 27-3 introduces a few of the numerous smartphone apps of which health care professionals should be aware. Additional discussion of mobile technology in drug information is addressed in Chapter 28. The mHealth era is just one

TABLE 27–3. EXAMPLES OF MOBILE HEALTH AND FITNESS APPLICATIONS[43–60]

Health and Fitness Applications	Description	Smartphone Availability	Fee
Apple Health	A Health app that consolidates data from your iPhone, Apple Watch, and third-party apps you already use. Overall health progress can be tracked in one convenient place. See your long-term trends, or dive into the daily details for a wide range of health metrics.	iOS	Free
Asthma MD	Allows users to log their asthma activity, medications, causes, and triggers of their asthma in the form of a diary. In addition, this information regarding their asthma activities can be shared with their physicians to be included in their medical records	iOS and Android	Free
Calm	An app specifically designed to help users lower stress, sleep better, and manage anxiety. Calm's mission is to make the world healthier and happier, through tutorials, videos, music, sleep stories, and much more; this app is focused on better sleep, meditation, and relaxation for the user	iOS and Android	Free Paid: premium version
First Aid	This app provides immediate first aid information to help with a variety of common emergencies. It is available through the American Red Cross	iOS and Android	Free
Flo Period and Ovulation Tracker	An evidence-based app focused on elevating women's health through their entire reproductive period	iOS and Android	Free Paid: premium version
GlucoseBuddy	An application designed for patients with diabetes who can monitor blood glucose levels, record when they take medication, and track food intake and physical activity	iOS and Android	Free Paid: premium version
Google Fit: Health and Activity Tracking	Tracks health information and coaches users to a healthier and more active lifestyle. Much like the Apple Health app, Google Fit works with many health apps and devices to provide a more holistic approach	iOS and Android	Free
Headspace	Officially launched in 2010, this app offers users education on the benefits of mindfulness and meditation. Exercises and techniques are provided to help patients with everything from stress to sleep	iOS and Android	Free trial Monthly: $12.99 Annually: $69.99

continued

TABLE 27–3. EXAMPLES OF MOBILE HEALTH AND FITNESS APPLICATIONS[43–60] (CONTINUED)

Health and Fitness Applications	Description	Smartphone Availability	Fee
Lose It!	Users looking to lose weight download this app in order to set daily calorie goals, track physical activity, find new exercises, and search for new health conscious recipes. Progress reports are also available for the consumer as well as the ability to share accomplishments via social media	iOS and Android	Free
MapMyRun	This app not only tracks the runners' exact path but also records other aspects of a workout like speed, distance, pace, and calories burned. The runner can also share their run data via social media. Versions also exist for walking, hiking, biking, and triathlons	iOS and Android	Free: lite version Paid: full version
MyFitnessPal	A popular app that gives users the ability to track their daily activity and food intake. Another feature making this a unique download is the searchable food database providing nutritional information on over two million items. The app even comes with a bar code scanner so users can easily upload nutritional data anywhere. Users can also get support from friends with similar health goals and track each other's progress	iOS and Android	Free
MyPlate	A calorie tracker app developed by LiveStrong.com that gives users access to largest database of nutritional information on food and restaurant items. It provides personalized daily calorie and water intake goals as well as allows the user to update others of their progress via social media	iOS and Android	Free: lite version Paid: full version
MyQuitCoach	This app put out by Livestrong.com helps smokers quit the habit gradually or right away. Users trying to quit can track their progress and will receive motivational tips and inspirational messages to help them remain strong	iOS	Free: lite version Paid: full version
PainScale	An app for patients with chronic pain conditions that allows them to track pain intensity, medications, symptoms, activity, mood, and sleep. Using this data, patients can create detailed pain reports to share with their providers	iOS and Android	Free
RunKeeper	Developed for the runner, this app tracks the progress of a workout and the global positioning system (GPS) lets users know where they are running, how fast they are going, and how many calories they have burned. Similar to MapMyRun, this app allows users to share statistics via social media. Other versions track activities like walking and cycling	iOS and Android	Free

TABLE 27–3. EXAMPLES OF MOBILE HEALTH AND FITNESS APPLICATIONS[43–60]

Health and Fitness Applications	Description	Smartphone Availability	Fee
TravWell	Brought to you by the Centers for Disease Control and Prevention (CDC), this app provides assistance to travelers who are looking for guidance on how to prepare for travel internationally. Some features include destination-specific vaccine recommendations, packing lists, emergency services phone numbers, as well as travel tips for a safe and healthy vacation	iOS and Android	Free
WebMD®	Few users are unfamiliar with WebMD and all it has to offer. This mobile app provides much of the same information found online such as popular symptom checker. It also provides first aid information that is available without a wireless connection in emergency instances where Internet access is unavailable. WebMD Pain Coach and WebMD Baby are also available	iOS and Android	Free
ZocDoc	An application developed to provide users a way to peruse reviews of local doctors and dentists while also conveniently booking appointments	iOS and Android	Free

1207

facet of a more global shift to **connected health**, also known as **technology-enabled care (TEC)**. Connected health or TEC converges health technology, digital media, and mobile devices in order to enable patients, caregivers, and health care professionals to access data and information more easily, thus improving quality and health outcomes.[42] Health care professionals must adapt to and understand these transformative innovations in technology to better serve their patients.

The idea that health care professionals are medically prescribing health apps for their patients has been defined as "prescribed **digital therapeutics**." Many of these apps do not just track health data, but function as a mechanism for patients to manage various disease states.[61] For example, WellDoc® was one of the first health care companies to gain FDA approval for their smartphone health app as a medical device. The app gathers data on meals, carbohydrates, blood sugar levels, insulin doses, exercise, and medication about specific patients. The app, BlueStarDiabetes®, advises the patient how to treat episodes of low blood sugar. It can also send medical data and clinical recommendations to the health care provider. In 2014, the Intercontinental Medical Statistics (IMS) Institute for Health Care Informatics found that one-third of physicians had prescribed mHealth apps to patients. Thirty-day adherence rates to medications and lifestyle changes were 10% higher for apps prescribed by a physician compared with apps that patients downloaded on their own. Additionally, adherence rates were 30% higher for fitness apps when prescribed by a physician.[62,63] In 2016, iPrescribeApps was created by a team of physicians in order to enable providers to prescribe health apps to their patients.[64] The American Medical Association (AMA) promotes the use of safe and effective mobile health applications and related devices in clinical care.[65] The number of health apps being developed to function as medical devices is increasing and more apps are entering the market. Mobile health technology opportunities continue to improve with the use of **"bio-sensing" wearables** which include a range of sensors that monitor changes in physiology such as glucose and blood pressure. These devices also conveniently provide real-time access to health care data and information for the patient and provider.[31] This has created a need for guidelines regarding the regulation required for mHealth apps and clarification of the role of the FDA in the approval process. Currently, many developers of mHealth apps provide several disclaimers with their apps to avoid FDA evaluation of their apps as medical devices, which would require submission of a medical device application.[66] Criteria for what the FDA considers a mobile medical app requiring regulation can be found at https://www.fda.gov/medical-devices/digital-health/mobile-medical-applications.[67] Additional resources and guidelines for all things related to digital health can be found under the section "Suggested Readings" at the end of the chapter.

With health care shifting into this era of health information exchange, the role of the practitioner must also evolve and transform. As with health information found on the Internet, the lack of efficacy and safety information for most mobile health applications

TABLE 27–4. AREAS OF EVALUATION FOR CONSUMER MOBILE HEALTH APPLICATIONS[70]

Areas of Evaluation	Questions to Consider
Credibility of app	Are credentials of app suitable?
	Are authors/publishers clearly listed?
	Is the app promoting a product?
	Is the organization that developed the app reputable?
Accuracy of information	Is it peer-reviewed?
	Is the information current and/or frequently updated?
	Are recent and reputable guidelines used to support recommendations made?
	Are references cited?
Evidence-based medicine	Are recommendations evidence-based?
	Do recommendations target a specific audience or are they general in nature?
	Are opinion statements clearly marked?
	Are users directed to a health care professional before making changes to health care routine?
Ease-of-use	Does the app fit to the screen?
	Is the setup of the app well designed and organized?
	Is the app easily navigated?
	Does the app have a search function?
	Is there a main menu that helps clearly lay content out?
Health literacy	Is medical jargon used? Is it easy for the lay reader to understand?
	Is font and setup of app easy to read?
	Does app gear information toward the consumer?

means health care professionals have a duty to warn patients to proceed with caution. This is an area that pharmacists especially can make an important impact. Sifting through the plethora of mobile health apps can be overwhelming for patients and health care professionals, but there are several platforms available that rate, evaluate, and certify mobile health apps. For example, the IMS Institute for Healthcare Informatics offers AppScript Score. It evaluates mHealth apps and includes physician input and patient feedback into their ratings.[68] An alternative mHealth app rating tool can be found via iMedical Apps, an online publication led by physicians that provides reviews for patients and medical professionals on available mobile medical technology.[69] A 2014 survey identified the top characteristics convincing patients and caregivers to use mHealth apps on a regular basis. Characteristics included that the app must provide trustworthy and accurate information, be easy-to-use, secure personal data, be of little to no cost, include no advertisements, be effective and consistent, ability to network with peers, and not be packed with a lot of detail.[31] Other considerations for evaluation of mobile health apps by health care professionals and patients are presented in Table 27-4.

Case Study 27–2

You are providing discharge counseling to a patient who was admitted to the emergency department for a severe hypoglycemic episode. He brings up the fact that 4 or 5 months ago, he downloaded the most amazing app for his smartphone that allows him to more easily manage his diabetes. He shares that the app does things like track his blood glucose levels, food intake, and physical activity. The app also adjusts his insulin dose based on his specific data. He swears by the app and is convinced his diabetes is better controlled and that he has never felt better. He believes his current hypoglycemic episode was a result of forgetting to track a few meals over the past few days and promises this won't happen again. You are unfamiliar with the app he is talking about.

- *What initial follow-up questions do you have for this patient?*
- *What guidance do you have for this patient navigating the mobile health arena?*

Case Study 27–3

During the patient's next office visit with his primary care provider, he is sure to mention the diabetes app that he has been using, following his discussion with you (refer to Case Study 27-2). The provider is unsure what process he should be using to evaluate this app for his patient. He has contacted and asked for you to provide some guidelines to help him evaluate this app as well as other apps that his patients are using to manage various disease states.

- *What suggestions do you have to help the physician in evaluating mobile health apps?*
- *What are the characteristics that make mHealth apps the most attractive to patients and caregivers?*

A New Model of Drug Information

According to a 2014 Pew Research Center report, even with the explosion of online and mobile CHI opportunities, a majority of people still turn to a health care professional before using the Internet to find information. For the moment, it appears most patients still view the Internet's role as supplemental and are looking to health care professionals to guide them in their search.[71,72] However, this trend is shifting and pharmacists should anticipate patients may likely seek health information before talking to their health care provider. For instance, 93% of millennials use social media to seek advice from peers who may be experiencing the same health-related concerns, in lieu of annual preventative wellness visits with their doctor. This falls in line with the growing trend of budget-conscious and convenience-seeking lifestyles.[73] This can be a dangerous practice, as many patients are ill-equipped to find and understand all the information they need to address their health care situation. Pharmacists have an option to either ignore the fact that patients can seek health information elsewhere, acknowledge this fact but discourage use of all other health information resources, or embrace the opportunity to collaborate with their patients as they seek and use information to improve their health and quality of life. As part of the screening process, pharmacists should ask their patients where they get health information and what their preferred method is to obtain such information. Inquiring about a patient's degree of access and use of online health information should become as routine as gathering vital signs at an office visit. The answer to these simple questions can open the door to more specific education about how the patient can obtain useful, quality health information. Pharmacists must be aware of the wide range of CHI sources and how and why their patients use them. ❽ *Pharmacists should discuss with their patients why they remain an important source of drug information. Patients can be encouraged not to see CHI as a replacement for personal interaction with a health care provider, but as an extension of care and a way to improve communication.* Pharmacists can direct patients to quality CHI sites tailored to their situation and teach them how to seek information from the Web. This skill is important as three out of four patients report just using a general search engine to seek out health information online versus a more specific site that specializes in health information. In addition, one-third of patients report using the Internet as a diagnostic tool.[16] Pharmacists may consider developing a list of online resources that have their seal of approval as providing high-quality information. Pharmacist recommended websites can be shared in a variety of different ways ranging from pamphlets, bulletin boards, social media, and space provided on the pharmacy website. Such a service is something relatively easy and quick to do and goes a long way to helping patients avoid low-quality or risky information. When providing resources, it is imperative they are monitored and updated on a consistent basis; otherwise, potential exists for these same resources to become yet another avenue that low-quality CHI reaches patients. Patients will also need tips on how to navigate the range of information sources, as well as how to decide what information is relevant to their individual situation. Not only does this include aiding the navigation of health information found on the web, but also in other resources, such as brochures and patient leaflets given out with prescriptions. The success of a website in delivering meaningful information is heavily reliant upon the consumers' ability to identify, interpret, and apply information that is relevant to their situation. If the patient does not understand their health condition, they may use the wrong information for their situation, even if it is of good quality. A study in the Journal of the American Medical Informatics Association gave patients a scenario describing angina symptoms, but not the actual diagnosis. They used MedlinePlus® to find information on the condition. The authors found that searches yielded information leading patients to draw incorrect conclusions 70% of the time. The authors concluded that patients and/or family and friends of patients searching the Web for information without a diagnosis most likely are confronted with a wealth of information and are unable to sift through what is relevant versus irrelevant.[74]

❾ *Patients often have difficulty finding accurate information in response to their specific health concerns on the Internet.*

Additionally, pharmacists may offer classes to teach patients how to use CHI to their advantage. Patients can be taught about the Health On the Net Foundation (HON). This nonprofit, nongovernmental organization's mission is to assess and stringently review those Internet sites and mHealth apps offering health information. Sites and apps passing inspection receive HON certification and are given the HON symbol to place on a visible area of their website for patients to see, giving assurance the website provides reliable and appropriate information. Unfortunately, as the number of health Internet sites and apps increase, there are more and more places patients will find their health information and many may not have the HON seal of approval. The National Institutes of Health (NIH) has also developed a website for both consumers and health care professionals to better determine quality of health information found online. This information can be found at https://nccih.nih.gov/health/webresources.[75] The FDA and Agency for Healthcare Research and Quality (AHRQ) also provide guidelines for reviewing health information found online.[76,77] Furthermore, patients can be referred to the National Library of Medicine's tutorial through MedlinePlus®. It is specifically dedicated to giving patients instruction on how to evaluate health information they find on the Web and is located at http://www.nlm.nih.gov/medlineplus/webeval/webeval.html.[78]

EVALUATING THE QUALITY OF HEALTH INTERNET WEBSITES

Questions have been raised about current standards for evaluating the quality of health and medical information on the Internet; many health care professionals feel proxy measures for evaluating the quality of such websites are less than ideal. One study suggests that even sites certified with the HON code may be questionable, with little correlation between certification and accuracy or completeness of information.[17] Table 27-5 is an example of the aforementioned current standards in health Internet evaluation recommended by the NIH.

TABLE 27–5. EXAMPLE OF CURRENT STANDARDS USED TO EVALUATE THE QUALITY OF HEALTH INFORMATION ON THE INTERNET[45]

Considerations When Determining Whether or Not Health Information on the Internet is Reliable
Who is responsible for the website? Does the website provide this information? Is the sponsor a government agency, a medical school, or a reliable health-related organization?
Is the only purpose of the website to provide information or is the website trying to sell something?
If the website inquires about personal information, does it offer a reason why and give an explanation about what it will do with that information once collected?
Is health information provided on the website backed up with evidence? Are there references to support recommendations being made?
Does the website give the source of their health information? If so, is that source credible? Does the website provide explanation about whether or not health information is reviewed and by whom?
Is health information provided in an unbiased and objective manner? Is material written in a way that would be understandable to most patients no matter their health literacy level?
Does health information on the website get updated regularly? Is material provided current?
Does health information on the website seem reasonable and credible overall?
Is information provided by site to allow visitors to contact website owners with feedback, problems, and questions?

The NIH current standards for evaluating health information on the Internet focus on structural design of a website, who the site sponsor is (e.g., government, nonprofit, academic institution), and whether or not the site lists its sources, but little emphasis is placed on actual content made available to consumers. The concern is most health information available on the Internet is not monitored for quality or accuracy. It appears there is no real efficient and effective method in place to evaluate the quality of health information online. The only real way is for the pharmacist to individually review each website or app and evaluate health information content provided before they recommend them to patients. Sites devoted to a particular disease state tend to be much more complete and more accurate than sites that attempt to cover multiple health topics, but there are still no guarantees. Complete regulation of all health content on the Internet is improbable, but health care providers can attempt to help patients by selecting and evaluating a handful of sites to recommend for patients.[42]

HEALTH LITERACY—FINAL KEY TO THE PATIENT'S SUCCESSFUL USE OF INFORMATION

🔟 *Once patients identify or are given quality health information, they still may face barriers in being able to use it to improve their health.* **Health literacy** is the capability of patients to read or hear health information, understand it, and then act upon it. Health literacy is a subset of literacy, which is the capability to read and understand.[79] The Office of Disease Prevention

TABLE 27–6. GUIDELINES FOR IDENTIFYING INTERNET SITES ADHERING TO PRINCIPLES OF HEALTH LITERACY[84,85]

• Designed for old hardware and software	• Link clearly defined
• Simple home page	• Printer friendly option
• Information prioritized	• Audio option
• Minimal text per screen	• Site map easy to find
• Navigation simple and consistent	• Contact information easy to find
• Searching simplified	• Content uses other principles of health literacy
• Scrolling need minimized	

and Health Promotion estimates that nearly 90% of adults lack the ability to use the U.S. health system sufficiently due to their poor health literacy skills.[80] Patients with poor health literacy may have trouble recognizing when health information is needed, identifying or obtaining access to health information resources, determining the quality of health information resources or understanding that quality is even a problem, and even more so analyzing and understanding information found.[81] Studies show a strong correlation with adults who report having poor health as also having the most limited literacy, numeracy, and health literacy skills. Health literacy even affects those patients who otherwise have no problems with normal literacy issues in their daily life. As a result of health literacy issues being unfamiliar to most people, many patients find themselves struggling with unfamiliarity of medical terms and how their bodies work, being unable to accurately judge risk versus benefit for their particular health situation, being challenged to follow complicated treatment plans, as well as being scared and confused when diagnosed with a serious condition.[82]

Pharmacists must consider a patient's health literacy when they provide information and education to their patients. Studies show that simplifying websites, and providing clear layouts and familiar language improves the experience of all users, not just those with limited literacy skills.[83] Table 27-6 describes the qualities of websites that can be used by pharmacists to screen for health literacy as they identify websites for their patients. Visit the AHRQ website (http://www.ahrq.gov/professionals/quality-patient-safety/quality-resources/tools/literacy-toolkit/tool3a/index.html) for additional detail about health literacy standards and the role health care professionals can play in helping their patients.

PARTICIPATORY MEDICINE

❶ *Participatory medicine refers to a recent movement for a new model of cooperative health care. In this model, patients no longer play a passive part when it comes to their health care but an active role alongside the health care provider. Patients are seen as valuable health* *care resources, and providers are encouraged to view them as equal partners.* By fostering a sense of patient/provider engagement, and patient education and empowerment, the Society for Participatory Medicine hopes to improve health outcomes along with increasing patient satisfaction among other measures. Studies show that nearly 90% of patients believe that working with their health care professional as a partner will help them to enhance their overall health.[86] Participatory medicine is a concept that is not new to most patients. Many have sought to be a part of the decision-making process when it comes to their health for quite some time. It is evident now more than ever that patients desire to equip themselves with the proper tools to be a valued part of the conversation regarding their health. Seeking health information online is a major way that patients feel invested, and with health care in the midst of a technology revolution in which the availability of health information is accelerating at an extraordinary rate, it is important that health care professionals do everything they can to ensure patients are accessing accurate and quality information. The U.S. Department of Health and Human Services even recognizes the importance of where health care professionals are going in terms of health communication and health information technology for patients. Through HealthyPeople 2020 (https://health.gov/healthypeople), it is their mission to deliver health information to patients that is accurate, targeted, and tailored for the individual, as well as to increase health literacy skills and advance health communication efforts online. This includes having a more active role in disease state self-management tools that can be accessed via mobile devices, which is a popular avenue for patients to take an active part in their health. According to a Society for Participatory Medicine survey, 84% of patients think sharing health data they have tracked themselves with their health care professionals between visits would greatly help them to better manage their health. It was also found that 76% would use a monitoring device to track personal clinical data, with 81% of those patients saying that they would be more likely to use the device if their health care professional recommended it.[86]

Participatory medicine encompasses both the patient and the health care professional, asking both to work together in making the best possible health care decisions for the patient. From asking more useful questions of physicians and other health care providers to more effectively managing conditions and participating in their own treatment, participatory medicine may help patients have more control over their lives in terms of their health. Pharmacists should encourage their patients to be engaged in their health care as it leads to patient empowerment and self-motivation.

Conclusion

Vast choices exist for both patients and health care professionals when it comes to obtaining and using health information. It is vital that health care professionals position themselves to be integral in their patients' approach to gaining an understanding of their health. Especially for pharmacists, as traditional roles change, new opportunities to get involved in managing patients' health care are presenting themselves. It has been the responsibility of health care professionals, especially pharmacists, for decades to educate and provide patients with quality drug information. In the end, it is up to health care professionals to design this new role and demonstrate value to the patient so that they continue to be used as a key ally in providing patient care.

Self-Assessment Questions

1. Which of the following are limitations a pharmacist faces when delivering drug information to their patients?
   a. Lack of readability of most patient leaflets given with prescription
   b. Pharmacists appear too busy and unavailable
   c. Counseling has become a passive process where patient education is only given if requested
   d. Pharmacists' lack of understanding in regards to patient's desire to take control of their own health
   e. All of the above

2. Patient education is best described by the following:
   a. Delivered by health care professional verbally only
   b. Occurs with the pickup of new prescriptions only
   c. Unplanned activity
   d. b and c only
   e. None of the above

3. Consumer health information (CHI) is best described by the following:
   a. Tailored to a patient's specific situation
   b. Actively sought by patients
   c. Created in response to patient's need for more information about their health
   d. b and c only
   e. None of the above

4. Which of the following site(s) is considered a consumer health information or social media site?
   a. WebMD®
   b. PatientsLikeMe®

   c. Everyday Health®

   d. b and c only

   e. All of the above

5. Through social media sites, patients share a wealth of personal information regarding their disease states and conditions. Examples of personal information shared includes all of the following *EXCEPT*:

   a. Treatment successes

   b. Treatment failures

   c. Adverse effects

   d. Opinions

   e. All of the above are examples of personal information that may be shared

6. All of the following are reasons why some patients prefer the collective wisdom of a group over the advice of an expert individual *EXCEPT* for:

   a. Patients are provided with a feeling of camaraderie and support.

   b. Patients may not trust their health care professional.

   c. Patients are more inclined to trust a person like them.

   d. Patients are not as willing to rely on a single expert for their information.

   e. All of the above are reasons some patients prefer wisdom of the group over advice of an expert.

7. Which of the following is *NOT* a useful strategy for pharmacists to employ when helping patients to empower themselves and effectively use consumer health information (CHI)?

   a. Ask patients where else they get health information besides their health care professional.

   b. Encourage patients to quit seeking information online regardless of the source.

   c. Become familiar with the range of CHI resources available.

   d. Develop a list of mobile health apps that are pharmacist-recommended.

   e. Discuss with patients why pharmacists still remain an important DI source.

8. Which of the following is an appropriate question to ask when evaluating consumer mobile health applications?

   a. Are authors/publishers clearly listed?

   b. Is the information current and/or frequently updated?

   c. Are users directed to a health care professional before making changes to health care routine?

   d. a and b only

   e. All of the above

9. Which of the following questions is NOT a consideration for evaluating the quality of a consumer health information site?
    a. Who is responsible for the website?
    b. Is health information provided on the website backed up with evidence?
    c. How long has the website been operational?
    d. Does health information on the website seem reasonable and credible overall?
    e. Is health information provided in an unbiased and objective manner?

10. Which mobile health and fitness application focuses on providing better sleep, meditation, and relaxation for its users?
    a. MyPlate
    b. Flo Period and Ovulation Tracker
    c. MyFitnessPal
    d. TravWell
    e. Calm

11. The American Red Cross developed which of the following mobile health and fitness application(s)?
    a. ZocDoc
    b. First Aid
    c. TravWell
    d. b and c only
    e. All of the above

12. Which mobile health and fitness application helps its users with smoking cessation?
    a. WebMD
    b. MyQuitCoach
    c. Lose It!
    d. First Aid
    e. TravWell

13. Which type of social media is best defined as "thoughts and ideas are shared and open discussion takes place via various mediums"?
    a. Online forums
    b. Blog
    c. Social network
    d. b and c only
    e. None of the above

14. Which of the following characteristics make an Internet site of high quality and accessible to patients of varying levels of health literacy?
    a. Simple home page
    b. Information prioritized
    c. Searching simplified
    d. Scrolling need minimized
    e. All of the above

15. Which of the following terms best describes a new model of cooperative health care where patients no longer play a passive part when it comes to their health but an active role alongside their health care provider?
    a. Participatory medicine
    b. Social media
    c. Medication therapy management
    d. a and c only
    e. None of the above

REFERENCES

1. California HealthCare Foundation. The wisdom of patients: health care meets online social media [Internet]. Oakland (CA): California HealthCare Foundation; c2009 [2008 Apr; cited 2009 Nov 10]. Available from: http://www.chcf.org/.

2. Fox S, Duggan M. Health online 2013 [Internet]. Washington (DC): Pew Research Center; 2013 Jan [cited 2016 Sep 8]; [1 p.]. Available from: http://www.pewinternet.org/2013/01/15/health-online-2013/.

3. Fox S, Duggan M. Part two: sources of health information [Internet]. Washington (DC): Pew Research Center; 2013 Nov [cited 2016 Sep 8]; [6 p.]. Available from: http://www.pewinternet.org/2013/11/26/part-two-sources-of-health-information/.

4. National Community Pharmacists Association. Project Destiny executive summary [Internet]. American Pharmacists Association, National Association of Chain Drug Stores, National Community Pharmacists Association; 2008 Feb [cited 2013 Jul 14]; [5 p.]. Available from: http://www.ncpanet.org/pdf/projectdestinyexecsummary.pdf

5. National Alliance of State Pharmacy Associations. Executive summary: an action plan for implementation of the JCPP future vision of pharmacy practice [Internet]. Joint Commission of Pharmacy Practitioners; 2007 Nov [updated 2008 Jan; cited 2013 Jul 14]; [19 p.]. Available from: https://pcms.ouhsc.edu/ams/common/docs_oac/ViewOAC_img_blobs.asp?DocID=091276228348

6. Watanabe JH, Mcinnis T, Hirsch JD. Cost of prescription drug-related morbidity and mortality. Ann Pharmacother. 2018;52(9):829-37.

7. Enhancing Prescription Medicine Adherence: A National Action Plan [Internet]. National Counsel on Patient Information and Education; 2007 Aug [cited 2012 Dec 20];

[35 p.]. Available from: http://www.scriptyourfuture.org/hcp/download/fact_sheet/Medication%20Adherence%20National%20Action%20Plan.pdf

8. Project Destiny Summary [Internet]. American Pharmacists Association. [2008 Aug; cited 29 May 2020]. Available from: https://www.pharmacist.com/sites/default/files/files/mtm_project_summary_prjdestiny.pdf

9. Anderson S. Pharmacy outlook 2016. Arlington (VA): National Association of Chain Drug Stores; 2016.

10. Here's the truth about why people aren't choosing your independent pharmacy [Internet]. Elements Magazine. [2017 Oct 26; cited 7 Oct 2019]. Available from: https://www.pbahealth.com/how-consumers-choose-pharmacies-and-how-to-market-to-them/

11. Omnibus Budget Reconciliation Act of 1990, Pub. L. 101-508, 104 Stat.1388 (Nov. 5, 1990).

12. Consumer Reports [Internet]. Yonkers (NY): Can you Read this Drug Label; 2011 Jun [cited 2016 Sep 8]. Available from: http://www.consumerreports.org/cro/2011/06/can-you-read-this-drug-label/index.htm

13. The Joint Commission. Transitions of care: the need for a more effective approach to continuing patient care. Joint Commission Center for Transforming Healthcare; 2012:1-8.

14. Malone PM, Malone MJ, Park S. Drug information: a guide for pharmacists. 6th ed. New York: McGraw-Hill; 2018.

15. Massengale L. Resources for Quality Health Information Online. Proceedings of the 119th Annual Meeting of the American Association of Colleges of Pharmacy. 2008 Jul 19-23; Chicago, IL.

16. Fox S, Duggan M. Information triage [Internet]. Washington (DC): Pew Research Center; 2013 Jan [cited 2016 Sep 8]; [11 p.]. Available from: http://www.pewinternet.org/2013/01/15/information-triage/

17. Felkey BG, Fox BI, Thrower MR, editors. Health care informatics: a skills-based resource. 1st ed. Washington (DC): American Pharmacists Association; 2006.

18. American Cancer Society [Internet]. c2020 [cited 2020 Jun 3]. Available from: https://www.cancer.org/.

19. Cleveland Clinic Health Library [Internet]. c2020 [cited 2020 Jun 3]. Available from: https://my.clevelandclinic.org/health

20. Drugs.com [Internet]. c2000-2020 [cited 2020 Jun 3]. Available from: https://www.drugs.com/

21. GoodRx [Internet]. c2011-2020 [cited 2020 Jun 3]. Available from: https://www.goodrx.com/

22. Consumer Reports Health [Internet]. c2004-2012 [cited 2012 Dec 12]. Available from: http://www.consumerreportshealth.org

23. Mayo Clinic [Internet]. c1998-2020 [cited 2020 Jun 3]. Available from: https://www.mayoclinic.org/

24. MedlinePlus [Internet]. c2020 [cited 2020 Jun 3]. Available from: https://medlineplus.gov/

25. Healthfinder [Internet]. c2012 [cited 2012 Dec 18]. Available from: http://www.healthfinder.gov

26. PatientsLikeMe [Internet]. c2005-2012 [cited 2012 Dec 12]. Available from: http://www.patientslikeme.com

27. Everyday Health Group, LLC [Internet]. c2012 [cited 2012 Dec 12]. Available from: http://www.everydayhealth.com

28. WebMD [Internet]. c2005-2012 [cited 2012 Dec 12]. Available from: http://www.webmd.com

29. Ventola CL. Social media and health care professionals: benefits, risks, and best practices. Pharm Therapeut. 2014;39(7):491–9.

30. Social Media Fact Sheet [Internet]. Washingon (DC): Pew Research Center; 2019 Jun [cited 2019 Sep 6]; [6 p.]. Available from: https://www.pewinternet.org/fact-sheet/social-media/

31. Fox S, Duggan M. Peer-to-peer health care [Internet]. Washington (DC): Pew Research Center; 2013 Jan [cited 2016 Sep 8]; [5 p.]. Available from: http://www.pewinternet.org/2013/01/15/peer-to-peer-health-care/

32. Tapscott D. Grown up digital: how the net generation is changing your world. New York: McGraw-Hill; 2009.

33. Edelman. 2008 Edelman Trust Barometer [Internet]. 2008 Jan 22 [cited 2009 Nov 10]. Available from: https://www.edelman.com/sites/g/files/aatuss191/files/2018-10/2008-Trust-Barometer-Executive-Summary.pdf

34. Fox S. Medicine 2.0: peer-to-peer healthcare [Internet]. Washington (DC): Pew Research Center's Internet & American Life Project; 2011 Sep [cited 2017 Feb 28]; [10 p.]. Available from: http://www.pewinternet.org/2011/09/18/medicine-2-0-peer-to-peer-healthcare/

35. Outstanding statistics on how social media has impacted health care [Internet]. Physician Referral Management and EConsult Software referral MD. 2015 [cited 2016 Sep 9]. Available from: https://getreferralmd.com/2013/09/healthcare-social-media-statistics/

36. Social media "likes" healthcare: From marketing to social business [Internet]. PwC Health Research Institute; 2012 Apr [cited 2019 Sep 6]. Available from: https://www.pwc.com/us/en/industries/health-industries/library/health-care-social-media.html

37. Smith A. U.S. smartphone use in 2015 [Internet]. Washington (DC): Pew Research Center; 2015 Apr [cited 2016 Sep 9]. Available from: http://www.pewinternet.org/2015/04/01/us-smartphone-use-in-2015/

38. Mobile Fact Sheet [Internet]. Washington (DC): Pew Research Center; 2019 Jun [cited 2019 Sep 6]. Available from: https://www.pewinternet.org/fact-sheet/mobile/.

39. 58% of smartphone owners download, use mobile health apps [Internet]. mHealthIntelligence. 2015 [cited 2016 Sep 9]. Available from: http://mhealthintelligence.com/news/58-of-smartphone-owners-download-use-mobile-health-apps

40. Safavi K, Kalis B. Accenture 2018 consumer survey on digital health [Internet]. Accenture; 2018 [cited 2019 Sep 6]. Available from: https://www.accenture.com/us-en/insight-new-2018-consumer-survey-digital-health?utm_source=newsletter&utm_medium=email&utm_campaign=newsletter_axiosvitals&stream=top-stories

41. Mobile Health (mHealth) App Market—industry trends, opportunities and forecasts to 2023. Research and Markets; 2017 Nov [cited 2019 Sep 6]; [80 p.]. Available from: https://www.researchandmarkets.com/research/pv554v/28_32_billion?w=5

42. Taylor K. Connected health: how digital technology is transforming health and social care [Internet]. London: Deloitte Centre for Health Solutions; 2015 Apr [cited 7 Oct 2019]; [38 p.].

Available from: https://www2.deloitte.com/uk/en/pages/life-sciences-and-healthcare/articles/connected-health.html

43. Apple Health [Internet]. c2020 [cited 2020 Jun 3]. Available from: https://www.apple.com/ios/health/

44. AsthmaMD [Internet]. c2009-2018 [cited 2020 Jun 3]. Available from: https://www.asthmamd.org/

45. Calm [Internet]. c2019 [cited 2019 Sep 9]. Available from: https://www.calm.com/

46. First Aid [Internet]. c2016 [cited 2016 Sep 9]. Available from: http://www.redcross.org/get-help/prepare-for-emergencies/mobile-apps

47. Flo Period & Ovulation Tracker [Internet]. c2019 [cited 2019 Sep 9]. Available from: https://flo.health/

48. GlucoseBuddy [Internet]. c2011-2012 [cited 2012 Dec 18]. Available from: http://www.glucosebuddy.com

49. Google Fit [Internet]. c2020 [cited 2020 Jun 3]. Available from: https://www.google.com/fit/

50. Headspace [Internet]. c2020 [cited 2020 Jun 3]. Available from: https://www.headspace.com/

51. Lose It! [Internet]. c2008-2012 [cited 2012 Dec 12]. Available from: http://www.loseit.com/

52. MapMyRun [Internet]. c2005-2012 [cited 2012 Dec 18]. Available from: http://www.mapmyrun.com

53. MyFitnessPal [Internet]. c2005-2012 [cited 2012 Dec 18]. Available from: http://www.myfitnesspal.com

54. MyPlate [Internet]. c2011-2012 [cited 2012 Dec 18]. Available from: http://www.livestrong.com/calorie-counter-mobile/

55. MyQuitCoach [Internet]. c2012 [cited 2012 Dec 18]. Available from: http://www.livestrong.com/quit-smoking-app/

56. PainScale [Internet]. c2017 [cited 2020 Jun 3]. Available from: https://www.painscale.com/

57. RunKeeper [Internet]. c2012 [cited 2012 Dec 18]. Available from: http://runkeeper.com/

58. TravWell [Internet]. c2014 [cited 2016 Sep 9]. Available from: http://wwwnc.cdc.gov/travel/page/apps-about

59. WebMD [Internet]. c2005-2012 [cited 2012 Dec 18]. Available from: http://www.webmd.com/mobile

60. ZocDoc [Internet]. c2012 [cited 2012 Dec 18]. Available from: http://www.zocdoc.com/

61. What is digital therapeutics and what is its potential in population health? [Internet]. Personal Connected Health Alliance; 2019 Jan [cited 2019 Oct 7]. Available from: https://www.pchalliance.org/news/what-digital-therapeutics-and-what-its-potential-population-health

62. Terry K. Number of health apps soars, but use does not always follow [Internet]. Medscape; 2015 Sep [cited 2019 Sep 6]. Available from: https://www.medscape.com/viewarticle/851226

63. A physician's guide to prescribing mobile health apps [Internet]. Medical Economics; 2014 Oct [cited 2019 Sep 6]. Available from: https://www.medicaleconomics.com/health-care-information-technology/physicians-guide-prescribing-mobile-health-apps

64. iPrescribeApps [Internet]. iPrescribeApps. [Cited 2019 Oct 7]. Available from: https://iprescribeapps.com/

65. AMA adopts principles to promote safe, effective mHealth applications [Internet]. American Medical Association; 2016 Nov [cited 2019 Sep 9]. Available from: https://www.ama-assn.org/press-center/press-releases/ama-adopts-principles-promote-safe-effective-mhealth-applications

66. Brustein J. Coming next: using an app as prescribed. New York Times (New York ed.). 2012 Aug 20:Sect. B:1.

67. Mobile Medical Applications [Internet]. Mobile Medical Applications. [Cited 2016 Sep 9]. Available from: http://www.fda.gov/medicaldevices/digitalhealth/mobilemedicalapplications/default.htm

68. AppScript Score [Internet]. AppScript Score. [Cited 2020 May 29]. Available from: https://www.appscript.net/score-details

69. iMedicalApps [Internet]. iMedicalApps. [Cited 2019 Oct 7]. Available from: https://www.imedicalapps.com/about/#

70. Pope A, Bryant P, Pace H, Sperry M. Evaluation and ranking of consumer health and drug information smart phone applications. Poster session presented at: American Society of Health System Pharmacists Midyear Meeting; 2011 Dec 4-8; New Orleans, LA.

71. Fox S. The social life of health information [Internet]. Washington (DC): Pew Research Center's Internet & American Life Project; 2011 May [cited 2012 Dec 20]; [19 p.]. Available from: http://pewinternet.org/Reports/2011/Social-Life-of-Health-Info.aspx

72. Fox S. The social life of health information [Internet]. Washington (DC): Pew Research Center's Internet & American Life Project; 2014 Jan [cited 2020 May 29]. Available from: https://www.pewresearch.org/fact-tank/2014/01/15/the-social-life-of-health-information/

73. Arnold, A. Can social media have a positive impact on global healthcare? [Internet]. Forbes Media LLC; 2018 Jun [cited 2019 Oct 7]. Available from: https://www.forbes.com/sites/andrewarnold/2018/06/05/can-social-media-have-a-positive-impact-on-global-healthcare/#5887102818a0

74. Keselman A, Browne AC, Kaufman DR. Consumer health information seeking as hypothesis testing. J Am Med Inform Assoc. 2008;15(4):484–95.

75. Finding and Evaluating Online Resources | NCCIH [Internet]. U.S National Library of Medicine. U.S. National Library of Medicine; [cited 2016 Sep 9]. Available from: https://nccih.nih.gov/health/webresources

76. U.S. Food and Drug Administration. How to evaluate health information on the internet: information for consumers [Internet]. Silver Spring (MD): U.S. Health and Human Services; 2010 Mar 9. [cited 2013 Jun 28]. Available from: http://www.fda.gov/Drugs/ResourcesForYou/Consumers/BuyingUsingMedicineSafely/BuyingMedicinesOvertheInternet/ucm202863.htm#resources

77. Agency for Healthcare Research and Quality. Assessing the quality of internet health information [Internet]. Rockville (MD): U.S. Health and Human Services; 1999 Jun. [cited 2013 Jun 28]. Available from: http://www.ahrq.gov/research/data/infoqual.html

78. Medline Plus. Evaluating Internet health information: a tutorial from the national library of medicine [Internet]. Bethesda (MD): National Library of Medicine; 2007 [cited 2009 Jan 12]. Available from: http://www.nlm.nih.gov/medlineplus/webeval/webeval.html

79. Kutner M, Greenberg E, Jin Y, Paulsen C. The health literacy of America's adults: results from the 2003 national assessment of adult literacy. Washington (DC): National Center for Education Statistics; 2003. Report No.: NCES 2006-483. Supported by the U.S. Department of Education.

80. Health literacy online: a guide for simplifying the user experience [Internet]. Office of Disease Prevention and Health Promotion. [2016 Jun 8; cited 2020 Jun 3]. Available from: https://health.gov/healthliteracyonline/

81. Nielsen-Bohlman L, Panzer AM, Kindig DA. Health literacy: a prescription to end confusion, Committee on Health Literacy, Board on Neuroscience and Behavioral Health. Institute of Medicine. Washington (DC): The National Academies Press; 2004. 41 p. Available from: http://hospitals.unm.edu/health_literacy/pdfs/HealthLiteracyExecutiveSummary.pdf

82. Understanding literacy and numeracy [Internet]. Centers for Disease Control and Prevention; 2015 [cited 2016 Sep 9]. Available from: http://www.cdc.gov/healthliteracy/learn/understandingliteracy.html

83. Why design easy-to-use web sites? [Internet]. U.S. Department of Health and Human Services. [Cited 2020 May 29]. Available from: https://health.gov/healthliteracyonline/2010/why.htm

84. Agency for Healthcare Research and Quality. Accessible health information technology (IT) for populations with limited literacy: a guide for developers and purchasers of health IT. 2007 Oct [cited 2013 Jan 15]. Available from: http://healthit.ahrq.gov/sites/default/files/docs/page/LiteracyGuide_0.pdf

85. Health literacy online: a guide to writing and designing easy-to-use health web sites [Internet]. Washington (DC): U.S. Department of Health and Human Services; 2010 [cited 2020 Jun 3]. Available from: https://health.gov/healthliteracyonline/2010/Web_Guide_Health_Lit_Online.pdf

86. Sands D. Evidence! New S4PM survey shows people want to collaborate with their doctors and co-produce their clinical data [Internet]. Society for Participatory Medicine; 2016 Feb [cited 2019 Sep 9]. Available from: https://participatorymedicine.org/epatients/2016/02/s4pm-survey-shows-people-want-to-collaborate-w-docs-and-co-produce-clinical-data.html

SUGGESTED READINGS

1. Agency for Healthcare Research and Quality (AHRQ)—Health Literacy: Hidden Barriers and Practical Strategies. Available from: http://www.ahrq.gov/professionals/quality-patient-safety/quality-resources/tools/literacy-toolkit/tool3a/index.html

2. Consumer and Patient Health Information Section (CAPHIS). Available from: https://www.mlanet.org/caphis

3. U.S. Food and Drug Administration (FDA). Available from: https://www.fda.gov/medical-devices/digital-health, https://www.fda.gov/medical-devices/digital-health/digital-health-criteria, https://www.fda.gov/medical-devices/digital-health/mobile-medical-applications

4. iMedicalApps. Available from: http://www.imedicalapps.com/#

5. MedlinePlus®—Evaluating Health Information. Available from: http://www.nlm.nih.gov/medlineplus/evaluatinghealthinformation.html

6. MedlinePlus®—Guide to Healthy Web Surfing. Available from: http://www.nlm.nih.gov/medlineplus/healthywebsurfing.html

7. National Institutes of Health—Finding and Evaluating Online Resources. Available from: https://nccih.nih.gov/health/webresources

8. National Institutes of Health—Mobile (mHealth) Health Information and Resources. Available from: http://www.fic.nih.gov/ResearchTopics/Pages/MobileHealth.aspx

9. Participatory Medicine. Available from: http://participatorymedicine.org/

10. VUCA Health. Available from: www.vucahealth.com.

Chapter Twenty-Eight

Pharmacy Informatics I: Systems and Technology for Patient Care

Brent I. Fox • Joshua C. Hollingsworth

Learning Objectives

After completing this chapter, the reader will be able to:

- List the activities that occur at each step of the medication-use process.
- Define pharmacy informatics and other core informatics terms.
- Discuss the role of pharmacy informatics at each step of the medication-use process.
- Describe challenges regarding effective utilization of computerized provider order entry (CPOE).
- Describe the components of an e-prescribing system.
- Describe the role of the three primary components of a clinical decision support system (CDSS).
- Describe limitations of health information technology (HIT) that is used during the order verification step of the medication-use process.
- Compare and contrast the health information technology used during dispensing in acute care and community pharmacy settings.
- Define the role of bar code medication administration (BCMA).
- Describe the role of the three primary components of a clinical surveillance system.
- Describe the importance and application of the Internet of Things (IoT) and digital health to the emerging health care delivery system.
- Describe the changing role of the patient in the U.S. health care system.
- Explain the importance of interoperability to the future of the U.S. health care system, including the role of the U.S. government.
- Describe the federal government's role in driving health information technology adoption and use.

- Compare and contrast privacy, security, and confidentiality as they relate to protected health information (PHI).
- Define cyber security and describe methods to protect against cyber breaches.

Key Concepts

1 The medication-use process is a system of interconnected parts that work together to achieve the common goal of safe and effective medication therapy.

2 All pharmacists are affected by the electronic information systems that make up pharmacy informatics in virtually every aspect of practice.

3 The two broad categories of information used in pharmacy informatics, as well as other clinical informatics domains, are patient-specific information and knowledge-based information.

4 The vision of health care is becoming more patient-centric.

5 The IoT and digital health are enabling technologies as the U.S. health care system moves to patient-centric model of care.

6 The current health care system is decentralized and fragmented. Because of this, significant communication gaps exist when multiple health care institutions provide care for the same patient. Substantial evidence suggests that more effective communication would improve patient care and reduce medical errors, such as adverse drug events (ADEs).

7 The desired result of interoperable systems and electronic health records (EHRs) is to readily provide all health practitioners in all locations, including the pharmacy, with access to information about a patient's care, as needed.

8 To drive adoption and use of EHRs, the federal government leveraged its position as policy maker and purchaser of health care through two programs focused on incentives and payments to providers and hospitals.

9 As interoperability and digital health advances and more patient data are shared across providers and organizations, the issues of security, privacy, and confidentiality of PHI inevitability arise.

Introduction

Health care practitioners of today have a multitude of responsibilities within their scopes of practice. Regardless of discipline and practice setting, health care providers must be able to input, access, share, evaluate, and utilize information to support their efforts in patient care. For pharmacists, whether verifying and filling prescriptions, compounding medications, advising patients on proper medication use, or collaborating with other practitioners in the care of patients, the core responsibility lies on the safe and effective use of medication therapy. Clinicians aim to maximize patient safety while minimizing medication misadventures, such as medication errors and adverse drug events, which are covered in Chapters 19 and 20. Given the sheer amount of information involved and available to take care of patients today, this focus on the safety and effectiveness of medication use can only be reasonably obtained via clinicians' effective management of the information and related information systems involved. In other words, drug information is vital to the medication-use process.

Medication-Use Process

❶ *The medication-use process is a system of interconnected parts that work together to achieve the common goal of safe and effective medication therapy.* The interconnected parts include the people, systems, procedures, and policies that manage medications and related information in patient care. It should be noted here that Chapter 18 further covers a portion of the medication-use process, specifically in the context of quality improvement. The medication-use process is cyclical in nature and begins with the **prescribing** stage (Figure 28-1). In this stage, the practitioner assesses whether medication therapy is warranted and, if so, orders therapy accordingly. The health information technology (HIT) utilized at the prescribing stage includes computerized provider order entry (CPOE), electronic prescribing (e-prescribing), and clinical decision support systems (CDSS), including various medication references.

In the next stage of the medication-use process, the **order-verification or transcribing** stage, the ordered medication enters the pharmacy computer system, a pharmacist assesses the appropriateness of the order, and any issues or discrepancies are addressed. CDSS is the primary HIT tool used at the order-verification stage. Various drug information references, often electronic in nature, may be used and may be built into the systems (e.g., drug interaction screening system, links to product-specific monographs, clinical practice guidelines, or seminal journal articles).

Next is the **dispensing** stage. Here, the medication is prepared and distributed from the pharmacy, either directly to the patient or to a health care provider such as a nurse. There are many HIT tools utilized in the dispensing stage, including bar code verification, automated dispensing cabinets (ADC), syringe fillers, total parenteral nutrition compounders, and other robotics.

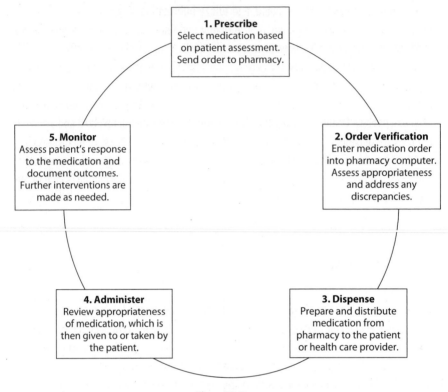

Figure 28–1.

Following the dispensing stage is the **administration** stage in which the medication is reviewed for appropriateness and then administered to, or taken by, the patient. Health care providers, caregivers, the patient, and the patient's family may be involved in the administration stage, depending on the setting. HIT tools used here have traditionally included point-of-care bar coding, electronic medication administration records (eMARs), and intelligent infusion (smart) pumps. Today, technologies allow patients to monitor parameters—such as blood glucose—and adjust dosing accordingly. Additionally, adherence monitoring technologies such as medication event monitoring systems (MEMS) can be used to track patient medication usage, by capturing each time a medication is self-administered. To do so, MEMS utilize computer chips embedded in specialized medication bottle caps. The computer chip records each time the cap is removed, which serves as an indicator that the medication was taken by the patient. The final stage in the medication-use process is **monitoring**. At the monitoring stage, the patient's response to the medication therapy is assessed, outcomes are documented, and interventions are made, as necessary. HIT tools used here include ADE surveillance, antibiotic/drug surveillance, rules engines, and smartphone apps/devices that allow patients to monitor symptoms and treatment response. As described above, some of these monitoring tools feed back to the administration stage to inform subsequent medication dosing, as is the case with diabetes. The following is a brief description of some of the HIT tools mentioned above in alphabetical order:[1]

- **Adverse drug event (ADE) monitoring:** Computer programs that use electronic data and predetermined rules to identify when an ADE may have occurred or is about to occur to a patient within a health care setting. This is separate from such programs as MedWatch (see Chapter 19) which is used to report adverse effects to the U.S. Food and Drug Administration (FDA).

- **Automated dispensing cabinets (ADCs):** Automated devices with a range of functions. Core capabilities include medication storage and retrieval for administration to patients, especially in patient care areas, as well as audit trails of cabinet access. Other functions can include medication charging and automated inventory management.

- **Bar code verification:** The use of bar code scanning to ensure that the correct drug, strength, and dosage form were dispensed in the drug selection process and to ensure that the six rights of medication administration (i.e., right patient, right drug, right dose, right route, right time, right documentation) are followed at the point-of-care.

- **Clinical decision support systems (CDSS):** Computer programs that augment clinical decision-making by combining referential information with patient-specific information to prevent negative actions and update clinicians of patient status.

- **Computerized provider order entry (CPOE):** A process allowing health care providers to electronically enter orders for medications, laboratory tests, consultations, radiography, etc., for the treatment of patients who are under their care in an acute/inpatient setting.

- **Electronic medication administration record (eMAR):** An electronic version of the traditional medication administration record. It supports patient safety by incorporating clinical decision support and bar coded medication administration. It also enables real-time documentation and billing of medication administration.

- **Electronic health record (EHR):** A digital compilation of a patient's health data originating from all clinicians involved in the patient's care and that allows these data to be shared across providers and institutions.

- **Electronic prescribing (e-prescribing):** The electronic process in which a medication prescription is created in an electronic format and then sent electronically to a community pharmacy for verification and dispensing. Prescriptions created electronically sent via fax are not electronic prescriptions.

- **Intelligent infusion (smart) pumps:** Infusion pumps containing software designed to help eliminate pump programming errors (e.g., an extra zero resulting in a 10-fold dosing error) through the use of standardized drug data-bases and dosing parameters.

- **Rules engines**: Computer programs, similar to ADE monitoring systems, with built-in, logic rules designed to aid in monitoring specific aspects of patient care. For example, a rule developed in an attempt to prevent hypoglycemia in patients receiving insulin may require documentation of the patient's meal being delivered prior to the patient receiving mealtime insulin.

Pharmacy Informatics

The term "informatics" simply refers to the use of computers to manage data and infor-mation. Informatics exists at the intersection of people, information, and technology.[2] Pharmacy informatics refers to a form of clinical informatics that is applied to the dis-cipline of pharmacy. More specifically, **pharmacy informatics** focuses on the use of information, information systems, and automation technology to ensure safe and effective medication usage. ❷ *All pharmacists are affected by the electronic information systems that make up pharmacy informatics in virtually every aspect of practice.* For example, patient records, medication administration and usage information, insurance information, as well as laboratory tests and results are just a few of the categories of information that are man-aged in electronic environments.

❸ *The two broad categories of information used in pharmacy informatics, as well as other clinical informatics domains, are* **patient-specific information** *and* **knowledge-based information.**[3] Patient-specific information, which is created and applied in the process of caring for individual patients, includes medication and medical histories, lab-oratory test results, radiology interpretations, immunization histories, physical assess-ments, and other information that is unique to the specific patient. Today, this information is generated and housed in health care facilities, such as pharmacies, hospitals, and clin-ics. **Consumer health informatics**, a rapidly growing field, has created an environment in which patients themselves are also generating and managing health-related informa-tion in addition to and outside of these traditional settings. Aspects of consumer health informatics can include **digital health technologies**, Internet-based direct-to-consumer advertising (see Chapter 25), and research activities.

Knowledge-based information, on the other hand, forms the scientific basis of health care and includes referential information (about medications, procedures, disease states, etc.), clinical practice guidelines, as well as many other domains of health and medical knowledge.[3] All health care providers make patient care decisions based on a combina-tion of patient-specific and knowledge-based information, a process that can often be a real challenge. Informatics addresses this challenge by using information technology (IT) to manage information, and the medication-use process is the context in which pharmacists work to promote safe and effective medication therapy. The following sections describe the role of pharmacists, pharmacy informatics, and other HIT in the medication-use process.

Much of this chapter focuses on systems that support pharmacists' and other providers' activities. Implementation and adoption of these systems is usually accompanied by change in individuals' daily workflow. Over the years, several principles have emerged as key to ensuring a smooth change in workflow. First, strong leadership from formal leaders (e.g., executives, managers) within the implementation setting establishes the organization's direction. Second, leadership from champions (well-respected colleagues) is important to generate adoption among users impacted by the change. Third, changes in workflow brought about by any new system must be addressed. Last, individuals who have previous experience with the system being implemented should be leveraged to support new users. Drug information specialists responsible for implementing such systems should work with these and other key stakeholders to ensure that their needs are met and changes to efficient workflows are minimized.

Order Entry (Prescribing Stage)

In the 1999 report, *To Err Is Human: Building a Safer Health System*, the Institute of Medicine (IOM; now called the National Academy of Medicine) estimated that 44,000–98,000 deaths occur each year in U.S. hospitals due to medical errors.[4] A study published in 2016 by researchers at Johns Hopkins Medicine indicates that this number is likely much higher, estimating that 210,000–400,000 deaths occur each year among U.S. hospital patients due to medical errors. This makes medical errors the third leading cause of death in the United States, behind heart disease and cancer.[5] ADEs resulting from medical errors undoubtedly make a significant contribution here. Chapters 19 and 20 provide a closer examination of ADEs and the larger topic of medication misadventures; brief statistics are provided here. Nineteen percent of the ADEs were deemed to be due to medication errors, by far the largest category of adverse events noted in the IOM report. The causes of errors and patient injury related to order entry identified in the report included illegible handwritten reports, manual order entry, and the use of nonstandard abbreviations.[6] Further, a study by Bates and associates,[7] which looked at more than 4000 hospital admissions over a 6-month period, found that errors resulting in preventable ADEs occur most often (i.e., 56% of cases) at the prescribing stage of the medication-use process. This same study judged 28% of ADEs as preventable. As such, it is imperative that pharmacists identify and prevent ADEs at this early stage in the medication-use process. The three

HIT tools that can aid in doing so include CPOE, e-prescribing, and CDSS, all of which must be maintained and updated by drug information specialists on an ongoing basis.

COMPUTERIZED PROVIDER ORDER ENTRY (CPOE)

CPOE, described earlier, is the process allowing electronic creating and sharing of medical provider orders for the treatment of patients under a provider's care in an acute or inpatient care setting. Orders for medications, laboratory tests, consultations, radiography, etc., entered via a CPOE system are communicated to the medical staff and appropriate departments over a computer network. CPOE eliminates illegible handwriting, decreases medical errors as well as the delay in order completion, improves patient care, and is, therefore, an important component in health care information systems.[8,9] Although features of a CPOE system may vary, ideal features are described here:

- Provider orders should be standardized across the organization (see Chapter 15), but may also be individualized based on the provider or the provider's specialty through the use of order sets. Orders should be communicated via the patient's EHR to all departments and health care providers involved in the patient's care.
- Patient-centered decision support, including display of the patient's medical history, current test results, and evidence-based guidelines to support treatment options, should be readily available. Site-specific policies and procedures, such as formularies, recommended therapeutic interchanges, and drug shortage alerts, may also be incorporated.
- CPOE systems must support clinical workflows through **algorithms** that provide clear, concise, and actionable advice and warnings. The order entry process should be simple and allow efficient use by new or infrequent users.
- Access must be secure, and a permanent record of access needs to be created with an electronic signature (i.e., any legally recognized means of indicating that a person accepts the contents of an electronic message).
- The CPOE system should be portable, accepting and managing orders from all departments through various devices, including desktop and laptop computers, smartphones, and tablets, whether onsite (e.g., at the hospital) or offsite (e.g., working from home).
- Data should be collected for training, planning, and analysis of patient safety events as part of ongoing quality initiatives.
- Diagnoses should be linked to orders at the time of order entry to support drug-condition checking, improve documentation, and support appropriate charges.
- Like all HIT systems, appropriate backup and downtime procedures should be established and routinized.

Despite having the ability to decrease ADEs, CPOE also potentially introduces new types of errors.[10] Inexperienced providers and staff using CPOE may cause slower order entry and person-to-person communication, especially at first. Alerts and warnings that appear too frequently may lead to **alert fatigue**, a situation in which a provider ignores or overrides CDSS messages without giving them appropriate consideration, due to their sheer volume. CPOE can also cause automation bias where prescribers over-rely on the CPOE and CDSS. Many other types of errors can occur, serving as a strong reminder that all health care providers share responsibility to ensure safe use of CPOE and other HIT systems.

Given these issues, as well as providers' resistance to change and the costs involved, adoption of this technology by providers and hospitals in the United States was slow for many years. However, use of CPOE increased dramatically as more hospitals became aware of the financial benefits of EHRs and CPOE and as hospitals complied with **Meaningful Use** criteria, a set of standards defined by the CMS as the use of certified EHR technology to (1) improve quality, safety, and efficiency; (2) engage patients and their families; (3) improve care coordination, as well as public and population health; and (4) maintain privacy and security of PHI. A study by RAND Health found that the U.S. health care system could save $70 billion or more annually, reduce ADEs, and improve the quality of care if CPOE and other HIT were widely adopted.[11] Similarly, a 2013 study reported the findings of a systematic review, generating a pooled estimate of the effects of CPOE implementation on medication errors. The study concluded that CPOE implementation decreases the likelihood of a medication error by 48%. Based on CPOE adoption in hospitals at the time, this translated into over 17 million medication errors averted in the United States in 1 year.[12]

ELECTRONIC PRESCRIBING (E-PRESCRIBING)

E-prescribing is commonly defined as the creation and transmission of an electronic structured order in the ambulatory setting. A more precise definition would be a medication prescription entered by a prescriber directly into an electronic format using agreed-upon standards that is securely transmitted to the pharmacy that the patient chooses. E-prescriptions predominantly transmit orders for medications, but other emerging uses include prescriptions for mobile apps. Faxes and printed prescriptions are not e-prescriptions. One of the primary early challenges to nationwide e-prescribing was a network on which to transfer prescriptions. A small number of vendors provide connection networks, which includes verification between prescribers, insurance providers, and pharmacies. The National Council for Prescription Drug Programs (NCPDP), which is accredited by the American National Standards Institute, provides the standards for provider identification and telecommunication of pharmacy claims in this process.[13]

Components of e-Prescribing

Aside from the prescriber, the e-prescribing network, and the pharmacy, there are many other components that make up an e-prescribing system. These components include:

- Specific computer software
- The hardware needed to run the software
- The organizations that support transmission and sharing of data
- Data standardization
- Authorization of payment
- Communications to the pharmacy
- The processing of prescriptions within the pharmacy.

The e-prescribing software should provide functionality to support accurate, efficient, and safe entry and transmission of prescriptions. The U.S. government provided incentives to health care providers who implemented e-prescribing and EHRs meeting certain minimum requirements in their functionalities. Examining sample functionality requirements indicate a focus on safety, efficacy, and cost:

- Generating a complete medication list
- Supporting prescription ordering, printing, and electronic transmission
- Including alerts for unsafe conditions (e.g., allergies)
- Providing information on lower cost, therapeutic alternatives
- Providing information on formulary and patient eligibility based on the patient's drug plan[14]

The overall functionality of the e-prescribing software depends on the management of multiple **databases**.

- A **drug database** is necessary and should include decision support functions, such as drug-drug and drug-disease interactions, dose range checking, and allergy warnings.
- A **pharmacy database**, which supports selection of and communication with the patient's specific pharmacy, is needed.
- A **user database**, consisting of a list of prescribers and their authority to prescribe, National Provider Identifier (NPI), Drug Enforcement Agency (DEA) number, and other identifiers (like address and phone number), is also needed.
- A **patient database**, listing a prescriber's patients and all pertinent patient information to support e-prescribing functions, must be included and managed.
- Other databases that are necessary include medication insurance plans/formularies and medication profile information for individual patients.

Depending on the functionality of the e-prescribing software, additional clinical information may also be available, such as laboratory results, patient problems and diagnoses, and information from prior visits.

Workflow in e-Prescribing

To fully comprehend the functionality of an e-prescribing system, an understanding of prescribing workflow is necessary. The first step is patient registration and eligibility verification, which generally occurs prior to or at the time the patient arrives for an appointment. Here, the patient's insurance coverage and address are verified, and the patient is put on a readily available selection list within the e-prescribing system for prescribers. The patient's medication history and prescription eligibility information are made available to prescribers.

Following this is the medication entry step. Since prescription entry workflow may vary between and within practices due to prescriber preferences, the e-prescribing system should support quickly transitioning between patients, data gathering, and ordering. Portable devices and the ability to quickly log into an immobile device (e.g., desktop computer) are needed to support this type of workflow. Although not yet addressed by federal regulations, delegating the task of medication entry to support staff introduces the potential for errors as reading and translating written prescriptions is often involved in this approach. The next step in the prescribing workflow is prescriber selection of the pharmacy to which the prescriptions should be sent. A common error at this stage is selection of the wrong pharmacy from the list of available pharmacies. Once the pharmacy is selected, the prescription is transmitted to the pharmacy using standard NCPDP SCRIPT interface transactions.

One area that has great potential for improvement with e-prescribing is the renewal authorization process (i.e., authorization by the prescriber for additional refills). Prior to e-prescribing, renewal authorization required multiple telephone calls and was highly interruptive. Now, pharmacies can initiate electronic renewal requests, which can be electronically processed and returned by the prescriber.

e-Prescribing of Controlled Substances

Federal law now allows e-prescriptions for controlled substances. However, both the prescriber's and the receiving pharmacy's e-prescription systems must first be verified by a DEA-approved third-party organization prior to their use. These systems are also subject to audit to ensure compliance with regulations. Although federal law began allowing electronic prescribing of controlled substances (EPCS) in June 2010, adoption was slow.[15] It was not until September of 2015 that all 50 U.S. states allowed for the EPCS in Schedules II-V, with Vermont being the last state to fully adopt this practice. Like many other states, Vermont authorized electronic prescribing of Schedule III-IV drugs prior to allowing electronic prescribing of Schedule II drugs.[16,17] Transitioning from *authorizing* to *requiring* EPCS, over half of the states have passed legislation requiring e-prescribing for opioids, controlled substances, or all prescriptions, and the proposed Federal Substance Use-Disorder Prevention that Promotes Opioid Recovery and Treatment for Patients and Communities Act (SUPPORT Act) will require EPCS covered under Medicare, beginning January 1, 2021.[18,19] Nationally, 31% of prescriptions for controlled substances were sent electronically in 2018, a 10% increase over 2017. Additionally, 95% of pharmacies are enabled for EPCS, as are 32% of prescribers, a 46% increase (22–32%) from 2017 to 2018.[20] Nationwide EPCS is expected to greatly decrease prescription fraud and abuse. In fact, progress in terms of allowing EPCS is closely linked with states' efforts to combat the current opioid epidemic, especially as it relates to stolen or forged prescriptions.[21]

CLINICAL DECISION SUPPORT SYSTEMS (CDSS)

According to the American Medical Association, clinical decision support (CDS) is described as "providing clinicians, patients or individuals with knowledge and person specific or population information, intelligently filtered or presented at appropriate times, to foster better health processes, better individual patient care, and better population health."[22] A CDSS is a computing system that provides CDS. The three basic components of a CDSS include (1) an inference engine, (2) a knowledge base, and (3) a communication mechanism. The **inference engine**, also known as the reasoning engine, forms the brain of the CDSS, working to link patient-specific information with information in the knowledge base. It evaluates the available information and determines what to present to the user. The **knowledge base** is composed of varied clinical knowledge, such as treatment guidelines, diagnoses, and drug-drug or drug-disease interactions. The communication mechanism allows entry of patient information and is responsible for communicating relevant information back to the clinician. A CDSS that checks a patient's age and immunization history against vaccination guidelines and presents recommendations to a provider serves as a useful example.

CDS can be generated in a variety of forms, including alerts, reminders, information displays, CPOE, electronic templates, and guidelines. CDSS have been employed in many clinical care domains and can support a wide range of complex decisions at various stages in the patient care process. In terms of preventive care, CDSS can provide reminders for vaccinations, cancer screenings, cardiovascular risk reduction, and other preventive measures. A study by Shea and associates found a 77% increase in the use of preventive practices when computer reminders were used.[23] There are several CDSS that have been designed to help clinicians diagnose based on the signs and symptoms exhibited by a patient. These systems have the potential to reduce diagnostic errors and should be linked with an EHR to achieve their full potential.[24] CDSS are used to provide evidence-based treatment at the point of care, often drawing upon evidence-based guidelines, which are covered in Chapter 8.

Medication Decision Support

Medication decision support is a large portion of the knowledge base for any CDSS. Basic support in this area includes drug-allergy checking, basic dosing guidance, formulary decision support, duplicate therapy checking, and drug-drug interaction checking. In the case of formulary decision support, CDSS can prompt prescribers of the preferred medications (according to the hospital's or insurer's formulary) at the point in time in which they are selecting from available medications. In addition, any restrictions placed on the ordering of the medication can be presented. This allows prescribers to implement agreed-upon formularies (see Chapter 15) within their practice settings with minimal disruption. More advanced decision support may include dosing suggestions for geriatric patients or patients with renal insufficiency, guidance for medication-related laboratory testing, drug-disease and drug-lab interaction checking, and drug-pregnancy contraindication checking. CDSS are also used for follow-up or corollary orders as well as adverse event monitoring. In fact, a study by Overhage and associates showed a 25% improvement in corollary orders (orders that are routine under certain situations, such as a stool softener when a patient is receiving a narcotic) with the use of CDSS.[25] The main benefits of CDSS use include the ability to decrease ADEs, costs, and length of patient stay as well as improve **clinical workflow**, provide useful information at the point of care, draw attention to possible drug interactions, and provide reminders of warranted follow-up interventions.

CDSS also have their limitations. For instance, developing and maintaining a comprehensive knowledge base is time consuming and resource intensive. For instance, at many institutions, pharmacists working in drug information services spend hours after each P&T meeting updating formularies, order sets, guidelines, etc., to align with new recommendations. CDSS need to communicate with other clinical information systems, such as EHRs, CPOE systems, and pharmacy systems. Additionally, excessive alerting can lead to alert fatigue and clinicians ignoring the warnings. In an attempt to minimize alert fatigue, drug information specialist can work to reduce repetitive warnings in the system, hold meetings to discuss the importance of the warnings currently in place, and remove warnings that are deemed to be clinically insignificant.

Case Study 28–1

While on a pharmacy informatics rotation, you as a pharmacy student attend rounds with medical students to gain insight into the use of health information technology from a physician's standpoint. After the physician leading rounds illustrates the use of the hospital's CPOE and CDS systems, she mentions the challenges that the hospital faced when implementing their CPOE system. The discussion then turns to the potential problems, limitations, and benefits of CPOE and CDS systems. Since the physician knows that you are on a pharmacy informatics rotation, she asks for your input.

- *What is the difference between CPOE and e-prescribing systems?*
- *What are the challenges with CPOE maintenance?*
- *What is a CDS system and what role does it play in CPOE and e-prescribing systems?*
- *What are the potential problems, limitations, and benefits of these two systems to users?*

Order Verification

Order verification occurs when prescribed medications are transferred, either manually (in a limited number of locations) or electronically, to the pharmacy. Once received, pharmacists must interpret the medication order and make an assessment regarding any drug-related problems. The goal of this process is to transform the order into a dispensable form that can be safely and correctly interpreted at the administration step. Pharmacists may use CDSS, pharmacy computer systems, and evidence-based medicine tools at this stage to perform their cognitive and administrative functions.

Pharmacists have traditionally relied upon CDSS within the pharmacy information system to support safe and efficacious decision-making regarding the filling of prescriptions. Although the use of CDSS at the prescribing stage helps improve the quality of orders received by the pharmacy, problems still exist with orders originating from CPOE systems and e-prescriptions. For instance, CPOE systems, while reducing certain errors, have been found to increase other types of errors. A study by Koppel and associates found that a widely used CPOE system actually facilitated 22 types of medication error risks, including pharmacy inventory displays being mistaken for dosage guidelines, fragmented CPOE displays that prevent full view of a patient's medications, and inflexible ordering formats that result in wrong orders.[10] As such, pharmacists must remain diligent in their review of orders prior to dispensing.

One of the main aspects of support provided by pharmacy CDSS software is information pertaining to drug-drug interactions (DDIs). This information is meant to augment and increase pharmacists' ability to detect clinically significant interactions. However, a study by Saverno and associates, which analyzed the ability of pharmacy CDSS to detect DDIs at 64 Arizona pharmacies, indicated that many perform suboptimally in terms of identifying well-known, clinically relevant interactions. Specifically, only 28% of the participating pharmacies accurately identified the interactions and noninteractions involved in the study's fictitious patient medication orders. The authors speculated that the variability in performance may be due to differences in knowledge bases, the occurrence of alert fatigue, and attempts to minimize alert fatigue, such as customizing CDSS software to limit drug-interaction warnings.[26] This further reiterates the point that pharmacists, all of whom rightly rely on the drug information systems and resources at their disposal, must remain diligent when reviewing orders to be dispensed.

Dispensing

Medications are prepared and distributed to patients in the dispensing stage of the medication-use process. The actual activities involved at this step vary depending on the setting: inpatient (institutional, acute care) versus outpatient care (community). However, there are many similarities shared between the two settings, including acquiring medications from a supplier, stocking medications based on needs, and safely and accurately preparing and dispensing medications based on the verified order. Further, there are many HIT tools utilized at the dispensing stage in both settings. That said, the two settings also have their differences when it comes to dispensing and the HIT tools used in the process. While processes and procedures may initially seem to drive this stage, the foundation for safe dispensing is optimal use of patient and knowledge-based information to inform decision-making.

ACUTE CARE PHARMACY SETTING

Many aspects related to dispensing from an acute care pharmacy (i.e., institutional pharmacy) can be automated by HIT. All automated systems utilized must be able to (1) uniquely identify managed products, (2) receive structured medication orders, (3) perform appropriate dose calculations as needed, and (4) report transactions to other automated systems for billing or other purposes.

For this to occur, all prescription medication packaging must be marked with an assigned, 10-digit National Drug Code (NDC), a requirement by the FDA. All NDCs consist of three segments: a labeler code, a drug code, and a package code in one of the following configurations: 4-4-2, 5-4-1, or 5-3-2, representing labeler (first 4 digits in the 4-4-2 configuration)-drug (second 4 digits in the 4-4-2 configuration)-package (last 2 digits in the 4-4-2 configuration). The labeler code is assigned by the FDA and identifies the vendor responsible for the final packaging of the drug. The drug code, which is assigned by the vendor, identifies the drug form and strength of the product. Lastly, the package code, also assigned by the vendor, identifies the packaging level type and size (e.g., unit, box, case). It should be noted that, due to a Health Insurance Portability and Accountability Act (HIPAA) standard, 10-digit NDCs must be converted into an 11-digit format in a 5-4-2 configuration for billing purposes.[27,28] The FDA maintains a central repository of NDCs. However, although manufacturers are required to report NDCs to the FDA, approval is not required. For automation to work properly, the pharmacy and related automated systems must maintain a current and accurate list of known NDCs.

Carousel cabinets, ADCs, robotic cart filling systems, and sterile compounding devices are some of the other prominent HIT tools used in automated drug distribution systems in acute care pharmacies. Carousel cabinets contain shelves that are attached to a carousel, which rotates shelves for medication selection. Benefits of carousel cabinets include ensuring selection of the prescribed medication, freeing up of floor space, reduced walking associated with drug distribution, and more accurate accounting of inventory.

ADCs are similar to carousels, except they do not use rotating shelves. ADCs, which may be located either in the pharmacy or on patient-care units, maintain inventory and audit trails as well as perform charging functions. Access to inventory contained in ADCs requires the user to log in, maintaining an audit trail of receiving and dispensing activity. ADCs can be configured with a variety of different drawers so that specified users may only have access to certain drawers or even specific drawer sections. Despite being able to limit access in this way, none of the drawers control the amount of product removed, which can be seen as a limitation. In some situations, like emergencies, override functions are permitted. Despite the obvious benefit of override access, this practice has also been associated with medication errors, such as obtaining the wrong strength of medication, obtaining the wrong medication, and obtaining a medication after it has been discontinued.[29–31]

While not as common as ADCs, robotic cart filling systems are commonly found in hospital settings as well. They utilize bar coding to locate, obtain, package, and deliver medications to a specified location (e.g., pediatric nursing unit). This is done by filling unit-dose carts and most often requires significant repackaging efforts because the medications must be in containers that can be manipulated by the device.

The preparation of sterile products for administration can also be automated. The FDA classifies the devices that automate sterile dose preparations as pharmacy compounding devices.[32] Total parenteral nutrition (TPN) compounders are an example of this type of device. TPN compounders first compute a TPN formulation based on clinical requirements, and then drive a machine to deliver the correct ingredients in the correct amounts and sequence. Chemotherapy preparations which include medications hazardous to pharmacy personnel can also be compounded by an automated system. Such automation enhances patient safety by prohibiting improper dosing (e.g., incompatible calcium and phosphorus concentrations in a TPN), while also freeing up drug information pharmacists' time, that would have otherwise been spent verifying such orders, to focus on enhancing patient care or to research more challenging questions.

COMMUNITY PHARMACY SETTING PHARMACY INFORMATION MANAGEMENT SYSTEM

In the community pharmacy, pharmacy information management systems (PIMS) serve as the core piece of HIT that supports pharmacy operations, managing all data associated with prescriptions, patients, and prescribers. They contain key data files, such as drug files, DEA and national provider identifier numbers, physician contact information, prescription pricing tables, third-party plan details, and patient profiles. The PIMS software and related databases commonly reside on a server in the pharmacy, but they may be located on a central server, allowing access from multiple sites. In the **software as a service (SaaS)** or **application service provider (ASP)** options, both the data and software are hosted offsite. PIMS may also have integrated workflow systems with multiple workstations assigned specific tasks (e.g., intake, processing, and verifying of prescriptions). For instance, faxed and paper prescriptions are scanned during intake, making the then digitized prescription available at the filling and verification steps (Note: this is not an e-prescription). The goal of digitization is to reduce the amount of paper handled and provide a faster way to file, index, share, and search for information. Bar code scanning is also an integral component of this workflow, which allows the tracking of every prescription through the filling queue. Such workflow systems provide efficiency and are usually found in high-volume pharmacies.[1]

Other HIT utilized in the community pharmacy setting includes automated counting systems and robotics, interactive voice response (IVR) systems (i.e., the automated menu that a caller is prompted through using the phone number pad), e-prescribing, real-time inventory management, and electronic signature capture. Refill requests are commonly routed into the PIMS filling queue via IVR, which guides patients in entering in their refill information. This practice reduces the number of phone calls that must be made and handled by pharmacy staff and gives patients the ability to submit refills after hours. The Internet is also being utilized for patient entered refill requests to the same effect. Further, IVR systems, along with text messaging, are being utilized to automate outbound contact with patients, such as prescription pick-up reminders and other, informative messages. Another method by which new or refill prescriptions can enter the PIMS queue is via e-prescribing. E-prescribing is a core feature of PIMS.[1]

Bar-Coded Verification System

Through the use of counting systems or robotic dispensing systems, the majority of a community pharmacy's prescription volume can be automated. Counting systems include countertop devices and stand-alone cabinets while robotic dispensing fills and labels vials. Bar codes are used in the dispensing process to match (1) the medication with the prescription (avoiding an incorrect medication selection) and (2) the patient with the prescription (avoiding an incorrect patient selection) as entered in the computer system. This use of bar codes allows multiple checks as an additional layer of safety. Further, bar codes on will-call bags are scanned when bags are hung. This information is updated in the pharmacy computer system for quick retrieval when the patient arrives, using light to identify the hanging bag in some instances.

Administration

Depending on the setting, medications may be administered by a health care provider, such as a physician, nurse, or pharmacist, by a caregiver, or by the patient themselves. Three important HIT tools being used in hospital settings at this stage of the medication-use process are **bar code medication administration (BCMA)** systems, eMARs, and smart pumps. Drug information specialists ensure these tools are properly implemented and maintained. BCMA systems are used typically by nurses at the point of care to ensure that the six rights of medication administration are followed. While use of these systems has been increasing steadily, there is a major issue that hinders implementation. While most products used in the inpatient care setting have bar codes, there are some products (e.g., unit-dose packets) that still require pharmacy to create and attach the bar code, which is labor-intensive. Also, products that are compounded for local use, such as intra-venous antibiotics, need special bar codes to store data (e.g., concentration, stability, proper storage conditions, applicable warnings) that are not supported by the basic linear bar-coding format due to limits regarding physical and digital space. Two-dimensional bar codes (e.g., QR codes), which take up less physical space and hold more data, can at least partly solve this issue.

Alongside BCMA systems, the use of eMARs replaces paper records used by nurses to document medication administration. eMARs decrease the potential for errors by eliminating the need to handwrite changes in medications and allowing a medication change to be updated in real time in the patient's medical record.[1] They also automati-cally document the time at which medications are administered (i.e., scanned). This is especially important for evaluating the timing of administration of critical medications (e.g., antimicrobials).

Whereas BCMA commonly covers the administration of oral and topical dosage forms, intelligent infusion devices are increasingly being deployed in institutional settings to increase the safety of intravenous medication administration. Smart pumps, as they are commonly called, include drug libraries that contain standardized concentrations of drugs used in the institution, agreed-upon maximum and minimum dosing limits for continuous and bolus doses, and rate and volume limits. The development and refinement of the standardized information (e.g., libraries, dosing limits) found in smart pumps is an important opportunity for pharmacists to leverage their drug information expertise to support institutional-wide decisions that impact direct patient care. Managing this information is an ongoing process. For instance, updates may be necessary when an applicable new drug is approved, an existing drug secures approval for a new indication at a significantly different dose, or when drug or supply shortages occur. Additional benefits of the incorporation of standardized information in smart pumps include: (1) a double check of programming when nursing staff prepares a medication for administration, (2) soft and hard stops that can temporarily pause or suspend administration, and (3) an electronic audit trail.

A closed-loop medication administration system allows individuals responsible for a patient's care to have access to the same information at the same time. Being fully electronic, these systems collate data from CPOE, BCMA, smart pumps, EHRs, and other sources across the continuum of care at all steps of the medication-use process via seamless documentation. Closed-loop medication administration systems allow health care providers access to nearly all activities related to a patient's care in real-time, with decision support incorporated as needed. The primary focus of these systems is patient safety, and they have been shown to significantly reduce medication errors.

Monitoring

Clinicians' monitoring activities vary greatly depending on their work setting and available resources. No matter the setting however, monitoring activities should result in clinical interventions, when necessary. A clinical intervention is the act of interceding with the intent of modifying the medication-use process. The broad categories of monitoring activities, and therefore clinical interventions, performed by health care providers include activities that promote safety, activities that promote quality, and activities that promote efficiency and cost-effectiveness. For instance, a pharmacist may intercept a medication ordered, for which the patient has an allergy, or a pharmacist may identify a less expensive, therapeutic alternative to the prescribed medication in order to decrease costs for the patient.

In the hospital setting, clinical surveillance systems are at the core of monitoring efforts. These systems exist as stand-alone applications and as components of integrated systems. Clinical surveillance refers to active surveillance or watchful waiting that includes a collection and analysis of patient-specific information that is then used to drive decisions. These systems are most often used by pharmacy to monitor information from the pharmacy system (i.e., medication lists), laboratory results, and patient demographics from the admission/discharge/transfer system. Rules are built to identify potential problems. Rules can be built locally by drug information specialist or included by vendors with other information systems components. Often, pharmacy or others charged with medication safety will assume responsibility for monitoring algorithm construction and investigation. For example, an algorithm may monitor all patients for orders of naloxone, which is used to treat opioid overdose. Another algorithm may monitor for all patients receiving ranitidine, whose platelet count has decreased to less than 50% of the previous value, suggesting an occurrence of rare thrombocytopenia. Patients meeting these criteria are presented to pharmacy staff for follow-up and evaluation.

Once a need is established and a clinical intervention has taken place, the intervention must be well documented. The purpose of clinical intervention documentation is multifaceted. One primary purpose is to demonstrate the cost and quality impact of programs, such as clinical pharmacy services. Documenting clinical interventions can also be used for staff performance improvement as well as quality improvement activities. Documentation gives insight into what clinical staff members are doing, and therefore allows constructive feedback to be provided. Similarly, clinical intervention documentation can be utilized to improve workflow.

There are certain basic elements that a good documentation system should have.

- It should be easy to use and fit into the existing workflow as much as possible.
- It should allow for quick documentation that includes sufficient details. Specifically, the system should have the capability to add or modify interventions, manage drug and prescriber databases, and mirror the organization's security policies.
- All documentation should be searchable as structured text.
- The system should provide a complete record of all clinical activities.
- The computer system should collect and document as much of the information as possible, leaving only the information that must be documented by a pharmacist.

Ideally, all practitioners providing care to the same patient would document all monitoring and intervention activities in a shared record. However, a common challenge is inconsistency in where information is documented across disparate systems. The record would then be accessible by all other providers who are also caring for that particular patient. In fact, a primary objective of the Pharmacy HIT Collaborative, a multiorganizational group focused on the role of pharmacists in the emerging EHR landscape, is to ensure that this is the case for the patient care efforts of pharmacists.[33] Reporting, which is the critical output of the documentation system, should be quick and easy. It should allow real-time selection and inclusion of any combination of documented fields in the system.[1]

Case Study 28-2

You are still on your pharmacy informatics rotation, and after your discussion on the potential problems/limitations of CPOE and e-prescribing systems from the physician's standpoint, the medical students with whom you are rounding ask you how pharmacists interface with CPOE and e-prescribing systems. The physician then illustrates the use of the hospital's BCMA system. The medical students inquire as to the purpose of the BCMA system. They also ask if health information technology is used to actively monitor patients. Again, the physician leading rounds asks for your input.

- *How do pharmacists interface with CPOE and e-prescribing systems?*
- *What is a BCMA system and what is its purpose?*
- *What health information technology is used to actively monitor patients and how does it do so?*

PRESCRIPTION DRUG MONITORING PROGRAMS (PDMPS)

Monitoring of prescription narcotics, especially opioids, has become increasingly important in recent years. While efforts to address the opioid epidemic have recently demonstrated decreases in deaths due to all opioids and synthetic opioids, deaths involving prescription opioids remain stable nationally.[34] **Prescription drug monitoring programs (PDMPs)** are central databases of statewide prescribing and dispensing records for controlled drugs and other drugs with high potential for abuse.[35] PDMPs are managed at the state level; there is not a national PDMP. However, most states have agreements allowing pharmacists from other states to search PDMPs other than the state in which the pharmacist is practicing. At the time of publication, all states maintained an operational statewide PDMP, except Missouri where the state Senate passed legislation in March 2020 to establish a statewide PDMP.

There are several PDMP vendors who develop and maintain the majority of states' databases. Access and reporting privileges and requirements vary among states. While the typical pharmacist may not have hands-on experience with the technical aspects of their state's PDMP, because of their access to PDMPs and to patients, pharmacists have an important role in curbing misuse of prescription medications. It is up to the pharmacist to review and act on the data found in their PDMP in those situations where concerns of abuse exist. Reviewing includes looking for indicators that patients may intentionally or unintentionally receive unnecessary or excessive prescriptions for controlled substances, including opioids. Indicators include prescriptions for the same controlled substance from multiple providers and filling prescriptions for the same controlled substance at different pharmacies. One of the challenges impacting pharmacists' use of PDMPs is workflow integration. Specifically, PDMP software is not incorporated into prescription processing software by default, requiring pharmacists to use separate software for searching. This functionality does exist, but often requiring additional fees.

Case Study 28–3

You are a student pharmacist completing an inpatient pharmacy administration rotation. Through your rotation experiences, you have observed and interacted with a variety of health information technologies and automation used to manage medications within the institution. Your preceptor gives you the following assignment.

- *What is the medication-use process, and what health technologies are used at each stage of the medication-use process to ensure safe and efficacious medication therapy?*

The Future: Informatics in the U.S. Health Care System

4 *The vision of health care is becoming more patient-centric.* Health care is transitioning from industrial age medicine—which places focus on professional care and is segmented and also highly expensive—to a new approach, alternatively described as information age health care, which encourages lower cost individual care, getting friends and family involved, and using self-help networks as first-line approaches.[36] This transformation has been given the label, patient-centric or (participatory) care, in that the new approach involves patients as highly active, decision-making members of their own care team. More information regarding drug information in the ambulatory and community settings can be found in Chapters 26 and 27.

As an example, **personal health records (PHRs)** allow patients increased opportunity to participate in the collection, maintenance, and sharing of their personal health-related information through a web-based environment. All the information is patient-maintained, and PHRs should be designed as a lifelong resource for the patient's health information. PHRs are ideally kept in a web-accessible, electronic format that is not only secure and private but also universally available to providers treating the patient. Further, the ability to move information from a patient's EHR, which is maintained by a health care organization, to the patient's PHR increases patient involvement in their own health care. Along with this ability, patients should also have the ability to annotate the information coming in from their providers or EHR. It should be noted here that the PHR does not and is not meant to replace the legal record of any provider.[37] In order for PHRs to be interoperable and share data with other systems as described, standards of data communication must be established and utilized. Current agreed upon standards include Continuity of Care Record (CCR) and Extensible Markup Language (XML). Strong levels of data encryption and passwords are also required. Although still evolving, there are dozens of PHRs available today. **Patient portals** are closely related to PHRs. The distinction is that patient portals are hosted and maintained by health institutions (e.g., hospitals, clinics, pharmacies). Features vary across portals, but in general, they provide patients a single location to access and review information related to the care they have received in that institutions.

INTERNET OF THINGS

The **Internet of Things (IoT)** refers to connecting everyday physical objects or devices to each other and the Internet, enabling them to share information and communicate with other devices. This has been enabled by the increasing availability of broadband Internet, decreasing technology costs, and an increasing number of devices with built-in sensors, Bluetooth, and Wi-Fi capabilities. The possibilities in terms of the types of devices that could take part in the IoT are endless. Current examples range from light bulbs to glucose monitors to toothbrushes. IoT-enabling technology is rapidly maturing. Over the next decade, more than 250 billion devices are expected to connect to the Internet.

Commonly, the devices that communicate via the IoT are called "smart devices," indicating their ability to communicate with other devices (usually wirelessly) as well as their ability to operate autonomously. Examples include consumer electronics devices like activity trackers (e.g., FitBit®) that share information with smartphones, smart watches that monitor health parameters such as pulse oximetry, and glucose monitoring devices that regulate insulin dosing through real-time data collection and smartphone integration.

DIGITAL HEALTH

Digital health is a broad field that has been defined as, *"the cultural transformation of how disruptive technologies that provide digital and objective data accessible to both caregivers* *and patients leads to an equal level doctor-patient relationship with shared decision-making and the democratization of care.*[38] Digital health is related to the IoT/smart devices and is composed of several domains:

- **Mobile health (mHealth)**—the use of mobile phones and other devices in health care
- **Digital therapeutics**—delivery of evidence-based interventions, driven by software programs[39]
- Devices, sensors, and wearables—consumer devices that track various health and non-health-related metrics
- **Telehealth**—the delivery of health-related services and information over distance with the aid of electronic devices
- Social media—the use of web-based applications that allow the creation and sharing of user-generated content

mHealth applications, when used in conjunction with devices, sensors, and wearables, allow patients to capture their personal biometric data, which can then be automatically or manually shared with health care providers. Digital therapeutics are exemplified by the delivery of cognitive behavioral therapy on someone's smartphone. The important distinction is that software applications are the central method for delivering digital therapeutic interventions. Digital therapeutics can be used alone or in conjunction with other treatment methods. Devices, sensors, and wearables play a central role in digital health efforts by capturing data. Often the focus is on data generated during the patient's regular, daily routine. While telehealth has existed for decades, recent advancements have expanded its use to activities including virtual visits with providers, including pharmacists, on smartphones and monitoring patients remotely. The COVID-19 pandemic, which prompted the U.S. Department of Health and Human Services to temporarily ease restrictions allowing the use of common, non-HIPAA compliant apps (e.g., FaceTime®, Zoom, Skype®), further accelerated the adoption and use of telehealth. ❺ *The IoT and digital health are enabling technologies as the U.S. health care system moves to patient-centric model of care.*

Given these and many more potential uses of IoT in the field, health care is seen by some as one of the most promising applications of the IoT. According to a 2019 report, the health care IoT market is expected to reach $537 billion by 2025.[40] Convergence is an important concept in the digital health landscape, as illustrated in the examples above. As another example, remote patient monitoring (a type of telehealth) relies on devices or sensors to capture data that are shared with providers. Additionally, a digital therapeutic activity that includes delivering an intervention via a smartphone app is also classified as mHealth. Data, devices, and interventions are converging in the care of patients. It is important to recognize that privacy, authentication, and integrity are requisite when dealing with protected health information (PHI).

Among the digital health domains, social media (e.g., Facebook®, Twitter®, Instagram®) is one of the primary drivers of shared decision-making by enabling patients and nonprofessional caregivers to engage professionals and nonprofessionals in collaborative efforts to improve care. Social media enables this reality by fostering interactions that may not necessarily have occurred in the absence of social media, by providing broader access to information, and by promoting connections for peer support. The primary challenge with social media in health care relates to validity and reliability of information.[41]

Despite the relevance of challenges related to privacy, security, etc., as they relate to digital health, one of the most significant challenges is incorporation, use, and impact of these data on the patient-provider dynamic. Imagine a patient who diligently records their blood glucose readings between visits to their pharmacist or doctor. Through the use of a smart monitoring device, these data are all available to share with their providers electronically. Does the provider have time or inclination to review potentially hundreds or thousands of data points? Even if the data are presented in aggregate, does the provider trust the data? Furthermore, what are the medical liability implications of the provider reviewing (or not reviewing) those data? This is not a scenario to be imagined. It is today's reality, and these questions remain to be answered.

Case Study 28–4

Your preceptor approaches you one morning and tells you about a new committee within the hospital that she has been asked to chair. The committee's role is to explore the emerging digital health domain and identify potential ways that the hospital can become involved. The committee is also interested in how the hospital can incorporate the IoT in ways that may benefit visitors, patients, and personnel. Knowing that you are a tech savvy person, your preceptor asks you to help conduct some of the initial research into the digital health domain and potential uses of the IoT. You are given the following assignment.

- *What are the primary journals that address the digital health domain?*
- *Suggest a few ways the hospital can use popular digital health tools to engage patients.*
- *Suggest a few ways the hospital can use IoT applications and devices.*

INTEROPERABLE ELECTRONIC HEALTH RECORDS

⑥ *The current U.S. health care system is decentralized and fragmented. Because of this, significant communication gaps exist when multiple health care institutions provide care for the same patient. Substantial evidence suggests that more effective communication would improve patient care and reduce medical errors, such as ADEs.*[5] Beyond the clinical improvements, there are also major financial benefits to be had. Projections indicate that greater health information exchange and interoperability could save the U.S. health care system $30–$77 billion annually.[42,43]**Interoperability** is the ability of disparate computer systems to exchange information in a manner that allows the information to be used meaningfully.[44]**⑦** *The desired result of interoperable systems and EHRs is to readily provide all health practitioners in all locations, including the pharmacy, with access to information about a patient's care, as needed.* As such, new health information systems (HIS) should focus on ensuring effective communication of data between and within institutions, which includes a focus on data transfer across applications, devices, and geographical locations. From a community pharmacy perspective, this communication should include the ability for pharmacist's medication-related contributions to be included in the patient's EHR. Efforts are underway to incorporate pharmacists' care activities into their patients' records (see the "Current Standards" section). Communication standards are necessary to achieve this desired level of meaningful data exchange.

CURRENT STANDARDS

Several health care standards exist today. For instance, the NCPDP developed an e-prescribing standard, NCPDP SCRIPT, for the transmission of prescription information, along with relevant medical history information, electronically between prescribers, pharmacies, and payers. Mentioned previously, NDCs, created by manufacturers and the FDA, with whom they are registered, are used as a standard way to signify the drug manufacturer, the drug formulation, and the packaging type. RxNorm, produced by the National Library of Medicine (NLM), is a standard for supporting **semantic interoperability** between pharmacy systems and drug terminologies by providing a standardized naming system for generic and branded drugs.[45] In other words, RxNorm provides a standardized system for communicating clinical drug names across the various drug databases that are found in pharmacy computer systems. **Unified Medical Language System (UMLS)**, also maintained by the NLM, enables interoperability between computer systems, such as EHRs, by providing a set of files and software that bring together many medical vocabularies and standards.[46] Contained within the UMLS is the**Logical Observation Identifiers Names and Codes (LOINC)** terminology for laboratory test results and procedures, which is maintained by the Regenstrief Institute. Another important medical terminology version also contained within UMLS is the **Systematized Nomenclature of Medicine-Clinical Terms (SNOMED CT)**. SNOMED CT maps to diagnosis and billing codes known as the International Classification of Disease-tenth revision (ICD-10). Further, **Current Procedural Terminology (CPT®)** codes, produced by the American Medical Association (AMA), provide medical nomenclature used to report medical procedures and services performed under private and public health insurance plans.[47]

The United States' transition to electronic health records highlights an important limitation for pharmacy practice, especially in the community setting. In the current community pharmacy practice model, pharmacists do not have access to their patients' medical records, other than the records in their pharmacy software. This prevents pharmacists from reviewing other providers' documentation, and it prevents pharmacists' contributions to patient care from being shared with other providers. Fortunately, standards-setting bodies have developed an electronic documentation and communication standard that addresses both limitations, known as the "Pharmacist eCare Plan." At the time of this writing, the standard is under review for eventual publication.[48]

THE GOVERNMENT'S ROLE IN INTEROPERABILITY

Technical standards are one piece of the interoperability puzzle. Other challenges include finding an organization or group to lead the charge through associated business, administrative, and financial considerations. The U.S. government led these efforts, beginning in 2004 when President George W. Bush targeted computerizing health records in his State of the Union Address. That same year, President Bush established the Office of the National Coordinator for Health Information Technology (ONC) within the Office of the Secretary of Health and Human Services (HHS).[49] The two major initial goals of the ONC were widespread adoption of EHRs by 2014 and the creation and implementation of an interoperable health information infrastructure.

❽ *To drive adoption and use of EHRs, the federal government leveraged its position as policy maker and purchaser of health care through two programs focused on incentives and payments to providers and hospitals.* First, the Centers for Medicare & Medicaid Services (CMS) developed a monetary incentive program, the Meaningful Use program. This program incentivized hospitals and physicians to use EHRs to achieve specific outcomes, which may be process-oriented or patient-oriented. The goals of the Meaningful Use program were to (1) improve quality, safety, and efficiency; (2) engage patients and their families; (3) improve care coordination, as well as public and population health; and (4) maintain privacy and security of PHI. For example, 60% of medication orders should be entered electronically or >50% of patients should have electronic access to their medical information within 36 hours after discharge. The central premise was that the adoption of and compliance with Meaningful Use would result in better clinical outcomes, improved population health, increased health care transparency and efficiency, more robust data for research, and the empowerment of individuals and patients.[50]

The Meaningful Use program was followed by the current Merit-based Incentive Program (MIPS), which began in 2017. MIPS focuses on four performance categories that result in a score for qualifying clinicians: quality, promoting interoperability, improvement activities, and cost. This score determines payment to clinicians for Medicare patients.[51] More information on MIPS is found in Chapter 18.

EHR adoption increased steadily, beginning in 2010. In 2017, 99% of hospitals with more than 300 beds had certified EHRs while small, rural hospitals had the lowest rate of adoption (93%). EHR adoption also demonstrated progress among physicians with 86% of office-based physicians adopting an EHR and 80% adopting a certified EHR by 2017.[52]

Despite this progress, the projected health and savings benefits of interoperable health IT systems was slow to fully realize. This was due to many factors, including slower than expected adoption, adoption of systems that are neither interoperable nor easy to use, and failure to redesign health care approaches to take full advantage of health IT.[53] In terms of the current MIPS program, small and rural practices face unique challenges, which include technical (e.g., EHR operation, lack of EHR vendor support) and nontechnical aspects (e.g., lack of financial resources to hire adequately strained staff, some measures do not align with patient care).[54]

When practice sites already have computerized management systems (e.g., to capture patient information, schedule appointments, perform billing tasks), as most sites do, choosing an EHR or other health IT to implement can be difficult. These sites can choose to either integrate their existing management system with the EHR or adopt a completely new, integrated system. With the former approach, often referred to as a "best-of-breeds" system, the EHR is selected based on its inherent qualities. Often, especially when the software applications are obtained from different vendors, interfaces must be built for them to exchange data. Integrated databases, on the other hand, share the same database, eliminating the need to build interfaces. Integrated systems also offer the convenience of having a single point of contact for technical support. However, the "best-of-breeds" approach is not without its advantages. It allows sites to keep their current, familiar software in place. This, combined with being able to choose an EHR based on its own merits, can make the choice between this approach and an integrated system a difficult one.

Case Study 28–5

You are wrapping up your rotation, and your preceptor comes to you with a final assignment. She has been tasked with representing the Pharmacy Department on the hospital committee responsible for health information technology (HIT) in the hospital. Your preceptor knows little about the topic and gives you several questions to answer to help her get up to speed.

- *What are EHRs and how do they differ from PHRs?*
- *What federal agency is responsible for overseeing national efforts related to health information technology?*
- *What role does the federal government play in driving HIT adoption?*
- *What are the primary concerns related to patients' protected health information? How is cyber security related to PHI?*

SECURITY, PRIVACY, AND CONFIDENTIALITY OF PROTECTED HEALTH INFORMATION

❾ *As interoperability and digital health advances and more patient data are shared across providers and organizations, the issues of security, privacy, and confidentiality of PHI inevitability arise.* **Protected health information (PHI)** includes any information that can be used to identify a person, including information about medical conditions, payment for care, or actual care delivered.[1] Privacy refers to being free from unauthorized intrusions and the protection of PHI. Health care organizations create policies that drive privacy measures that determine how and what information is gathered, stored, and used, and how patients are involved in the process. Security here refers to restricting access to patient health data to everyone except those with authorized access. This is accomplished using electronic tools, such as login identifications, password protection, dual authentication, and other measures. Confidentiality here refers to the provider-client privilege that, under most circumstances, any health-related information communicated between a provider and a patient is private. PHI can be in any form (e.g., written, oral, or electronic), and examples include patient name, address, Social Security number, email address, or any other part of a medical record that could be used to identify a patient.[1]

Health care providers need to be aware of the existing and emerging regulations that apply to the security, privacy, and confidentiality of PHI. For instance, the Health Breach Notification Rule, passed into law in 2009, requires that covered entities provide notice to patients following a breach in security. Also, the Patient Safety and Quality Improvement Act of 2005 (Patient Safety Act) establishes a framework that allows providers to report patient safety events voluntarily and confidentially to Patient Safety Organizations for aggregation and analysis purposes.[55]

Cyber security threats are a related and increasingly important topic in this space. In health care, cyber security threats most often take the form of unauthorized use of electronic patient information. Cyber security breaches lead to both direct and indirect costs. Direct costs include the actions taken to resolve a breach (e.g., notifications, fines, lawsuits), while indirect costs include lost revenue due to a breach (e.g., loss of patient trust). On average, health care data breaches cost $408 per record, which is three times the cross-industry average of $148 per record.[56] Methods to minimize the opportunity for cyber security breaches include routinely applying software patches and updates to critical information systems and using least privileged user access, which limits individual user's access to only the systems necessary to complete their job responsibilities. Other methods include routine education of employees, the use of encryption, and collaborating with an external entity to conduct a threat assessment to identify opportunities for security breaches.[57] The COVID-19 pandemic resulted in a shift to remote work, which heightened the need for measures to minimize cyber security risks.

HEALTH INSURANCE PORTABILITY AND ACCOUNTABILITY ACT (HIPAA)

Another major piece of legislation with which health care providers need to be intimately familiar is the Health Insurance Portability and Accountability Act (HIPAA), passed into law in 1996. The main component of concern here is the HIPAA Privacy Rule, which establishes how medical information should be handled. The major goal of the Privacy Rule is to ensure proper protection of individuals' health information while also allowing the flow of health information needed to provide high-quality health care. As such, the law defines PHI, describes how health care organizations can use and disclose PHI, and outlines the requirements of health organizations to protect PHI from inappropriate disclosure and misuse. For instance, the Privacy Rule specifies that PHI can be transmitted and used for treatment, payment, and operations (TPO) processes (i.e., general health care operational use).

As it is not intended to prevent providers from meaningfully discussing the treatment of their patients, the rule specifies that some incidental disclosures of PHI are permitted. That said, reasonable safeguards, such as speaking in a low voice, not discussing patient care in the presence of others, and closing patient charts after use—including electronic charts and records, should be used to limit such incidental disclosures. There are also certain disclosures, permitted by law, which may be made to governmental agencies for such purposes as law enforcement, research, workers' compensation, and organ donation. Further, the HIPAA Privacy Rule requires that health care organizations notify patients of their rights when receiving care and provides them with a process to exercise those rights. Also, patients should be given the opportunity to agree or object to disclosures of their PHI while under the care of a health care organization.[1,58]

There is also the HIPAA Security Rule that covers electronic PHI (ePHI). ePHI is simply PHI stored in electronic form. Health care organizations are required by the

Security Rule to ensure the integrity, confidentiality, and availability of all ePHI created, received, maintained, or transmitted by the organization. As such, almost all organizations have fax, Internet, and email policies that outline appropriate use to protect ePHI.[59] Measures to secure ePHI include data encryption and access control measures limiting access to PHI and the networks it traverses. Networks themselves can also serve as security tools through physical isolation of hardware and software. Network monitoring can also identify potential and real risks to information security.

Conclusion

Pharmacy informatics is the scientific discipline found at the intersection of people, data, and technology systems. It is governed by business, technical, and regulatory standards to ensure optimal use of patient-specific and knowledge-based information. Health care providers rely on informatics to support their activities associated with the medication-use process. Pharmacy informaticists must synthesize and manage much of the drug information utilized by the HIT tools at their institution. This is an ongoing process that requires frequent attention and updating due to the never-ending stream of new drug approvals, guideline updates, drug, and supply shortages, etc. In addition, pharmacists specializing in drug information must be able to effectively communicate with other health care providers as well as patients, whether in-person or via telehealth solutions, to promote medication utilization that helps control costs, improves outcomes, and maximizes patient safety. As the U.S. health care system continues to advance, relying more and more on the effective and efficient use of drug information, health care providers will continue to see a growing role of informatics in their practice, regardless of the setting.

Self-Assessment Questions

1. Which of the following represents the correct order of the medication-use process?
   a. Monitoring, prescribing, order verification, administration, follow-up
   b. Prescribing, order verification, dispensing, administration, monitoring
   c. Order verification, dispensing, administration, monitoring, documentation
   d. Assessment, prescribing, order verification, administration, monitoring
   e. None of the above

2. Pharmacy informatics includes:
   a. People
   b. Information
   c. Technology
   d. a and b
   e. a, b, and c

3. The two primary types of information used in pharmacy informatics include:
   a. Patient-specific and clinical expertise
   b. Clinical expertise and knowledge-based
   c. Patient-specific and knowledge-based
   d. Referential and guidelines
   e. None of the above

4. The primary similarity between CPOE and e-prescriptions is they:
   a. Are easy to implement because they do not disrupt workflow
   b. Both address the dispensing stage of the medication-use process
   c. Eliminate illegible prescriptions
   d. Eliminate all errors related to prescribing
   e. c and d

5. Which of the following provides a structured method to identify drug products?
   a. Current Procedural Terminology (CPT)
   b. National drug code (NDC)
   c. Prescription Drug Monitoring Programs (PDMP)
   d. Internet of Things (IoT)

6. The three components of clinical decision support systems include:
   a. CPOE system, transmission network, transmission standards
   b. Knowledge base, e-prescription network, transmission standards
   c. Communication mechanism, knowledge base, CPOE system
   d. Inference engine, knowledge base, communication mechanism
   e. None of the above

7. The main benefits of CDSS include the ability to decrease:
   a. ADEs
   b. Costs
   c. Length of stay
   d. All of the above
   e. a and b

8. Prescriptions created electronically (by CPOE and e-prescribing) have already undergone clinical review by CDSS when they reach the pharmacists for order verification. Research suggests that:
   a. These prescriptions are ready for dispensing, requiring no additional review.
   b. Problems still exist with prescriptions created electronically.
   c. Pharmacists must remain diligent when reviewing all prescription orders.
   d. Physicians do not rely on the information presented to them by CDSS.
   e. b and c.

9. Which of the following is an example of patient-generated health data?
   a. Electronic health records
   b. Patient portal
   c. A hospital's Facebook page
   d. Personal health records

10. Which technology includes drug libraries that contain standardized concentrations of drugs for dosing purposes?
    a. Carousel cabinets
    b. Automated dispensing cabinets
    c. Robotic cart filling systems
    d. Smart pumps
    e. BCMA

11. Which of the following are challenges facing HIT?
    a. Cyber breaches of PHI
    b. Integrating patient-generated data in clinician decision-making
    c. Federal legislation that prohibits electronic prescribing of controlled substances
    d. A lack of connectivity between devices to share information
    e. a and b

12. Which of the following are challenges to the use of patient-generated data in clinical decision-making?
    a. Workflow integration
    b. Trust in the data
    c. Lack of devices to record data
    d. a and b

13. Which Digital Health domain delivers evidence-based interventions with the use of software programs?
    a. mHealth
    b. Digital therapeutics

   c. Devices, sensors, and wearables
   d. Telehealth

14. Methods to prevent against cyber breaches include Which of the following?
   a. Least privilege user access
   b. Routine software patch installation
   c. Education of employees
   d. The use of encryption
   e. All of the above

15. Which of the following is the primary purpose of prescription drug monitoring programs?
   a. Decrease health care costs
   b. Increase Meaningful Use
   c. Decrease prescription drug abuse and fraud
   d. Decrease errors in the medication-use process
   e. None of the above

REFERENCES

1. Fox BI, Thrower MR, Felkey BG, editors. Building core competencies in pharmacy informatics. Washington (DC): American Pharmacists Association; 2010.
2. Hersh W. A stimulus to define informatics and health information technology. BMC Med Inform Decis Mak. 2009;9(1):24.
3. Hersh W. Medical informatics: improving health care through information. JAMA. 2002;288:1955-8.
4. Kohn LT, Corrigan JM, Donaldson MS, editors. To err is human: building a safer health system. Washington (DC): National Academies of Science; 2000: 1-5.
5. Makary MA, Daniel M. Medical error: the third leading cause of death in the US. BMJ. 2016;353:i2139.
6. Kohn LT, Corrigan JM, Donaldson MS, editors. To err is human: building a safer health system. Washington (DC): National Academies of Science; 2000:1-5.
7. Bates DW, Cullen DJ, Laird N, Petersen LA, Small SD, Servi D, Laffel G, Sweitzer BJ, Shea BF, Hallisey R, Vander Vliet M, Nemeskal R, Leape LL. Incidence of adverse drug events and potential adverse drug events. Implications for prevention. ADE Prevention Study Group. JAMA. 1995;274(1):29-34.
8. Kaushal R, Shojania KG, Bates DW. Effects of computerized physician order entry and clinical decision support systems on medication safety: a systematic review. Arch Intern Med. 2003;163(12);1409-16.
9. Bates DW, Leape LL Cullen DJ, Laird N, Petersen LA, Teich JM, Burdick E, Hickey M, Kleefield S, Shea B, Vander Vliet M, Seger DL. Effect of computerized physician order entry and a team intervention on prevention of serious medication errors. JAMA. 1998;280(5):1311-6.

10. Koppel R, Metlay JP, Cohen A, Abaluck B, Localdo AR, Kimmel SE, Strom BL. Role of computerized physician order entry systems in facilitating medication errors. JAMA. 2005;293(10):1197-1203.

11. Hillestad R, Bigelow JH. Health Information Technology. Can HIT lower costs and improve quality? [Internet]. California: RAND Corporation; 2005 [cited 2016 Sep 16]. Available from: http://www.rand.org/pubs/research_briefs/RB9136.html

12. Radley DC, Wasserman MR, Olsho LE, Shoemaker SJ, Spranca MD, Bradshaw B. Reduction in medication errors in hospitals due to adoption of computerized provider order entry systems. J Am Med Inform Assoc. 2013;20(3):470-6.

13. National Council for Prescription Drug Programs [Internet]. Scottsdale (AZ): National Council for Prescription Drug Programs; About—Contact Us; [cited 2016 Sep 16]; [about 1 screen]. Available from: https://www.ncpdp.org/About-Us

14. Centers for Medicare and Medicaid Services [Internet]. Baltimore (MD): Centers for Medicare and Medicaid Services; Electronic Prescribing (eRx) Incentive Program; 2013 May 28 [cited 2016 Sep 16]; [about 3 screens]. Available from: http://www.cms.hhs.gov/ERxIncentive

15. U.S. Department of Justice Drug Enforcement Administration, Office of Diversion Control [Internet]. Springfield (VA): Drug Enforcement Administration; Electronic Prescribing for Controlled Substances (EPCS); [cited 2016 Sep 16]; [about 2 screens]. Available from: http://www.deadiversion.usdoj.gov/ecomm/e_rx/index.html

16. Bonner L. Controlled substance e-prescribing now legal in all 50 states [Internet]. Washington (DC): Pharmacy Today; 2016 Jan [cited 2016 Jul 1]; [1 p.]. Available from: http://www.pharmacytoday.org/article/S1042-0991(15)00020-1/pdf

17. Administrative rules of the Board of Pharmacy [Internet]. Montpelier (VT): Vermont Board of Pharmacy; 2015 Jul 8 [cited 2016 Aug 4]; [89 p.]. Available from: https://www.sec.state.vt.us//media/690234/6-RX-Rules-2015-Final-Proposed-LCAR-Annotated-June-24-2015.pdf

18. US reaches major milestone with half of all states requiring the use of technology to combat the opioid crisis [Internet]. Alexandria (VA): Surescripts; 2019 Jul 1 [cited 2020 Nov 4]. Available from: https://surescripts.com/news-center/press-releases/!content/u.s.-reaches-major-milestone-with-half-of-all-states-requiring-the-use-of-technology-to-combat-the-opioid-crisis

19. Medicare program: Electronic prescribing of controlled substances; Request for information (RFI) [Internet]. Baltimore (MD): Centers for Medicare and Medicaid Services; [cited 2020 Nov 4]. Available from: https://www.federalregister.gov/documents/2020/08/04/2020-16897/medicare-program-electronic-prescribing-of-controlled-substances-request-for-information-rfi

20. 2018 National Progress Report [Internet]. Alexandra (VA): Surescripts; 2019 [cited 2019 Oct 7]. Available from: https://surescripts.com/news-center/national-progress-report-2018/

21. Uhrig P. Laws requiring the e-prescribing of opioids have gained momentum, but prescriber adoption is playing catch up [Internet]. Alexandra (VA): Surescripts; 2019 Jan 2 [cited 7 Oct 2019]. Available from: https://surescripts.com/news-center/intelligence-in-action/opioids/laws-requiring-the-e-prescribing-of-opioids-have-gained-momentum-but-prescriber-adoption-is-playing-catch-up/

22. Osheroff JA, Teich JM, Middleton B, Steen EB, Wright A, Detmer DE. A roadmap for national action on clinical decision support. J Am Med Inform Assoc. 2007;14(2):141-5.

23. Shea S, DuMouchel W, Bahamonde L. A meta-analysis of 16 randomized controlled trials to evaluate computer-based clinical reminder systems for preventive care in the ambulatory setting. J Am Med Inform Assoc. 1996;3(6):399-409.

24. Berner ES. Clinical decision support systems: theory and practice. 2nd ed. New York: Springer; 2007.

25. Overhage JM, Tierney WM, Zhou XH, McDonald CJ. A randomized trial of "corollary orders" to prevent errors of omission. J Am Med Inform Assoc. 1997;4(5):364-75.

26. Saverno KR, Hines LE, Warholak TL, Grizzle AJ, Babits L, Clark C, Taylor AM, Malone DC. Ability of pharmacy clinical decision-support software to alert users about clinically important drug–drug interactions. J Am Med Inform Assoc. 2011;18(1):32-7.

27. National drug code database background information [Internet]. Rockville (MD): U.S. Department of Health and Human Services, Food and Drug Administration. 2012 Jun 6 [cited 2020 Jul 22]; [4 p.]. Available from: https://www.fda.gov/drugs/development-approval-process-drugs/national-drug-code-database-background-information

28. National drug code (NDC) conversion table [Internet]. Baltimore (MD): Department of Health and Mental Hygiene; [cited 2016 Aug 4]; [1 p.]. Available from: http://phpa.dhmh.maryland.gov/OIDEOR/IMMUN/Shared%20Documents/Handout%203%20-%20NDC%20conversion%20to%2011%20digits.pdf

29. Oren E, Griffiths LP, Guglielmo BJ. Characteristics of antimicrobial overrides associated with automated dispensing machines. Am J Health-Syst Pharm. 2002;59(15);1445-8.

30. Kester K, Baxter J, Freudenthal K. Errors associated with medications removed from automated dispensing machines using override function. Hosp Pharm. 2006;41: 535-537.

31. Safety enhancements every hospital must consider in the wake of another tragic neuromuscular blocker event [Internet]. Horsham (PA): Institute for Safe Medication Practices; 2019 Jan 17 [cited 2020 Nov 4]. Available from: https://www.ismp.org/resources/safety-enhancements-every-hospital-must-consider-wake-another-tragic-neuromuscular

32. Pharmacy Compounding Systems—Final Class II Special Controls Guidance Document for Industry and FDA [Internet]. Rockville (MD): U.S. Department of Health and Human Services, Food and Drug Administration, Centers for Devices and Radiological Health; 2001 Mar 12 [cited 2020 Jul 22]; [9 p.]. Available from: https://www.fda.gov/medical-devices/guidance-documents-medical-devices-and-radiation-emitting-products/pharmacy-compounding-systems-final-class-ii-special-controls-guidance-document-industry-and-fda

33. Pharmacy Health Information Technology Collaborative Home page [Internet]. Alexandria (VA): Pharmacy Health Information Technology Collaborative; c2011 [cited 2016 Aug 30]. Available from: http://www.pharmacyhit.org/.

34. Wilson N, Kariisa M, Seth P, Smith HIV, Davis NL. Drug and opioid-involved overdose deaths—United States, 2017–2018. MMWR Morb Mortal Wkly Rep. 2020;69:290-7.

35. Prescription drug monitoring programs (PDMPs) [Internet]. Atlanta (GA): Centers for Disease Control and Prevention, National Center for Injury Prevention and Control, Division of Unintentional Injury Prevention; 2016 Mar 23 [cited 2016 Jul 20]; [1 p.]. Available from: http://www.cdc.gov/drugoverdose/pdmp/

36. Smith R. Information technology and consumerism will transform health care worldwide. BMJ. 1997;314:1495.

37. AHIMA e-HIM Personal Health Record Work Group. The role of the personal health record in the EHR. J AHIMA. 2005;76(7):64A-64D.

38. Mesko B, Drobni Z, Benyei E, Gergely B, Gyorffy Z. Digital health is a cultural transformation of traditional healthcare. mHealth. 2017;3:38.

39. What are digital therapeutics? Industry overview [Internet]. Digital Therapeutics Alliance. [Cited 2019 Oct 7]. Available from: https://www.dtxalliance.org/dtx-solutions/

40. Bayern M. Health IoT will drive digital health market to $537B by 2025 [Internet]. TechRepublic; 2019 Feb 4 [cited 7 Oct 2019]. Available from: https://www.techrepublic.com/article/health-iot-will-drive-digital-health-market-to-537b-by-2025/

41. Moorhead A, Hazlett DE, Harrison L, Carroll JK, Irwin A, Hoving C. A new dimension of health care: systematic review of the uses, benefits, and limitations of social media for health communication. J Med Internet Res. 2013(4):e85.

42. Walker J, Pan E, Johnson D, Adler-Milstein J, Bates DW, Middleton B. The value of health care information exchange and interoperability [Internet]. Bethesda (MD): Health Affairs; 2005 Jan 19 [cited 2016 Sep 16]; [8 p.]. Available from: http://content.healthaffairs.org/content/suppl/2005/02/07/hlthaff.w5.10.DC1

43. The value of medical device interoperability: improving patient care with more than $30 billion in annual health care savings [Internet]. San Diego (CA): West Health Institute; 2013 Mar [cited 2020 Nov 4]. Available from: http://www.westhealth.org/wp-content/uploads/2015/02/The-Value-of-Medical-Device-Interoperability.pdf

44. The National Alliance for Health Information Technology report to the Office of the National Coordinator for Health Information Technology on defining key health information technology terms [Internet]. Department of Health and Human Services; 2008 Apr 28 [cited 2016 Aug 1]; [40 p.]. Available from: http://cdm16064.contentdm.oclc.org/cdm/singleitem/collection/p266901coll4/id/2086/rec/10

45. U.S. National Library of Medicine [Internet]. Bethesda (MD): U.S. National Library of Medicine; 1993 Oct 10 [updated 2013 Jul 3]. RxNorm Overview; 2005 May 5 [updated 2013 Mar 5; cited 2012 Dec 29]; [about 14 screens]. Available from: https://www.nlm.nih.gov/research/umls/rxnorm/overview.html

46. U.S. National Library of Medicine [Internet]. Bethesda (MD): U.S. National Library of Medicine; 1993 Oct 10 [updated 2013 Jul 3]. UMLS Quick Start Guide; 2011 Mar 30 [updated 2012 Jul 27; cited 2012 Dec 29]; [about 2 screens]. Available from: http://www.nlm.nih.gov/research/umls/quickstart.html

47. American Medical Association. CPT® overview and code approval [Internet]. Chicago (IL): American Medical Association; [cited 2020 Nov 4]. Available from: https://www.ama-assn.org/practice-management/cpt/cpt-overview-and-code-approval

48. Pharmacy eCare Plan Initiative [Internet]; Pharmacy HIT Collaborative; [cited 2020 Nov 4]. Available from: https://www.ecareplaninitiative.com

49. Bush GW. Executive Order 13335—incentives for the use of health information technology and establishing the position of the National Health Information Technology Coordinator [Internet]. Washington (DC): Federal Register; 2004 Apr 27 [cited 2012 Dec 29]; [3 p.]. Available from: http://www.gpo.gov/fdsys/pkg/FR-2004-04-30/pdf/04-10024.pdf

50. HealthIT.gov [Internet]. Washington (DC): The Office of the National Coordinator for Health Information Technology; Meaningful Use Definitions and Objectives; [cited 2012 Dec 29]; [about 1 screen]. Available from: http://www.healthit.gov/providers-professionals/meaningful-use-definition-objectives

51. MIPS overview [Internet]. Baltimore (MD): Centers for Medicare and Medicaid Services; [cited 2020 Nov 4]; [about 2 screens]. Available from: https://qpp.cms.gov/mips/overview

52. Office-based physician electronic health record adoption [Internet]. Washington (DC): The Office of the National Coordinator for Health Information Technology; 2017 [cited 4 Nov 2020]. Available from: https://dashboard.healthit.gov/quickstats/pages/physician-ehr-adoption-trends.php

53. Kellermann AL, Jones SS. What it will take to achieve the as-yet-unfulfilled promises of health information technology. Health Affairs. 2013;32(1):63-8.

54. Rosenberg J. Challenges in previous incentive programs will continue under MIPS for small, rural practices [Internet]. 2018 Jul 12 [cited 2020 Nov 4]. Available from: https://www.ajmc.com/view/challenges-in-previous-incentive-programs-will-continue-under-mips-for-small-rural-practices

55. Summary of selected federal laws and regulations addressing confidentiality, privacy and security [Internet]. Washington (DC): The Office of the National Coordinator for Health Information Technology; 2010 Feb 18 [cited 2012 Dec 29]; [12 p.]. Available from: http://www.healthit.gov/sites/default/files/federal_privacy_laws_table_2_26_10_final_0.pdf

56. Cost of a data breach report [Internet]. Armonk (NY): IBM Security; 2019 [cited 8 Oct 2019]. Available from: https://www.ibm.com/security/data-breach

57. 10 tips to prevent a healthcare data breach [Internet]. San Diego (CA): Managed solution; 2018 Dec 13 [cited 2019 Oct 8]. Available from: https://www.managedsolution.com/10-tips-to-prevent-a-healthcare-data-breach/

58. Summary of the HIPAA Privacy Rule [Internet]. Washington (DC): U.S. Department of Health and Human Services; 2003 May [cited 2012 Dec 29]; [25 p.]. Available from: https://www.hhs.gov/hipaa/for-professionals/privacy/laws-regulations/

59. HIPAA Administrative Simplification [Internet]. Washington (DC): U.S. Department of Health and Human Services; 2013 Mar [cited 2016 Aug 5]; [101 p.]. Available from: https://www.hhs.gov/sites/default/files/hipaa-simplification-201303.pdf

SUGGESTED READINGS

1. Fox BI, Thrower MR, Felkey BG, editors. Building core competencies in pharmacy informatics. Washington (DC): American Pharmacists Association; 2010.

2. The Office of the National Coordinator for Health Information Technology [Internet]. Washington (DC): U.S. Department of Health and Human Services; [updated 2011 Feb 18; cited 2012 Dec 12]. Available from: https://www.healthit.gov/

3. Journal of the American Medical Informatics Association. Available from: http://jamia.bmj.com/

4. ACI—Applied Clinical Informatics. Available from: https://www.thieme.com/books-main/clinical-informatics/product/4433-aci-applied-clinical-informatics

5. Friedman C. A "fundamental theorem" of biomedical informatics. JAMIA. 2009;16:169-70

6. Pew Internet and American Life Project. Available from: http://www.pewinternet.org/

7. American Society of Health-System Pharmacists. Technology-enabled practice: a vision statement by the ASHP Section of Pharmacy Informatics and Technology. Am J Health-Syst Pharm. 2009;66:1573-7.

8. Journal of Medical Internet Research. Available from: http://www.jmir.org

9. Journal of Participatory Medicine. Available from: http://www.jopm.org

10. Journal of Biomedical Informatics. Available from: http://www.sciencedirect.com/science/journal/15320464

11. Dumitru D, editor. The pharmacy informatics primer. Bethesda (MD): American Society of Health-System Pharmacists; 2009.

12. Siska MH, Tribble DA. Opportunities and challenges related to technology in supporting optimal pharmacy practice models in hospitals and health systems. Am J Health-Syst Pharm. 2011;68(12):1116-26.

Pharmacy Informatics II: Big Data

Marc A. Willner • Eric D. Vogan

Learning Objectives

● *After completing this chapter, the reader will be able to:*

- Describe how relational databases collate and store data.
- Explain how Structured Query Language (SQL) is used to interact with relational databases to select and filter data.
- Illustrate data analysis techniques and methodology used to evaluate data sets.
- Define the differences between "little data" and "big data."
- Define the "5 V's" of big data.
- Explain the concept of a data warehouse and its relation to reporting and analytics.
- Explain the differences between and limitations of predictive analytics and machine learning.
- Describe basic concepts of different machine learning methodologies.
- Describe examples of machine learning used in health care, as well as potential future directions for machine learning in health care.

Key Concepts

❶ A relational database is a type of database that collects and stores data in structured formats called tables that are related to one another.

❷ SQL is a comprehensive, text-based language that allows the user to define and manipulate data in relational databases using four primary operators: projection, filter, join, and aggregate.

❸ Data analysis is methodically taking large amounts of raw data from databases and aggregating it in such a way to reveal hidden, meaningful information.

❹ "Little data" stems from patients and end users, whereas "big data" is an aggregation of data from all sources of little data.

❺ Big data is characterized by the "5 V's": volume, velocity, variety, veracity, and value.

❻ Analysis of big data typically requires use of data warehouses for reporting and analytical methods.

❼ The ultimate goal of using big data is to take raw data from sources, such as electronic medical records, and translate that to make meaningful decisions or provide insight or intelligence to change the scope of patient care for current and future patients.

❽ Machine learning differs from a predictive analytics model, in that machine learning will change its decision dynamically in a programmatic fashion utilizing different statistical methodologies, such as logistic regression, and is considered to be a new frontier in the way that patient care will unfold within the next few decades.

Introduction

The advent and increasing adoption of the electronic health records (EHR) has led to an explosion in the quantity of patient data. With this, there is an increased need for subject matter experts trained in the use, extraction, and analysis of data generated from an EHR. These experts can assist clinicians in providing information to make data-based decisions. Along with the need of proper data extraction and analysis, the amount of data available to lead to changes in the health care landscape is unprecedented, yet questions remain about how to use this data in a reliable way to conduct research and make clinical and operational decisions. This chapter will cover various aspects of data reporting, data management, **data mining** artificial intelligence, and the ultimate end-use of this vast amount of data pertaining to patients.

Reporting and Analytics

The breadth of electronic applications and software utilized to organize and manage the different processes and procedures across today's health care systems provide ample opportunity for engagement with data generated by those systems. They are increasingly used to document and store patient data, including demographic information, clinical notes, prescriptions, lab results, allergies, vaccination status, risk levels, surgical cases, and so on. When knowledge and known information are used in conjunction with data, previously unknown information can be generated to support research efforts and guide decision-makers at all levels of health care organizations. Once clinicians and leadership engage with analysts, their respective skill sets create the potential to intelligently use data through a partnership that removes ambiguity and promotes discovery. Timely *ad hoc* reporting, longitudinal retrospective analyses, predictive modeling, and other methods of analysis can attain meaningful results when organizations employ the tools and practices necessary to utilize data effectively.

RELATIONAL DATABASES

Data generated in health care system applications that are deposited and stored in a database can be queried and retrieved for analysis. This means that the clicks and entries performed in the EHR get translated into data stored neatly and orderly in a database. To get data from the database one must perform a **query** defined as "a request for data or information from a database."[1] The **relational database** model is the most widely used database type and is the model used for the top three database management systems in the world: Oracle, MySQL, and Microsoft SQL Server, listed according to their popularity.[2] It is also considered to be the most efficient and adaptable type of database and thus is widely used among industry leaders.[3] Other database types include object-oriented databases, distributed databases, and NoSQL or nonrelational databases.[3]

❶*A relational database is a type of database that collects and stores data in structured formats called tables that are related to one another.*[3] Relational databases store data in rows, with each row containing a unique identifier known as the **primary key** further referred to as the "key." The primary key allows the user to exclusively refer to an entire record of data stored within the individual rows. The rows are then stored in separate tables depending on the data's attributes. Data with the same attributes, or data of the same type (e.g., medication orders), are stored in the same table.[3] Large-scale EHRs may store upwards of 18,000 tables of data.[4] **Tables** organize the data they contain by associating the data for each record with its primary key. Think of the table as a set of rows and columns, much the same as a spreadsheet would look. The rows each contain a unique record defined by its key and the columns storing different pieces of data of the same type for each record. Made up of many tables, relational databases provide access to data stored in different locations across the database by allowing for relationships between tables using the key or a combination of keys. In the example below, relationships are built between the tables which allow the analyst to combine related data from one or more tables by associating the key from one table to the next. The "relationships" between the tables are known as joins and are represented by lines that create a connection using

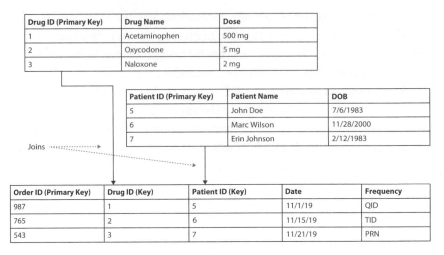

Figure 29–1. Relational database structure.

common keys. See Figure 29-1 for an example relational database structure. Here the bottom table containing Order ID also houses the drug and patient IDs. In order to include relevant information in a report based on the medication orders, joins are created between the tables on the respective keys to allow the drug name, dose, patient name, and date of birth (DOB) to be incorporated in an output, with the different pieces of information being obtained from separate tables.

DATA TYPES

When conducting a research study or using data to gain insight into everyday operational challenges, it is important to understand the different data types and characteristics associated with data, which will be described below. These groups are also described in Chapter 6, although there is further information in this chapter about how they apply to computer data.

    Categorical data, also known as nominal data, are data that can be parsed and separated into discrete categories and further divided into two (**dichotomous**—two categories) or multiple groups (polytomous—more than two categories). **Dichotomous data** fall into only one of two categories and are thus considered binary.[5–9] Many clinical measurements or statuses can be documented using a dichotomous descriptor. For example, patient mortality, allergic reaction, or 30-day readmission status are dichotomous data. **Polytomous data** is similar except that it is nonbinary categorical data, meaning the data is associated with more than two groupings.[5–7,10,11] Examples of these are eye color (blue/green/brown/hazel), race (White, Black, Hispanic/Latino, American Indian/Alaska Native, Asian/Pacific Islander, Multiracial/Multicultural, Native Hawaiian/Pacific Islander), and blood type (A, B, O, or AB).[5-8,10,11]

Discrete data are another form of categorical data that is not mutually exclusive of the other two forms: dichotomous and polytomous. Discrete categorical data are data that neatly fit into a group or interval, in that they can only take on certain specific values.[5] Both patient mortality and admissions in a month are examples of discrete categorical data as they have distinct and definite values. In this example, patient mortality can only be classified as "Alive" or "Deceased," and admissions in a particular month is one, singular number.

Ordinal data are data that are logically oriented and ordered by rank, typically a numerical rank. The primary characteristic of ordinal data is that even though they are ranked in order by numbers, the difference between ranks cannot be considered to be equal. Take, for example, a pain scale that measures pain from 0 (none) to 10 (unbearable). It cannot be assumed that a patient who measures their pain at 5 is in 50% less pain than a patient who considers their pain to be 10.[5-7,10,11]

Continuous data are measured on a numeric range similar to ordinal data but differ in two distinct ways. First, continuous data can occupy any number on a range and be divided into smaller and smaller increments based on the precision of the measurement instrument. Second, the intervals between the measurements equate to the differences in the property being measured.[5-8,12] For example, a 0.1 difference between 2.5 and 2.6 international normalized ratio (INR) values is the same as another 0.1 difference between 3.1 and 3.2 INR value.

STRUCTURED QUERY LANGUAGE

The American National Standards Institute (ANSI) identifies **Structured Query Language** (SQL) as the standard language for communicating with relational databases.[13] To begin, a database manager writes the code to obtain data from the database. The code that is prepared is known as an SQL statement. This allows the user to extract and obtain related pieces of information from the database by listing the data points desired, the location(s) of said data, describing the relationships between the data (joins), and any pertinent criteria to "filter" the data and attain the desired results. The result table is the final product of processing an SQL statement and contains the output of the tables specified in the standardized code.[14] ❷ *SQL is a comprehensive, text-based language that allows the user to define and manipulate data in relational databases using four primary operators: projection, join, filter, and aggregate,*[15] which will be explained below.

Projection

Often referred to as the **SELECT** statement or clause, this makes up the initial portion of an SQL statement and involves listing the items to include in the output. Rather than including all items from all tables in the query, you can specify only the items you wish to see. For example, a table comprised of all the patient's demographics likely contains more information than is needed for a medication orders report. So instead of reporting out items, such as zip code, marital status, and email address, the SELECT statement allows the user to define only the desired columns to include in the data set, such as patient name, medical record number, and date of birth.

Join

Joins make up the second section of an SQL statement and are used to combine records from multiple tables. A join is performed by connecting tables through a common key shared between them. For example, a table containing patient information can be joined to a table with medication orders information using the patient's ID as we would expect the patient ID to be a part of the patient record as well as the record of the medication order. These are necessary when there is a need to bring in data from more than one table.

Filter

In this section, the user must incorporate the**WHERE** clause to identify the records to include (or exclude) to filter the data so that only the desired output results. For example, filtering data set can mean specifying a date range, excluding patients who are less than 18 years of age, or only looking for patients who have been admitted for a cardiac surgery procedure. This allows the user to tailor the results to meet their specific needs.

Aggregate

Aggregating data is the process of collecting information and compiling and summarizing it for the purpose of reporting or analysis. Aggregating your data set may not be necessary if the goal is only to obtain raw, detailed data. However, applying statistical inferences to the data set can provide the user with valuable information right at their fingertips. For example, using an aggregation-based function such as SUM or COUNT could allow the user to get the total number of prescriptions dispensed each month over the course of a year. These functions can be especially useful and can transform the data from a raw, untouched format to a simplified, aggregated format.

In conclusion, intelligent SQL coding in combination with other tools can provide the end user with automated reports on a scheduled, periodic basis. Reports such as these can allow management, leadership, or practitioners to track trends and make predictions about important operational changes or clinical challenges. Additionally, SQL provides organizations with the ability to carry out retrospective analyses. For example, a 2017 study utilized SQL to retrospectively analyze inpatient pharmacist compliance with standardized dosing guidelines when verifying systemic antibiotic orders. This analysis allowed leadership to provide the education and resources needed to make a statistically significant improvement in guideline compliance.[16]

DATA ANALYSIS

❸ *Data analysis is methodically taking large amounts of raw data from databases and aggregating it in such a way to reveal hidden, meaningful information.*[17] Essentially, data analysis involves methodically examining and aggregating data to reveal hidden information in order to gain insight to make informed clinical or business decisions. Statistical approaches involve employing standardized methods to summarize data in a logical and meaningful way although certain levels of in-depth analysis may not have a clear, predetermined roadmap and call for critical thinking to achieve meaningful results.[5]

Statistics

An in-depth look at the statistics pertaining to statistical methodology is covered in Chapter 6; however, this chapter will provide a reminder of various types of statistics to better reinforce statistical analysis methodologies.

Descriptive statistics are used to calculate and describe data in an ordered and efficient way. They are generally reported numerically using graphs, tables, and figures, and are regarded as able to answer the five basic W questions: who, what, why, when, and where.[6,18-20] Common examples of descriptive statistics are mean, median, and mode, along with standard deviation.[18]

Inferential statistics involve using data to make an estimate (inference) about the corresponding cohort within the data based on randomized cause and effect outcomes.[5] Inferential statistics are often used in research studies in an attempt to apply "statistical significance" to a hypothesis. This often means, for example, that researchers are looking for p values, or the calculated probability, below a threshold to either prove or disprove the study's hypothesis.

Methodology

When analyzing data, establishing a clear goal helps to clarify the purpose and create a guide for obtaining accurate data and how to proceed with the analysis. As the clinical expert who is directly involved with the workflow of patient care, the pharmacist is an integral part of this process. It is the clinician that provides the guideposts for data generation and develops the protocol for research or analysis. For example, a practitioner wants to perform a longitudinal retrospective analysis to assess the 30-day readmission rate of patients who have received either drug A or drug B for a particular diagnosis while admitted to the hospital intensive care unit (ICU) in the past year. Working directly with an informatics expert allows them to construct a clear and precise reporting plan.

In this case, the initial step for the reporting analyst would be to query the inpatient medication administration record for patients who received either of these drugs in the past year. The second step would be to verify that these medications were administered while the patient was in the ICU. Since it can be assumed that the patient location at the time of administration is stored in the medication administration record, the first two steps can in effect be performed at the same time. This will yield an initial subset of patients who will then be queried to verify that they had said diagnosis at the time they received the medication. For simplicity, assume this phase decreases the "*N*" from 1000 patients (received drug A or drug B in the ICU in the past year) to 750 patients (received drug A or drug B in the ICU in the past year *and* had a pertinent diagnosis). There are now 750 patients who need to be assessed for an unplanned admission that occurred within 30 days of the discharge date of their index encounter. At this point each of the patients will likely have a different discharge date leading to potentially having 750 different 30-day date ranges that need to be queried for an unplanned admission but creatively using SQL code will prevent the need to run 750 separate queries. After this is achieved, patients with an unplanned admission are flagged appropriately and the 30-day readmission rate can be calculated.

Case Study 29-1

You are a pharmacist that would like to conduct research on the effects of a vancomycin dosing service and need to enter in a report request with your Pharmacy Informatics team. Within your hospital's EHR, a vancomycin dosing consult order is placed by a licensed independent practitioner. This order remains within the patient's medical record throughout the admission. For the vancomycin dosing service, pharmacists can adjust vancomycin dosing based on patient weight, trough, and renal function. Additionally, pharmacists can order vancomycin trough levels, as well as adjust due times within the EHR. This service is available for both adult and pediatric patient populations, but you are only going to evaluate the adult patients. After a pharmacist adjusts a vancomycin dose or orders a vancomycin trough level, they are required to enter in a note documenting their actions for transparency to other health care professionals.

- *What criteria would you provide to a reporting analyst to construct a report? Which criteria would you want to include, and which criteria would you want to exclude?*
- *What data would you request to be extracted from the report?*

Big Data

The definition of **big data** has taken many forms, but a few trends outline big data as data sets so large, complex, multisource, and multifaceted that conventional software and storage solutions are unable to analyze and create meaningful visualizations of the data, in addition to a specialized skill set being necessary to gather, run, and perform data analyses.[21,22] Big data started to come to a forefront in health care with the advent of EHRs and constant data generation from day-to-day patient care. For example, a single data set of orders data from a large academic medical center's EHR can easily surpass the 1,048,576 row limit of Microsoft® Excel®.[23]

LITTLE DATA VERSUS BIG DATA

❹ *"Little data" stems from patients and end users, whereas "big data" is an aggregation of data from all sources of little data.* An example of little data is the collection of data points from a specific patient's medical record. An example of big data would be the aggregation of all data from various integrated systems sued within a hospital, such as the EHR, radiology systems, laboratory systems, and pharmacy systems. As technology changes, various sources of data are shared between systems, and patients generate data, the amount of little data feeding into big data grows. For example, with the advent of wearable technologies, information gathered on a device such as a fitness tracker may very well feed into an EHR. Patients now can log into a patient-facing application and view the information gathered by an external source such as a fitness tracker. As the sources of data and the expansion of EHR use increases, big data has developed a number of characteristics differentiating it from what we would historically consider little data, known below as the "Five V's".

THE FIVE V'S

❺ *Big data is characterized by the "5 V's": volume, velocity, variety, veracity, and value.* Below we will go more in-depth with these definitions, as they each warrant their own explanation to grasp the scope of big data in health care.[21,24]

Volume

One of the defining characteristics of big data is volume, as indicated in the aforementioned definition of big data, the sheer scope of data that is already available is reaching petabyte (10^{15} bytes) and at times exabyte (10^{18} bytes) size.[21,24] This is far beyond the storage capabilities of conventional personal storage, requiring sophisticated storage solutions for systems attempting to analyze this data. It is projected that data generated by the United States health care system will reach zettabyte (10^{21} bytes) and yottabyte (10^{24} bytes) size in the near future; though from a practicality standpoint, it is unlikely that this amount of data would need to be generated for the purposes of an individual institution.[21] Even the most complicated report pulls from a single EHR would be unlikely to exceed a few hundred gigabytes. With the ever-expanding amount of data generated, gone are the traditional methods of extraction of data on a single personal workstation and exporting to spreadsheet applications. The extraction and analysis of this amount of data requires employment of specific infrastructure, such as **data warehouses** that are designed specifically for analytical purposes. To better understand this, we must differentiate between the concept of a database and data warehouse. ❻ *Analysis of big data typically requires use of data warehouses for reporting and analytical methods.* A database can be thought of as a site's EHR, which stores all data from one application. When adding data from this database, which would involve entering any data on a patient record, such as writing notes, entering orders, etc., the methodology of updating this data is through an **online transaction processing** (OLTP) system. An OLTP is used to add, edit, or delete data from the database, and is not routinely used for analytical purposes, as speed and performance are of the utmost importance to maintain expeditious patient care. Alongside the EHR the health system likely has other systems with disparate databases, which in turn multiply the amount of data available for analysis. For example, an institution may have separate databases for radiology, lab, and billing information, apart from the main EHR. With disparate systems, all need to interface and communicate with each other. In addition to this, as EHR vendors work toward the sharing of electronic medical data between health systems, the numbers of databases from which to pull data is continually increasing. The concept of a data warehouse is that of an application that receives data from various sources, stores said data, and allows analysts to extract data more efficiently than if they were to do so from the individual data sources. Data warehouses are typically segregated from the databases used for patient care, as data will flow into the data warehouse on a schedule, but not out of the data warehouse back to the EHR. Since the purpose of the data warehouse is simply storage, it is not necessary for the data to flow back to the EHR. This allows for better performance when queries are made from data warehouses.

Velocity

Velocity can be defined as the rate in which data is added to a database, in this case, an EHR or its ancillary systems. As data is constantly flowing into an EHR's database, or ancillary systems are generating image, instrumentation, and device data, the increase in data generated within the system is increasing at a rapid pace. Though there is no specific threshold for when the rate of increase in data would constitute as "big data," data generated at high rates leads to interesting challenges, both within the aspect of day-to-day decision-making, and the potential for research derived from EHR data.[25] Traditionally, new scientific evidence has been generated from standardized processes for research, with a prospective randomized controlled trial as research methodology with the highest strength. With data growing at such speeds, the future may hold that extraction and analysis of big data becomes a standard method of generating new scientific findings, rather than randomized controlled trials.[25] As we will cover in the "Artificial Intelligence" section within this chapter, the goal of using this data is ultimately for decision-making, and as the rate of data generation grows, we may find that large data analyses may drive medical practices.

Variety

Variety can be defined as the differences in sources of data from an EHR and its ancillary systems. The traditional source of patient data is that of the EHR; however, as EHRs become more sophisticated, other ancillary systems communicate with the EHR, and more sources of "little data" interoperate with the EHR, there is an increase in the types of data that can be stored for extraction and analysis. Though there is no distinct quantitative threshold between data variety crossing from little data to big data, the difference comes down to the number of different sources of data that a centralized EHR gathers. For example, as EHRs are now able to provide radiological images, this information is available for analysis along with final reads from a radiologist. In just a few year's past, health care providers would need to track down a patient's X-rays, or patients would need to be provided with a CD containing X-ray images to take to other health care providers, but now, EHRs are able to store and provide that information from different health care sites.

Veracity

This fourth "V" of big data can also be defined as the assurance of data accuracy. As data sets grow, so does the chance of issues with data integrity. This issue of integrity may occur due to the manual nature of data entry within the EHR, for example, miscoding or failure to update the status of diagnoses on a patient's problem list. The accuracy of much of the data contained within an EHR is at the mercy of the person entering the data. Due to the speed and amount in which data is generated, therein lies an issue with the ability to ensure that data is clean and precise.[21]

Value

The last "V" of big data, value, indicates the worth of the data in decision-making.[26] If the data provided does not lead to meaningful decisions, or does not provide enough information to lead to any decision, then the value of the data is marginal, or the data was not analyzed properly. Value is subjective to the recipient, wherein the true utility of the data may differ from person to person. This does not mean that the data presented may lead to an undesired outcome. This is why analyses occur in the first place. Additionally, a recipient of a finalized data analysis may have some bias as to what an expected outcome might be based on preconceived notions or experiences. If the data provides information that is contrary to these beliefs/experiences, then they may value the data less than someone who received good news from their data.

TRANSLATING DATA INTO INTELLIGENCE

❼ *The ultimate goal of using big data is to take raw data from sources, such as electronic medical records, and translate that to make meaningful decisions or provide insight or intelligence to change the scope of patient care for current and future patients.* A way to visualize the transformation of data into intelligence is known as the "DIKI pyramid" (Figure 29-2), which illustrates that the amount of raw data is meaningless unless it is translated into data that can lead to decision-making. At the bottom of the pyramid, we have the raw data, which is provided in the most copious amount. As the data is refined and transformed into information, then knowledge, intelligence, its specificity and complexity increases as well, but the amount generated is the least.

To put this concept into a clinical example, consider the situation if a clinician wants to determine if timing of first antimicrobial administration when presenting to the emergency department in patients with suspected sepsis leads to a change in readmission risk. Here, data points, such as admission time, antimicrobial administration time, and diagnosis codes on the patient's medical record, would be extracted from the EHR. The

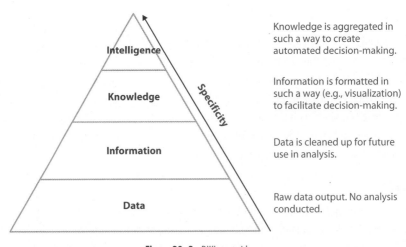

Figure 29–2. DIKI pyramid.

raw data contained within the medical record constitutes the "Data" aspect of the DIKI pyramid. Once those raw data points are extracted from the EHR and imported onto a spreadsheet software, this would constitute the "Information" aspect of the DIKI pyramid. Taking the information from a spreadsheet, performing analysis, and providing visualizations such as tables and/or graphs would constitute the "Knowledge" aspect of the DIKI pyramid. Finally, the process of taking the data, extracting additional points, and running the information through software which is able to predict which patient-specific variables would lead to an increased risk of readmission would constitute the "Intelligence" aspect of the DIKI pyramid.

Case Study 29–2

You receive your data pertaining to your study (see the preceding case study in this chapter) from the pharmacy informatics team and review your spreadsheet. It contains thousands of lines of data, which is not very meaningful at face value. You need to take this data, analyze it, and create outcomes from the data for your study.

• *Using the concepts contained within the DIKI pyramid, describe how the data is formatted in current state and what steps you might need to take to make the data more meaningful.*

USING BIG DATA

The use of big data within health care has demonstrated significant benefits.[27] When analyzing and applying big data to specific patient populations, it is recommended that clinical subject matter experts, technical experts, and statisticians be engaged through the process of gathering, analyzing, and making decisions from the big data sources.[27] The engagement of these experts in the process of design, extraction, and analysis early in the development process can expedite accurate reporting and analysis, as well as preventing rework.

Examples within Health Care

Studies have shown that leveraging big data may be useful in decision-making for common medication-related issues, both from a patient-level and from a health system-level in certain complex clinical scenarios, such as opioid and diabetes management.[27]

Another target of big data is within the growing field of pharmacogenomics. A patient's genome is yet another source of information that can contribute to the vast array of data that can ultimately drive patient care, as it contains a vast amount of data that can be leveraged to make therapeutic decisions mitigating risk for adverse drug reactions or preventing lack of medication efficacy. There are a number of challenges that lay ahead to utilize a patient's genome, mainly stemming from the ability to take raw genetic information, store it within an EHR, and then translate that raw genetic information into meaningful genotypes and phenotypes. At the current rate of patients having their genome sequenced, it is projected that 2–40 exabytes of storage will be generated per year.[28] To put this into perspective, this is higher than the storage capacity of about a billion home computers. Pharmacogenomics organizations such as the Clinical Pharmacogenomics Implementation Consortium (https://cpicpgx.org/) are leading the way to create meaningful drug therapy recommendations based on patient data, as well as educate health care providers on the role of pharmacogenomics. Data supports that utilization of genomic big data has led to positive patient outcomes, such as decreased adverse events or increased medication efficacy, particularly with individual gene-drug pairs.[29–32] In other words, raw genetic data (the "big data" in this situation) will eventually be able to be translated into meaningful information that may lead to a customized medication profile for individual patients. However, implementation of these gene-drug pairs are on a case-by-case basis, and challenges still lie ahead of development of a comprehensive automated genomic decision support system using raw genomic data.[33] Regardless, genomic data has one advantage that other conventional laboratory results do not have: permanence. A patient's genomic markers will not change over time as would laboratory data, such as potassium, creatinine, or hemoglobin A1c. Even if genomic data continues to be gathered in the same piecemeal fashion, through individual tests versus a comprehensive genomic profile, the data will remain for the rest of the patient's life.

Artificial Intelligence

Artificial intelligence leverages big data to make decisions and meaningful information, and is the peak and most specific aspect of the DIKI pyramid. As data analysis and models generate intelligent, meaningful decisions about patients, many forms of artificial intelligence are taking shape. Below is a description of a few forms of artificial intelligence and their applicability to health care.

PREDICTIVE ANALYTICS

One of the most commonly leveraged forms of artificial intelligence in the health care space is that of predictive analytics, which uses big data to create intelligence from historical patient data, conducting statistical analysis, such as logistic regression models against many (upwards of a few hundred) patient-specific variables, and then removing variables that do not lead to a significant change in a model's predictability. For predictive analytics and artificial intelligence models, a common statistical marker of predictability is the **C-statistic**, also known as the concordance statistic. The C-statistic predicts the risk of a patient having an event (e.g., risk of 30-day readmission) compared to a patient that does not have the event. The range of a C-statistic is between 0.5 and 1, where 0.5 indicates a very poor predictive model (i.e., no better than a coin flip), and 1 indicates perfect predictability. Generally, a predictive model with a C-statistic around 0.75 is considered a high-performance model. As a statistician develops the predictive model and adds different variables that would be considered significant to changing the predictability of the model, it may get to a point where additional significant variables lead to a marginal and impractical change in the model's C-statistic. For example, if a predictive analytics model with 20 different patient-specific variables has a C-statistic of 0.7524562, and the same model has the 20 variables, as well as 80 additional variables, for a total of 100 variables, and the C-statistic is 0.7524573, it is more practical to conclude that the predictive model has 20 significant variables versus 100.

As big data continues to grow in scope and size, a fundamental issue lies with a static predictive analytics model: once the model is developed it is already outdated. This is because patient data changes over time. Upon the initial development of the predictive model, a statistician may use as much data as possible, but the farther back the data goes, and the longer period elapses between the endpoint of the data and the current time, the higher the risk of the predictive model losing its validity.

Many examples of predictive analytics models have been developed and validated within medical literature.[34-42] One of the most commonly cited and analyzed predictive analytics model is the LACE index, which provides a patient's risk of 30-day readmission based on the following variables[34,43]:

- Length of stay
- Acuity (e.g., whether the patient was admitted through the emergency department [ED])
- Comorbidities
- ED visits within the previous 6 months

If resources and capacity are limited to address all patients' transitions of care needs, this model can be used to prioritize the patients at highest risk for readmission.

Another number of predictive analytics scores have been demonstrated in the literature, attempting to predict other risks, such as stroke, bleeding from oral anticoagulants, heart failure exacerbation, QT prolongation, and hyperkalemia.[35,36,38,40-42] Though these models have been developed and validated, literature indicating a successful operationalization into clinical workflows is limited.

MACHINE LEARNING

❽ *Machine learning differs from a predictive analytics model, in that machine learning will change its decision dynamically in a programmatic fashion utilizing different statistical methodologies, such as logistic regression, and is considered to be a new frontier in the way that patient care will unfold within the next few decades.*[44–47] For example, a predictive analytics model for readmission risk using logistic regression may have analyzed a number of variables that lead to a significant risk of readmission, with each variable having a specific weight in which it contributes to readmission risk. As a result, these variable weights are static, as the variables that lead to a significant risk of readmission have been defined beforehand and are unchanged unless the entire predictive model is rebuilt. With a machine learning model, simply put, the variables and their associated contribution to a decision's weighting will dynamically change over time. As machine learning comes to the forefront, other less familiar statistical methods may begin to surface in literature and methodologies of machine learning model development, such as **decision trees**, **random forests**, **neural networks**, and **deep learning**.[44,48] These concepts will be covered in more detail later.

The development of a machine learning model typically undergoes two steps: first, a training data set is used to apply selected statistical methodologies; and second, a validation data set is run independently using the same methods to look for measures of validity from the training data set.[44] These steps are typically performed by a data scientist or statistician. There is typically a limited role in this validation step for clinicians. In addition to this, there are technical and computational hardware and software considerations, which may include[44]:

- Computer equipment with the ability to perform the required high-level statistical analysis needed
- Software with the ability to deploy machine learning models
- A programmer and/or statistician knowledgeable in regard to programming and running a machine learning algorithm

Machine learning comes in many forms and various levels of complexity. The use of machine learning models is complex and requires a level of expertise that is beyond the scope of the practice of pharmacy. However, as machine learning models become more prevalent, pharmacists may benefit from a high-level knowledge of some machine learning methodologies. Below are some basic concepts of select machine learning algorithms.

Decision Trees and Random Forest

Decision trees are simple graphical representations of a number of variables and the selected outcomes of such combinations of decisions. These are used to map out various combinations, different variable's outcomes, and a simpler machine learning methodology. Within the decision tree, various "nodes" represent stages of a decision problem,

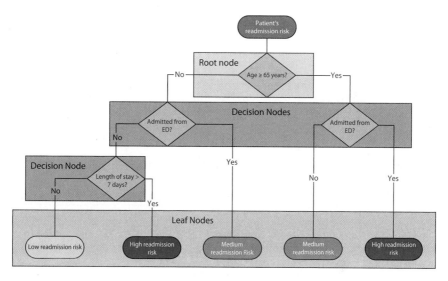

Figure 29–3. Decision tree.

with all various outcomes illustrated on termini.[49] Python is a common programming language that utilizes decision trees for machine learning algorithms, where the "root node" represents the start of a decision, "interior nodes" represent various decision points along the decision tree's path, and the "leaf node" represents the end point of the decision tree.

An example of the use of decision trees is outlined in Figure 29-3, which pertains to readmission risk. In this example, a patient is admitted to the ED, and certain variables are put through the decision tree. In this case, the variables serve as the "nodes." The decision tree model runs through all the select variables, and the patient's risk for readmission is classified based on how they meet the criteria specified in each node.

Random forest algorithm uses a network of decision trees and a strength-in-numbers approach, undergoing various permutations of outcomes known as an **ensemble**.[50] The prediction from the model is based on the most common outcome of the various decision trees, performed by a majority vote by the computational model, after all potential outcomes are evaluated.[50] See Figure 29-4 for an example of the random forest approach; however, the various decision tree formats contained within the random forest network serve as illustrative purposes only. An example of this can be applied to the readmission risk example above, where a patient's readmission risk is the final outcome to be determined. Here, the various decision trees may constitute different types and numbers of variables, and after all decision trees are analyzed, the random forest model will perform majority voting, and the most common outcome is determined to be the model's decision. The major difference between a decision tree model and a random forest model is that random forest employs what is known as a **"black box"** approach to machine learning,

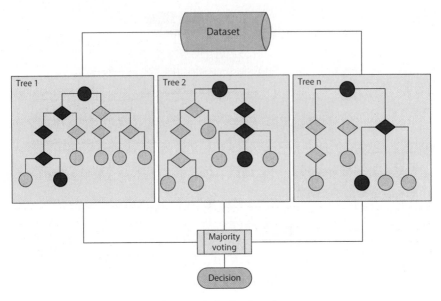

Figure 29–4. Random forest plot.

wherein the inputs to the machine learning model are known, but the decision point and permutations used to arrive at an outcome are unknown. Utilizing this approach is challenging in the health care environment, as transparency is paramount to making a decision that could alter a patient's well-being. Clinicians may find themselves hesitant to trust or employ these models without knowing how a program arrived at a decision.

Neural Networks

Neural networks take the opposite shape of decision trees. Decision trees take the start of one point and then arrive at multiple potential outcomes.[51] In contrast, neural networks take an approach where in multiple inputs are added to the data model, various weights and biases for each variable are assigned, and then fewer outputs are made.[51] Neural networks are useful when attempting to create a machine learning model wherein a program is able to identify an outcome. This is done by inputting data into a training set of data that contains the outcome that the model is looking for, and the neural networks identify common characteristics of the outcome. For example, if you wanted a neural network to be able to identify a patient with sepsis, the training of this model would involve inputting the medical records of patients with diagnosed sepsis. After a while, the model will be able to pick up on common characteristics of a sepsis and identify that a patient may be septic upon admission. As with the random forest models, neural networks also employ a black box approach with how the program arrives at an outcome, which again is an inherent issue when making health care-related decisions. One major difference between random forest and neural network is that random forest models may only employ text-based data, whereas neural networks may leverage images and audio data.

Deep Learning

Deep learning is the next frontier of machine learning capabilities, wherein the data model will constantly re-run itself through thousands of permutations, which will become more and more refined based on the different scenarios presented to it, eventually arriving at the most optimal outcome.[51] Examples of deep learning have already been utilized in the health care space, such as applications for the use of natural language processing and reading radiograms.[52,53] Since deep learning is one of the newest methods of machine learning, it is currently unclear which clinical applications can utilize a deep learning algorithm. As deep learning models lack transparency as to how certain clinical decisions are made, clinicians must also develop trust in these models.

Tying this concept to the practice of drug information, the increasing use of artificial intelligence may lead to advanced literature searching capabilities or generalized question-asking in a database, where the use of artificial intelligence is able to provide answers to questions rather than search results. Machine learning models that scan medical literature may also lead to dynamic drug monographs that are able to update information in real time as studies are published, rather than requiring manual literature reviews and monograph compositions.

Will Machine Learning Make Health Care Professionals Obsolete?

With the advent of this new machine learning technology, there are large unknowns as to what this may lead to in health care. One such question that is posed is whether machine learning models make certain tasks and types of health care professionals obsolete? For example, can a machine-learning platform become intelligent enough to perform a diagnosis, or conduct a prospective medication review? An analysis was conducted in the United Kingdom in 2013, reviewing the probability of computerization of 702 occupations.[54] The analysis looked at factors that would lend an increase or decrease in probability of an occupation becoming computerized, such as repetitive tasks, amount of labor needed, and levels of cognition, background education, and creativity.[54] Fortunately, of the 702 occupations analyzed, physicians and surgeons, registered nurses, and pharmacists ranked 15th, 46th, and 54th in the probability of the occupation not becoming computerized, respectively, with probabilities of computerization of 0.0042, 0.009, and 0.012, respectively.[54]

The practice of pharmacy is no stranger to the incorporation of technology into its workflows, with the incorporation of automated devices into traditional dispensing practices in hospitals (e.g., automated dispensing cabinets, dispensing robots, and carousels, IV preparation software and robotics). While dispensing practices have largely seen automation drive workflows, the practice of clinical pharmacy has largely been untouched outside of the use of clinical decision support methodologies in the EHR (e.g., active alerts). Will artificial intelligence replace clinical pharmacy practice, such as with active alerting or autonomous order verification? It is unlikely that artificial intelligence will completely replace clinical pharmacy; there will likely be opportunities for enhancements to clinical workflows, such as proactive patient monitoring, predictive scores, and smarter, patient-specific alerts. Given that artificial intelligence models work in a "black box" and clinicians will likely not be able to validate the steps that an artificial intelligence model arrives at a recommendation for a specific patient, it is more likely that artificial intelligence will provide recommendations for decisions, rather than absolute decisions, such as automatic diagnoses or decisions on medication therapy.

If trust in big data and machine learning models is eventually gained, there may be a significant benefit to clinical and operational aspects of pharmacy practice. The extent to which big data may be applied may depend on the ability to report and extract data from a local EHR. As analytical models are applied, we may see increased or smarter features within the EHR, such as the aforementioned medication-related alerts, or enhanced monitoring tools to provide pharmacists with optimized therapy recommendations. From an operational side, predictive models may be used to predict inventory or cost trends, or even provide real-time feedback to enhance pharmacy staffing levels.

When it comes to the application of big data and machine learning to the practice of drug information, this currently is largely unknown, and may vary based on the size, type, and resources of specific institutions. Hospital-based drug information specialists may find themselves leveraging large amounts of data from within the EHR to review prescribing trends for formulary decisions and cost-savings opportunities. Drug information staff based out of academia or private industry may find that big data and machine learning models will eventually be able to quickly scan and analyze literature, leading to enhanced tertiary drug information databases. An added benefit to this concept would be the autonomous updating of drug databases based on new literature, unlike current practice which requires manual review and updating.

Conclusion

As sources and amounts of data continue to grow and become more sophisticated, it is important to grasp methodologies for data extraction and analysis. This large-scale data generation has led to the concept of big data, which involves large-scale amounts of data that can be leveraged for analysis. Predictive analytics and machine learning are two methods to leverage big data to make meaningful clinical decisions. Though there is uncertainty in the health care field regarding the future use of these tools, it is unlikely they will replace human clinicians.

Self-Assessment Questions

1. Data loaded into a relational database is stored in the following format:
   a. Spreadsheets and cells
   b. Folders and files
   c. Tables and rows
   d. Databases and tables
   e. Queries and folders

2. These are the unique identifiers in relational databases that help organize data:
   a. Locks
   b. IDs
   c. Keys
   d. Headers
   e. None of the above

3. The "relationships" formed between tables in relational databases are known as:
   a. Joins
   b. Extractions
   c. Links
   d. Lines
   e. Associations

4. The projection operator of an SQL query:
   a. Determines search criteria of a report
   b. Reformats the data for analysis
   c. Defines the tables to include in the output
   d. Both a and c
   e. All of the above

5. The WHERE clause of an SQL query determines:
   a. Data to include in the return
   b. Data to exclude in the return
   c. Where to find the data in the database
   d. Both a and b
   e. None of the above

6. An inner join in an SQL query performs the following operation:
   a. Will pull all data from both tables
   b. Will pull data from both tables only when there is a match

   c. Will pull all data from the left table and only data from the right table where there is a match

   d. Will pull all data from the right table and only data from the left table where there is a match

   e. Will pull data from both tables regardless of whether there is a match or not

7. Which of the following is an example of ordinal data?
   a. Eye color
   b. Blood type
   c. Serum creatinine
   d. Milliliters of medication administered
   e. Educational level

8. Calculating a patient's average INR over the course of treatment would involve using:
   a. Descriptive statistics with continuous data
   b. Descriptive statistics with discrete data
   c. Inferential statistics with continuous data
   d. Descriptive statistics with ordinal data
   e. Inferential statistics with dichotomous data

9. Which of the following machine learning methods involves not knowing the process of how the data input is analyzed?
   a. Black box
   b. White cube
   c. Black cube
   d. White box
   e. Grey box

10. Which of the following machine learning methods involves taking many inputs, evaluating weight and bias, and then generating results from those many inputs?
   a. Predictive analytics
   b. Decision trees
   c. Random forest
   d. Neural networks
   e. None of the above

11. Which of the following is not one of the 5 V's of big data?
   a. Volume
   b. Velocity

    c. Value

    d. Vector

    e. Variety

12. Which of the following is not a component of the DIKI pyramid?

    a. Data

    b. Intelligence

    c. Interpretation

    d. Knowledge

    e. Information

13. Which of the following statements regarding C-statistics is false?

    a. C-statistics have a range from 0 to 1.

    b. A C-statistic of 0.5 has the same predictability as a coin flip.

    c. The C-statistic is a method of statistical analysis for predictive analytics models.

    d. C-statistic compares the probability of a patient having a specific outcome event compared to a patient that does not have the event.

    e. All of the above are true.

14. Which of the following statements pertaining to data warehouses is false?

    a. Data warehouses receive a one-way data feed.

    b. Data warehouses are optimized for data analysis.

    c. It is more efficient to extract data from individual data sources rather than a data warehouse.

    d. Data warehouses are a conglomeration of databases.

    e. All of the above are true.

15. Which of the following statements pertaining to artificial intelligence is true?

    a. Predictive analytics is a dynamic method of artificial intelligence.

    b. Machine learning will likely enhance, not replace, the ability for a clinician to care for patients.

    c. Newer machine learning models only require a training data set.

    d. Machine learning models are currently not sophisticated enough to have health care applications.

    e. Artificial intelligence analysis can be conducted using conventional spreadsheet software.

REFERENCES

1. Techopedia.com [Internet]. Query. c2020 [cited 2020 Feb 18]. Available from: https://www.techopedia.com/definition/5736/query

2. DB-Engines [Internet]. DB-Engines ranking. [cited 2020 Feb 18]. Available from: https://db-engines.com/en/ranking

3. Oracle [Internet]. What is a database? Oracle; [cited 2020 Feb 18]. Available from: https://www.oracle.com/database/what-is-database.html

4. Penn Medicine. [Internet]. Data analytics center: Epic Clarity. Penn Medicine; [cited 2020 Feb 18]. Available from: https://www.med.upenn.edu/dac/epic-clarity-data-warehousing.html

5. Vetter TR. Fundamentals of research data and variables: the devil is in the details. Anesth Analg. 2017 Oct;125(4):1375-80.

6. Urdan TC. Statistics in plain English. 4th ed. London (UK): Routledge Press; 2016. 1-12 p.

7. Field A. Discovering statistics using IBM SPSS Statistics: and sex and drugs and rock'n' roll. 4th ed. Los Angeles (CA): Sage; 2013. 1-39 p.

8. StatSoft Inc. Overview of elementary concepts in statistics. Tulsa (OK): StatSoft; 2013.

9. Maciejewski ML, Diehr P, Smith MA, Hebert P. Common methodological terms in health services research and their synonyms [correction of symptoms]. Med Care. 2002 Jun;40(6):477–84.

10. Campbell MJ, Swinscow TDV. Statistics at square one. 11th ed. Chichester (UK), Hoboken (NJ): Wiley-Blackwell/BMJ Books; 2009. 1-13 p.

11. Hulley Stephen B, Newman TB, Cummings SR. Designing clinical research. 4th ed. Philadelphia (PA): Wolters Kluwer Health/Lippincott Williams & Wilkins; 2013. 32-42 p.

12. Motulsky H. Intuitive biostatistics: a nonmathematical guide to statistical thinking. 3rd ed. New York (NY): Oxford University Press; 2014. 72-76 p.

13. American National Standards Institute [Internet]. SQL: American national standard adoptions by INCITS; 2018 [cited 2020 Feb 18]. Available from: https://blog.ansi.org/2018/10/sql-incits-american-national-standard/

14. IBM Knowledge Center [Internet]. Armonk (NY): IBM. Structured query language; [cited 2020 Feb 18]. Available from: https://www.ibm.com/support/knowledgecenter/ssw_ibm_i_71/db2/rbafzsqlcon.htm

15. Oracle [Internet]. SQL—the natural language for analysis; 2015 [cited 2020 Feb 18]. Available from: https://www.oracle.com/technetwork/database/bi-datawarehousing/wp-sqlnaturallanguageanalysis-2565840.pdf

16. Trinh LD, Roach EM, Vogan ED, Lam SW, Eggers GG. Impact of a quality-assessment dashboard on the comprehensive review of pharmacist performance. Am J Health-Syst Pharm. 2017 Sep 1;74(17 Supplement 3):S75-S83.

17. Office of Research Integrity. Responsible conduct in data management [Internet]. Rockville (MD): Department of Health and Human Services; c2003-2004 [cited 2020 Feb 18]. Available from: https://ori.hhs.gov/education/products/n_illinois_u/datamanagement/datopic.html

18. Vetter TR. Descriptive statistics: reporting the answers to the 5 basic questions of who, what, why, when, where, and a sixth, so what? Anesth Analg. 2017;125(5):1797-1802.

19. Salkind NJ. Statistics for people who (think they) hate statistics. 6th ed. Thousand Oaks (CA): Sage Publications; 2016.

20. Mendenhall W, Beaver RJ, Beaver BM. Introduction to probability and statistics. 14th ed. Boston (MA): Cengage Learning; 2013.

21. Raghupathi W, Raghupathi V. Big data analytics in healthcare: promise and potential. Health Inf Sci Syst. 2014 Jul;2(3):1-10.

22. Hernandez I, Zhang Y. Using predictive analytics and big data to optimize pharmaceutical outcomes. Am J Health-Syst Pharm. 2017 Sep 15;74(18):1494-1500.

23. Microsoft Support. Excel specifications and limits [Internet]. Redmond (WA): Microsoft Corporation; [cited 2020 Feb 18]. Available from: https://support.office.com/en-us/article/excel-specifications-and-limits-1672b34d-7043-467e-8e27-269d656771c3

24. McAfee A, Brynjolfsson E. Big data: the management revolution [Internet]. Harvard Business Review; 2014 [cited 2020 Feb 18]. Available from: https://hbr.org/2012/10/big-data-the-management-revolution

25. Weil AR. Big data in health: a new era for research and patient care. Health Aff (Millwood). 2014 Jul;33(7):1110.

26. Marr B. The 5 V's of big data [Internet]. Data Science Central; 2015 [cited 2020 Feb 18]. Available from: https://www.datasciencecentral.com/profiles/blogs/the-5-v-s-of-big-data-by-bernard-marr

27. Jones LK, Pulk R, Gionfriddo MR, Evans MA, Parry D. Utilizing big data to provide better health at lower cost. Am J Health-Syst Pharm. 2018 Jan;75(7):427-35.

28. Gebelhoff R. Sequencing the genome creates so much data we don't know what to do with it [Internet]. The Washington Post. WP Company; 2015 [cited 2020 Feb 18]. Available from: https://www.washingtonpost.com/news/speaking-of-science/wp/2015/07/07/sequencing-the-genome-creates-so-much-data-we-dont-know-what-to-do-with-it/

29. Clinical Pharmacogenomics Implementation Cosortium [Internet]. CPIC; 2020 [cited 2020 Feb 18]. Available from: http://www.cpicpgx.org/

30. Hicks JK, Stowe D, Willner MA, Wai M, Daly T, Gordon SM, Lashner BA, White R, Teng K, Moss T, Erwin A, Chalmers J, Eng C, Knoer S. Implementation of clinical pharmacogenomics within a large health system: from electronic health record decision support to consultation services. Pharmacotherapy. 2016 Aug;36(8):940-8.

31. Hicks JK, Dunnenberger HM, Gumpper KF, Haidar CE, Hoffman JM. Integrating pharmacogenomics into electronic health records with clinical decision support. Am J Health-Syst Pharm. 2016 Jan;73(23):1967-76.

32. O'Donnell PH, Wadhwa N, Danahey K, Danahey K, Borden BA, Lee SM, Klammer C, Hussain S, Siegler M, Sorrentino MJ, Davis AM, Sacro YA, Nanda R, Polonsky TS, Koyner JL, Burnet DL, Lipstreuer K, Rubin DT, Mulcahy C, Strek ME, Harper W, Cifu AS, Polite B, Patrick-Miller L, Yeo K-Tj, Leung Eky, Volchenboum SL, Altman RB, Olopade OI, Stadler WM, Meltzer DO, Ratain MJ. Pharmacogenomics-based point-of-care

clinical decision support significantly alters drug prescribing. Clin Pharmacol Ther. 2017 Nov;102(5):859-69.

33. Barrot C-C, Woillard J-B, Picard N. Big data in pharmacogenomics: current applications, perspectives and pitfalls. Pharmacogenomics. 2019 Jun;20(8):609-20.

34. van Walraven C, Dhalla IA, Bell C, Etchells E, Stiell IG, Zarnke K, Austin P-C, Forster A-J. Derivation and validation of an index to predict early death or unplanned readmission after discharge from hospital to the community. CMAJ. 2010 Apr 6;182(6):551-7.

35. Hincapie-Castillo JM, Staley B, Henriksen C, Saidi A, Lipori GP, Winterstein AG. Development of a predictive model for drug-associated QT prolongation in the inpatient setting using electronic health record data. Am J Health-Syst Pharm. 2019 Jul 11;76(14):1059-70.

36. Krittanawong C, Zhang H, Wang Z, Aydar M, Kitai T. Artificial intelligence in precision cardiovascular medicine. J Am Coll Cardiol. 2017 May 30;69(21):2657-64.

37. Lee SK, Kang B-Y, Kim H-G, Son Y-J. Predictors of medication adherence in elderly patients with chronic diseases using support vector machine models. Healthc Inform Res. 2013 Mar;19(1):33-41.

38. van den Ham HA, Klungel OH, Singer DE, Leufkens HG, Staa TPV. Comparative performance of ATRIA, CHADS2, and CHA2DS2-VAScr risk scores predicting stroke in patients with atrial fibrillation. J Am Coll Cardiol. 2015 Oct 27;66(17):1851-9.

39. Winterstein AG, Staley B, Henriksen C, Xu D, Lipori G, Jeon N, Choi Y, Li Y, Hincapie-Castillo J, Soria-Saucedo R, Brumback B, Johns T. Development and validation of a complexity score to rank hospitalized patients at risk for preventable adverse drug events. Am J Health-Syst Pharm. 2017 Dec 1;74(23):1970-84.

40. Li Y, Staley B, Henriksen C, Xu D, Lipori G, Winterstein AG. Development and validation of a dynamic inpatient risk prediction model for clinically significant hypokalemia using electronic health record data. Am J Health-Syst Pharm. 2019 Mar 29;76(5):301-11.

41. Yao X, Gersh BJ, Sangaralingham LR, Kent DM, Shah ND, Abraham NS, Noseworthy PA. Comparison of the CHA2DS2-VASc, CHADS2, HAS-BLED, ORBIT, and ATRIA risk scores in predicting non-vitamin K antagonist oral anticoagulants-associated bleeding in patients with atrial fibrillation. Am J Cardiol. 2017 Nov 1;120(9):1549-56.

42. Yeh RW, Secemsky EA, Kereiakes DJ, Normand S-LT, Gershlick AH, Cohen DJ, Spertus JA, Gabriel PS, Cutlip DE, Rinaldi MJ, Camenzind E, Wijns W, Apruzzese PK, Song Y,J Massaro JM, Mauri L. Development and validation of a prediction rule for benefit and harm of dual antiplatelet therapy beyond 1 year after percutaneous coronary intervention. JAMA. 2016 Apr 26;315(16):1735-49.

43. Linzey JR, Nadel JL, Wilkinson DA, Rajajee V, Daou BJ, Pandey AS. Validation of the LACE index (length of stay, acuity of admission, comorbidities, emergency department use) in the adult neurosurgical patient population. Neurosurgery. 2020 Jan 1;86(1):E33-7.

44. Flynn A. Using artificial intelligence in health-system pharmacy practice: finding new patterns that matter. Am J Health-Syst Pharm. 2019 Apr 17;76(9):622-7.

45. Domingos P. A few useful things to know about machine learning. Commun ACM. 2012 Oct 1;55(10):78-87.

46. Beam AL, Kohane IS. Translating artificial intelligence into clinical care. JAMA. 2016 Dec 13;316(22):2368-9.

47. Chen JH, Asch SM. Machine learning and prediction in medicine—beyond the peak of inflated expectations. N Engl J Med. 2017 Jun 29;376(26):2507-9.

48. Son YJ, Kim HG, Kim EH, Choi S, Lee SK. Application of support vector machine for prediction of medication adherence in heart failure patients. Healthc Inform Res. 2010 Dec;16(4):253-9.

49. Kaminski B, Jakubczyk M, Szufel P. A framework for sensitivity analysis of decision trees. Cent Eur J Oper Res. 2018;26(1):135-59.

50. Yiu T. Understanding random forest [Internet]. Medium. Towards Data Science; 2019 [cited 2020 Feb 18]. Available from: https://towardsdatascience.com/understanding-random-forest-58381e0602d2

51. Nielsen, AM. Neural networks and deep learning [Internet]. Determination Press; 2015 [cited 2020 Feb 18]. Available from: http://neuralnetworksanddeeplearning.com/chap1.html

52. Bresnick J. What is deep learning and how will it change healthcare? [Internet]. HealthITAnalytics; 2019 [cited 2020 Feb 18]. Available from: https://healthitanalytics.com/features/what-is-deep-learning-and-how-will-it-change-healthcare

53. Miotto R, Wang F, Wang S, Jiang X, Dudley JT. Deep learning for healthcare: review, opportunities and challenges. Brief Bioinform. 2018 Nov 27;19(6):1236-46.

54. Frey CB, Osborne MA. The future of employment: how susceptible are jobs to computerisation? Technologic Forecast Social Change. 2017;114:254-80.

SUGGESTED READINGS

1. McAfee A, Brynjolfsson E. Big data: the management revolution [Internet]. Harvard Business Review; 2012. Available from: https://hbr.org/2012/10/big-data-the-management-revolution

2. Sheriff S. Understanding the 5 V's of big data [Internet]. Acuvate; 2019. Available from: https://acuvate.com/blog/understanding-the-5vs-of-big-data/

3. Porter ME, Heppelmann JE. HBR's 10 must reads on AI, analytics, and the new machine age. Boston (MA): Harvard Business Publishing Corporation; 2019.

4. McKeown R. 50 best resources for learning SQL in 2020 [Internet]. LearnSQL.com; 2020. Available from: https://learnsql.com/blog/ultimate-resources-for-learning-sql-2020/

5. Morkar T. Beginner-friendly resources for machine learning [Internet]. Towards Data Science; 2020. Available from: https://towardsdatascience.com/beginner-friendly-resources-for-machine-learning-fd198f844dc3

6. Motulsky H. Intuitive biostatistics: a nonmathematical guide to statistical thinking. 4th ed. Oxford (UK): Oxford University Press; 2017.

30

Chapter Thirty

Drug Information Education and Training

Michelle W. McCarthy

Learning Objectives

After completing this chapter, the reader will be able to:

- Determine fundamental drug information skills for all pharmacy students.
- Identify settings where drug information skills can be developed and refined.
- Define the recommended training path for drug information specialists.
- Describe job responsibilities of contemporary drug information specialists.
- Formulate a strategy by which interested candidates can learn about available drug information residencies and fellowships.

Key Concepts

1. Information retrieval, evaluation, and application skills represent a significant component of the core skill set each pharmacist must possess.

2. Drug information skills are core concepts incorporated in pharmacy curricula.

3. The majority of foundational skill development should occur prior to student participation in advanced pharmacy practice experiences (APPEs).

4. Drug information rotations may occur in institutional and nontraditional settings (e.g., pharmaceutical industry, managed care, group purchasing organization), a reflection of the expanding role of drug information in contemporary pharmacy practice.

⑤ Pharmacy residency training standards include core drug information retrieval and evaluation skills for both postgraduate year one (PGY1) and postgraduate year two (PGY2) programs.

⑥ Consistent with the profession-wide model for specialist training, the preferred training model for a drug information specialist is a PGY1 residency program, followed by completion of a PGY2 residency in Medication-Use Safety and Policy (formerly Drug Information).

⑦ The American Society of Health-System Pharmacists (ASHP), the organization charged with accrediting pharmacy residency programs, has developed competency areas, goals, and objectives that must be incorporated into ASHP-accredited PGY2 Medication-Use Safety and Policy residency programs.

⑧ PGY2 programs in Medication-Use Safety and Policy are not limited to health systems, as programs exist in academic, industrial, and managed care settings.

⑨ Fellowship programs emphasize skills beyond those provided in residency training programs especially related to research.

Introduction

❶ *Information retrieval, evaluation, and application skills represent a significant component of the core skill set each pharmacist must possess.*[1] As the medication experts of the health care team, drug information skills are important for all pharmacists to possess. In addition to the basic skills for all pharmacists, opportunities to specialize in drug information practice also exist. Practice scope for those who practice specifically in drug information has evolved from a focus on literature retrieval, evaluation, and application to specific organizational needs and patient care situations such as therapeutic policy management, oversight of safe medication practices including information systems, and promotion of health and wellness. The dynamic health care environment and expanded practice responsibilities were traditionally linked to drug information practices (e.g., medication-use policy); developing and maintaining practitioners with expertise in such activities is critically important.[2,3] This chapter will focus on key drug information education and training needs for all pharmacists, especially those necessary for practitioners specializing in drug information practice.

Drug Information in Pharmacy Curriculum

❷ *Drug information skills are core concepts incorporated in pharmacy curricula.*[2] Pharmacy curricula must be designed to prepare graduates in the knowledge, skills,

TABLE 30–1. CENTER FOR ADVANCEMENT OF PHARMACY EDUCATION (CAPE) EDUCATIONAL OUTCOMES (2013)[2]

Select learning objectives that correlate with drug information knowledge and skills

Domain 1: Foundational Knowledge

Subdomain 1.1 Learner: Develop, integrate, and apply knowledge from the foundational sciences (i.e., pharmaceutical, social/behavioral/administrative, and clinical sciences) to evaluate the scientific literature, explain drug action, solve therapeutic problems, and advance population health and patient-centered care.

Example learning objectives:

- 1.1.5 Critically analyze scientific literature related to drugs and disease to enhance clinical decision-making.
- 1.1.6 Identify and critically analyze emerging theories, information, and technologies that may impact patient-centered and population-based care.

Domain 2: Essentials for Practice and Care

Subdomain 2.2 Medication-use systems management: Manage patient healthcare needs using human, financial, technological, and physical resources to optimize the safety and efficacy of medication-use systems.

Example learning objectives:

- 2.2.2 Describe the role of the pharmacist in impacting the safety and efficacy of each component of a typical medication-use system (e.g., procurement, storage, prescribing, transcription, dispensing, administration, monitoring, and documentation).
- 2.2.3 Utilize technology to optimize the medication-use system.
- 2.2.6 Apply standards, guidelines, best practices, and established processes related to safe and effective medication use.
- 2.2.7 Utilize continuous quality improvement techniques in the medication-use process.

Domain 3: Approach to Practice and Care

Subdomain 3: Communication: Effectively communicate verbally and nonverbally when interacting with an individual, group, or organization.

Example learning objectives:

- 3.6.8 Develop professional documents pertinent to organizational needs (e.g., monographs, policy documents).

abilities, behaviors, and attitudes necessary to apply the foundational sciences to the provision of patient-centered care.[3] The expectation of the Accreditation Council for Pharmacy Education (ACPE) accreditation standards is that students will develop the comprehensive knowledge base to be "practice and team-ready" and be able to retain, recall, build upon, and apply knowledge to deliver quality patient care in a variety of entry-level practice settings.[4] Educational outcomes of contemporary professional degree programs include four broad domains and 15 subdomains. The four domains are foundational knowledge, essentials for practice and care, approach to patient care, and personal and professional development. Table 30-1 lists the educational outcomes, domains, subdomains, and example learning objectives that correlate to drug information practice.[2]

DRUG INFORMATION IN DIDACTIC CURRICULUM

The accreditation standards for professional degree programs identify required didactic elements for Doctor of Pharmacy curricula. The required didactic elements are written as broad learning outcomes to provide the comprehensive knowledge base required for entry-level practice. The goal of the latest ACPE standard is to ensure that critical areas of learning are included in pharmacy curricula; however, individual programs have the flexibility to determine how lessons are structured and delivered. The required didactic content that aligns with traditional and contemporary drug information skills are as follows[3]:

- Biostatistics (see Chapter 6)
- Health care systems
- Pharmacoeconomics (see Chapter 7)
- Pharmacy law and regulatory affairs (see Chapters 11 and 24)
- Practice management
- Professional communication (see Chapter 13)
- Research design (see Chapters 4 and 5)
- Health informatics (see Chapters 28 and 29)
- Health information retrieval and evaluation (see Chapters 2–5)
- Natural products and alternative and complementary therapies (see Chapters 3 and 5)
- Medication dispensing, distribution, and administration
- Patient safety (see Chapters 19 and 20)

Case Study 30–1

You have been hired as a drug information faculty member in a new school of pharmacy. You and your colleagues are evaluating how you will incorporate drug information skills into the curricula to ensure graduates are practice and team ready by providing evidence-based drug information to patients and other members of the health care team.

- *What methods may be used for incorporating drug information into the curricula?*
- *What structures can be used for teaching literature evaluation and when might this be taught?*

TABLE 30-2. ESSENTIAL DRUG INFORMATION CONCEPTS FOR PROFESSIONAL DEGREE CURRICULA[4]

- Apply medical information to specific patient situations
- Counterdetail and appropriately interact with the pharmaceutical industry
- Create effective and efficient literature searching strategies
- Critically evaluate marketing and promotional materials and advertisements
- Critically evaluate medical literature
- Describe the process of drug regulation in the United States
- Distinguish statistical versus clinical significance
- Discern and communicate appropriate health information for patient education
- Evaluate drug use policies and procedures
- Identify, evaluate, and utilize key print (text) sources of medical information
- Identify, manage, report, and prevent adverse drug events
- Incorporate principles and practices of evidence-based medicine (EBM) into pharmaceutical care
- Locate and critically evaluate medical information on the Internet
- Prepare, present, and participate in journal clubs
- Provide verbal and written responses to drug information requests
- Summarize basic biostatistics and research design methods
- Understand the creation, maintenance, and management of a drug formulary
- Use electronic medical information databases and other technologically enhanced references and resources in an effective and efficient manner to advance pharmaceutical care

The American College of Clinical Pharmacy (ACCP) Drug Information Practice and Research Network (DI PRN) published an opinion paper to ensure that drug information education and practice is designed to meet the needs of the changing health care environment. This paper recommended specific core drug information concepts that should be formally taught and evaluated in all colleges of pharmacy (see Table 30-2).[5] Other topic areas closely aligned with drug information practice include alternative medicine, adverse drug event surveillance, drug shortage management and mitigation, formulary management, oversight of Risk Evaluation Mitigation Strategies (REMS), medical writing, informatics, and investigational drug services.

A number of pedagogical approaches may be used to build drug information associated skills in the didactic setting. A 2012 survey conducted by the ACCP DI PRN summarized the methods by which colleges of pharmacy include drug information, literature evaluation, and biostatistics content into the curricula. Survey responses represented 50% of the pharmacy schools listed in the American Association of Colleges of Pharmacy (AACP) online directory. Instructional methodologies used included didactic lectures, small-group learning, Internet-based learning, and other formats. Survey respondents indicated using online course management programs, audience response systems,

TABLE 30–3. ACCREDITATION COUNCIL FOR PHARMACY EDUCATION (ACPE) GUIDANCE FOR PREADVANCED PHARMACY PRACTICE EXPERIENCE (APPE) CORE COMPETENCIES[7]

Ability statement:
Assess information needs of patients and health providers and apply knowledge of study design and literature analysis and retrieval to provide accurate, evidence-based drug information

Example performance competencies:

- Collect accurate and comprehensive drug information from appropriate sources to make informed, evidence-based, patient-specific, or population-based decisions
- Recognize the type of content that is available in tertiary (general), secondary, and primary information sources
- Collect, summarize, analyze, and apply information from the biomedical literature to patient-specific or population-based health needs
- Demonstrate utilization of drug information resources
- Describe the type of content in commonly used drug and medical information resources
- Collect and interpret accurate drug information from appropriate sources to make informed, evidence-based decisions
- Use effective written, visual, verbal, and nonverbal communication skills to accurately respond to drug information questions

YouTube, online blogs, tweets, and wikis to teach drug information, literature evaluation, and biostatistics content.[6] The availability of instructional technologies and focus on active-learning components in the professional program provide many opportunities for instructors to engage learners through incorporation of practical, practice-oriented scenarios.

More recently, another survey of school of pharmacy faculty evaluated how and when medical literature evaluation skills were taught within the curriculum. The survey found that medical literature evaluation is a major topic taught in pharmacy schools. The most common response was that medical literature evaluation was taught in a stand-alone course (49% of respondents), and this course was placed within the second professional year (43%). However, teaching medical literature evaluation was also embedded within a drug information course for 37% and taught through laboratory-based courses for 11%.[7]

DRUG INFORMATION IN EXPERIENTIAL EDUCATION

❸ *The majority of foundational skill development should occur prior to student participation in advanced pharmacy practice experiences (APPEs).* Integration of practice-related activities in the introductory pharmacy practice experiences (IPPEs) are also important activities supported by ACPE. Table 30-3 provides core competencies pharmacy students must possess prior to APPE experiences which may include IPPEs.[2,8] Having the opportunity to

TABLE 30–4. DRUG INFORMATION ACTIVITIES INCLUDED IN ADVANCED PHARMACY PRACTICE EXPERIENCE (APPE) CURRICULA[3]

- Deliver evidence-based care through the retrieval, evaluation, and application of findings from the scientific and clinical literature
- Participate in the health system's formulary process
- Participate in the management of medication-use systems and applying the systems approach to medication safety
- Conduct a drug utilization review
- Participate in the management of the use of investigational drug products
- Participate in therapeutic protocol development
- Perform prospective and retrospective financial and clinical outcomes analyses to support formulary recommendations and therapeutic guideline development

complete "real" drug information–specific activities (e.g., responding to drug information requests, medication-use evaluation, formulary class review or monograph, evaluation of adverse drug events) following completion of didactic coursework provides students with even greater opportunities to apply pharmacotherapeutic, pharmacokinetic, legal and ethical principles learned earlier to their approach to providing drug information. Drug information historically was a required learning experience for each Doctor of Pharmacy (PharmD) student. The growth in the number of colleges of pharmacy and the pharmacy student population, combined with reductions in the number of formal drug information centers, has resulted in an inadequate number of teaching sites to support completion of required drug information APPEs for every student.[9] While some colleges have developed their own formalized centers, others provide only elective drug information APPEs.[2,9] ❹ Drug information rotations may also occur in nontraditional settings (e.g., pharmaceutical industry, managed care, group purchasing organization), a reflection of the expanding role of drug information in contemporary pharmacy practice.

The new ACPE standard guidance document includes APPE activities to foster student drug information skill development (see Table 30-4).[7] Students require adequate supervision and oversight to ensure the quality of service they provide, as well as to provide them valuable feedback to subsequently improve their performance. Practice sites often realize that incorporation of students into the site may expand the capacity of services provided, including responding to more drug information requests, preparing analyses of drug policy or safety issues for consideration by various health system committees (e.g., pharmacy and therapeutics committee), and conducting medication-use evaluations or adverse drug reaction surveillance. Other advanced practice experiences beyond those labeled as drug information (e.g., pharmacy management, informatics, and medication safety) also provide opportunities beneficial to building skills in drug information.

You practice in a community hospital and regularly provide both IPPE and APPE hospital experiences to PharmD students. Based upon organizational priorities and your responsibilities associated with formulary management and medication safety, you are considering providing an elective APPE experience in drug information. You are preparing your rotation description for submission to the school of pharmacy experiential education office.

- *Do you need a call center in order to provide a drug information APPE?*
- *What types of activities will you provide for students completing this rotation?*

Postgraduate Training in Drug Information

❻ *Pharmacy* **residency** *training standards include core drug information retrieval and evaluation skills for both* **postgraduate year one (PGY1)** *and* **postgraduate year two (PGY2)** *programs.*[10,11] All PGY1 residency graduates are required to complete basic drug information activities such as completion of a drug monograph and medication-use evaluation. As early as 1966, the need for pharmacists with advanced skills in drug information was documented.[12] For those seeking to practice as a specialist in drug information, the preferred training model for a drug information specialist is a PGY1 residency program, followed by completion of a PGY2 residency in Medication-Use Safety and Policy (formerly Drug Information). This training model is also supported by drug information specialist members of ACCP.[3]

SHORTAGE OF TRAINED DRUG INFORMATION SPECIALISTS

Although there is long standing recognition regarding the importance of advanced training, a 2009 survey identified that 40% of drug information pharmacists had completed such training and the remaining 60% developed skill in their position responsibilities through on-the-job training.[13] This may reflect an imbalance in pharmacists with advanced training and available job openings. A relative lack of popularity or desirability of the specialty to students and new trainees, or pressures on employers to fill positions with applicants who lack the desired formal training may have contributed to this imbalance; no formal assessment of these or other factors has been conducted. The number of available PGY2 Drug Information residency programs has been decreasing, and there is fluctuation in the number of interested applicants. This could be due to misconceptions regarding the activities of drug information residents and specialists. Drug information has evolved from merely providing responses to drug information queries to serving as organizational leaders in medication-use policy and safety.[14,15] As a result of overlapping responsibilities, and to ensure there are adequately trained candidates to meet the needs of the changing health care environment, the American Society of Health-System Pharmacists (ASHP), with the input of representatives practicing in both drug information and medication-use safety, merged the educational goals and objectives for Medication-Use Safety and Drug Information residency programs into Medication-Use Safety and Policy. This nomenclature now replaces "Drug Information" when referring to residency training.[3,14]

A 2006 survey (published in 2009) of United States pharmacists with presumed drug information practices was conducted to determine the perceptions regarding drug information practice and training.[13] The survey was sent to members of the ACCP DI PRN, participants of a drug information practice listserv, and pharmacists employed by drug information centers; because of this methodology, the sample may not reflect all pharmacists with drug information responsibilities particularly those practicing in pharmaceutical industry, managed care, etc. The most common job responsibilities of those surveyed were instructing pharmacy students and staff (64%), maintaining formal drug information center operations (63%), responding to drug information queries (59%), conducting original research (53%), providing pharmacy and therapeutics committee support (46%), providing medication safety support (41%), publishing pharmacy-related newsletters (38%), and developing medication-use policy (35%). Respondents generally felt prepared to undertake their responsibilities in relation to the extent of postgraduate training they received. However, areas in which pharmacists felt less prepared included information systems support (41%), pharmacoeconomic evaluations (32%), and clinical outcomes research (19%). Approximately 80% of those who had completed postgraduate training felt adequately prepared overall for their job roles. Preparing for practice changes and innovations is a focus of residency training and perhaps was reflected in the greater sense of preparedness reported by residency-trained pharmacists.[13] A 2011 survey of pharmacy residents and fellows identified that a new motivator of pharmacy students to pursue residency and **fellowship** training is that these additional training programs are prerequisites for certain jobs.[16]

ACCREDITATION STANDARDS FOR POSTGRADUATE TRAINING IN MEDICATION-USE SAFETY AND POLICY

❼ *ASHP, the organization charged with accrediting pharmacy residency programs, has developed competency areas, goals, and objectives that must be included in ASHP-accredited*

PGY2 residency programs.[9] In 2015, ASHP approved a new PGY2 Accreditation Standard where outcomes were replaced by competency areas.[17] ASHP has worked systematically with practice experts to update the required and elective competency areas, goals, and objectives from the 2007 PGY2 Drug Information program and those from the PGY2 Medication-Use Safety residency program.[18] The resultant outcome is a combined set of competency areas, goals, and objectives for PGY2 residencies in Medication-Use Safety and Policy. The required competency areas include the following:

- Assessing safe and effective medication-use systems and policies
- Medication-use data collection and analysis
- Designing safe and effective medication-use systems/policies
- Drug shortages and supply interruptions
- Medication-use technology
- Medication-use research
- Leadership and management
- Teaching, education, and dissemination of knowledge[9]

The purpose of PGY2 residency programs is to "build on Doctor of Pharmacy (PharmD) education and PGY1 pharmacy residency programs to contribute to the development of clinical pharmacists in specialized areas of practice. PGY2 residencies provide residents with opportunities to function independently as practitioners by conceptualizing and integrating accumulated experience and knowledge and incorporating both into the provision of patient care or other advanced practice areas. Residents who successfully complete an accredited PGY2 pharmacy residency are prepared for advanced patient care, academic, or other specialized positions, along with board certification, if available."[16] As noted in the 2006 survey (published in 2009), contemporary drug information specialists should be prepared to utilize technology and advance population-based approaches (e.g., data mining, pharmacoepidemiology, pharmacovigilance) to support a safe and effective medication-use process.[13] These tools and approaches may include information systems support, clinical outcomes research, pharmacoeconomic evaluations, and other such techniques that are also consistent with the Institute of Medicine's (IOM) focus on evidence-based medicine, technology, and quality assurance as core competencies for health care practitioners.[19]

OPPORTUNITIES FOR POSTGRADUATE RESIDENTS

❽ *PGY2 programs in Medication-Use Safety and Policy are not limited to health systems, as programs exist in academic, industrial, and managed care settings.* The ASHP required competency areas, goals, and objectives of PGY2 Medication-Use Safety and Policy residency programs provide opportunity for development of an advanced skill set that can be applied to many practice settings. Residency graduates who are actively engaged in the practice environment of their training program and then become employed in the same type of practice environment should be well equipped to effectively contribute to the drug information needs of their new organization, and the time to effectively transition from resident to independent practitioner may be shortened. For example, a graduate of an ASHP-accredited PGY2 Medication-Use Safety and Policy residency in an academic medical center would likely be a highly desirable candidate for drug information or medication-use policy specialist positions within other hospitals and health systems. However, the skills afforded by advanced training in any setting are transferable and beneficial to other settings since having a greater understanding of the operations of an alternate setting may improve decision making in the new environment. For example, fellowship training in pharmaceutical industry can better inform a pharmacist of the Food and Drug Administration (FDA) regulations and internal policies that may shape the manner in which a manufacturer can provide information about an investigational drug or suspected adverse effects of a marketed drug.

Case Study 30-3

A Doctor of Pharmacy student has expressed interest in pursuing a career in drug information. The individual is seeking information about various practice settings and responsibilities. As the faculty advisor for the student, you have volunteered to identify shadowing opportunities for various drug information positions.

- *What positions may individuals with expertise in drug information hold?*
- *In what settings may these individuals practice?*
- *What advice regarding postgraduate training would you recommend for this student?*

POSTGRADUATE FELLOWSHIP IN DRUG INFORMATION

❾ *Fellowship programs emphasize skills beyond those provided in residency training programs especially related to research.* Drug information fellowships are focused in a number of subspecialty areas including evidence-based practice, medical communications, medication-use policy, medication safety, pharmacoepidemiology, and pharmacoeconomics. As with therapeutic specialties, fellowship training in drug information should focus on expanding the fellow's research abilities. These postgraduate experiences are highly variable and may not have prerequisites beyond the PharmD for entry. There are no accreditation standards for fellowship programs, so the application requirements (completion of a residency or not), structure, duration and delivery are guided by the program director.[20] Given the growing complexity and cost of health care, the need for practice-focused researchers has grown more vital. Drug information fellowships that focus on research skills in pharmacoepidemiology, pharmacoeconomics and comparative effectiveness, or the role of informatics to support a safe and effective medication-use system, would be well suited to fill this need.[3,13,16]

Pursuing Specialty Training

Identifying potential residency or fellowship programs that may meet an individual's training needs should begin with a search of available training directories such as the ASHP Online Residency Directory and the ACCP Directory of Residencies and Fellowships.[20] Different factors may be important to individual applicants as they evaluate available programs. Beyond traditional drug information activities, like responding to queries and providing formulary management, factors that may be important to individual candidates include the ability to gain experience working with students in didactic and experiential settings, co-precepting PGY1 residents, performing contract work, extensive opportunities to manage drug policy across a health system, and intensive training in medical writing. Regardless of the special features or characteristics, there should be opportunities that will prepare the individual for the type of practice envisioned for him or herself. Residents completing PGY2 Medication-Use Safety and Policy residencies will be well prepared for positions in both medication-use policy and medication safety, regulatory/quality, drug policy, and medical writing. Settings in which positions may be available include hospitals and health systems, managed care organizations, group purchasing organizations, government organizations, pharmaceutical industry, and academia. A directory of accredited or accreditation-pending residency programs can easily be accessed from the ASHP Online Residency Directory (https://accred.ashp.org/aps/pages/directory/residencyProgramSearch.aspx).[21] In addition to employment (e.g., salary, benefits) and contact information, each program's listing includes a description of the practice site, key program features, application information, and a hyperlink to the program's website. More detailed information such as schedules, learning experience descriptions, and accomplishments of program graduates may be found on the websites of the individual programs. Residency programs, including those that are not accredited, may also be identified through a review of the Directory of Residencies, Fellowships, and Graduate

Programs hosted on the ACCP website (http://www.accp.com/resandfel/).[20] This directory is also the primary catalog of possible fellowship options. Fellowship programs may be identified by searching drug information or medication-use safety and policy. The program listings also provide descriptions of a secondary specialty, if applicable. Descriptions of secondary specialty may continue to evolve as programs morph to meet the demands of the changing health care environment.

Conclusion

All pharmacists, regardless of practice setting, require drug information skills in order to provide evidence-based, patient-centered care and appropriately support other health care professionals. Equipping pharmacists with those skills begins in professional degree programs, continues into residency training, and may extend into fellowship programs. Additionally, pharmacists may continue to expand drug information skill development throughout their careers by involvement in continuing professional development and on-the-job training. Each of these important elements of education and training should continue to evolve to meet contemporary practice and research needs and to prepare future practitioners to be "practice and team ready" to provide innovative services grounded in principles of evidence-based medicine.

Self-Assessment Questions

1. During your college's review of its professional degree program, a committee member recommends to eliminate a course entitled "Drug Information Skill Development." When asked to justify the recommendation, the faculty member replies, "The accreditation standards don't require a drug information course." What is a factual response to the statement?
   a. The standards *do not* prescribe specific concepts that must be taught in professional degree curricula.
   b. The standards *do* require the inclusion of concepts generally categorized as drug information, in addition to related concepts.
   c. Drug information concepts *are* required to be taught only during advanced pharmacy practice experiences (APPEs).
   d. All of the above.
   e. None of the above.

2. Although ACPE does not require pharmacy school graduates to have completed a drug information course or rotation, which of the following educational subdomains correlate with drug information knowledge and skills:
   a. Manage patient health care needs using human, financial, technological, and physical resources to optimize the safety and efficacy of medication-use systems.
   b. Develop, integrate, and apply knowledge from foundational sciences to evaluate the scientific literature, explain drug action, solve therapeutic problems, and advance population health and patient centered care.
   c. Effectively communicate verbally and nonverbally when interacting with an individual, group, or organization.
   d. All of the above.
   e. None of the above.

3. Which specific drug information concept is **NOT** recommended by ACCP to be formally taught and evaluated in all colleges of pharmacy?
   a. Creating drug policies and procedures
   b. Critically evaluating medical literature
   c. Understanding the creation, maintenance, and management of a drug formulary
   d. Preparing, presenting, and participating in journal clubs

4. In which activity can you engage pharmacy students enrolled in a drug information course to demonstrate the broad applicability of drug information skills, using an example from the popular media?
   a. Critiquing the accuracy of a local television news reporter's segment about a newly approved prescription drug
   b. Crafting a letter to the editor describing the role pharmacists play in preventing medication errors, in response to an article about the national impact of medication errors published in the local newspaper
   c. Evaluating a front page article from the New York Times regarding a recently published drug study
   d. All of the above
   e. None of the above

5. The college of pharmacy in which you work is unable to provide drug information APPEs in a traditional drug information setting. Which alternate APPE settings also provide opportunities to build drug information skills?
   a. Pharmacy management/administration
   b. Pharmacy informatics

    c. Medication safety

    d. All of the above

    e. None of the above

6. Which unique educational methods have been used to teach drug information concepts to pharmacy students?

    a. Small-group hands-on assignments

    b. Online blogs, tweets, and wikis

    c. Audience response systems

    d. All of the above

    e. None of the above

7. The preferred credentials for a drug information specialist practicing in a hospital, health system, or school of pharmacy are:

    a. Pharmacy degree

    b. Pharmacy degree + Postgraduate Year One Pharmacy Residency

    c. Pharmacy degree + Pharmacoeconomics Fellowship

    d. All of the above

    e. None of the above

8. What role(s) can postgraduate year two (PGY2) Medication-Use Safety and Policy residents play in teaching, educating, and disseminating knowledge?

    a. Provide a continuing education presentation to providers regarding a new medication.

    b. Provide classroom instruction about literature evaluation skills to doctor of pharmacy students.

    c. Prepare an article summarizing recently released therapeutic guidelines.

    d. All of the above.

    e. None of the above.

9. What activities support the required competency areas, goals, and objectives of ASHP-accredited PGY2 Medication-Use Safety and Policy residencies?

    a. Develop treatment guidelines for a select agent(s) used within an organization.

    b. Assess the impact of a drug shortage for the organization including the impact on patient care and medication safety.

    c. Collaborate with information technology personnel to incorporate a new or revised medication-use process into the appropriate order set, electronic health record, and/or technology-based software.

    d. All of the above.

    e. None of the above.

10. What types of positions may individuals completing an ASHP-accredited PGY2 Medication-Use Safety and Policy residency pursue?
    a. Drug information or medication-use policy specialist in hospital/health system
    b. Editor at medical communications company
    c. Medication safety pharmacist
    d. All of the above
    e. None of the above

11. Drug information and associated fellowships may be desired by individuals interested in the following:
    a. Extensive research-related activities
    b. Pharmacoeconomics
    c. Pharmacoepidemiology
    d. All of the above
    e. None of the above

12. Where would you be able to find the employment paths that graduates of PGY2 Medication-Use Safety and Policy residencies have pursued over the last 5 years?
    a. The individual training program's website
    b. The ACCP Online Residency Directory
    c. The ASHP Online Residency Directory
    d. All of the above
    e. None of the above

13. What job responsibilities are performed by contemporary drug information specialists?
    a. Supporting pharmacy and therapeutics committees
    b. Educating health care providers and health care providers in training on medication therapy
    c. Ensuring safe and effective use of medications through the use of technology
    d. Developing medication-use policies
    e. All of the above

14. In what settings are drug information residencies and fellowships conducted:
    a. Hospitals/health systems
    b. Schools of pharmacy
    c. Pharmaceutical industry
    d. Managed care organizations
    e. All of the above

15. Which of the following statements is correct?
    a. Drug information APPEs are required for all pharmacy school graduates.
    b. Drug information practice has evolved from merely responding to drug information queries to serving as organizational leaders in medication-use safety.
    c. AACP recommends drug information skills be taught only in didactic lectures.
    d. ASHP is the only organization that accredits drug information residency and fellowship programs.

REFERENCES

1. Wang F, Troutman WG, Seo T, Peak A. Rosenberg JM. Drug information education in doctor of pharmacy programs. Am J Pharm Educ. 2006;70(3):1–7.
2. Medina MS, Plaza CM, Stowe CD, Robinson ET, DeLander G, Beck DE, Melchert RB, Supernaw RB, Roche VF, Gleason BL, Strong MN, Bain A, Meyer GE, Dong BJ, Rochon J, Johnston P. Report of the 2012-13 Academic Affairs Standing Committee: Revising the Center for the Advancement of Pharmacy Education (CAPE) educational outcomes 2013. Am J Pharm Educ. 2013;77(8):Article 162.
3. Accreditation Council for Pharmaceutical Education. Accreditation standards and key elements for the professional program in pharmacy leading to the doctor of pharmacy degree. Chicago; 2015 [cited 2016 Jul 22]. Available from: https://www.acpe-accredit.org/pdf/Standards2016FINAL.pdf.
4. Bernknopf AC, Karpinski JP, McKeever AL, Peak AS, Smith KM, Smith WD, Timpe EM, Ward KE. Drug information: from education to practice. Pharmacotherapy. 2009;29(3):331–46.
5. Phillips JA, Gabay MP, Ficzere C, Ward KE. Curriculum and instructional methods for drug information, literature evaluation, and biostatistics: survey of US pharmacy schools. Ann Pharmacother. 2012;46(6):793–801.
6. O'Sullivan TA, Phillips J, Demaris K. Medical literature evaluation education at US Schools of Pharmacy. Am J Pharm Educ. 2016;80(1): article 5.
7. Accreditation Council for Pharmacy Education. Guidance for the accreditation standards and key elements for the professional program in pharmacy leading to the doctor of pharmacy degree. Chicago; 2015 [cited 2016 Aug 31]. Available from: https://www.acpe-accredit.org/pdf/GuidanceforStandards2016FINAL.pdf.
8. Cole SW, Berensen NM. Comparison of drug information practice curriculum components in US colleges of pharmacy. Am J Pharm Educ. 2005;69(2):240–4.
9. American Society of Health-System Pharmacists. Required competency areas, goals, and objectives for postgraduate year two (PGY2) medication-use safety and policy pharmacy residency. [cited 2019 Aug 7]. Available from: https://www.ashp.org/-/media/assets/professional-development/residencies/docs/pgy2-medication-use-safety.ashx.

10. American Society of Health-System Pharmacists. Required competency areas, goals and objectives for postgraduate year one (PGY1) pharmacy residencies. [cited 2019 Aug 22]. Available from: https://www.ashp.org/-/media/assets/professional-development/residencies/docs/required-competency-areas-goals-objectives.

11. Walton CA. Education and training of the drug information specialist. Drug Intell. 1967;1:132-7.

12. Gettig JP, Jordan JK, Sheehan AH. A survey of current perceptions of drug information practice and training. Hosp Pharm. 2009;44(4):325-31.

13. Vanscoy GJ, Gajewski LK, Tyler LS, Gora-Harper ML, Grant KL, May JR. The future of medication information practice: a consensus. Ann Pharmacother. 1996;30(7-8):876-81.

14. Ghaibi S, Ipema H, Gabay M. ASHP guidelines on the pharmacist's role in providing drug information. Am J Health-Syst Pharm. 2015;72(7):573-7.

15. McCarthy BC, Weber LM. Update on factors motivating pharmacy students to pursue residency and fellowship training. Am J Health-Syst Pharm. 2013;70(16):1397-1403.

16. American Society of Health-System Pharmacists. ASHP accreditation standard for post-graduate year two (PGY2) pharmacy residencies. [cited 2020 May 28]. Available from: https://www.ashp.org/Professional-Development/Residency-Information/Residency-Program-Resources/Residency-Accreditation/Accreditation-Standards-for-PGY2-Pharmacy-Residencies.

17. American Society of Health-System Pharmacists. Accreditation Services Division. PGY2 goals and objectives revision update. The Communiqué. 2016;19(1):5.

18. Institute of Medicine: executive summary. In: Greiner AC, Knebel E, editors. Health professions education: a bridge to quality. Washington (DC): National Academy Press; 2003:1-18.

19. American College of Clinical Pharmacy Directory of Residencies, Fellowships and Graduate Programs [Internet]. Lenexa: American College of Clinical Pharmacy; 2016 [cited 2019 Aug 23]. Available from: http://www.accp.com/resandfel/index.aspx.

20. American Society of Health-System Pharmacists Online Residency Directory [Internet]. Bethesda (MD): American Society of Health-System Pharmacists; 2019 [cited 2019 Aug 23]. Available from: https://accreditation.ashp.org/directory/#/program/residency.

SUGGESTED READINGS

1. Bernknopf AC, Karpinski JP, McKeever AL, Peak AS, Smith KM, Smith WD, Smith WD, Timpe EM, Ward KE. Drug information: from education to practice. Pharmacotherapy. 2009 Mar;29(3):331-46.

2. Cole SW, Berensen NM. Comparison of drug information practice curriculum components in U.S. colleges of pharmacy. Am J Pharm Educ. 2005;69:240-4.

3. Phillips JA, Gabay MP, Ficzere C, Ward KE. Curriculum and instructional methods for drug information, literature evaluation, and biostatistics: survey of US pharmacy schools. Ann Pharmacother. 2012;46:793-801.

4. Gettig JP, Jordan JK, Sheehan AH. A survey of current perceptions of drug information practice and training. Hosp Pharm. 2009;44:325–31.

5. American Society of Health-System Pharmacists. Required competency areas, goals, and objectives for postgraduate year two (PGY2) medication-use safety and policy pharmacy residency. [cited 2019 Aug 7]. Available from: https://www.ashp.org/-/media/assets/professional-development/residencies/docs/pgy2-medication-use-safety.ashx.

Appendices

Appendix 2–1

Example of Drug Information Consult Documentation Form

DRUG CONSULTATION REQUEST FORM
DRUG INFORMATION SERVICE
NATIONAL INSTITUTES OF HEALTH

LOG# _____
Final QA Check _____

REQUESTER INFORMATION

Date Received _____

Time Received _____ AM / PM *(circle one)*

Name _____

Phone# _____

FAX# _____

Pager# _____

e-mail _____

INTERNAL:
☐ MD ☐ DDS
☐ RN
☐ Pharmacist
☐ Other Professional _____
☐ NIH Patient
☐ Other _____

EXTERNAL:
☐ Pharmacist
☐ Physician
☐ General Public
☐ Other Healthcare Professional _____
☐ Other Professional/Organization _____

AFFILIATION CATEGORY:
☐ Institute _____
☐ Clinic _____
☐ Pt Care Unit _____
☐ Other _____

HOW RECEIVED: ☐ Phone ☐ Voice Mail ☐ E-Mail ☐ Mail ☐ FAX ☐ In Person ☐ Referred by _____
PRIORITY: ☐ Urgent ☐ High Priority ☐ Routine ☐ Low Priority

ORIGINAL QUESTION / REQUEST

CLEAR STATEMENT(S) OF ACTUAL DRUG INFORMATION NEED

PERTINENT PATIENT DATA / BACKGROUND INFORMATION

Name _____

Pt Care Unit/Clinic _____ ☐ Inpatient ☐ Outpatient

Age _____ Race _____ ☐ Male ☐ Female

Height _____ cm _____ ft _____ in   Weight _____ lb _____ kg

Primary Diagnosis _____

Allergies/Intolerances _____

End-Organ Function _____

Special Circumstances _____

CC:
HPI:
PMH:
FH:
SH:
ROS:
Meds:
PE:
Labs:
Diagnostics:
Problem List:

LOG# _____

CLASSIFICATION(S) OF REQUEST

☐ Administration (Routes/Methods)
☐ Adverse Effects/Intolerances
☐ Allergy/Cross Reactivity
☐ Alternative Medicine
☐ Biotechnology/Gene Therapy
☐ Clinical Nutrition/Metabolic Support
☐ Compatibility/Stability/Storage
☐ Contraindications/Precautions
☐ Cost/Pharmacoeconomics
☐ Dose/Schedule
☐ Drug Delivery Devices/Systems/Forms
☐ Drug Interactions (Drug-Drug, Drug-Food)
☐ Drug of choice/Therapeutic Alternatives/Therapeutic Use
☐ Drug Standards/Legal/Regulatory
☐ Drug Use in Special Populations
   (Effects of Age, Organ System Function, Disease,
   Extracorporeal Circulation, etc.)
☐ Excipients/Compounding/Formulations

☐ Investigational Products (Pre-Clinical and Clinical)
☐ Lab Test Interferences (Drug-Lab Interactions)
☐ Monitoring Parameters
☐ Nonprescription Products
☐ Patient Information/Education
☐ Pharmacokinetics (LADME/TDM)
☐ Pharmacology/Mechanisms/Pharmacodynamics
☐ Physicochemical Properties
☐ Poisoning/Toxicology (Environmental/Occupational Exposure,
   Mutagenicity, Carcinogenicity)
☐ Pregnancy/Lactation/Teratogenicity/Fertility
☐ Product Availability/Status
☐ Product Identification (Tablet/Capsule)
☐ Product Identification (Generic, Brand, Orphan,
   Foreign, Chemical Substances, Discontinued Products, etc.)
☐ Product Information
☐ Study Design/Protocol Development/Research Support
☐ Other _____

REQUEST CATEGORY

☐ Patient Care   ☐ Research   ☐ Other _____

RESPONSE (Referenced)

REFERENCES (Numbered)

TRACKING / FOLLOW-UP

Request Received By_____   Reviewed By_____
Response Formulated By_____   Response Communicated By_____
                                                          Time Required to Answer_____

☐ Documents/Literature Provided   ☐ Verbal Response   ☐ E-Mail   ☐ Written Response/Consult

OUTCOME / FOLLOW-UP

Appendix 2–2

Standard Questions for Obtaining Background Information from Requestors

Regardless of the type or classification of the question, the following information should be obtained:

1. The requestor's name.
2. The requestor's location and/or page number.
3. The requestor's affiliation (institution or practice), if a health care professional.
4. The requestor's frame of reference (i.e., title, profession/occupation, rank).
5. The resources the requestor has already consulted.
6. If the request is patient-specific or academic.
7. The patient's diagnosis and other medications.
8. The urgency of the request (negotiate time of response).

The following questions should be asked when appropriate for specific requests*.

Availability of Dosage Forms
1. What is the dosage form desired?
2. What administration routes are feasible with this patient?
3. Is this patient alert and oriented?
4. Does the patient have a water or sodium restriction?
5. What other special factors regarding drug administration should be considered?

Identification of Product
1. What is the generic or trade name of the product?
2. Who is the manufacturer? What country of origin?
3. What is the suspected use of this product?
4. Under what circumstances was this product found? Who found the product?
5. What is the dosage form, color markings, size, etc.?
6. What was your source of information? Was it reliable?

General Product Information
1. Why is there a particular concern for this product?
2. Is written patient information required?
3. What type of information do you need?
4. Is this for an inpatient, outpatient, or private patient?

Foreign Drug Identification

1. What are the drug's generic name, trade, manufacturer, and/or country of origin?
2. What is the dosage form, markings, color, strength, or size?
3. What is the suspected use of the drug? How often is the patient taking it? What is the patient's response to the drug? Is the patient male or female?
4. If the medication was found, what were the circumstances/conditions at the time of discovery?
5. Is the patient just visiting, or are they planning on staying?

Investigational Drug Information

1. Why do you need this information? Is the patient in need of the drug or currently enrolled in a protocol?
2. If a drug is to be identified, what is the dosage form, markings, color, strength, or size of the product?
3. Why was the patient receiving the drug? What is the response when the patient was on the drug? What are the patient's pathological conditions?
4. If a drug is desired what approved or accepted therapies have been tried? Was therapy maximized before discontinued?

Method and Rate of Administration

1. What dosage form or preparation is being used (if multiple salts available)?
2. What is the dose ordered? Is the drug a one-time dose or standing orders?
3. What is the clinical status of the patient? For example, could the patient tolerate a fluid push of XX mL? Is the patient fluid or sodium restricted? Does the patient have congestive heart failure or edema?
4. What possible delivery routes are available?
5. What other medications is the patient receiving currently? Are any by the same route?

Incompatibility and Stability

1. What are the routes for the patient's medications?
2. What are the doses, concentrations, and volumes for all pertinent medications?
3. What are the infusion times/rates expected or desired?
4. What is the base solution or diluent used?
5. Was the product stored and handled appropriately, based on requirements?
6. When was the product compounded/prepared?

Drug Interactions

1. What event(s) suggest that an interaction occurred? Please describe.
2. For the drugs in question, what are the doses, volumes, concentrations, rate of administration, administration schedules, and length of therapies?
3. What is the temporal relationship between the drugs in question?
4. Has the patient received this combination or a similar combination in the past?
5. Other than the drugs in question, what other drugs is the patient receiving currently? When were these started?

Drug-Laboratory Test Interference

1. What event(s) suggest an interaction occurred? Please describe.
2. For the drug in question, what is the dose, volume, concentration, rate of administration, administration schedule, and length of therapy?
3. What is the temporal relationship between drug administration and laboratory test sampling?
4. What other drugs is the patient receiving?
5. Has clinical chemistry (or the appropriate laboratory) been contacted? Are they aware of any known interference similar to this event?
6. Was this one isolated test or a trend in results?

Pharmacokinetics

1. Which product (e.g., drug, dose, brand) is being used?
2. What are the dose and route of the drug?
3. What are the patient's age, sex, height, and weight?
4. What are the disease being treated and the severity of the illness?
5. What are the patient's hepatic and renal functions?
6. What other medications is the patient receiving?
7. What physiologic conditions exist (e.g., pneumonia, severe burns, or obesity)?
8. What are the patient's dietary and ethanol habits?

Therapeutic Levels

1. Is the patient currently receiving the drug? Have samples already been drawn? At what time?
2. What is the disease or underlying pathology being treated? If infectious in nature, what is the organism suspected/cultured?
3. If not stated in the question, what was the source of the sample (blood, urine, saliva; venous or arterial blood)?
4. What was the timing of the samples relative to drug administration? Over what period of time was the drug administered and by what route?
5. What were the previous concentrations for this patient? Was the patient receiving the same dose then?
6. How long has the patient received the drug? Is the patient at steady state?

Therapy Evaluation/Drug of Choice

1. What medications, including doses and routes of administration, is the patient receiving?
2. What are the patient's pathology(ies) and disease(s) severity?
3. What are the patient's specifics: age, weight, height, gender, organ function/dysfunction?
4. Has the patient received the drug previously? Was response similar?
5. Has the patient been adherent?
6. What alternative therapies has the patient received? Was therapy maximized for each of these before discontinuation? What other therapies are being considered?
7. What monitoring parameters have been followed (serum concentrations/levels, clinical status, other clinical lab results, objective measurements, and subjective assessment)?

Dosage Recommendations

1. What disease is being treated? What is the extent/severity of the illness?
2. What are the medications (all) being prescribed? Has the patient been adherent?
3. Does the patient have any insufficiency of the renal, hepatic, or cardiac system?
4. For drugs with renal elimination, what are the serum creatinine/creatinine clearance, blood urea nitrogen (BUN), and/or urine output? Is the patient receiving peritoneal dialysis or hemodialysis?
5. For drugs with hepatic elimination, what are the liver function tests (LFTs), bilirubin (direct and indirect), and/or albumin?
6. For drugs with serum-level monitoring utility, characterize the most recent levels per timing relative to dose and results.
7. Are these lab values recent? Is the patient's condition stable?
8. Does this patient have a known factor that could affect drug metabolism (ethnic background or acetylator status)?

Adverse Events

1. What is the name, dosage, and route for all drugs currently and recently prescribed?
2. What are the patient specifics (age, sex, height, weight, organ dysfunction, and indication for drug use)?
3. What is the temporal relationship with the drug?
4. Has the patient experienced this adverse relationship (or a similar event) with this drug (or similar agent) previously?
5. Was the suspected drug ever administered before? Why was it discontinued then?
6. What were the events/findings that characterize this adverse drug reaction (include onset and duration)?
7. Has any intervention been initiated at this time?
8. Does the patient have any food intolerance?
9. Is there a family history for this ADR and/or drug allergy?

Toxicology Information

1. What is your name, relationship to the patient, and telephone number?
2. What are the patient specifics (age, sex, height, weight, organ dysfunction, and indication for drug use)?
3. Is this a suspected ingestion or exposure?
4. What is the product suspected to have been ingested? What is the strength of the product and the possible quantity ingested (e.g., how much was in the bottle)?
5. How long ago did the ingestion occur?
6. How much is on the patient or surrounding area?
7. How much was removed from the patient's hands and mouth? Was the ingestion in the same room where the product was stored?
8. What has been done for the patient already? Has the Poison Control Center or emergency department been called?

9. Do you have Syrup of Ipecac available (only if recommended by a poison control center)? Do you know how to give it properly?
10. What is the patient's condition (sensorium, heart rate, respiratory rate, temperature, skin color/turgor, pupils, sweating/salvation, etc.)?
11. Does the patient have any known illnesses?

Teratogenicity/Drugs in Pregnancy

1. What is the drug the patient received and what was the dose? What was the duration of therapy?
2. Is the patient pregnant or planning to become pregnant?
3. When during pregnancy was the exposure (trimester or weeks)?
4. What are the patient specifics (age, height, weight, sex)?
5. Was the patient adherent?
6. For what indication was the drug being prescribed?

Drugs in Breast Milk/Lactation

1. What is the drug the patient received and what was the dose? What was the duration of therapy?
2. How long has the infant been breast feeding?
3. Has the infant ever received nonmaternal nutrition? Is bottle feeding a plausible alternative?
4. What is the frequency of the breast feeds? What is the milk volume?
5. How old is the infant?
6. Does the mother have hepatic or renal insufficiency?
7. What was the indication for prescribing the drug? Was this initial or alternate therapy?
8. Has the mother breast fed previously while on the drug?

*Specific questions for only selected types of requests presented; other specific questions would be appropriate for other types of requests.

3–1

Appendix 3–1

Performing a PubMed Search

PubMed Search

PubMed is a database maintained by the U.S. National Library of Medicine. It is available free to the public online at: https://www.ncbi.nlm.nih.gov/PubMed. The information indexed by PubMed includes MEDLINE, OldMEDLINE (articles from the 1950s to the mid-1960s), and citations from additional life science journals.

This database is especially helpful when looking for off-label uses of medications when tertiary resources do not contain pertinent information. For example, if a prescriber contacts you asking for information about the efficacy of fluoxetine in the treatment of anorexia nervosa, it may be appropriate to seek information from the primary literature. Users can begin a search using just one keyword (e.g., fluoxetine). As Figure 1 shows, only using the term "fluoxetine" yields 10,310 results. Users can narrow results by adding a second keyword, such as anorexia nervosa, and combining the two terms with the BOOLEAN operator AND.

While adding a second term (see Figure 2) narrowed the results, there are still 88. Users can now consider narrowing results further by exploring the limit options within the database. Databases allow users to limit search results based on a variety of factors, including: language of publication, species, year of publication, type of article (e.g., human study, review, case report), or by type of journal where publication is found. There are many other limits available depending on the database. Since the requestor is seeking efficacy data in the fluoxetine example, we can limit the search results to clinical trials.

Users can identify a more manageable number of possibly useful citations by limiting the results to only human clinical trials published in English (23 citations of possible interest vs. 88; see Figure 3). Now a user can review the abstracts for these citations (Figure 4) and determine if these are helpful in answering the provider's question. Users can view an abstract by clicking on the blue hyperlinked title of an article. The abstract summarizes the information in the article and provides complete citation information for that article. Sometimes the information contained in an abstract may not represent the data in the full-text article; in some cases, you may exclude pertinent articles if only abstracts are reviewed. If the publisher's website offers full text of an article, a link is provided at the top of the page to the journal website. Some journals charge a fee for access to full-text articles, while others do not (i.e., open-access journals). Articles from open-access journals are clearly marked as "free full text." You can then select that icon and go directly to a full-text PDF or html of the desired article.

One additional helpful feature offered by PubMed is the "Similar articles" tab. The database will first identify the keywords or Medical Subject Headings (MeSH) headings associated with the article selected and then identify secondary words and terms. The database will compare these terms (both primary and secondary) with other articles indexed in PubMed to determine which include similarly ranked terms, and therefore, might be of interest.

The best way to effectively search this database is by gaining experience. PubMed also offers a tutorial to help teach users how to effectively conduct literature searches within the database. This interactive tutorial is available at https://learn.nlm.nih.gov/documentation/training-packets/T0042010P/.

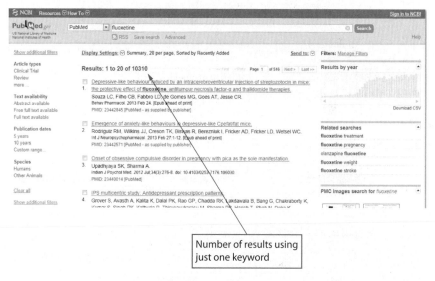

Figure 1. Keyword search.

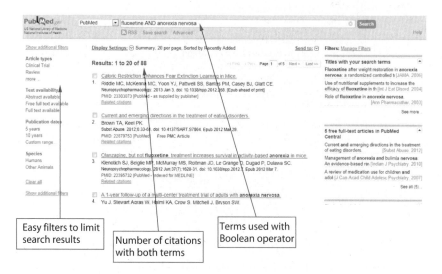

Figure 2. Multiple keyword search.

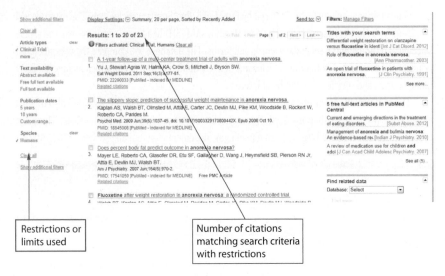

Restrictions or limits used

Number of citations matching search criteria with restrictions

Figure 3. Results of search with restrictions.

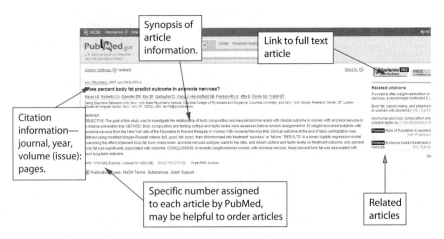

Synopsis of article information.

Link to full text article

Citation information—journal, year, volume (issue): pages.

Specific number assigned to each article by PubMed, may be helpful to order articles

Related articles

Figure 4. PubMed abstract.

Appendix 3–2

Selected Primary Literatures Sources

Journal Title	Publisher	ISSN	Areas Covered
American Journal of Health-System Pharmacy (AJHP)	American Society of Health-System Pharmacists (ASHP)	1079-2082 (print) 1535-2900 (online)	Clinical and managerial areas of pharmacy practice in health systems
American Journal of Pharmaceutical Education (AJPE)	American Association of Colleges of Pharmacy (AACP)	0002-9459 (print) 1553-6467 (online)	Scholarship and advancement of pharmacy education
Annals of Internal Medicine	American College of Physicians	0003-4819 (print) 1539-3704 (online)	Internal medicine, including management of disease states
Annals of Pharmacotherapy	SAGE Publications	1060-0280 (print) 1542-6270 (online)	Safe, effective, and economical use of drugs
Antimicrobial Agents and Chemotherapy	American Society for Microbiology	0066-4804 (print) 1098-6596 (online)	Information regarding the use of antimicrobial agents
The BMJ (formerly British Medical Journal)	BMJ	0959-8138 (print) 1756-1833 (online)	A wide range of primary and tertiary papers regarding human health and includes a suite of journals focusing on specialty care
Chest	American College of Chest Physicians	0012-3692 (print) 1931-3543 (online)	A wide range of research papers related to pulmonary and respiratory conditions, critical care, imaging, and cardiovascular diseases
Circulation	American Heart Association	0009-7322 (print) 1524-4539 (online)	Topics related to cardiovascular and cerebrovascular research, including clinical practice guidelines
Clin-Alert	SAGE Publications	0069-4770 (print) 1530-812X (online)	Focus on adverse drug reactions, drug-drug and drug-food interactions, and medication errors

Journal Title	Publisher	ISSN	Areas Covered
Clinical Pharmacokinetics	Adis International	0312-5963 (print) 1179-1926 (online)	Focus on pharmacokinetic and pharmacodynamic properties of drugs
Clinical Pharmacology & Therapeutics	Wiley	0009-9236 (print) 1532-6535 (online)	The effect of drugs on the human body
Drug Topics	MJH Life Sciences	0012-6616 (print) 1937-8157 (online)	Clinical topics, issues impacting both community pharmacy and health systems, and new drug therapies
Drugs	Adis International	0012-6667 (print) 1179-1950 (online)	Pharmacotherapeutic aspects of both new and established drugs
Hospital Pharmacy	SAGE Publications	0018-5787 (print) 1945-1253 (online)	Issues related to pharmacy in institutional settings
International Journal of Pharmaceutical Compounding	International Journal of Compounding Pharmacy, Inc.	1092-4221 (print) 1943-5223 (online)	Pharmaceutical compounding including recipes and stability data
JACCP: Journal of the American College of Clinical Pharmacy	Wiley	2574-9870 (online)	Published by American College of Clinical Pharmacy and focused on clinical pharmacy services, education and training, practice models, and outcomes
JAMA (The Journal of the American Medical Association)	American Medical Association	0098-7484 (print) 1538-3598 (online)	New research and review information that impacts health care
Journal of Cardiovascular Pharmacology	Wolters Kluwer Health	0160-2446 (print) 1533-4023 (online)	New information about the treatment of cardiovascular disease
The Journal of Clinical Pharmacology	Wiley	0091-2700 (print) 1552-4604 (online)	Clinical information about the safety, tolerability, efficacy, therapeutic use, and toxicology of drugs
Journal of Pharmaceutical Sciences	Elsevier	0022-3549 (print) 1520-6017 (online)	Application of physical and analytical chemistry to pharmaceutical sciences
The Journal of Pharmacology and Experimental Therapeutics	American Society for Pharmacology and Experimental Therapeutics	0022-3565 (print) 1521-0103 (online)	Covers interaction between chemicals and biological systems as well as metabolism, distribution, and toxicology

continued

Journal Title	Publisher	ISSN	Areas Covered
Journal of Pharmacy and Pharmacology	Wiley	0022-3573 (print) 2042-7158 (online)	Addresses a variety of practice areas including: drug delivery systems, biomaterials and polymers, and implications of human genome on drug therapies
Journal of The American Pharmacists Association	American Pharmacists Association	1544-3191 (print) 1544-3450 (online)	News, information, and research in the area of pharmacotherapeutic management
The Lancet	Elsevier	0140-6736 (print) 1474-547X (online)	New topics and research related to human health and include a suite of journals that focus on specialty areas of health care
Mayo Clinic Proceedings	Elsevier	0025-6196 (print) 1942-5546 (online)	A variety of articles related to health research, policy, and meeting reports as well as clinical practice recommendations
The Medical Letter	The Medical Letter, Inc.	0025-732X (print) 1523-2859 (online)	Provides information on new drug therapies and drugs of choice for disease management
New England Journal of Medicine	Massachusetts Medical Society	0028-4793 (print) 1533-4406 (online)	Results of recent research considered important to the practice of medicine
P&T	MMMM Group LLC	1052-1372 (print)	Focus on managed care and hospital formulary management
Pharmaceutical Research	Springer US	0724-8741 (print) 1573-904X (online)	Emphasis on drug delivery, drug formulation, pharmacokinetics, pharmacodynamics, and drug disposition
PharmacoEconomics	Adis International	1170-7690 (print) 1179-2027 (online)	Information regarding the economical use of drug therapies
Pharmacological Reviews	American Society of Pharmacology and Experimental Therapeutics	0031-6997 (print) 1521-0081 (online)	Current topics of interest including: cellular pharmacology, drug metabolism and disposition, renal pharmacology, and neuropharmacology
Pharmacotherapy	Wiley	0277-0008 (print) 1875-9114 (online)	Published by American College of Clinical pharmacy and focused on original research in clinical practice

continued

Journal Title	Publisher	ISSN	Areas Covered
Pharmacy Times	Pharmacy & Healthcare Communications, LLC	0003-0627 (print) 2168-7234 (online)	Focus on new drug therapies and patient counseling as it relates to community pharmacy
PLoS ONE	Public Library of Science (PLOS)	1932-6203	First multidisciplinary open-access journal, covering diverse topics of primary research and systematic reviews
Therapeutic Drug Monitoring	Wolters Kluwer Health	0163-4356 (print) 1536-3694 (online)	Fosters exchange of knowledge between fields of pharmacology, pathology, toxicology, and analytical
Therapeutic Innovation & Regulatory Science	SAGE Publications	0092-8615 (print) 2164-9200 (online)	Technology related to disseminating drug information. Official journal of the Drug Information Association
U.S. Pharmacist	Jobson Medical Information LLC	0148-4818 (print) 2331-3501 (online)	Information regarding the practice of academic, ambulatory, community, and institutional pharmacy

Appendix 4–1

Drug Literature Assessment Questions for Clinical Trials

OVERALL ASSESSMENT

- Was the article published in a reputable, peer-reviewed journal?
- Are the investigator's training/education/practice sites adequate for the study objective?
- Can the funding source bias the study?

TITLE/ABSTRACT

- Was the title unbiased?
- Did the abstract contain information not found within the study?
- Did the abstract provide a clear overview of the purpose, methods, results, and conclusions of the study?

INTRODUCTION

- Did the authors provide sufficient background information to demonstrate the rationale for the study? What research gap does it fill?
- Were the study objectives clearly identified?
- What were the major null hypothesis and alternate hypothesis?

METHODS

- Was an appropriate study design used to answer the question?
- Were reasonable inclusion/exclusion criteria presented to represent an appropriate patient population?
- Was a selection bias present?
- Was subject recruitment described? If so, how were subjects recruited? Was the method appropriate?
- Was IRB approval obtained?
- Was subject informed consent obtained?
- Were the intervention and control regimens appropriate?
- What type of blinding was used? Was this type appropriate?

- Was randomization included? If so, what type was used? Was this appropriate?
- Who generated the allocation sequence, enrolled participants, and assigned participants to groups? Was this appropriate?
- Which ancillary treatments were permitted? Would they have affected the outcome?
- Was a run-in period included? How does this affect the results?
- Did the investigators measure compliance? How was compliance measured? Was compliance adequate?
- Was the primary endpoint appropriate for the study objective?
- Were secondary endpoints measured? If so, were they adequate for what was being studied?
- Were subgroup analyses specified a priori? If so, were they appropriate?
- Was the method used to measure the primary endpoint appropriate?
- What type of data best describes the primary endpoint?
- Were data collected appropriately?
- How many patients were needed for the primary endpoint to detect a difference between groups (power analysis)? Was the necessary sample size calculated? Were there enough patients enrolled to reach this endpoint?
- What were the alpha (α) and beta (β) values? Were these appropriate?
- Were the statistical tests used appropriate?

RESULTS

- Were the numbers of patients screened, enrolled, administered treatment, completing, and withdrawing from the study reported? Were reasons for subject discontinuations reported? Were withdrawals handled appropriately?
- Was the trial adequately powered?
- Were the subject demographics between groups similar at baseline? If not, were the differences likely to have an effect on the outcome data?
- Were data presented clearly?
- Were the results adjusted to consider confounding variables?
- Was intention-to-treat analysis used? Was this appropriate?
- Were estimated effect size, p values, and confidence intervals reported?
- Were the results statistically significant? Clinically different?
- Was the null hypothesis accepted or rejected?
- Can the trial results be extrapolated to the population?
- Based on the results, could a Type I or Type II error have occurred?
- Are subgroup analyses presented? Are these appropriate?
- Was ancillary therapy included? Did this affect the study results?
- Were therapy adverse effects included?

CONCLUSIONS/DISCUSSION

- Did the information appear biased, and did the trial results support the conclusions?
- Were trial limitations described?

- Did the investigators explain unexpected results?
- Are the results able to be extrapolated to the population?
- Were the study results clinically meaningful?

REFERENCES

- Were the references listed well represented (e.g., current, well-representing the literature)?
- Is a comprehensive list of published articles related to the trial objective presented?

Drug Literature Assessment Questions for Other Study Designs

CASE REPORT/CASE SERIES

- Did the term "case report" or "case series" appear in the title?
- Was enough background information presented that relates to the particular case?
- Was the appropriate patient information included (e.g., demographics, symptoms, history)?
- Were the important clinical findings described?
- Were important dates and times relating to the case mentioned?
- Was the diagnostic assessment appropriate?
- Was the therapeutic intervention described in detail?
- Were follow-up and outcomes of the patient described?
- Was there a discussion of the strengths/limitations of the case?
- Were there any conclusions drawn or "take home" points mentioned?

CROSS-SECTIONAL, CASE-CONTROL, AND COHORT STUDIES

Title, Abstract, and Introduction

- Did the title and abstract contain the appropriate information?
- Was the research question clearly stated?

Methods

- Was the design of the study appropriate?
- How were the patients selected?
- Was matching used to create the groups?
- How was the sample size determined?
- Were the exposures and outcomes clearly defined?
- Were the statistical tests appropriate for the outcomes?
- What steps were taken to identify and address confounders?
- Were sources of bias identified?

Results

- Was the number of patients mentioned at each stage of the study?
- Was the duration/follow-up of the study appropriate?
- What were the patient characteristics at baseline?
- Were the results for all primary outcomes provided?
- Were other results for additional analysis provided?

Discussion, Conclusion, and Funding

- Were the main findings summarized appropriately?
- Did the authors mention the strengths and limitations of the study?
- Was the conclusion appropriate?
- Was funding or conflicts of interest mentioned?

NARRATIVE (NONSYSTEMATIC) REVIEWS

- Was the review balanced and objective?
- Was the search for studies comprehensive?
- Was the population clearly defined?
- Did the included studies use valid research methods?
- Were the outcomes of included studies clinically important?
- Were differences in the results and conclusions of included studies explored?
- Were benefits and risks of the drug therapy considered?

SYSTEMATIC REVIEWS (QUALITATIVE AND QUANTITATIVE)

Title, Abstract, and Introduction

- Was the title appropriate?
- Was the abstract appropriate?
- Was the introduction appropriate?
- Was the objective clearly stated?

Methods

- Was the search for studies comprehensive?
- Were the eligibility criteria appropriate?
- Was the quality of included studies assessed?
- Were the processes for data collection appropriate?
- Was the principal summary measure appropriate?
- Was the degree of heterogeneity assessed?
- If quantitative, what model was used to pool data?
- If quantitative, was the risk of publication bias assessed?
- Were additional analyses planned?

Results

- Was the number of studies identified, screened, eligible, and included provided?
- Were the important characteristics of included studies provided?
- Were the results for all main analyses provided?
- Was the quality of included studies acceptable?
- If quantitative, was the risk of publication bias acceptable?
- Were the results for all additional analyses provided?

Discussion, Conclusion, and Funding

- Were the main findings summarized?
- Were the strengths identified?
- Were the limitations identified?
- Was the conclusion appropriate?
- Was the source of funding disclosed?

N-OF-1 TRIALS

- Was assignment of active and control treatment to study periods randomized?
- Was the study blinded?
- Were multiple observation periods used?
- Were study endpoints clearly defined?
- Was the washout period between study periods adequate?

HEALTH OUTCOMES RESEARCH

- Were HR-QOL instruments validated?
- If a series of HR-QOL measurements were used, did this result in a valid HR-QOL battery?
- Were HR-QOL instruments sensitive to changes in the patients' status as the trial progressed?
- Were important aspects of patients' lives measured, as determined by patients themselves?
- Was timing of HR-QOL measurements to answer the research questions appropriately related to anticipated timing of the clinical effects?
- Were sequences of HR-QOL assessments conducted in the same order for all patients?
- Was mode of data collection (self-report vs. trained interviewer) appropriate for type of questions being asked?
  - If mode of data collection was a trained interviewer, could the interview location lead to biased answers?
- Were response rates to questionnaires reported?
- Was there missing data?
  - If there was missing data, was there a specific pattern that suggested author manipulation providing desired results (missing data could have countered author's hypothesis)?
- If a multicenter trial, did all sites evaluate HR-QOL?
- Was the HR-QOL instrument valid for examining the specific disease in question?
- Were both positive and negative findings reported?
- Were adverse drug events and HR-QOL measurements considered separately?

- Was impact of treatment effects included with HR-QOL measurements?
- Was there evidence that culturally defined factors may have impacted patient HR-QOL measurements and/or the assessment of these measurements?
- Did there appear to be a bias on the part of the study researchers?
- Were general measures of quality of life evaluated?

STABILITY STUDIES

- Were study methodologies and test conditions clearly defined?
- Were validated assays used?
- Were assays validated using time-zero measurements and an adequate number of test samples taken?

BIOEQUIVALENCE STUDIES

- Did the protocol define the characteristics of the subjects?
- Were confounding factors (e.g., smoking, alcohol use) identified and controlled?
- Was a crossover design used?
- Was the study randomized and blinded?

POSTMARKETING STUDIES

- Was a large enough sample studied to reflect current uses of and side effects associated with the new drug therapy?
- Were appropriate methods used to measure clearly defined endpoints?

QUALITY IMPROVEMENT RESEARCH

- What study design was utilized to assess the QI initiative and how likely was it to introduce bias?
- Was the QI study designed to target clinicians? If so, was their performance directly evaluated?
- Were the outcomes measured appropriate? Were patient-centered outcomes considered?
- Were staff trained to appropriately collect data and was there oversight of these processes?
- Were missing data considered and reported?
- Was flow of participants reported?
- Have the study findings been demonstrated in any other research?
- Can this initiative be successful in the setting where the reader practices?
- What are the cost and potential unintended consequences of introducing the initiative?

SURVEY RESEARCH

- Was there a good chance for most members of the population to be included in the sample?
- How were potential participants recognized and recruited?
- What sampling method was used?
- What steps were used to make sure the sample was representative of the population? Were they effective?
- Did the authors address sampling error?
- Was the sample representative of the target population?

- Were data quantifiable?
- Was the sample size large enough to detect a difference between groups?
- Was response rate high enough to reflect results that would be expected of the target population?
- Did the investigators determine whether nonresponders differed from responders?
- Were adjustments made for nonresponse and, if so, how did these affect results?
- How was the survey administered?
- Was the survey objective and carefully planned? Were questions unbiased and clear?
- Was the survey instrument valid and reliable? Was a pretest or pilot test conducted on the survey instrument?
- Were any steps taken to ensure respondents were truthful? Were any respondents removed from the field?
- How long was the survey in the field?
- Were incentives offered to participate?
- What is the reputation and record of the organization conducting the survey?

EDUCATIONAL RESEARCH

- Does the study fill an existing knowledge gap?
- Does the study design selected support the rationale for the research?
- Did the investigators use objective data that demonstrates learning as the primary outcome? If not, were investigators assessing metacognition (i.e., student evaluation of their own knowledge) or motivation?
- Does the report provide enough detail that the research can be replicated?
- Does the research describe methods and results, including interventions, outcomes, participants, and settings, that are relevant and generalizable to you or your institution?

NATURAL MEDICINES MEDICAL LITERATURE

Botanicals

- What plant species was used? Which plant part?
- Was a standardized extract used and was it appropriate?
- Was the study product stability ensured?
- Was the dose appropriate? What about dosage form and/or route of administration (especially important for cannabis trials)?
- Was blinding ensured and evaluated?
- Was the trial length appropriate to perceive treatment effects or differences?
- Was sample size sufficient to detect a difference between groups if one exists?

Nonbotanicals

- Was a specific salt form used and was it appropriate?
- Was the dose appropriate?
- Was the trial length appropriate to perceive treatment effects or differences?
- Was sample size sufficient to detect a difference between groups if one exists?

Appendix 8–1

Grade Evidence Profile: Antibiotics for Children with Acute Otitis Media

Quality Assessment						Summary of Findings					
Number of studies (Design)	**Limitations**	**Inconsistency**	**Indirectness**	**Imprecision**	**Publication bias**	**Number of patients**		**Relative risk (95% CI)**	**Absolute risk**		**Quality**
						Placebo	**Antibiotics**		**Control risk**[a]	**Risk difference (95% CI)**	
Pain at 24 hours											
5 (RCT)	No serious limitations	No serious inconsistency	No serious indirectness	No serious imprecision	Undetected	241/605	223/624	RR 0.9 (0.78–1.04)	367/1000	Not significant	⊕⊕⊕⊕ High
Pain at 2–7 days											
10 (RCT)	No serious limitations	No serious inconsistency	No serious indirectness	No serious imprecision	Undetected	303/1366	228/1425	RR 0.72 (0.62–0.83)	257/1000	72 fewer per 1000 (44–98)	⊕⊕⊕⊕ High
Hearing, inferred from the surrogate outcome abnormal tympanometry—1 month											
4 (RCT)	No serious limitations	No serious inconsistency	Serious indirectness (because of indirectness of outcome)	No serious imprecision	Undetected	168/460	153/467	RR 0.89 (0.75–1.07)	350/1000	Not significant	⊕⊕⊕○ Moderate
Hearing, inferred from the surrogate outcome abnormal tympanometry—3 months											
3 (RCT)	No serious limitations	No serious inconsistency (because of indirectness of outcome)	Serious indirectness	No serious imprecision	Undetected	96/398	96/410	RR 0.97 (0.76–1.24)	234/1000	Not significant	⊕⊕⊕○ Moderate
Vomiting, diarrhea, or rash											
5 (RCT)	No serious limitations	Serious inconsistency (because of inconsistency in absolute effects)	No serious indirectness	No serious imprecision	Undetected	83/711	110/690	RR 1.38 (1.09–1.76)	113/1000	43 more per 1000 (10–86)	⊕⊕⊕○ Moderate

[a] The control rate is based on the median control group risk across studies.

GRADE = Grading of Recommendations Assessment, Development, and Evaluation; RCT = randomized controlled trials; CI = confidence interval; RR = risk ratio.

Reproduced from Journal of Clinical Epidemiology, Vol 64, Gordon Guyatt, Andrew D. Oxman, Elie A. Akl, Regina Kunz, Gunn Vist, et al. Grade guidelines: Introduction GRADE evidence profiles and summary of findings tables. p. 383–394, Copyright 2011, with permission from Elsevier.

12–1

Appendix 12–1

Code of Ethics for Pharmacists[1]

Pharmacists are health professionals who assist individuals in making the best use of medications. This Code, prepared and supported by pharmacists, is intended to state publicly the principles that form the fundamental basis of the roles and responsibilities of pharmacists. These principles, based on moral obligations and virtues, are established to guide pharmacists in relationships with patients, health professionals, and society.

I. A pharmacist respects the covenantal relationship between the patient and pharmacist.

Considering the patient-pharmacist relationship as a covenant means that a pharmacist has moral obligations in response to the gift of trust received from society. In return for this gift, a pharmacist promises to help individuals achieve optimum benefit from their medications, to be committed to their welfare, and to maintain their trust.

II. A pharmacist promotes the good of every patient in a caring, compassionate, and confidential manner.

A pharmacist places concern for the well-being of the patient at the center of professional practice. In doing so, a pharmacist considers needs stated by the patient as well as those defined by health science. A pharmacist is dedicated to protecting the dignity of the patient. With a caring attitude and a compassionate spirit, a pharmacist focuses on serving the patient in a private and confidential manner.

III. A pharmacist respects the autonomy and dignity of each patient.

A pharmacist promotes the right of self-determination and recognizes individual self-worth by encouraging patients to participate in decisions about their health. A pharmacist communicates with patients in terms that are understandable. In all cases, a pharmacist respects personal and cultural differences among patients.

IV. A pharmacist acts with honesty and integrity in professional relationships.

A pharmacist has a duty to tell the truth and to act with conviction of conscience. A pharmacist avoids discriminatory practices, behavior or work conditions that impair professional judgment, and actions that compromise dedication to the best interests of patients.

V. A pharmacist maintains professional competence.

A pharmacist has a duty to maintain knowledge and abilities as new medications, devices, and technologies become available and as health information advances.

1341

VI. A pharmacist respects the values and abilities of colleagues and other health professionals.

When appropriate, a pharmacist asks for the consultation of colleagues or other health professionals or refers the patient. A pharmacist acknowledges that colleagues and other health professionals may differ in the beliefs and values they apply to the care of the patient.

VII. A pharmacist serves individual, community, and societal needs.

The primary obligation of a pharmacist is to individual patients. However, the obligations of a pharmacist may at times extend beyond the individual to the community and society. In these situations, the pharmacist recognizes the responsibilities that accompany these obligations and acts accordingly.

VIII. A pharmacist seeks justice in the distribution of health resources.

When health resources are allocated, a pharmacist is fair and equitable, balancing the needs of patients and society.

Adopted by the membership of the American Pharmacists Association, October 27, 1994.

REFERENCE

1. American Pharmacists Association. Code of ethics 1994 [updated 1994 Oct 27; 2010 Mar 26]. Available from: http://www.pharmacist.com/code-ethics.

13–1

Appendix 13–1

Question Example

DRUG INFORMATION CENTER

St. Anywhere Hospital

Name of Inquirer:	Dr. Meghan J. Malone	Date: XX/XX/XX
Address:	2184 Fall St. Seneca Falls, NY 13148	Time Received: XX:XX am/pm
		Time Required: 5 hours
		Nature of Request: Therapeutics
Telephone Number:	(315)555-1212	Type of Inquirer: Pharmacist

QUESTION

A young, adult male patient recently arrived from Japan and presented to the physician with sparse medical records indicating he is suffering from Tsutsugamushi disease. Because of the language difficulties, little is known about the patient, other than he is taking drug X for the illness. Physical exam reveals a patient in some discomfort with elevated temperature, swollen lymph glands, and red rash. All other findings appear to be normal. (*Note:* the person answering this question obtained as much background as possible about the patient.) The physician has little information on the disease and would like to know if that drug X is the most appropriate treatment.

ANSWER

Tsutsugamushi disease is an acute infectious disease seen in harvesters of hemp in Japan.[1] It is caused by *Rickettsia tsutsugamushi*. Common symptoms of the disease include fever, painful swelling of the lymph glands, a small black scab in the genital region, neck or axilla, and large dark-red papules. The disease is known by a number of other names, including akamushi disease, flood fever, inundation fever, island disease, Japanese river fever, and scrub typhus.[2-4] (*Note:* background information presented.) The standard treatment of the disease includes either drug X or drug Y, although there are several other less effective treatments.[5-7] In the remainder of this paper, a comparison of the two major drugs will be presented. (*Note:* clear objective for paper is presented.)

A thorough search of the available literature was conducted. Unfortunately, there were few textbooks available on this disease. A search of MEDLINE® (1966 to present) and Embase® Drugs and Pharmacology (1980 to present) produced a number of articles that were obtained and are reviewed below. (*Note:* This documents the type of search and acts as a lead-in to the remainder of the body of the paper.)

Smith and Jones[8] performed a double-blind, randomized comparison of the effects of drug X and drug Y in patients with Tsutsugamushi fever. Patients were required to be between 18 and 70 years old, and could not have any concurrent infection or disorder that would affect the immune response to the disease (e.g., neutropenia, AIDS). Twenty patients received 10 mg of drug X three times a day for 15 days. Eighteen patients received 250 mg of drug Y twice a day for 10 days. The two groups were comparable, except that the patients receiving drug X were an average of 5 years younger ($p < 0.05$). Drug X was shown to produce a cure, both in terms of symptoms and cultures in 85% of patients, whereas drug Y only produced a cure in 55.5% of patients. The difference was statistically significant ($p < 0.01$). No significant adverse effects were seen in either group. Although it appears that drug X was the better agent, it should be noted that drug Y was given at its minimally effective dose, and may have performed better in a somewhat higher dose or longer regimen. (*Note:* evaluative comments made about article.)

(*Note:* Other articles would be described at this point.)

Based on the literature found, it appears that drug Y is generally accepted as the better agent, except in those patients with severe renal insufficiency. Because this patient does not appear to be suffering from that problem, it is recommended that he receive a 3-week course of drug Y at a dose of 500 mg three times a day. Renal function should be monitored weekly. The patient should receive an additional week of therapy, if the symptoms have not been gone for the final week of therapy. (*Note:* This patient's situation was specifically addressed, rather than just presenting a general conclusion.)

Signature: _____ Date: March 20, 2019

        Mia Q. Pharmacist, PharmD, BCPS

REFERENCES

(References used in answering the above question would be provided here. The citation numbers in the above paragraphs are for example only and do not refer to actual references in this example.)

Appendix 13–2

Abstracts

Abstracts are a synopsis (usually 250 words or less) of the most important aspect of an article. They should be clear, concise, and complete enough for readers to have a reasonable understanding of the important portions of the article.[1] Since they are the most commonly read part of an article, they must be accurate and avoid the three most common errors: differences in information presented in the abstract and in the body of the article, information given in the abstract that was not presented in the article, and conclusions presented in the abstract that are not supported by information in the abstract.[2-4]

There are basically three types of abstracts that are seen in the literature. The first two (descriptive and informational) are somewhat traditional; however, they do not convey as much information as structured abstracts. Structured abstracts were originally designed to convey more information, and have been in use since the 1980s. The type of abstract to be used depends on the type of information and the requirements of the place the work is being submitted or used.

In addition to writing an abstract, some journals ask that indexing terms (sometimes called key words) be submitted. Whenever possible, Medical Subject Headings (MeSH) from the National Library of Medicine should be used for the indexing terms (they may be found at https://www.nlm.nih.gov/mesh/MBrowser.html). Each of the abstracts will be discussed in more detail in the following sections.

DESCRIPTIVE ABSTRACTS

A descriptive abstract, as its name implies, simply describes the information found in an article. Few specific details are given, and it is primarily used in a review article. An example of this type of abstract is as follows:

> Lists of references that should be available, depending on location of the drug information service, are presented. These lists are specific to community, hospital, long-term care facility, and academic sites. Included are general references, indexing and abstracting services, and journals. Specialty references that would be useful in specific circumstances are also presented. In addition, the equipment and software necessary to access the computerized resources are shown for the individual references.

INFORMATIONAL ABSTRACTS

Informational abstracts concisely summarize the factual information presented in a study. This type of abstract is more applicable to clinical studies.

1345

Key points in an informational abstract include:

- Study design (e.g., double-blind, crossover)
- Purpose
- Number of patients and other demographic aspects
- Dosages
- Results
- Conclusions

An example of this type of abstract is as follows:

A double-blind, randomized comparison of the effects of drug X and drug Y was performed in patients with Tsutsugamushi disease, in order to determine whether either drug was superior in efficacy or safety. Twenty patients received 10 mg of drug X three times a day for 15 days. Eighteen patients received 250 mg of drug Y twice a day for 10 days. The two groups were comparable, except that the patients receiving drug X were an average of 5 years younger ($p < 0.05$). Drug X was shown to produce a cure, both in terms of symptoms and cultures in 85% of patients, whereas drug Y only produced a cure in 55.5% of patients. The difference was statistically significant ($p < 0.01$). No significant adverse effects were seen in either group. Drug X was shown to be significantly better than drug Y in the treatment of tsutsugamushi fever.

STRUCTURED ABSTRACTS

Due to perceived deficiencies in abstracts,[5] including lack of sufficient information,[6] another type of abstract was presented in 1987[7] and later updated in 1990.[8] The most recent version of this was published in 2008.[9] This structured abstract was designed to present more information about clinical studies and possibly laboratory studies, as compared to the informational abstract presented earlier.[10,11] This type of abstract is not meant for case reports, studies of tissues or animals, opinion articles, and position papers.[8] Abstracts following this standard have gained popularity[12] and have been mandated by an influential group of journals (e.g., New England Journal of Medicine,[13] Annals of Internal Medicine,[8] JAMA: Journal of the American Medical Association,[10] BMJ,[14] Canadian Medical Association Journal,[15] CHEST[16]), sometimes in a somewhat modified form (e.g., the PICO model used by BMJ[17] and their newer, shorter print abstract[18]), although this type of abstract may not be used in the majority of articles found in popular medical journals.[19] This type of abstract has also been suggested in the pharmacy literature.[20] Although the overall acceptance and approval of this format of abstract appears to be good, there are some who disapprove.[21–23] Also, there is some data suggesting that structured abstracts do not always contain as much information as they should, if the published rules are followed,[24] and that they do not necessarily contain any more useful information than informational abstracts.[25]

It is worth noting that articles with structured abstracts are indexed with a greater number of terms in MEDLINE®, which may make it easier to find such articles in a computer search.[26]

An abstract following this procedure would contain the following subheadings and information:

- *Title*—The title should be descriptive and identify the study as being randomized.
- *Authors*—This should provide contact details for the corresponding author, including such things as mail address, email address, and phone numbers. Please note that this item is specific to conference abstracts only.

- *Trial Design*—The basic design of the study (e.g., randomized, double-blind, crossover, placebo-controlled, parallel, prospective vs. retrospective, noninferiority).
- *Methods*
  - *Participants*—Description of the eligibility requirements for those participating in the study and also the setting for data collection.
  - *Intervention(s)*—A brief description of any treatment(s) or intervention(s) for each group.
  - *Objective*—The main objective or hypothesis of the study and key secondary objectives.
  - *Main outcome measure(s)*—The primary study outcome, as planned before data collection was begun (*a priori*).
  - *Randomization*—How the study subjects were allocated to the interventions.
  - *Blinding (masking)*—Identify who, if anyone, was blinded to the group assignment, including the patient (single-blind), patient and caregivers (double-blind), or even other additional people (triple-blind).
- *Results*
  - *Numbers randomized*—The number of subjects randomized to each group.
  - *Recruitment*—This should indicate whether the trial is still ongoing, closed to recruitment, or closed to follow-up. The first two categories indicate whether this is an interim analysis.
  - *Numbers analyzed*—Provides the number of subjects analyzed in each group.
  - *Outcome*—The result for each group for the primary outcome, including its estimated effect size and precision.
  - *Harms*—Any important adverse effects.
- *Conclusion(s)*—The key conclusion(s) directly supported by the evidence presented in the study and their clinical application(s).
- *Trial registration*—The registration number and trial register name.
- *Funding*—Source of funding.

An example of this type of abstract is as follows:

Title—A randomized study to compare the safety and efficacy of drug X and drug Y in the treatment of Tsutsugamushi disease.

Authors—Correspondence to: Dr. Mia D. Labrador, Grammie's Place Clinic, 198 Fall St., Seneca Falls, NY 13148, USA. Tel: +1(315)555-6147; Fax: +1(315)555-5689; email: mial@gpc.org.

Trial Design—Randomized, parallel group trial.

Methods

Participants—Trial conducted between June 20XX and December 20XX at a tertiary care, military hospital located on Guam. Male patients between 18 and 50 years old with tsutsugamushi fever were randomly assigned to receive drug X and drug Y.

Interventions—Patients received either 10 mg of drug X three times a day for 15 days or 250 mg of drug Y twice a day for 10 days.

Objective—To compare the effectiveness of drug X and drug Y in the treatment of tsutsugamushi fever.

Outcome—Physician and patients' global assessment of disease activity; five-point scale from 0 (no symptoms) to 5 (severe disability). Cure was defined as absence of organism on laboratory specimens.

Randomization—Random computer-generated randomization of patients to one of two groups.

Blinding—Patients, caregivers, and those assessing study outcomes were blinded to group assignment.

Results

Numbers randomized—Sequential sample of 40 young (age 20–37 years old), otherwise healthy male patients with tsutsugamushi fever randomly allocated to receive 10 mg of drug X three times a day for 15 days (n = 20) or 250 mg of drug Y twice a day for 10 days (n = 20).

Recruitment—Trial is closed to follow-up.

Numbers analyzed—Of 40 patients entered into study, 38 were included in analysis, 20 received drug X, and 18 received drug Y. Two patients were removed from the drug Y group, due to transfer to U.S. mainland hospitals.

Outcome—Drug X was shown to produce a cure, both in terms of symptoms and cultures in 85% of patients, whereas drug Y only produced a cure in 55.5% of patients. The difference was statistically significant ($p < 0.01$). A level of significance was set at less than or equal to 0.05, using X^2 test.

Harms—No significant adverse effects were seen in either group.

Conclusions—Drug X was shown to produce significantly higher cure rates than drug Y in the treatment of tsutsugamushi fever, with no difference in adverse effects.

Trial registration—www.clinicaltrials.gov; Identifier: NCT03089731.

Funding—Tsutsugamushi Research Foundation.

The Preferred Reporting Items for Systemic Reviews and Meta-Analysis (PRISMA) contains directions for abstracts for systemic reviews that are similar to the above. Further information can be found at http://www.prisma-statement.org/.

A method to prepare a structured abstract for a review article differs from the first example.[27] This method would only be applicable in specific situations, where a number of similar studies were evaluated together. It would not be useful in a situation where a number of dissimilar articles dealing with the same topic were discussed (e.g., a review of all therapies for a particular disease). This method was last updated in 2013.[28] Such an abstract would consist of the following items:

- *Title*—Identifies the report as a systematic review, meta-analysis, or both.
- *Objective*—The research question, including such things as participants, interventions, comparators, and the outcomes.
- *Methods*
  - *Eligibility criteria*—Characteristics of study or report that are used as the criteria for inclusion.
  - *Information sources*—A brief summary of data sources and the time periods covered.

- ○ *Risk of bias*—Provides the methods of assessing any bias risk.
- • Results
  - ○ *Included studies*—The number of studies covered in the article and how they were selected for inclusion, including characteristics, with reasons for excluding other studies.
  - ○ *Synthesis of results* — The results for main outcomes. Preferably will indicate the number of studies and participants in each. In the case of meta-analysis, should include summary measures and confidence intervals.
  - ○ *Description of the effect*—Direction and size of the effect in meaningful clinical terms.
- • Discussion
  - ○ *Strengths and limitations of evidence*—Summarize the strength and limitations of the evidence.
  - ○ *Interpretation*—Result interpretation and important implications.
- • *Funding*—Primary source for funding.
- • *Registration*—Registration name and number

An example of this type of abstract would be as follows:

Title—Systematic analysis and meta-analysis of drug X on symptoms of allergic reactions.
Objective—To evaluate the effect of the antihistamine, drug X, on symptoms of allergic reactions, as determined by physicians' and patients' global symptom assessment.
Methods

Eligibility criteria—Randomized control trials evaluating drug X in the treatment of patients with allergies.

Information sources—Studies published from January 1980 to December 2019 were identified by computer searches of MEDLINE® and Embase®—Drugs and Pharmacology and hand searching of bibliographies of the articles identified via the computer search.

Risk of bias—Bias was assessed in regards to randomization, blinding, lack of outcome data, and selective reporting.
Results

Included studies—Fifty-three studies (n = 10,234 patients) evaluating the effects of drug X in the treatment of allergies were located.

Synthesis of results—Fifty-three studies (n = 10,234 patients) showed a significant reduction in allergic symptoms, relative risk 0.78, 0.56–0.89.

Description of the effect—Subjective and objective measures of effectiveness demonstrated that drug X decreased or eliminated allergy symptoms approximately 80% of the time in a variety of patient types (e.g., seasonal allergic rhinitis, perennial allergic rhinitis, anaphylaxis). The only adverse effects seen were dryness of mucous membranes and sedation, seen in approximately 5% and 2% of patients, respectively.
Discussion

Strengths and limitations of evidence—Four of the studies were open label. Duration of 11 studies was only 2 weeks.

Interpretation—Drug X is an effective agent for the treatment of allergic reactions. It has a low incidence of typical antihistamine adverse effects. Further studies should be performed to verify the effectiveness of drug X in comparison to other drugs commonly used for anaphylaxis.

Funding—This study was not funded by any outside organization.

Registration—PROSPERO 2019:CRD123456789012.

A version of a structured abstract has also been proposed for use in describing clinical practice guidelines (see Chapter 8 for more information about such guidelines).[29] The format is as follows:

Objective—Provides the primary objective of the guideline. This must include the health problem, along with the targeted patients, providers, and settings.

Options—This includes the various clinical practice options that were considered when the guideline was formulated.

Outcomes—Presents the significant health and economic outcomes that were considered when the alternative practices were considered.

Evidence—Describes how and when the evidence was gathered, selected for use, and synthesized.

Values—Describes how values were assigned to the potential outcomes, along with who was involved in doing so.

Benefits, Harms, and Costs—Provides both the type and magnitude of the benefits, harms, and costs that might be expected from using the guideline.

Recommendations—Provides a summary of the key recommendations.

Validation—Describes any external validation of the guidelines that was conducted.

Sponsors—Provides a list of the people who developed, funded, and/or endorsed the guideline.

An example of this type of abstract would be as follows:

Objective: To determine the best initial therapy for allergic rhinitis. This guideline is intended for physicians and pharmacists to determine the best way to start therapy, particularly in the community.

Options: Different nonprescription medications are considered first (antihistamines, decongestants [systemic and local], cromolyn), with the place for intranasal steroids in initial therapy.

Outcomes: The major outcomes evaluated are relief of symptoms, adverse effects, and direct cost to the patient.

Evidence: All randomized, controlled clinical trials published in English found in MEDLINE from 1990 to 2019 were considered. In regard to costs, the average retail cost of the medication and the cost of a physician visit (for prescription medications) were calculated, based on what therapy was used in the studies.

Values: A group of three board-certified allergy physicians and three pharmacists board-certified in pharmacotherapy or ambulatory care were appointed by the American Academy of Allergy, Asthma & Immunology to review and evaluate the studies and pharmacoeconomic data. Patients were not represented.

Benefits, Harms, and Costs: Use of a second-generation antihistamine (e.g., loratadine, cetirizine) provides the greatest efficacy with the least cost. Decongestants may be of value in the first few days, but are contraindicated in hypertensive patients. All other therapies have less effectiveness or greater cost.

Recommendations: Patients suffering from allergies should begin therapy with an intranasal steroid spray, preferably at least a week prior to anticipated allergen exposure. If therapy cannot be started early, pseudoephedrine may be used for up to 3 days as part of initial therapy in patients without hypertension or other contraindications. If this therapy is not sufficient, patients should add a second-generation antihistamine.

Validations: This recommendation was reviewed by three reviewers in the normal peer-review process established by the American Academy of Allergy, Asthma & Immunology.

Sponsors: Development of this recommendation was funded by the American Academy of Allergy, Asthma & Immunology.

REFERENCES

1. Staub NC. On writing abstracts. Physiologist. 1991;34:276–7.
2. Pitkin RM, Branagan MA. Can the accuracy of abstracts be improved by providing specific instructions? A randomized controlled trial. JAMA. 1998;280:267–9.
3. Pitkin RM, Branagan MA, Burmeister LF. Accuracy of data in abstracts of published research articles. JAMA. 1999;281:1110–1.
4. Winker MA. The need for concrete improvement in abstract quality. JAMA. 1999;281:1129–30.
5. Huth EJ. Structured abstracts for papers reporting clinical trials. Ann Intern Med. 1987;106:626–7.
6. Narine L, Yee DS, Einarson TR, Ilersich AL. Quality of abstracts of original research articles in CMAJ in 1989. CMAJ. 1991;144:449–53.
7. Ad Hoc Working Group for Critical Appraisal of the Medical Literature. A proposal for more informative abstracts of clinical articles. Ann Intern Med. 1987;106:598–604.
8. Haynes RB, Mulrow CD, Huth EJ, Altman DG, Gardner MJ. More informative abstracts revisited. Ann Intern Med. 1990;113:69–76.
9. Hopewell S, Clarke M, Moher D, Wager E, Middleton P, Altman DG, Schutz KF, CONSORT Group. CONSORT for reporting randomized controlled trials in journal and conference abstracts: explanation and elaboration. PLoS Med. 2008 Jan;5(1):0048-56.
10. Rennie D, Glass RM. Structuring abstracts to make them more informative. JAMA. 1991;266:116–7.
11. Haynes RB. Dissent. More informative abstracts: current status and evaluation. J Clin Epidemiol. 1993;46:595–7.
12. Ripple AM, Mork JG, Knecht LS, Humphreys BL. A retrospective cohort study of structured abstracts in MEDLINE, 1992-2006. J Med Libr Assoc. 2011;99(2):160–3.
13. Relman AS. New "Information for Authors"—and readers. NEJM. 1990;323:56.
14. Lock S. Structure abstracts. Now required for all papers reporting clinical trials. BMJ. 1988;297:156.
15. Squires BP. Structured abstracts of original research and review articles. CMAJ. 1990;143:619–22.

16. Soffer A. Abstracts of clinical investigations. A new and standardized format. Chest. 1987;92: 389–90.

17. New format for BMJ research articles in print. BMJ. 2008;337:a294 6.

18. Restructured abstracts for research in The BMJ. BMJ. 2015;351:h5499.

19. Nakayama T, Hirai N, Yamazaki S, Naito M. Adoption of structured abstracts by general medical journals and format for a structured abstract. J Med Libr Assoc. 2005;93(2):237242.

20. Kane-Gill S, Olsen KM. How to write an abstract suitable for publication. Hosp Pharm. 2004;39:289–92.

21. Spitzer WO. Second thoughts. The structured sonnet. J Clin Epidemiol. 1991;44:729.

22. Heller MB. Dissent. Structured abstracts: a modest dissent. J Clin Epidemiol. 1991;44:739–40.

23. Heller MB. Structured abstracts [letter]. Ann Intern Med. 1990;113:722.

24. Froom P, Froom J. Variance and dissent. presentation. Deficiencies in structured medical abstracts. J Clin Epidemiol. 1993;46:591–4.

25. Scherer RW, Crawley B. Reporting of randomized clinical trial descriptors and use of structured abstracts. JAMA. 1998;280:269–72.

26. Harbourt AM, Knecht LS, Humphreys BL. Structured abstracts in MEDLINE®, 1989–1991. Bull Med Libr Assoc. 1995:83(2):190–5.

27. Mulrow CD, Thacker SB, Pugh JA. A proposal for more informative abstracts of review articles. Ann Intern Med. 1988;108:613–5.

28. Beller EM, Glasziou PP, Altman DG, Hopewell S, Bastian H, Chalmers I, Gotzsche PC, Lasserson T, Tovey D, PRISMA for Abstracts group. PRISMA for abstracts: reporting systematic reviews in journal and conference abstracts. PLoS Med. 2013;10(4):1–8.

29. Hayward RS, Wilson MC, Tunis SR, Bass EB, Rubin HR, Haynes RB. More informative abstracts of articles describing clinical practice guidelines. Ann Intern Med. 1993;118:731–7.

Appendix 13-3

Bibliography

Although there seems to be a different method to prepare a bibliography for every English class ever given, there is fortunately a standardized method to prepare a bibliography in medical writing. This method is used by the National Library of Medicine and has been incorporated into the Recommendations for the Conduct, Reporting, Editing, and Publication of Scholarly Work in Medical Journals[1] and published in Citing Medicine;[1-3] it has been used widely since the 1970s in both journals and other medical writing. This method will be presented here, although some other methods are sometimes employed in the literature.

References in the bibliography are usually placed in the order they are first cited in the text of a document, and each reference is assigned a consecutive Arabic number. Two acceptable variations involve citing the references at the end in alphabetical order by author. In one of those cases, the citations are numbered in that order and the number appears in the text. In the other, the citation in the text includes the author's name and year (e.g., Jones 2017).[3] Those cited only in tables or figures are numbered according to the place the table or figure is identified in the text. References are not listed multiple times in the bibliography, if they are cited more than once in the text of the document. Instead, subsequent citations to the same reference use the original reference number. The reference number in the text will be the Arabic number in superscript. This number is often cited after the sentence that contains the fact being referenced. If there are several references used to prepare a specific sentence, they may be listed at the end of the sentence or throughout the sentence. Also, if the sentence is a lead-in to an abstract, the authors' names are commonly listed followed by the reference number. See the sentences below for examples.

- Drug X has been shown to cause green rash with purple spots.[2,3]
- Drug Y is useful in the treatment of hypertension,[4] congestive heart failure,[5] and arrhythmias.[6]
- Smith and Jones[7] studied the effects of...
- Brown *et al.*[9] treated...(please notice on this example, *al.* is followed by a period since it is an abbreviation, whereas *et* is a full Latin word, and there is no need for a comma after the first author's name. The term *et al.* is italicized because it is Latin.)
- Brown and associates[9] treated... (this is used the same way as the previous example, but is preferred by some people over the use of *et al.*)

Before getting into the method for listing references and examples, it should be mentioned that there are a number of general rules to be followed. They are:

- Citations are often not found in conclusions of documents. The conclusions are based on the information presented, and cited, earlier in the article.
- Avoid using abstracts as references, if at all possible. Sometimes the information is only published as an abstract, so it is necessary to cite the abstract in this situation.
- Avoid using unpublished observations or personal communications as references. In the latter case, it is proper to insert references to communications in parentheses in the text only and indicate that it will not be formally referenced at the end of publication. Permission must be obtained from the author for the use of this material and this should only be used if the material is not available from a public source of information. A note should be made at the end of the publication, stating that permission was given.
- If reference is made to an article that has been accepted by a journal, but not yet published, the phrase Forthcoming followed by the year of planned publication should be inserted where the volume and page numbers would normally be listed. It is usually necessary to get permission to cite this type of article, since the publisher may have strict confidentiality rules, and verification of acceptance by the journal should be obtained if that is the case.
- Today the Internet is used very frequently, so it is important to use the correct citation based on where the reference is found.
- Only place a period at the end of a web address if a slash is the last character in the address.
- For items such as wikis, blogs, and databases, when they are still open (people can still add something), use a hyphen with three spaces following it for date of publication. If they are closed (people can no longer add something), list the range of dates it was open.
- Do not include any headers, such as "news" or "case report" unless the table of contents of the journal indicates that is officially part of the article title.
- Cite the name of the journal that was used when that journal was published. For example, British Medical Journal became BMJ in 1988 or Annals of Pharmacotherapy at various times has been known as Drug Intelligence and Clinical Pharmacy and DICP: the Annals of Pharmacotherapy.

Examples and some general templates of the above mentioned and other types of references used in a bibliography are provided in the remaining part of this appendix. Please note that these should provide adequate information on how to cite most publications. However, if detailed directions and further examples are needed, the reader is referred to Citing Medicine, which is available free on the Internet at http://nlm.nih.gov/citingmedicine.[3]

JOURNAL ARTICLES

To cite a journal article, the following information should be given:

- Last name of author(s) and initials (maximum of two) each separated by commas, with a period at the end. Please note that some publications will list only three or six authors followed by the phrase *et al.*; however, according to the standard, all authors must be listed regardless of how many unless space is limited. If an author's name has a suffix, such as Jr, that is inserted at the end (e.g., Smith AB Jr), but degrees are not listed. If a study group name is included after a specific author, separate that name from the individual authors using a semicolon.

- Title of article (do not use quotation marks, capitalize only the initial word of title and proper nouns in English) followed by a period with the exception when punctuation is already at the end of the title—for example, if a title ends with a question mark or exclamation point, use that instead of the period.
- Journal Title (abbreviated as found in the International Organization for Standardization [ISO] 4 List of Title Word Abbreviations [LTWA] that is found at http://www.issn.org/services/online-services/access-to-the-ltwa/ or the National Library of Medicine [NLM] catalog at https://www.ncbi.nlm.nih.gov/nlmcatalog/journals) followed by a period. Do not italicize the journal name. If this is an Internet article, put [Internet] after the journal name. Other types of medium would similarly be indicated (e.g., [microfiche], [microfilm]).
- Date of Publication (year, month (three-letter abbreviation), and day of month [if available]) followed by a semicolon.
- Volume number (listing the issue number in parenthesis) followed by a colon.
- Page numbers (If continuous, use first and last pages separated by a hyphen. Keep page numbers concise (e.g., 561–569 should be 561–9). If separate pages, list the pages separated by a comma and a space. If a combination of continuous and separate pages, use both (e.g., 18–29, 33, 40) followed by a period. If an Internet article does not have page numbers, put the actual number of pages in square brackets, followed by p. (e.g., [20 p.]). If the article is in unpaginated format (e.g., html, xml), precede the number with the word about (e.g., [about 10 screens] or [about 15 p.]). If a journal uses an article numbering scheme for Internet articles, be sure to use that number instead of a page number.

Generally speaking, if a piece of information listed above is not given by the publisher, it is simply omitted from the citation.

A condensed version of the above information is as follows:

Author(s). Title of article. Journal Title. Date of Publication;Volume Number (Issue Number): Page Number(s).

Journal on the Internet:

Author(s). Title of article. Journal Title [Internet]. Date of Publication [Date of Update; Date of Citation]; Volume Number(Issue Number):Page Number(s) or [Length of Article]. Available from: Web Address

Example Journal Citations

Standard Journal Article

Smythe M, Hoffman J, Kizy K, Dmuchowski C. Estimating creatinine clearance in elderly patients with low serum creatinine concentrations. Am J Hosp Pharm. 1994 Jan 15;51:198–204.

Beck DE, Aceves-Blumenthal C, Carson R, Culley J, Noguchi J, Dawson K, Hotchkiss G. Factors contributing to volunteer practitioner-faculty vitality. Am J Pharm Ed. 1993 Apr;57:305–12.

Journal Article on the Internet

Robinson ET. The pharmacist as educator: implications for practice and education. Am J Pharm Ed [Internet]. 2004 Aug 5 [cited 2016 Jul 24];68(3):Article 72 [4 p.]. Available from: http://www.ajpe.org/doi/pdf/10.5688/aj680372

Nemecz G. Evening primrose. US Pharmacist [Internet]. 1998 Nov [cited 1998 Dec 10];23: [about 1 p.]. Available from: http://www.uspharmacist.com/NewLook/Docs/1998/Nov1998/Evening Primrose.htm

Organization as Author

Task Force on Specialty Recognition of Oncology Pharmacy Practice. Executive summary of petition requesting specialty recognition of oncology pharmacy practice. Am J Hosp Pharm. 1994 Jan 15;51:219–24.

Personal Authors and Organization as Author

Wiencke K, Louka AS, Spurkland A, Vatn M; The IBSEN Study Group; Schrumpf E. Association of matrix metalloproteinase-1 and -3 promoter polymorphisms with clinical subsets of Norwegian primary sclerosing cholangitis patients. J Hepatol. 2004 Aug;41(2):209–14.

No Author Given

N.Y. court rules against Medicaid co-pay. Drug Topics. 1994 Mar;138(3):6.

Article Not in English

Translate into English and put the translation in square brackets; note that the language is stated at the end.

Antoni N. [For criticism of the erroneously called tendon- and periostreflex]. Acta Psychiatrica Neurologica. 1932;VII:9–19. German.

Volume with Supplement

Nayler WG. Pharmacological aspects of calcium antagonism: short term and long term benefits. Drugs. 1993 Apr;46 Suppl 2:40–7.

Issue with Supplement

Graves NM. Pharmacokinetics and interactions of antiepileptic drugs. Am J Hosp Pharm. 1993 Dec;50(12 Suppl A):S23–9.

Volume with Part

Katchen MS, Lyons TJ, Gillingham KK, Schlegel W. A case of left hypoglossal neurapraxia following G exposure in a centrifuge. Aviat Space Environ Med. 1990 Sep;61(Pt 2):837–9.

Issue with Part

Dudley MN. Maximizing patient outcomes of antiinfective therapy. Pharmacotherapy. 1993 Mar-Apr;13(2 Pt 2):29S–33S.

Issue with no Volume

Slaga TJ, Gimenez-Conti IB. An animal model for oral cancer. Monogr J Nat Cancer Instit. 1992;(13):55–60.

No Issue or Volume

Payne R. Acute exacerbation of chronic cancer pain: basic assessment and treatments of break-through pain. Acute Pain Sympt Manage. 1998:4–5.

Pagination in Roman Numerals

Koretz RL. Clinical nutrition. Gastroenterol Clin North Am. 1998 Jun;27(2):xi–xiii.

Expressing Type of Article (as desired; optional)

Goldwater SH, Chatelain F. Taking time to communicate [letter]. Am J Hosp Pharm. 1994 Feb 1;51:232, 234.

Talley CR. Reducing demand through preventive care [editorial]. Am J Hosp Pharm. 1994 Jan 1;51:55.

Saritas A, Cakir Z, Emet M, Uzkeser M, Akoz A, Acemoglu F. Factors affecting the b-type natriuretic peptide levels in stroke patients [abstract]. Ann Acad Med Singapore. 2010 May;39(5):385.

Article Containing a Retraction

Brown MD. Retraction. Am Heart J. 1986;111:623. Retraction of: Slutsky RA, Olson LK. Am Heart J. 1984;108:543–7.

Article Retracted

Slutsky RA, Olson LK. Intravascular and extravascular pulmonary fluid volumes during chronic experimental left ventricular dysfunction. Am Heart J. 1984 Sep;108:543–7. Retraction in: Am Heart J. 1986 Mar;111:623.

Article with Published Erratum

Reitz MS Jr, Juo HG, Oleske J, Hoxie J, Popovic M, Read-Connole E. On the historical origins of HIV-1 (MN) and (RF) [letter]. AIDS Res Hum Retroviruses. 1992 Aug;8:1539–41. Erratum in: AIDS Res Hum Retroviruses 1992 Aug;8:1731.

Item (e.g., Table, Figure, Box, Image, or Appendix) in Article

Hohnloser SH, Pajitnev D, Pogue J, Healey JS, Pfeffer MA, Yusuf S, Connolly SJ. Incidence of stroke in paroxysmal versus sustained atrial fibrillation in patients taking oral anticoagulation or combined antiplatelet therapy: an ACTIVE W substudy. J Am Coll Cardiol. 2007 Nov 22;50(22):2156–61. Table 4, Incidence of stoke or non-CNS systemic embolism in patients with paroxysmal versus persistent/permanent AF treated with aspirin plus clopidogrel or OAC; p. 2159.

Unpublished Article

Malone PM. Topics in informatics. Adv Pharm. Forthcoming 2004.

BOOKS

To cite a book, which can include manuals, brochures, or fact sheets, the following information should be given:

- Last name of author(s) and a maximum of two initials for each author separated by a comma and followed by a period. Some publications will list only three authors followed by the phrase *et al.*; however, all authors should be listed unless otherwise specified by the publication or if space is limited.
- Title of book (capitalize only the initial word of title and proper nouns in English) followed by a period with the exception that punctuation is already at the end of the title—for example, if a title ends with a question mark or exclamation point, use that instead of the period.
- Edition, other than the first, followed by period.
- Place of publication (city) followed by colon (if the location is not clear with just a city name, the state or country abbreviation may be placed in parenthesis after the city name and before the colon). If place of publication is not explicitly stated, but is implied based on the location of publisher then add square brackets around place of publication.
- Name of publisher followed by semicolon.
- Year of publication followed by period.

Please note: If place of publication, name of publisher, or year of publication cannot be found, then in square brackets, it should be stated that one or more of these are unknown (e.g., [date unknown] or [place, publisher, date unknown]).

A condensed version of the above information is as follows:

Author(s). Title of Book. Edition. Place of Publication: Publisher; Date of Publication.

Book on the Internet:

Author(s). Title of Book [Internet]. Place of Publication: Publisher; Date of Publication [Date of Update; Date of Citation]. Available from: Web Address

Example Book Citations

Standard Book

Albright RG. A basic guide to online information systems for health care professionals. Arlington (VA): Information Resource Press; 1988.

Book on the Internet

DiPiro JT, Talbert RL, Yee GC, Matzke GR, Wells BG, Posey LM, editors. Pharmacotherapy: a pathophysiologic approach [Internet]. 10th ed. New York: McGraw-Hill Education; 2017 [cited 2019 Jul 24]. Available from: https://accesspharmacy.mhmedical.com/book.aspx?bookID=1861

Lexicomp online [Internet]. [place unknown]: Wolters Kluwer; 2019 [cited 2019 Jun 24]. Available from: http://online.lexi.com/lco/action/home

Editor(s) as Author

Chisholm-Burns MA, Schwinghammer TL, Malone PM, Kolesar JM, Lee KC, Bookstaver PB, editors. Pharmacotherapy principles and practice. 6th ed. New York: McGraw-Hill Education; 2022.

No Specific Editor(s), Compiler, or Author Identified
Drug facts and comparisons 1999. St. Louis: Facts and Comparisons; 1998.

Organization as Author and Publisher
United States Pharmacopeial Convention, Inc. USAN and the USP dictionary of drug names. Rockville: United States Pharmacopeial Convention, Inc.; 1993.

Volumes (Same Author(s)/Editor(s))
United States Pharmacopeial Convention, Inc. USP dispensing information. 22nd ed. Vol. 2, Advice for the patient: drug information in lay language. Greenwood Village (CO): Micromedex; 2002.
If on the Internet, use the following format:

Author(s). Title of Book. Volume Number, Volume Title [Internet]. Place of Publication: Publisher; Date of Publication [Date of Update, Date of Citation]. Available from: Web Address

Ross IA. Medicinal plants of the world. Vol. 3, Chemical constituents, traditional and modern medicinal uses [Internet]. Totowa (NJ): Humana Press, Inc.; 2005 [cited 2010 Jun 23]. Available from: http://metis.findlay.edu:2080/xtf-ebc/search?keyword=pharmacy

Portion of a Book (e.g., Chapter, Table, Figure, or Appendix) With Author(s) Writing Entire Book
Bauer LA. Applied clinical pharmacokinetics. 2nd ed. New York: McGraw-Hill Education; 2008. Chapter 6, Digoxin; p. 301–55.

If on the Internet, use the following format:

Author(s). Title of Book [Internet]. Edition. Place of Publication: Publisher; Date of Publication [Date of Update of Book]. Portion Number, Portion Title; [Date of Update of Portion; Date of Citation]; Page Number(s) or [Length of Portion]. Available from: Web Address

Bauer LA. Applied clinical pharmacokinetics [Internet]. 2nd ed. New York: McGraw Hill; c2008. Chapter 6, Digoxin; [cited 2010 Jun 23]; [about 20 screens]. Available from: http://accesspharmacy.mhmedical.com/content.aspx?bookid=510&sectionid=40843080

Contribution to Book (Portions of Book Written by Different Authors)
Malesker MA, Morrow LE. Fluids and electrolytes. In: Chisholm-Burns MA, Schwinghammer TL, Malone PM, Kolesar JM, Lee KC, Bookstaver PB, editors. Pharmacotherapy principles and practice. 6th ed. New York: McGraw-Hill Education; 2022. p. 433–46.
If on the Internet, use the following format:

Chapter Author(s). Chapter Title. In: Author(s)/Editor(s). Title of Book [Internet]. Place of Publication: Publisher; Date of Publication [Date of Citation]. Available from: Web address

Malone PM, Malone MJ. Professional writing. In: Malone PM, Malone MJ, Park SK, editors. Drug information: a guide for pharmacists [Internet]. 6th ed. New York: McGraw-Hill Education; c2014 [cited 2016 Jun 23]. Available from: http://accesspharmacy.mhmedical.com/book.aspx?bookID=981

Unpublished Book

Malone PM, Malone MJ, Witt BA, Peterson DM, editors. Drug information: a guide for pharmacists. 7th ed. New York: McGraw-Hill Education. Forthcoming 2022.

Book on CD-ROM or DVD

Haux R, Kulikowski C. Yearbook 04 of medical informatics—towards clinical bioinformatics [CD-ROM]. Stuttgart (Germany): Schatteuer; 2004.

Video Clip, Videocast, or Podcast Associated with Book

Author(s). Title of Book [Internet]. Place of Publication: Publisher; Date of Publication [Date of Citation]. Videocast or Podcast: Length of Video. Available from: Web Address

Brunton LL, Hilal-Dandan R, Knollmann BC, editors. Goodman and Gilman's: the pharmacological basis of therapeutics [Internet]. 13th ed. New York: McGraw-Hill Education; 2018 [cited 2019 Jul 25]. Videocast: 1 min. Available from: https://accesspharmacy.mhmedical.com/MultimediaPlayer.aspx?MultimediaID=13551242

OTHER MATERIAL (IN ALPHABETICAL ORDER)

Format and Example Citations

Conference Proceedings

Editor(s). Book Title. Conference Title; Date(s) of Conference; Conference Location. Place of Publication: Publisher; Date of Publication.

Allebeck P, Jansson B, editors. Ethics in medicine: individual integrity versus demands of society (Karolinska Institute Novel Conference Series). Proceedings of the 3rd International Congress on Ethics in Medicine; 1989 Sep 13–15; Stockholm. New York: Raven Press; 1990.

If on the Internet, use the following format:

Editor(s). Book Title [Internet]. Conference Title; Date(s) of Conference; Conference Location. Place of Publication: Publisher; Date of Publication [Date of Citation]. [Length of Publication]. Available from: Web Address

Allebeck P, Jansson B, editors. Ethics in medicine: individual integrity versus demands of society (Karolinska Institute Novel Conference Series) [Internet]. Proceedings of the 3rd International Congress on Ethics in Medicine; 1989 Sep 13–15; Stockholm. New York: Raven Press; 1990 [cited 2010 Jun 23]. [8 p.]. Available from: http://jmp.oxfordjournals.org/cgi/issue_pdf/backmatter_pdf/13/4.pdf

Conference Paper

Author(s) of Conference Paper. Title of Paper. In: Editors of Conference Proceedings. Conference Title; Date(s) of Conference; Conference Location. Place of Publication: Publisher; Date of Publication. Pages.

Keyserlingk E. Ethical guidelines and codes: can they be universally applicable in a multi-cultural world? In: Allebeck P, Jansson B, editors. Ethics in medicine: individual integrity versus demands of society (Karolinska Institute Novel Conference Series). Proceedings of the 3rd International Congress on Ethics in Medicine; 1989 Sep 13–15; Stockholm. New York: Raven Press; 1990. p. 137–49.

If on the Internet, use the following format:

Author(s) of Conference Paper. Title of Paper [Internet]. In: Conference Title; Date(s) of Conference; Conference Location. Place of Publication: Publisher; Date of Publication [Date of Citation]. [Length of Paper]. Available from: Web Address

Keyserlingk E. Ethical guidelines and codes: can they be universally applicable in a multi-cultural world? In: Allebeck P, Jansson B, editors. Ethics in medicine: individual integrity versus demands of society (Karolinska Institute Novel Conference Series) [Internet]. Proceedings of the 3rd International Congress on Ethics in Medicine; 1989 Sep 13–15; Stockholm. New York: Raven Press; 1990 [cited 2010 Jun 23]. [about 2 p.]. Available from: http://jmp.oxfordjournals.org/cgi/issue_pdf/backmatter_pdf/13/4.pdf

Dictionary Definition

Dictionary Name. Edition. Place of Publication: Publisher; Date of Publication. Word Being Defined; Page Number.

Stedman's medical dictionary. 27th ed. New York: Lippincott Williams & Wilkins; 2000. Asthenia; p. 158.

If on the Internet, use the following format:

Dictionary Name [Internet]. Place of Publication: Publisher; Date of Publication. Word Being Defined; [Date of Citation]. Available from: Web Address

Merriam-Webster Online [Internet]. Springfield (MA): Merriam-Webster, Inc.; c2010. Blood pressure; [cited 2010 Jun 23]. Available from: http://www.merriam-webster.com/dictionary/blood%20pressure

Dissertation/Thesis

Author(s). Title [dissertation or master's thesis]. [Place of Publication]: Publisher; Date of Publication.

Wellman CO. Pain perceptions and coping strategies of school-age children and their parents: a descriptive-correlational study [dissertation]. [Omaha (NE)]: Creighton University; 1985.

If on the Internet, use the following format:

Author(s). Title [dissertation or master's thesis on the Internet]. Place of Publication: Publisher; Date of Publication [Date of Citation]. Pages p. Available from: Web Address

Mil JW. Pharmaceutical care, the future of pharmacy: theory, research, and practice [dissertation on the Internet]. Groningen (Netherlands): University of Groningen; 2000 Feb 1 [cited 2010 Jun 23]. 264 p. Available from: http://dissertations.ub.rug.nl/faculties/science/2000/j.w.f.van.mil/?pLanguage=en&pFullItemRecord=ON

Encyclopedia Entry

Author(s). Name of Encyclopedia. Place of Publication: Publisher; Date of Publication. Name of Entry; Page Number.

If on the Internet, use the following format:

Author(s). Name of Encyclopedia [Internet]. Place of Publication: Publisher; Date of Publication [Date of Update; Date of Citation]. Available from: Web Address

Encyclopedia Britannica Online [Internet]. Chicago: Britannica; c2010 [cited 2010 Jun 23]. Available from: http://www.britannica.com/EBchecked/topic/569347/stroke

Legal Documents

Please consult: Harvard Law Review; Columbia Law Review; Yale Law Review. The bluebook: a uniform system of citation. 21th ed. [Cambridge (MA)]: Harvard Law Review Association; 2020.

Newspaper Article

Author(s). Title of Article. Newspaper Title (Edition). Date of Publication; Section: Page Number (Column Number).

Fein EB. Rise in fetal tests prompts ethical debate. New York Times (National Ed.). 1994 Feb 5; Sect. A:1(col. 2).

If on the Internet, use the following format:

Author(s). Title of Article. Newspaper Title [Internet]. Date of Publication [Date of Update; Date of Citation]; Section: Page Number or [Length of Article]. Available from: Web Address

Painter K. Your health: feet bear the strain of extra weight. USA Today [Internet]. 2010 Jun 20 [cited 2010 Jun 23]; Health and Behavior:[about 2 screens]. Available from: http://www.usatoday.com/news/health/painter/2010-06-21-yourhealth21_ST_N.htm

Package Insert

Package inserts are commonly cited in professional writing; however, the standards do not address the format to use. The following is a common format that is similar to those presented in this appendix.

Medication Name [package insert]. Place of Publication: Publisher; Date of Publication.

Prilosec® (omeprazole) delayed-release capsules [package insert]. Wayne, PA: Astra Merck; 1998 Jun.

If on the Internet, use the following format:

Medication Name [package insert on the Internet]. Place of Publication: Publisher; Date of Publication [Date of Update; Date of Citation]. Available from: Web Address

omeprazole [package insert on the Internet]. Bethesda (MD): U.S. National Library of Medicine; 2009 Aug [updated 2009 Dec; cited 2010 Jun 23]. Available from: http://dailymed.nlm.nih.gov/dailymed/drugInfo.cfm?id=14749

Meeting Presentations of Paper and Poster Sessions

Author(s). Title of Paper or Poster. Paper or Poster session presented at: Conference Title; Date(s) of Conference; Conference Location.

Ciaccia V, Hinders C, Malone M, Morales R, Sanchez A. Comparison of evidence based hypertension guideline model to an alternative model. Poster session presented at: The University of Findlay Symposium for Scholarship and Creativity; 2010 Apr 13; Findlay, OH.

Patent

Inventor(s); Assignee. Title. Patent Country patent Country Code Patent Number. Date patent issued.

Schwartz B, inventor; New England Medical Center Hospital, Inc., assignee. Method of and solution for treating glaucoma. United States patent US 5,212,168. 1993 May 18.

Personal Communication

Normally in-text citation only (e.g., Letter from or Conversation with; unreferenced, see Notes Section).

Author. Letter to or Conversation with: Recipient (Recipient Affiliation). Date. Located at: Location of Letter.

In Notes Section, state that permission was given to reference the letter or conversation.

Jones, Max. Letter to: Charlie Smith. 2005 Feb 14. Located at: Veterinary Medicine Division, College of Pharmacy, University of Findlay, Findlay, OH; Cabinet 1, Drawer 2, Folder 10.

Scientific or Technical Report

Author(s). Title. Place of Publication: Publisher; Date of Publication. Report No.: Report Number.

Issued by funding/sponsoring agency:

Shekelle P, Morton S, Maglione M (Southern California Evidence-Based Practice Center/RAND, Santa Monica, CA). Ephedra and ephedrine for weight loss and athletic performance enhancement: clinical efficacy and side effects. Vol. 1, Evidence report and evidence tables. Rockville (MD): Agency for Healthcare Research and Quality; 2003 Mar. (Evidence report/technology assessment; no. 78). Report No.: AHRQPUB03E022. Contract No.: AHRQ-290-97-001.

Issued by performing agency:

Shekelle P, Morton S, Maglione M. Ephedra and ephedrine for weight loss and athletic performance enhancement: clinical efficacy and side effects. Vol. 1, Evidence report and evidence tables. Santa Monica: Southern California Evidence-Based Practice Center/RAND; 2003 Mar. (Evidence report/technology assessment; no. 78). Report No.: AHRQPUB03E022. Contract No.: AHRQ-290-97-001. Supported by the Agency for Healthcare Research and Quality.

If on the Internet, use the following format:

Author(s). Title [Internet]. Place of Publication: Publisher; Date of Publication [Date of Citation]. Pagination. Report No.: Report Number. Available from: Web Address

Qureshi N, Wilson B, Santaguida P, Carroll J, Allanson J, Culebro CR, Brouwers M, Raina P. Collection and use of cancer family history in primary care [Internet]. Rockville (MD): Agency for Healthcare Research and Quality; 2007 Oct [cited 2010 Jun 23]. [about 2 screens]. (Evidence reports/technology assessments no. 159) Report No.: AHRQPUB08E001. Contract No.: 290-02-0020. Available from: http://www.ncbi.nlm.nih.gov/bookshelf/br.fcgi?book=erta159

OTHER ELECTRONIC MATERIAL (IN ALPHABETICAL ORDER)

Format and Example Citations

Part of a Blog (Only One Author)

Since this is personal communication, as above, it usually is done as an in-text citation only (Posting on given date from author on given blog; unreferenced, see Notes Section). In Notes Section, state that permission was given to reference the blog post. Otherwise, follow the format below:

Author of Blog. Title of Blog [blog on the Internet] or [Internet] if the word blog is part of title of blog. Place of Publication: Publisher. Start Date of Blog- . or End Date if blog is closed- Title of Part; Date of Publication [Date of Citation]; [Length of Part]. Available from: Web Address

Please note: if a piece of information is implied, but cannot be confirmed, place that information in square brackets, and if it is unknown, state that in square brackets (e.g., [publisher unknown]).

Daria. Living with Cancer [blog on the Internet]. Edmonton (AB): Daria. 2008 Aug- 2011 Jan Chemo went well; 2010 Jun 12 [cited 2016 Jul 31]; [about 1 screen]. Available from: http://daria-living-withcancer.blogspot.com/.

Part of a Blog (Multiple Authors)

Since this is personal communication, as above, it usually is done as an in-text citation only (Posting on given date from author on given blog; unreferenced, see Notes Section). In Notes Section, state that permission was given to reference the blog post. Otherwise, follow the format below:

Author of Comment. Title of Blog Comment. Date of Publication of Comment [Date of Citation]. In: Author of Blog. Name of Blog [blog on the Internet] or [Internet] if the word blog is part of title of blog. Place of Publication: Publisher. Date of Publication- . or End Date if blog is closed [Length of Comment]. Available from: Web Address

Please note: if a piece of information is implied, but cannot be confirmed, place that information in square brackets, and if it is unknown, state that in square brackets (e.g., [publisher unknown]).

Smith J. Dialysis. 2010 Jun 16 [cited 2010 Jun 16]. In: Kidney Coaching Foundation, Inc. KCF Blog and News [Internet]. Raleigh (NC): Kidney Coaching Foundation, Inc. c2005-2010- . [about 1 paragraph]. Available from: http://www.thekcf.org/bn/.

Database on the Internet

Title of Database [Internet]. Place of Publication: Publisher. Initial Date of Publication- (list end date if database closed) [Date of Citation]. Available from: Web Address

<u>Please note</u>: if a piece of information is implied, but cannot be confirmed, place that information in square brackets, and if it is unknown, state that in square brackets (e.g., [publisher unknown]).

PubMed [Internet]. Bethesda (MD): National Library of Medicine. 2004- [cited 2016 Jul 31]. Available from: https://www.ncbi.nlm.nih.gov/pubmed

DRUGDEX [Internet]. [place unknown]: Truven Health Analytics. c2012-2016 [cited 2016 Jul 31]. Available from: https://www.micromedexsolutions.com/home/dispatch/ssl/true

Part of a Database on the Internet (e.g., a single drug monograph out of a publication)

Title of Database [Internet]. Place of Publication: Publisher. Initial Date of Publication- (list end date if database closed). Record Identifier, Title of Part; [Date of Citation]; [Length of Part]. Available from: Web Address

<u>Please note</u>: if a piece of information is implied, but cannot be confirmed, place that information in square brackets, and if it is unknown, state that in square brackets (e.g., [publisher unknown]).

MeSH Browser [Internet]. Bethesda (MD): National Library of Medicine. 2004- . ID: D015201, Phenytoin; [cited 2004 Aug 18]; [about 670 p.]. Available from: http://www.nlm.nih.gov/mesh/MBrowser.html

DRUGDEX [Internet]. [place unknown]: Truven Health Analytics. c2012-2016. Amiodarone; [cited 2016 Jul 31]; [about 8 screens]. Available from: https://www.micromedexsolutions.com/home/dispatch/ssl/true

Electronic Mail

Since this is personal communication, as above, it usually is done as an in-text citation only (Email on given date from sender to recipient; unreferenced, see Notes Section). In Notes Section, state that permission was given to reference the email. Otherwise, follow the format below:

Author. Title of Email [Internet]. Message to: Recipient(s). Date of Message [Date of Citation]. [Length of Email].

Malone, Patrick. Drug information textbook [Internet]. Message to: John Stanovich; Mark Malesker. 2010 Jun 14 [2010 Jun 16]. [3 paragraphs].

LISTSERV

Since this is personal communication, as above, it usually is done as an in-text citation only (Posting on given date from sender to given LISTSERV; unreferenced, see Notes Section). In Notes Section, state that permission was given from the sender to reference the email. Otherwise, follow the format below:

Author. Title of Message. In: Name of LISTSERV [Internet]. Place of Publication: Publisher; Date of Message [Date of Citation]. [Length of Message].

Malone PM. CAMIPR—discussion forum for medication information specialists. In: CAMIPR [Internet]. Iowa City: Consortium for the Advancement of Medication Policy and Research; 2010 May 6 [cited 2010 Jun 18]. [about 1 p.].

Video Clip, Videocast, or Podcast

Author(s). Title of Homepage [Internet]. Place of Publication: Publisher; Date of Publication of Homepage. [Video or Videocast or Podcast], Title of Video; Date of Publication of Video Clip, Videocast, or Podcast [Date of Update; Date of Citation]; [Length of Video Clip, Videocast, or Podcast]. Available from: Web Address

Gulseth MP, Messler JC. ASHP Advantage [Internet]. Bethesda (MD): American Society of Health-System Pharmacists; c2010. [Podcast], Multidisciplinary approach to identifying patients at risk for VTE; 2010 May 4 [cited 2016 Jul 31]; [45 min.]. Available from: http://www.ashpadvantage.com/podcasts/.

Website Homepage

Author(s). Title of Homepage [Internet]. Place of Publication: Publisher; Date of Publication [Date of Update; Date of Citation]. Available from: Web Address

American Society of Health-System Pharmacists [Internet]. Bethesda (MD): American Society of Health-System Pharmacists; c1997-2004 [updated 2004 Aug 18; cited 2004 Aug 18]. Available from: http://www.ashp.org/.

Part of a Website

Title of Homepage [Internet]. Place of Publication: Publisher; Date of Publication of Homepage. Title of Part; Date of Publication of Part (if different from Homepage) [Date of Update; Date of Citation]; [Length of Part]. Available from: Web Address

American Society of Health-System Pharmacists [Internet]. Bethesda (MD): American Society of Health-System Pharmacists; c2019. Compounding Resource Center; [updated 2019 Jul 25; cited 2019 Jul 19]; [about 1 screen]. Available from: https://www.ashp.org/Pharmacy-Practice/Resource-Centers/Sterile-Compounding#

Part of a Wiki

Since this is personal communication, as above, it usually is done as an in-text citation only (Posting on given date from author on given wiki; unreferenced, see Notes Section). In Notes Section, state that permission was given from the author to reference the wiki. Otherwise, follow the format below:

Author(s) of Part. Title of Part of Wiki. Date of Posting [Date of Update; Date of Citation]. In: Title of Wiki [Internet]. Place of Publication: Publisher. Start Date of Wiki- . (list end date if wiki closed) [Length of Part]. Available from: Web Address

If no author for part:

Title of Wiki [Internet]. Place of Publication: Publisher. Start Date of Wiki- . (list end date if wiki closed) Title of Part of Wiki; [Date of Update; Date of Citation]; [Length of Part]. Available from: Web Address

Please note: if a piece of information is implied, but cannot be confirmed, place that information in square brackets, and if it is unknown, state that in square brackets (e.g., [publisher unknown]).

Wiki Public Health [Internet]. [place unknown]: WikiPH. [date unknown]- . Health care; [updated 2007 Mar 27; cited 2010 Jun 16]; [about 2 screens]. Available from: http://wikiph.org/index. php?title=Health_care

REFERENCES

1. International Committee of Medical Journal Editors. Uniform requirements for manuscripts submitted to biomedical journals: writing and editing for biomedical publication [Internet]. Philadelphia: International Committee of Medical Journal Editors. 2009 Nov. [cited 2010 Nov 16]. Available from: http://www.icmje.org/index.html.
2. International Committee of Medical Journal Editors. Uniform requirements for manuscripts submitted to biomedical journals: sample references [Internet]. Philadelphia: International Committee of Medical Journal Editors; 2003 [updated 2011 Jul 15; cited 2012 May 15]. Available from: http://www.nlm.nih.gov/bsd/uniform_requirements.html
3. Patrias K. Citing medicine: the NLM style guide for authors, editors, and publishers [Internet]. 2nd ed. Wendling DL, technical editor. Bethesda (MD): National Library of Medicine (US); 2007 [updated 2015 Oct 2; cited 2016 Jun 24]. Available from: http://nlm.nih.gov/ citingmedicine

Pharmacy and Therapeutics Committee Procedure

This appendix includes two policy and procedure operational statements. The first is specifically written to centralize the formulary decision process for a multihospital health system: a Formulary Committee. The second, and closely related, operational statement is written as a model to function as the traditional Pharmacy and Therapeutics Committee for a Hospital's Medical Staff. Both operational statements describe the functions of their related committees based on a certain degree of autonomy. Their membership is ultimately chosen by an administrative leader as a means to best isolate the committee from organizational as well as economic influences. The decision process for each operational statement is intended to create predictability and transparency. To implement this set of operational statements, each Executive Committee of the hospitals in a multihospital system would pass the following resolution:

> The Medical Staff of Alpha Hospital delegates its Pharmacy and Therapeutic Committee responsibilities to ALPHAOMEGA HEALTH based on the policy and procedures for a "Hospital Formulary System" and a "Hospital Pharmacy and Therapeutics Committee."

The two operational statements can also be combined to reflect the traditional functions of a single hospital, medical staff-based pharmacy and therapeutics committee. Also, there may be other arrangements where the two operational statements could provide the organizational environment for a closed health system, a pharmacy benefits manager, or one of the new organizational structures created by Federal Legislation in 2004 for the new financing of drug coverage in the United States.

POLICY TITLE: HOSPITAL FORMULARY SYSTEM

I. PURPOSE

To maintain a **HOSPITAL FORMULARY** and a Formulary Committee for all ALPHAOMEGA HEALTH Hospitals as a means to enhance the quality of health care for all patients served by ALPHAOMEGA HEALTH.

II. POLICY

A. The Formulary Committee of ALPHAOMEGA HEALTH periodically evaluates its performance as a means to improve its ability to support the Vision and Mission of ALPHAOMEGA HEALTH.

B. ALPHAOMEGA HEALTH maintains one Formulary Committee and a Pharmacy and Therapeutics Committee (P&T COMMITTEE) at each ALPHAOMEGA HEALTH Hospital to implement this POLICY in accord with the applicable Medical Staff Bylaws and this POLICY.

C. The Formulary Committee of ALPHAOMEGA HEALTH maintains a standard format for a **HOSPITAL FORMULARY** that is based on the provisions of this POLICY.

D. The Formulary Committee develops and continually revises a list of therapeutic products, a **HOSPITAL FORMULARY,** which reflects the current clinical judgment of the Medical Staff of ALPHAOMEGA HEALTH Hospitals regarding the selection of the best therapeutic products for the health care of hospitalized patients. The Formulary Committee evaluates the various alternative therapeutic products available and develops the **HOSPITAL FORMULARY** based on an evaluation of each therapeutic product's indications, effectiveness, risks, patient safety, and overall impact on health care costs.

E. The Formulary Committee collaborates with the P&T Committee at each ALPHAOMEGA HEALTH Hospital to monitor compliance with the provisions of the **HOSPITAL FORMULARY.**

F. The Formulary Committee supports the quality improvement functions of ALPHAOMEGA HEALTH where necessary to improve the use of the **HOSPITAL FORMULARY.**

III. PROCEDURE

A. FORMULARY COMMITTEE DEVELOPMENT

1. The Formulary Committee recommends, when appropriate, amendments to this POLICY AND PROCEDURE to the Chief Medical Officer of ALPHAOMEGA HEALTH. After revisions to any of these proposed amendments by the Chief Medical Officer, in collaboration with the Formulary Committee, the Chief Medical Officer submits the amendments to the Executive Committee of the Medical Staff at each ALPHAOMEGA HEALTH Hospital for final approval.

2. The Officers of the Formulary Committee prepare an Annual Membership Report to the Chief Medical Officer of ALPHAOMEGA HEALTH regarding participation of its Members and any recommendations that may be important to maintain the expertise necessary for the affairs of the Formulary Committee.

3. The Officers of the Formulary Committee prepare an Annual Report and submit it to the Professional Affairs Committee of ALPHAOMEGA HEALTH for approval. As a result of this review, the Professional Affairs Committee may make recommendations to the Formulary Committee for consideration regarding its affairs or to the Chief Medical Officer regarding amendments to this POLICY AND PROCEDURE.

B. FORMULARY COMMITTEE ORGANIZATION

1. REGULAR MEMBERS

a. MEDICAL STAFF MEMBERS

i. Up to 16 Medical Staff members are nominated annually by the Chief Medical Officer of ALPHAOMEGA HEALTH, each President or Chief of Staff from the Medical Staff of an ALPHAOMEGA HEALTH Hospital, or the Officers of the

Formulary Committee. A Medical Staff nominee must demonstrate an active interest in evidence-based therapeutics, a willingness to be an active participant in the affairs of the Formulary Committee, and represent as a group, whenever possible, the specialties of: Family Practice, Internal Medicine, Pediatrics, Obstetrics and Gynecology, Hematology and Oncology, Cardiology, Infectious Disease, Pulmonology, and General Surgery.

   ii. From any Nominees, 12–16 are selected by the Chief Medical Officer of ALPHAOMEGA HEALTH on the basis of maintaining a reasonable balance among the following factors: hospital and outpatient-based physicians, primary care and disease focused physicians, physician liaison to the Medical Staff Executive Committee or P&T Committee of each ALPHAOMEGA HEALTH Hospital, and a balanced representation from the Medical Staffs of the ALPHAOMEGA HEALTH Hospitals.

  b. ADMINISTRATION MEMBER—The Chief Medical Officer of ALPHAOMEGA HEALTH, or designee who is a Medical Staff Member of an ALPHAOMEGA HEALTH Hospital, is a Member of the Formulary Committee.

2. SPECIAL MEMBERS AND SOURCE OF SELECTION

  a. The Chief Medical Officer of ALPHAOMEGA HEALTH selects Special Members as may be needed to provide administrative or technical support for the affairs of the Formulary Committee. The Special Members includes, at a minimum:

   i. any pharmacist recommended by the Pharmacist in charge at a Hospital Pharmacy of ALPHAOMEGA HEALTH and

   ii. at least one Registered Nurse from among the Nursing Staff of an ALPHAOMEGA HEALTH Hospital.

  b. The Chairperson of the Formulary Committee selects one or more Special Members from the personnel of ALPHAOMEGA HEALTH or the Medical Staff of any ALPHAOMEGA HEALTH Hospital on a temporary basis as may be necessary for:

   i. technical support for the activities of the Formulary Committee or any Ad Hoc Subcommittee of the Formulary Committee or

   ii. information for the deliberations of the Formulary Committee regarding a proposal to add or delete an individual therapeutic product listed on the **HOSPITAL FORMULARY.**

3. FORMULARY COMMITTEE OFFICERS

  a. The CHAIRPERSON is selected by the Chief Medical Officer of ALPHAOMEGA HEALTH from among the Regular Members of the Formulary Committee. The Chairperson:

   i. manages the affairs of the Formulary Committee in a manner to

     I) support the active, positive involvement of each Regular and Special Member,

     II) acknowledge any conflict of interests,

     III) initiate a replacement appointment of any Officer, Regular Member, or Special Member becoming inactive during a calendar year,

     IV) appoint temporary Special Members, and

     V) select the location for Meetings of the Formulary Committee;

       ii. prepares the Annual Membership and Self-Evaluation reports; and

      iii. appoints an Ad Hoc Committee when necessary to study decisions in greater depth or to arrive at consensus recommendations for consideration by the Formulary Committee whose membership includes

          I) six or less members from the Medical Staffs of the ALPHAOMEGA HEALTH Hospitals,

          II) at least one member who is a Regular Member of the Formulary Committee, and

          III) the Secretary, or designee, of the Formulary Committee.

    b. The VICE CHAIRPERSON is selected by the Chief Medical Officer of ALPHAO-MEGA HEALTH from the Regular Members of the Formulary Committee. The Vice chairperson assumes the duties of the Chairperson during their absence.

    c. The SECRETARY is selected by the Chief Medical Officer of ALPHAOMEGA HEALTH from among the Regular or Special Members of the Formulary Committee. The Secretary assists the Chairperson in managing the affairs of the Formulary Committee by:

      i. preparing the minutes for each meeting of the Formulary Committee or any of its Ad Hoc Committees,

      ii. sending an Agenda to the Members prior to each meeting of the Formulary Committee,

      iii. maintaining a schedule for the annual regular review by the Formulary Committee of all therapeutic products listed on the **HOSPITAL FORMULARY**, and

      iv. coordinating the preparation of any Drug Monograph or any other report necessary for a meeting of the Formulary Committee by a Pharmacist in Charge, or designee, at an ALPHAOMEGA HEALTH Hospital.

4. TERM OF APPOINTMENT

    a. The Regular and Special Members are appointed or reappointed each January for 1 year.

    b. Each Officer is appointed or reappointed each January for 1 year.

5. VOTING

    a. Each Regular Member has one vote, and each Special Member does not have a vote.

    b. Any two Regular Members present during a Meeting of the Formulary Committee constitutes a quorum.

    c. Based on attendance, the Regular Members of the Formulary Committee may delay voting, when the appropriate expertise is not available during a meeting of the Formulary Committee.

    d. A simple majority of Regular Members voting is required for any action of the Formulary Committee. Any abstention on the basis of a conflict of interests is noted in the minutes for the meeting.

6. LIAISON—A Regular or Special Member may be appointed by the Chief Medical Officer of ALPHAOMEGA HEALTH to report on the affairs of the Formulary Committee during the deliberations of any other Committee of ALPHAOMEGA HEALTH.

7. MEETINGS—The meetings of the Formulary Committee are:

    a. scheduled once a month for 1 hour or as may be planned by the Members of the Formulary Committee,

    b. attended by Regular and Special Members only, and

    c. convened at a location arranged by the Chairperson, but may be attended through secure electronic access.

8. COMMITTEE PROTOCOLS—The Formulary Committee may also arrange for the:

    a. definitions applicable to the resignation and replacement of any Regular Member, Special Member, or Officer during a calendar year;

    b. management of any potential or actual conflict of interests affecting the participation of a Regular or Special Member during a meeting of the Formulary Committee;

    c. use of ALTERNATIVE MEDICATION for the health care of a patient at any ALPHA-OMEGA HEALTH Hospital;

    d. information necessary to request a change in the list of therapeutic products or other information described in the **HOSPITAL FORMULARY**;

    e. contents of a DRUG MONOGRAPH that must be prepared before a therapeutic product not listed on the **HOSPITAL FORMULARY** and

    f. management of any shortage of a therapeutic product listed in the **HOSPITAL FORMULARY** by the:

        i. timely notification of the Medical Staff at each ALPHAOMEGA HEALTH Hospital listing the specific dosage forms in limited or unavailable supply,

        ii. development of alternative strategies for a patient's health care using therapeutic products currently available on the **HOSPITAL FORMULARY** when a therapeutic product becomes either not available or in limited supply,

        iii. collaboration with the appropriate expertise within the Medical Staff of ALPHAO-MEGA HEALTH Hospitals when a rationing protocol is necessary for a critical therapeutic product in limited supply, and

        iv. review of any proposal for a rationing protocol by the Ethics Council of ALPHAO-MEGA HEALTH when the Formulary Committee requests assistance before final approval to ensure that the appropriate ethical standards have been considered.

C. HOSPITAL FORMULARY FORMAT

    1. Any therapeutic product used in the health care of a patient is eligible for the **HOSPITAL FORMULARY.** This includes samples, prescription drugs as defined by the Food and Drug Administration, herbal or other alternative therapies administered topically or enterally, nutraceuticals, nonprescription drugs, vaccines, diagnostic or contrast agents, radioactive agents, respiratory products, parenteral or enteral nutrients, blood products, intravenous solutions, and anesthetic gases. A therapeutic product may not be considered for the **HOSPITAL FORMULARY** if it would normally be considered a medical device, durable medical equipment, or implant.

    2. The **HOSPITAL FORMULARY** lists the therapeutic products approved by the Formulary Committee in a format approved by the Formulary Committee. The format

for the **HOSPITAL FORMULARY** reflects the recommendations of nationally recognized organizations and includes certain attributes, where appropriate, as described below.

  a. Any restricted use provision is defined by credentialing categories in use by the Medical Staffs of ALPHAOMEGA HEALTH Hospitals and be implemented when necessary to monitor or limit the use of a **HOSPITAL FORMULARY** therapeutic product known to be associated with:

   i. an increased risk of a substantial adverse patient reaction,

   ii. a highly specific therapeutic indication, or

   iii. an unusual impact on the overall cost of health care.

  b. Specific patient education provisions are added for any **HOSPITAL FORMULARY** therapeutic product known to require:

   i. special nutritional adjustments,

   ii. prevention of substantial adverse effects or noncompliance, or

   iii. unique requirements for informed consent.

  c. Continuing education provisions are added when a Medical Staff Member or qualified Hospital employee requires specialized knowledge prior to or during the administration of a given **HOSPITAL FORMULARY** therapeutic product. This is particularly applicable in the professional areas of oncology and cardiology.

  d. Special information may be added to assist the Medical Staff at each ALPHAOMEGA HEALTH HOSPITAL when necessary to improve the:

   i. level of compliance with prescribing only therapeutic products listed on the **HOSPITAL FORMULARY**,

   ii. acceptance of rational therapeutic concepts as a basis for planning health care intervention strategies, and

   iii. acceptance of therapeutic interchange strategies involving therapeutic products not listed on the **HOSPITAL FORMULARY**.

 3. The Formulary Committee may establish a provision for inventory control of a **HOSPITAL FORMULARY** therapeutic product.

D. HOSPITAL FORMULARY MAINTENANCE

 1. A proposal for a change in a single therapeutic product listed on the **HOSPITAL FORMULARY** requires a specific set of steps before final approval by the Formulary Committee. These steps are defined below. The Formulary Committee may make a temporary exception to this provision when necessary to improve the quality of health care to patients at an ALPHAOMEGA HEALTH Hospital.

  a. timely submission of a completed Formulary Request form to any pharmacist at an ALPHAOMEGA HEALTH Hospital by a Medical Staff member of an ALPHAOMEGA HEALTH Hospital or other professional employee of ALPHAOMEGA HEALTH,

  b. review of the Formulary Request by a pharmacist in charge, or designee, of an ALPHA-OMEGA HEALTH Hospital's Pharmacy to be sure that it has been fully completed,

  c. preparation of a Drug Monograph, as may be arranged by the Secretary of the Formulary Committee if a new therapeutic product has been proposed by the Formulary Request for the **HOSPITAL FORMULARY**,

    d. preliminary review of the Formulary Request and any associated Drug Monograph by representative specialists affected by any proposed change in the **HOSPITAL FORMULARY**,

    e. initial approval or disapproval of the Formulary Request at one meeting of the Formulary Committee, followed by review for comments at each ALPHAOMEGA HEALTH Hospital's P&T Committee, before final approval or disapproval including any amendments to the Formulary Request at a subsequent meeting of the Formulary Committee.

2. The Formulary Committee annually reviews therapeutic products listed on the **HOSPITAL FORMULARY** according to a schedule of therapeutic classes as may be arranged throughout a calendar year by the Secretary of the Formulary Committee. The review of each class of therapeutic products requires a specific set of events before final approval. These steps are defined below.

    a. review of a class of therapeutic products preliminarily by the pharmacists in charge, or designees, of the ALPHAOMEGA HEALTH Hospital Pharmacies prior to a meeting of the Formulary Committee regarding the possible need to:

      i. initiate a Formulary Request for a new addition to the **HOSPITAL FORMULARY,**

      ii. deletion of a therapeutic product because of production defects, non-use, non-availability, recall, or replacement by another therapeutic product, or

      iii. a need to change information included in the **HOSPITAL FORMULARY** such as patient education, professional education, therapeutic interchange, or a restricted use provision;

    b. preliminary review of the proposed revisions to the **HOSPITAL FORMULARY** by representative specialists affected by the proposed revisions;

    c. initial approval or disapproval of the therapeutic product class review at one meeting of the Formulary Committee, followed by review for comments at each ALPHAOMEGA HEALTH Hospital's P&T Committee, before final approval or disapproval including amendments to the class review at a subsequent meeting of the Formulary Committee.

3. The Formulary Committee may authorize certain strategies by the ALPHAOMEGA HEALTH Hospital pharmacies that are necessary to offer the most appropriate therapeutic products for hospitalized patients. The Formulary Committee may authorize these special strategies when supported by its own decision and the support of each ALPHAOMEGA HEALTH Hospital's P&T Committee. Certain specific strategies to be authorized by this POLICY AND PROCEDURE are listed below.

    a. A class review of **HOSPITAL FORMULARY** therapeutic products as described above may also be initiated when there is a Formulary Request for a therapeutic product that substantially affects the inclusion or supplementary information of other therapeutic products currently listed in the **HOSPITAL FORMULARY.**

    b. The pharmacist in charge, or designee, at all ALPHAOMEGA HEALTH Hospital Pharmacies arranges to prepare a preliminary or full Drug Monograph before any therapeutic product is dispensed that has not previously been ordered for a hospitalized patient at any ALPHAOMEGA HEALTH Hospital.

c. The Formulary Committee may provide for automatic therapeutic interchange between a therapeutic product that is not listed for another therapeutic product that is listed on the **HOSPITAL FORMULARY** when supported by appropriate scientific evidence and appropriately considered standards of practice.

d. The Formulary Committee may also select certain therapeutic products for the **HOSPITAL FORMULARY** that are dispensed for certain indications or any indication even if prescribed with a "Do Not Substitute" designation. The Formulary Committee uses the same process for this designation as defined above for a new change in the **HOSPITAL FORMULARY.**

E. HOSPITAL FORMULARY COMPLIANCE

1. The P&T Committee of each ALPHAOMEGA HEALTH Hospital is responsible for monitoring each Medical Staff physician's orders for a therapeutic product that is:

   a. not listed or does not have an automatic therapeutic interchange with a therapeutic product listed on the current **HOSPITAL FORMULARY,**

   b. for an indication not permitted by the **HOSPITAL FORMULARY**, or

   c. for an indication having a restricted use provision.

2. Any ALPHAOMEGA HEALTH Hospital's P&T Committee may establish a Special Formulary as a means to temporarily support the efforts of its Medical Staff in the health care of hospitalized patients having special requirements that are unique to that Hospital. The Special Formulary therapeutic products are selected using the same process defined above for a change in the **HOSPITAL FORMULARY**. For a Special Formulary, the other Committees of the Hospital's Medical Staff provide a consent process. For any therapeutic product listed on an ALPHAOMEGA HEALTH Hospital's Special Formulary for 1 year or more, continued use of the Special Formulary status for the therapeutic product requires the approval of the Formulary Committee.

3. If a P&T Committee votes to not accept a decision of the Formulary Committee, the Chairperson, or designee, of the P&T Committee is invited to a subsequent meeting of the Formulary Committee. At this Formulary Meeting, the Formulary Committee attempts to develop a strategy for resolving the conflict between the original decision of the Formulary Committee and the respective P&T Committee. In the event that a resolution is not achieved, the issue may be appealed by either Committee to the Professional Affairs Committee for a final decision within 3 months of the appeal.

F. QUALITY IMPROVEMENT

1. The Formulary Committee maintains access to the decisions of other hospital's Formulary or P&T Committees as a resource for the basis in managing difficult decisions regarding the **HOSPITAL FORMULARY.** The hospitals chosen should reflect regional as well as national locations.

2. The Formulary Committee assesses the pending availability of new therapeutic products in the future that may require the preparation of a Formulary Request and Drug Monograph.

3. The Formulary Committee monitors the possible evolution of a shortage involving the availability of a therapeutic product listed on the **HOSPITAL FORMULARY.**

4. The Formulary Committee may recommend to each P&T Committee certain quality improvement projects, such as a Drug Use Evaluations for a certain product that would reflect the health care at all ALPHAOMEGA HEALTH Hospitals.

5. The Formulary Committee monitors all black box warnings or other Advisories issued by the Food and Drug Administration or pharmaceutical manufacturing company. The Formulary Committee uses the monitoring process as a basis to collaborate with each ALPHAOMEGA HEALTH Hospital's P&T Committee as a means to promote patient safety.

6. The Formulary Committee maintains a newsletter regarding its decisions and distribute it to each member of the Medical Staff of all ALPHAOMEGA HEALTH Hospitals.

7. The Formulary Committee collaborates with the P&T Committee at each ALPHAOMEGA HEALTH Hospital to develop educational strategies for the ALPHAOMEGA HEALTH professional employees and each Hospital's Medical Staff that builds support for the principles and priorities used to maintain the **HOSPITAL FORMULARY.**

8. The Formulary Committee offers consultation when requested or directed by the Board of Directors of ALPHAOMEGA HEALTH, its Committees, or any other ALPHAOMEGA HEALTH Committee regarding therapeutic products in the investigation, protocols, standard order sets, or quality assessment of health care.

9. The Formulary Committee offers a means to coordinate the standardization of POLICY AND PROCEDURE's for the Pharmacy Departments of ALPHAOMEGA HEALTH Hospitals.

POLICY TITLE: HOSPITAL PHARMACY AND THERAPEUTICS COMMITTEE

I. PURPOSE

To maintain a Pharmacy and Therapeutics Committee as a means to enhance the quality of health care for all patients served by the Alpha Medical Center.

II. POLICY

A. The Pharmacy and Therapeutics Committee of Alpha Medical Center periodically evaluates its performance as a means to improve its ability to support the Vision and Mission of ALPHAOMEGA HEALTH.

B. The Alpha Medical Center maintains a Pharmacy and Therapeutics Committee (P&T committee) to implement this POLICY in accord with the applicable Medical Staff By-Laws and this POLICY.

C. The P&T Committee may maintain a SPECIAL FORMULARY at the Alpha Medical Center based on the provisions of the Hospital Formulary System POLICY AND PROCEDURE of ALPHAOMEGA HEALTH.

D. The P&T Committee monitors compliance with the provisions of the **HOSPITAL FORMULARY.**

E. The P&T Committee supports the quality improvement functions of ALPHAOMEGA HEALTH where necessary to improve the use of the **HOSPITAL FORMULARY.**

F. The P&T Committee reviews and approves any POLICY AND PROCEDURE of the Alpha Medical Center Pharmacy.

III. PROCEDURE

    A. PHARMACY AND THERAPEUTICS COMMITTEE DEVELOPMENT

        1. The P&T Committee recommends, when appropriate, amendments to this POLICY AND PROCEDURE to the Administrator of Alpha Medical Center. After revisions to any of these proposed amendments by the Administrator, in collaboration with the P&T Committee, the Administrator submits the amendments to the Executive Committee of the Alpha Medical Center Medical Staff for final approval.

        2. The Officers of the P&T Committee prepare an Annual Membership Report to the Administrator of the Alpha Medical Center regarding participation of its Members and any recommendations for changes in its membership that may be important to maintain the expertise necessary for the affairs of the P&T Committee.

        3. The Officers of the P&T Committee prepares an Annual Report and submits it to the Executive Committee of the Alpha Medical Center Medical Staff for approval. As a result of this review, the Executive Committee may make recommendations to the P&T Committee for consideration regarding its affairs or to the Administrator regarding amendments to this POLICY AND PROCEDURE.

    B. FORMULARY COMMITTEE ORGANIZATION

        1. REGULAR MEMBERS AND SOURCE OF SELECTION

            a. MEDICAL STAFF MEMBERS

                i. There may be up to eight Medical Staff members nominated annually by the Administrator, or designee, of Alpha Medical Center, the President of the Medical Staff of the Alpha Medical Center, or the Officers of the P&T Committee. Any Medical Staff nominee should demonstrate an active interest in evidence-based therapeutics, a willingness to be an active participant in the affairs of the P&T Committee, and represent as a group, whenever possible, the specialties of: Family Practice, Internal Medicine, Pediatrics, Obstetrics and Gynecology, Hematology and Oncology, Cardiology, Infectious Disease, Pulmonology, and General Surgery.

                ii. From any nominees, eight are selected by the Administrator, or designee, of Alpha Medical Center on the basis of maintaining a reasonable balance among the following factors: hospital and outpatient-based physicians, primary care and disease focused physicians, physician continuity from year to year, and physician liaison to the Medical Staff Executive Committee of the Alpha Medical Center or the Formulary Committee of ALPHAOMEGA HEALTH.

            b. PHARMACY MEMBERS—The Administrator, or designee, of Alpha Medical Center selects two pharmacists and includes the Pharmacist In Charge of the Hospital's Pharmacy.

            c. NURSING SERVICE MEMBER—The Administrator, or designee, of Alpha Medical Center selects one registered nurse from the Nursing Service.

        2. SPECIAL MEMBERS AND SOURCE OF SELECTION

            a. The Administrator, or designee, of Alpha Medical Center may select Special Members as needed to provide administrative or technical support for the affairs of the P&T Committee.

    b. The Chairperson of the Formulary Committee may select one or more Special Members from the personnel of the Alpha Medical Center or its Medical Staff on a temporary basis as may be necessary for:

        i. technical support for the activities of the P&T Committee or any Ad Hoc Subcommittee or

        ii. information for the deliberations of the P&T Committee regarding a proposal to add or delete an individual therapeutic product listed on the **HOSPITAL FORMULARY.**

3. P&T COMMITTEE OFFICERS AND SOURCE OF SELECTION

    a. The CHAIRPERSON is selected by the Administrator, or designee, of the Alpha Medical Center from the physician Regular Members of the P&T Committee. The Chairperson:

        i. manages the affairs of the P&T Committee in a manner to:

            I) support the active, positive involvement of each Regular and Special Member,

            II) acknowledge any conflict of interests,

            III) initiate a replacement appointment of any Officer, Regular Member, or Special Member becoming inactive during a calendar year,

            IV) appoint temporary Special Members,

            V) select the location for Meetings of the P&T Committee;

        ii. prepares the Annual Membership and Self-Evaluation reports; and

        iii. appoints an Ad Hoc Committee when necessary to study decisions in greater depth or to arrive at consensus recommendations for consideration by the P&T Committee whose membership includes

            I) six or less members from the Medical Staff of the Alpha Medical Center,

            II) at least one member who is a physician Regular Member of the P&T Committee, and

            III) the Secretary, or designee, of the P&T Committee.

    b. The VICE CHAIRPERSON is selected by the Administrator of the Alpha Medical Center from among the physician Regular Members of the P&T Committee. The Vice chairperson assumes the duties of the Chairperson during their absence.

    c. The SECRETARY is selected by the Administrator of the Alpha Medical Center from among the Regular or Special Members of the P&T Committee. The Secretary assists the Chairperson in managing the affairs of the P&T Committee by:

        i. preparing the minutes for each meeting of the P&T Committee or any of its Ad Hoc Committees,

        ii. sending an Agenda to the Members prior to each meeting of the P&T Committee,

        iii. maintaining liaison with the other Committees of the Medical Staff,

        iv. maintaining a schedule for the annual Quality Assurance activities of the P&T Committee, and

        v. assisting in the preparation of any Drug Monograph or any other report necessary for a meeting of the Formulary Committee of ALPHAOMEGA HEALTH.

4. TERM OF APPOINTMENT

    a. The Regular and Special Members are appointed or reappointed each January for 1 year.

    b. Each Officer is appointed or reappointed each January for 1 year.

5. VOTING
   a. Each Regular Member has one vote, and each Special Member does not have a vote.
   b. Any two physician Regular Members present during a Meeting of the Formulary Committee constitutes a quorum.
   c. Regular Members present at a meeting of the P&T Committee may delay voting, when the appropriate expertise is not available during a meeting of the P&T Committee.
   d. A simple majority of Regular Members voting is required for any action of the P&T Committee. Any abstention on the basis of a conflict of interests is noted in the Minutes for the meeting.
6. LIAISON—A Regular or Special Member is appointed by the Administrator to report on the affairs of the P&T Committee during the deliberations of any other Committee of the Alpha Medical Center.
7. MEETINGS—The meetings of the P&T Committee are:
   a. scheduled once a month for 1 hour or as may be planned by the Members of the P&T Committee,
   b. attended by Regular and Special Members only,
   c. convened at a location arranged by the Chairperson.
8. COMMITTEE PROTOCOLS—The P&T Committee may also arrange for the:
   a. use of definitions applicable to the resignation and replacement of any Regular Member, Special Member, or Officer during a calendar year as may be established by the Formulary Committee of ALPHAOMEGA HEALTH and
   b. management of any potential or actual conflict of interests affecting the participation of a Regular or Special Member during a meeting of the P&T Committee as may be determined by the Formulary Committee of ALPHAOMEGA HEALTH.

C. HOSPITAL FORMULARY DEVELOPMENT
   1. The P&T Committee reviews, for comment at each meeting, any therapeutic product recommended for addition or deletion to the **HOSPITAL FORMULARY** by the Formulary Committee of ALPHAOMEGA HEALTH.
   2. The P&T Committee reviews, for comment at each meeting, any class review of therapeutic products by the Formulary Committee of ALPHAOMEGA HEALTH and their recommendations for changes in the **HOSPITAL FORMULARY.**

D. HOSPITAL FORMULARY COMPLIANCE
   1. The P&T Committee monitors each Medical Staff physician's orders for a therapeutic product that is:
      a. not listed or does not have an automatic therapeutic interchange with a therapeutic product listed on the current **HOSPITAL FORMULARY,**
      b. for an indication not permitted by the **HOSPITAL FORMULARY,** or
      c. for an indication having a restricted use provision.
   2. The P&T Committee may establish a Special Formulary for therapeutic products not listed on the **HOSPITAL FORMULARY** as means to temporarily support the efforts of the Medical Staff for hospitalized patients having special requirements that are unique to Alpha Medical Center. The Special Formulary therapeutic products is selected using the same process defined by the ALPHAOMEGA HEALTH Formulary Committee for the

HOSPITAL FORMULARY. For any therapeutic product listed on Special Formulary for 1 year or more, continued use of the Special Formulary status for the therapeutic product will require the approval of the Formulary Committee.

3. If the Alpha Medical Center P&T Committee votes to not accept a decision of the Formulary Committee, the Chairperson, or designee, of the P&T Committee attends a subsequent meeting of the Formulary Committee. At this Formulary Meeting, the Formulary Committee attempts to develop a strategy for resolving the conflict between the original decision of the Formulary Committee and the P&T Committee of the Alpha Medical Center. In the event that a resolution is not achieved, the issue may be appealed by either the Formulary Committee or the Alpha Medical Center P&T Committee to the Professional Affairs Committee for a final decision within 3 months of the appeal.

E. QUALITY IMPROVEMENT

1. The P&T Committee regularly reviews the decisions of the ALPHAOMEGA HEALTH Formulary Committee as a means to evaluate any issues requiring the development of carefully considered implementation requirements at the Alpha Medical Center, such as the shortage of a therapeutic product.

2. The P&T Committee maintains an annually revised schedule for Drug Use Evaluations as may be established through consultation with other Medical Staff Committees.

3. The P&T Committee or an Ad Hoc Committee reviews Medication Error Reports.

4. The P&T Committee quarterly reviews Adverse Medication Reaction Reports.

5. The P&T Committee participates in the development of standard order sets as may be requested by a Member, a group of Members, or a Committee of the Medical Staff.

6. The P&T Committee prepares an annual report to the Executive Committee regarding the overall level of prescribing compliance with the **HOSPITAL FORMULARY.**

7. The P&T Committee in collaboration with the Formulary Committee monitors black box warnings or other advisories issued by the Food and Drug Administration or pharmaceutical manufacturing company. The Formulary Committee uses the monitoring process as a basis to collaborate with each P&T Committee of ALPHAOMEGA HEALTH as a means to promote patient safety.

8. The P&T Committee suggests information to the Formulary Committee for inclusion in the **HOSPITAL FORMULARY** newsletter.

9. The P&T Committee may make recommendations to the Medical Staff of Alpha Medical Center regarding the health care of hospitalized patients regarding the use of the **HOSPITAL FORMULARY** based on the outcome of certain studies undertaken by the P&T Committee. These studies exclude any direct identification of patient names or medical records.

F. PHARMACY DEPARTMENT POLICY AND PROCEDURE

1. The P&T Committee periodically reviews and approves the POLICY AND PROCEDURES of the Alpha Medical Center Pharmacy Department.

2. The review and approval is coordinated with the operational statements of the other Pharmacy Departments of ALPHAOMEGA HEALTH Hospitals.

Appendix 15-2

Formulary Request Form

PHARMACY AND THERAPEUTICS COMMITTEE
FORMULARY ADDITION REQUEST

NOTE: This entire form must be completed in order for consideration by the **Formulary Committee** at its next regularly scheduled meeting. You may submit additional information based on the outline of this **request** if more space is required. If you are not a member of the committee, you must also complete a Conflict of Interest Statement and attach it to this request.

Generic Name _____ **Brand Name** _____

Indications—Describe the FDA approved or potential off-label uses which have prompted this **request.** _____

_____

_____

_____

Dosing—Describe the specific strength and administration form of this product necessary for this **request.** _____

_____

_____

_____

_____

Comparative Efficacy—Describe how this agent relates to other products in terms of effectiveness. Please include citations to any clinical trials or other publications that the P&T committee should consider. _____

_____

_____

_____

Contraindications and Warnings—Describe any substantial issues related to this product, including REMS. _____

_____

_____

_____

Adverse Effects—List any substantial issues related to this product. _____
_____
_____
_____
_____

Expected Outcomes—Describe how this product would substitute or add to the current **Formulary** products. _____
_____
_____
_____

Cost of Therapy—Describe how this product would change the overall cost of medical care. _____
_____
_____
_____
_____

Impact on Inpatient Care Processes—Describe any special requirements on the hospital for use of this product such as nursing/medical staff education, standards of care, discharge planning, certification, or standard order sets. _____
_____
_____
_____

Impact on Outpatient Care Processes—Describe any special requirements on ambulatory care for use of this product such as compliance, follow-up, or monitoring. _____
_____
_____
_____

Conflict of Interest—Describe conflicts of interest for the requester regarding medication or its manufacturer. _____
_____
_____
_____

Other Considerations—Describe any information not applicable to the above categories (e.g., need for order set, guideline, or policy and procedure). _____
_____
_____
_____

Requested By—Must be a **Formulary Committee Member** or **Hospital Medical Staff Member.**

Printed Name _____

Signature _____

Response—For record keeping by the **Formulary Committee**.

Received by a **Formulary Committee Member date** _____

Initial **Formulary Committee** consideration **date** _____

Final **Formulary Committee** consideration **date** _____

Action Taken _____

Notification of Medical Staff Member submitting request date _____

15-3

Appendix 15–3

P&T Committee Meeting Attributes[1-3]

I. TIMING

A. Regular—The choice is often between monthly or bimonthly. Overall, a long-term commitment to one schedule that does not vary is ideal. An atypical but practical variation might include monthly meetings except August and December, in order to adjust for times when it is difficult to get quorum, because of vacations and holidays. To support a regular meeting cycle, any cancellation on a sudden, unexpected basis must be avoided virtually without exception. Finally, a 2- to 3-year experience with a given schedule would be necessary to permit members an opportunity to work membership commitment into their own schedule.

B. Monthly work cycle—Virtually all holidays occur in association with the first or last week of any month during the calendar year. Similarly, Mondays and Fridays frequently have distractions caused by these associated weekend demands. Thus, the second or third Tuesday-Wednesday-Thursday of the calendar month are often the best choice for a regular meeting.

C. Daily work cycle—Given the character of the discussion above, the start of the morning or afternoon would be ideal for a meeting. The afternoon timing could be associated with a light lunch prior to starting the meeting.

II. MEETING ROOM CHARACTER

A. Location—A location that minimizes the travel barriers encountered by all the members of the committee is best. In a multihospital organization, this choice may not be ideal if a perception of interhospital territoriality would create a perception of bias in the decisions of the committee. There have also been suggestions regarding the use of teleconferencing.[4] As this becomes a more widely accepted professional tool, the barriers of travel time can be eliminated as a means to incorporate a higher degree of expertise within the members of the committee.

B. Size—The room should have a rectangular table, or tables set up in a U shape if there are too many members for a single table, with chairs on all sides and enough room for additional chairs next to the walls for guests who might be attending a meeting. The room should allow a comfortable fit for a table that is large enough for the usual attendance as well as appropriate audiovisual equipment. Overall, the room or table should not be so large that the usual attendees might feel isolated and thus less engaged in the agenda of any meeting. Similarly, a full turnout would crowd the room, giving greater emphasis to the character of the deliberations. If it is necessary for a portion of the attendees to do so virtually, it may be necessary to set the room up to take advantage of the necessary equipment.

C. Seating—This can be highly defined as is seen in cases with assigned seats having a name card displayed on the table for each member. The benefits of universal identity of the members would thus be enhanced, especially if they are generally unknown to each other because of the size of an institution or hospital group. More commonly, there could be no fixed seating arrangements for a more informal tradition that could better support collaboration and open discussion. A decision by the chairperson to sit in different locations would further emphasize this approach to a seating tradition. It is also often good for pharmacy personnel to disperse themselves throughout the room to avoid a feeling of us/them in discussions.

D. Electronic Access—With the implementation of health care system committees, it is likely that members may be scattered over a wide geographic area, making face-to-face meetings impractical, at least for some members. Because of that, it may be necessary to have an electronic system to distribute materials, allow online discussion in the meeting, and electronic voting.[5]

It may also be necessary to have electronic votes between regular meetings for minor issues or issues that must be resolved quickly before a meeting can be convened.

REFERENCES

1. Doyle M, Straus D. How to make meetings work: the new interaction method. New York: Berkeley Publishing Group; 1993.
2. Nair KV, Coombs JH, Ascione FJ. Assessing the structure, activities, and functioning of P&T committees: a multisite case study. P&T. 2000;25(10):516–28.
3. Balu S, O'Connor P, Vogenberg FR. Contemporary issues affecting P&T committees. Part 2: beyond managed care. P&T. 2004;29:780–3.
4. Boedeker B. Virtual pharmacy & therapeutics meetings [Internet]. The Harry S. Truman VA Hospital experience. Columbia (MO): Harry S. Truman Memorial Veteran's Hospital; 1999 Mar [cited 2004 Jan 27]. Available from: http://www.gasnet.org/esia/1999/march/virtual.html
5. Al-Jedai AH, Algain RA, Alghamidi SA, Al-Jazairi AS, Amin R, Bin Hussain IZ. A P&T committee's transition to a complete electronic meeting system—a multisite institution experience. P&T. 2017 Oct;42(10): 641–6, 651.

15-4

Appendix 15-4

Example P&T Committee Minutes[*]

ORGANIZATION, INC.

PHARMACY AND THERAPEUTICS COMMITTEE MEETING

January 21, 20XX

SCHEDULED AT 0700

THESE MINUTES ARE PRIVILEGED AND NOT SUBJECT TO DISCLOSURE OR LEGAL DISCOVERY PROCEEDINGS UNDER (STATUTE NUMBER)

I. Call to order

The members or Guests present or members absent are indicated below:

(legal names, usually with degrees)

The meeting was called to order by the chairperson at 7:00 A.M. The physician members present represented a quorum. The minutes for the previous meeting were presented to the members. The section regarding a report of the chairperson from a discussion with the executive committee about unapproved abbreviations was specifically reviewed by the chairperson. The minutes did not describe the executive committee's request that the P&T committee quarterly forward five to eight examples of physician progress notes that reflect this issue. The executive committee decided to have the president of the medical staff have individual contact with the medical staff members involved. A motion was made to approve the amended minutes and seconded. There being no further discussion, the motion was approved unanimously. After the vote, there was a brief discussion of the impending transition to a total electronic medical record with physician order entry and its ability to reduce transcribing errors. The physician members expressed concern regarding the ease of order entry. No further action was taken.

II. Pharmacy and Therapeutics Committee Organizational Affairs

A. Policy and Procedure Amendments—The chairperson submitted a draft revision of the entire policy and procedure for the P&T committee in response to new standards of TJC and previously discussed requirements for the functions of the committee. The committee reviewed the proposed draft and agreed informally to reconsider it at the next meeting after the chairperson has had a chance to meet with the Chief Medical Officer regarding any other amendments that may be necessary.

---

[*]Minutes listed in this Appendix follow a paragraph format. Use of a table or bullet points to provide a more concise minute review is done in some places.

B. Committee Procedures
   1. Conflict of Interest Disclosure—The chairperson gave the Members the forms necessary to declare any potential or actual conflicts of interest according to the procedure established previously by the committee. The chairperson briefly reviewed this process and emphasized that conflicts of interest were only unacceptable when not acknowledged or no action is taken to resolve them during a meeting of the committee.
   2. Formulary Request format—no change
   3. Alternate Medication Use—no change
   4. Drug Monograph—no change
C. Committee membership—no action; end of year report due December 31st
D. Annual Report—Draft Report due January 5th
E. Ad hoc committees—none currently
F. Budget—reports due February, May, August, November
III. Formulary System
A. Formulary Maintenance
   1. Formulary additions/deletions
      a. sodium zirconium cyclosilicate (LOKELMA®)—Approved Formulary
      b. coagulation factor Xa (recombinant) (Andexxa)—Not approved—Nonformulary
      c. meropenem and vaborbactam (VABOMERE®)—Approved Formulary with restrictions or guidelines or policy and procedure
   2. Formulary Class Reviews
      28:04 General anesthetic agents
      72:00 Local anesthetic agents
      86:00 Smooth muscle relaxants
      24:00 Cardiovascular agents
   3. Nonformulary usage report
   4. Review of standard order sets/guidelines
      TPN order sheet
IV. Drug Use and Quality Improvement
A. Medication error report—No report
B. Adverse medication reaction report—No report
C. Drug Usage Evaluation report—No report
D. Medication recall—No report
V. Hospital Pharmacy Policies—No report
VI. Current Medication Shortages
VII. Medications in the pipeline

Appendix 15–5

Chairperson Skills

I. Experience

A. Knowledge of formulary issues—This occurs ideally as a result of prior experience on the committee for several years. P&T committee meetings are often associated with an individual hospital, group of hospitals, a staff model health maintenance organization, or an insurance-related pharmacy benefit management (PBM) process. A chairperson's experience in each of these areas would be ideal.

B. Professional practice—It could be suggested that at least 10 years is required for a pharmacist, nurse, administrator, or physician to have a sense of the overall trends evolving within health care. Within a P&T committee, the chairperson would need this background to best respond to the biases that each member might bring to the deliberations. It is beneficial if the members have had mutual experience with the chairperson at a direct patient care level.

C. Leadership—The chairperson is likely to be the most essential person for the overall success of a P&T committee. This is most directly related to the organization truism that it is nearly impossible to hold a committee responsible for anything except when a committee is acting as the ultimate authority for an organization. Thus, the value of a P&T committee is related to its ability to serve the common interests of the entire organization affected by its actions. If the costs of the P&T committee members' time are considered, the committee's activities are the result of a very expensive effort. To best utilize this expertise, a chairperson must be skilled at mobilizing these resources in a manner that best supports the overall efforts of the organization to which it is attached. A previously demonstrated ability to create this role for a committee is the most valuable attribute for use in choosing a committee's chairperson.

II. Meeting Strategies

A. Punctuality—Given the busy schedules of the members, it is necessary to start and end on time. To open a meeting, it is best to lay out the agenda including any new additions and briefly discuss any items that will require a special discussion. Within

2–3 minutes, the chairperson and each member should understand the scope of the meeting ahead.

B. Fairness—Often the health care process vacillates unpredictably between deductive and inductive reasoning processes. External observers are often baffled by this interplay. Related to this, it is suggested that a strict use of the Robert's Rules of Order for a meeting agenda may not facilitate the spontaneity for a committee's members that usually underlies their involvement in the character of health care. It is the responsibility of the chairperson to guide this process and seek out the opinions that the members have for a given issue. Also, if the knowledge necessary to make the best judgment for a given issue does not exist for a decision on the issue, it is important that the chairperson be able to facilitate a consensus that develops a means to rectify the deficiency.

C. Involvement—Some members may not normally wish to participate spontaneously during a meeting. It is up to the chairperson to ask these members a specific question that would allow them a meaningful opportunity to participate in a given discussion. Occasionally, the chairperson might ask each member present about their opinion for a final decision being faced by the committee. This strategy should begin at one place around the table moving to each member present clockwise around the meeting room.

15–6

Appendix 15–6

Conflict of Interest Declaration

FORMULARY ADDITION REQUEST CONFLICT OF INTEREST STATEMENT

NOTE: This must be submitted along with the actual **Request** form if the person submitting the **Request** is not a member of the Formulary Committee. A copy of the Formulary Committee's Policy on Conflict of Interest Management is attached.

Generic Name _____ Trade Name _____

Substantial Involvement with a Competing Organization— ☐ Yes ☐ No
Please describe if:

1) A member of a health insurance company or another health system Pharmacy and Therapeutics Committee.
2) Another health system medical staff officer.
3) A member of a group practice primarily affiliated with another health system.

Substantial Involvement with a Company Which Manufactures the Product or Competes with the Product's Company— ☐ Yes ☐ No
Please describe if:

1) Receiving financial income or support in the last 12 months of more than $5000 for research, attendance at a **company** supported seminar, travel to an out-of-town meeting, or participation in a **company** sponsored speaker's bureau.
2) Receiving pharmaceutical products from the **company in** the last 12 months for personal or family use, gifts for family or personal use, or samples for use other than as a courtesy for patients.
3) Maintaining in the last 12 months a substantial ownership of stock (>10% of outstanding shares) in the **company** having >30% of its revenue from sales to **this organization,** its affiliated organizations, or another local health system.

Substantial Inside Information—☐ Yes ☐ No
Please describe if there are other outside relationships for which involvement in this **request** may be actually or potentially perceived as affecting the decision of the committee such as:

1) Having a substantial position of authority in another organization which might affect a member of the committee for employment or medical staff privileges.

2) Disclosing information about this **request** to another organization directly or indirectly which might give **this organization,** the other organization, or the requester an unfair advantage.

3) Receiving substantial assistance from the company or its representative which manufactures the requested product in the preparation of this **Formulary Addition Request.**

16-1

Appendix 16-1

Format for Drug Monograph

INSTITUTION/ORGANIZATION NAME HEADING

Generic Name: Can include other common, non-official names—e.g., TPA for alteplase.

Trade Brand Name: If more than one, indicate company that each is from.

Manufacturer (or source of supply): Include website address.

Therapeutic Category: e.g., Thrombolytic Agent for alteplase.

Classification: Note—other classifications, such as the VA Class, can also be used.

- AHFS Number and Classification (if not in the book yet, see the list in the front of AHFS Drug Information book and determine the most appropriate classification) or USP-DC.
- FDA Classification (include specific FDA website URL concerning approval).
- Status—Prescription, Nonprescription, and/or Controlled Substance Schedule (if applicable); note that there may be a discrepancy between federal and state laws.

Similar agents: A list of common treatments used for the same indication(s).

Summary: Includes a short summary of advantages and disadvantages of the drug, particularly in relation to other drugs or treatments used for each major indication, and any other significant information. Must include indications allowed in the institution.

Recommendations: Indicate whether or not the drug should be added to the drug formulary of an institution, including specifying the indications that it is approved for use in the institution, assuming they would have patients that would be treated for illnesses where this drug might be used. Also indicate specific formulary status for the drug (e.g., uncontrolled, monitored, restricted, conditional—see ASHP guidelines) and whether the drug will replace any other product that might already be on the formulary. In addition, any information on how the drug is to be placed in any clinical guidelines. For third-party payer monographs, information will need to be included on the payment tier.

Page one of the drug monograph consists of the above information.

Pharmacological Data:

- Mechanism of Action (usually brief)
- Bacterial Spectrum (if applicable)

Therapeutic Indications:

- FDA-Approved Indications (see package insert)—Clearly state which indications are FDA approved.
- Potential Unlabeled Uses (list only if they are considered to be acceptable medical practice, although it is allowable to mention others that are early in investigation with a statement that the drug should not be used for them or that they require more study)—Clearly indicate they are not FDA approved.
- How the drug, and similar drugs, fit into clinical guidelines.
- Clinical Comparison (abstract at least two studies; see Appendix 13-2 for more guidelines. Include human efficacy studies and, where available, studies comparing the product to standard therapy. Note: if there are other supportive studies for an indication, they can be covered briefly along with the major study covered in detail. Be sure to note any deficiencies in the studies). Also, pharmacogenomic information may need to be included here and elsewhere.

Bioavailability/Pharmacokinetics:

A table summarizing the following, in comparison to the gold standard can be very useful.

- Absorption
- Distribution
- Metabolism
- Excretion

Dosage Forms:

- Forms and Strengths—compare to other agents (consider a table), since new products often have a limited number of dosage forms/routes as compared to established products. Purity and composition information should be included for herbal and alternative medications.
- Explain any special information needed for preparation and storage, in comparison to other products. Sometimes a product will be so difficult to prepare or have such a limited shelf-life after preparation that it is not worth stocking.

Dosage Range:

- Adults
- Children
- Elderly
- Renal or Hepatic Failure

- Special Administration Requirements
- Any anticipated problems in supplies (i.e., shortages) or restrictions in distribution (e.g., prescriber certification required)

Known Adverse Effects/Toxicities:

- Frequency and Type (a table comparing the drug to others can be a clear and concise way of expressing this information)
- Prevention of Toxicity
- Risk and Benefit Data

Special Precautions: Usually includes pregnancy and lactation.

Contraindications:

Drug Interactions:

A simple one or two sentence statement for each—usually separate various interactions into separate short paragraphs and compare to other drugs; may also be presented as a table.

- Drug-Drug
- Drug-Food
- Drug-Laboratory

Patient Safety Information:

Includes medication error information and product safety information from outside sources (e.g., Institute for Safe Medication Practices [ISMP], MedWatch, FDA Patient Safety News, United States Pharmacopeia Patient Safety Program, National Institute for Occupational Safety and Health [NIOSH]).

Patient Monitoring Guidelines:

Include effectiveness, adverse effects, compliance, and other appropriate items.

Patient Information:

- Name and description of the medication
- Dosage form
- Route of administration
- Duration of therapy
- Special directions and precautions
- Side effects
- Techniques for self-monitoring
- Proper storage
- Refill information
- What to do if dose is missed

Guideline/Order Set:

Guideline(s) or order set(s) needed and how operations will be affected if the drug is added to formulary. This will include any pharmacoinformatics issues and IV pump library issues.

Cost Comparison:

Use AWP and institutional prices, and make sure there is a comparison with any similar products at equivalent doses—a pharmacoeconomic analysis (see Chapter 7) is the best method of comparing drugs in this section; remember to include any required concomitant therapy. Providing a spreadsheet file with information to consider different patient circumstances that can change may be helpful.

List different costs for each hospital if part of a multihospital health system (consider group purchasing organization costs, 340b program costs, retail pharmacy account costs, or other discounted pricing).

Reimbursement:

If a primarily outpatient medication, especially for an infusion center.

Consider patient costs after insurance/Medicare benefits, for ambulatory medications.

Date Presented to pharmacy and therapeutics committee, and name and title of the person preparing the document

REFERENCES:

Follow guidelines as described in Appendix 13-3.

Appendix 16–2

Example Drug Monograph

Note: This example is based on fictional products and is condensed. It shows examples of most sections in a real drug monograph, but often does not go into all of the details (e.g., a table of adverse effects is seen, but only a couple items are listed, whereas a full drug monograph would list at least all common and/or serious reactions).

St. Anywhere Medical Center (St. AMC)
Pharmacy & Therapeutics Committee
Drug Evaluation Monograph

Generic Name:	Artiblood
Brand Name:	MegaBlood
Manufacturer:	MegaPharmics
Therapeutic Category:	Blood substitute
Classification:	AHFS 16:00 Blood Derivatives
	FDA Classification: 1A
	Status: Prescription Only
Similar Agents:	Fakered

Summary:

Artiblood is a new perfluorocarbon that has many similarities to the only other product in its class, fakered. Both products have the ability to temporarily replace the oxygen-carrying function of red blood cells in patients in whom use of whole blood or packed red blood cells is impossible due to medical or religious reasons. In general, artiblood was found to be more efficacious than fakered; however, it also has been shown to produce a greater number of adverse effects. The adverse effects are mostly gastrointestinal in nature; however, the increased INR can be a problem in some patients. Artiblood is not metabolized in the body, whereas fakered is approximately 50% metabolized to inactive components. These differences are generally not clinically significant, since the dose of either product is unlikely to need adjustment. Fakered is available in several different volume bags, allowing the dose to be matched more closely to the anticipated patient need. While the cost of fakered appears to be lower, a pharmacoeconomic analysis shows that artiblood would produce the greatest cost savings for the institution.

Recommendations:

It is recommended that artiblood be added to the Drug Formulary for use restricted to those who cannot use natural blood replacement products because of religious reasons or because suitable blood types are not available, including for use in cardiac catheterization procedures. It is not approved for use as a volume expander, except when in conjunction with the previous indications.

Pharmacologic Data:

Artiblood is a type of perfluorocarbon, similar to fakered. These products have the unique ability to freely bind with or give up oxygen, depending on the partial pressures of the gas where the product is located (i.e., in the lungs there is an abundance of oxygen, so the product adsorbs oxygen; in the tissues there is a relative deficiency of oxygen, so the product gives up the gas).[1,2] The products do not have direct immunologic properties, nor do they have the ability to aid in blood clotting, although there may be some effect on blood clotting (either interference by coating platelets or precipitation of the clotting pathway mechanism).[3]

In addition to oxygen-carrying capabilities, the products have some plasma volume expansion properties. Artiblood has an effect similar to Dextran 40,[1] whereas fakered's properties are relatively insignificant.[4] Maximum plasma volume expansion occurs within several minutes of administration and lasts for approximately 1 day in normal patients. This results in increased central venous pressure, cardiac output, stroke volume, blood pressure, urinary output, capillary perfusion, and pulse pressure. Microcirculation is improved.

Therapeutic Indications:

Indications:

Artiblood is FDA approved for the short-term replacement of the oxygen-carrying capabilities of blood in patients who cannot use normal whole blood.[1] In addition, the product has been used successfully in cardiac catheter procedures, although this use is not FDA approved.[5] There is some early research into the use of the product as a plasma expansion product, but there is not enough information to support this use.[6]

Fakered is approved only for use in cardiac catheterization,[2] although it is commonly used as a blood replacement product in patients who cannot or will not use whole blood products.[7]

Evidence-Based Clinical Guidelines:

A search of the literature was performed to identify evidence-based clinical guidelines. This included Medline, Embase Drugs and Pharmacology, the ECRI Guidelines Trust website, the American College of Cardiology website, and approximately a dozen Internet search engines; however, no applicable guidelines were identified.

Clinical Studies:

Max and Sugar[6] conducted a comparison trial of artiblood (500 mL/day administered once daily to over 1 hour to 80 patients) and fakered (750 mL administered once over 90 minutes to 82 patients) in patients (18–80 years of age) suffering from massive blood loss (>1 L), who could not use whole blood due to religious beliefs (e.g., Jehovah's Witnesses). In the artiblood group, all patients were undergoing open-heart surgery, as were 78 of the patients in fakered group. The remainder of the fakered group consisted of gunshot patients. Patients with renal insufficiency (creatinine clearance < 50 mL/min) or diagnosed with liver dysfunction were eliminated from consideration. Both groups were similar, except that the artiblood group had more smokers, which may have had an effect on oxygen requirements. Withdrawals from the artiblood group were for the following reasons: death due to failure of heart-lung machine (one patient), noncompliance with protocol (ten patients), worsening symptoms (three patients), and side effects (one patient—vomiting). The authors noted that protocol compliance problems were due to inappropriate staff education and were not related to the drug itself. In the fakered group, withdrawals were due to side effects (one patient—diarrhea, one patient—nausea, one patient—abdominal cramps) and noncompliance with protocol (two patients). The patients were assessed on the following items: oxygen and carbon dioxide content of the blood (samples drawn immediately before and after administration, and every 4 hours for 24 hours), coagulation profile of patient (drawn within 2 hours before and after administration), effect on normal blood chemistry profiles (SMA-20) (drawn within 2 hours before and after administration), and time to discontinuation of supplemental oxygen to the patient. Adverse effects were also noted. Results were analyzed using appropriate statistical methods. Artiblood was found to increase the oxygen-carrying capabilities of the blood in comparison to fakered ($p < 0.01$), although fakered did significantly improve oxygen-carrying capabilities over baseline ($p < 0.05$). While fakered had minimal effect on blood chemistry and coagulation profile, it was noted that INRs were increased in patients receiving artiblood ($p < 0.001$). Other adverse effects, mostly gastrointestinal in nature, were more common with fakered, although the symptoms typically disappeared within 2 hours of administration. Other measured characteristics seemed similar between the two groups. The authors concluded that artiblood was the superior agent, due to increased oxygen-carrying capabilities. The authors downplayed adverse effects, although the effects on INRs do appear worrisome.

[Other studies would be covered here for all likely uses within an institution.]

There were no studies found that demonstrated any effects of genome on either artiblood or fakered therapy.

Bioavailability/Pharmacokinetics[16–18]:

Absorption:

Absorption is not applicable, since these agents are administered by IV infusion.

Distribution:

Artiblood is found in the blood stream, with little being distributed to the tissues. Approximately 5% of fakered is found in the liver, with the rest being in the bloodstream.

Metabolism:

Artiblood is not metabolized in the body, whereas approximately 50% of fakered is broken down to inactive components and is excreted in the bile. Patients with a genotype that is associated with ultra-rapid metabolism of CYP2D6 substrates quickly and more completely metabolize fakered to inactive components and, therefore, may need a higher dose of the product for a therapeutic result.

Elimination:

Artiblood has a half-life of 5–15 hours. It is excreted unchanged in the urine. The longer half-life is seen in patients with renal insufficiency. Since the drug is usually given as a single dose, renal insufficiency does not pose a significant problem. Fakered has a half-life of 4–7 hours in normal patients. Significant renal or hepatic impairment may double the half-life.

Dosage Forms:

Large Volume Parenteral:

- Artiblood—500 mL IV bags
- Fakered—500, 750, and 1000 mL IV bags

No other forms or strengths available. This product will have limited availability for the next 6 months due to the ability of the manufacturer to produce an adequate amount to satisfy demands. No problems in availability are expected after that point. Due to the restrictions on indicated uses in the institution, this is not expected to cause any difficulties and, therefore, no specific procedures are being mandated to address a possible shortage.

Dosage Range:

The normal dose of artiblood for blood replacement is 500 mL, which may be repeated once after 4 hours. Doses may be cut in half for patients weighing less than 50 kg. No dosage adjustments are necessary in renal or hepatic impairment. The product has not been tested in patients younger than 12 years of age and is not recommended in that population. No dosage adjustment is necessary in the elderly.[1]

Fakered is given in doses of 500 mL–1 L, with a maximum daily dose of 1.5 L. The dose is adjusted based on clinical response of the patient. The product can be used in patients as young as 6 years of age; however, the initial dose is 250 mL.[2]

Known Adverse Effects/Toxicities:

The two agents are compared in the following table:

Adverse Effect	Artiblood (% of Patients)	Fakered (% of Patients)
Gastrointestinal		
Nausea	20	7
. . .	. . .	. . .

Special Precautions:

Neither drug has been studied long-term; therefore, the effects are not known.

Both products are considered Pregnancy Category C. Tests in pregnant animals have shown adverse effects and no adequate, well-controlled studies have been conducted in humans. There is no information available on the excretion of the drug in human milk. Overall, when considering use in pregnant or lactating women, the physician must consider the benefits versus the risks.

Safety and effectiveness of artiblood in children have not been established, although fakered may be used in children at least 6 years old.

Contraindications:

Both agents are contraindicated in patients with hypersensitivities to the drug or any component of the dosage form.

Drug Interactions:

Drug-Drug Interactions:

Heparin—Effects of heparin or low-molecular-weight heparins may be significantly increased by either artificial blood replacement agent, although the effect by artiblood tends to be greater. There is no effect on either artiblood or fakered, although the heparin may improve circulation of the products to underperfused tissues.

[Other interactions for both drugs would be listed and compared.]

Drug-Food Interactions:

None are known or expected, since these agents are given intravenously and do not undergo entero-hepatic recirculation.

Drug-Laboratory Test Interactions:

INR—INRs can be increased by both agents, although the effect is more noticeable with artiblood.

[Other interactions for both drugs would be listed and compared.]

Patient Safety:

This product has a good patient safety profile, with relatively minor adverse effects (e.g., nausea). Since the product has no coagulation or immunologic activity, health care providers must be aware that it is only used for temporary help in oxygen-carrying capabilities. Other specific safety concerns include:

- Patients on warfarin must have a baseline INR and one each day for the 2 days following administration.
- The product has been on the market less than 6 months and information is limited.
- Product must be refrigerated until approximately 30 minutes prior to infusion.

Patient Monitoring Guidelines:

Monitor patient for objective evidence of effectiveness (e.g., oxygen content of blood and clinical effects). Obtain baseline INR and normal chemistry values, and monitor regularly. Monitor for adverse effects.

Patient Information:

In a patient receiving the product due to trauma, it is likely that he or she will not be able to be given information. In that case, provide the information to the next of kin or guardian. Inform patients that the product is an intravenous product that does not contain any blood products. The patient or family should know that he or she may receive this product once or more during the first day after surgery. The patient or family should be informed that the drug has few noticeable adverse effects other than some gastrointestinal upset; however, the physician or pharmacist should be consulted if anything unusual occurs. The patient or family should know that some blood tests will be regularly performed to exclude the possibility of adverse effects. The nurse will keep the drug refrigerated until approximately 30 minutes before infusion. Warnings about missed doses are irrelevant.

Guideline or Order Set:

None anticipated, other than addition to IV pump library for up to 1 L per hour.

Cost Comparison:

General Pricing Information:

	AWP	Daily Dose*	St. AMC	Daily Dose*
Artiblood 500 mL	$2500/bag	$2500	$2310/bag	$2310
Fakered 500 mL	$1000/bag	$1000	$800/bag	$800
Fakered 750 mL	$1500/bag	$1500	$1200/bag	$1200
Fakered 1000 mL	$2000/bag	$2000	$1600/bag	$1600

*Assume used one bag of each strength.

Pharmacoeconomic Analysis:

- *Problem definition*—The objective of this analysis is to determine which artificial blood product should be included on the St. AMC drug formulary.
- *Perspective*—This will be from the perspective of the institution.
- *Specific treatment alternatives and outcomes*—There are two drugs to be compared, artiblood and fakered. It will be assumed that natural blood products are not an alternative, since the ability to use natural products would preclude consideration of the artificial products. The outcomes to be measured are hospital costs.
- *Pharmacoeconomic model*—A cost-benefit analysis will be performed. A cost-utility analysis would be desirable, but insufficient information is available. Note—no published pharmacoeconomic analysis is available. The following is based on information obtained from the literature concerning efficacy, adverse effects, monitoring, etc., and uses St. AMC costs, since outside prices would be irrelevant.

	Cost per Patient	Benefit-to-Cost Ratio	Net Benefit
Cost of artiblood (including administration, monitoring, adverse reactions, etc.)	$5120	$7430/$5120 = 1.45:1	$7430 − $5120=$2310
Benefits of artiblood (money save by early patient discharge from ICU)	$7430		
Cost of fakered (including administration, monitoring, adverse reactions, etc.)	$4000	$4500/$4000 = 1.125:1	$4500 − $4000 =$500
Benefits of fakered (money saved by early patient discharge from ICU)	$4500		

[Note to reader—the above information is a summary of information, including averages, decision analysis, and sensitivity analysis that would be used in a pharmacoeconomic evaluation. While the details could be presented here, it may be distracting and confusing to some readers—a decision must be made as to whether all of the details will be presented. See Chapter 7 for details on how to prepare a pharmacoeconomic analysis of a drug being evaluated by the P&T committee.]

Presented by Mia M. Labrador, PharmD, to the Pharmacy and Therapeutics committee on February 30, 20XX.

REFERENCES

[References would be listed in the order in which they are cited in the text—see Appendix 13-3 in the Professional Communication of Drug Information chapter for format and details.]

Appendix 16–3

Biosimilar Monograph

HOSPITAL/ORGANIZATION NAME

Biosimilar
Brand Name® (Company)
Reference product

Summary (1 page maximum)

- Market approval date
- Requester & why
- Expected # of patients
- Does the biosimilar cover all indications as the reference? Y/N, implications
- Do the studies show the biosimilar is highly similar to the reference? Y/N
- Safety—major safety concerns
- Do the major payors and PBMs cover the medication?
- Operation issues
  - USP 800 Assessment of Risk
  - Risk Evaluation and Mitigation Strategies—Y/N
  - Alaris Y/N
  - High alert Y/N
- Formulary recommendation
  - Therapeutic interchange
  - Primary product?
- Formulary recommendation
- Annual cost savings:
- Other?

MONOGRAPH

Introduction

- *Pertinent disease state considerations for the medication*
- *Current guideline recommendations*
- *Formulary request (by which medical group and in what population)*

Indications and Usage

- *FDA indications comparison with reference product. Highlight differences.*

FDA indications covered by reference	FDA indications covered by biosimilar

Dosage and Administration

- *FDA dosing comparison with reference product. Highlight differences.*

FDA dosing for reference	FDA dosing for biosimilar

CLINICAL EFFICACY

Analytical study

- *List important point(s) from the analytical studies demonstrating highly similar with no clinically meaningful differences.*

Animal study

- *List important point(s).*

Clinical study

- *List important point(s) for safety, purity, potency (pharmacology, pharmacokinetics, immunogenicity).*
- *Is the biosimilar considered interchangeable by the FDA?*
- *Which indication(s) has the biosimilar been studied for?*

FDA clinical review

- *List any pertinent points.*

Safety considerations

Include any safety considerations from the original reference product.

- *FDA Medwatch*
- *ISMP*
- *Potential for error*
- *Black box warnings*
- *Pregnancy/lactation issues*
- *Adverse effects different from the reference product*
- *Drug interactions different from reference product*

Coverage Review

PBM and Insurance coverage assessment

Reimbursement information for outpatient infusion center medications

[Substitute 106% WAC for ASP in the calculations above if no ASP is available yet.]

Abbreviations: WAC, wholesale acquisition cost.

https://www.cms.gov/Medicare/Medicare-Fee-for-Service-Part-B-Drugs/McrPartBDrugAvgSales
Price/index.html

Payor information for outpatient infusion center medications

Do our top payors cover the medication?

- *Medicare* https://www.cms.gov/medicare-coverage-database/overview-and-quick-search.aspx?
CoverageSelection=Both&ArticleType=All&PolicyType=Final&s=Ohio&KeyWord=spravato
&KeyWordLookUp=Title&KeyWordSearchType=And&bc=gAAAAAAAAAAA&=&

Operational needs

- *If reference product has an IV guideline, include biosimilar.*
- *If reference product is considered hazardous or nonhazardous (USP 800), include the same classification for biosimilar.*
- *If the reference product has a REMS program, assess if biosimilar is included. Create REMS language similar to reference product for UHCare.*

Availability and Cost

Table. Number. Table title.

	Strength	Quantity	Cost
Biosimilar			
Reference			

Summary

- *Formulary recommendation*
- *Format: Recommend addition or rejection/removal of medication name [doses] for disease state to/from system adult or pediatric formulary based on supporting efficacy and safety data*
- *Categories*
  - Determine if biosimilar will be preferred product for formulary *Formulary categories*

Date Prepared: *Month date, year*
Prepared by: *Name and credentials (Position)*
Edited by: *Name and credentials (Position)*—This can be another pharmacist or physician.

REFERENCES

1. Follow NLM citation format (http://www.nlm.nih.gov/bsd/uniform_requirements.html)

Appendix 18–1

Tools Used in Quality Assurance

FLOW CHARTS

Flow charts illustrate the steps of a process and how the steps are related to each other. It can be used to describe the process, to increase a team's knowledge of the entire process, to identify weaknesses or breakdown points in the current process, or to design a new process. An example of a flow chart outlining how adverse drug reactions might be addressed within an organization is provided below.

Flowchart: suspected adverse drug reactions

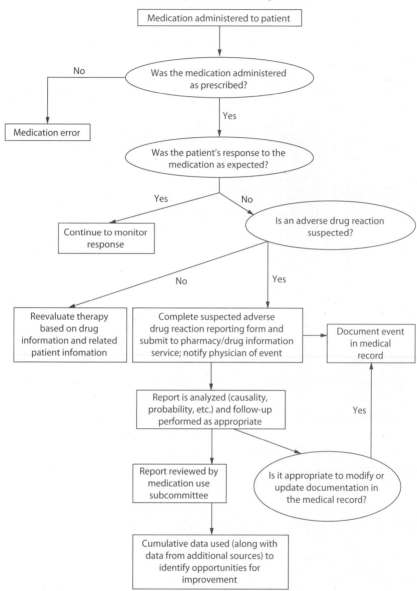

PARETO CHART

Pareto charts are vertical bar graphs with the data presented so that the bars are arranged from left to right on the horizontal axis in their order of decreasing frequency. This arrangement helps to identify which problems to address in what order. By addressing the data represented in the tallest bars (e.g., the most frequently occurring problems or contributing factors), efforts can be focused on areas where the most gain can be realized. Pareto charts are commonly used to identify issues to address, delineate potential causes of a problem, and monitor improvements in processes. An example of a Pareto chart appears below. This example illustrates frequently occurring factors contributing to improper dose medication errors. By focusing on transcription errors as a contributing factor on which to focus quality improvement (QI) efforts, the QI team will generally gain more than by tackling the smaller bars.

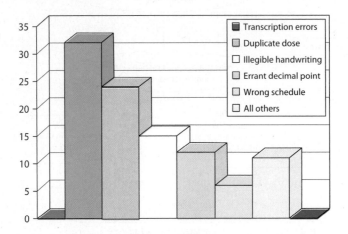

FISHBONE OR CAUSE-AND-EFFECT DIAGRAM

Fishbone or cause-and-effect diagrams represent the relationship between an outcome (represented at the head of the fish) and the possible causes of the outcome (represented as the bones of the fish). The bones of the fish should represent causes and not symptoms of the issue. Fishbone diagrams are commonly used to identify components of a process to address, delineate potential causes of a problem, or identify practitioner groups that participate in producing an outcome and should be represented in the group addressing quality issues in the process(es). An example of a Fishbone chart appears below.

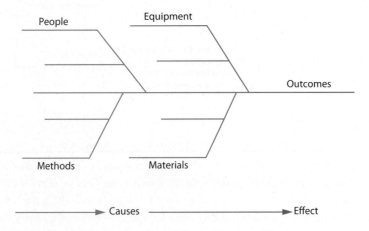

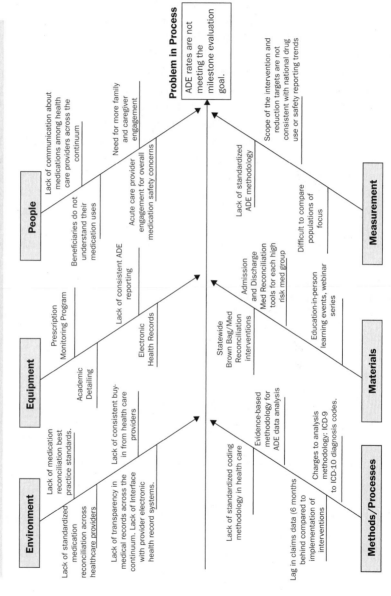

Medication Safety and Adverse Drug Events (ADEs)

A completed example of a medication safety and adverse drug event reduction fishbone is completed below.

CONTROL CHARTS

Control charts are run charts or line graphs with defined allowable limits of variation. Data are plotted on the graph as they become available with new data points connected to older data by a continuous line. The x-axis is usually a measure of time. The control limits help to identify which variations in data are important. Control limits are statistically determined based on average ranges and sample size. Fluctuation in data points above and below the average is expected and is referred to as common variation or common cause if they remain between the control limits. Data points above the upper control limit or below the lower control limit are referred to as special variation or special cause. Special cause variation indicates that something different is going on outside the normal operation of the process. Also, a series of data points above or below average may indicate a trend in performance that may need to be addressed. As variability in a process is reduced by quality improvement efforts, control limits should be recalculated (and narrowed) based on ongoing data. An example of a control chart appears below. Calls from pharmacists to prescribers in response to questions or issues related to new medication orders are represented over a 6-month period. Data from the month of July indicates a significant increase in the number of calls made. A quality improvement team evaluating this data would then attempt to identify what contributed to this increase. A potential cause in many institutions might be the influx of new medical house staff into the organization each July. One potential intervention to reduce this special cause is to improve the orientation of new practitioners to the medication use process within the organization.

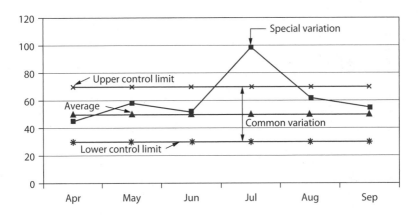

18-2

Appendix 18–2

Example of Criteria and Request for Approval

MEDICATION USE EVALUATION CRITERIA

Antiemetic Use in the Prophylaxis of Chemotherapy-induced Nausea and Vomiting

Request for Approval by Medication Use Evaluation Committee

Purpose of evaluation: The purpose of this Medication Use Evaluation (MUE) is to evaluate the use of antiemetic therapy in the prevention of chemotherapy-induced nausea and vomiting. This therapeutic class was selected for evaluation based on its essential role in the management of this patient population, potential inappropriate use, and increased cost relative to other antiemetic agents. This class of medications has not been evaluated within the organization for at least 5 years.

Criteria: A multidisciplinary group including physicians, clinical nurse specialists, staff nurses from the oncology unit, and pharmacists developed the attached criteria. They are submitted for approval by the MUE Committee.

[The actual criteria would be listed here.]

Data Collection: Data will be collected on all patients with orders for this agent written throughout a period of approximately 30 days beginning in mid-January 20XX. A minimum of 50 cases will be reviewed. Pharmacists and clinical nurse specialists will collect data concurrently from the medical record. Patients will be identified by means of the clinical information system.

Results: Results will be presented to this Committee. Information will also be shared with the Cancer Care Committee and Health System Performance Improvement Council. Prescriber-specific results will be confidentially provided to Medical Staff Support for use in the reappointment/recredentialing process.

18–3

Appendix 18–3

Example of Medication Use Evaluation (MUE) Results

MEDICATION USE EVALUATION

Summary of Overall Results

Antiemetic: January–February 20XX

Background: This topic was selected based on high use, potential misuse, and high cost of these agents. Criteria for this evaluation were approved at the MUE Committee's December 20XX meeting. Please refer to attached criteria for additional information.

Total Patients Evaluated (All Indications for Use) = 52

ELEMENT	STANDARD	RESULTS	COMPLIANCE
PRESCRIBING			
Indication for use	95%	OVERALL RESULTS	
		Treatment/prevention of nausea/ vomiting (N/V) associated with chemotherapy	100% (52/52)
		Highly emetogenic chemotherapy	46/46
		Anticipatory N/V associated with chemotherapy	6/6
DISPENSING/ADMINISTERING			
Dosing	95%	OVERALL RESULTS	71% (37/52)
		Highly emetogenic chemotherapy	31/46
		Anticipatory N/V associated with chemotherapy	6/6
MONITORING			
Adverse drug reaction(s)	<10–25% (varies with ADR)	OVERALL RESULTS	4% (2/52)
		Headache: 1 patient	
		Constipation: 1 patient	

continued

ELEMENT	STANDARD	RESULTS	COMPLIANCE
OUTCOME			
Prevention of nausea and emesis	95%	OVERALL RESULTS	92% (46/50)*
		Highly emetogenic chemotherapy	41/44
		Anticipatory N/V associated with chemotherapy	5/6
Chemotherapy course not interrupted	95%	OVERALL RESULTS (ALL INDICATIONS)	100% (52/52)

*Includes only patients in whom outcome was documented. Outcome was not assessed in two patients who were discharged immediately following administration of chemotherapy.

SUMMARY OF RESULTS

Prescribing: Criteria for indication for use were met in all cases.

Dispensing/Administering: Criteria for dosing was met in 37 of 52 cases with all cases involving anticipatory nausea and vomiting meeting criteria.

In 15 cases, patients receiving the antiemetic prior to highly emetogenic chemotherapy received doses not included in the approved criteria. Five of these patients received doses based on an investigational protocol. This dose is now under consideration by the FDA for approval, and preliminary results (available only in abstract form) were recently presented at the American Society of Clinical Oncology meeting. Results with the new dosing regimen have been comparable to those with the currently approved doses.

In seven cases not meeting dosing criteria, patients received a single dose prior to chemotherapy consistent with the criteria. However, an additional dose was administered 24 hours after the first dose. These orders were written by two prescribers.

Two cases did not meet dosing criteria because the dose was not adjusted based on renal dysfunction. In both cases, the estimated creatinine clearance was between 20 and 25 mL/min and nephrotoxic drugs were not being administered concurrently. In both cases, the estimated creatinine clearance increased to 30 mL/min or more by day 2 of the admission (probably due to rehydration of the patient). Neither patient experienced adverse effects.

One dose was not administered within the appropriate timeframe. In this case, the antiemetic dose was administered just 5 minutes prior to the initiation of chemotherapy administration. The nurse administering the antiemetic documented its administration on the way to the patient's room. When she arrived, the patient was not in the room. The dose was administered after he was located, approximately 25 minutes later. The nurse did not correct the actual administration time until after the chemotherapy was administered by a second nurse.

Recommendations:

1. Add new dosing regimen to dosing criteria.
2. Send letters to prescribers giving extra dose.
3. Renal dosing was not significantly outside guidelines. Mention findings in report to be published in quality improvement newsletter but do not take prescriber-specific action.

4. The dose administered late was reported via an incident report; no further action by this group is required at this time.

Monitoring: The rate of adverse drug reactions was less than that reported in the literature. This might be reflective of underreporting and underdocumenting of adverse drug events.

Recommendations:

1. The Adverse Drug Event Task Force is currently implementing a new process to improve reporting and documentation. No specific action by this group is required at this time.

Outcome: Ninety-two percent of patients did not experience nausea or vomiting. Outcome was assessable in 50 patients; two patients were discharged immediately following the administration of chemotherapy.

The patient who received his antiemetic dose just 5 minutes prior to chemotherapy experienced moderate nausea and no vomiting. Otherwise, the occurrence of nausea and vomiting was not related to problems with administration or dosing.

Recommendations:

1. Ninety-two percent success rate is acceptable based on literature; no action is necessary.

General Recommendations:

1. After approval, implement recommendations presented above.
2. Publish results in the Quality Improvement Newsletter following review by the Cancer Care Committee and the Quality Improvement Committee.
3. Perform a follow-up evaluation focusing on dosing issues.
4. Initiate planned assessment of this agent's use in postoperative nausea and vomiting as soon as possible.

Appendix 18–4

Evaluation Form for Drug Information Response

Request #		Date of Request		
Response by (circle one):		DI Staff	Resident	Student
Caller (circle type):	MD	RPh	Nurse	Other:

Assessment of Search and Response to Request	Yes	No	NA	Standard %*
1. Is requestor's demographic information complete?				100%
2. Background information is:				100%
A. Thorough				
B. Appropriate to request				
3. Is the question clearly stated?				100%
4. Search Strategy/References:				100%
A. Appropriate references were used				
B. Search was sufficiently comprehensive				
C. Is search strategy clearly documented				
5. Response was:				100%
A. Appropriate for the situation				
B. Sufficient to answer the question				
C. Provided in a timely manner				
D. Integrated with available patient data				
E. Supported by appropriate materials supplied to requestor				
6. If complete response could not be provided within timeframe requested, was requestor advised as to the status of their request and the anticipated delivery of the final response?				100%

*If performance falls below 90% in any category during any month, the service director will coordinate an assessment of the process, and findings and actions will be reported to the P&T committee.

Comments:

Reviewed By: _____

19-1

Appendix 19–1

Kramer Questionnaire*

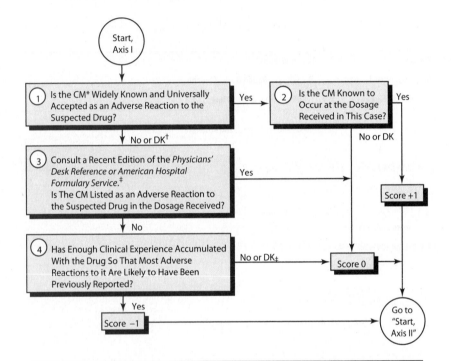

*Abbreviation CM indicates clinical manifestation, the abnormal sign, symptom, or laboratory test, or cluster of abnormal signs, symptoms, and tests, that is being considered as a possible adverse drug reaction.

† Abbreviation DK indicates do not know. This answer should be given when no data are available for the question being answered or when the quality of the data does not allow a firm "Yes" or "No" response.

‡ When these are not available, an equivalent reference source may be used.

Figure 1. Axis I. Previous general experience with drug.

*Kramer MS, Leventhal JM, Hutchinson TA, Feinstein AR. An algorithm for the operational assessment of adverse drug reaction: I. background, descriptions, and instructions for use. JAMA 1979; 242(7):623–32.

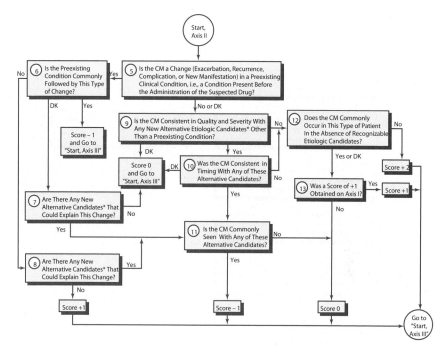

Figure 2. Axis II. Alternative etiologic candidates. For explanation of abbreviations, see Axis I.

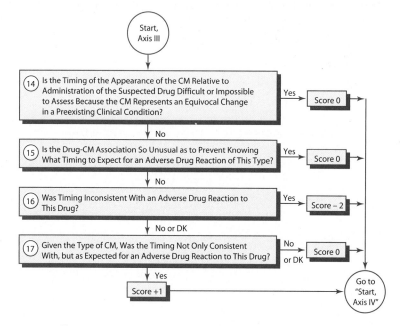

Figure 3. Axis III. Timing of events. For explanation of abbreviations, see Axis I.

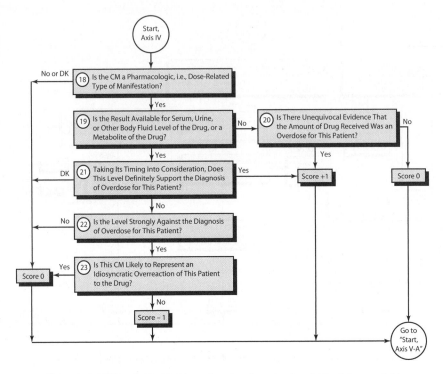

Figure 4. Axis IV. Drug levels and evidence of overdose. For explanation of abbreviations, see Axis I.

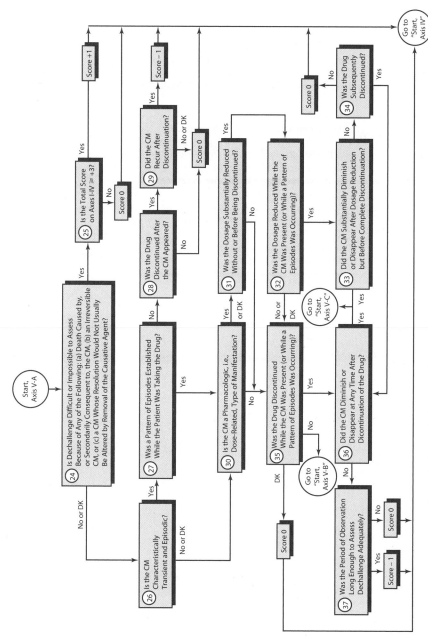

Figure 5A. Axis V-A. Dechallenge: difficult assessments. For explanation of abbreviations, see Axis I.

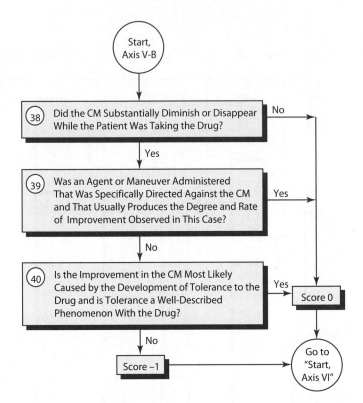

Figure 5B. Axis V-B. Dechallenge: absence of dechallenge. For explanation of abbreviation, see Axis I.

1420

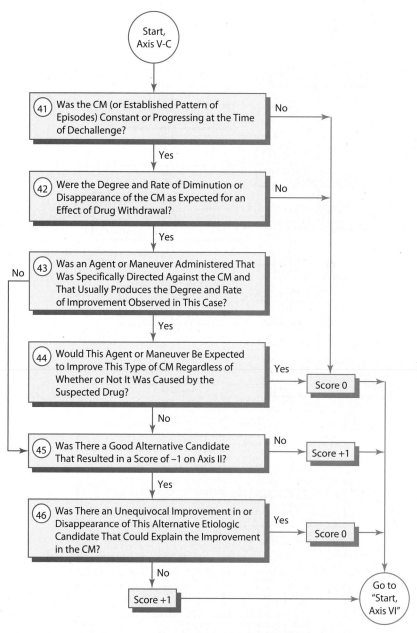

Figure 5C. Axis V-C. Dechallenge: improvement after dechallenge. For explanation of abbreviation, see Axis I.

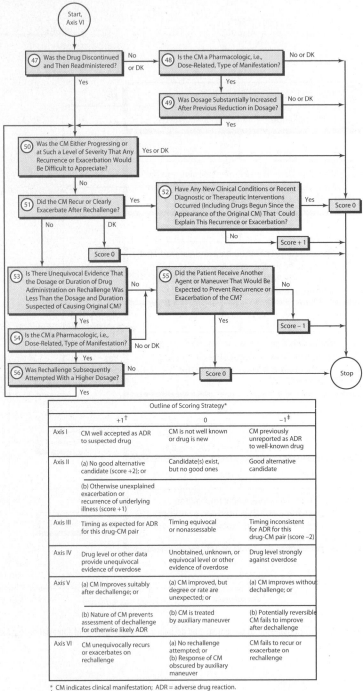

Figure 6. Axis VI. Rechallenge. For explanation of abbreviation, see Axis I.

Appendix 19–2

Naranjo Algorithm[*]

To assess the adverse drug reaction, please answer the following questionnaire and give the pertinent score.

	Yes	No	Don't know	Score
1. Are there previous conclusive reports on this reaction?	+1	0	0	
2. Did the adverse event appear after the suspected drug was administered?	+2	−1	0	
3. Did the adverse reaction improve when the drug was discontinued or a specific antagonist was administered?	+1	0	0	
4. Did the adverse reaction reappear when the drug was readministered?	+2	−1	0	
5. Are there alternative causes (other than the drug) that could on their own have caused the reaction?	−1	+2	0	
6. Did the reaction reappear when a placebo was given?	−1	+1	0	
7. Was the drug detected in the blood (or other fluids) in concentrations known to be toxic?	+1	0	0	
8. Was the reaction more severe when the dose was increased, or less severe when the dose was decreased?	+1	0	0	
9. Did the patient have a similar reaction to the same or similar drugs in any previous exposure?	+1	0	0	
10. Was the adverse event confirmed by any objective evidence?	+1	0	0	
			Total Score_____	

Score Interpretation

___Definite: ≥9

___Probable: 5 to 8

___Possible: 1 to 4

___Doubtful: ≤0

_____

[*]Naranjo CA, Busto U, Sellers EM, Sandor P, Ruiz I, Roberts EA, et al. A method of estimating the probability of adverse drug reactions. Clin Pharmacol Ther. 1981;30(2):239–45.

19-3

Appendix 19–3

Jones Algorithm[*]

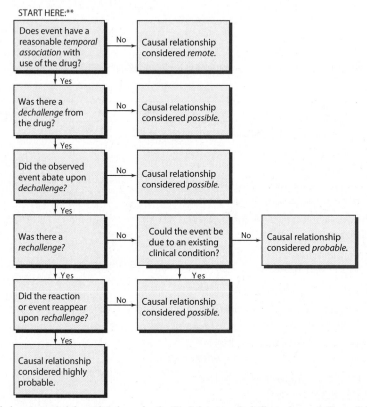

START HERE:**

Does event have a reasonable *temporal association* with use of the drug? — No → Causal relationship considered *remote.*

↓ Yes

Was there a *dechallenge* from the drug? — No → Causal relationship considered *possible.*

↓ Yes

Did the observed event abate upon *dechallenge?* — No → Causal relationship considered *possible.*

↓ Yes

Was there a *rechallenge?* — No → Could the event be due to an existing clinical condition? — No → Causal relationship considered *probable.*

↓ Yes   ↓ Yes

Did the reaction or event reappear upon *rechallenge?* — No → Causal relationship considered *possible.*

↓ Yes

Causal relationship considered highly probable.

**Each drug is carried through independently; if > 1 drug was dechallenged or rechallenged simultaneously, causality for all is ≤ possible.

QUESTIONS:

1. Did the reaction follow a reasonable temporal sequence?
2. Did the patient improve after stopping the drug?
3. Did the reaction reappear on repeated exposure (rechallenge)?
4. Could the reaction be reasonably explained by the known characteristics of the patient's clinical *state?*

---

*Jones JK. Adverse drug reactions in the community health setting: approaches to recognizing, counseling, and reporting. Clin Comm Health. 1982;5(2):58–67.

Appendix 19-4

Liverpool ADR Causality Assessment Tool

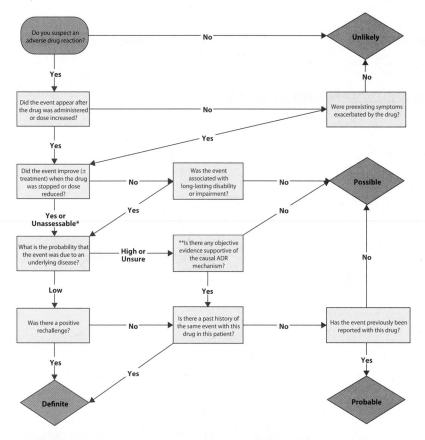

*Unassessable refers to situations where the medicine is administered on one occasion (e.g., Vaccine), the patient receives intermittent therapy (e.g., Chemotherapy), or is on medication which cannot be stopped (e.g., Immunosuppressants).

** Examples of objective evidence: positive laboratory investigation of the causal ADR mechanism (not those merely confirming the adverse reaction), supra-therapeutic drug levels, good evidence of dose-dependent relationship with toxicity in the patient.

Published with permission. Gallagher RM, Kirkham JJ, Mason JR, Bird KA, Williamson PR, Nunn AJ, et al. (2011) Development and Inter-Rater Reliability of the Liverpool Adverse Drug Reaction Causality Assessment Tool. PLoS ONE 6(12): e28096. doi:10.1371/journal.pone.0028096

19-5

Appendix 19-5

MedWatch Form

Reset Form

U.S. Department of Health and Human Services
Food and Drug Administration

MEDWATCH

FORM FDA 3500 (2/19)
The FDA Safety Information and
Adverse Event Reporting Program

For VOLUNTARY reporting of
adverse events, product problems
and product use/medication errors

Page 1 of 2

Form Approved: OMB No. 0910-0291, Expires: 11-30-2021
See PRA statement on reverse.

FDA USE ONLY
Triage unit sequence #
FDA Rec. Date

Note: For date prompts of "dd-mmm-yyyy" please use 2-digit day, 3-letter month abbreviation, and 4-digit year; for example, 01-Jul-2018.

A. PATIENT INFORMATION

1. **Patient Identifier**

2. **Age**
   - [ ] Year(s) [ ] Month(s)
   - [ ] Week(s) [ ] Day(s)
   - or Date of Birth (e.g., 08 Feb 1925)
   - In Confidence

3. **Gender** (check one)
   - [ ] Female
   - [ ] Male
   - [ ] Intersex
   - [ ] Transgender
   - [ ] Prefer not to disclose

4. **Weight**
   - [ ] lb
   - [ ] kg

5. **Ethnicity** (check one)
   - [ ] Hispanic/Latino
   - [ ] Not Hispanic/Latino

6. **Race** (check all that apply)
   - [ ] Asian
   - [ ] American Indian or Alaskan Native
   - [ ] Black or African American
   - [ ] White
   - [ ] Native Hawaiian or Other Pacific Islander

B. ADVERSE EVENT, PRODUCT PROBLEM

1. **Type of Report** (check all that apply)
   - [ ] Adverse Event
   - [ ] Product Problem (e.g., defects/malfunctions)
   - [ ] Product Use/ Medication Error
   - [ ] Problem with Different Manufacturer of Same Medicine

2. **Outcome Attributed to Adverse Event** (check all that apply)
   - [ ] Death   Date of death (dd-mmm-yyyy):
   - [ ] Life-threatening
   - [ ] Disability or Permanent Damage
   - [ ] Hospitalization (initial or prolonged)
   - [ ] Congenital Anomaly/Birth Defects
   - [ ] Other Serious or Important Medical Events
   - [ ] Required Intervention to Prevent Permanent Impairment/Damage

3. **Date of Event** (dd-mmm-yyyy)

4. **Date of this Report** (dd-mmm-yyyy)

5. **Describe Event, Problem or Product Use/Medication Error**

(Continue on page 2)

6. **Relevant Tests/Laboratory Data**   **Date** (dd-mmm-yyyy)

(Continue on page 2)

7. **Other Relevant History, Including Preexisting Medical Conditions** (e.g., allergies, pregnancy, smoking and alcohol use, liver/kidney problems, etc.)

(Continue on page 2)

C. PRODUCT AVAILABILITY

1. **Product Available for Evaluation?** (Do not send product to FDA)
   - [ ] Yes [ ] No [ ] Returned to Manufacturer on (dd-mmm-yyyy)

2. **Do you have a picture of the product?** (check yes if you are including a picture)   [ ] Yes

D. SUSPECT PRODUCTS

1. **Name, Strength, Manufacturer/Compounder** (from product label).
   Does this report involve cosmetic, dietary supplement or food/medical food?
   - #1 [ ] Yes
   - #2 [ ] Yes

#1 – Name and Strength	#1 – NDC # or Unique ID
#1 – Manufacturer/Compounder	#1 – Lot #
#2 – Name and Strength	#2 – NDC # or Unique ID
#2 – Manufacturer/Compounder	#2 – Lot #

2. **Dose or Amount**   **Frequency**   **Route**

#1		
#2		

3. **Treatment Dates/Therapy Dates** (give best estimate) of length of treatment (start/stop) or duration.)
   - #1 Start
   - #1 Stop
   - Is therapy still on-going? [ ] Yes [ ] No
   - #2 Start
   - #2 Stop
   - Is therapy still on-going? [ ] Yes [ ] No

4. **Diagnosis for Use** (Indication)
   - #1
   - #2

5. **Product Type** (check all that apply)
   - #1 [ ] OTC   #2 [ ] OTC
   - [ ] Compounded   [ ] Compounded
   - [ ] Generic   [ ] Generic
   - [ ] Biosimilar   [ ] Biosimilar

6. **Expiration Date** (dd-mmm-yyyy)
   - #1
   - #2

7. **Event Abated After Use Stopped or Dose Reduced?**
   - #1 [ ] Yes [ ] No [ ] Doesn't apply
   - #2 [ ] Yes [ ] No [ ] Doesn't apply

8. **Event Reappeared After Reintroduction?**
   - #1 [ ] Yes [ ] No [ ] Doesn't apply
   - #2 [ ] Yes [ ] No [ ] Doesn't apply

E. SUSPECT MEDICAL DEVICE

1. **Brand Name**

2a. **Common Device Name**	2b. **Procode**

3. **Manufacturer Name, City and State**

4. **Model #**	**Lot #**	5. **Operator of Device**
Catalog #	Expiration Date (dd-mmm-yyyy)	[ ] Health Professional [ ] Patient/Consumer
Serial #	Unique Identifier (UDI) #	[ ] Other

6a. **If Implanted, Give Date** (dd-mmm-yyyy)	6b. **If Explanted, Give Date** (dd-mmm-yyyy)

7a. **Is this a single-use device that was reprocessed and reused on a patient?** [ ] Yes [ ] No

7b. **If Yes to Item 7a, Enter Name and Address of Reprocessor**

8. **Was this device serviced by a third party servicer?** [ ] Yes [ ] No [ ] Unknown

F. OTHER (CONCOMITANT) MEDICAL PRODUCTS

1. **Product names and therapy dates** (Exclude treatment of event)

(Continue on page 2)

G. REPORTER (See confidentiality section on back)

1. **Name and Address**

Last Name:	First Name:
Address:	
City:	State/Province/Region:
ZIP/Postal Code:	Country:
Phone #:	Email:

2. **Health Professional?** [ ] Yes [ ] No

3. **Occupation**

4. **Also Reported to:**
   - [ ] Manufacturer/Compounder
   - [ ] User Facility
   - [ ] Distributor/Importer

5. **If you do NOT want your identity disclosed to the manufacturer, please mark this box:** [ ]

FORM FDA 3500 (2/19)   Submission of a report does not constitute an admission that medical personnel or the product caused or contributed to the event.
* Please see instructions

ADVICE ABOUT VOLUNTARY REPORTING

Detailed instructions available at: http://www.fda.gov/medwatch/report/consumer/instruct.htm

Report adverse events, product problems or product use errors with:

- Medications (drugs or biologics)
- Medical devices (including diabetes glucose-test kit, hearing aids, breast pumps, and many more)
- Combination products (medication & medical devices)
- Blood transfusions, gene therapies, and human cells and tissue transplants (for example, tendons, bone, and corneas)
- Special nutritional products (dietary supplements, medical foods, infant formulas)
- Cosmetics (such as moisturizers, makeup, shampoos and conditioners, face and body washes, deodorants, nail care products, hair dyes and relaxers, and tattoos)
- Food (including beverages and ingredients added to foods)

Report product problems – quality, performance or safety concerns such as:

- Suspected counterfeit product
- Suspected contamination
- Questionable stability
- Defective components
- Poor packaging or labeling
- Therapeutic failures (product didn't work)

Report SERIOUS adverse events. An event is serious when the patient outcome is:

- Death
- Life-threatening
- Hospitalization (initial or prolonged)
- Disability or permanent damage
- Congenital anomaly/birth defect
- Required intervention to prevent permanent impairment or damage
- Other serious (important medical events)

Report even if:

- You're not certain the product caused the event
- You don't have all the details
- Just fill in the sections that apply to your report

How to report:

- Use section D for all products except medical devices
- Attach additional pages if needed
- Use a separate form for each patient
- Report either to FDA or the manufacturer (or both)

How to submit report:

- To report by phone, call toll-free: 1-800-FDA (332)-1088
- To fax report: 1-800-FDA(332)-0178
- To report online: www.fda.gov/medwatch/report.htm

If your report involves a serious adverse event with a device and it occurred in a facility outside a doctor's office, that facility may be legally required to report to FDA and/or the manufacturer. Please notify the person in that facility who would handle such reporting.

If your report involves an adverse event with a vaccine, go to http://vaers.hhs.gov to report or call 1-800-822-7967.

Confidentiality:

The patient's identity is held in strict confidence by FDA and protected to the fullest extent of the law. The reporter's identity, including the identity of a self-reporter, may be shared with the manufacturer unless requested otherwise.

The information in this box applies only to requirements of the Paperwork Reduction Act of 1995.

The burden time for this collection of information has been estimated to average 40 minutes per response, including the time to review instructions, search existing data sources, gather and maintain the data needed, and complete and review the collection of information. Send comments regarding this burden estimate or any other aspect of this collection of information, including suggestions for reducing this burden to:

Department of Health and Human Services
Food and Drug Administration
Office of Chief Information Officer
Office of Chief Information Officer
Paperwork Reduction Act (PRA) Staff
PRAStaff@fda.hhs.gov

Please DO NOT RETURN this form to the PRA Staff e-mail above.

OMB statement:

"An agency may not conduct or sponsor, and a person is not required to respond to, a collection of information unless it displays a currently valid OMB control number."

U.S. DEPARTMENT OF HEALTH AND HUMAN SERVICES
Food and Drug Administration

U.S. Department of Health and Human Services
Food and Drug Administration

MEDWATCH

FORM FDA 3500 (2/19) *(continued)*
**The FDA Safety Information and
Adverse Event Reporting Program**

(CONTINUATION PAGE)
For VOLUNTARY reporting of
adverse events, product problems
and product use/medication errors

Page 2 of 2

B.5. **Describe Event or Problem** *(continued)*

Back to Item B.5

B.6. **Relevant Tests/Laboratory Data** *(continued)*

	Date *(dd-mmm-yyyy)*	Relevant Tests/Laboratory Data	Date *(dd-mmm-yyyy)*

Additional comments

Back to Item B.6

B.7. **Other Relevant History** *(continued)*

Back to Item B.7

F.1. **Concomitant Medical Products and Therapy Dates** *(Exclude treatment of event) (continued)*

Back to Item F.1

1428

Appendix 21–1

Policy Example: High-Alert Medications

I. PURPOSE:

This policy outlines the process for the safe use of high-alert medications.

II. DEFINITIONS:

When used in this policy, these terms have the following meanings:

A. High-alert medications: Medications that have a higher risk of causing harm when an error occurs.

B. Independent double verification (IDV):

1. Is performed by two staff members (as appropriate to the task, e.g., blood administration, breast milk retrieval) in the same proximity but separately, without prompting by another, as an independent cognitive task.

2. Both professionals will dialog to confirm what was checked independently prior to administration.

3. IDV of a medication also includes the following steps in addition to the two steps above:

   a. Performed by two professionals (e.g., nurse/pharmacist/physician [within the approved LPN scope of practice]) in the same proximity but separately, without prompting by another, as an independent cognitive task.

   b. Each professional must check: the actual prescriber's order, drug, calculation, concentration, and other information specific to the medication.

   c. Each professional performing the verification performs all calculations independently without knowledge of any prior calculations and documents the verification in the medical record.

III. POLICY:

It is the policy of the health system that:

A. All systems and data repositories relating to medication use (medication error reports, adverse drug event reports, etc.) shall be systematically evaluated on an ongoing basis to identify those medications in the hospital formulary determined to be high-alert medications.

B. Medications being added to the hospital formulary shall be evaluated for their high-alert potential.

C. Medications identified as high-alert shall be targeted for specific error reduction interventions.

D. The following three principles shall be followed to safeguard the use of high-alert medications:

1. Reduce or eliminate the possibility of error (e.g., limit the number of high-alert medications on the hospital formulary; remove high-alert medications from the clinical areas).

2. Make errors visible by detecting serious events before they reach the patient (e.g., follow the five rights and when appropriate utilize the independent double verification process).

3. Minimize the consequences of errors (e.g., stock high-alert medications in smaller volume units of use, minimizing the error effect if the medication was administered in error).

E. Engineering safety controls shall be used as appropriate.

IV. PROCEDURE:

A. The Pharmacy and Therapeutics Committee will approve all medications added to the formulary.

B. The following processes for safeguarding high-alert medication use have been implemented:

1. Build in system redundancies (e.g., unit dose drug distribution).

2. Use fail-safes (e.g., pumps with locking mechanisms).

3. Reduce options (e.g., limit concentration available).

4. Utilize engineering safety controls (e.g., oral syringes that will not fit IV tubing, computer systems that force the order of standardized products).

5. Externalize or centralize error-prone processes (e.g., centralize IV solution preparations).

6. Use differentiation (e.g., identify and isolate look-alike and sound-alike products, use generic names).

7. Store medications appropriately (e.g., separate potentially dangerous drugs with similar names or similar packaging).

8. Screen new products (e.g., inspect all new drugs and drug delivery devices for poor labeling and/or packaging).

9. Standardize and simplify order communication (e.g., only approved abbreviations will be used, all verbal orders will be read back verbatim to the ordering physician).

10. Limit access (e.g., high-alert medications will be securely stored).

11. Use of constraints (e.g., pharmacy will screen all medication orders, automatic stop orders, or duration limits).

12. Standardize or automate dosing procedures (e.g., use of standard dosing charts rather than calculating doses based on weight or renal function when appropriate).

C. When initiating any high-alert medication by any route, and for those high-alert medications administered via pump, and with all subsequent bag/syringe changes and with dose changes requiring pump adjustment, the following must occur:

1. Independent double verification, each professional will independently:
   a. Review/verify the physician order in the medical record (i.e., on the physician's order sheet or in the clinical information system).
   b. Verify the correct medication, dose (all required dosage calculations must be done independently by each nurse), frequency/rate/titration, and route against the order.
      i. Note: After the initial IDV, ongoing titration in Level I areas is exempt from the IDV process for each continuing adjustment.
      ii. Some medications require IDV of pump settings at change of shift (e.g., insulin).
      iii. Additional information regarding medication-specific IDV requirements is available in the IDV Policy and Procedure.
2. The nurse administering the medication will:
   a. Identify the patient using two acceptable identifiers.
   b. Verify the correct connection/patient access when administering the medication via an intravenous drip, trace the flow of the medication from the bag > to the pump > to the patient access, prior to hanging the medication.
   c. Document the verification.

D. When an infusion device with prebuilt infusion parameters is used and pre-set infusion parameters are not available for a high-alert medication (e.g., when the medication is new and not yet added to the library), independent double verification of the medication parameters programmed into the pump must occur prior to initiation of the infusion.

V. DOCUMENTATION:

As appropriate in the medical record or clinical information system.

VI. REFERENCES:

A. Institute for Safe Medication Practices (ISMP); ISMP's list of high-alert medications. 2008.
B. Patient Care Policy and Procedure #0282, Independent Double Verification.
C. Patient Care Policy and Procedure #0500, Verbal Orders.
D. Patient Care Policy and Procedure #0700, Abbreviations.
E. Patient Care Policy and Procedure #0282, IDV.
F. Patient Care Policy and Procedure #5010, Anticoagulant Safety.
G. Patient Care Policy and Procedure #5020, Chemotherapy: Oncology/Hematology.
H. Patient Care Policy and Procedure #5070, Electrolyte Infusions.
I. Patient Care Policy and Procedure #5117, Insulin Intravenous Infusions.
J. Patient Care Policy and Procedure #5130, Medication Administration.
K. Patient Care Policy and Procedure #5131, Medfusion Syringe Infusion Pump.
L. Patient Care Policy and Procedure #5140, Medication Use Analysis/Error Prevention.
M. Patient Care Policy and Procedure #5150, Moderate/Deep Sedation/Analgesia.

VII. ATTACHMENTS:

High-Alert Medications/Classes, one page.

Source: Used by permission from Orlando Health, Orlando, FL. www.orlandohealth.com.

High-Alert Medications/Classes	Safeguards, Etc.
Chemotherapy agents (all routes, includes antineoplastic, biological, immunological agents used for malignant oncology and hematology diagnoses)	Chemotherapy Policy and Procedure outlines requirements for independent double verification (IDV) of order, laboratory parameters, body surface area, medication, dose, route, frequency, etc.
	Chemotherapy order form (or electronic equivalent) required
	Only attending physicians with chemotherapy privileges may write orders
	No verbal or telephone orders allowed (except to clarify as outlined in policy)
	Only Chemo-verified RN's may administer (exceptions are made for some oral agents, refer to the Chemotherapy Policy and Procedure for details)
IV Electrolytes (i.e., potassium chloride and phosphate, concentrated sodium chloride, magnesium sulfate, calcium chloride, and calcium gluconate)	Independent double verification required (IDV not required for 1000 mL premixed IV solutions)
	No concentrated products outside Pharmacy (*Rare exceptions exist, but only with specific safeguards*)
	Electrolyte policy provides specific administration parameters and limits
	Electrolyte replacement protocol includes dosing and monitoring parameters
	Standard concentrations/premixes
Intravenous/subcutaneous anticoagulants (i.e., heparin, lepirudin, enoxaparin, argatroban, bivalirudin—excluding flushes)	Independent double verification required
	Weight-based protocol for heparin. The prescriber must designate the specific protocol (e.g., cardiac, noncardiac) to be implemented
	Duplication warning in Clinical Information System
	Standardized order review requirements for enoxaparin and fondaparinux
	Standardized laboratory assessments for heparin, enoxaparin, and fondaparinux for treatment of deep vein thrombosis/pulmonary embolism
	Premixed heparin solutions in standard concentrations
Neuromuscular blocking agents	IDV required
	Availability limited to specific units and access limited on these units (e.g., emergency department, operating room, intensive care unit)
	Special labeling of packages
	Standard concentrations established

continued

High-Alert Medications/Classes	Safeguards, Etc.
Insulin	IDV required (Note: verification of the insulin product is not required when insulin is supplied directly from pharmacy in patient-specific units of use [e.g., prefilled syringes versus vials])
	Floor stock limited to specific agents and pharmacy removes unused patient-specific vials from patient care units daily
	Resources include the Insulin Infusion Policy and the IV push insulin parameters defined within policy
	Sliding scale order sets create a consistent process
Anesthetic agents used outside the OR (e.g., propofol, ketamine, methohexital, etomidate, dexmedetomidine)	IDV required
	Guidelines for use and administration of propofol
	These agents have been added to the Moderate-Deep Sedation Policy with defined safeguards for use
Warfarin	IDV required
	Standard administration time to allow access to International Normalized Ratio (INR) results prior to daily dosing
	Laboratory monitoring standards and standardized order review processes
	Critical value—clinical laboratory calls with INR results >5
	Automated dispensing cabinet (ADC) inquiry—nurse is asked if he/she knows the patient's current INR as warfarin is being taken from ADC for administration to the patient
	Pharmacy monitoring of at-risk patients

22-1

Appendix 22–1

Example of a Project Charter

GOALS

The primary goal of this IV workflow improvement project is to eliminate all preventable patient harm when compounding medications. It is believed that by accomplishing the following secondary goals, significant progress toward improving patient safety will also be made:

1. Ensure correct ingredients in each compound.
2. Ensure correct quantities of admixtures in each compound.
3. Create standard compounding processes in conjunction with the electronic health record (EHR) system.
4. Ensure a retrievable historical compounding record to reference in scenarios of patient safety concern.
5. Facilitate the ability for pharmacists to remotely verify compound accuracy.
6. Facilitate compounding standards adoption.
7. Implement an automation solution that ensures the other goals are met.
8. Track and measure waste.

Through the research and selection process, Compounding Software X has been determined to be the best available automation solution for these specific needs. Within the next 12 months, the goal is to implement Software X at all hospitals throughout the health care system.

SUCCESS CRITERIA

This IV workflow improvement project will be considered a success when the following has been achieved:

Goal	Success Criteria
1 Ensure correct ingredients in each compound.	Create a standard list of compounded products.
2 Ensure correct quantities of admixture in each compound.	Create a standard list of recipes and procedures for compounding.
3 Create standard compounding processes in conjunction with the electronic health record system.	Create a list of drugs, and all associated data points, for use in compounding.

continued

1434

	Goal	Success Criteria
4	Ensure a retrievable historical compounding record to reference in scenarios of patient safety concern.	Develop, build, and integrate within the enterprise data warehouse repository.
5	Facilitate the ability for pharmacists to remotely verify compound accuracy.	Create a practice model, procedure, roles, and responsibilities for remote and collocated verification.
6	Facilitate compounding standards adoption.	Finalize, communicate, and enforce a benchmark percentage of compounded drugs and high-risk compounds to be created using automation technology.
7	Implement an automation solution that ensures the other goals are met.	All hospitals within the health system are using Software X for IV compounding.
8	Track and measure waste.	Finalize, communicate, and enforce a benchmark percentage of waste reduction that can be tracked and monitored using automation technology.

DELIVERABLES

The high-level deliverables for this project are as follows:

	Success Criteria	Deliverables
1	Create a standard list of compounded products.	1.1 Collaborate with facility teams to identify list of compounds to standardize. 1.2 Create a workflow for maintenance within the hospital formulary. 1.3 Create a workflow for maintenance of the software formulary. 1.4 Create governance process for standard compounded products list.
2	Create a standard list of recipes and procedures for compounding.	2.1 Create a list of standard compounds and identify the piece of technology on which each solution will be created. 2.2 Create a downtime procedure for standard compounding without the software technology. 2.3 Standardize recipe, drug data, and process for each compound. 2.4 Ensure new standards align with system standards and the hospital formulary.
3	Create a list of drugs, and all associated data points, for use in compounding.	3.1 Create a bidirectional interface between the electronic health record and the IV compounding software. 3.2 Populate the database with standard compounds.
4	Develop, build, and integrate within the enterprise data warehouse repository.	4.1 Build a method to facilitate data transfer from the Software X server to the enterprise data warehouse. 4.2 Create reporting and data analysis requirements to inform the data transfer method. 4.3 Define storage parameters.
5	Create a practice model, procedure, roles, and responsibilities for remote and collocated verification.	5.1 Create a workflow for collocated verification. 5.2 Create a workflow for remote verification. 5.3 Create a downtime procedure for remote verification. 5.4 Create formal education for pharmacy team members. 5.5 Create formal education for nonpharmacy team members.

continued

Success Criteria	Deliverables
6 Finalize, communicate, and enforce a benchmark percentage of compounded drugs and high-risk compounds to be created using automation technology.	6.1 Update the compounding policies, procedures, and guidelines.
7 All hospitals within the health system are using Software X for IV compounding.	7.1 Create an installation readiness matrix and assess each location for installation. 7.2 Implement Software X at three hospitals.
8 Finalize, communicate, and enforce a benchmark percentage of waste reduction that can be tracked and monitored using automation technology.	8.1 Create reporting and data analysis requirements to inform the data extract and load.

SCOPE

In Scope: These items will be addressed by this project.	Out of Scope: These items will not be addressed by this project.
Development of batch processing workflow with the IV compounding software	Infusion Center compounding practices
Electronic health record interface	Parenteral nutrition
IV admixtures, nonhazardous	Premixed IV medications (including minibags)
IV admixtures, hazardous	New hospitals that are planned but construction is not complete
	Oral nonsterile extemporaneous compounds

KEY STAKEHOLDERS

Name	Org./Dept./Title	Role	Contact Information
John Washington	Hospital Pharmacy Operations Director	Executive Sponsor	XXX-XXX-XXXX
Kathryn Morris	Medication Policy & Outcomes Director	Executive Sponsor	XXX-XXX-XXXX
Robert Henry	Pharmacy Automation and Technology Manager	Project Owner	XXX-XXX-XXXX
Eliot Cogan	Drug Information Manager	Subject Matter Expert	XXX-XXX-XXXX
Natalie Smyth	Project Manager	Project Manager	XXX-XXX-XXXX
Emily Garfield	Automation and Technology Pharmacy Technician	Subject Matter Expert	XXX-XXX-XXXX
Michael Kline	National Strategic Accounts Manager, Software Company X	Software X account representative	XXX-XXX-XXXX

PROJECT BUDGET

Funds have been secured to implement the IV workflow at each hospital. As with most new technology, there are significant upfront costs for both the software and hardware ($10,000 per workstation). When fully implemented, the annual maintenance fees will be $75,000 per year with an unlimited number of workstations within the health care system. Projections have identified the need for 50 workstations for the enterprise. In this regard, the annual maintenance fees will be approximately $1500 per workstation per year. In contrast, the request for proposal (RFP) from the company not selected was listed as $15,500 per workstation per year until the organization reached 50 workstations, and then the cost dropped to $9000 per workstation per year. At full capacity, the annual maintenance for the selected product is significantly less than the competitor. The company has also agreed to price protection in the contract. The hardware costs include scales, bar code scanners, cameras, monitors, and a keyboard (specifically designed to be in a cleanroom).

Contract Funding

Purchase Costs	Year #1	Year #2	Each Additional Year
Service Fees or License Fees	$400,000		
Implementation	$175,000		
Training Costs	$25,000		
Hardware	$800,000		
Maintenance Fees		$75,000	$75,000
Total Cost	**$1,400,000**	**$75,000**	**$75,000**

Hardware Funding Per Facility

Hospital	No. of Workstations	Cost per Workstation	Hardware Cost
Hospital 1	5	$10,000	$50,000
Hospital 2	8	$10,000	$80,000
Hospital 3	4	$10,000	$40,000
Total Hardware Costs Year #			**$170,000**

CONSTRAINTS, ASSUMPTIONS, AND RISKS

Constraints

- The initial project scope will not encompass all compounded products. The expansion of the system to include all compounded products will happen during optimization.
- An installation readiness assessment will be conducted for each installation site at every location. Each site must meet the readiness criteria for installation to begin.

Assumptions

- Use of a software solution during IV compounding is not currently a standard practice at the hospitals. The assumption is that staff will adopt this practice to accommodate the project and mitigate patient risk in compounding.

Risks

- Installation of power and data was not factored into the original budget. Hospitals will need to fund the construction required to pull power and data.
- If approved for a site, augmenting the barrier isolators will require contract labor, the cost of which was not included in the original budget.

Appendix 22–2

Stakeholder Matrix—IV Compounding Software Project

Name	Position	Role	Contact Information	Requirements	Expectations	Classification
Stakeholder's name	*Position in the organization*	*The function they perform on the project*	*Communication and correspondence information*	*High-level needs or wants for the project/ product*	*High-level expectations from the project/product*	*See classification table below**
John Washington	Hospital Pharmacy Operations Director	Primary Executive Sponsor	Weekly meetings	Improved IV workflow	Patient safety improvement and operational efficiency	C
Kathryn Morris	Medication Policy and Outcomes Director	Secondary Executive Sponsor	Weekly email	Formulary and recipe standardization	System-wide standardization and improved patient safety	C
Robert Henry	Pharmacy Automation and Technology Manager	Project Owner	Weekly meetings	Implementation system wide	Patient safety improvement and operational efficiency	D
Gregory Smith	Drug Information Specialist	Project participant	Weekly meetings	Formulary and recipe validation and standardization	System-wide standardization and improved patient safety	D
Dean Kipling	Inpatient Pharmacy Operations Manager	Interested in project	Monthly email	Improved IV workflow	Improved patient safety and operational efficiency	B

*A = monitor; B = keep informed; C = keep satisfied; D = manage closely/key stakeholder.

Appendix 22–3

Example PESTLE analysis—IV Compounding Software Project

Categories	Factors	What Does It Affect?	Probability of Impact (Rate 1–5)*	Severity of Impact (Rate 1–5)*	Score (Add Previous Two Columns)	Potential Responses	Who Will Monitor This Factor?
1 Political	Pharmacy Services	Hospital leadership reorganization may result in Key Stakeholders changes to include Central Entities hospital representation. This may ultimately impact the priorities of the project.	3	2	5	Prioritize the project as requested	Project owner
2 Economic	Unplanned Funding	Completing the facility work required to prepare an installation site for implementation may require leaders from that location to acquire additional funding. The facility work (including running data and power, adding data switches, buying biosafety cabinets, and/or remodeling clean rooms) was not budgeted in the original project cost estimates.	4	5	9	Inquire with Central Entities if they could support funding for the site(s)	Project owner
3 Social	Front-line staff response	The successful completion of this project is dependent upon a significant amount of standardization. Front-line staff will likely have a variety of responses to the new technology, application permissions, and compounding recipes as well as the new governance process.	4	3	7	Develop a communication plan outlining benefits to patient safety	Project owner
4 Technological	Cyber Security	All software must be reviewed and cleared through Cyber Security. Because data are stored in a cloud on an external server, there may be delays in receiving approval or barriers to moving forward if servers do not meet security requirements.	2	5	7	Work upfront with external vendor to ensure data security standards are met	Informatics

continued

	Categories	Factors	What Does It Affect?	Probability of Impact (Rate 1–5)*	Severity of Impact (Rate 1–5)*	Score (Add Previous Two Columns)	Potential Responses	Who Will Monitor This Factor?
5	Legal	Contracting	The organization and external vendor may not be able to reach an agreeable contractual arrangement, thereby delaying or preventing implementation	3	3	6	Determine essential legal requirements for contract negotiations	Legal counsel
6	Environmental	Raw materials	Ongoing natural disasters may cause shortages of technological components necessary for the IV compounding equipment (scanners, chips, gravimetric scales, etc.)	1	2	3	Discuss risks with the external vendor	Project owner

* 1 = lower likelihood; 5 = higher likelihood.

Appendix 22–4

Example Work Breakdown Structure (WBS)—IV Compounding Software Project

WBS ID	Action Item	Predecessor	Individual Responsible	Start Date	Effort	Duration
1.0	**Create governance process for identifying and managing system standard compounded products**		**Robert Henry**		**9 days**	**9 days**
1.1	Determine, document, and communicate that pharmacy team members throughout the system need to participate on this committee	—	Robert Henry		1 day	1 day
1.2	Determine, document, and communicate the frequency with which this committee needs to meet	—	Robert Henry		1 day	1 day
1.3	Determine, document, and communicate the decisions, rights, and reporting structure for this new committee	—	Robert Henry		1 day	1 day
1.4	Determine, document, and communicate a system leader for this committee	—	Robert Henry		1 day	1 day
1.5	Develop and document a committee charter	—	Robert Henry		5 days	5 days
2.0	**Create system standards for compounded products**		**Eliot Cogan**		**24 days**	**184 days**
2.1	**Identify initial compounds to standardize**		**Eliot Cogan**		**5 days**	**92 days**
2.1.1	Create a criteria matrix for compounds that can and will be created using the IV software	—	Robert Henry		1 day	1 day
2.1.2	Review inventory provided by Pharmacy Informatics team of all compounds created throughout system	—	Eliot Cogan		1 day	1 day
2.1.3	Assess all compounds created throughout system against criteria matrix	2.1.1	Eliot Cogan		1 day	30 days
2.1.4	Committee will approve and document compounding opportunities	2.1.3	Eliot Cogan		1 day	30 day
2.1.5	Request feedback and elaboration from hospital pharmacies on the compounds they are creating (as needed)	2.1.4	Eliot Cogan		1 day	30 days

continued

2.2	Create a standard list of recipes and procedures for compounding		Eliot Cogan	19 days	92 days
2.2.1	Review inventory provided by Pharmacy Informatics team of all compound recipes created throughout system	—	Eliot Cogan	1 day	1 day
2.2.2	Evaluate tertiary and primary references to validate compounds and associated information (i.e., beyond use date); Verify that best practice aligns with system formulary	2.1.3	Eliot Cogan	15 day	50 days
2.2.3	Committee will review and approve best practice for each compound	2.2.2	Eliot Cogan	2 days	40 days
2.2.4	Record and communicate best practice for each compound	2.2.3	Eliot Cogan	1 day	1 day

Appendix 24–1

Example REMS Template for Writing Participant Information

REMS Template for Writing Participant Information

Risk Evaluation and Mitigation Strategy (REMS) Document
[Drug/Class Name (Generic Name)] REMS Program

I. Administrative Information

Application Number(s): NDA/BLA [application number(s)]
Application Holder: [applicant name]
Initial [Shared System] REMS Approval: [MM/YYYY]
Most Recent REMS Update: [MM/YYYY]

II. REMS Goal(s)

[This section describes the overall, safety-related health outcome that the REMS is designed to achieve (e.g., mitigate the risk of a particular serious adverse event) and the intermediate, measurable objectives. In many cases, it is not possible to measure a risk mitigation goal directly; therefore, it is important to include one or more intermediate, measurable objectives that, if achieved, indicate that the program is meeting its goal.]
[Overall REMS goal]

1. [REMS objective]
2. [Other REMS objectives, as needed]
3. REMS Requirements

III. REMS Participant Requirements

[Applicant] must ensure that [List the participants who have requirements under this REMS, e.g., health care providers/pharmacies/health care settings/patients/wholesalers-distributors] comply with the following requirements:

1. Health Care Providers who prescribe [drug/class name] must:
2. Patients who are prescribed [drug/class name] must:
3. [Health care settings/prescribers/pharmacies] that dispense [drug/class name] must:
4. Wholesalers that distribute [drug/class name] must:

REMS Materials

[This section should include a consolidated list of all materials mentioned in the REMS Participant Requirements section.]

The following materials are part of the [drug/class name] REMS and are appended:

Enrollment Forms:

Prescriber:

1. [Prescriber Enrollment Form]

Patient:

2. [Patient Enrollment Form]
3. If the REMS includes different enrollment forms for different patient populations, include them as follows:

[Patient Enrollment Form for [type of patient]]

Pharmacy:

4. [Pharmacy Enrollment Form]
5. If the REMS includes specific enrollment forms for different types of pharmacies, include them as follows:

[[Type of pharmacy] Pharmacy Enrollment Form]

For example:

[Independent Pharmacy Enrollment Form]

[Inpatient Pharmacy Enrollment Form]

Health Care Setting:

6. [Health Care Setting Enrollment Form]
7. [Other setting-specific Enrollment Forms, as needed]

Other Enrollment Form(s): Include the names of other enrollment forms here

Training and Educational Materials

Prescriber:

8. [Prescriber Education]
9. [REMS Program Overview]
10. [Knowledge Assessment]

Pharmacy:

11. [Pharmacy Education]
12. [REMS Program Overview]
13. [Knowledge Assessment]

Patient Care Form(s)

14. [Patient Care Form] Include the names of forms used in patient care (other than enrollment forms), such as forms used to support patient monitoring or to document safe use conditions

Communication Materials

15. [Dear Health Care Provider letter]
16. [Professional Society REMS letter]
17. [Journal Information Piece]
18. [Fact Sheet]

Other Materials

19. [REMS Program website]

[Administrative forms and materials] Include any administrative forms or materials here, as well as materials that don't fit into the above categories
(Adapted from: https://www.fda.gov/media/77846/download)

Appendix 24–2

Response Letter Drug A—Incidence of Yellow Stripes

DRUG A—Adverse Event—Yellow Stripes

Dear Dr. Smith,

Thank you for your inquiry. The following information is provided in response to your question regarding the use of DRUG A and the incidence of yellow stripes appearing on the skin. Please note that the information provided is not intended to advocate the use of our product in any manner other than as described in the enclosed full prescribing information.

INDICATION(S)

DRUG A is indicated for the relief of moderate to severe hiccups in patients 18 years of age or older.[1]

PRESCRIBING INFORMATION

Please refer to the following sections of the enclosed Full Prescribing Information that are relevant to your inquiry: ADVERSE REACTIONS, WARNINGS, PRECAUTIONS.[1]

LITERATURE SEARCH RESULTS

A literature search of MEDLINE databases (and other resources) pertaining to the incidence of yellow stripes appearing on the skin associated with the use of DRUG A was conducted through September 20XX.

CLINICAL STUDIES

In phase III efficacy and safety studies of DRUG A for the relief of moderate to severe hiccups, yellow stripes appearing on patients skin was reported in 7% of patients (see Table 1).[2]

TABLE 1. INCIDENCE OF YELLOW STRIPES APPEARING ON SKIN[2]

Adverse Event	Drug A	Placebo
Yellow stripes on skin	7%	7%

In a 12-month long-term safety study, the incidence of yellow stripes appearing on the skin was evaluated. DRUG A users reported yellow stripes on their skin with an incidence rate of 9% (see Table 2).[3]

TABLE 2. INCIDENCE OF YELLOW STRIPES APPEARING ON SKIN—LONG-TERM STUDY[3]

Adverse Event	Drug A	Placebo
Yellow stripes on skin	9%	8%

Multiple case reports were identified reporting yellow stripes appearing on patient's skin. In a report by Jones *et al.*, a 90-year-old woman suffering from severe hiccups reported yellow stripes appearing on the skin within 4 days of starting treatment. She was treated with DRUG FIX-IT and her yellow stripes resolved immediately.[4]

In a report by Owens *et al.*, a 20-year-old man suffering from moderate hiccups reported yellow stripes on his skin within 2 minutes of starting treatment. The patient did not seek treatment, continued taking DRUG A, and the yellow stripes resolved.[5]

ADVERSE EVENT REPORTING

Please see the enclosed Prescribing Information for the complete safety and drug interaction information on our product. In order to monitor the safety of our products, we encourage clinicians to report adverse events by calling 1-800-555-9999 from 9 am to 9 pm Mountain Time, Monday through Sunday. Adverse events may also be reported to the FDA MedWatch program by phone (1-800-FDA-1088), fax (1-800-FDA-0178), or email (http://www.fda.gov/medwatch). To view a description of ongoing clinical trials for our products, please visit www.clinicaltrials.gov.

REFERENCES

1. DRUG A [package insert]. Awesome Drugs R Us, Inc. Any Town, USA; 2019.
2. Jones Z, Smith Y, Miller T. Efficacy and safety of DRUG A® in the treatment of hiccups. JAHA. 2009;6542:735–46.
3. Davis C, Jones Y, Rodriguez J. Long-term safety of the use of DRUG A® in severe hiccups. JAHA. 2009; 6543:887–96.
4. Jones A, Haines R, Lane K. 90-year old woman with yellow stripes. Hiccup Central. 2009;78(4):232–5.
5. Owens C, Cooper S, Jones B. 20-year-old male with resolved yellow stripes. Hiccup Central. 2010;83(3):196–9.

Glossary

340b program A program created by the U.S. government and managed by the Health Resources and Services Administration that requires drug manufacturers to provide significant discounts to qualifying health organizations for outpatient medications.

a priori Determining specific study criteria prior to study initiation.

Abbreviated New Drug Application (ANDA) A version of a new drug application that is submitted to the FDA for the review and potential approval of a generic drug product.

absolute liability See strict liability.

absolute risk reduction The difference in the percentage of subjects developing the adverse event in the control group versus subjects in the intervention group. Also refers to the number of subjects spared the adverse event by taking the intervention compared to the control.

abstracting A literature cataloging activity that includes a brief description (or abstract) of the information provided by the article or resource cited.

abstracts A synopsis (usually of 250 words or less) of the most important aspect(s) of an article.

academia Pertaining to a college, school, or other educational institution.

academic detailing A process by which a health care educator visits physicians to provide a 15 to 20 minute educational intervention on specific topics. Information provided is based on prescribing patterns and evidence-based medicine.

accountable care organization (ACO) A collaborative group of hospitals, doctors, and other providers of health care who coordinate their patient care efforts for Medicare patients. An emphasis is placed on minimizing duplication of effort and on preventing medical errors, in particular, for the chronically ill.

ACO See accountable care organization.

action-guides A term coined by Beauchamp and Childress to refer to a hierarchical approach to analysis of an ethical issue when forming particular judgments about the issue.

active control A standard therapy or procedure (but not a placebo) used in a study to determine the difference in effect produced by the study intervention.

active pharmaceutical ingredient (API) The active portion of a medication, sometimes known as the "raw material."

adaptive clinical trial A trial design, also known as group sequential design, that allows adaptation of various components such as inclusion/exclusion criteria, dosing, efficacy outcomes, and duration of trial based on continuously emerging knowledge throughout the study.

1451

ADC   See automated dispensing cabinet.

ADE   See adverse drug event.

adjunctive therapy   A therapy (e.g., medication, exercise, diet) that all subjects within a study receive; it is not considered a study bias since the effect of this therapy occurs among all subjects within the study.

ADR   See adverse drug reaction.

adverse drug event (ADE)   An ADE is defined as an injury from a medicine or lack of intended medicine. An ADE refers to all adverse drug reactions (ADRs), including allergic or idiosyncratic reactions, as well as medication errors that result in harm to a patient.

adverse drug event (ADE) monitoring   Computer programs that use electronic data and predetermined rules to identify when an ADE may have occurred or is about to occur. May be done by manual methods in some places.

adverse drug event (ADE) trigger tool   An augmented chart review method that uses automated systems to identify alerts or triggers to efficiently identify patients with potential ADEs. The triggers are cues that a patient may have experienced an error and/or adverse event. When these triggers are identified, it is suspected that the patient may have experienced a medication error. The patient's chart is reviewed for evidence of error and/or level of harm and data is collected and collated to determine potential common causes.

adverse drug reaction (ADR)   Defined broadly, any unexpected, unintended, undesired, or excessive response to a medicine. Many national and international organizations, including the U.S. Food and Drug Administration (FDA) and World Health Organization (WHO), as well as individual facilities or institutions, have their own definitions of what constitutes an adverse drug reaction. Defined by WHO as "any response that is noxious, unintended, or undesired, which occurs at doses normally used in humans for prophylaxis, diagnosis, therapy of disease or modification of physiological function."

adverse event   Any undesirable experience associated with the use of a medical product in a patient. This includes death, life-threatening, initial, or prolonged hospitalization, disability or permanent harm, birth defects, required intervention to prevent permanent impairment or damage, or other serious medical events.

after-action review   Provides a structured framework, often using a facilitator, for the project team to reflect on strengths, weaknesses, and opportunities for improvement after a project is completed.

aggregate   To collect and compile data and/or information and present it in a summarized format.

aggregate indicators   Provide a summary of the frequency, or timeliness, of a process by aggregating numerous cases.

AGREE II instrument   See Appraisal of Guidelines for Research and Evaluation II instrument.

AHFS classification   See American Hospital Formulary Service classification.

alert fatigue   A situation in which a provider becomes desensitized and therefore ignores or overrides clinical decision support system (CDSS) messages because of the large number of frequent alerts.

algorithm   A set of rules to be followed by a computer program when performing calculations or other operations.

alpha (α)   A value (usually 0.05) that is set prior to the beginning of a study and in which the p value is compared at the end of the study to determine if a statistical difference is present in the outcome being measured. A *p* value less than alpha (e.g., $0.001 < 0.05$) is interpreted as a statistical difference between the intervention and control groups of a study. Alpha also represents the amount of error researchers are willing to accept that a false-positive (Type I error) result is identified between the study intervention and control groups (e.g., alpha of 0.05 is up to a 5% chance of a false-positive result).

alternative hypothesis   See research hypothesis.

American Hospital Formulary Service (AHFS) classification   A classification that can be found in the *AHFS Drug Information* reference, published by the American Society of Health-System Pharmacists. It groups agents by use and/or drug class into specific numbered categories (e.g., 24:32.04 Angiotensin-Converting Enzyme Inhibitors).

analysis   The critical assessment of the nature, merit, and significance of individual elements, ideas, or factors. Functionally, it involves separating the information into its isolated parts so that each can be critically assessed. Analysis requires thoughtful review and evaluation of the quality and overall weight of available evidence.

ancillary therapy   A therapy (e.g., medication, exercise, diet) that is disproportional in use among the subjects in the groups of a study and has an effect on the outcome being measured; this can lead to a difference in effect between the groups which can bias the study results.

ANDA   See Abbreviated New Drug Application.

antibiogram   A report that shows the susceptibility of pathogen strains to various antibiotics. It is commonly prepared for each specific institution.

API   See active pharmaceutical ingredient.

application service provider   See software as a service.

Appraisal of Guidelines for Research and Evaluation (AGREE) II instrument   A structured instrument to assess guideline quality, provide a methodological strategy for guideline development, and inform what information and how information ought to be reported in guidelines.

article proposal   A letter asking the publisher whether he or she would be interested in possibly publishing something on a topic written by the person(s) who are inquiring.

aspect of care   A term used in quality assurance programs to indicate the title that describes the area being evaluated.

assay sensitivity   If noninferiority is established for the test drug, further concluding the test drug is effective can only be made if the reference drug's efficacy has been confirmed with high-quality clinical trials against placebo.

assumption of the risk   A defense in the law of torts, which bars a plaintiff from recovery against a negligent party if the defendant can demonstrate that the plaintiff voluntarily and knowingly assumed the risks at issue inherent to the dangerous activity in which he or she was participating at the time of his or her injury.

attributable risk   A statistical technique used in follow-up studies to determine the risk associated with exposure to a certain factor on disease state development. Attributable risk estimates the number of disease cases per number of exposures to the factor. This is primarily used in cohort studies and is considered an epidemiological term.

automated dispensing cabinet (ADC)   Automated device with a range of functions. Core capabilities include medication storage and retrieval for administration to patients, especially inpatient care areas, as well as audit trails of cabinet access. Other functions can include medication charging and automated inventory management.

autonomy   Autonomy is the personal rule that is free from both controlling interferences by others and from personal limitations that prevent meaningful choice. Autonomous individuals act intentionally, with understanding, and without controlling influences.

bar code medication administration (BCMA)   The use of bar code scanning to ensure the appropriate drug is administered to the appropriate patient at the appropriate time and via the appropriate route.

bar code verification   The use of bar code scanning to ensure that the correct drug, strength, and dosage form were dispensed in the drug selection process and to ensure that the five basic patient rights (i.e., right patient, right drug, right dose, right route, right time) are followed at the point of care.

BCMA   See bar code medication administration.

beneficence   A basic principle of consequentialist theory that expresses the duty to promote good.

Berkson's Bias   A type of selection bias noted in case-control studies that is produced when the probability of hospitalization of cases and controls differ. This probability can be increased based on the specific exposure being studied and increases the chance of hospital admission.

beta   The probability of a false-negative result in a study.

bias   An intentional or unintentional systematic error in the way a study is designed, conducted, analyzed, or reported.

bibliography   A list of references, usually placed at the end of a piece of professional writing.

big data   Large-scale amounts of data collected from various sources, which is characterized by the five Vs: volume, velocity, variety, veracity, value.

biocreep   Phenomenon by which a new treatment is eventually no more efficacious than placebo due to conclusions of noninferiority made from sequential noninferiority studies, usually from comparing the new treatment to a somewhat inferior active treatment.

bioequivalence study   Research that evaluates whether products are similar in rate and extent of absorption.

Biologics License Applications (BLA)   A biologics license application is a submission that contains specific information on the manufacturing processes, chemistry, pharmacology, clinical pharmacology, and the medical effects of the biologic product. It is a request for permission to introduce, or deliver for introduction, a biologic product into interstate commerce.

bio-sensing wearables   An on-body or in-body accessory that enhance user experience by use of a biosensor.

biosensor   An analytical device which converts a biological response into an electrical signal.

biosimilar   A highly similar biologic product that has no meaningful differences from an existing product. Typically, this means the active ingredient is identical, but there may be some minor differences between inactive ingredients.

BLA   See Biologics License Applications.

black box   In artificial intelligence, an analytical approach wherein inputs are known, but the methodology and path to arrive at an outcome is unknown.

black letter rules   Principles of law that are known generally to all and are free from doubt and ambiguity. Also known as hornbook law, since they are in a format that would probably be enunciated in a hornbook.

blinding   Study technique used in research to reduce bias by minimizing the risk that study subject assignment is known by the study subjects and/or investigators.

CAM   See complementary and alternative medicine.

case report   A descriptive observational study design that involves a clinical observation in a single patient. If a small group of patients is described, it may be referred to as a case series. A case report/case series does not involve a control group.

case report form (CRF)   A paper or electronic questionnaire specifically used in clinical trial research. The case report form is the tool used by the sponsor of the clinical trial to collect data from each participating patient.

case study   A record of descriptive research that documents a practitioner's experiences, thoughts, or observations related to the care of a single patient. Not useful to test a hypothesis but can serve to generate pilot information to design future controlled trials.

case-control study   An analytical observational study design in which researchers identify a group of patients with and without an outcome (often a disease) and follow data backward in time to determine if they were exposed to a risk factor (often a drug). Case-control studies are retrospective.

categorical data or variable   A variable measured on a nominal or ordinal scale. This data can be parsed and separated into discrete categories and further divided into two groups: dichotomous (two categories) or polytomous (more than two categories).

CBA   See cost-benefit analysis.

CCA   See cost-consequence analysis.

CDS   See clinical decision support.

CDSS   See clinical decision support system.

CEA   See cost-effectiveness analysis.

Centers for Medicare and Medicaid Innovation (CMMI)   Also called the CMS Innovation Center, supports the development and testing of innovative health care payment and service delivery models.

central limit theorem   The central limit theorem states when equally sized samples are drawn from a non-normal distribution, the plotted mean values from each sample will approximate a normal distribution if the non-normality was not due to outliers.

CER   See cost-effectiveness ratio.

CFL promotional communication   A term FDA uses to refer to Consistent with FDA-Required Labeling Communication. A three-factor test is applied to determine if the communication is false or misleading, possibly leading to enforcement action.

CHI   See consumer health information.

civil liability   Negligent acts and/or omissions, other than breach of contract, normally independent of moral obligations for which a remedy can be provided in a court of law. This form of liability is imposed under civil laws and processes, not criminal law. For example, a person injured in someone's home can bring suit under civil liability law.

clinical decision support (CDS)   A variety of information technology tools to assist with patient care decision-making.

clinical decision support system (CDSS)   Computer programs that augment clinical decision-making by combining referential information with patient-specific information to prevent negative actions and update providers of patient status.

clinical guideline   See clinical practice guidelines.

clinical investigation   Any experiment in which a drug is administered or dispensed to one or more human subjects. An experiment is any use of a drug (except for the use of a marketed drug) in the course of medical practice. Although there are many other definitions, this is the FDA's definition and would seem the appropriate one to use, given the nature of this topic. Please note that the FDA does not regulate the practice of medicine, and prescribers are (as far as the agency is concerned) free to use any marketed drug for off-label use.

clinical practice guidelines   Recommendations for optimizing patient care developed by experts systematically reviewing evidence and assessing the benefits and harms of health care interventions.

clinical response letter   Written correspondence that contains company-approved content in response to an unsolicited request for medical information.

Clinical Safety Officer (CSO)   Also known as the Regulatory Management Officer (RMO). This will be the sponsor's Food and Drug Administration contact person. Generally, the CSO/RMO assigned to a drug's Investigational New Drug Application will also be assigned to the New Drug Application.

clinical significance   The clinical importance of data generated in a study, irrespective of statistical results. Usually refers to the application of study results into clinical practice. Also, can be called clinical meaningfulness.

clinically significant   A result large enough to cause an effect on an efficacy outcome measure that noticeably changes a patient's condition.

clinical workflow   The sequence of events normally carried out in the delivery of clinical services.

closed formulary   A drug formulary that restricts the drugs available within an institution or available under a third-party plan.

CMA   See cost-minimization analysis.

CMMI   See Centers for Medicare and Medicaid Innovation.

CMR   See comprehensive medication review.

coauthor   Any individual who writes a portion of an article, chapter, book, etc. This includes individuals other than the primary author, whose name is normally listed first on a publication.

cohort study   An analytical observational study design in which researchers identify a group of patients exposed and not exposed to a risk factor (often a drug) and follow data forward in time to determine if they develop an outcome (often a disease). Cohort studies may be retrospective (use previously collected data) or prospective (gather new data starting in the present and going into the future).

COI   See conflict of interest.

commercial IND   An IND for which the sponsor is usually either a corporate entity or one of the institutes of the National Institutes of Health (NIH). In addition, CDER may designate other INDs as commercial, if it is clear the sponsor intends the product to be commercialized at a later date.

community rule   See locality rule.

comparative negligence   The allocation of responsibility for damages incurred between the plaintiff and defendant, based on the relative negligence of the two.

compendia   Collections of concise but detailed information about particular subjects (e.g., summaries of drug information compiled by experts).

complementary and alternative medicine (CAM)   An approach to health care outside conventional medicine. Complementary medicine, also known as integrative medicine, refers to using a nonmainstream approach *together with* conventional medicine. Alternative medicine refers to using a nonmainstream approach *in place of* conventional medicine.

compliance   A measure of how well instructions are followed. In a study, compliance refers to how well a patient follows instructions for medication administration and how well the investigator follows the study protocol.

composite outcome   An endpoint where multiple endpoints are combined into one (e.g., the incidence of death, recurrent myocardial infarction, or recurrent stroke).

composite score   A score calculated when adding two or more scores together. For example, a prescription drug that reports efficacy outcomes as a composite score assesses how well the medication works for the two outcomes added together (not individual outcomes).

comprehensive medication review (CMR)   An essential element of medication therapy management (MTM). A CMR is a systematic process of collecting patient-specific information, assessing medication therapies to identify medication-related problems, developing a prioritized list of medication-related problems, and creating a plan to resolve them with the patient, caregiver, and/or prescriber.

computer-based clinical decision support systems   software that is designed to assist clinical decision-making which utilizes both patient-specific information and clinical knowledge to make assessments or recommendations in clinical practice.

computerized provider order entry (CPOE)   A process allowing medical provider instructions to be electronically entered for the treatment of patients who are under a provider's care.

concurrent indicator   An indicator used in any quality assurance program that determines whether quality is acceptable while an action is being taken or care is being given.

concurrent negligence   The wrongful acts or omissions of two or more persons acting independently, but causing the same injury.

confidence interval   Range calculated for a study result in which the true value for the population exists. The percentage association with the range (e.g., 95%) indicates the confidence in which the true population value is within the range. For instance, the investigators are 95% confident that the mean blood pressure lowering effect of the medication for the population is between −8 to −12 mmHg for the 95% confidence interval of (−8 to −12 mmHg).

confidentiality   A moral rule, related to the principle of autonomy, which specifically addresses the individual client's right to give or refuse consent relative to release of privileged information.

confirmation bias   The natural tendency to accept new information that confirms ones' beliefs and reject evidence that goes against them.

conflict of interest (COI)   A situation in which the interests of an investigator conflict with the study purpose, design, and/or result interpretation. An investigator may be a stockholder of and/or speaker for a pharmaceutical company; the study may be designed to produce favorable results and/or these be interpreted or promoted with a bias to use the study intervention.

confounder   A variable, other than the one being researched, that may influence the outcome in analytical observational study designs.

consent   A moral rule related to the principle of autonomy which states that the client has a right to be informed and to freely choose a course of action.

consequential damages   Also called special damages; damages claimed and/or awarded in a lawsuit which were caused as a direct foreseeable result of wrongdoing. Consequential damages occur with injury or harm that does not ensue directly and immediately from the act of a party, but only from some of the results of such act, and that is compensable by a monetary award after a judgment has been rendered in a lawsuit.

consequentialist   An ethical theory which holds that the rightness or wrongness of decisions or actions is determined by the total of good that is achieved or harm that is prevented.

constancy assumption   That historical studies and a new noninferiority study should be as identical as possible regarding important characteristics.

consumer health informatics   A branch of medical informatics focused on analyzing consumers and empowering them to manage their own health through the use of consumer education, consumer-friendly language, personal health records, and other strategies.

consumer health information (CHI)   Information actively sought by the patient in response to their need for more information about their health. Information is not individualized for a specific patient but rather general health information.

continuous data or variable   A variable measured on an interval or ratio scale.

continuous indicators   Provide a simple count, or time estimate, related to a process (e.g., average turnaround time on medication orders).

continuous quality improvement (CQI)   The term given to the methodologies used in the process of Total Quality Management. Efforts to improve quality are part of each participant's responsibilities on an ongoing basis.

contract research organization (CRO)   An individual or organization that assumes one or more of the obligations of the sponsor through an independent contractual agreement.

control group   The group of test animals or humans that receive a placebo (a dosage that does not contain active medicine) or active (a dosage that does contain active medicine) treatment. For most preclinical and clinical trials, the FDA will require that this group receive placebo (commonly referred to as the placebo control). However, some studies may have an active control, which generally consists of an available (standard of care) treatment modality. An active control may, with the concurrence of the FDA, be used in studies where it would be considered unethical to use a placebo. A historical control is one in which a group of previous patients is compared to a matched set of patients receiving the new therapy. A historical control might be used in cases where the disease is consistently fatal (i.e., acquired immunodeficiency syndrome [AIDS]).

control limits   Horizontal lines on a graph, often set at plus or minus three standard deviations from the mean to determine whether a process is out of control.

controlled clinical trial   Research design that prospectively and directly compares, measures, and quantifies differences in outcome between an intervention and control. This is the best study design to determine a cause and effect relationship between an item under investigation and an outcome.

co-payment   Payment made by an individual who has health insurance at the time the service is received to offset the cost of care. Copayments may vary depending on the service rendered.

cost-benefit analysis (CBA) A study where monetary value is given for both costs and benefits associated with a drug or service. The results are expressed as a ratio (benefit-to-cost), and the ratio is used to determine the economic value of the drug or service.

cost-consequence analysis (CCA) An informal variant of a cost-effectiveness analysis (CEA). The costs and various outcomes are listed but no evaluations are conducted.

cost-effectiveness analysis (CEA) A study where the cost of a drug or service is compared to its therapeutic impact. Cost-effectiveness studies determine the relative efficiency of various drugs or services in achieving desired therapeutic outcomes.

cost-effectiveness ratio (CER) The CER is the ratio of resources used per unit of clinical benefit, and implies that this calculation has been made in relation to doing nothing or no treatment.

cost-minimization analysis (CMA) A study that compares costs of drugs or services that have been determined to have equivalent therapeutic outcomes.

cost-utility analysis (CUA) A study that relates therapeutic outcomes to both costs of drugs or services and patient preferences, and measures cost per unit of utility. Utility is the amount of satisfaction obtained from a drug or service.

counterfeit drugs Medications that do not contain the correct active ingredient or the correct amount.

covenant An ethical covenant in medical ethics suggests an implicit contract between client and health care provider that broadly describes the relationship involved whenever a health care service is provided, including the provision of information. Within this contract the service recipient has a right to competently provided service, as well as respectful treatment. The service recipient also has an obligation to provide needed information to the provider in a respectful manner.

coverage error Form of bias occurring when the sample population actually surveyed does not coincide with the target population intended for the survey.

coverage rules Criteria for specific drugs determined by the health plan in conjunction with the pharmacy and therapeutics committee that is used to determine if a prescription is covered. Criteria are based on evidence-based medicine.

CPOE See computerized provider order entry.

CPT® See Current Procedural Terminology.

CQI See continuous quality improvement.

CRF See case report form.

criteria Definitions of safe and effective use of medications used to assess components of the medication use process that are endorsed by the organization within which they are to be applied. Criteria summarize an organization's definition of appropriate or acceptable use of the medication.

critical appraisal The process of systematically and critically evaluating a scientific study for relevance and value within a specific context.

CRO See contract research organization.

crossover study A study where each subject receives all study treatments, and endpoints during the various treatments are compared.

cross-sectional Data that is measured one time.

cross-sectional study An analytical observational study design in which researchers identify a group of patients with and without an outcome (often a disease) and determine if they have been exposed to a risk factor (often a drug) at a single point in time. Cross-sectional studies involve concurrent data collection.

C-statistic Also known as the concordance statistic. The C-statistic predicts the risk of a patient having an event (e.g., risk of 30-day readmission) compared to a patient that does not have the event.

CUA See cost-utility analysis.

Current Good Manufacturing Practices (CGMP or CGMPS) Regulations enforced by the FDA to assure proper design, monitoring, and control of manufacturing processes and facilities.

Current Procedural Terminology (CPT®) A standard for documenting and billing medical procedures and services, primarily used by physicians.

customer response center A pharmaceutical company's first-line response team for unsolicited requests for medical information from patients and providers.

cybermedicine A concept broader than telemedicine that includes the marketing, relationship creation, advice, prescribing, and selling pharmaceuticals and devices in cyberspace.

data mining The process of discovering patterns in large data sets.

data warehouse An application that receives and stores data from various sources. Data warehouses also serve as a data reporting application, which allows analysts to more expeditiously extract data rather than from individual applications.

database A computer program containing data in a structured manner.

Dear Health Care Provider Letter A letter from a manufacturer to highlight critical information for health care providers about new or updated information about a medication.

dechallenge In relation to adverse drug reactions (ADRs), this occurs when the drug is taken away and the patient is monitored to determine whether the ADR abates or decreases in intensity.

decision analysis A tool that can help visualize a pharmacoeconomic analysis. It is the application of an analytical method for systematically comparing different decision options. It graphically displays choices and performs the calculations needed to compare these options.

decision tree A machine learning model which starts with an initial variable, and generates all various permutations of a specific outcome.

deep learning A machine learning model in which the analytical model constantly runs through permutations and becomes more refined over time using previous permutations.

deep pocket Practical consideration that involves the naming of additional codefendants in personal injury lawsuits to provide assurance to the plaintiff that there will be sufficient assets to pay the judgment.

degrees of freedom The number of data points that are free to vary.

deliverable Term used in project management, referring to a tangible component produced in order to achieve predefined success criteria.

delta (δ) The amount of difference that the investigators wish to detect between intervention and control groups in a study.

deontological An ethical theory that seeks to establish what is a right or wrong decision or action on the basis of prioritizing specific recognized ethical rules or principles.

descriptive statistics   A summarization of data in order to summarize characteristics in an ordered and efficient way (e.g., patient gender, race). They include mean, median, mode, variance, and standard deviation.

detailing   Promotions made directly from pharmaceutical industry to health care professionals, generally in one-on-one or small group meetings.

dichotomous data or variable   A variable that has two mutually exclusive categories.

digital health   The cultural transformation of how disruptive technologies that provide digital and objective data accessible to both caregivers and patients leads to an equal level doctor-patient relationship with shared decision-making and the democratization of care. Using technology such as EHR, wearable devices, or mobile health apps to improve individuals' health and wellness.

digital health technologies   Technologies, such as mobile health (mHealth) apps and wearable devices, that may be used for general wellness or as actual medical devices.

digital therapeutics   A subset of digital health, evidence-based therapeutic interventions driven by high-quality software programs to prevent, manage, or treat a medical disorder or disease.

direct medical costs   One of four categories of costs in pharmacoeconomic studies. These are the medically related inputs used directly in providing the treatment.

direct non-medical costs   One of four categories of costs in pharmacoeconomic studies. These are costs directly associated with treatment, but are not medical in nature. Examples include travel, food, and lodging to get to a place of treatment.

direct to consumer advertising (DTCA)   Promotion of prescription medications to consumers via magazines, newspapers, radio, television, direct mailing, or other means.

DIS   See drug information service.

disaggregated   Data elements broken into component or independent groups, such as age range groupings of the study population to assist in analysis of differences in outcomes of subgroups versus the aggregate, summary results of an entire study population.

discount rate   A financing term which approximates the cost of capital by taking into account both the projected inflation rate and the interest rates of borrowed money, and then estimates the time value of money.

discrete data   Data that fit neatly into a group or interval, in that they can only take on certain specific values.

DMF   See drug master file.

double-blind peer review   A type of peer review in which the author and reviewer are both blinded to each other's identity.

drug class review   A drug evaluation monograph comparing all products in a particular class of drugs. It is used to determine what products will be preferred or available for use.

drug database   A database of drugs that should ideally include decision support functions, such as therapeutic categories, drug-drug and drug-disease interactions, dose range checking, and allergy warnings.

drug evaluation monograph   A structured document covering all aspects of a particular drug product or class of drugs. It compares similar agents and is used to determine which products will be preferred or available for use.

drug formulary   See formulary.

drug formulary system   See formulary system.

drug informatics   A technologically advanced version of drug information. This often denotes the electronic management of drug information.

drug information   Facts or advice on drugs (including chemicals that have medicinal, performance-enhancing, or intoxicating effects) regarding a specific patient or a group of patients, based on the most current and accurate evidence.

drug information center (DIC)   A physical location where pharmacists have the resources (e.g., books, journals, computer systems, etc.) to provide drug information. This area is generally staffed by a pharmacist specializing in drug information, but may be used by a variety of the pharmacy staff or other individuals.

drug information service   A professional service providing drug information. This service is normally located in a drug information center.

drug interaction   The Food and Drug Administration defines this as "a pharmacologic response that cannot be explained by the action of a simple drug, but is due to two or more drugs acting simultaneously."

drug master file (DMF)   A submission to the FDA that may be used to provide confidential detailed information about facilities, processes, or articles used in the manufacturing, processing, packaging, and storing of one or more human drugs.

drug product   The final dosage form prepared from the drug substance.

drug promotion   Information provided by pharmaceutical industry through advertising, detailing, and other printed material intended to increase sales of a medication.

drug substance   An active ingredient that is intended to furnish pharmacological activity or other direct effect in the diagnosis, cure, mitigation, treatment, or prevention of disease or to affect the structure or any function of the human body.

drug use (or utilization) review (DUR)   A program related to outpatient pharmacy services designed to educate physicians and pharmacists in identifying and reducing the frequency and patterns of fraud, abuse, gross overuse, or inappropriate or medically unnecessary care. DUR frequently is retrospective in nature and utilizes claims data as its primary source of information. DUR may also be concurrent or prospective.

drug use evaluation (DUE)   Concurrent evaluation of prescribing and outcome only. Multidisciplinary involvement.

DTCA   See direct to consumer advertising.

DUE   See drug use evaluation.

DUR   See drug utilization review.

EBM   See evidence-based medicine.

editorial   A commentary, usually written by an expert, that describes study strengths and limitations and the application of the study results into practice. This is published in the same journal issue as the study. Not all studies have an accompanying editorial.

educational research   The practice of evaluating various educational aspects in the interest of creating better practices in the hopes of advancing knowledge and benefiting society.

effectiveness   The response to an intervention under "real world" conditions. Effectiveness is typically associated with intention-to-treat analyses and external validity.

efficacy   The response to an intervention under ideal conditions. Efficacy is typically associated with per-protocol analyses and internal validity.

EHR   See electronic health record.

electronic health record (EHR)   A digital compilation of a patient's health data originating from all clinicians involved in the patient's care and that allows these data to be shared across providers and institutions.

electronic mail (email)   Brief messages sent from one computer to another, similar in use to interoffice memos. This serves as a quick, informal method of written communication. Also, email may be used to send other items, such as word processing files, graphics, video, etc., to others.

electronic medication administration record (eMAR)   An electronic version of the traditional medication administration record. It supports patient safety by incorporating clinical decision support and bar coded medication administration. It also enables real-time documentation and billing of medication administration.

electronic prescribing (e-prescribing)   Prescription entered by a prescriber directly into an electronic format using agreed-upon standards that is securely transmitted to the pharmacy that the patient chooses. Faxes and printed prescriptions are not e-prescriptions.

email   See electronic mail.

eMAR   See electronic medical administration record.

Emtree terms   A set of specific biomedical keywords or phrases organized by broader and narrower terms for the purpose of indexing articles within Embase®.

endpoint, primary   An outcome measured by the study investigators that quantifies the difference in effect between the intervention and control of the clinical trial. The results of this outcome measurement are used to answer the primary study objective. This outcome is used by the study investigators to determine other study methods (e.g., sample size, statistical tests, duration, dose, patient type to enroll).

endpoint, secondary   An outcome measured by the study investigators that quantifies the difference in effect between the intervention and control of a clinical trial but is not considered the focus of the study. The results of this outcome measurement are used to answer secondary study objectives. For example, a study compares a statin to placebo to determine if the statin can reduce the risk of having a stroke (primary endpoint); change in LDL-C levels also are compared between the two groups (secondary endpoint).

ensemble   A machine learning model that generates its output by use of many different data models.

e-prescribing   See electronic prescribing.

error type I   Rejecting the null hypothesis instead of failing-to-reject (i.e., accepting) the null hypothesis; also known as a false-positive result or alpha-error; chance is the reason for this to occur.

error type II   Failing-to-reject (i.e., accepting) the null hypothesis instead of rejecting the null hypothesis; also known as a false-negative result or beta-error; chance or small sample size are reasons for this to occur.

ethical theories   Integrated bodies of principles and rules that may include mediating rules that govern cases of conflicts.

ethics   The philosophical inquiry of the moral dimensions of human conduct. An ethical issue involves judgments between right and wrong human conduct or praiseworthy and blameworthy human character.

evidence-based medicine (EBM)   A systematic approach to clinical problem solving which allows the integration of the best available research evidence with clinical expertise and patient values.

exclusion criteria   Characteristics of subjects defined prior to starting the study that are used as parameters to disqualify subjects from enrolling into the study (e.g., patients with cancer, lactating females, patients receiving corticosteroid therapy).

exculpatory clause   The part of an agreement which relieves one party from liability. It is a provision in a contract which stipulates: (1) one party is relieved of any blame or liability arising from the other party's wrongdoing, or (2) one party (usually the one that drafted the agreement) is freed of all liability arising out of performance of that contract. An exculpatory clause will not be enforced when the party protected by the clause intentionally causes harm or engages in acts of reckless, wanton, or gross negligence or when found to be unreasonable under the particular circumstances (e.g., a restaurant checks a person's coat but the ticket states they are not responsible for loss or damage).

expected variation   Allowable and anticipated variation observed inside of control limits within a process as by statistical analysis of the normal distribution expected variation is plus or minus three standard deviations from the mean.

external validity   See validity, external.

failure modes and effects analysis (FMEA)   FMEA is a structured proactive method of evaluating a process to identify the gaps—how the process might fail. The process includes identification of the likelihood of each of the failures along with its relative impact to the patient. This provides a prioritization of action plans to drive improvement and reduce the likelihood of failure.

fair balance   A quality of drug promotions where similar attention is given to safety risks (e.g., contraindications, precautions/warnings, adverse effects) and efficacy benefits.

false negatives   Individuals with the disease that were incorrectly identified as being disease-free by the test.

false positives   Individuals without the disease that were incorrectly identified as having the disease by the test.

fatal flaw   A significant deficiency in a manuscript, often related to methodology, that renders the manuscript unpublishable.

FDA   See Food and Drug Administration.

FDA Form 483   A report issued after an inspection if investigators observe any violations of the Food Drug and Cosmetic Act and other FDA Acts.

FDS   See formulary decision support.

fellowship   A directed, highly individualized postgraduate training program designed to prepare the participant to function as an independent investigator. The purpose of fellowship training programs is to develop competency and expertise in the scientific research process, including hypothesis generation and development, study design, protocol development, grantsmanship, study coordination, data collection, analysis and interpretation, technical skills development, presentation of results, and manuscript preparation and publication. A fellowship candidate is expected to possess appropriate practice skills relevant to the knowledge area of the fellowship. Such skills may be obtained through prior practice experience or completion of a residency program.

fidelity   A principle of moral duty in deontological theory that addresses the responsibility to be trustworthy and keep promises.

field-based outcomes liaisons   A field-based role within a pharmaceutical company responsible for demonstrating the value of a product to managed care organizations (e.g., accountable care organizations), pharmacy benefit managers (PBMs), or other HCPs in similar decision-making roles through the generation of outcomes data. Otherwise known as managed market specialists.

filter   The process of using specific design and criteria to limit resultant information when querying datasets.

first author   See primary author.

FMEA   See failure modes and effects analysis.

follow-up study   A study where subjects exposed to a factor and those not exposed to the factor are followed forward in time and compared to determine the factor's influence on disease state development. Also called a cohort study.

Food and Drug Administration (FDA)   The agency of the U.S. government that is responsible for ensuring the safety and efficacy of all drugs on the market.

forest plot   The preferred method to display the results from a systematic review. It includes the point estimate and confidence interval (usually expressed as the 95% confidence interval) for the outcome of each included study, and if the review is quantitative (i.e., a meta-analysis), it will also include the pooled results.

formulary   A continually revised list of medications that are readily available for use within an institution or from a third-party payer (e.g., insurance company, government) that reflects the current clinical judgment of the medical staff or the payer. Restrictions on this list may be placed that indicate certain drugs will not be reimbursed by insurance, or will only be reimbursed if several other alternatives are tried first.

formulary decision support (FDS)   A program (often software) used to enhance compliance with formulary by guiding the prescriber to preferred formulary drugs over those considered nonformulary.

formulary system   A method used to develop a drug formulary. It is sometimes even thought of as a philosophy.

funnel plot   A scatterplot that relates the estimate of effect size to the weight of each individual study in a quantitative systematic review (i.e., meta-analysis). It is used for detecting publication bias.

futility   Stopping a trial because of recognition of the inability of that study to achieve its objectives.

galley proofs   A copy of a written work as it is to be published. The purpose of this document is to allow the author(s) to make a final check to ensure everything is correct before actual publication. They are sometimes referred to as page proofs.

Gantt chart   Project management tool used to provide a visual progression and overall timeline for a project.

gap analysis   A process used to measure the difference between expected versus actual performance or knowledge.

GCP   See Good Clinical Practice.

gender bias   Showing favoritism or discrimination toward a selected gender.

Good Clinical Practice (GCP)   A standard for the design, conduct, monitoring, analyses, and reporting of clinical trials that provides assurance that the results are credible and accurate, and that the rights of study subjects are protected.

GPO   See group purchasing organization.

GRADE   See Grading of Recommendations, Assessment, Development, and Evaluation system.

Grading of Recommendations, Assessment, Development, and Evaluation (GRADE) system   A standardized system for grading evidence quality and the strength of recommendations in clinical practice guidelines.

gray literature   Documents provided in limited numbers outside the formal channels of publication and distribution. The concern with these documents is that they may include inaccurate information (not completely correct information), misinformation (incorrect information), and disinformation (false information deliberately provided in order to influence opinions) that can confound the meta-analysis results.

group purchasing organization (GPO)   An organization that assists health care providers or organizations by aggregating purchase volume to negotiate cost savings from suppliers.

guideline   Document that provides suggestions or advice for a particular activity. Guidelines are evidence-based recommendations but should not replace professional judgment. Guidelines are not prescriptive in nature.

HCEI   See Health Care Economic Information.

health applications (apps)   Software for devices designed to manage various aspects of health for the specific user.

Health Care Economic Information (HCEI)   Defined by the FDA as "any analysis (including clinical data, inputs, clinical or other assumptions, methods, results, and other components underlying or comprising the analysis) that identifies, measures, or describes the economic consequences, which may be based on the separate or aggregated clinical consequences of the represented health outcomes, of the use of the drug."

health equity   Attainment of the highest level of health for all people. Achieving health equity requires valuing everyone equally with focused and ongoing societal efforts to address avoidable inequalities, historical and contemporary injustices, and the elimination of health and health care disparities.

health literacy   The capability of patients to read or hear health information, understand it, and then act upon health information.

health maintenance organization (HMO)   Form of health insurance whereby the member prepays a premium for the HMO's health services, which generally include inpatient and outpatient care.

health outcomes research   A systematic investigation which seeks to identify, measure, and evaluate the end results of health care services. It may include not only clinical and economic consequences, but also outcomes, such as patient health status and satisfaction with their health care.

Health Plan Employer Data and Information Set (HEDIS)   A set of performance measures used to compare managed health care plans.

health-related quality of life (HR-QOL or HRQL) The value assigned to the duration of a patient's life when altered by various impairments, functional states, perceptions, and social opportunities that have been modified by disease, injury, treatment, and social policy.

help-seeking advertisement A type of direct-to-consumer advertisement that describes a disease or condition but does not recommend or suggest a treatment medication.

heterogeneity The extent of dissimilarity among individual study results in a systematic review. It is desirable for heterogeneity to be not statistically significant and low in magnitude in a quantitative systematic review (i.e., meta-analysis).

Hippocratic Oath A central ethical tradition of Western medicine that is committed to producing good for one's patient and protecting that patient from harm. There is a special emphasis placed on the responsibility of the medical professional to the specific patient.

historical data Data used in research that was collected prior to the decision to conduct the study (e.g., medical records, insurance information, Medicaid databases).

Historical Evidence of Sensitivity to Drug Effects (HESDE) In noninferiority trials, this concept applies to appropriately designed and conducted past trials using the reference drug and regularly exhibiting the reference drug to be superior to placebo.

HMO See Health Maintenance Organization.

homogenicity tests Tests used when conducting a meta-analysis to determine the similarity of studies whose results were combined for the analysis.

homoscedasticity In correlation and regression, the variability around the best fit line of the linear relationship is constant across all data points.

HRQL see health-related quality of life.

HR-QOL see health-related quality of life.

hyperlink Also called a link; is a word, group of words, or image that can be clicked on to jump (link) to another place within the same document or to an entirely different document. When you move the cursor over a link in a website, the arrow will turn into a little hand. Hyperlinks are the most essential ingredient of all hypertext systems, including the Internet.

hypothesis The researchers' assumptions regarding probable study results. The research hypothesis or alternative hypothesis (H_A) is the expectations of the researchers in terms of study results. The null hypothesis (H_0) is the no difference hypothesis, which assumes equality among study treatments. The null hypothesis is the basis for all statistical tests and must be rejected in order to accept the research hypothesis.

ICER See incremental cost-effectiveness ratio.

ICUR See incremental cost-utility ratio.

IDE See Investigational Device Exemption.

IDMC See independent data monitoring committee.

impact factor The number of times a journal is cited in the literature relative to its number of publications within the same timeframe; used to determine the relative prestige of a journal.

in vitro   Experiments conducted using components of an organism that have been isolated from their usual biological surroundings. These types of experiments are also referred to as "test tube experiments."

in vivo   Experiments conducted in living organisms in their intact state.

inattentional blindness   The failure to see the obvious because attention is focused on a different task.

incidence rate   Measures the probability that a healthy person will develop a disease within a specified period of time. It is the number of new cases of disease in the population over a specific time period.

inclusion criteria   Characteristics of subjects defined prior to starting the study that are used as parameters to enroll participants into the study (e.g., males and females between 50 and 75 years of age with a prior myocardial infarction).

increment medical costs   One of four categories of costs in pharmacoeconomic studies. Indirect costs involve costs that result from the loss of productivity due to illness or death.

incremental cost-effectiveness ratio (ICER)   Ratio calculated by the difference in costs divided by the difference in clinical outcomes (e.g., patients cured, patients under control of disease, lab values that indicate health level).

incremental cost-utility ratio (ICUR)   Ratio calculated by the difference in cost divided by the difference in utilities (usually measured using quality-adjusted life years—QALYs).

INDA   See Investigational New Drug Application.

independent data monitoring committee (IDMC)   Group of individuals who monitor an ongoing study protocol to ensure subjects' safety and uphold study design integrity.

indexing   A literature cataloging activity to tag articles to specific keywords that are a major or minor focus of the publication. Using indexing terms when performing a literature search will tailor search results to relevant and specific research questions. The search results consist of bibliographic citation information (e.g., title, author, and citation of the article) and may include abstract and/or full text of the publication.

indexing service   A searchable database of biomedical journal citations.

indexing term   A specific keyword or phrase used to catalogue articles within a secondary database. Examples include Emtree and Medical Subject Headings (MeSH).

indicator   A statement of a measurable item in the area being evaluated which signals whether the area being evaluated is or is not of sufficient quality. They can focus on structure, process, or outcomes.

indicator drug   A drug that, when prescribed, may offer evidence that an adverse effect to a drug may have occurred. Pharmacists can then investigate further to determine whether there really was an adverse effect.

indirect medical costs   One of four categories of costs in pharmacoeconomic studies. Indirect costs involve costs that result from the loss of productivity due to illness or death.

inference engine   Also known as the reasoning engine, this forms the brain of the clinical decision support system, working to link patient-specific information with information in the knowledge base. It evaluates the available information and determines what to present to the user.

inferential statistics   Statistical methods that allow prediction from data (e.g., *t* test). Inferential statistics are used to determine the probability that a true difference is present between two or more groups.

informatics specialist   An individual that has advanced medication information skills with a keen understanding of computer and information technology.

information therapy   Evidence-based patient education and/or medical information presented at an appropriate time to most effectively assist the patient in making a specific health decision or change in their behavior.

informed consent   The document signed by a subject, or the subject's representative, entering into a trial that informs him or her of his or her rights as a research subject, plus potential benefits and risks of the trial. This document indicates that the person is willing to participate in the study.

inherent drug risks   Are unique to the drug and usually identified in the package insert, but do not include probable or common side effects.

injunction   A judicial remedy issues in order to prohibit a party from doing or continuing to do a certain activity.

institutional ethics committee   See institutional review board.

institutional review board (IRB)   A group of individuals from various disciplines (e.g., lay people, physicians, pharmacists, nurses, clergy), who evaluate protocols for clinical studies to assess risks to the research participants and benefits to society. Approval by an IRB is necessary prior to initiation of a clinical study involving patients. It is known outside of the United States as the institutional ethics committee.

intangible costs   Intangible costs extend beyond the monetary costs of goods and services and include other sequelae that reflect decreased enjoyment of life because of illness. Such costs are associated with functional limitations, pain, psychological distress, and decreased social interaction because of an illness or the treatment of an illness.

integrative medicine   See complementary and alternative medicine.

intelligent infusion pumps   Infusion pumps containing software designed to help eliminate pump programming errors. Also referred to as smart pumps.

intention-to-treat (ITT)   Study design technique used to include results of all subjects in the final analysis even when the subject does not complete the entire study.

interim analysis   Evaluation of data at specified time points before scheduled termination or completion of a study.

internal validity   Refers to how well an experiment is done, especially whether it avoids confounding factors that could affect the results.

Internet   A worldwide computer network.

Internet of Things (IoT)   The connected network of electronic devices that collect and share data with other devices via the Internet.

interoperability   The ability of disparate computer systems to exchange information in a manner that allows the information to be used meaningfully.

interval data or scale   A scale of measurement that has rank ordered data with meaningful distance between two ranks, but no natural zero (e.g., temperature on a Celsius or Fahrenheit scale). A value of zero does not indicate absence of the characteristic.

interventional study   A study where the investigator introduces a factor and examines the factor's influence on certain variables or outcomes.

intranet   A computer network with restricted access, as within a health system.

Inverse Variance Test A statistical test commonly used to combine continuous data in meta-analyses.

Investigational Device Exemption (IDE) An approved IDE means that the IRB (and FDA for significant risk devices) has approved the sponsor's study application and all requirements under 21CFR812 are met. It allows the use of a device in a clinical investigation to collect safety and effectiveness data.

Investigational New Drug A drug, antibiotic, or biological that is used in a clinical investigation. The label of an investigational drug must bear the statement: "Caution: New Drug-Limited by Federal (or United States) law to investigational use."

Investigational New Drug Application (INDA) The application by the study sponsor to the FDA to begin clinical trials in humans.

investigator The individual responsible for initiating the clinical trial at the study site. This individual must treat the patients, assure that the protocol is followed, evaluate responses and adverse reactions, solve problems as they arise, and assure proper conduct of the study.

IoT See Internet of Things.

IRB See institutional review board.

ITT See intention-to-treat.

JCAHO Joint Commission on Accreditation of Healthcare Organizations—a previous name for The Joint Commission. See The Joint Commission.

join A SQL clause used to combine data from two or more tables using a common data point.

joint and several liability Refers to the sharing of liabilities among a group of people collectively and also individually. If the defendants are "jointly and severally" liable, the injured party may sue some or all of the defendants together, or each one separately, and may collect equal or unequal amounts from each.

journal club A group of individuals who meet regularly to discuss and critically evaluate the biomedical literature.

Just Culture A term coined by David Marx, which is a structured accountability model that supports patient safety and a learning culture. It is intended to balance recognition and understanding of system contribution to errors with an understanding of human error concepts to facilitate an accountability process that is valued by leadership and staff. When applied consistently and fairly, it is also a proactive approach to identifying gaps in system processes.

justice A concept that relates to fairness and tendering what is due, resource allocation and providing that to which the individual is entitled.

key opinion leaders Health care professionals considered to be experts in their area by their peers. Key opinion leaders are often highly regarded for their expertise in publications, speaking engagements, and influential value in the medical community.

knowledge base One of the three main components of clinical decision support systems (CDSS); composed of varied clinical knowledge, such as treatment guidelines, diagnoses, and drug-drug or drug-disease interactions.

knowledge-based human performance Performance that utilizes prior knowledge, understanding, and experience with a situation or task. Knowledge-based errors can occur when an individual is in a situation to which he or she has never been exposed, has a lack of required knowledge, or no preprogrammed rules to apply.

knowledge-based information Clinical information that forms the scientific basis of health care, including referential information (about medications, procedures, disease states, etc.), clinical practice guidelines, and other domains of health and medical knowledge.

kurtosis Refers to how flat or peaked the curve appears. A curve with a flat or board top is referred to as platykurtic while a peaked distribution is described as leptokurtic.

landmark trial A clinical trial that significantly shapes medical practice or provides important new knowledge where gaps previously existed.

language bias Occurs when only specific articles are included in a review or study that are published in a specific language such as the review author's native language. The issue is that potentially important articles are eliminated from the review.

law Involves written rules set by the whole society, or its representatives, that address the responsibilities of that society's members.

Learned Intermediary Doctrine A doctrine of products liability law and personal injury law; the manufacturer of a prescription drug fulfills its duty to warn of potentially harmful effects of the drug by informing the prescribing physician and is not also obligated to warn the user. The prescribing physician acts as a learned intermediary between manufacturer and consumer and has the primary responsibility of warning patients of the hazards of prescribed pharmaceutical products. This doctrine is an exception to the rule that one who markets goods must warn foreseeable ultimate users of dangers inherent in their products.

learning organization An organization that uses insights gained over time to modify its behavior and enhance patient safety.

letter to the editor A written piece to the editor of a medical journal or other publication expressing opinions or concerns of the reader.

level of evidence A scale used to categorize the overall quality of a specific clinical trial. The reliability of the results can be inferred from the category given a trial.

life table methods In the context of cohort study life tables, data are collected by following patients throughout their lives or a specific duration of their life and then compiled into tables for such uses as survival or mortality analyses comparing exposed to nonexposed situations.

little data Data that stems from individual data sources, such as patient records or single applications.

locality rule Legal doctrine created in the latter part of the nineteenth century that stated that the local defendant practitioner would have his or her standard of performance evaluated in light of the performance of other peers in the same or similar communities. Also known as community rule.

Logical Observations Identifiers Names and Codes (LOINC) A standardized language for communicating laboratory test and observation data between computer systems.

logical operator A term such as AND, OR, NOT, NEAR, or WITH that can be used in searching a computer database.

logit See log-odds.

log-odds A linear transformation of probability. That is, probability is bounded between 0 and 1, log-odds transform probability to a continuous scale ranging from $-\infty$ to $+\infty$. The log-odds become the dependent variable in logistic regression.

LOINC See Logical Observations Identifiers Names and Codes.

longitudinal Data that is measured repeatedly over time.

machine learning An approach to data analytics wherein various methodologies are employed to generate a most accurate result, in which the analytical model dynamically changes over time to arrive at an optimal outcome.

macro Level of decision-making that sets policy for the health system, as a standard established for an entire profession, or through government as law/regulation for the society as a whole.

major statement Used in broadcast (TV or radio) advertisements for prescription medications in which the drug's most important risks are verbally presented.

managed care organization (MCO) Health care provider who contracts with participating providers to provide a variety of services to enrolled members.

managed market specialists See field-based outcomes liaisons.

Mantel-Haenszel test A statistical test commonly used to combine categorical data in meta-analyses.

marginal (or incremental) cost-utility ratio Is the gain in a benefit from an increase, or loss from a decrease, in a good or service, such as the QALY. Calculated to estimate the added cost for an added benefit, not calculated when the added benefit comes at a lower cost.

marginal cost-effectiveness ratio The additional cost of one unit expansion of a single intervention.

matching A technique that may be used in analytical observational study designs so that patients share similar characteristics at baseline.

material issue of fact Genuine issue of material fact is a legal term often used as the basis for a motion for summary judgment. A summary judgment is proper if there is no genuine issue of material fact and the movant is entitled to a judgment as a matter of law. Such a motion will be granted if the party making the motion proves there is no genuine issue of material fact to be decided. When the moving party makes a prima facie showing that no genuine issue of material fact exists, the burden shifts to the nonmoving party to rebut the showing by presenting substantial evidence creating a genuine issue.

MCO See managed care organization.

mean The arithmetic average of a set of numbers.

Meaningful Use A set of standards defined by the Center for Medicare and Medicaid Services as the use of certified electronic health record technology to (1) improve quality, safety, and efficiency, (2) engage patients and their families, (3) improve care coordination, as well as public and population health, and (4) maintain privacy and security of protected health information.

measurement error Occurs when the collection of data is influenced by the interviewer or when the survey item itself is unclear from the respondent's point of view.

measures of association Calculation and interpretation of nominal study results using relative risk (RR), relative risk reduction (RRR), absolute risk reduction (ARR), and number needed to treat (NNT).

median The absolute middle value of a set of number.

medical executive committee A committee that acts as the administrative body of a medical staff in an institution. It is responsible for overseeing all aspects of care within the institution. This committee may be known by other names at specific institutions.

Medical Literature Analysis and Retrieval System (MedLARS) The computerized information retrieval system at the National Library of Medicine.

medical science liaison A field-based role (typically a health care provider such as a physician or pharmacist) within a pharmaceutical company responsible for providing medical information to health care provider regarding the company's marketed drugs and making connections to key opinion leaders.

Medical Subject Heading (MeSH) terms A set of specific biomedical keywords or phrases that the U.S. National Library of Medicine uses to define or categorize a topic for the purpose of indexing articles in MEDLINE®.

medication error Any preventable event that may cause or lead to inappropriate medication use or patient harm while the medication is in the control of the health care professional, patient, or consumer. Such events may be related to professional practice, health care products, procedures, and systems, including prescribing; order communication; product labeling, packaging, and nomenclature; compounding; dispensing; distribution; administration; education; monitoring; and use.

Medication Guides Information for drug and biological products that FDA determines pose a serious and significant public health concern requiring the distribution of Food and Drug Administration-approved patient medication information that is necessary to patients' safe and effective use of the drug products.

medication information Facts or advice on medicines regarding a specific patient or a group of patients.

medication misadventure Any iatrogenic hazard or incident associated with medications that is an inherent risk when medication therapy is indicated; is created through either omission or commission by the administration of a medicine or medicines during which a patient may be harmed, with effects ranging from mild discomfort to fatality; may be attributable to error (human or system, or both), immunologic response, or idiosyncratic response; is always unexpected or undesirable to the patient and the health professional; and whose outcome may or may not be independent of the preexisting pathology or disease process It includes adverse drug events (ADEs), adverse drug reactions (ADRs), and medication errors.

medication therapy management (MTM) Medication therapy management is a distinct service or group of services that optimizes drug therapy with the intent of improved therapeutic outcomes for individual patients.

medication tier status a designation by the payer for prescriptions, as to whether a medication is a preferred agent within its class (i.e., first tier), second choice (second tier), third choice (third tier) or not covered. Each "tier" is generally associated with decreasing payment from the payer and increasing patient responsibility for the cost of the drug, with "not covered" (or nonformulary) being entirely the patient's responsibility to pay.

medication usage patterns Trends and patterns of drug use. Often influenced by reimbursement decisions and formularies of insurance companies, Medicare and Medicaid, direct-to-consumer-advertising, etc.

medication use evaluation (MUE) A part of the overall performance improvement program within institutional settings that provides in-depth assessment of the medication use process including prescribing, order verification, dispensing, administering, monitoring, and outcome. Multidisciplinary involvement.

medication use process The steps involved in providing medications to patients including prescribing, order verification, dispensing, administering, and monitoring to determine outcomes.

MedLARS   see Medical Literature Analysis and Retrieval System.

MedWatch   FDA's safety information and adverse event reporting program that takes reports from either health care professionals or patients.

meso   Level of decision-making variably described as occurring at the institutional/organizational level or at community/regional levels of health care.

meta-analysis   Results of previously conducted similar clinical trials are combined, statistically analyzed, and new data is created for interpretation. Meta-analyses are especially useful when previous studies are inconclusive or controversial. They are also useful where sample size of multiple similar studies are too small to detect a statistically significant difference, but combining them will provide adequate sample size to meet a set power.

mHealth   See mobile health.

micro   Level of health care–related decision-making, which involves decisions made at the individual professional–patient level of health care.

middle technical style   A writing style used by professionals addressing professionals in other fields. It tends to be formal and avoids use of the first person (e.g., I, us). Technical jargon is avoided in this writing style.

mobile apps   Software applications intended for use on mobile platforms, or web-based software applications tailored to mobile platforms, but executed on a server.

mobile health (mHealth)   Medical and public health practice supported by mobile devices, patient monitoring devices, personal digital assistants, and other wireless devices.

mode   The most frequently occurring data point in a set of numbers.

modified systematic approach   A seven-step approach to answering drug information requests that includes (1) secure demographics of requestor, (2) obtain background information, (3) determine and categorize ultimate question, (4) develop strategy and conduct search, (5) perform evaluation, analysis, and synthesis, (6) formulate and provide response, and (7) conduct follow-up and documentation.

morbidity   Detrimental consequences (other than death) related to a treatment, exposure, or disease state.

MTM   See medication therapy management.

MUE   See medication use evaluation.

multicollinearity   Two or more variables have extremely high correlations (e.g., >0.90) indicating that they are redundant or that they are measuring the same construct.

narrative review   A summary of previously conducted research that lacks systematic methods such as formal criteria for selection of studies. Also called a nonsystematic review.

narrow therapeutic index   Used to describe a drug with small differences in dose or blood concentration that may lead to dose and blood concentration dependent serious therapeutic failures or adverse drug reactions.

National Committee for Quality Assurance (NCQA)   An organization dedicated to assessing and reporting on the quality of managed care plans; it surveys and accredits managed care organizations much like The Joint Commission accredits hospitals.

National Patient Safety Goals (NPSGs)   Program established and updated by The Joint Commission to assist health care organizations to address safety concerns related to patient safety.

NCQA   see National Committee for Quality Assurance.

NDA   See New Drug Application.

negative formulary   A drug formulary that starts out with every marketed drug product and specifically eliminates products that are considered inferior, unnecessary, unsafe, too expensive, etc.

negligence   Failure to exercise that degree of care that a person of ordinary prudence or a reasonable person would exercise under the same circumstances. Elements of a negligence case include: (1) Duty breached, (2) Damages, (3) Direct causation, and (4) Defenses absent.

negligent misrepresentation   Occurs when the defendant carelessly makes a representation or statement without reasonable basis to believe it to be true. The burden of proof that is required passes to the person who made the statement who must prove that the statement was either not one of fact but opinion and that he or she had reasonable ground to believe and did believe that the facts represented were true.

network analysis   Also known as multiple treatment comparison or mixed treatment meta-analysis. A network meta-analysis simultaneously compares and ranks a "network" of treatments in which subsets have been compared in individual studies.

neural network   A machine learning methodology in which multiple inputs are entered into the model, and a specific outcome is generated.

New Drug Application (NDA)   The application to the FDA requesting approval to market a new drug for human use. The NDA contains data supporting the safety and efficacy of the drug for its intended use.

New Molecular Entity (NME)   A compound that can be patented and has not been previously marketed in the United States in any form.

NME   See New Molecular Entity.

N-of-1 trial   A study design similar to a crossover study design conducted in a single patient who receives treatments in pairs (one period of the experimental therapy and one period of either alternative treatment or placebo) in random order.

nominal data or scale   A scale of measurement that places data into mutually exclusive categories without reference to rank order (e.g., male or female gender).

noninferiority   Usually referring to a type of study design in which researchers seek to prove that a new treatment is not less efficacious than a standard treatment within a prespecified amount (i.e., delta or noninferiority margin).

noninferiority margin   a prespecified amount of effect used to show the test drug's treatment effect is not worse than the reference drug by more than this specific degree.

noninherent drug risks   Are created by the particular drug in combination with some extrinsic factor that the pharmacist should reasonably know about.

nonmaleficence   A basic principle of consequentialist theory that encompasses the duty to do no harm.

nonparametric tests   Statistical tests that do not assume a conditional normal distribution.

nonpharmacologic   Treatment options focusing on a holistic approach to patient care (e.g., nutrition and exercise-related interventions).

nonpublic unsolicited requests   A nonpublic unsolicited request is an unsolicited request that is directed privately to a firm using a one-on-one communication approach.

nonresponse bias   Can result in surveys where the answers of respondents differ from the potential answers of those who did not answer.

nonresponse error   Occurs when a significant number of subjects in a sample do not respond to the survey.

nonsystematic review   See narrative review.

NPSG   See National Patient Safety Goals.

null hypothesis   Statement of no difference in outcome between the intervention and control; created before the beginning of a study. This statement is either rejected or failed-to-be-rejected (i.e., accepted) at the end of the study based upon the p value compared to the alpha.

number needed to treat (NNT)   A measure used to determine the effectiveness of an intervention. This measure states the average number of patients who need to be treated with the intervention to prevent one additional negative outcome such as a myocardial infarction. The higher the value, the less effective is the intervention. NNT is calculated as the reciprocal of absolute risk reduction.

observational study   A study where the investigator analyzes naturally occurring events.

observer bias   tendency for observer/investigator to consciously or unconsciously distort what they see and record as the effect in a clinical trial situation. In other words, seeing what they expect to see.

odds ratio   A ratio of the odds (events / nonevents) between two groups that is most appropriate for prevalence and typically reported from case-control studies.

off-label   Information that originates from sources (e.g., clinical studies, case reports) outside of the FDA-approved prescription drug labeling. The use of a drug for indications, dosage forms or regimens, or other use parameter not stated in the product labeling approved by the FDA.

OLTP   See online transaction processing.

omission negligence   Consulting the correct source, but failure to locate the correct answer(s) when providing information.

omnibus test   A statistical test of an overall difference. That is, the test indicates if at least one difference or relationship is statistically significant.

one-tailed test   A hypothesis that makes claim to the direction of the difference or relationship.

online transaction processing (OLTP)   An online system used to add, edit, or delete data from a database.

open formulary   A formulary that allows any marketed drug to be ordered in an institution or under a third-party plan. Can be considered an oxymoron.

open peer review   A type of peer review in which the identities of the author and reviewer are not concealed from one another.

operation   Term used in project management to define routine, day-to-day activities without a clear beginning and end.

ordinal data or scale   A scale of measurement that has rank order, but makes no reference to the distance between ranks (e.g., pain scale).

outcome indicators   Quality assurance indicators that review whether the final desired result was obtained from whatever action was being reviewed.

outcomes   A change in a patient's health status (e.g., recovery, death, disability, disease, discomfort, and dissatisfaction) that can be attributed to the care provided.

outcomes research   A systematic investigation which seeks to provide evidence about which interventions are best for certain types of patients and under certain circumstances. An attempt to identify, measure, and evaluate the end results of health care services. It may include not only clinical and economic consequences, but also outcomes, such as patient health status and satisfaction with their health care.

overview   A general term for a summary of the literature. Includes nonsystematic (narrative), systematic (qualitative), and quantitative (meta-analysis) reviews.

p **value**   The probability of obtaining a test statistic as large or larger than the one actually obtained, conditional on the null hypothesis being true. It is the remaining area under a given probability distribution. When this number is less than the alpha (α), it is interpreted as the probability of rejecting a true null hypothesis or the probability of chance being the reason that a difference in the results between the two groups was calculated.

P&T committee   See pharmacy and therapeutics committee.

page proofs   See galley proofs.

pair-wise analysis   The pair-wise approach is the traditional method to compile a meta-analysis by synthesizing the results of different trials to obtain an overall estimate of the treatment effect of one intervention relative to the control.

parallel forms   Alternatively worded survey items placed throughout a survey used to increase reliability of survey research.

parallel study   A study where two or more groups receive different treatments and the outcomes are compared.

parameter negligence   Failure to consult the correct source in providing information.

parametric tests   Statistical tests that assume a conditional normal distribution.

parenteral admixtures   Solutions containing drug products for intravenous administration.

participatory medicine   A new model of cooperative health care where patients no longer play a passive part when it comes to their health but an active role alongside the health care provider.

patient-centered medical home (PCMH)   A care delivery model led by a physician or other primary care provider that includes multiple other types of providers, including pharmacists, and coordinates patient treatment to ensure necessary care and optimized patient outcomes.

patient database   A database of patients based on prescriber and that includes all pertinent patient information to support e-prescribing functions.

patient education   Written or verbal drug information through a planned activity initiated by a health care provider with the goal of changing patient behavior, improving adherence, and ultimately improving health.

patient pocket formulary   Pocket-sized drug formulary listing top therapeutic drug classes, preferred products within those classes, cost index for the products, and other pertinent information.

patient portals   Web sites that allow patients secure access to their medical records at any time. Portals may also include tools to communicate with providers.

Patient Safety Organization (PSO)   The Patient Safety and Quality Improvement Act of 2005 (Patient Safety Act) authorized the creation of a nationwide network of Patient Safety Organizations (PSOs) to improve safety and quality through the collection and analysis of data on patient events.

patient-by-treatment interaction   Describes the variation in response to therapy due to the heterogeneity of multiple patients' individual characteristics. This heterogeneity can be reduced somewhat with inclusion and exclusion criteria. The best method to minimize patient-by-treatment interaction is to use the patient as their own control such as in a crossover trial design.

patient-specific information   Information created and applied in the process of caring for an individual patient, including medication and medical histories, laboratory test results, radiology interpretations, immunization histories, physical assessments, and other information that is unique to the specific patient.

PBM   See pharmacy benefit management companies does not need to be capitalized.

PCMH   See patient-centered medical home.

PDMP   See prescription drug monitoring program.

peer review   The critical evaluation of a manuscript that has been submitted for publication, performed by a content expert who serves as a neutral party between the publisher and the manuscript author.

performance indicators   Items used to measure quality as part of the check function of quality improvement. The indicators typically focus on the process or outcomes of a care system, although they can also focus on structure.

per-protocol   Study design technique to analyze the study results of only those subjects who completed the entire duration of the study.

personal health record (PHR)   Web-based software application that provides the patient increased opportunity to participate in the collection, maintenance, and sharing of their personal health-related information through a web-based environment.

perspective   A pharmacoeconomic term that describes whose costs (such as the insurer, or the patient) are relevant based on the purpose of the study.

PESTLE analysis   A type of external environment analysis used in project management that encompasses political, economic, social, technological, legal, and environmental factors that may influence a project.

PGY1 residency   See postgraduate year one residency.

PGY2 residency   See postgraduate year two residency.

PGY3 residency   See postgraduate year three residency.

pharmacists' patient care process   A patient-centered, evidence-based approach by pharmacists in collaboration with other providers on the health care team to optimize patient health and medication outcomes.

pharmacoeconomics   The description and analysis of the costs of drug therapy to health care systems and society—it identifies, measures, and compares the costs and consequences of pharmaceutical products and services.

pharmacoepidemiologic trials   A type of trial that combines clinical pharmacology and epidemiology design concepts to study the use of and the effects of drugs in large numbers of people.

pharmacogenomics Using knowledge of a person's genes to develop effective, safe medications and doses tailored to an individual's genetic makeup.

pharmacovigilance The process of preventing and detecting adverse effects from medications.

pharmacy and therapeutics (P&T) committee An interdisciplinary group in an institution or company that oversees any and/or all aspects of drug therapy for that institution or company. In hospitals, it is usually a subcommittee of the Medical Staff. May be known by a variety of similar names, such as pharmacy and formulary committee, drug and therapeutics committee (DTC), or formulary committee.

pharmacy benefit management (PBM) companies Organizations that manage pharmaceutical benefits for managed care organizations, medical providers, or employers.

pharmacy database A database of available pharmacies which supports selection of and communication with the patient's specific pharmacy.

pharmacy informatics A subspecialty of clinical informatics focusing on the management and integration of medication-related data, information, and knowledge across systems that support the medication use process.

pharmacy informatics specialist an individual who has advanced drug information skills with a keen understanding of computer and information technology.

PHI See protected health information.

PHR See personal health record.

pivotal trial A clinical trial that provides the data that serves as the basis of FDA approval or guideline recommendations.

placebo A pharmaceutical preparation that does not contain a pharmacologically active ingredient, but is otherwise identical to the active drug preparation in terms of appearance, taste, and smell.

placebo creep See biocreep.

placebo effect A phenomenon where the patient has a perceived or actual improvement in their medical condition after receiving placebo treatment.

poison information A specialized area of drug information. By definition, it is the provision of information on the toxic effects of an extensive range of chemicals, as well as plant and animal exposures.

poison information center A place that specializes in research, management, and dissemination of toxicity information. A physician usually directs it, although a pharmacist directs many on a day-to-day basis. Often, pharmacists and nurses provide staffing of these centers.

policy Document that ensures consistency, establishes expectations, and sets minimum standards. Policies change infrequently and address the "what," "who," and "why," laying the foundation for a procedure. Policies are prescriptive in nature.

polytomous data Data that falls into more than two categories.

popular technical style A writing style used by professionals addressing laypeople. This is less formal than writing addressed to professionals.

population Every individual in the entire universe with the characteristics or disease states under investigation. Since entire populations are generally very large, a sample representative of the population is usually selected for an investigation.

portfolio   Term used in project management to define various programs, projects, and operations aimed at meeting an overall strategic objective.

positive formulary   A drug formulary that starts out with no drug products and specifically adds products, after appropriate evaluation, that are needed by the institution or company.

post hoc   In clinical trial design this distinguishes something that is done after the study is completed.

postgraduate year one (PGY1) residency   An organized, directed, accredited program that builds upon knowledge, skills, attitudes, and abilities gained from an accredited professional pharmacy degree program. The first-year residency program enhances general competencies in managing medication use systems and supports optimal medication therapy outcomes for patients with a broad range of disease states.

postgraduate year three (PGY3) residency   An organized, directed, accredited program that builds upon the competencies established in postgraduate year two of residency training. The third-year residency program is focused on a subspecialty area of practice.

postgraduate year two (PGY2) residency   An organized, directed, accredited program that builds upon the competencies established in postgraduate year one of residency training. The second-year residency program is focused on a specific area of practice. The PGY2 program increases the resident's depth of knowledge, skills, attitudes, and abilities to raise the resident's level of expertise in medication therapy management and clinical leadership in the area of focus. In those practice areas where board certification exists, graduates are prepared to pursue such certification.

post-hoc tests   A set of statistical tests that follow omnibus tests, such as ANOVA, that determine which groups are statistically different.

postmarketing study   A type of phase IV study mandated by a regulatory authority to examine efficacy and/or safety following approval of the drug.

postmarketing surveillance   The process of continually monitoring and reviewing suspected adverse reactions associated with medications once they reach the market and are available to the public. Legislation mandates this activity for pharmaceutical manufacturers and the U.S. Food and Drug Administration (FDA), but health care providers can also participate by reporting adverse drug events, adverse drug reactions, and medication errors to the FDA and other regulatory bodies.

postpublication peer review   Peer review that occurs following publication. This contrasts with traditional peer review which occurs prior to publication.

power   The ability of a study to detect a difference between a study intervention and control, if a difference exists. Usual minimum target value is 80%; power increases by increasing sample size which also decreases the probability of a Type II or beta error.

power analysis   A statistical procedure conducted by the investigators to determine a sample size for the trial.

practice document   General term referring collectively to a policy, procedure, guideline. or other similar document (e.g., manual).

preferred drug product   Specific drug product within a specific therapeutic class selected as the most appropriate to treat a specific disease or condition as determined by the pharmacy and therapeutics committee.

preferred therapeutic class   Specific drug class selected as the most appropriate to treat a specific disease or condition as determined by the pharmacy and therapeutics committee.

prescribability   The ability of a drug to be prescribed for the first time.

prescription drug monitoring program (PDMP)   A state-level electronic database of controlled substances dispensed for residents of that state.

prevalence   Measures the number of people in the population who have the disease at a given time.

prima facie   A fact presumed to be true unless it is disproved. That is evidence that is sufficient to raise a presumption of fact or to establish the fact in question unless rebutted.

primary author   The author listed first on a publication. Sometimes referred to as the "first author."

primary endpoint   See endpoint, primary.

primary key   The unique identifier for a record of data in a relational database.

primary literature/resource   A resource that contains original information such as a clinical trial protocol, case reports, trial data, dissertation, and descriptive reports.

principles   In ethical analysis, a principle is relatively broad and fundamental in scope, and guides ethical decision-making or actions.

prior authorization   Authorization from the health plan or pharmacy benefit manager in conjunction with the pharmacy and therapeutics committee for specified medications or specified quantities of medications. Request is reviewed against pre-established criteria which are based on evidence-based medicine.

privacy   A rule within the principle of autonomy, more generally relating to the right of the individual to control his or her own affairs without interference from or knowledge of outside parties.

probabilistic sensitivity analysis   A sensitivity analysis allows one to determine how the results of an analysis would change when best guesses or assumptions are varied over a relevant range of values. In pharmacoeconomic analyses, probability distributions are created for each factor about which there is uncertainty. By simulating the results of random samplings from these distributions, it enables judgments to be formed about the decisions in relation to each factor.

procedure   Document that outlines the steps or specific actions to be taken to achieve an objective or implement a policy. Procedures focus on the "how" and are more flexible and subject to change than policies. Procedures are prescriptive in nature.

process   The set of activities that occur between patient and provider, encompassing the services and products that are provided to patients and the way the services are provided.

process change   Making a change to routine process. It may be through changes in policy or procedures, implementation of new services, acquisition of new equipment, changes in staffing, generation of regular notifications, or other methods. It is used to correct practice when quality assurance/drug usage evaluation/medication usage evaluation shows a deficiency.

process mapping   Developing a detailed diagram or flowchart of all steps required to accomplish a task or process.

product claim advertisement/full product promotion   A type of direct-to-consumer advertisement that includes the name of the medication, the indication, and a balanced overview of the risks and benefits.

product label   The information affixed to the product and used to identify the contents.

product labeling   Product information including prescribing information.

professional writing   Any written communication prepared in the fulfillment of the practice of a profession.

program   Term used in project management to describe a group of related projects that are managed in a coordinated way. Programs have their own goals and objectives that ultimately support the main strategic objective of a portfolio.

project   Finite endeavors with a distinct beginning and end, which are also progressively elaborated.

project charter   Project management tool guidepost used to outline the scope, goals and success criteria, final deliverables, stakeholders, budgets, quality assessments, and constraints of a project.

project constraints   Term used to describe factors that could limit or constrain a project; constraints typically include the scope, time, and available resources (funding, personnel, etc.).

project management   A discipline or science that is goal-oriented, organized, detailed, and has built-in accountability.

project quality   Project management term that refers to how good the end result or accomplishment is. Quality is often thought of as a function of time, scope, and resources.

projection   The initial portion of an SQL statement, commonly including the SELECT clause.

propensity scoring   An advanced technique that may be used in analytical observational study designs to perform matching based on all observed baseline characteristics.

prospective indicator   An indicator used in any quality assurance program that determines whether quality is acceptable before an action is taken or care is given.

prospective study   A study where data are collected forward in time from date of study initiation.

protected health information (PHI)   A term under the HIPAA Privacy Rule, which refers to individually identifiable health information which can be linked to a particular person. Specifically, this information can relate to the individual's past, present, or future physical or mental health or condition; the provision of health care to the individual; or the past, present, or future payment for the provision of health care to the individual. Common identifiers of health information include names, social security numbers, addresses, and birth dates.

protopathic bias   When a treatment for the first symptoms of a disease or other outcome appears to cause the outcome. In this case the first symptoms of the outcome of interest are the reason for the treatment under study and not the outcome itself. For instance, early symptoms of pancreatic cancer can be the symptoms of diabetes since beta cells are being destroyed by the cancer.

proximate cause   Cause which immediately precedes and produces the effect, as distinguished from the remote or intervening cause.

PSO   See Patient Safety Organization.

public unsolicited request   An unsolicited request made in a public form, whether directed to a firm specifically or to a forum at large.

publication bias   A type of bias that occurs when the decision to publish a study is based on the magnitude, direction, or statistical significance of the results. It is assessed in quantitative systematic reviews (i.e., meta-analyses) by creating a funnel plot.

pure technical style   A writing style used by professionals addressing other professionals in the same field. It tends to be formal and avoids use of the first person (e.g., I, us). Technical jargon can be used in this writing style.

QALY   See quality-adjusted life years.

QIN-QIO   See Quality Innovation Network–Quality Improvement Organization.

QIO   See Quality Improvement Organization.

QR (Quick Response) codes   A type of two-dimensional bar code that provides more information than is possible with a standard UPC barcode. It is common to find these codes on advertisements or items available for purchase, where the code can be scanned by an application on a smartphone to link to a website where further information may be found on something of interest.

qualitative systematic review   See systematic review.

quality   Project management term that refers to how good the end result or accomplishment is. Quality is often thought of as a function of time, scope, and resources.

quality assessment and assurance committee   A committee found in long-term care facilities to evaluate quality of care, including drug usage evaluation.

quality assurance   Activities that prevent deficiencies along the process.

quality control   Activities that ensure the value of the final product/deliverable.

Quality Improvement Organization (QIO)   The QIO Program is one of the largest federal programs dedicated to improving health quality at the community level for people with Medicare. Each state has a QIO that works with health care providers, community partners, beneficiaries, and caregivers on data-driven initiatives designed to improve the quality of care for people with specific health conditions.

quality improvement research   Studies designed to assess clinical interventions with the goal of changing clinician behavior to ultimately improve patient care and outcomes.

Quality Innovation Network–Quality Improvement Organization (QIN-QIO)   In 2014, contracts for QIOs from the Centers for Medicare & Medicaid Services required building regional improvement networks with state QIOs joining together to provide the assistance and services previously contained within the state borders. There were 14 regional QIN-QIOs awarded contracts in 2014–2019, and the number of regional QIN-QIOs is 12 for 2019–2024. In the ever-changing CMS health care programs landscape, the QIN-QIO program will continue to evolve.

quality measure   When this term is used in health care, it is used to indicate methods of quantifying the type of care a patient received (indicators may include details about processes and organization structure, overall patient outcomes, and even patients' perceptions of the quality of the care received).

quality of life   This is an evaluation of a patient's living situation based on the patient's environment, family life, financial situation, education, and health. It is used in quality assurance programs when developing indicators. In some cases, quality-of-life aspects will take precedence over the absolute best treatment. For example, a quick cure to a disease state may not be as desirable when it costs so much that a family is bankrupted in the process.

quality-adjusted life years (QALY)   A QALY is a health utility measure combining quality and quantity of life, as determined by some valuations process.

quantitative systematic review   See meta-analysis.

quantity limits   Set quantity of drug that can be prescribed that is determined by the health plan in conjunction with the pharmacy and therapeutics committee that is usually based on FDA prescribing guidelines.

query   A request for data or information from a database.

random error   See sampling error.

random forest   A machine learning model consisting of more than one decision tree models.

randomization   Process used in a study in which all subjects enrolled in the study have an equal opportunity to be in any of the study groups. This is used to reduce bias, enable the groups to be as similar as possible at baseline, and is required to validate certain statistical tests.

randomized clinical trial   See controlled clinical trial.

range   The difference between the highest data value and the lowest data value.

rate-based indicators   Usually measure the proportion of activities, or patients, that conform to a desired standard (e.g., the proportion of stat orders that are dispensed within 15 minutes).

ratio data or scale   A scale of measurement that has rank ordered data with meaningful distance between ranks and a natural zero.

RCA   See root cause analysis.

reasonable or due care   Also called ordinary care; conduct that an ordinarily prudent or reasonable person would normally exercise in a particular situation to avoid harm to another, taking the circumstances into account. The concept of due care is used as a test of liability for negligence and usually made on a case by case basis where each juror has to determine what a reasonable man or woman would do.

reasoning engine   See inference engine.

rechallenge   In relation to adverse drug reactions, this occurs when the drug is discontinued and, after the adverse drug reaction abates, the patient is given the same medication drug in an attempt to elicit the response again.

referee   An expert in a specific area who reviews a written document to determine whether it is appropriate for publication.

refereed publication   A publication in which the editors have experts in the appropriate field review items submitted for possible publication to determine whether those items are of suitable quality.

regulatory project manager (RPM)   This will be the sponsor's primary FDA contact person. Each application that is submitted is assigned an RPM. Contact information for the RPM is provided in the letter sent to the applicant acknowledging receipt of the application. If the RPM is changed during the course of the review, the applicant is notified by the new RPM.

relational database   A relational database is a type of database that collects and stores data in structured formats called tables that are related to one another.

relative risk   A ratio of the risks (events / population at risk) between two groups; typically reported from cohort studies.

reminder advertisement   A type of direct-to-consumer advertisement that provides a medication's name but does not include or imply the medication's indication.

REMS   See Risk Evaluation and Mitigation Strategy.

requirements matrix   A project management tool used to align the requirements of a project with the goals in the charter.

research hypothesis   Also known as the alternative hypothesis or hypothesis (H_a). A statement of difference between the therapy under investigation and the control.

residual value   The difference between the model predicted dependent variable and the actual dependent variable value.

respondeat superior   Refers to the proposition that the employer is responsible for the negligent acts of its agents or employees.

response bias   See measurement error.

Restatement (Second) of Torts   "An attempt by the American Law Institute to present an orderly statement of the general common law of the United States, including in that term not only the law developed solely by judicial decision, but also the law that has grown from the application by the courts of statutes..." It takes into account other factors, such as the modern trend of the law according to influential jurisdictions and well-thought out opinions.

retrospective indicator   An indicator used in any quality assurance program that determines whether quality was acceptable after an action was taken or care was given.

retrospective study   A study that analyzes historical data (e.g., previously collected data such as medical records or insurance information).

Risk Evaluation and Mitigation Strategy (REMS)   A risk management plan required by the FDA that goes beyond requirements in the drug prescribing information to manage serious risks associated with a drug.

Risk Minimization Action Plans (RiskMAPs)   A strategic safety program designed to meet specific goals and objectives in minimizing known risks of a product while preserving its benefits.

RiskMAPs   See risk minimization action plans.

robustness   The ability of the statistical test to produce correct test statistics and parameter estimates in the presence of assumption violations.

root cause analysis (RCA)   A retrospective evaluation conducted by organizations to better understand why an error happened by identifying underlying system vulnerabilities that contributed to the error, then generate and implement an action plan to improve the system and reduce the risk of error recurrence.

RPM   See regulatory project manager.

rule   In ethical analysis, a rule guides ethical decision-making or actions, but is relatively specific in context and restricted in scope.

rule-based human performance   Applying a past solution that solved a problem previously. Rule-based errors arise from misapplication of a good rule, failure to apply a rule, or application of a bad rule.

rules engines   Computer programs, similar to adverse drug effect monitoring systems, with built-in, logic rules designed to aid in monitoring specific aspects of patient care.

run-in phase   A short duration of patient assessment that occurs prior to subject enrollment into the study. Various reasons exist for this phase including: assessment of medication compliance; meet inclusion criteria (e.g., LDL-C less than 130 mg/dL); and allow medication wash-out.

SaaS   See software as a service.

sample   A group of subjects, taken from the population, who are enrolled in a study. These individuals should represent the population so that study results may be extrapolated to the population.

sample frame   A term describing the population that will actually be drawn from to make up the survey sample.

sampling error   Refers to the difference between the estimate derived from a sample survey and the true value that would result if a census of the entire target population were taken under the same conditions.

scope   Project management term that refers to the amount of work that is to be done, as well as what the project will and will not entail.

scope statement   Part of a document that clarifies applicability of the document based on factors such as practice area, department, or location.

secondary endpoint   See endpoint, secondary.

secondary literature/resource   A resource mainly in the form of searchable database that enables location and retrieval of primary or tertiary resources. This category of resources is similar to an old cataloging system.

SELECT   An SQL clause that indicates and determines the items to be included in the output.

selection bias   Occurs when researchers intentionally or unintentionally exclude certain patients from participating in studies whether through nonadherence to inclusion/exclusion criteria or by defining inclusion and exclusion criteria so narrowly that only ideal patients are enrolled.

SEM   See standard error of the mean.

semantic interoperability   The ability of computers to share and use information in a meaningful manner as it relates to the content of electronic messages.

sensitivity   The probability an individual with a disease will have a positive test result.

sensitivity analysis   Tests that are undertaken to determine the influence of various criteria or conditions on study results. Sensitivity analyses are commonly used in meta-analyses and pharmacoeconomic research.

sentinel event   The Joint Commission defines a sentinel event as an unexpected occurrence involving death or serious physical or psychological injury, or the risk thereof. Serious injury specifically includes loss of limb or function. The phrase "or the risk thereof" includes any process variation for which a recurrence would carry a significant chance of a serious adverse outcome. Such events are called "sentinel" because they signal the need for immediate investigation and response.

sentinel indicators   Reflect the occurrence of a serious event that requires further investigation (e.g., adverse drug–related event, death).

side effect   The American Society of Health-System Pharmacists (ASHP) defines a side effect as any common and predictable reaction that results in minor or no change to the drug therapy regimen.

single-blind peer review   A type of peer review where the author is blinded to the reviewer's identity, but the reviewer is not blinded to the author's identity.

skewness   The measure of symmetry of a curve.

skill-based human performance   Reliance on action or execution to prevent an error. Skill-based errors occur during familiar and routine tasks. The action can be intentional or unintentional. Errors occur when the action is not carried out or executed according to plan—too soon, too late, omitting a step, performing a task in the wrong direction, or forgetting a step.

smart pumps   A programmable device used to control and administer intravenous drugs. By using a library of medications' doses and infusion rates, error can be prevented.

smartphone   a cellular device that has Internet capabilities and supports various software functions.

SNOMED CT   See Systemized Nomenclature of Medicine-Clinical Terms.

social media   Form of electronic communication allowing interactions with users to share information, messages, and other various forms of content. Consists of social networking sites, content-sharing sites, and blogs.

software as a service (SaaS)   A computing model in which an organization's data and software are hosted by an off-site vendor who is responsible for maintaining data storage as well as the equipment on which it is stored.

special protocol assessment   A statement from the U.S. Food and Drug Administration that an uninitiated or ongoing Phase III trial's design, clinical endpoints, and statistical analyses are adequate for FDA approval.

special variation   Data points above the upper control limit or below the lower control limit which indicate that something different is going on outside the normal operation of a process. Variation that can be attributed to an identified event or assignable cause (e.g., the laboratory glucose analysis of quality control standards identifies a lower result outside control). The analyst identifies new reagents were started at the same time as the change in results and determines recalibration is required.

specialty drugs   These are high-cost medications used to treat complex chronic conditions. They require special handling, may be difficult to administer, and need ongoing clinical assessment.

specificity   The probability an individual without a disease will have a negative test result.

sponsor   An organization (or individual) who takes responsibility for and initiates a clinical investigation. The sponsor may be an individual or pharmaceutical company, government agency, academic institution, private organization, or other organization.

sponsor-investigator   An individual who both initiates and conducts a clinical investigation (i.e., submits the IND and directly supervises administration of the drug as well as other investigator responsibilities).

SQL   See Structured Query Language.

stability study   A study designed to determine the stability of drugs in various preparations or environmental conditions.

stakeholder   Term used in project management to describe anyone who is involved in, interested in, or affected by a project.

stakeholder impact analysis   A systematic process to help recognize people affected by a project and estimate their ultimate impact on the work.

stakeholder matrix   Project management tool used to identify stakeholders, as well as their involvement, expectations, interest, and engagement for a given project.

standard   A term used in quality assurance program that indicates how often an indicator must be complied with. The level of compliance will be set at either 0% (i.e., never done) or 100% (i.e., always done). A threshold, which allows compliance of between 0% and 100%, has sometimes been used instead of a standard.

standard deviation (1) A measurement of the range of data values (i.e., variability) around the mean. (2) The measure of the average amount by which each observation in a series of data points differs from the mean. In other words, how far away is each data point from the mean (dispersion or variability) or the average deviation from the mean.

standard error of the mean (SEM) Estimates the variability between sample means when multiple samples are taken from the same population. The standard error of the mean estimates the variability between samples whereas the standard deviation measures the variability within a single sample.

standard gamble One method used for measuring health preferences. Each subject is offered two alternatives. Alternative one is treatment with two possible outcomes: either the return to normal health or immediate death. Alternative two is the certain outcome of a chronic disease state for life. The probability of dying is varied until the subject is indifferent between alternative one and alternative two. Used to assess his or her QALY estimate.

statistic A measurement that describes part of a sample.

statistical significance The impact of a study in terms of the outcome of statistical tests conducted on the data. A study is said to be statistically significant when statistical tests demonstrate a difference between treatment groups.

statute Written law enacted by a legislature other than that of a municipality.

step therapy Prescribing guidelines set by the health plan in conjunction with the pharmacy and therapeutics committee that specify which drugs should be prescribed first before more expensive drugs will be covered. Guidelines are based on evidence-based medicine.

stratification An advanced type of randomization to produce study groups as similar as possible; considers baseline demographic information of the subjects selected for the study.

stratified Data elements identified by groupings or subgroupings to assist in analysis of differences in outcomes, such as the differences of outcomes by race and ethnicity population subgroups versus the aggregate, summary outcomes of an entire population.

strict liability Also called absolute liability; the legal responsibility for damages, or injury, even if the person was not at fault or negligent. Strict liability has been applied to certain activities, such as holding employers absolutely liable for the torts of their employees, but it is most commonly associated with claims for injuries resulting from defectively manufactured or designed products. A successful plaintiff need only show that the product was in fact defective in design or manufacture, rendering it unreasonably dangerous and the cause of injury.

structure Refers to the characteristics of providers, the tools and resources at their disposal, and the physical or organizational settings in which they work.

structure indicators Quality assurance indicators based on the presence or absence of items, such as staffing patterns, available space, equipment, resources, or administrative organization.

Structured Query Language (SQL) A comprehensive, text-based language to link relational databases that allows the user to define and manipulate data in relational databases using four primary operators: projection, filter, join, and aggregate.

study objective A brief statement of the goals and purpose of a research study.

subgroup analysis Evaluation of study results within a subset of subjects enrolled in the study according to specific demographic (e.g., age, gender, disease state).

subject An individual who participates in a clinical investigation (either as the recipient of the investigational drug or as a member of the control group).

success criteria Term used in project management to describe quantifiable measures that indicate when a project goal has been accomplished.

summary judgment A party moving (applying) for summary judgment is attempting to avoid the time and expense of a trial when the outcome is obvious. A party may also move for summary judgment in order to eliminate the risk of losing at trial, and possibly avoid having to go through discovery (i.e., by moving at the outset of discovery), by demonstrating to the judge, via sworn statements and documentary evidence, that there are no material factual issues remaining to be tried. If there is nothing for the factfinder to decide, then the moving party asks rhetorically, why have a trial? A dispute over a material fact (see above) upon which the outcome of a legal case may rely, and which therefore must be decided by a judge or jury; a dispute which precludes summary judgment.

surrogate endpoint An effect that can be easily measured to correlate a clinical outcome that is more difficult and/or time-consuming to measure (e.g., reducing LDL-C levels [measured effect] should result in less cardiovascular events [predicted outcome] such as myocardial infarction, stroke, or death).

survey instrument Questionnaire used for the survey.

survey research Research in which responses to questions asked of subjects are analyzed to determine the incidence, distribution, and relationships of sociological and psychological variables.

SWOT analysis A type of internal environment analysis used in project management that encompasses strengths, weaknesses, opportunities, and threats.

synthesis Synthesis is the careful, systematic, and orderly process of integrating varied and diverse elements, ideas, or factors into a coherent response. This process relies not only on the type and quality of the data gathered, but also on how the data are organized, viewed, and evaluated. Synthesis, as it relates to pharmacotherapy, involves the careful integration of critical information about the patient, disease, and medication along with pertinent background information to arrive at a judgment or conclusion.

systematic review A summary of previously conducted studies that involves systematic methods such as formal criteria for selection of studies. They may be qualitative, in which data are not statistically combined, or quantitative, in which data are statistically combined. A systematic review that is quantitative is also called a meta-analysis.

Systemized Nomenclature of Medicine-Clinical Terms (SNOMED CT) A clinical terminology that enables sharing of clinical terminology between electronic systems.

tables In relational databases, tables are a collection of data stored in memory as a series of records, each defined by a unique key.

target drug program A program that evaluates the use of a medication or group of medications on an ongoing basis. Within these programs, interventions are usually made at the time of discovery based on established criteria or guidelines.

target population The entire group a researcher is interested in because this is the population that the findings of the survey are meant to generalize and the researcher wishes to make inferences and draw conclusions.

targeted medication review (TMR)   A scheduled (quarterly, monthly) targeted medication review to focus on identified issues/problems with medications that require patient or prescriber's attention.

TEC   See technology-enabled care.

technology-enabled care (TEC)   The use of technology to enhance the quality and cost-effectiveness of care and support and improve outcomes for individuals through the application of technology as an integral part of the care and support process.

telehealth   The delivery of health-related services and information over distance with the aid of electronic devices.

telemedicine   The use of telecommunications and interactive video technology to provide health care services to patients who are at a distance.

teratogenicity   Toxicity of drugs to the unborn fetus.

tertiary literature/resource   A resource that reviews, summarizes, compares, and reports what has already been published as primary literature. This includes narrative and systematic reviews as well as clinical practice guidelines. Examples include textbooks and review articles.

The Joint Commission (TJC)   An organization that accredits health care organizations and programs in the United States.

third-party payer   Organization, such as an insurance company or the government, that pays for or underwrites coverage for health care expenses for another entity.

third-party plan   A method of reimbursement for medical care in which neither the care provider nor the patient is charged. Third-party payers include insurance, health maintenance organizations, and government entities.

threshold   A term used in quality assurance program that indicates how often an indicator must be complied with. Unlike standards, thresholds can be set at any level of compliance from 0% to 100%.

tiered copayment benefit   A pharmacy benefit design that encourages patients to use generic and formulary drugs, by requiring the patient to pay progressively higher copayments for brand name and nonformulary drugs.

time-trade-off   A method for measuring health preferences. The subject is offered two alternatives. Alternative one is a certain disease state for a specific length of time t, the life expectancy for a person with the disease, then death. Alternative two is being healthy for time x, which is less than t. Time x is varied until the respondent is indifferent between the two alternatives. The proportion of the number of years of life a person is willing to give up $(t - x)$ to have his or her remaining years (x) of life in a healthy state is used to assess his or her QALY estimate.

TJC   See The Joint Commission.

TMR   See targeted medication review.

tort liability   Civil wrongs recognized by law as grounds for a lawsuit.

total quality management (TQM)   A management concept dealing with the implementation of continuous quality improvement.

TQM   See total quality management.

treatment effect   A mean difference in the outcome measure over time between two drugs (i.e., drug – placebo or test drug – reference drug).

treatment order effect A situation where the order in which patients receive the treatment in a trial (generally a crossover design) affects the results of that trial.

treatment-by-time interaction Chance that the effects associated with each treatment might vary over time.

trohoc study See case-control study.

true experiment A study where researchers apply a treatment and determine its effects on subjects.

true negatives Individuals without the disease that were correctly identified as being disease-free by the test.

true positives Individuals with the disease that were correctly identified as diseased by the test.

two-tailed test A hypothesis that does not claim a direction of the difference or relationship.

type I error Rejecting the null hypothesis instead of failing-to-reject (i.e., accepting) the null hypothesis; also known as a false-positive result or alpha-error. Chance is the reason for this to occur.

type II error Failing to reject (i.e., accepting) the null hypothesis instead of rejecting the null hypothesis; also known as a false-negative result or beta-error. Chance or small sample size are reasons for this to occur.

UMLS See Unified Medical Language System.

unexpected drug reaction The Food and Drug Administration defines this as "one that is not listed in the current labeling for the drug as having been reported or associated with the use of the drug. This includes an ADR that may be symptomatically or pathophysiologically related to an ADR listed in the labeling but may differ from the labeled ADR because of greater severity or specificity (e.g., abnormal liver function vs. hepatic necrosis)."

Unified Medical Language System (UMLS) Software that enables computer system interoperability through inclusion of multiple controlled vocabularies.

uniform resource locator—URL An Internet address (e.g., http://druginfo.creighton.edu).

unsolicited requests Requests initiated by persons or entities that are completely independent of the relevant firm.

URAC® Organization that accredits community pharmacies, specialty pharmacies, telehealth providers, and other health programs in the United States.

user database A database consisting of a list of prescribers and other users along with their authority to prescribe, National Provider Identifier (NPI), Drug Enforcement Agency (DEA) number, and other identifiers (e.g., address and phone number).

utility Utility is the amount of satisfaction obtained from a drug or service.

validity The truthfulness of study results. Internal validity refers to the extent to which the study results reflect what actually happened in the study (i.e., appropriate and sound study methods). External validity is the degree to which the study results can be applied to patients routinely encountered in clinical practice.

validity filter A type of term or limit used to narrow a search to only the highest quality studies, such as randomized controlled trial or double-blind.

validity, external   Quality of the study design that allows the result to be applied into practice. Study results are meaningful to practitioners and can be used for patient care.

validity, internal   Quality of the study design that produces accurate results. Strong study design should translate into reliable results.

value   Has been assigned many definitions, but within health care; it usually reflects the ratio of quality and costs (value = quality/cost).

variables   Factors (characteristics that are being observed or measured) that are the focus of a study. The independent variable (e.g., treatment) causes change in the dependent variable (e.g., outcome).

variance   A measurement of the range of data values (i.e., variability) about the mean. Variance is the square of the standard deviation.

veracity   This term addresses the obligation to truth telling or honesty.

vicarious liability   Also called imputed liability or imputed negligence; the doctrine that attaches responsibility upon one person for the failure of another, with whom the person has a special relationship (such as parent and child, employer and employee, husband and wife, or owner of vehicle and driver), to exercise such care as a reasonably prudent person would use under similar circumstances. Ordinarily, the independent negligence of one person is not imputable to another person.

virtual journal club   A journal club conducted through a web-based platform.

virtual private network (VPN)   A method to connect computers over a distance, for example, over the Internet, that allows secure transmission of confidential data.

warning letter   An official message from the FDA to a pharmaceutical manufacturer, identifying rule violations such as not following CGMP.

warranty   An assurance by one party to a contract of the existence of a fact upon which the other party may rely, intended to relieve the promisee of any duty to ascertain the fact for himself or herself. Amounts to a promise to indemnify the promisee for any loss if the fact warranted proves untrue. Warranties may be expressed (made overtly) or implied (by implication).

WHERE   A SQL clause that allows for specific restrictions of the data to be included in the output.

white bagging   Receiving a medication from the pharmacy (usually specialty pharmacy) and taking it to the physician's office for administration.

wikis   Websites which allow its users to add, modify, or delete its content via a web browser usually using a simplified markup language or a rich-text editor. Wikis are powered by wiki software, are created collaboratively, and can be community websites and intranets, for example. Some permit control over different functions (levels of access). For example, editing rights may permit changing, adding, or removing material. Others may permit access without enforcing access control.

work breakdown structure   Project management tool used to identify and collate tasks needed to complete a deliverable.

workflow software solutions   A computer program used to coordinate and track steps in the document management process. It may also organize documents into a searchable repository.

z-score   The distance a data point is from its variable's mean in standard deviation units.

Case Study Answers

Chapter 3

CASE STUDY 3-1

Common side effects would be included in all major compendia (e.g., IBM® Micromedex®, Clinical Pharmacology, or Lexicomp®) which would be a good initial search. In addition, some of the adverse effect specific resources (e.g., Meyler's Side Effects of Drugs) would be appropriate to consult for less common side effects. The package insert will also contain detail on common side effects based on results of clinical trial(s) leading to FDA approval.

CASE STUDY 3-2

- There are a variety of resources that could be consulted for this information including LactMed, Drugs in Pregnancy and Lactation, or the major compendia (possibly, IBM® Micromedex® or Clinical Pharmacology).
- Practitioners should review multiple resources to determine if there are additional pertinent data. If there are concerns with fluconazole, the practitioner can review the disease state to determine other possible treatment options.

CASE STUDY 3-3

- The student might start a search for general information in a toxicology text such as Goldfrank's Toxicologic Emergencies. She could then search in Lexicomp® or IBM® Micromedex® to find some general toxicology information, and within the POISINDEX® component of IBM® Micromedex® for comprehensive information on this topic.
- The student would do best to identify relevant MeSH terms prior to searching (e.g., gabapentin, opioid-related disorders, substance-related disorders). Identifying appropriate search terms can help the student find results involving the correct drug and patient population.

CASE STUDY 3-4

- Since this would be an off-label use, there may be fewer data in the tertiary resources. However, AHFS® DI, DRUGDEX® (part of IBM® Micromedex®), and Lexicomp® may contain information on off-label uses. In this case, related treatment guidelines may also contain information on the use of this combination prior to hematopoietic stem cell transplant. A literature search may be

appropriate if the tertiary resources do not contain adequate data. MEDLINE® and Embase, using MeSH and Emtree terms, respectively, are good places to start.
- Initially conducting a search with no restrictions/limits ensures that valuable information is not missed.
- If the initial search yields a significant number of results, then a restriction to human clinical trials may be beneficial. It is important to realize that the term "Hematopoietic Stem Cell Transplantation" has changed over time in the MeSH database, so a more general search for stem cell transplant will give more results. In addition, searching for the specific drugs fludarabine and busulfan will yield useful data, but expanding the search using the class of drugs will provide more data.

CASE STUDY 3–5

- Tertiary resources could provide a good overview on how a treatment might work in a large patient population, appropriate dosing, as well as provide a quick summary of safety data. The disadvantage is the lag time from when the information is updated until it is published, so recently discovered safety or efficacy information might not be included in that type of resource.
- Primary literature would provide very timely information, but in a case like this, the volume of primary literature may be extensive and time-consuming to navigate and accurately assess.

CASE STUDY 3–6

Since the patient specifically mentioned hearing about this in the news, going directly to the Internet page for the news source would be an excellent start. You could also search LexisNexis® and perform a general Internet search if you are unable to find the story on the news source page.

Chapter 4

CASE STUDY 4–1

- The intention-to-treat principle is a way of viewing data for analysis. This analytical method includes the data points (i.e., endpoints) of every subject included in the study protocol. This method of analysis gives the reader a "worst-case scenario" of medication therapy performance in the general population. Intention-to-treat analysis is desired in a controlled clinical trial designed to determine superiority of one treatment versus another. The fact that a medication can demonstrate significant efficacy in a "worst-case scenario" implies that the medication is more likely to be efficacious even though some patients may not be as adherent to their medication as necessary in real practice. Alternatively, a per-protocol analysis only uses the data points (i.e., endpoints) of subjects who complete the study "per study protocol." This method of analysis can be considered a "best case scenario" approach to viewing study results. Per-protocol data are helpful in studies that have high rates of subject attrition, as the intention-to-treat data set may reflect artificially lower medication efficacy results.
- The individual outcomes within the primary efficacy endpoint in this study were cardiovascular death, nonfatal myocardial infarction, nonfatal stroke, coronary revascularization, and unstable angina. A composite endpoint includes several, individual events, and the occurrence of one individual event qualifies as one event within the composite primary endpoint. For example, in the current study, if a subject experienced a nonfatal myocardial infarction and another subject

experienced unstable angina, both subjects would be counted as having experienced the primary efficacy endpoint. This type of endpoint is usually reserved for studies that analyze health events that are negative or undesired and have an observed pathophysiological association (e.g., cardiovascular death, myocardial infarction, stroke). Use of composite endpoints makes it easier for a subject to attain the endpoint because study investigators do not have to wait on a subject to experience one health event, but rather, one of several associated health events. Use of composite endpoints may shorten the duration of a study. In addition, fewer subjects are often needed to achieve sufficient statistical power when using composite endpoints. A disadvantage of a composite endpoint is the potential for a disproportionate number of subjects experiencing one of the qualifying endpoints over the remaining endpoints within the composite, and this effect may preclude a straightforward interpretation of the results. It is important for the reader to closely analyze outcome rates within studies that use composite endpoints to ensure the distribution of event rates among qualifying events is somewhat similar, and if not, that any statistically significant differences between individual outcome rates receive comment in the discussion section of the article.

- If the authors had sought 85% power instead of 90% power, the estimated sample size would have likely been lower since statistical power and sample size are directly related, i.e., the lower the desired power, the fewer subjects that are needed. Conversely, if the authors sought to detect a smaller difference in the primary composite endpoint (i.e., 10% instead of 15%), a larger sample of subjects would likely have been necessary since smaller treatment effects are more difficult to detect than larger treatment effects.

- $p < 0.001$ indicates that there is less than a 0.1% probability for a false-positive conclusion (i.e., Type I error) with respect to the primary endpoint result. The p value of 0.001 is less than the predetermined α of 0.0437 (i.e., 4.37%) which indicates that the primary endpoint result is statistically significant and leads the investigators to reject the null hypothesis. A p value this low implies that it is highly unlikely that the result is due to random chance alone.

- Subgroup analyses improve the ability of researchers to provide additional context to the primary endpoint through the lens of variables that may be important to health care professionals. Additionally, subgroup analyses may act as a springboard for future research into a variable's influence on outcomes. The results of subgroup analyses enable researchers to generate new, testable hypotheses.

  Disadvantages of subgroup analyses include the potential for results to be misleading or over-interpreted in certain circumstances. For example, if a statistically significant difference is identified in the primary endpoint, a subgroup analysis should not be performed on this endpoint. In addition, the list of planned subgroup analyses should be explicitly stated in the protocol *a priori*, and all planned subgroup analysis results should be disseminated, regardless of statistical significance.

  The patients in the secondary prevention cohort appeared to experience more benefit from the use of icosapent ethyl than patients in the primary prevention cohort. This is evidenced by the hazard ratio (HR) (95% CI) of the primary efficacy composite endpoint in each of these subgroups. The HR (95% CI) of the primary efficacy composite endpoint was 0.73 (0.65 – 0.81) in the secondary prevention subgroup, whereas it was 0.88 (0.70 – 1.10) in the primary prevention subgroup. The reduction of the composite primary efficacy endpoint is statistically significant in the secondary prevention subgroup because the 95% CI of the HR does NOT include 1. This is not the case for the primary prevention subgroup. However, there does not appear to be a significant difference in the composite primary efficacy endpoint BETWEEN the two subgroups as evidenced by the p value for interaction which was greater than α at 0.14. Icosapent ethyl may be more effective in secondary prevention patients than primary prevention patients, but this study was not powered to detect a difference between these subgroups, so this research may act as a pilot for future research that compares efficacy of the medication in primary versus secondary prevention specifically.

CASE STUDY 4-2

- Double-dummy blinding is a sophisticated blinding scheme that is used in select situations. Double-dummy means that both the intervention and control arm receive "dummy" doses of the opposing therapy. Use in the case of this study was necessary in order to conceal therapies, as this study used therapies that come in different dosage forms and dosing schedules (i.e., daily subcutaneous injection vs. once weekly oral tablet). Use of a double-dummy approach in a trial that has an active control is desired and increases the internal validity of the study by reducing the potential for confounding due to subjects being able to identify their assigned therapy.

- The fact that the study was performed in over 100 study centers in multiple countries around the world generally enhances the external validity of the results. By including diverse subjects across diverse geographic locations in the sample, the results are able to be extrapolated more broadly to different patient populations. It is important to note that the study was not conducted in Asia, Africa, or Australia, so extrapolating results to patients on those continents may be more questionable.

  On the other hand, including a broad array of subjects across many countries could negatively affect internal validity. Recall that internal validity is the extent to which study results reflect what actually happened in the study. Each additional study center inherently increases variability in the way subjects are assessed, diagnosed, and monitored, even if researchers take precautions to minimize these inconsistencies.

- RR teriparatide vs. risedronate = 5.4% / 12.0% = 0.45

  This quotient value is less than 1, indicating a protective benefit conferred to the recipient of teriparatide versus risedronate for the prevention of new vertebral fractures in patients with severe osteoporosis within the given study sample. In other words, the quotient value of 0.45 could be utilized to indicate that use of teriparatide is associated with 45% of the risk of new vertebral fractures that is associated with risedronate.

- RRR = 1 − RR = 1 − 0.45 = 0.55 = 55%

  This value indicates that 55% of baseline risk of the occurrence of new vertebral fractures is removed by receiving teriparatide versus risedronate. This result indicates that teriparatide reduces new vertebral fracture risk versus risedronate.

- ARR = %C − %I = 12.0% − 5.4% = 6.6%

  This value indicates that 6.6% of subjects were spared from experiencing new vertebral fractures by receiving teriparatide versus risedronate. This result indicates that teriparatide reduces new vertebral fracture risk versus risedronate.

- NNT = 1/ARR (in decimal format) = 1 / 0.066 = 15.2 (round up to 16)

  This result indicates that the investigators would have to treat 16 patients for approximately 24 months (mean trial follow-up period) to prevent one new vertebral fracture that otherwise would occur with receipt of risedronate. It is customary to round NNTs up to the nearest integer as not to overstate the efficacy of the intervention. [Note the converse is true about NNHs, which are customarily rounded down to the nearest integer as not to understate safety concerns with the intervention.] Lower NNT values are preferred. The best possible NNT value is one which implies 100% effectiveness rate with respect to the primary endpoint.

- The HR for the first nonvertebral fragility fracture in this sample is 0.66, and the investigators are 95% confident that the true HR in the general population lies between 0.39 and 1.10. The value of equality (one) is contained in this range, indicating that the difference in this outcome is not statistically significant between the groups. Investigators fail to reject the null hypothesis with respect to the comparison of teriparatide and risedronate in the context of nonvertebral fragility fractures.

CASE STUDY 4-3

- Yes, any study enrolling human subjects requires IRB approval. The IRB approval is needed to protect the enrolled subjects.
- The type of data being evaluated for the FDA's primary efficacy endpoint is nominal data which is represented by an endpoint that is "yes/no" or dichotomous in nature. For the study under consideration, the endpoint of overall success falls into this category. [Note: "overall success" is a composite endpoint of clinical cure and microbial eradication.] Either someone achieves overall success or does not.

A benefit of nominal endpoints is that they represent an objective outcome and are driven by clinical events (e.g., occurrence of "event x" or no occurrence of "event x"). With nominal endpoints, there is no ranking or scaling of endpoint results. Outcomes cannot be influenced by personal perception or opinion. Furthermore, measures of association (i.e., RR, ARR, RRR, NNT) can be calculated from nominal endpoints. Thus, such endpoints are good for comparing objective outcomes between treatments.

- Null hypothesis: The mean treatment difference and 95% CI associated with that treatment difference fails to exhibit noninferiority (within a 15% margin) for meropenem-vaborbactam compared to piperacillin-tazobactam regarding the primary efficacy endpoint of overall success. In other words, the study results would be inconclusive.

  Alternative hypothesis: The mean treatment difference and 95% CI associated with that treatment difference exhibits noninferiority (within a 15% margin) for meropenem-vaborbactam compared to piperacillin-tazobactam regarding the primary efficacy endpoint of overall success.

- Meropenem-vaborbactam is noninferior to piperacillin-tazobactam regarding the treatment of complicated UTIs, including pyelonephritis.

- Performing a superiority analysis after noninferiority has been established is acceptable and appropriate. Per the study, "If noninferiority was demonstrated in FDA or EMA primary end points, the protocol and statistical analysis plan included an assessment of superiority using the CI to determine whether the lower bound of the two-sided 95% CI was greater than 0." Conversely, it is generally not acceptable or appropriate to seek the conclusion of noninferiority from a failed superiority trial.

Chapter 5

CASE STUDY 5-1

- Selection bias may occur from recruiting nurses who may have healthier lifestyles than the general population leading to lower risk for endometrial cancer (e.g., more active, decreased rates of obesity/diabetes/high blood pressure). Also, because no matching or propensity scoring was used initially to create groups of coffee drinkers, groups may be somewhat dissimilar in terms of baseline characteristics. Therefore, nurses consuming four or more cups of coffee may be made up of healthier subjects than the group of women consuming less than one cup of coffee per day.

- Some unknown factors may be playing a protective role in those women who had an associated reduction in endometrial cancer risk. This might include immune system health, genetic familial effects, and exposure to environmental factors that may be causing the cancer. Other things like types of coffee (e.g., levels of caffeination, brewing method) or alcohol/tobacco consumption may confound the results. A healthier lifestyle (e.g., lower body mass index) or increased age could also be a factor relating to endometrial cancer risk. Even though this study evaluated a specific age range of nurses, older patients (>60 years of age) were not considered.

- Stratification of groups could be considered. They could be grouped/stratified based on age range, daily activity, alcohol/tobacco use, body mass index, and/or types of coffee ingested (e.g., flavored, cold, brewed).

- Because this is a prospective cohort study, a cause-effect relationship cannot be determined. In order to truly say that drinking four or more cups of coffee per day leads to lower rates of endometrial cancer in women (e.g., nurses), a randomized controlled trial would need to be undertaken.

CASE STUDY 5-2

- A well-constructed strategy will use various terms, which may include acronyms, synonyms, and singular and plural forms of words. To capture all studies involving statin therapy, the following are some terms that should be used: statin, statins, HMG-CoA reductase inhibitor, HMG-Co-A reductase inhibitors, atorvastatin, fluvastatin, lovastatin, pitavastatin, pravastatin, rosuvastatin, and simvastatin.
- The participants are patients with elevated lipid levels, the intervention is a statin, the comparator is a placebo, the outcome is diabetes, and the study design is a randomized controlled trial. In addition, this meta-analysis had criteria for sample size (at least 1000 patients) and duration (at least 1 year).
- The statistical significance and magnitude of heterogeneity were assessed. The results were desirable because the p value was not statistically significant at a value of 0.32 (values < 0.1 are typically considered statistically significant for heterogeneity) and the I^2 value was low in magnitude at a value of 11.7% (values of 0–40% are typically not important). Because the results for assessments of heterogeneity were desirable, one can be reasonably confident in the pooled result.
- Publication bias was assessed by visual inspection of a funnel plot and a statistical test for asymmetry. The results were desirable because the plot was described as symmetrical (asymmetry suggests that publication bias is possible) and the p value from an Egger's test was not statistically significant at a value of 0.67 (values < 0.05 are typically considered statistically significant for asymmetry). Because the results for assessments of publication bias were desirable, one can be reasonably confident in the pooled result.

CASE STUDY 5-3

- Both products are from "colostrum," but have two major differences. First, Colostrinin® is a specific polypeptide complex with one component extracted from whole colostrum, while the store product is concentrated whole colostrum. Second, Colostrinin® is prepared from ovine, or sheep, colostrum, while the store product consisted of bovine, or cow, colostrum. Though some components of colostrum may be similar across species, these two products are so different that clinical trial results for one cannot be extrapolated to the other.
- The majority of natural medicine trials are conducted in Europe and Asia. Appropriateness of generalizability of results to a practitioner's own patient population must always be considered, just as with standard drug trials. This is especially true of trials when the treatment under investigation is added to any standard treatments the subjects may be receiving, as both available drugs and recommended treatment regimens could differ.
- Small subject population is a common flaw with natural medicine trials. This study utilized a small number of patients, especially considering they were divided into three groups and then were further subdivided into illness severity strata. The fact that statistical power was not calculated means that it is more difficult to interpret the results within any strata that had nonsignificant results. In addition, more serious adverse reactions can be overlooked in smaller groups versus a larger one, as they may have a much lower occurrence rate.

Chapter 6

CASE STUDY 6-1

- There are two populations of interest: (1) patients recently discharged with STEMI and (2) patients who had routine discharge.
- Because this was a single-institution study, a convenience sample was used. It could be argued that anyone could randomly need the hospital, but at the very least, the sample is a convenience on a

regional level. The randomness of the convenience sample is determined by the demographics of the patients, where hospitals in bigger cites may have a more generalizable sample.
- The DV is 30-day or 90-day hospital readmission for any cause. For both DVs, there are two levels—readmit versus no readmit. The scale of measurement is nominal, binary, or dichotomous.
- For both outcomes, the appropriate measure of central tendency is the mode because the data are nominal. This data should be presented as frequency count and percentage.
- The IV is treatment group. There are two levels—treatment versus control. The scale of measurement is nominal, binary, or dichotomous.
- Confounding variables are considered as sources of error. There are numerous sources of error applicable to the patient, hospitalist, pharmacist, or nurse.
  - Patient—length of stay prior to discharge, severity of disease state, comorbid disorders, concomitant medications, demographic characteristics (e.g., age, gender, race, family history, support system), among others.
  - Healthcare practitioners—years of experience, level of training (e.g., resident, fellow), number of patients seen daily, demographic characteristics, among others.
- As phrased, the control group is inadequate because patients with routine discharges could be at higher or lower risk of readmission based on their discharge diagnosis. A better method would be to match patients based on various demographic and clinical characteristic (e.g., age, sex, comorbidities). Alternatively, a randomized control trial might be possible which would randomize STEMI patients to treatment or control at discharge. Secondary question: would IRB allow an RCT to be conducted?
- The binomial distribution should be used, because there is one mutually exclusive outcome and the study is analyzed retrospectively (i.e., although the study was conducted prospectively, the analysis assesses the overall occurrence of 30-day and 90-day readmissions retrospectively). You may think the Poisson distribution could be used, and this would have been correct if the study was interested in the number (or rate) of readmissions within 30 or 90 days.
- An odds ratio is the most appropriate epidemiological statistic as this is essentially a case-control study. If an RCT was conducted, a (relative) risk ratio would be appropriate.

CASE STUDY 6–2

- This is a crossover design because the patients were randomized to one clopidogrel dose and after a washout period receive the other clopidogrel dose.
- The length of the washout period is approximately 2 weeks (14 days).
- Statistical power of 90% indicates that there is a 90% probability of detecting a 15% difference in impedance change, given that it actually exists.
- No. The stated hypothesis speaks to detecting a difference in impedance change, but not a direction of that difference. As such, a two-tailed hypothesis test is more appropriate. Further, the one-tailed test will have a higher Type I error rate.
- This is called an interim analysis.
- Several limitations must be considered. First, there will be bias in impedance change difference as it will likely be either under- or over-estimated. Second, given that only 75% of the required sample size was enrolled, the study is underpowered, which will result in either inflated Type I or Type II error rates.
- Small p values (no matter how small) provide absolutely no information about the size of the difference or whether the difference is clinically meaningful. Further, small p values do not provide any information about how likely the results are to replicate. In isolation, a p value is not enough to stop a clinical trial (or any study for that matter). Aside from p values, the researcher should present the mean difference, an estimate of effect size for the difference (e.g., Cohen's d), and a 95% confidence interval around the size of the difference.

CASE STUDY 6–3

- The DV is achievement of therapeutic INR. The scale of measurement is not explicitly stated but it is presumed that it is nominal, binary, or dichotomous.
- The IV for this study is whether the patient was pharmacist or physician managed. This IV has two levels.

- The chi-square test would answer whether there is a difference in the rate of achieving therapeutic INR between patients who were pharmacist-managed vs. physician-managed.
- Logistic regression would answer whether there is a difference in the odds of achieving therapeutic INR between patients who were pharmacist-managed vs. physician-managed.
- The Kaplan-Meier method would answer whether there is a difference in the time-to-achieve therapeutic INR between patients who were pharmacist-managed vs. physician-managed. We would need to know the number of days required to achieve therapeutic INR as well as whether the time metric should be censored or not. Censoring could be at a chosen inpatient day (e.g., day 5) and/or at discharge.
- The Cox proportional-hazards model would answer whether there is a difference in the risk of achieving therapeutic INR between patients who were pharmacist-managed vs. physician-managed. Similar to the Kaplan-Meier method, we would need to know the number of days required to achieve therapeutic INR as well as whether the time metric should be censored or not. Censoring could be at a chosen inpatient day (e.g., day 5) and/or at discharge.
- This could happen because the chi-square test and Cox proportional-hazards model answer two different questions. It could be that by inpatient day 5, the rates of achieving therapeutic INR are similar in both the pharmacist-managed and physician-managed groups, but that patients in the pharmacist-managed group tend to achieve therapeutic INR more quickly than patients in the physician-managed group (e.g., median time to therapeutic INR could be 2 days for the pharmacist-managed group vs. 4 days for the physician-managed group). This highlights the importance of understanding the types of research questions answered by any given statistical test.

Chapter 8

CASE STUDY 8-1

Establish transparency. The Institute of Medicine (IOM) proposed eight standards for the evaluation of the transparency of guideline development (see Table 8-1). You can use these standards to see if the details and guideline development steps are easily replicated or followed. You should evaluate whether limitations to the guidelines exist (e.g., validity, conflicts of interest, bias).

Consider whether the specific disease conditions for which the clinical practice guidelines are evaluated possess the maximum potential for benefit from the implementation of a clinical practice guideline. Do the conditions have a high prevalence, frequency, or severity? Is there evidence available to support a reduction in morbidity and mortality? Is it feasible and cost-effective to implement? Is there proof of nonoptimal practices or practice variations? Are personnel, expertise, and resources available to implement the practice guidelines?

Management of conflicts of interest. Before selecting the clinical practice guidelines, think about how the guideline panels managed conflicts of interest. Determine whether the individuals considered for membership on each panel are asked to declare in writing all potential conflicts of interest. These conflicts of interest not only may have included financial conflicts, but also possibly intellectual conflicts, institutional conflicts, and patient-public activities.

How the multidisciplinary guideline development group was established. Determine if the guideline development group was multidisciplinary. Look to see if patients were involved, since patient involvement is critical in the formulation and prioritization of questions addressed by the guidelines. Additionally, look to see if a member of the panel had expertise in the content area.

Consider if a systematic search for evidence was conducted. As a health care practitioner, recognize that conducting a systemic review of the available literature is essential. Recognize that before the development of a clinical practice guideline, the clinical questions to be addressed are stated. Consider if the study selection criteria were determined before any systematic search was conducted. See if the clinical practice guideline describes how studies were appraised and the body of evidence was synthesized.

Consider how studies were selected. This evaluation includes types of published or unpublished research that were considered. Look to see if the panel included evidence from previous guidelines, meta-analyses, systematic reviews, randomized controlled trials, observational studies, diagnostic studies, economic studies, and qualitative studies.

Evaluate if specialized database searches were performed. Furthermore, determine whether available bibliographic resources were used. Citations listed in published bibliographies, textbooks, and identified literature should have been reviewed in the identification of evidence not produced from database searches. Remember that search terms should be easily identifiable from clinical questions addressed by the clinical practice guideline.

The guideline development panels should have appraised individual studies in efforts to identify issues that exist in studies for potential inclusion, such as with trial design or potential biases that would affect internal or external validity. Consider whether details of trial design, sample size, statistical power, selection bias, inclusion/exclusion criteria, choice of a control group, randomization methods, comparability of groups, definition of exposure or intervention, definition of outcome measures, accuracy and appropriateness of outcome measures, attrition rates, data collection methods, methods of statistical analysis confounding variables, unique study population characteristics, and adequacy of blinding were provided.

Consider how the information was summarized to develop conclusions. Look for clinical practice guidelines formatted to consider individual studies, consistency of results between studies, scope of evidence, and size of treatment effects.

CASE STUDY 8-2

In consideration of how the clinical questions addressed were defined, remember that a process or format of framing questions addressed by clinical practice guidelines is critical. Describe this to your health care system administrators and explain that guideline development groups use such formats as PICO to frame the clinical question of focus. The "P" stands for patients or problems considered. The "I" represents the treatment intervention to be considered and the "C" stands for comparison or alternatives compared to the intervention. The "O" stands for the outcome of focus and greatest importance to patients. Examples of outcomes of focus include mortality, morbidity, complications, physical function, quality of life, costs, and other outcomes.

CASE STUDY 8-3

The seven categories of guideline implementation barriers that limit or restrict complete prescriber adherence include lack of awareness, lack of familiarity, lack of agreement, lack of self-efficacy (disbelief that the guideline recommendations could be performed), lack of outcome expectancy (doubt that expected outcomes would occur), motivation to change current practice (inertia of current practice) and external barriers. External barriers include patient resistance, patient embarrassment, lack of reminder system, the cost to the patient, and lack of time.

CASE STUDY 8-4

Establishing plans for updating the guideline is essential. Recognize the importance of establishing plans for updating the guideline. In a review of a clinical practice guideline, explain that the publication date and dates of systematic reviews used should be clear. It is important to have a plan to update a guideline to identify new technology or evidence that may affect the guideline. A review interval to update a guideline should always be established. The duration of the interval is dependent upon the topic and existence of ongoing studies. A plan also should be made for expiring a guideline.

Chapter 9

CASE STUDY 9-1

Many practitioners find article discussions more interesting when they can relate the information to a previous or current patient care scenario. One method may be to solicit topics from staff to gather opinions for exciting topics. Another method may be to base the journal club on a recent notable clinical case within the service or health system to spark interest in the topic. Additionally, articles should be sent out in advance of the discussion so that participants have the opportunity to review and come prepared. If feasible, providing snacks or food has been shown to lead to increased participation. The preceptor may also consider changing the expectations of participants, the setting, or the format. For example, switching the setting to a more comfortable location, or changing the format to a discussion or debate format may make the activity more engaging for learners and staff.

CASE STUDY 9-2

Inviting a drug information specialist or another clinician with advanced training in this area can help address issues relating to study design and methodology. Including a content expert in the condition that is being studied can help provide greater clinical context and insight. If concerns still exist after a drug information specialist or content expert has weighed in, the pharmacist may consider promoting participants to write letters to the editor to express their concerns with the study methodology.

CASE STUDY 9-3

It is possible to host using the virtual journal club format. The pharmacist may choose a synchronous, asynchronous, or hybrid approach to best engage all interested parties. For example, synchronous sessions can be hosted and recorded for viewers to watch at a later date. Optionally, participants can also engage via an asynchronous platform, where participants post their critiques online via an online forum at their availability.

Chapter 10

CASE STUDY 10-1

- One of the best ways to acquire peer review skills is to work with a mentor who already participates in peer review. Because many of your colleagues fit this description, it is likely that one of them would be willing to help you as a mentor. There is no need to feel embarrassed about your lack of experience and understanding of the process. Just identify someone with similar areas of interest or expertise, or someone with whom you have a good relationship, and ask them. In the absence of a mentor, or while waiting for your chosen mentor to receive a peer review invitation, you can read review articles about peer review (see Suggested Readings) or locate and read the peer review instructions for a journal you follow.

- Assuming you have a mentor who already performs peer review for a journal you're interested in reviewing for, you can just ask the mentor to provide a referral. The journal may also have an online application that you can fill out to request consideration as a peer reviewer. Other options include sending an email request to the editor of the journal or visiting the journal's exhibitor booth at a professional conference.

CASE STUDY 10-2

- This situation represents a potential conflict of interest. Although you can often identify conflicts of interest from the abstract included in the invitation to review a manuscript, sometimes the conflict of interest is not apparent until you see the full manuscript. In this situation you should notify the editor about your potential conflict of interest as soon as possible, and the editor can help you identify the best course of action. Confidentiality is especially important in this case, since you and the author share a lot of mutual contacts. To protect confidentiality, the details of the manuscript should not be shared with other coworkers.

CASE STUDY 10-3

- The very first step is to read the invitation closely to determine the scope of the manuscript, the due date, and to look for any potential conflicts of interest. If the scope of the manuscript falls within your areas of expertise, you have sufficient time to meet the deadline, and you have no conflicts of interest, then go ahead and accept the invitation. If you identify any potential problems related to the scope, deadline, or conflicts of interest, you should either decline the invitation, or let the editor know about the potential problem and seek their advice on how to proceed. For instance, if the article is a good fit but your schedule will not allow you to complete the review until a few days after the deadline, the editor may be willing to extend the deadline by a few days.
- Before reading the manuscript, it is a good idea to review the journal's instructions for reviewers. Usually these instructions will be included in the invitation email or on the journal's website. It is also important to review the submission form for the peer review assignment to see if there are any specific questions or areas of focus that the journal is asking you to respond to. Once you have done those things, it is a good idea to give the manuscript a quick initial read to provide you with an overview of the article, help to identify any major flaws, and double-check for any conflicts of interest. A thorough review of a manuscript usually requires reading the manuscript two or three times. The second read of the manuscript will serve as a more detailed examination of the manuscript.

Chapter 11

CASE STUDY 11-1

- Factors that favor finding the pharmacist liable for negligence:
  - Pharmacist is a specialist (e.g., BCACP).
  - Anticoagulation pharmacist.
  - Reasonable pharmacist should know that an INR of 5.2 in a patient on warfarin places the patient at increased bleeding risk.

- ○ Reasonable pharmacist would question the use of the two medications together and document the same. For example, enoxaparin may be used for bridging anticoagulation when initiating warfarin but the INR of 5.2 would not indicate warfarin initiation.
- • No. While combining these two drugs may increase the risk of serious or life-threatening bleeding complications, enoxaparin and warfarin may be used together to treat acute deep vein thrombosis with or without pulmonary embolism. However, where the pharmacist possesses special knowledge of the patient's condition, there is a responsibility to the patient to clarify the order.
  - ○ If there is any protocol or guideline used at the clinic which was not followed.
  - ○ If there was no follow-up or documentation of the rationale for the combo.
- • Yes. The courts would hold a specialist to a higher standard. The fact that the pharmacist is the anticoagulation clinic pharmacist and is board certified places this individual into a higher liability category. If there was a collaborative practice agreement, it would be seen as a voluntary undertaking to provide expanded services to the physician and patient.
- • All three would be liable—the pharmacist, physician, and the clinic under the theory of *respondeat superior* for actions of employee.

CASE STUDY 11-2

- • The pharmacist fell below the standard of care. A health-system pharmacist has access to the patient's renal function tests. Dispensing metformin without checking renal function falls below the standard. Not following a pharmacy department policy which requires both checking and documenting the patient's creatinine clearance prior to dispensing metformin also falls below the standard of care.

  Looking at the elements of negligence: (1) duty was breached; (2) damages resulted; (3) the damages would seem to be directly caused by the breach of the duty; and (4) defenses to not checking the renal function or following the policy are absent.

CASE STUDY 11-3

- • Several activities occurring in this case violate the copyright law.
  - ○ Mere listing of all drugs which should not be crushed—derived from published references.
  - ○ Not classroom use.
  - ○ Permission must be obtained to use material that is paraphrased, abridged, or condensed. However, a new table created from data that is copyrighted sources would probably not require permission in this case. Copy work is informational.
  - ○ Unless the reference was government materials, permission must be obtained. In looking at Fair Use, a four-pronged test is used—the nature of work; the amount copied; commercial use; effect on market would all be considered.
  - ○ You take several direct sentences without providing a source reference. One of the references is out of print. One factor in copying infringement is the amount copied. Even though only several sentences were copied, there is no minimal amount or threshold quantity standard where fair use would be presumed.
  - ○ The fact that some of the material is out of print does not mean the material is in the public domain. Out of print does not necessarily mean out of copyright. The rights revert to the author, and the underlying copyright remains unaffected.

CASE STUDY 11-4

- • HIPAA prohibits:
  - ○ The pharmacist sharing PHI and diagnosis in an area where it was easily overheard by others.
  - ○ PHI faxed to a fax machine in an unsecured area where many people have access.
- • Safeguards:
  - ○ Private area for discussing patient information
  - ○ Fax machine should be in a private area

- Reasonable steps
  - ° Fax machine should be in a private and secure location
  - ° Reasonable steps may include programming, testing, and double-checking numbers; using a fax cover sheet with an erraneous transmission statement; and checking confirmations

Chapter 12

CASE STUDY 12-1

- Assessment of whether this drug information request constitutes a potential ethical dilemma:
  - ° What does it mean to you if confronting an ethical dilemma for such judgments of right or wrong to be ultimate/fundamental?
  - ° How do you interpret what it means for an ethical issue to be universal, in your own words?
  - ° Who are the various parties whose welfare could be impacted by the resolution to this situation, if indeed it does constitute an ethical dilemma?
- Background information to obtain to clarify this information request:
  - ° What are the facts of this case that you will want to learn more about before reaching a determination of whether it is indeed an ethical dilemma?
  - ° Considering who is affected is really a continuation of item #1.3 above defining an ethical dilemma. However, it may help you further to consider specific people involved in the case at hand—the study subject, the family members of the study subject, and the study team.
- Given that a specific patient's welfare must be addressed, this case certainly involves a micro level of ethical decision-making; however, as is often the case with ethical dilemmas, it might be argued that there are also meso level decision-making issues to be considered—What standards and policies does the organization have to address in informing study subjects of IGFs?
- Refer to the listing of Rules and Principles provided in the chapter—Which if any seem to have relevance to this case? For example, how do you think the principles of "Confidentiality" and "Privacy" impact this case?
- Remember that Rules often apply best to more narrow cases, and may be reasonably limited in some circumstances to meet the demands of more fundamental ethical principles. Decisions about competing principles will often rely on the decision maker's priorities relative to primacy of anticipated good/bad consequences of the action (For the individual only? How about for society?) versus for instance certain core beliefs about fundamental rights (e.g., deontological principle prioritizing "respect for persons").
- What kinds of standards, policies, or procedures might be useful to help the study team with ethical decision-making?

Refer to the article "Management and return of incidental genomic findings in clinical trials" by C Ayuso and associates for further information regarding IGF during clinical trials.[1]

CASE STUDY 12-2

- Assessment of whether this drug information request constitutes a potential ethical dilemma:
  - ° What does it mean to you if confronting an ethical dilemma for such judgments of right or wrong to be ultimate/fundamental?
  - ° How do you interpret what it means for an ethical issue to be universal, in your own words?
  - ° Who are the various parties whose welfare could be impacted by the resolution to this situation, if indeed it does constitute an ethical dilemma?

- Background information to obtain to clarify this information request:
  - ° What are the facts of this case that you will want to learn more about before reaching a determination of whether it is indeed an ethical dilemma? (For example: What is the clinical condition of the patient in question? and, What standards or patient care commitments has your institution established for addressing patient pain issues?)
  - ° Considering who is affected is really a continuation of item #1.3 above defining an ethical dilemma. However, it may help you further to consider specific people involved in the case at hand—the patient himself; the supervising physician; the various other staff and trainees who must try to meet this patient's needs under the circumstances at hand, and may learn to address future patients' needs based on their experience; family members of the patient who will observe their loved ones' suffering; the future patients who will be treated in similar or different ways based on the accumulating experience from this case.
  - ° What cultural perspectives might be at work for the prescribing physician (imagine, for instance, an older practitioner or one who is trained in a particular perspective relative to standards of pain control)? Likewise, what is the culture in the case environment relative to lines of authority, or freedom to question authority, or approaches to patient rights?
- Given that a specific patient's welfare must be addressed, this case certainly involves a micro level of ethical decision-making; however, as is often the case with ethical dilemmas, it might be argued that there are also meso level decision-making issues to be considered—What standards is the organization held to in meeting the pain control needs of its patients? What policies are established within the organization regarding supervision/accountability of practitioners charged with patient care relative to specified standards?
- Refer to the listing of Rules and Principles provided in the chapter—Which, if any, seem to have relevance to this case?
- Remember that Rules often apply best to more narrow cases, and may be reasonably limited in some circumstances to meet the demands of more fundamental ethical principles. Decisions about competing principles will often rely on the decision maker's priorities relative to primacy of anticipated good/bad consequences of the action (For the individual only? How about for society?) versus, for instance, certain core beliefs about fundamental rights (e.g., deontological principle prioritizing "respect for persons").
- What kinds of standards, policies, or procedures might be useful to this nurse specialist, both to aid in her ethical decision-making and to provide support in her dealings with the prescriber and other involved staff as well as the patient/family?

Refer to the article "Ethical dilemmas: controversies in pain management" by Janet Brown to read the analysis of a similar case.[2]

REFERENCES

1. Ayuso C, Millan JM, Dal-Re R. Management and return of incidental genomic findings in clinical trials. Pharmacogenomics J. 2015;15:1-5.
2. Brown J. Ethical dilemmas: controversies in pain management. Adv Nurse Pract. 1997:69-72.

CASE STUDY 12-3

- First recognize and understand the meaning of these characteristics as they apply to this specific case. However, final determination of whether they apply will require the reader to first address other steps of analysis below.
- There are a number of important factual questions that Dr. Blake is honor bound to address before deciding on any ethical dimensions of this case:
  - ° Examples: What is the drug in question? How available is it, other than relative to cost?
  - ° What is the level of evidence supporting or refuting the agent's efficacy and safety when used for the requested purpose?

     - At a macro level of decision making, cost-effectiveness is often deemed another appropriate factor to consider in recommendations for use at a population level.

     - However, the pharmacy and therapeutics committee will need to assess the safety and efficacy of the medication in question.

    ° How do the formulary management policies instruct the pharmacy and therapeutics committee regarding making formulary considerations?

    ° What kind of checks and balances are there in the institution regarding conflicts of interests? What kind of recusal of decision-making policies is in place to prevent situations like the one described in this case?

- Certainly, the professional must address this dilemma at a meso level. His/her decision making may be improved if s/he also thinks about what his responsibility is to the individual patients who will undoubtedly be impacted by the decision, as well as overall macro (system or societal) level consequences of policies established by this and similar organizations.

- How do you think the principles of "Veracity" or "Fidelity" might apply to this case? How do you think Justice Theory might speak in favor of or in opposition to restrictions?

- Please imagine a specific product and case in order to personally determine how you would prioritize the various pertinent rules and principles in order to decide in such a case as this. Do you think that you would be justified in simply acting on the orders from your job supervisor, regardless of the factual circumstances and possible ethical issues of the case?

- Organizational strategies that might best prepare this pharmacist to most effectively respond to ethical dilemmas:

    ° What organization policies or standards do you think should be established in health care systems to support ethical decision-making pertinent to cases such as this one?

    ° Do you think there are laws or regulations that should be in place at the governmental level to guide health care systems in providing ethical service to their patients? If so, what measures do you think could be useful?

CASE STUDY 12–4

- First recognize and understand the meaning of these characteristics as they apply to this specific case. However, final determination of whether they apply will require the reader to first address other steps of analysis below.

- There are a number of important factual questions that the physician is honor bound to address before deciding on any ethical dimensions of this case:

    ° Examples: What is the compounded product in question? What data other than anecdotal are there to support the use of this compounded product?

    ° What is the level of evidence supporting or refuting the efficacy and safety of the compounded product when used for the requested purpose?

     - At a macro level of decision making, cost-effectiveness is often deemed another appropriate factor to consider in recommendations for use at a population level.

     - Ultimately, the use of the compounded product would be the decision of the pharmacy and therapeutics committee. This committee will assess the safety and efficacy of the medication in question. However, if new legislation is approved by the state then it may not be relevant what the committee decides.

- The health care professionals must address this dilemma at a meso level initially. Their decision making may be improved if they also think about their responsibility to the individual patients who will undoubtedly be impacted by the decision. Another aspect of this case is the macro level (system or societal) consequences of policies should the state legislature change pharmacy law.

- How do you think the principles of "Consent" and "Veracity" might apply to this case? How do you think Justice Theory might speak in favor of or in opposition to restrictions?

- Please imagine a specific product and case in order to personally decide how you would prioritize the various pertinent rules and principles in order to decide in such a case as this.

- Organizational strategies that might best prepare this pharmacist to most effectively respond to ethical dilemmas:

- ° What organization policies or standards do you think should be established in health care systems to support ethical decision-making pertinent to cases such as this one?
- ° Do you think there are laws or regulations that should be in place at the governmental level to guide health care systems in providing ethical service to their patients? If so, what measures do you think could be useful?

Chapter 13

CASE STUDY 13-1

- Since the topic is known, it is possible to skip the first step listed in this chapter. You will need to find out if anyone else is to work with you (e.g., perhaps someone very involved with the use of that product) and get that person involved, if only as a reviewer. Also, it is known where it will be published—in the policy and procedure section of the institutional intranet. So, the next thing to do is review the institution's standard format of policies and procedures, to determine what needs to be written. As a part of this, determine that it needs to be written in the middle technical style, since it is being aimed at a variety of health care practitioners. Then, it is necessary to do research into the topic.
- First, organize the material. This can be done in conjunction with preparation of an outline of the order in which the material needs to be covered. That outline can be done on a word processor and serve as the template for the document. In many cases, the way the institution lays out its policy and procedure documents can serve as a good part of the outline. Perhaps even a preexisting template can be used as the outline. Then proceed to write the policy and procedures. At this stage, simply make sure everything necessary is recorded in the document. The document can be written in order of the topics, or each individual section may be written separately, in whatever order is easiest. Also, remember to cite material as the document is written, preferably using the endnote feature in the word processor (some institutions may also have other programs available to help in this). Besides being appropriate to give credit, it is also useful for the future when someone may have to come back to revise the document after several years and may not otherwise be able to tell the origin of some of the information.
- Some would say to just present it to the pharmacy and therapeutics committee, but there are a couple of things that need to be done first. To start, the author should reread and edit the document. Then, get others who have expertise in the area to read and edit the document. These others should include one or more representatives from each group affected by the document (e.g., pharmacist, physician, nurse). An effort must be made to make sure the document is in a logical order, covers all aspects of the topic, and is understandable. Then incorporate any necessary revisions. This process may need to be done several times (e.g., some chapters in this book went through a dozen versions before being submitted to the publisher). Sometimes, there will even be a meeting of key members of a committee to look over things briefly prior to an official committee meeting in order to make sure everything is appropriately addressed.

CASE STUDY 13-2

First, clarify who the website is addressing—the audience. It will be different for patients versus other health care practitioners. Sometimes it will be both groups. Then, in relationship to the above, determine what information or features need to be on the website. It may simply be a reference site, but also may provide much more information and communication. There may need to be certain functions built in to provide specific services. Then determine what equipment (e.g., computer hardware and software) and budget are available to prepare the website. It will also be necessary to learn the software. At that point, it would be necessary to go into specific functions and information that would be available on the website and how it is to be organized. After that, it is possible to start working on the website itself.

CASE STUDY 13-3

First, be sure to prepare slides on something that is compatible with the software used at the meeting. Then determine what information needs to be on the slides. Generally, assume that each slide should be shown for a minute or two. Keep each slide simple, with a maximum of five bullet points and five words per bullet point, so that attendees can concentrate on the message and read it from the back of the room. Also, remember that the speaker is not to read directly from the slides, but use them just as a jumping-off spot for the presentation and to organize thoughts and to engage the audience. In addition, be sure to make them look attractive and professional. Graphics may help, if they do not make the slide too busy and if they can be used without copyright infringement.

Chapter 14

CASE STUDY 14-1

- Is this a real recall? If so, why is there a recall? Does the FDA or the company have any specific instructions for patients? What will be the key message in trying to balance not scaring patients unnecessarily, but providing good information?

CASE STUDY 14-2

- Is this something you feel you can speak to? If so, first talk to your public relations department before responding to get permission if needed and to help develop your key messages. When you frame your key messages, make sure to think about not only the general facts, but also how a patient might react.

CASE STUDY 14-3

- Think about how your hospital is currently managing the situation as this type of story could be perceived as negative for the organization. Craft key messages about how your organization is doing extra work to keep patients safe despite the shortage.

Chapter 15

CASE STUDY 15-1

- Determining if the medication is on formulary or in the review queue is important.
- If the medication has not been reviewed, provide guidance on how the provider may request a nonformulary case evaluation. If the medication is also needed for formulary addition, provide guidance on how the provider may request a full formulary evaluation.
- Depending on the patient needs for this new medication (FDA indicated for anemia due to beta thalassemia), this medication may need full formulary evaluation. Being a new agent approved by the FDA

(approved less than 1 month before the question was posed), determining when to evaluate will be based on patient need and process support. Prioritizing P&T functions is important for the secretary.

CASE STUDY 15–2

- The P&T committee should consider indication coverage and dosing comparisons between the biosimilar(s) and their reference product. Clinical efficacy, including analytical, animal, clinical, and FDA clinical review studies, should be assessed. A safety analysis of adverse effects, drug interactions, and black box warnings also needs to be included. Of importance is the reimbursement and payor analysis. Reviewing the main payors covering patients at the institution and how they cover the biosimilar(s) and reimbursement calculations from Medicare ASP pricing is imperative.
- The P&T committee may choose to keep the reference product on formulary due to payor coverage and add the other biosimilar(s) based on payor analysis and indication coverage. Some institutions may choose to convert over to one product. If this is a recommendation, indication and dosing coverage as well as payor coverage need to be confirmed. In the event the reference product has an orphan indication, the biosimilars will not cover that indication. Determining how payors will address that indication is important to investigate.
- Education flyers, therapeutic interchange tables in the online formulary, newsletters, electronic implementation in the online ordering system, and transparent communication between informatics, pharmacy operations, pharmacy distributor conversations, and contracting.

CASE STUDY 15–3

- The restriction can be built into the electronic ordering system and added to the online formulary with links to the guideline describing the restriction on the hospital Internet page. All providers have access to this and are guided during prescribing on the restriction.
- The minutes at the anti-infective or antimicrobial medication subcommittee and P&T committee should reflect the discussion and approval of the restriction.
- Information can be shared in a monthly newsletter to providers, included in the medication executive committee report, and shared at the next month's meeting during the review of the minutes.

CASE STUDY 15–4

- Review the ASHP and FDA shortage database, check with the hospital wholesaler on shortage information, and review availability of stock in the hospital.
- Develop a recommendation. Since the hospital has a therapeutic interchange between IV esomeprazole and IV pantoprazole, during the shortage the hospital could use esomeprazole IV.
- The recommendation is reviewed with the P&T committee chair and pharmacy director. A memorandum is drafted and provided to staff to indicate the practice change until the shortage is lifted.

Chapter 16

CASE STUDY 16–1

- Steps to add this drug to the formulary:
  - ○ Review nonformulary utilization and indications for use.
  - ○ Review utilization of similar agents in the therapeutic class (if applicable) that are on the formulary.

- ° Seek input from the appropriate specialists who would have knowledge of the product or recommendations for formulary status.
- ° Review available literature to evaluate clinical evidence.
- ° Consider discussions with pharmacists at other hospitals.
- ° Determine financial implications of product addition by reviewing cost information with purchasing agent and contract information from wholesaler and manufacturer.
- ° Prepare a drug monograph.
- Essential elements of a medication monograph:
  - ° Generic name (Trade name)
  - ° Approval rating
  - ° Therapeutic class
  - ° Sound/Look-alike
  - ° Indications/Place in therapy
  - ° Pharmacogenomics
  - ° Adverse effects
  - ° Drug interactions
  - ° Recommended monitoring
  - ° Dosing
  - ° Product dosage form, availability, and storage
  - ° Efficacy analysis (i.e., clinical trial evaluation)
  - ° Drug safety/REMS
  - ° Comparative pricing information/pharmacoeconomic analysis
  - ° Operational considerations, including pharmacoinformatic and legal considerations
  - ° Formulary implications/Conclusion/Recommendation
  - ° References
- Sources of information to develop a complete, evidence-based, medication monograph:
  - ° Current published clinical studies and abstracts
  - ° Nonpublished data or data awaiting publication (contact manufacturer)
  - ° Current package labeling
  - ° Obtaining a formulary kit from the manufacturer may be helpful for double checking information, but this should not be the primary reference source for your monograph
  - ° Check current evidence-based clinical guidelines

CASE STUDY 16–2

- Each of the following would be necessary, with comparison to other similar products. Essentially, it will be a quick comparison of the major similarities and differences, which can be fit on a single page.
  - ° Generic name and trade name
  - ° Indications/Therapeutic use/Pharmacogenomics
  - ° Clinical pharmacology
  - ° Pharmacokinetics
  - ° Adverse reactions
  - ° Drug interactions
  - ° Dosing
  - ° Product availability and storage
  - ° Drug safety/REMS
  - ° Evidence-based clinical guidelines
  - ° Recommendation
- The following information should be included:
  - ° All of the previous mentioned items
  - ° Defined tier status for copayments
  - ° Restrictions—such as prior approvals
  - ° REMS
  - ° Outpatient medication acquisition cost and if covered by Medicare or other key local pharmacy benefits management organizations

- Different types of formulary status recommendations:
  ° Added for uncontrolled use by the entire medical staff.
  ° Added for monitored use—No restrictions placed on use, but the drug will be monitored via a quality assurance study (e.g., drug use evaluation and medication use evaluation) to determine appropriateness of use. This is a tie-in to the institution's quality assurance/drug use evaluation process. Please note: this category does not mean that the patient is monitored, since that is necessary for every drug. It means that the quality and appropriateness of how the drug is used is monitored.
  ° Added with restrictions—The drug is added to the drug formulary, but there are restrictions on who may prescribe it and/or how it may be used (e.g., specific indications, certain physicians or physician groups, and certain policies to be followed).
  ° Conditional—Available for use by the entire medical staff for a finite period of time.
  ° Not added/deleted from formulary—The product can be ordered as a nonformulary product, but will not be routinely stocked in the pharmacy. Nonformulary products may take up to 24 hours or longer to obtain.
  ° Therapeutic interchange with a preferred agent for the organization's formulary.

CASE STUDY 16-3

- The financial components of this medication in a complex health system with different medication pricing can best be calculated with a spreadsheet program and one method of calculating this is summarized in the below table:

	Vial Cost	Cost per Patient	Medicare Payment	Patient Charge	Private Insurance Payment	Medicare Margin	Private Insurance Margin	Blended Margin
GPO Price	$10,000	$30,000	$28,500	$60,000	$31,800	$1,500	$1,800	$150
340b Price	$9,000	$27,000	$28,500	$60,000	$31,800	$1,500	$4,800	$3,150

	Patients	Doses	Total Spend	Total Charges	Total Margin
GPO Price	63	28	$52,920,000	$105,840,000	$264,600
340b Price	7	28	$5,292,000	$11,760,000	$617,400
Total	70		$58,212,000	$117,600,000	$882,000

The cost impact of adding this medication to formulary, given the high cost of the medication, the number of patients predicted to need the medication, and the number of doses they would receive, is significant. This medication has the potential to add up to $58,212,000 of total drug expenses to the health system.
- Reimbursement varies significantly between Medicare and private insurers. For this medication, the health system will on average lose $1500 per Medicare patient at hospital buying the drug at GPO pricing and will make $1500 on Medicare patients at 340b pricing. For private insurances, hospital with GPO pricing will make $1800 and hospitals with 340b pricing will make $3150 in margin. The total impact of adding this medication could be up to a positive net margin of $882,000.

- Medication pricing is dynamic. Medicare reimbursement changes quarterly for medications and there is a trend toward payment reform and even bundled pricing which may change the way pharmacies are reimbursed for medications.

Hospitals that evaluate the price of a medication and note that reimbursement is less than cost, resulting in a net loss for the medication, must evaluate their medication pricing and evaluate contracting opportunities to lower the acquisition cost of the drug.

CASE STUDY 16–4

- The P&T committee should consider indication coverage and dosing comparisons between the biosimilar(s) and their reference product. Clinical efficacy, including analytical, animal, clinical, and FDA clinical review studies, should be assessed. A safety analysis of adverse effects, drug interactions, and black box warnings also needs to be included. Of importance is the reimbursement and payor analysis. Reviewing the main payors covering patients at the institution and how they cover the biosimilar (s) and reimbursement calculations from Medicare ASP pricing is imperative.
- The hospital should set standards on payor coverage acceptance, if a biosimilar is not covered by Medicare and all major commercial payors.
- The cost analysis should include at least an annualized review of reference product purchasing compared to what that annualized use would be if using the biosimilar. This comparison helps to evaluate cost savings to the institution on a base level. Once this is evaluated, reimbursement using Medicare ASP or 106% of WAC can help understand how much is reimbursed to the hospital when using a biosimilar or reference product.

CASE STUDY 16–5

- Important items to consider for the monograph:
  - ° Safety, efficacy, data on effectiveness or ineffectiveness, amount of waste that would be permitted
  - ° Creation of an operational procedure and record keeping
  - ° Collaboration with Finance to ensure ordering the medication is feasible and confirming reimbursement
- Implementation of medication:
  - ° Using a set procedure
  - ° Working with informatics to build the medication into the order entry system and ensuring the cost can be included (some systems cannot accept a charge at such a high cost)
  - ° Confirming insurance coverage
- Monitoring of medication:
  - ° Real-time DUE
  - ° Review outcome with physician and patient to assess if medication should stay on formulary
  - ° Review procedure

CASE STUDY 16–6

- Tools available to stay organized:
  - ° Project management software
  - ° Documentation forms
  - ° Annual accomplishment summary for P&T committee
- Prioritization of medication reviews:
  - ° Transparent communication to identify the need for patients, whether emergent or not, helps to prioritize the work.

- Ways to remain efficient:
  - ° Utilize layered learning to complete monographs.
  - ° Stay organized.
  - ° Provide clear communication on accomplishments, open projects, and goals.
    Set clear goals at the beginning of the year, each quarter, and each month to strategize and prioritize most important monographs.

Chapter 17

CASE STUDY 17-1

- Check both the ASHP and FDA drug shortage websites. Also check with the purchasing agents at your organization.

CASE STUDY 17-2

- Determine the clinical impact of the shortage—this is a potentially lifesaving drug and for some infections, there may not be clear alternatives. Contact the Infectious Diseases clinicians or the antimicrobial committee within the institution to get their management suggestions. Potential actions could include restricting the product for approval from Infectious Diseases or contacting the ethics committee and pharmacy and therapeutics committee to determine and approve a rationing strategy.

CASE STUDY 17-3

- Both substitutes pose patient-safety risks, but the most concerning is the dopamine substitution. Using a four times lower strength product will affect smart pumps and may not be appropriate for patients who are fluid-restricted. Without changes to the ordering system and smart pump libraries, patients could be given subtherapeutic doses of the medication. The heparin vials also pose potential risks. The sterile production room will have to prepare bags of heparin during a shortage of premixed bags. This will pose operational challenges and may also affect IV workflow technology. Convene a team to work through the management challenges that both of these shortages pose.

Chapter 18

CASE STUDY 18-1

In evaluating the current process on communicating to patients about their medications, the committee found the communications about medications is identified as a task assigned to nursing staff at patient discharge. The requirements for patient discharge tasks are numerous for nursing staff and the patients in many cases receive only a very brief communication about medications. The steps the committee should take to assess the communications about medication process include:

- Review medical/surgical units/floors for their HCAHPS survey results (if available). Are there some units performing significantly better than others? If so, review the difference in process compared to the lower performing units/floors for reasons for the better performance.
- Identify the process steps for providing communications about medications and identify the time of day for providing the communications and the amount of time spent by staff providing the communication.
- Conduct a sampling of nursing staff and patient interactions for observing and documenting the communications about medications task.
- Identify resources in use to facilitate the communications about medications, such as online medication information websites, pamphlets, medication reconciliation on discharge form, patient portal, or other resources.
- Summarize the results by floor/unit and by time in the hospital stay or discharge time (morning, afternoon, evening, or other) and the amount of time devoted to the task.
- If differences exist, investigate what the better performers utilize and how they accomplish the communication about medications and determine what solutions are applicable for the hospital to improve house-wide.

CASE STUDY 18–2

Enhanced MTM services can decrease medical expenses, including hospital admissions, emergency room visits, and medication nonadherence. Based on the results of the initial performance year of the enhanced MTM pilot, pharmacist will conduct targeted and comprehensive medication reviews for select patients with several targeted medication-related problems.

Policy and procedure for the enhanced MTM program:

- Identify the patients for review from the Medicare Part D Plan list of the patients receiving medications from your pharmacies and meeting criteria for MTM services.
- Flag the identified patients in your pharmacy information system and document in your pharmacy care plan software as enhanced MTM services.
- Identify any patients requiring the CMR and any medication-related problems with a focus on medication adherence for **targeted medication review (TMR)**.
- Contact the patients to inform them of the free service, one that will potentially save them from future medical expenses and visits; schedule an appointment within the month.
- Meet with the patient to provide either the CMR or the TMR.
- Provide the patient their medication record, their medication-related action plan, communicate with prescribers as necessary, document in the pharmacy care plan utilizing approved standardized coding.
- Follow up as necessary depending on the specific medication-related problem (medication adherence, high-risk medications, additional medications required, drug interactions, duplicate, unnecessary medications, nonachievement of therapeutic goals, other), and determine patient outcomes of utilization of medical services and any medication-related harm. Reassess with TMR to problem resolution or change in status. Document findings in the pharmacy care plan.
- Repeat the process each month.

CASE STUDY 18–3

Steps to assess medication reconciliation:

- Identify an appropriate sampling strategy to review medication reconciliation at admission.
- Include necessary demographic data elements to collect for each patient record reviewed (gender, age groups, race/ethnicity, preferred language, payor, other).

- Develop a data dictionary specifying each data element and where to locate the information in the patient record so each reviewer will obtain consistent results.
- Conduct the review by nursing staff and the consultant pharmacist.
- Summarize the results in aggregate and by demographic subgroup. If differences are found, investigate possible causes.

CASE STUDY 18-4

Specific items to review include:
- Prescriptions include the indication for use, acute or chronic pain—100% threshold.
- Opioid days' supply is limited to 7 days for initial opioid prescription (exceptions oncology, hospice)—100% threshold.
- Opioid dose as determined by calculating the morphine milligram equivalent (MME)—100% threshold:
  ° ≥ 50 MME patient is counseled on risk, especially identifying other sedating medications and clinical conditions; documentation in the patient care plan (EHRs and pharmacy information system care plan).
  ° ≥ 90 MME must receive prior authorization or approval.
- Concomitant benzodiazepines or other central nervous system sedating medications are identified by the prescriber, pharmacist, and to the patient with risk of harm documented in electronic health records (EHRs) and pharmacy information system care plan—100% threshold.
- Prescribers and dispensers must review the state prescription drug monitoring program (PDMP) prior to the initial prescription and every 90 days for continued prescriptions—100% threshold.

CASE STUDY 18-5

Possible responses include:
- Physicians (surgeons, medicine/family medicine, infectious disease specialists)
- Nurses from the perioperative areas, inpatient units, and home care areas
- Pharmacists
- Discharge planners/case managers who help to plan for discharge and arrange home care

CASE STUDY 18-6

Reponses include:
- Develop policies and protocols for use of anticoagulants based on evidence-based medical literature, to include appropriate selection.
- Diagnosis and indication for use.
- Age and weight considerations, including any changes.
- Dosing appropriate for age, weight, and renal and hepatic function.
- Identify drug-drug interactions, drug-food interactions.
- Identify additional disease states or factors.
- Identify appropriate monitoring parameters and duration of therapy.
- Baseline monitoring.
- Follow-up periodicity, monthly INR for warfarin and/or as clinical conditions change or steady state and for different DOACs for changes in renal function changes every 6 months and hepatic function every 6–12 months and/or if indicated specific Anti-Factor Xa (anti-Xa) assays.
- Identify assessment of overdose and emergent requirements for reversal agents and specifying dosing for which agent is applicable for each anticoagulant.
- Identify perioperative or procedural management (http://mappp.ipro.org/ and https://www.acc.org/tools-and-practice-support/mobile-resources/features/manageanticoag).
- Educate patients and inquire at each encounter to assess adherence, changes in use, drug-disease state changes, and adverse events.

- Document and report ADEs to the appropriate reporting system; in-house, FDA MedWatch, state reporting systems as applicable.
- Utilize electronic health records systems and clinical decision support for appropriate ordering and monitoring of anticoagulants when possible.

Chapter 19

CASE STUDY 19-1

- There was a dechallenge in this case.
- Yes. The patient's exposure to the drug precedes the suspected ADR.
- Yes, the patient's symptoms are consistent with the known pharmacology of *Keto-gone*. The product contains raspberry ketones, which have stimulant effects.
- Using clinical judgment, you can determine that the product is likely responsible for the side effects described. This is supported by the fact that the symptoms occurred after ingestion of the product and that the symptoms are consistent with the known pharmacology of the ingredients contained in the product. You could also complete one of the algorithms discussed above in order to assess the likelihood that this reaction was caused by *Keto-gone*.

CASE STUDY 19-2

- There are several options for reporting the reaction to the FDA. You can report this ADR to the FDA through the Department of Health and Human Services' online Safety Reporting Portal. Because this ADR involved a nonprescription natural supplement product, you also have the option of reporting the reaction through a third-party system like Natural MedWatch, or directly to the product's manufacturer or distributor. These entities will forward your ADR report to the FDA. Your patient can report the ADR through the Department of Health and Human Services' online Safety Reporting Portal.

CASE STUDY 19-3

- There are several options for reporting this suspected medical device event to the FDA such as MedWatch, Medical Device Reporting (MDR) page, or directly to the manufacturer.
- Since this is a suspected medical device-related event, MAUDE would be the appropriate database to search for similar reports involving medical devices.

Chapter 20

CASE STUDY 20-1

This is a much debated topic. While eliminating errors seems like our goal, it is important to understand and remember that it is not possible to eliminate all human errors. Humans err many times per day and fortunately, most of the time there is no consequence. Forgetting to attach an attachment to an email or putting the milk in the pantry is embarrassing, but not life-threatening. Understanding human error concepts is important in developing systems and barriers that will prevent a human error from reaching a patient. These barriers may include technology checking systems, pharmacist review of medications prior to administration, double-check, focusing techniques, checklists, or time outs. The goal is to work to reduce and eliminate events of harm by instituting reliable barriers to errors, building in layers designed to catch these errors, improving monitoring strategies such that an error can be detected rapidly, all of which are meant to reduce the potential harm to a patient. Quality improvement work should focus on knowing how humans commonly err in a process in order to develop both prevention and identification strategies. Defining and avoiding preventable harm may provide the most clarity and feel to be an achievable goal.

- Questions to ask the individual involved in the error:
  - It is important to ask staff to provide a description of the situation as they remember it, without leading questions. It is also very important to interview staff early to prevent unintentional alterations to the story based on fading memory or hearing other discussions related to the event.
  - Ask the pharmacist to describe what happened and what they remember.
- Type of error:
  - It depends on the information that is gathered during interviews and observation of the usual process. The system did not alert the physician nor pharmacist of the increased dose that was being ordered, which is a system opportunity. It is a human error, in that it was not an intentional action and the system set up the physician and pharmacist to potentially fail. It is considered a combination of both human error and system contributing cause.

CASE STUDY 20-2

- Error type is wrong rate and harm score is category E as the error caused temporary patient harm.
- An RCA was carried out by the medication safety pharmacist to investigate underlying system factors that contributed to the error.
- Latent failures included pharmacy laptop equipment failure, lack of preprogrammed CPOE order, and lack of smart infusion pump technology. Active failures included physician typing "12" instead of "120" and pharmacist not scrolling down to view the infusion rate on the order.
- Create preprogrammed CPOE order forms so physicians do not have to manually type in rates or doses; create a downtime plan for malfunctioning pharmacy computer equipment so staff do not have to use their own laptops; implement smart pump infusion technology with preprogrammed rate limits.

CASE STUDY 20-3

- System issues that contributed to the error:
  - Drug label displayed the concentration more prominently than the total drug in the bag, which does not conform to USP <7> drug label design principles. The infusion pump requires programming the total drug amount in the bag. Poor label design set the nurse up to program the pump incorrectly.
  - Lack of preset concentrations and hard limits in the infusion pump. Smart pump drug libraries with preset concentrations for each drug prevent manual nurse entry. If manual entry cannot be avoided, hard limits are more effective than soft limits to catch and correct programming errors.
- Just Culture application:
  - Were the actions as intended? Did the nurse intentionally program the pump incorrectly? No.
  - Was the person under the influence of unauthorized substances? No.

○ Did he or she knowingly violate a safe operating procedure? There was not a required double-check, and pump programming was taught to all staff upon institution of the new pumps. She did override a warning. Upon further inquiry, she asked her charge nurse about the situation, who recommended she override the warning. She did not make a conscious choice to skip steps within the process or subvert the process.

○ Do they pass the substitution test described above? When this was discussed with several other nurses, two of the three noted that they had made a similar error and/or caught a similar error. Would others have made the same decisions and, if so, less likely to be culpable? If not, were there deficiencies in training or experience? The training must be carefully considered. Providing didactic information without practice or competency testing is not the most appropriate method of teaching staff. Adequate practice is needed to develop good habits and skill-based actions. What is the role of the charge nurse and her recommendation to continue despite the warning? Further inquiry should include asking if she reviewed the programming prior to her recommendation.

○ Does the individual have a history of unsafe acts? This is the first error of this type that has been identified for this nurse. If not, again less likely to be culpable.

• Identifying potential system fixes:

○ The label design should match the entry in the pump if at all possible. Rearranging or increasing the visibility of the required information for programming is another option.

○ Add preset concentrations and hard limits to smart pump drug library.

○ Consider use of independent double-check when programming high-alert drips and/or when encountering pump warnings before overriding.

CASE STUDY 20–4

• Identifying system or process issues:

○ The epidural medication was brought into the patient's room before there was an order, at the request of the anesthesiologists. They wanted to have everything ready when the patient and team decided it was time for the epidural. This increases the risk of inadvertent administration due to availability.

○ How was the bupivacaine dispensed? Why/how was the medication accessible to the nurse prior to there being an order?

○ The nurse had not placed an identification band on the patient which is required for use of the medication barcode scanning process. Part of this was because of the lack of immediate availability of labels in the patient's room or upon admission, requiring the nurse to go searching for the identification band. A contributing factor was found to be a prior tolerance of not using the barcode scanning on this unit.

○ The nurse did not use the barcode scanning technology to verify the medication prior to administration. This would have detected the error prior to administration to the patient if used correctly. This was partly due to the lack of patient identification band and a unit tolerance to inconsistent use of this technology. This unit experienced a difficult implementation with this process which was ineffective at times, leading nurses to skip the process.

○ The nurse picked up the wrong medication, did not closely read the label, and administered the incorrect medication. Contributing factors to this human error include the similar bag size and look of the two medications, a rushed nature, and a low suspicion of risk—never having experienced an error or problem in the treatment of a laboring mother in this manner. This nurse was fatigued due to her work schedule and distracted, both of which increase the risk of a human error.

• The two types of technology that could have helped prevent this error:

○ BCMA—barcode scanning prior to medication administration could have alerted the nurse that the bag in her hand was bupivacaine and not penicillin.

○ Profiled ADCs—ADCs that interface with CPOE systems to limit nurse access to only medications for which a patient has an active order and help ensure correct drug, dose, and time.

• Key elements to successful implementation of new technology include the need for processes to support: engagement and buy-in into the implementation requiring change management techniques, standardization of processes prior to implementation, effective education and training that is timed in proximity to implementation, technologic and emotional support at go-live, efficient methods of feedback about problems with closed-loop communication back to the reporting individual, and development and adaptation of optimization process post-go-live for continued improvement. There are likely many others that can be identified but these are key processes.

- In a world of competing priorities, it is important to set expectations and standard work for key processes. Perhaps as important is how organizations monitor for compliance and opportunities to improve standard work, to be followed by accountability actions. Throughput and financial pressures may be perceived as more important than safety. If someone has a concern that needs to be raised and it is perceived that working toward a resolution is too time-consuming or is met with resistance by others, this important clarifying action may not occur. Supporting and providing positive feedback for prioritizing these behaviors is one strategy to build the culture of "Safety First." All professionals should be included and mentored in these expectations. It is critical that a "stop-the-line" process be supported by administrative and physician leadership to avoid significant events.

- Confirmation bias is a phenomenon in which humans are programmed into patterns of recognition, which may lead to inappropriate assumptions based on those patterns. One example is color-coding. This can be an effective technique for recognition purposes; however, there is no guarantee that there is only one "pink-capped drug." For example, if furosemide injectable was always in the pink cap and a generic heparin manufacturer starts to utilize a pink cap, human behavior may lead to a tragic error. Bar code scanning is designed to prevent these types of assumptions. However, assuring that the technology functions reliably and the culture supports the technology to include accountability measures are appropriate are critical to the use of the scanning process.

Chapter 21

CASE STUDY 21–1

- Steps used to approach this assignment:
  - Collect information on the background related to this formulary decision.
  - If unfamiliar with the role and development of an IV-to-PO conversion, engage in background readings to help understand this type of policy, including the strengths and limitations.
  - Determine what the standard format/template is for policies at the medical center.
  - Conduct a systematic search to determine comparative dosing, safety profiles, and cost considerations.
  - Review the information gathered in your search and consider this information in the context of the needs of the health system.
  - Solicit input from colleagues in similar institutions or professional organizations for sample policies.
  - Prepare a draft policy that is specific, succinct, and well referenced.
  - An IV-to-PO conversion should include specific guidance on how the IV product will be converted to the oral product(s) and should include all potential oral formulations and all usual prescribed regimens (i.e., drug, dose, route, frequency).
  - Convene a group of stakeholders and solicit input on the policy.
- A variety of resources can be used in this process. As discussed in Chapter 3 on Drug Information Resources, an appropriate search should begin with tertiary references and should progress to secondary resources and eventually to primary literature in this scenario. The safety and efficacy of the acetaminophen is well documented in the tertiary literature, and resources such as Micromedex®, AHFS® Drug Information, and textbooks (e.g., Pharmacotherapy Principles and Practice) are a good starting point for understanding a comparison of the formulations with respect to clinical efficacy, safety profile, and dosing and administration considerations, in addition to other parameters. Following a thorough search of the tertiary literature, it may be

appropriate to conduct a literature search in a secondary database (e.g., PubMed®) to identify primary literature that supports a conversion from the intravenous formulation to an oral formulation. Adequate clinical trials should be collected and evaluated to assess the appropriateness of an IV-to-PO conversion policy. Finally, cost should be obtained directly from the pharmacy department regarding institution-specific pricing to develop a cost comparison between the available formulations of acetaminophen.

- Once the information is collected from tertiary and primary resources, a thorough evaluation should be conducted. This will involve a critical assessment of the literature in the context of the needs of the organization.
- Defining stakeholder and identifying key stakeholders:
  - A stakeholder is an individual who has a vested interest in the matter and policy in question.
  - For the policy on an IV-to-PO acetaminophen conversion, the key stakeholders would be physicians in the specialties of surgery, pain, internal medicine, and critical care medicine. This policy would affect the pharmacy department and clinical pharmacists practicing in these specialties as well.
  - Once a draft policy is developed, it should be presented to key stakeholders for review and input prior to its presentation for approval by a pharmacy and therapeutics committee or medical director. This can be accomplished in several ways. Perhaps a formal meeting of the stakeholders could be convened (e.g., expert panel) or individual discussions and dissemination of the draft could be handled by the pharmacist responsible for drafting the policy.

CASE STUDY 21–2

- Regardless of the strategy chosen to disseminate and educate individuals, the policy should be readily accessible to frontline staff that would perform the IV-to-PO conversions. Depending on the institution, this may include verbal, digital, and/or printed dissemination and education to frontline staff (e.g., via email, team huddles, or department newsletters). References or hyperlinks to the policy could also be incorporated into a targeted section of the electronic health record. Staff could also be required to complete computer-based training modules or required to attend a continuing education seminar on the IV-to-PO practices.
- Exact groups that should be educated may vary by institution, but likely include pharmacists, pharmacy technicians, nurses, physicians, internal compliance personnel, informatics personnel, policy managers, and the pharmacy and therapeutics committee.
- The policy may be able to be implemented concurrently with changes to the electronic health record, such as alerts or other clinical decision support, which prompt pharmacists to evaluate eligible patients and/or medications for IV-to-PO conversions. Before implementation, follow-up compliance audits should also be proactively planned. This may include manual or automated reporting to identify if eligible patients were in fact assessed and appropriate actions executed after that assessment. The department could approach these assessments with continuous quality improvement methods, as discussed in Chapter 18, in order to iteratively improve the process, documentation, or compliance with the process. If the department identifies poor compliance, the policy, process, and/or education may need to be revisited with stakeholders.

Chapter 22

CASE STUDY 22–1

- Before undertaking this assignment, it would be helpful to clarify and narrow the project goal and scope. For example, is the purpose to evaluate the biosimilar medication compared only with the reference product, or in the context of all breast cancer therapies on the market? Similarly, is the ultimate goal of the formulary evaluation to encourage biosimilar use as a cost-savings lever, or to simply ensure that the existing formulary-preferred products are appropriate? It would also be useful to understand any previous work that has been done on this project, such as when the last time a class review was conducted. Additionally, it would be important to understand the urgency of this project and where it ranks in the overall priorities for your department.

- Recall that success criteria are quantifiable measures that define when the goal is accomplished, whereas a deliverable is a tangible component that is produced to achieve the success criteria. With this current project, one success criteria might be that a decision is voted upon by the hospital pharmacy and therapeutics committee. A corresponding deliverable might be to develop an evidence-based class review with a formulary recommendation that the committee can use. Another success criterion might be to increase utilization of biosimilar products for breast cancer treatment. Corresponding deliverables may include a monitoring dashboard to track biosimilar drug utilization, standardized order form that includes the biosimilar product, or therapeutic interchange to better ensure utilization of formulary products.
- Stakeholders may vary greatly depending on the size and scope of an organization. For this specific example, some stakeholders may include adult oncologists; adult clinical pharmacy specialists in oncology; nursing; informatics personnel (if an electronic medical record system is used); and drug sourcing or contracting personnel.
- Potential constraints may include limited time to dedicate to the project due to existing patient care responsibilities; time needed to conduct a proper contracting/sourcing evaluation with the biosimilar manufacturer; poor access to key physician stakeholders that prevents the gathering of timely input; and functionality limitations within an electronic health record system that may prevent using medication management strategies, such as automatic therapeutic interchanges.
- Major tasks that would inform the project timeline may include gathering primary and tertiary literature, synthesizing the evidence you identified, gathering input from stakeholders, undertaking contract negotiations; presenting recommendations to the pharmacy and therapeutics committee; and implementing final decisions (e.g., updating technology systems with any changes). It may also be reasonable to break down the project further by dividing work on the evidence review into sections (e.g., complete the background and FDA-indications section one day, then complete the adverse effects section another day, etc.).

Chapter 23

CASE STUDY 23–1

- Yes, the product is going to be used in a different patient population and be infused using a different route of administration. In both cases the risk profile is higher for the new usage and as such submission of a new IND is going to be required.

    The company may select to work with Dr. Smith's data to further develop the product, develop an appropriate protocol, and submit the IND to the FDA.

    Alternatively, the company may select to simply support Dr. Smith as he develops a protocol and IND for submission. In that case, the company will provide Dr. Smith with a letter of authorization to cross reference their regulatory submission in support of his IND application.

CASE STUDY 23-2

- A well-researched comparison of the risks of liver metastases as compared to the risks of cirrhosis will be needed to justify further development of this product using this route of administration. In addition, submission of an REMS will be crucial.

- Appropriate components of the REMS:
  ° Letters to health care providers
  ° Patient medication guide
  ° Patient registry to track enrollment of patients receiving the drug via this route of administration
  ° Patient monitoring of liver function tests

CASE STUDY 23-3

- The IRB is likely to determine that not only must this risk be included in the consent form, but that if the purpose of the new studies is to obtain further information about this risk, that must be explained to the subjects as part of the consent form.
- Children are considered a special population in clinical research. 45CFR46 specifies criteria for the evaluation of risk as compared to benefit when research is conducted in children. In this case it is likely that an IRB would still consider this study to be approvable since the product holds the promise of potential benefit to the patient in addition to the known risks. In children prior to the age of legal majority (as defined by state law), their guardians are responsible for making health care decisions for them. In some situations the agreement of one guardian is sufficient; however, if the IRB has determined that there is risk to the child and no direct benefit to them, the agreement of both guardians is required. In addition, the agreement of the child (referred to as assent) is also required.
- At the point at which a child reaches the age of majority, they must provide their own consent to participate in the study.

Chapter 24

CASE STUDY 24-1

- A 21st Century Cures Act section is included in FDA's Regulatory Information topic page. This section provides information on the Cures Act's goal, associated initiatives, implementation steps,andrelatedmaterials:https://www.fda.gov/regulatory-information/selected-amendments-fdc-act/21st-century-cures-act
- The Cures Act established two new expedited development programs: the Regenerative Medicine Advanced Therapy for certain biologic products and the Breakthrough Devices program for innovative medical devices.
- The OCE is an intercenter institute that collaborates across centers and offices within FDA. The mission of OCE is "to achieve patient-centered regulatory decision-making through innovation and collaboration," and OCE's vision statement reads "we seek to create a unified and collaborative scientific environment to advance the development and regulation of oncology products for patients with cancer."
- RWD is the data collected about a patient's health or the delivery of care he or she underwent and can come from a variety of sources including the electronic health record, billing claims, and disease registries. The evidence of a drug's benefits and risk derived from RWD is considered the RWE, and is generated by various study designs or analyses that collect RWD.

CASE STUDY 24-2

- The medical information department at Amazing Drugs LP should search the medical literature for any studies comparing their product to other compounds. They should evaluate the literature and create a standard response letter with the information.

- Amazing Drugs LP should anticipate receiving safety questions regarding the possible occurrence of DRUG A causing yellow stripes as it is similar to DRUG B, which is known to cause yellow stripes.

CASE STUDY 24-3

- Amazing Drugs LP must obtain information regarding the adverse event and document this information on form 3500A.
- Amazing Drugs LP is required to submit form 3500A to the FDA.

Chapter 25

CASE STUDY 25-1

- This help-seeking advertisement should describe hypertension's symptoms and risk factors. In addition, the images on the advertisement should depict the appropriate patient population at risk for hypertension and encourage patients to discuss their symptoms with their physician. The advertisement may contain the pharmaceutical company's name and provide a phone number that patients can call to obtain more information about hypertension.
- This help-seeking advertisement should not include references to particular hypertension treatments or images of drug products.
- Since specific medications are not referenced in help-seeking advertisements, they are regulated by the Federal Trade Commission (FTC) as opposed to the FDA. However, if the help-seeking advertisement's violation is that it recommends a particular treatment, the advertisement would be reclassified as a product claim advertisement and would be regulated by the FDA. The FDA accepts comments regarding product claim and violations through the BadAd program (Email: BadAd@FDA.gov; Phone: 855-RX-BADAD [855-792-2323]).

CASE STUDY 25-2

- It is very important to have a clear conflict of interest policy in place. This policy and procedure should guide who may meet with pharmaceutical industry, how often individuals should meet with industry representatives, what topics are discussed, and what types of information and/or items may be exchanged. It is also wise to have a system in place to track and document these visits. Finally, it is also beneficial to complete a training session or course regarding best practices for industry interactions.
- Prior to the visit, it is recommended to determine what medications will be discussed, either by directly asking the representative or reviewing their portfolio. Key evidence-based information from resources such as the prescription drug labeling will be used. It is also helpful to conduct a primary literature search and ensure you are up to date with current clinical literature regarding the medications.
- Be polite and professional but also use active listening skills to detect use of flawed logic (e.g., appeal to authority, red herring).

CASE STUDY 25-3

- Health care professionals should critically analyze all information presented at these programs for accuracy, reliability, and potential violations.

- Common violations likely to occur in this setting include the following: presenting inadequate risk information and minimizing risks, exaggerating benefits, presenting off-label or unapproved information, and making false or deceiving comparisons with other medications. In this instance, you would also want to be on the lookout for off-label promotion. The speaker can address off-label uses, but the industry representative, at the time of writing, should not engage in off-label promotion unless responding to a request from an audience member.
- Health care professionals can report advertising violations to the FDA through the Bad Ad program via email: BadAd@FDA.gov or by phone: 855-RX-BADAD (855-792-2323).

CASE STUDY 25–4

- Some type of needs assessment should be done prior to launching an academic detailing programing. Possible sources of data include review of prescribing practices, patient demographics, financial data, and survey of health care professionals and/or patients. It will be essential to the success of the program that you develop a very targeted intervention in order to yield the most positive outcome.
- Materials used in academic detailing should be developed using an evidence-based approach; they should draw from tertiary resources and primary literature. One organization that may provide validated materials is NaRCAD. Academic institutions may also serve as valuable partners. You could also consider networking with the Veterans Administration, SCORxE, or iDiS.
- The advantage of a one-on-one approach is that it may facilitate a more meaningful discussion as well as allow for privacy of the prescriber. However, a group approach has the advantage of potentially reaching a larger audience and require a lesser time investment (i.e., less pharmacy resources). Either approach could be considered depending on the scope, goals, and resources of the program. Given that you are already embedded in the organization, you could also employ both strategies, or even peer-to-peer academic detailing.
- Metrics should be specific to the intervention targets and actionable. For example, if a program was designed to promote evidence-based use of antihypertensives, prescribing patterns could be monitored with the goal of observing increased adherence to an institutional guideline. If increasing use of generic medications was a goal, prescription data could also be monitored to ensure effectiveness. Finally, humanistic data may also be collected in the form of a prescriber and/or patient survey.

Chapter 26

CASE STUDY 26–1

Accurate, reputable treatment guidelines may be quickly found in sources such as PubMed® as well as through databases such as UpToDate® or Dynamed®. The professional organizations such as the American Academy of Dermatology (https://www.aad.org) or the American Academy of Family Physicians (https://www.aafp.org) also have published clinical guidelines and recommendations on their websites.

CASE STUDY 26–2

- Drug information questions that PP has either requested or implied:
  ° What is meant by the term "not on formulary"?
  ° What *is* covered on this patient's prescription formulary?
- Dr. Collins might begin to answer each of these questions as follows:

- ° "Not on formulary" means that a medication is not listed in a prescription drug plan as being paid for or being provided at a discounted rate through a prescription insurance plan.
- ° Prescription formulary coverage information may be determined in a variety of ways, including visiting http://medicare.gov for Medicare recipients, by typing prescription insurance provider + formulary + the calendar year you desire (e.g., 2020) in an Internet search engine, searching select drug information databases such as Epocrates® or Lexicomp®, or within e-prescribing platform formulary decision support systems.
- Reputable databases with information geared specifically toward the patient, and with materials that have been reviewed and placed at the 8th grade reading level or below include Clinical Pharmacology®, Facts and Comparisons eAnswers®, Lexicomp®, and Micromedex®.
- Clinical Pharmacology®, Facts and Comparisons eAnswers®, and Lexicomp® each contain patient-oriented materials in both English and Spanish. In addition, the Lexicomp® database includes medication leaflets in up to 19 additional languages, and Micromedex®'s Patient Connect Suite includes medication information in up to 15 languages geared toward the patient (although the reading level for the additional languages in Lexicomp® and Micromedex® is not specified).

CASE STUDY 26-3

- In general, the most important thing to advise a patient or caregiver is to avoid flushing medication and avoid pouring them down the drain. Patients should be informed that certain pharmacies will now take back medications for disposal; the program is voluntary for pharmacies. Patients can mail their unused prescription medications in or they can place them in a pharmacy-maintained collection container or one found at several law enforcement agencies. Consumers should also be encouraged to take advantage of medication take-back collection days. Other methods for safe personal disposal of medications, including syringes, can be found on the Institute for Safe Medical Practice (ISMP) website (http://www.ismp.org), as well as the Pharmacist's Letter website (http://www.pharmacistsletter.com). A very small number of drugs may be flushed (due to the potential risk of inappropriate exposure), and these are listed online at http://www.fda.gov/downloads/Drugs/ResourcesForYou/Consumers/BuyingUsingMedicineSafely/EnsuringSafeUseofMedicine/SafeDisposalofMedicines/UCM337803.pdf, as well as in Table 26-1. In addition to the do not flush list, the FDA also has information on how to dispose of medications if no collections bins or take-back options are available (https://www.fda.gov/drugs/safe-disposal-medicines/disposal-unused-medicines-what-you-should-know). Finally, for sharps disposal, the caregiver should be encouraged to contact his local disposal company.
- While multiple governmental initiatives exist to promote the safe and appropriate disposal of unused, unwanted, and/or expired medications (e.g., The White House Office of National Drug Control Policy), these are not enforceable laws on the consumer.

CASE STUDY 26-4

- Examples of such quality indicators include, but are not limited to, efficiency (resource use), structure, process, intermediate outcomes, long-term outcomes, and patient centeredness. Newer measures may include those focused on medication-related patient safety (e.g., detecting/preventing medication errors and adverse drug reactions).
- Yes, it is, and it falls under the quality measure related to patient centeredness.
- Yes, the U.S. Department of Health and Human Services, as part of the Accountable Care Organization model, has specified and published 33 required quality measures that are evaluated to determine payment structure for patient care networks (including ambulatory care settings).

Chapter 27

CASE STUDY 27-1

- As a pharmacist in a busy pharmacy, it is important to triage the problems in front of you. In this situation, you have multiple things going on and you are the only pharmacist on duty. It is up to you to decide what takes priority. This patient may be making decisions about her health based solely on information found online. If the patient follows through on her plan to stop taking her antidepressants, she will be at risk of being harmed. This should make her your top priority.

    The patient in this particular case is actually seeking input from you in her attempt to have a dialogue about quitting her medication. You would be negligent in your duties if you did not choose to counsel the patient on the pros and cons of obtaining health information online, the danger of stopping antidepressant medications abruptly, and the risk of her severe depression reoccurring.

    As a pharmacist, you have a professional obligation to engage with your patients and provide them with the education and tools to obtain the best health care possible. Patients are increasingly using alternative sources beyond health care providers for advice and/or counseling, which makes it vital that pharmacists initiate even difficult conversations.

- First, the patient should be encouraged to continue to take an active role in her own health care. Patient empowerment has many positives for health outcomes. On the flip side, it is important to make the patient aware that when taking her health care into her own hands there can be negative consequences as well. It is crucial that she involves a health care practitioner if she decides to change her therapy in anyway.

    Second, agree with your patient that there are a lot of good places to find health information out there but that it is really important that they identify quality websites from which to obtain that information. Even then, every individual is different and the information they find on these websites may not necessarily be patient-specific, or applicable to his or her situation. For example, the patient in this case is deciding to discontinue her antidepressant medication based on other patients' opinions of the medication. These other patients quite possibly have an entirely different health situation. Encourage the patient to take these concerns to her primary care practitioner so that they may have a discussion on whether or not what she found online is relevant to her situation.

    Third, you review suggestions for determining a quality health information website, thereby ensuring she is obtaining information from reputable sources and bringing information to discuss with her health care practitioner that has value. In this specific case, you are extremely busy and unable to meet now so you should arrange a time to call the patient or make an appointment for her to come back in to discuss her plans.

    Our role as health care practitioners is to support the patient and their beliefs. Show respect and the desire to collaborate with them and you will gain their trust. If you trivialize what they bring to you and insist that the health care practitioner is the expert and the one who knows best, you may damage the relationship with the patient beyond repair.

- Safety first. If the patient has made up her mind that there is no stopping her from discontinuing her antidepressant immediately, advising her how to do so safely becomes your number one priority. First, direct the patient to see her primary care provider as soon as possible. Together they can work out a plan of action to taper her off the medication and possibly get her started on something she feels more comfortable taking.

    If you sense the patient will not consult her physician, it is important to counsel her on possible withdrawal symptoms she may experience as well as the consequences of quitting her medication all at once without tapering. Also arrange a follow-up time after your initial discussion to evaluate the control of her disease state and how well she tolerated stopping the medication.

CASE STUDY 27–2

- The first question that should come to mind as a health care professional is whether or not the patient has discussed the use of this particular app with his primary care provider. Although the tracking of health data to assist in the management of a disease state can be extremely helpful for the patient, it can become dangerous when an app is making clinical recommendations about treating a condition (i.e., adjusting insulin dosage) without the supervision of a health care professional.

  Second it is important to confirm the patient's diabetes truly has been under control over the past few months. Although the patient sings the app's praises because of the positive difference he feels in terms of his disease state since downloading it, you want to verify that his blood glucose levels are well controlled. Taking a look at the patient's chart and A1C can better help you determine whether or not the app has been harmful or helpful. It is also necessary to redirect the patient back to their primary care provider in order to ensure both the health care professional and patient are on the same page in regard to how the disease state is being managed. Encouraging communication between these two health care partners creates a perfect opportunity for patient and physician to discuss the mobile software and whether or not it will be a part of their treatment plan going forward.

  Finally, you should ask more questions about the particular app in question. Was it developed by a credible source? Are clinical recommendations based on evidence? Is the app capable of tailoring a recommendation to a specific patient? The answers to these questions and others may help you better guide the patient in whether the app is a reliable one or in some cases FDA approved as a medical device to use in managing a disease state.
- In this particular scenario, it seems the patient has not just dipped his toes into the mobile health arena but has jumped head first. The app he describes using puts him, the patient, in a position to be very reliant on a device to make therapeutic decisions that his physician would normally make. While it seems the application does factor in patient-specific data when making its decisions, without the supervision of a clinician, this is risky territory.

  The single best piece of advice you can give a patient who is interested or has been using mobile health apps is to always check with a health care professional before making any changes to their prescribed medication regimen. Use of mobile health software by a patient wanting to get more involved in their health should never be discouraged; in fact, the benefits seen in patients who use apps to keep track of health and fitness progress, find health information, and to stay connected with others in their health situation are infinite. The danger lies when patients start using apps as a sole resource to diagnose, manage their disease state, adjust their medication regimens, etc. Smartphone apps with these types of capabilities should be used in conjunction with a physician. In some cases, they may be medically prescribed.

CASE STUDY 27–3

In general, there are five key areas that are important to consider when evaluating a new mHealth app: credibility, accuracy, whether or not it is evidence-based, ease-of-use, and health literacy. There are several questions under each key area that are important to ask yourself as a reviewer of an app.

- Credibility of app
  - Are credentials of the app suitable?
  - Are authors/publishers clearly listed?
  - Is the app promoting a product?
  - Is the organization that developed the app reputable?
- Accuracy of information
  - Is it peer-reviewed?
  - Is the information current and/or frequently updated?
  - Are recent and reputable guidelines used to support recommendations made?
  - Are references cited?

- Evidence-based medicine
  - ○ Are recommendations evidence-based?
  - ○ Do recommendations target a specific audience or are they general in nature?
  - ○ Are opinion statements clearly marked?
  - ○ Are users directed to a health care professional before making changes to health care routine?
- Ease-of-use
  - ○ Does the app fit to the screen?
  - ○ Is the set-up of the app well designed and organized?
  - ○ Is the app easily navigated?
  - ○ Does the app have a search function?
  - ○ Is there a main menu that helps clearly lay content out?
- Health literacy
  - ○ Is medical jargon avoided? Is it easy for the lay reader to understand?
  - ○ Is font and set up of app easy to read?
  - ○ Does app gear information toward the consumer?

Unfortunately, even after thoroughly reviewing an mHealth app using the five key areas, there still may be some questions as to whether or not the app is capable of making therapeutic decisions for a patient. In these instances, it may be best to suggest contacting the developer of the software to better determine how their particular app arrives at therapeutic decisions.

- There are a variety of mHealth app characteristics that make patients more likely to use them regularly. In turn, patients are more likely to be adherent and have more success with the app. It has been shown patients want the following from their mHealth apps:
  - ○ Provides trustworthy and accurate information
  - ○ Easy-to-use, simple, and well-designed
  - ○ Guarantees personal data is secure
  - ○ Free of charge or inexpensive
  - ○ No advertisements
  - ○ Works effectively and consistent over time
  - ○ Allows networking with other people
  - ○ Uncomplicated

Chapter 28

CASE STUDY 28-1

- Computerized provider order entry (CPOE) systems allow medical provider instructions to be electronically entered for the treatment of patients who are under the provider's direct care in an acute care facility. This may include medication orders as well as orders for tests, procedures, and consultations. Electronic prescribing (e-prescribing) systems allow medical providers to electronically transmit a prescription for a medication, which is then verified and processed in an electronic format at an outpatient or community pharmacy.
- It can be a long and difficult process to integrate CPOE into a complex medical environment. Once implemented, however, challenges persist. The system will need routine maintenance to ensure features meet users' needs. Prebuilt orders will require updating and refinement to reflect changes in practice. Additionally, decision support content will require routine updating to reflect new knowledge from the literature. Collaboration with the CPOE vendor is critical to ensure maintenance needs are addressed. Leadership within the medical environment will also need to clearly define the group (or person) who is ultimately responsible for decision support governance.

- Clinical decision support systems (CDSS) are computer programs that augment clinical decision-making by combining referential information with patient-specific information. CDSS can provide alerts and messages in CPOE and e-prescribing systems that ultimately improve the safety, quality, efficiency, and cost-effectiveness of care.
- CPOE and e-prescribing systems may introduce new types of errors. For inexperienced users, order entry and therefore communication may be slower. CDSS-based alerts and warnings that appear too often may lead to alert fatigue for providers.

CASE STUDY 28-2

- Whereas providers are on the data entry end of these systems, which occurs at the prescribing stage of the medication use process, pharmacists are on the receiving end and interact with these systems at the order-verification stage of the medication use process. Once the order for a medication enters the pharmacy computer system through one of these systems, the pharmacist assesses the appropriateness of the order and addresses any issues or discrepancies before filling the order.
- Bar code medication administration (BCMA) systems are used in the hospital setting at the administration stage of the medication use process. The purpose of a BCMA system is to ensure that the six rights of medication administration are followed by electronically validating and documenting medications at the point of care.
- Clinical surveillance systems are used to actively monitor patients. Rules are built to identify potential problems. These rules, if met, then prompt medical providers to follow-up with or re-evaluate the patient.

CASE STUDY 28-3

- The medication use process is a cyclical process in which various interconnected parts—people, systems, procedures, and policies—work together to achieve the common goal of safe and effective medication therapy. The five stages of the medication use process as well as the technologies used at each stage are as follows:
  - **Order entry (prescribing)**—computerized provider order entry, clinical decision support systems, e-prescribing
  - **Order verification**—clinical decision support systems
  - **Dispensing**—automated dispensing cabinets, carousel cabinets, robotic cart filling systems, sterile compounding devices, bar code verification
  - **Administration**—bar code medication administration, electronic medication administration record, intelligent infusion pumps, medication event monitoring systems (MEMS)
  - **Monitoring**—clinical surveillance systems, clinical documentation systems

CASE STUDY 28-4

- Journal of Medical Internet Research, Journal of Participatory Medicine
- Initially, Facebook can be used to provide general information about services offered, to showcase the expertise of staff, and to provide basic health and medical information. As the institution's comfort with the technology grows, Facebook can be used for online question and answer sessions, to host videos of highly advanced procedures, and to provide patient perspectives on their experiences at the facility. Twitter can also be used to send the latest news about significant additions to the medical staff, to inform followers about upcoming clinical education classes, and to highlight the acquisition of high-tech tools for patient care. As resources become available and as patients express interest, Twitter may also be used for targeted messaging to remind patients of activities that encourage healthy behaviors. Ultimately, the information that is shared on Facebook, Twitter, or any other medium should address the needs of the institution's patients. The best way to find out what information patients want to receive or access electronically is to ask them. Additionally, the

hospital could start a patient-focused blog. Topics covered could be informed by patient input and feedback. The hospital could also recommend vetted PHRs for patient use on the blog site.
- The hospital could utilize the IoT for indoor navigation, allowing patients and visitors to use their smartphones to navigate to desired locations within the hospital. The IoT could also be used to keep track of devices, personnel, and patients.

CASE STUDY 28-5

- Electronic health records (EHRs) contain information related to a patient's care and are meant to be used by health practitioners. EHRs are maintained by health care organizations, whereas personal health records (PHRs) are maintained by patients themselves.
- The Office of the National Coordinator for Health Information Technology
- One of the primary methods the federal government drives HIT adoption is through its role as a purchaser of health care. In simplest terms, the government creates practice standards and metrics that providers must meet in their use of HIT to deliver care to Medicare patients. If providers meet these standards, their reimbursement is not negatively impacted. In other models, the government has provided financial support (i.e., reimbursement) to drive adoption of HIT.
- The primary concerns related to PHI is maintaining privacy and security of patients' information. Cyber security breaches are malicious acts to acquire unauthorized access to others information. Cyber security breaches are increasingly growing in importance for those in health care.

Chapter 29

CASE STUDY 29-1

- In this situation, you would want your inclusion criteria to be all patients that received an order for a pharmacy vancomycin dosing consult within the past 6 months. For exclusion criteria, you would want to indicate that patients with an age < 18 years old (or however you define "pediatric") would be excluded from the search criteria.
- This answer may be variable, but it is important to consider which data would allow analysis expeditiously. For example, consider patient demographic data (e.g., age, sex, weight, renal function, location within the hospital), ordering data (doses ordered, troughs ordered, timing of troughs, timing of vancomycin administrations), as well as documentation data (pharmacist notes).

CASE STUDY 29-2

- Data: The data is currently in raw format, which does not allow the end user to glean meaning from it.
- Information: To turn the vancomycin dosing consult data into information. We can take a few steps: (1) Utilize spreadsheet software to clean the data for use in a statistical software. (2) Create visualizations such as tables and graphs within the spreadsheet to create some descriptive statistics.
- Knowledge: After the data is cleaned, running the data through a statistical software program to determine the appropriate statistical outcomes is an appropriate step.
- Intelligence: Creation of artificial intelligence is likely beyond the scope of this project. To create artificial intelligence, many more data points would need to be extracted from the EHR.

Chapter 30

CASE STUDY 30-1

- Instructional methods to teach drug information include didactic lectures, small group learning, Internet-based learning including online course management programs (e.g., Blackboard, Canvas, Joule), audience response systems, YouTube, online blogs, tweets, and wikis.
  - ○ Literature evaluation is often taught in a stand-alone course placed in the second professional year. Other options include embedding within a drug information and teaching within laboratory-based courses.

CASE STUDY 30-2

- Drug information experiences can be provided in many practice settings beyond call centers.
  - ○ Activities that a student may be assigned include completion of a drug monograph or therapeutic class review, completion of a medication use evaluation, and investigation and assessment of adverse medication events.

CASE STUDY 30-3

- Individuals with expertise in drug information may work in many different roles beyond that of drug information specialist, including medication safety pharmacist, medication policy pharmacist, regulatory pharmacist, and medical writer/editor.
- These individuals may practice in a variety of settings including hospital, community, industry, government, medical publishing company, and schools of pharmacy.
- The recommended training for drug information specialists is completion of a postgraduate year one residency followed by a postgraduate year two medication-use safety and policy residency program.

Abbreviations

AACP—American Association of Colleges of Pharmacy
AAR—after-action review
ACA—Affordable Care Act
ACCME—American Council for Continuing Medical Education
ACCP—American College of Clinical Pharmacy or American College of Chest
   Physicians
ACE—angiotensin-converting enzyme
ACO—accountable care organization
ACPE—Accreditation Council for Pharmacy Education
ADC—automated dispensing cabinet
ADE—adverse drug effect or event
ADR—adverse drug reaction
AE—adverse effect or adverse event
AF—atrial fibrillation
AGA—American Gastroenterological Association
AGREE–Appraisal of Guidelines for Research and Evaluation
AHFS—American Hospital Formulary Service
AHFS CDI—AHFS® Clinical Drug Information™
AHRQ—Agency for Healthcare Research and Quality
AIDS—acquired immunodeficiency syndrome
AJHP—American Journal of Health-System Pharmacy
AMA—American Medical Association
AMCP—Academy of Managed Care Pharmacy
AMH—Accreditation Manual for Hospitals
ANDA—abbreviated new drug application
ANSI—American National Standards Institute
AP—action priority
API—active pharmaceutical ingredient, or Asian or Pacific Islanders
APM—Alternative Payment Model

ART—adverse reaction tracking
ASHP—American Society of Health-System Pharmacists
ASOP—Alliance for Safe Online Pharmacies
ASP—Academy of Student Pharmacists or application service provider
BCMA—bar code medication administration
BG—blood glucose
BLA—biologics license application
BMJ—British Medical Journal
BP—blood pressure
BUN—blood urea nitrogen
CAD—coronary artery disease
CAERS—Center for Food Safety and Applied Nutrition Adverse Event Reporting System
CAHPS—Consumer Assessment of Healthcare Providers and Systems
CAM—complementary and alternative medicine
CAMIPR—Consortium for the Advancement of Medication Information Policy and Research
CAPE—Center for the Advancement of Pharmaceutical Education
CAS—Chemical Abstracts Service
CAT—causality assessment tool
CBA—cost-benefit analysis
CBD—cannabidiol
CBER—Center for Biologics Evaluation and Research
CCA—Cochrane Clinical Answers or cost-consequence analysis
CCR—continuity of care record
CDC—Centers for Disease Control and Prevention
CDER—Center for Drug Evaluation and Research
CDRH—Center for Devices and Radiological Health
CDS—clinical decision support
CDSR—Cochrane Database of Systematic Reviews
CDSS—clinical decision support system
CE—continuing education
CEA—cost-effectiveness analysis
CENT—Consolidated Standards of Reporting Trials Extension for Reporting N-of-1 Trials
CENTRAL—Cochrane Central Register of Controlled Trials
CER—cost-effectiveness ratio
CFL—consistent with FDA required labeling
CFR—Code of Federal Regulations
CFSAN—Center for Food Safety and Applied Nutrition

CGMP—current good manufacturing practices
CHI—consumer health information
CHIP—Children's Health Insurance Program
CI—confidence interval
CINAHL—Cumulative Index to Nursing and Allied Health Literature
CITI—Collaborative Institutional Training Initiative
CMA—cost-minimization analysis
CME—continuing medical education
CMMI—Centers for Medicare and Medicaid Innovation
CMR—comprehensive medication review
CMS—Centers for Medicare and Medicaid Services
COI—conflict of interest
CONSORT—Consolidated Standards of Reporting Trials
CoP—conditions of participation
COSTEP—Commissioned Officer Student Training and Extern Program
COVID-19—coronavirus disease 2019. Now officially known as SARS-CoV-2 (severe acute respiratory syndrome coronavirus 2)
CPE—continuing pharmacy education
CPOE—computerized physician order entry
CPT—current procedural terminology
CQI—continuous quality improvement
CRO—contract research organization
CSIP—Center for Safe Internet Pharmacies
CTC—common toxicity criteria
CTCAE—Common Terminology Criteria for Adverse Events
CTEA—Copyright Term Extension Act
CUA—cost-utility analysis
CV—coefficients of variance
DAW—dispense as written
DDI—Division of Drug Information or drug-drug interaction
DEA—Drug Enforcement Administration
df—degrees of freedom
DHHS—Department of Health and Human Services
DI—drug information
DI PRN—Drug Information Practice and Research Network
DIC—drug information center
DIS—drug information service
DISCO—Drug Information Soundcast in Clinical Oncology
DM—diabetes mellitus

DMF—drug master files

DOB—date of birth

DSC—Drug Safety Communications

DSCSA—Drug Supply Chain Security Act

DTCA—direct to consumer advertising

DUE—drug utilization, usage or use evaluation

DUHS—Duke University Health System

DUR—drug use or utilization review

EBM—evidence-based medicine

ED—emergency department

EHR—electronic health record

eMAR—electronic medication administration record

EMR—electronic medical record

EPCS—electronic prescribing of controlled substances

ePHI—electronic protected health information

e-prescribing—electronic prescribing

ER—extended release or estrogen receptor

ESRD QIP—End-Stage Renal Disease Quality Incentive Program

ETASU—elements to assure safe use

FAERS—FDA adverse event reporting system

FBOL—field-based outcomes liaison

FCC—Federal Communication Commission

FDA—Food and Drug Administration

FDAAA—Food and Drug Administration Amendments Act of 2007

FDAMA—Food and Drug Administration Modernization Act

FDASIA—Food and Drug Administration Safety and Innovation Act

FDCA or FD&C Act—Food, Drug, and Cosmetic Act

FFS—Fee-for-Service

FMEA—failure mode and effects analysis

FOCUS-PDCA—Find, Organize, Clarify, Understand, Select, Plan, Do, Check, Act

FOIA—Freedom of Information Act

FPP—finished pharmaceutical product

GADIS—Global Alliance of Drug Information Specialists

GAO—Government Accountability Office

GCP—good clinical practice

GEDSA—Global Enteral Device Supplier Association

GP—general practitioner

GRADE—Grading of Recommendations, Assessment, Development, and Evaluation system

HAC—Hospital-Acquired Conditions
HCEI—Health Care Economic Information
HCP—health care professional
HDL—high-density lipoprotein
HEDIS—Healthcare Effectiveness Data and Information Set
HEOR—health economics and outcomes research
HF—human factors
HFE—human factors engineering
HHS—Health and Human Services
HIPAA—Health Insurance Portability and Accountability Act
HIS—health information system
HIT—health information technology
HIV—human immunodeficiency virus
HMO—health maintenance organization
HON—Health on the Net
HR—hazard ratio or heart rate
HRM—high-risk medication
HR-QOL—Health-related quality of life
HRRP—Hospital Readmission Reduction Program
HRSA—Health Resources and Services Administration
IB—International Baccalaureate
ICD-10—International Classification of Disease—tenth revision
ICER—incremental cost-effectiveness ratio
ICH—International Conference on Harmonization
ICMJE—International Committee of Medical Journal Editors
ICU—intensive care unit
IDE—investigational device exemption
IDSA—Infectious Diseases Society of America
IGF—incidental genomic finding
IHI—Institute for Healthcare Improvement
IMSN—International Medication Safety Network
IND—investigational new drug
INDA—investigational new drug application
INN—international non-proprietary names
INR—International Normalized Ratio
IOM—Institute of Medicine—now known as the National Academy of Medicine (NAM)
IoT—Internet of Things
IPA—International Pharmaceutical Abstracts
IRB—Institutional Review Board

ISMP—Institute for Safe Medicine Practices

ISMP MERP—Institute for Safe Medication Practices Medication Errors Reporting Program

ISPE—International Society for Pharmaceutical Engineering

IT—information technology

IV—intravenous

IVIG—intravenous immunoglobulin

IVR—interactive voice response

LDL—low-density lipoprotein

LOA—letter of authorization

LOINC—Logical Observation Identifiers Names and Codes

LST—large, simple trial

MACRA—Medicare Access and CHIP Reauthorization

MAUDE—Manufacturer and User Facility Device Experience

MBA—Master of Business Administration

MCO—managed care organization

MDR—Medical Device Reporting

MEADERS—Medication Error and Adverse Drug Event Reporting System

MEMS—medication event monitoring systems

MeSH—Medical Subject Headings

MHA—Master of Healthcare Administration

mHealth—mobile health

MI—myocardial infarction

MIPS—Merit-based Incentive Program or Merit-based Incentive Payment System

MIR—medical information request

MME—morphine milligram equivalent

MMWR—Morbidity and Mortality Weekly Report

MS—Master of Science

MSDS—material safety data sheet

MSL—medical science liaison

MTM—medication therapy management

MUE—medication use evaluation

NAM—National Academy of Medicine (once known as the Institute of Medicine [IOM])

NCBI—National Center for Biotechnology Information

NCC MERP—National Coordinating Council for Medication Error Reporting and Prevention

NCI—National Cancer Institute

NCPDP—National Council for Prescription Drug Programs

NCQA—National Committee for Quality Assurance

NDA—new drug application
NDC—National Drug Code
NDI—new dietary ingredient
NECC—New England Compounding Center
NHIS—National Health Interview Survey
NIH—National Institutes of Health
NLM—National Library of Medicine
NMBER™—Natural Medicines Brand Evidence-based Rating™
NME—new molecular entity
NPO—nothing by mouth
NQF—National Quality Forum
NQS—National Quality Strategy
NS—normal saline
NSAID—nonsteroidal anti-inflammatory drug
NY—New York
OHRP—Office of Human Research Subject Protection
OLTP—online transaction processing
OMH—Office of Minority Health
ONC—Office of the National Coordinator for Health Information Technology
OR—odds ratio
OSHA—Occupational Safety & Health Administration
OTC—over the counter
P&T—pharmacy and therapeutics
PA—physician assistant
PACU—post-anesthesia care unit
PBM—pharmacy benefit manager
PC—product complaint
PCMH—patient centered medical home
PDC—proportion of days covered
PDCA—Plan, Do, Check, Act
PDMP—prescription drug monitoring program
PDR—Physician's Desk Reference® / Prescribers' Digital Reference®
PDUFA—Prescription Drug User Fee Act
PE—pulmonary embolism
PGY1—postgraduate year one residency
PGY2—postgraduate year two residency
PGY3—postgraduate year three residency
PHI—protected health information
PHR—personal health record

PhRMA—Pharmaceutical Research and Manufacturers of America
PHSA—Public Health Service Act
PI—primary or principle investigator
PICO—patients, intervention, comparator, and outcome
PICOS—Participants, interventions, comparators, outcomes, and study designs
PIMS—pharmacy information management systems
PLOS—Public Library of Science
PO—by mouth
PPCP—Pharmacists' Patient Care Process
PPI—patient package insert
PQA—Pharmacy Quality Alliance
PRISMA—Preferred Reporting Items for Systemic Reviews and Meta-Analysis
PRISMA-IPD—PRISMA for Individual Patient Data systematic reviews
PRISMA-NMA—PRISMA for Network Meta-analyses
PROSPERO—International Prospective Register of Systematic Reviews
PSO—Patient Safety Organization
PSQH—Patient Safety and Quality Healthcare
PT—prothrombin time
PVBM—Physician Value-Based Modifier
QA—quality assurance
QALY—quality-adjusted life years
QAPI—quality assurance, performance improvement
QCT—qualifying clinical trial
QI—quality improvement
QIN-QIO—Quality Innovation Network–Quality Improvement Organization
QPP—Quality Payment Program
QPS—Quality Positions System
QRS—Quality Reporting System
RA—rheumatoid arthritis
RASA—renin angiotensin system antagonist
RCA—root cause analysis
RCA^2—root cause analysis and actions
RCT—randomized controlled trial
REaL—race, ethnicity, and language
REMS—risk evaluation and mitigation strategy
RF—rheumatoid factor
RFID—radio frequency identification
RPM—regulatory project manager
RPN—risk profile number

RR—relative risk
RR—respiratory rate
RWD—real-world data
RWE—real-world evidence
SA—sensitivity analysis
SaaS—software as a service
SBIA—Small Business and Industry Assistance
SCr—serum creatinine
SD—standard deviation
SDS—safety data sheet
SEA—Sentinel Event Alert
SNF QRP—Skilled Nursing Facility Quality Reporting Program
SNF VBP—Skilled Nursing Facility Value-Based Program
SNOMED-CT—Systematized Nomenclature of Medicine—Clinical Terms
SOP—standard operating procedure
SOW—scope of work
SPC—statistical process control
SQL—Structured Query Language
SQUIRE—Standards for Quality Improvement Reporting Excellence
SrLC—Drug Safety-related Labeling Changes
SRS—spontaneous reporting system
SSRI—selective serotonin reuptake inhibitors
STROBE—Strengthening the Reporting of Observational Studies in Epidemiology
SUPD—statin use in persons with diabetes
TCPA—Telephone Consumer Protection Act
TEC—technology enabled care
TG—triglycerides
THC—delta-9-tetrahydrocannabinol
TJC—The Joint Commission
TMR—targeted medication review
TPN—total parenteral nutrition
TPO—treatment, payment, and operations
TQM—total quality management
UI—user interface
UMLS—Unified Medical Language System
US—United States
USAN—United States Adopted Names
USP—United States Pharmacopeia
USPHS—United States Public Health Service

USP-NF—United States Pharmacopeia and National Formulary
UTI—urinary tract infection
VA—Veterans Affairs
VA ADERS—VA Adverse Drug Event Reporting System
VAERS—Vaccine Adverse Event Reporting System
VBP—value-based purchasing
VHA—Veterans Health Administration
VIPPS—verified Internet pharmacy practice sites
VM—Value Modifier
VUR—vesicoureteral reflux
WBC—white blood cells
WBS—work breakdown structure
WHO—World Health Organization
WHO PIDM—World Health Organization Programme for International Drug
    Monitoring
XML—extensible markup language

Answers for Self-Assessment Questions

Chapter 1

1. c	6. d	11. a
2. e	7. e	12. e
3. e	8. c	13. e
4. c	9. e	14. b
5. e	10. d	15. b

Chapter 2

1. c	6. d	11. b
2. c	7. d	12. d
3. b	8. a	13. a
4. a	9. c	14. d
5. a	10. c	15. c

Chapter 3

1. b	6. c	11. b
2. a	7. a	12. c
3. c	8. d	13. d
4. d	9. a	14. a
5. d	10. a	15. b

Chapter 4

1. d	6. e	11. b
2. a	7. a	12. a
3. c	8. b	13. e
4. a	9. a	14. e
5. a	10. d	15. c

Chapter 5

1. a	6. d	11. c
2. d	7. b	12. a
3. c	8. d	13. a
4. b	9. c	14. d
5. c	10. a	15. b

Chapter 6

1. c	6. a	11. b
2. a	7. d	12. b
3. a	8. d	13. b
4. b	9. c	14. d
5. c	10. c	15. a

Chapter 7

1. a	6. a	11. c
2. c	7. a	12. a
3. c	8. d	13. b
4. b	9. a	14. a
5. b	10. d	15. c

Chapter 8

1. e	6. c	11. d
2. c	7. b	12. d
3. d	8. d	13. c
4. d	9. b	14. a
5. d	10. d	15. b

Chapter 9

1. b	6. a	11. a
2. b	7. a	12. c
3. a	8. b	13. a
4. b	9. b	14. a
5. d	10. d	15. a

Chapter 10

1. c	6. d	11. b
2. b	7. d	12. d
3. b	8. c	13. c
4. a	9. e	14. a
5. d	10. d	15. c

Chapter 11

1. c	6. e	11. d
2. a	7. c	12. d
3. b	8. e	13. b
4. e	9. c	14. e
5. d	10. c	15. e

Chapter 12

1. a, c, and d	6. b, c, and d	11. a
2. a	7. a	12. a
3. b, c, d	8. a	13. c
4. d	9. b, c, and d	14. b
5. d	10. a, b, and d	15. b

Chapter 13

1. e	6. b	11. b
2. b	7. b	12. b
3. b	8. a	13. b
4. e	9. c	14. d
5. b	10. a	15. b

Chapter 14

1. b	6. b
2. c	7. d
3. b	8. a
4. c	9. b
5. d	10. c

Chapter 15

1. f	6. a	11. c
2. e	7. d	12. e
3. a	8. d	13. e
4. a	9. c	14. a
5. e	10. e	15. c

Chapter 16

1. a	6. d	11. e
2. a	7. a	12. b
3. e	8. a	13. b
4. a	9. b	14. d
5. d	10. b	15. d

Chapter 17

1. a	6. b	11. c
2. c	7. a	12. d
3. d	8. b	13. a
4. a	9. d	14. a
5. c	10. a	15. c

Chapter 18

1. a	6. d	11. a
2. d	7. e	12. e
3. d	8. b	13. c
4. c	9. e	14. b
5. d	10. a	15. f

Chapter 19

1. d	6. e	11. d
2. d	7. a	12. b
3. a	8. d	13. a
4. d	9. e	14. b
5. e	10. e	15. c

Chapter 20

1. c	6. b	11. d
2. a	7. b	12. d
3. c	8. a	13. b
4. d	9. c	14. a
5. c	10. a	15. b

Chapter 21

1. c	6. b	11. a
2. d	7. b	12. e
3. a	8. e	13. a
4. e	9. e	14. b
5. e	10. a	15. a

Chapter 22

1. b	6. d	11. b
2. b	7. a	12. c
3. d	8. d	13. b
4. a, c, d	9. a	14. d
5. a	10. a	15. b

Chapter 23

1. a	6. c	11. d
2. b	7. c	12. c
3. c	8. b	13. a
4. a	9. c	14. d
5. d	10. c	15. c

Chapter 24

1. b	6. d	11. a
2. b	7. c	12. e
3. d	8. d	13. e
4. a	9. b	14. a, c
5. c	10. a, b, d	15. e

Chapter 25

1. d	6. d	11. a
2. b	7. c	12. d
3. a	8. a	13. b
4. b	9. c	14. b
5. a	10. d	15. b

Chapter 26

1. a, c, d	6. d	11. b
2. e	7. d	12. b, c
3. c	8. c	13. b
4. a	9. b	14. b
5. e	10. d	15. a

Chapter 27

1. e	6. e	11. b
2. e	7. b	12. b
3. d	8. e	13. a
4. e	9. c	14. e
5. e	10. e	15. a

Chapter 28

1. b	6. d	11. e
2. e	7. d	12. e
3. c	8. e	13. b
4. c	9. d	14. e
5. b	10. d	15. c

Chapter 29

1. c	6. b	11. d
2. c	7. e	12. c
3. a	8. a	13. a
4. c	9. a	14. c
5. d	10. d	15. b

Chapter 30

1. b	6. d	11. d
2. d	7. e	12. a
3. a	8. d	13. e
4. d	9. d	14. e
5. d	10. d	15. b

Index